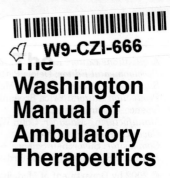

W9-CZI-666

The Washington Manual of Ambulatory Therapeutics

Department of Medicine
Washington University
School of Medicine
St. Louis, Missouri

Tammy L. Lin, M.D.
Scott W. Rypkema, M.D.
Editors

Robyn A. Schaiff, Pharm. D.
Associate Editor for
Pharmacotherapeutics

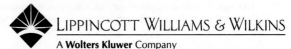

LIPPINCOTT WILLIAMS & WILKINS
A **Wolters Kluwer** Company
Philadelphia · Baltimore · New York · London
Buenos Aires · Hong Kong · Sydney · Tokyo

Acquisitions Editor: Richard Winters
Developmental Editor: Delois Patterson
Supervising Editor: Mary Ann McLaughlin
Production Editors: Erica Broennle Nelson and Shannon Allen, Silverchair Science + Communications
Manufacturing Manager: Colin Warnock
Cover Designer: Patricia Gast
Compositor: Silverchair Science + Communications
Printer: RR Donnelley, Crawfordsville

Library of Congress Cataloging-in-Publication Data
The Washington manual of ambulatory therapeutics / [edited by] Tammy L. Lin, Scott W. Rypkema.
     p. ; cm.
  Includes bibliographical references and index.
  ISBN 0-7817-2361-2 (spiral)
  1. Ambulatory medical care--Handbooks, manuals, etc. I. Title: Manual of ambulatory therapeutics. II. Lin, Tammy L. III. Rypkema, Scott W. IV. Washington University (Saint Louis, Mo.). School of Medicine.
  [DNLM: 1. Ambulatory Care--Handbooks. 2. Ambulatory Care--Outlines. WB 39 W319 2001]
  RC55 .W37 2001
  616--dc21

                                                                    2001038536

Care has been taken to confirm the accuracy of the information presented and to describe generally accepted practices. However, the authors, editors, and publisher are not responsible for errors or omissions or for any consequences from application of the information in this book and make no warranty, expressed or implied, with respect to the currency, completeness, or accuracy of the contents of the publication. Application of this information in a particular situation remains the professional responsibility of the practitioner.

The authors, editors, and publisher have exerted every effort to ensure that drug selection and dosage set forth in this text are in accordance with current recommendations and practice at the time of publication. However, in view of ongoing research, changes in government regulations, and the constant flow of information relating to drug therapy and drug reactions, the reader is urged to check the package insert for each drug for any change in indications and dosage and for added warnings and precautions. This is particularly important when the recommended agent is a new or infrequently employed drug.

Some drugs and medical devices presented in this publication have Food and Drug Administration (FDA) clearance for limited use in restricted research settings. It is the responsibility of health care providers to ascertain the FDA status of each drug or device planned for use in their clinical practice.

10 9 8 7 6 5 4 3 2 1

The Washington Manual of Ambulatory Therapeutics

To our families for their
unconditional love and support

Contents

Preface

We are proud to introduce the first edition of *The Washington Manual of Ambulatory Therapeutics*. It joins *The Washington Manual of Medical Therapeutics* and *The Washington Manual Internship Survival Guide* as the newest member of the Washington Manual series and recognizes the ever-increasing role that ambulatory care is assuming in health care. Rational yet practical diagnostic and therapeutic approaches in the ambulatory setting are critical, and we offer this manual to help fulfill this need.

Our focus is to provide a reference that covers common ambulatory medical problems encountered in each medical subspecialty. Recognizing that the approach to each may be handled differently, many of the subspecialties have separate symptom- and disease-based chapters. Many problems seen in the ambulatory setting fall outside traditional internal medicine subspecialties; we have included chapters on topics such as dermatology, neurology, ophthalmology, otolaryngology, and psychiatry to help address this. Each of these chapters benefits from being written by a subspecialist in the given field but with the primary care practitioner in mind. Recognizing the increasing importance of population-specific problems, we have included several pertinent appendixes and separate chapters on geriatrics and men's and women's health.

The diagnostic and therapeutic approaches presented reflect the current practices of physicians at the Washington University School of Medicine, although there may be several effective therapies for any disease process. Each author is a well-respected clinician and teacher. All have faced the challenges of a busy clinic and the degree of uncertainty inherent in the ambulatory setting.

An endeavor of this sort would not have been possible without the assistance and support of many people. We wish to thank the many fellows, house officers, medical students, and other colleagues at Barnes-Jewish Hospital who reviewed manuscripts and provided feedback. Jeff Blunt, Peter Crawford, Margaret Coplin, Anupam Goel, Grace Lin, Martin Maron, John Mohart, Toni Rastelli, William Read, Michael Riley, Gregory Sayuk, Dan Williams, and, particularly, Kevin Latinis were helpful in this regard. We thank Alice Lin and Joanne Shen for their input during manuscript review. Jeanne Wehner provided helpful assistance as well. From the Agency for Health Care Quality and Research, we thank Gregg Meyers for his contribution. We also thank the late John Eisenberg, a beloved friend of Washington University, for his contributions. The pharmacy staff from Barnes-Jewish Hospital was instrumental in reviewing drug dosages, and we would like to thank Robyn Schaiff for her expert assistance as Associate Editor for Pharmacotherapeutics.

From Lippincott Williams & Wilkins, we thank Katie Sharp, Kathy Neely, Delois Patterson, and Richard Winters for their excellent guidance and assistance. Erica Nelson, Shannon Allen, and Elizabeth Willingham from Silverchair Science + Communications were especially patient and helpful as we moved from manuscript to manual completion.

Erica Nelson deserves our special thanks and appreciation as she followed up every detail and treated this project as her own.

We received tremendous support throughout the Department of Medicine, and there are several people without whom this manual would not have been possible. Megan Wren and Thomas DeFer not only served as authors, but also provided encouragement and valuable assistance at key points. Daniel Goodenberger and Alison Whelan provided guidance, steadfast support, and the benefit of their experience on previous manuals. It was our pleasure to serve as chief residents under Kenneth Polonsky, Chairman of the Department of Medicine, whose enthusiasm for medical education allows innovative ideas to become realities.

Finally, we acknowledge those close to us for their support, especially the unwavering support of our families—George, Jean, Grace, and Alice; Amy, Keaton, Richard, and Elaine.

Tammy L. Lin
Scott W. Rypkema

The
Washington
Manual of
Ambulatory
Therapeutics

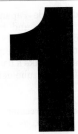

Approach to the Ambulatory Patient

Megan E. Wren
and John Min

I. **The goals of the ambulatory visit** are many, and the focus will vary from visit to visit.
   A. **Diagnosis and treatment of disease** are key elements of each visit. The clinician should evaluate the status of chronic diseases and watch for new problems. Because of time constraints, not every problem can be exhaustively analyzed at each visit. The most active or serious problems, or both, should receive the most attention, and the more stable problems can be reviewed more briefly. It is often necessary to schedule additional visits to investigate more fully all problems and complaints.
   B. **Explanation of and relief of symptoms** are key to the patient's satisfaction. The patient's chief complaint should never be forgotten! Relief of symptoms does not necessarily entail drug therapy but can include heat, ice, physical therapy, and changes in diet or activities. Reassurance that the symptoms do not represent serious disease may be all that some patients seek (e.g., that irritable bowel syndrome may cause pain but will not evolve into cancer).
   C. **Screening for asymptomatic disease** while in an early treatable stage. The clinician should keep a flowsheet to keep track of the schedule of screening tests. These may include screening for common cancers, hypertension, hypercholesterolemia, osteoporosis, and others.
   D. **Prevention of disease** can be accomplished through immunizations, risk factor modification (e.g., treatment of hypertension), and patient education. Patients seek reliable advice regarding a healthy lifestyle, including diet, exercise, sleep habits, and so forth.
   E. **An ongoing physician-patient relationship** provides an opportunity to become familiar with all of a patient's problems and how they interrelate and to understand them in the context of the patient's personality and life circumstances. If the physician is truly open to listening to a patient, mutual understanding and trust will grow as a therapeutic relationship develops. Patients will say that just talking to their physician makes them feel better.
II. **The periodic health examination.** Preventive medicine requires an individualized assessment tailored to each patient's age, sex, risk factors, and existing illnesses. Counseling about a healthy lifestyle is a critical component of health care at any age. See the individual sections for further details on cancer screening, immunizations, geriatrics, and so forth.
   A. **Adolescents and young adults** are at risk for serious morbidity and even mortality related to the risky behaviors that are common in this age group. The clinician should maintain an open and nonjudgmental attitude to encourage the adolescent to speak frankly. Confidentiality should be assured.
      1. **Important topics to discuss** include the avoidance of smoking, drinking, and illicit drug use; the use of bike helmets and car seatbelts; firearm safety; depression and suicide; the potential consequences of sexual activity and how to avoid them; healthy dietary habits and eating disorders; and appropriate exercise.
      2. **The physical examination** should include weight, BP, testicular or breast and pelvic examinations, and patient instruction on self-examination of

the breasts or testes. **Laboratory tests** should include Papanicolaou (Pap) smear, screening for chlamydia and gonorrhea, and targeted screening for syphilis, hepatitis B, and HIV infection.

3. **Preventive measures include updating immunizations,** especially rubella in women. Women of childbearing years should take a daily vitamin with 0.4 mg **folic acid** to reduce the risk of neural tube defects in their offspring.

B. **Midlife adults**

1. **Important topics to discuss** include continued reinforcement of the importance of healthy habits, especially diet, exercise, avoidance of tobacco, and moderation in alcohol.

2. **Physical and laboratory examinations** should include weight, BP, and screening for hyperlipidemia and common treatable cancers. In most women, annual mammography should begin at age 40. Men should be offered screening for prostate cancer beginning at age 50 (see Chap. 25), and all patients should be screened for colorectal cancer beginning at age 50 (see Chap. 13). Patients with high-risk factors, including a family history of disease, need more aggressive screening.

3. **Preventive measures at age 50** include starting annual influenza vaccination and assessing the need for a tetanus booster or pneumococcal vaccination. **Perimenopausal women** should be counseled about the risks and benefits of hormone replacement therapy and should be offered screening for osteoporosis.

C. **Older adults**

1. **Important topics to discuss** include continued reinforcement of the importance of healthy habits, especially diet, exercise, avoidance of tobacco, and moderation in alcohol. As patients age, it is important to **review medication lists** for avoidance of polypharmacy and surveillance for side effects, drug interactions, and the need for dose adjustments due to changes in age, weight, and renal or hepatic function.

2. **Physical and laboratory examinations** generally continue as for younger adults. Cessation of cancer screening is an individualized decision with no definite age and is based on patient preferences, age, comorbidities, functional status, and estimated life expectancy. Ongoing attention should be paid to minimizing the impact of deficits in vision, hearing, and mobility. Patients should be monitored for ability to perform **activities of daily living,** including the ability to take medications accurately.

3. **Preventive measures include** offering one-time pneumococcal and annual influenza **vaccinations.** Many elderly patients would benefit from a **daily multivitamin** to prevent micronutrient deficiencies as the daily caloric intake wanes with aging. Discussion of **home safety** may reduce the risk of falls. One should enlist family and community resources, which can provide essential support to enable the aging patient to remain as independent and active as possible.

III. **Compliance**

A. **Assessment of compliance requires a nonjudgmental attitude** and acknowledgment of the many challenges to compliance. **Open-ended questions** are more productive. **Pill counts** may occasionally be useful but may be insulting to the patient. The patient's pharmacist can provide information on the frequency of **refills.** Low **serum drug levels** may represent failure to take the medication, poor absorption, rapid metabolism, and/or large volume of distribution. **Noncompliance must be distinguished from noneffectiveness** of treatment.

B. **Presumed noncompliance** should be approached as for any other clinical symptom by forming a **differential diagnosis of possible etiologies.**

C. Strategies to enhance compliance

1. **Educate** patient about the medical condition, the risks and benefits of therapy, and alternatives, using understandable language.

2. **Collaborate** on the treatment plan; involve the patient in decision making to establish reasonable goals. Clarify expectations, and address fears and concerns.
3. **Consider the patient's perspective and keep an open nonjudgmental attitude.** The patient's health belief model includes acceptance of diagnosis, perceived seriousness of condition, perceived benefits of the treatment, perceived barriers, readiness for change, and the level of confidence in the ability to carry out the plan.
4. **Maintain contact** by follow-up visits and telephone calls.
5. **Keep care simple and inexpensive** by using generic drugs, once-daily or combination formulations, and drugs that are not affected by meals.
6. **Give written instructions.** Have the patient repeat the instructions to assess understanding.
7. **Encourage self-monitoring** so that the patient feels a sense of control over his/her own health (e.g., home BP, blood sugar, peak flows, exercise log).
8. **Identify and address barriers,** which can include limitations of time, money, transportation, functional illiteracy, social isolation or conflict, depression, mental illness, substance abuse, or cognitive dysfunction.
9. **Focus on the positive benefits** of treatment and reinforce the patient's efforts. Set small specific goals that are achievable by breaking large projects into smaller steps. A relapse is not a failure: Take a problem-solving approach to analyze causes and work out alternative strategies.
10. **Ask about side effects.**
11. **Discuss compliance strategies,** such as the use of medication logsheets, calendars, or daily pillboxes. A wristwatch alarm can provide reminders, or medication-taking can be tied to well-established daily routines such as meals or tooth-brushing. Help with lifestyle changes can include substitution of other activities to cope with cravings or stress and avoidance of situations that tempt old habits. Achievement of new behaviors should be celebrated with small frequent rewards, such as a new book, a movie, or an outing. Family and friends should encourage healthy new habits by joining smoking cessation attempts or new diet and exercise plans.

IV. **Lifestyle counseling.** The most important interventions for promoting good health center on changing personal health behaviors and habits rather than specific clinical interventions.
A. **Tobacco users should receive brief counseling at every visit** (see Tobacco Use and Cessation, sec. I).
B. **Regular physical activity** is important at all ages. Patients should be encouraged to be physically active, either through formal vigorous exercise (30 minutes 3–4 times/week) or by incorporating physical activity into the daily routine, with a goal of accumulating 30 minutes of moderate to vigorous activity on most or all days of the week. Activities can include walking, stair-climbing, gardening, and other "lifestyle exercise."
C. **Diet.** All patients should be counseled regarding a prudent low-fat diet with abundant fruits, vegetables, and whole grains. Some patients may benefit from decreased sodium intake. Women, particularly those at risk for osteoporosis, should be counseled to consume between 1000 and 1500 mg calcium each day (see Chap. 24), and women of childbearing years should consume at least 0.4 mg folic acid daily by diet or supplements.
D. **Safety precautions.** Patients should be advised to use lap/shoulder belts for themselves and their passengers, to use safety helmets when riding motorcycles or bicycles, and to avoid alcohol or sedating drugs when driving. Elderly patients should be advised regarding home safety (see Chap. 30).
E. **Other areas for counseling and screening** include alcohol use, dental health, domestic violence, unintended pregnancy, and sexually transmitted diseases (STDs).

    F. Alternative health care practices, including herbal medicines, chiropractic care, acupuncture, or hypnosis, should be asked about in a nonjudgmental manner.

V. Patient safety and medical errors are pertinent topics in the ambulatory setting, where pharmaceutical drugs are frequently prescribed. Adverse drug events can account for hospital admissions and significantly contribute to increased morbidity and mortality (*JAMA* 1995;274:29). Some simple actions can be easily incorporated into routine clinical practice to reduce the number of errors.

    A. Involve your patients and make them active participants in their care. This helps avoid misinterpretations of diagnostic or therapeutic plans and problems with compliance or follow-up. Involving other members of the health care team, including nurses, dietitians, and therapists, is vital. Ensure that the patient leaves with clear comprehensible written directions for whom to contact and how to do so if they have any questions.

    B. Know what medications your patients are taking. Ask them (or a family member) to bring all of the medicines and supplements (nutritional and alternative) they are currently taking to each visit. Always review and inquire about any new allergies or adverse reactions. Errors due to illegible handwriting are easily preventable, and ensuring that your patients know their medications is essential in case there is a mistake.

    C. Educating patients about their medications helps ensure their safety. Ask them to check with their pharmacist that the medication they receive is the one you meant to prescribe. Make sure that they know what the medication is prescribed for, the dosing schedule, how long they should take it, what to do about a missed dose, interactions with other medications and alcohol, any monitoring or screening that may be necessary, and the importance of compliance with the medication to their overall health.

    D. To minimize and prevent errors, use computerized order entry, a reminder or alert system when available, and attempt to identify and minimize systemic errors in your practice.

Screening for Disease

The benefit of screening depends on the prevalence of the disease, the sensitivity and specificity of the screening test, the ability to change the natural course of disease with treatment, and the acceptability of the test to the patient. Various professional organizations have made recommendations regarding screening for disease; these guidelines apply only to asymptomatic patients at average risk, and they must be individualized. Many areas of controversy exist, including ages to start and stop screening, which tests to use, or whether to screen at all. For many diseases, there is a lack of definitive research evidence regarding the effect of screening on morbidity and mortality.

I. Hypertension. All patients should have their BP measured every 1–2 years. A diastolic BP of greater than 90 mm Hg or a systolic BP of greater than 140 mm Hg (measured on more than one reading) is considered hypertension; a diastolic BP of 85–89 mm Hg is considered high normal and warrants annual follow-up. Initial therapy includes counseling on weight loss, aerobic exercise, limiting alcohol intake, and reduction of sodium intake. The decision as to whether to start drug therapy should depend on the severity of hypertension, the presence of other disease, and evidence of end-organ damage (see Chap. 4).

II. Cholesterol screening is recommended every 5 years for all adults older than 20 years of age. Initial therapy for patients with elevated cholesterol includes counseling to decrease consumption of fats and to promote weight loss in overweight patients (see Chap. 5).

III. Screening for diabetes mellitus (DM) is not routinely recommended, but screening of high-risk individuals should be considered at 3-year intervals. Risk factors include being overweight [body mass index (BMI) >27 kg/m^2], age older than 45 years, impaired glucose tolerance, history of gestational DM or delivery of babies over 9 lb, family history of DM, and patients of certain ethnic groups (e.g., African-Americans, Hispanic Americans, Native Americans, Asian Americans, Pacific Islanders). The test of choice is the fasting plasma glucose (FPG). The normal FPG is less than 110 mg/dl; levels of 110–125 mg/dl indicate impairment of glucose tolerance; a FPG of 126 mg/dl or greater on two occasions is diagnostic of DM. A random glucose greater than 160 mg/dl is considered a positive screening test and requires follow-up testing (see Chap. 18).

IV. Screening for thyroid disease is not routinely recommended, but clinicians should keep a low threshold for measurement of thyroid-stimulating hormone for subtle or nonspecific symptoms, especially in older women (see Chap. 17).

V. Screening for obesity. Periodic height and weight measurements are recommended for all patients. The BMI is calculated by dividing the body weight in kilograms by the square of the height in meters. A BMI of greater than 25 kg/m^2 is considered overweight; greater than 30 kg/m^2 is considered obese, and greater than 40 kg/m^2 is considered severely obese. Morbid obesity is obesity accompanied by medical complications (see Chap. 3).

VI. Screening for osteoporosis can be considered in women who are at high risk for osteoporosis, including Caucasian women, Asian-American women, women with low body weight, and women who have had a bilateral oophorectomy before menopause. All women should receive counseling regarding dietary calcium, vitamin D, weightbearing exercise, and smoking cessation (see Chap. 24).

VII. Screening for sexually transmitted diseases (see Chap. 19)
  A. Syphilis serologic testing is recommended for all pregnant women and for all patients at increased risk for infection.
  B. Routine screening for gonorrhea and chlamydia is recommended for all sexually active adolescents and in high-risk asymptomatic women, including commercial sex workers, or persons with a history of recurrent STDs or multiple sex partners.
  C. Counseling and screening should be offered to all patients at increased risk for HIV infection, including those with a history of STDs or injection drug use, patients who received transfusions between 1978 and 1985, homosexual men, persons who exchange sex for money or drugs, or patients who have had partners with HIV risk factors.

VIII. Screening for alcohol abuse and dependence is an important part of the routine checkup.
  A. Definitions (from the National Institute on Alcohol Abuse and Alcoholism at http://www.niaaa.nih.gov).
    1. Heavy or "at-risk" drinking is diagnosed in men who drink more than 14 drinks/week or more than 4 drinks/occasion or in women or the elderly who consume more than 7 drinks/week or more than 3 drinks/occasion. One "drink" is 12 g ethanol, the amount found in 12 oz of beer, 5 oz of wine, or 1.5 oz of distilled spirits.
    2. Alcohol abuse is a maladaptive pattern of use, manifest by continued or recurrent use despite failure in major role obligations at work, school, or home; use in physically hazardous situations; or use despite alcohol-related legal, social, or interpersonal problems.
    3. Alcohol dependence is marked by tolerance, the presence of withdrawal symptoms on cessation, impaired control (drinking more/longer than intended), persistent desire, and continued use despite physical or psychological problems related to alcohol.
  B. The "CAGE" questions are a useful screening tool. If a patient has one or more positive responses that occurred in the last year, she or he may be at risk for alcohol-related problems.
    1. Have you ever felt that you should **C**ut down on drinking?

      2. Have you ever been **A**nnoyed with people's criticism about your drinking?

      3. Have you ever felt **G**uilty about drinking?

      4. Have you ever needed an **E**ye-opener in the morning to relieve the shakes?

IX. Cancer screening recommendations have been issued by many organizations, including the American Cancer Society (ACS; http://www.cancer.org), the National Cancer Institute (http://www.nci.nih.gov), the American College of Physicians (ACP; http://www.acponline.org), the United States Preventive Services Task Force (USPSTF; http://www.ahrq.gov/clinic), and many specialty societies. Research evidence has been inadequate to reach definitive conclusions regarding how, when, whom, and if to screen for various cancers. The guidelines below are a synthesis of the recommendations of the major organizations.

    A. Breast cancer screening includes, at a minimum, annual clinical breast examination and mammography every 1–2 years for women who are 50–70 years old; the ACS recommends annual mammography. The ACS, National Cancer Institute, and ACP recommend that screening start at age 40, and the ACS recommends that women perform breast self-examinations starting at 20 years of age (see Chap. 24).

    B. Cervical cancer screening with the Pap smear is recommended for all women who have been or are sexually active and who have a cervix. Testing should begin at age 18 years or earlier if they are sexually active. Initial screening should be annual and, if results are repeatedly normal, the frequency of testing can be reduced. High-risk patients should continue annual testing, but low-risk women may prefer screening every 2–3 years. Risk factors include a history of abnormal Pap smears, STDs, or multiple sexual partners. The ACP and USPSTF suggest that screening may cease in patients older than age 65 who have had regular testing with no prior abnormal results (see Chap. 24).

    C. Colorectal cancer screening should be offered to all patients age 50 and older. Options include annual fecal occult blood testing (with three mail-in guaiac cards) with flexible sigmoidoscopy every 3–5 years or colonoscopy every 10 years. Any abnormalities on fecal occult blood testing or flexible sigmoidoscopy should be followed up with colonoscopy. Earlier screening (starting at age 40) is indicated in those with a family history of adenomatous polyps before age 60 or a family history of colorectal cancer (see Chap. 13).

    D. Lung cancer screening is not currently recommended by major organizations. All patients should be counseled about tobacco use. Promising results have been obtained from pilot projects using low-dose spiral CT scans for lung cancer screening in current and former smokers over age 60 [*Lancet* 1999;354(9173):99–105].

    E. Prostate cancer screening is controversial. The ACS recommends annual screening with digital rectal examination and prostate-specific antigen starting at age 50 in all men and age 40 in high-risk patients (African-American men or those with a family history of prostate cancer). The ACP and USPSTF do not recommend universal screening because of uncertainty regarding the relative weights of benefit and risk (see Chap. 25).

Tobacco Use and Cessation

Nearly one-fourth of American adults smoke, but an estimated 70% want to quit. Although only approximately 7% of patients are able to quit long term on their own, it is estimated that counseling and appropriate pharmacotherapy can increase the quit rate to 15–30%. A widely accepted approach to brief office-based counseling and pharmacotherapy was published as a U.S. Public Health Service Report (summarized in *JAMA* 2000;283:3244–3254).

I. **Brief counseling should be provided to all smokers at every visit.**
   Interventions as short as 3 minutes can increase quit rate significantly. The
   recommended five steps are as follows.
   A. **ASK about smoking status.** At each visit, every tobacco user should be
      identified. Some practices include smoking status as a vital sign.
   B. **ADVISE all smokers to quit.** The advice for smokers should be clear, strong,
      and personalized. Physicians' advice is a strong incentive to attempt smok-
      ing cessation.
   C. **ASSESS the smoker's willingness to quit.** The Prochaska model of stages
      of change provides a useful framework for targeting interventions to the
      smoker's readiness to attempt to quit (the same stages apply to any behav-
      ior change: quitting smoking or drinking, starting to exercise or follow a
      diet, etc.). The stages form a predictable cycle.
      1. **Precontemplation stage:** The smoker is unaware or underaware of the
         problem and has no intention of changing the behavior. The physician's
         role is to raise doubts in the patient's mind and to reinforce the need to
         quit smoking.
      2. **Contemplation stage:** The patient is aware that a problem exists but is
         not yet ready to make a commitment to take action. This stage may last
         for long periods of time. The physician's role is to strengthen the
         patient's self-confidence in ability to make the change and to offer assis-
         tance in helping the patient to quit.
      3. **Preparation stage:** The patient intends to take action in the next few
         months; this may be a brief stage. The physician should increase the
         intensity and specificity of counseling and help the patient determine a
         course of action.
      4. **Action stage:** This is the most visible stage, in which the addictive behav-
         ior is actually altered (for 1 day to 6 months). The physician should recom-
         mend nicotine replacement therapy (NRT) and monitor the efficacy.
      5. **Maintenance stage:** The patient maintains the change (smoking cessa-
         tion) and works to prevent relapse. This stage extends beyond 6 months
         and may last a lifetime. The physician should provide follow-up and
         continued support.
      6. **Relapse stage:** This can also be termed **recycle** because the patient
         again moves through the cycle and may achieve long-term success on
         subsequent cycles. The physician should assist the patient in renewing
         the process.
   D. **ASSIST the patient in quitting** by helping the patient with a quit plan. The
      patient should set a quit date in the next few weeks. He or she should antic-
      ipate challenges to quitting and enlist the aid of family and friends. Before
      the quit date the patient should start to break the habit by avoiding smok-
      ing in the usual places. The physician should offer NRT or bupropion and
      supplementary reading materials.
   E. **ARRANGE follow-up** by phone or in person within 1 week of the quit date
      and again within 1 month.
      1. Successful quitters should be congratulated and reminded to be on
         guard against tempting situations and cravings, which can persist for
         months to years.
      2. Those who did not try to quit should be assessed for willingness to change
         (step **C** above) and encouraged to again set a quit date when ready.
      3. Those who quit and have relapsed should be encouraged to learn from
         the experience. The physician should focus on the positive (congratulate
         for the days or weeks of abstinence) and help the patient feel empow-
         ered to try again by discussing strategies to cope with challenging situa-
         tions (see also Approach to the Ambulatory Patient, sec. **III.C**).
II. **Pharmacologic therapy** can double the quit rate and should be offered to all
    patients except in the presence of special circumstances (see sec. **II.C**). First-line
    treatments include sustained-release bupropion and NRT.

A. Sustained-release bupropion (bupropion SR) should be started 1–2 weeks before the quit date. Dosing should be 150 mg each morning for 3 days, then 150 mg bid for 7–12 weeks. Bupropion SR can be combined with NRT, but the NRT may not add to the effectiveness (*N Engl J Med* 1999;340:685–691). The most common side effects are dry mouth and insomnia. Contraindications include a history of a seizure disorder, eating disorder, or use of a monoamine oxidase inhibitor within 14 days.

B. Nicotine replacement therapy

1. Nicotine gum (polacrilex) is available over the counter in 2-mg and 4-mg strengths; the 4-mg strength is recommended for those who smoke more than 25 cigarettes/day. Because the nicotine is absorbed only through the buccal mucosa and absorption is decreased by acidic beverages, the patient should be instructed not to eat or drink while chewing the gum or 15 minutes before. The gum should be chewed slowly until a peppery taste emerges, then parked between cheek and gum for buccal absorption. The gum should be chewed slowly and intermittently for approximately 30 minutes or until the taste dissipates. Patients may be more successful on a fixed schedule: at least one piece every 1–2 hours for at least 1–3 months, then taper off. The maximum daily dose is 24 pieces. Side effects include mouth soreness, dyspepsia, and hiccups.

2. Nicotine patches are available over the counter in several strengths. Each morning a patch should be placed on a relatively hairless location on the trunk or upper arm; locations should be rotated to minimize skin irritation. Any of the patches may either be used overnight to minimize morning cravings or may be taken off at bedtime to minimize insomnia. A typical dosage schedule is to use the strongest patch for 2–4 weeks, then the intermediate strength for 2 weeks, and then the weakest strength for 2 weeks (e.g., 21-mg, then 14-mg, then 7-mg patches). Some patients choose to combine the patch and gum to provide continuous nicotine with intermittent boosts for "breakthrough" cravings. The most common side effects include insomnia and skin irritation.

3. Nicotine nasal spray is available by prescription only. Patients should use one spray in each nostril (for a total dose of 1 mg) and should use 1–2 doses/hour with a maximum of 40 doses/day. Treatment should last 3–6 months. The spray has a faster onset of action than the gum or patch and therefore has greater potential for dependence. The most common side effect is nasal irritation, which can be minimized by avoiding sniffing or inhaling while administering. The combination of the spray and patch may be more effective than the patch alone [*BMJ* 1999;318(7179):285–288].

4. The nicotine inhaler is available by prescription only and is less popular with patients. Each cartridge delivers 4 mg nicotine over 80 inhalations. Patients should use 6–16 cartridges daily for up to 6 months. Best effects are achieved by frequent puffing. Because the nicotine is absorbed only through the buccal mucosa and absorption is decreased by acidic beverages, the patient should be instructed not to eat or drink while using the inhaler or 15 minutes before. The most common side effects are irritation of the mouth and throat, coughing, and rhinitis.

C. Special circumstances

1. Pregnancy and lactation. Clinicians should provide intensive nonpharmacologic efforts to help pregnant and lactating women quit smoking. Nicotine gum is rated category C, and the patches are rated category D, but the circulating nicotine levels are usually less than those seen in pack-a-day smokers. NRT can be considered if prior attempts to quit have been unsuccessful and the patient continues to smoke more than 10–15 cigarettes/day; each patient should be informed about the presumed risks and benefits [*Int J Gynecol Obstet* 1997;60(240):71–82].

2. **Coronary artery disease.** Transdermal nicotine has been found to be safe for patients with stable coronary artery disease and actually decreased myocardial ischemia as measured by thallium imaging [*J Am Coll Cardiol* 1997;30(1):131–132] and by ambulatory ECG and exercise stress testing [*Cardiovasc Drugs Ther* 1998;12(3):239–244].

3. **Weight gain** is a significant concern for many would-be quitters. The average weight gain is only about 2–3 kg, but a minority may gain more than 12 kg. The use of NRT or bupropion may delay the weight gain, permitting time for the patient to focus on smoking cessation. Exercise will attenuate the weight gain. Patients should follow a prudent healthy diet, but the period of smoking cessation is not a good time for a stringent diet.

Adult Immunizations

I. **General considerations.** These are general guidelines, and manufacturer's information should be consulted regarding individual products. Each patient's clinical context should be considered and risks and benefits weighed. Guidelines are subject to change over time and according to local public health conditions (Table 1-1).

A. **Legal responsibilities of the provider**
   1. **Serious or unusual adverse events** must be reported to the Vaccine Adverse Events Reporting System, whether or not the provider thinks they are causally associated. Forms are available from the U.S. Food and Drug Administration (http://www.fda.gov) and the *Physicians' Desk Reference* or at 1-800-822-7967.
   2. **Vaccine Information Statements must be given** to all patients who receive measles, mumps, rubella (MMR); poliomyelitis; and diphtheria, tetanus, or pertussis (DPT and Td) vaccines. Copies are available from the Centers for Disease Control and Prevention (CDC) and state health authorities. The CDC has also developed important information statements for other vaccines (**http://www.cdc.gov**).
   3. **Permanent vaccination records** must be maintained by all vaccine providers.

B. **Timing of administration**
   1. **Specified times are minimum intervals**; delay or interruption in the immunization schedule does not require starting over or extra doses. Doses that are administered at shorter intervals may not result in adequate antibody response and should not be counted as part of a primary series.
   2. **Simultaneous administration** of multiple vaccines improves compliance. In general, inactivated (killed) and most live vaccines can be administered at the same time at separate anatomic sites; exceptions include cholera, parenteral typhoid, plague, and yellow fever vaccines. **Immune globulin preparations** can interfere with the response to live virus vaccines. **Tuberculin test response** can be inhibited by live virus vaccines. Tuberculin testing can be done on the same day as the vaccination or 4–6 weeks later.

C. **Hypersensitivity to vaccine components**
   1. Persons with a **history of anaphylactic reactions** to any vaccine component generally should not receive that vaccine, except under the supervision of an experienced allergist. Vaccines may have traces of egg protein or antibiotics; the manufacturer's insert should be carefully checked.
   2. Contact dermatitis to **neomycin** is a delayed-type (cell-mediated) immune response, not anaphylaxis, and is therefore not a contraindica-

Table 1-1. Dosages[a]

Vaccine	Dose/route	Schedule[b]					Contraindications
		First dose	Minimum interval between doses 1 and 2	Second dose	Minimum interval between doses 2 and 3	Third dose	
MMR	0.5 ml SC	X	≥4 wks	X			Immune compromise, pregnancy, anaphylaxis to eggs or neomycin
IPV	0.5 ml SC	X	4–8 wks	X	6–12 mos	X	Anaphylaxis to streptomycin, polymyxin B, neomycin
Td	0.5 ml IM	X	≥4 wks	X	≥6–12 mos	X	Urticarial or anaphylactic reaction to previous Td
Influenza	0.5 ml IM	X	Annual				Anaphylaxis to eggs
Pneumococcus	0.5 ml IM, SC	X	(5 yrs)	(X)			Severe reaction to previous dose (see text for indications for revaccination)
Hepatitis A	1.0 ml IM	X	≥6 mos	X			Hypersensitivity to alum or 2-phenoxyethanol
Hepatitis B[c]	1.0 ml IM	X	≥4 wks	X	≥5 mos	X	Administer in deltoid area only
Varicella	0.5 ml SC[d]	X	≥4–8 wks	X			Pregnancy, immune compromise
Haemophilus	0.5 ml IM	X					
Meningococcus	0.5 ml SC	X					Pregnancy, sensitivity to thimerosal

IPV, inactivated poliovirus vaccine; MMR, measles, mumps, rubella; Td, tetanus and diphtheria toxoids.
[a]See text for further details.
[b]Intervals are minimums to achieve adequate antibody response; longer intervals do *not* necessitate any additional doses.
[c]See text for schedule for hemodialysis patients.
[d]Keep frozen and use <30 mins after reconstitution.

tion to vaccine use. Hypersensitivity to **thimerosal** is usually a local delayed-type or an irritant effect.

3. **DPT, cholera, plague, and typhoid** are frequently associated with local or systemic adverse effects that are toxic rather than immunologic in nature.

II. Special groups

A. **Young adults (18–24 years of age)** should receive a primary series of diphtheria and tetanus toxoids (Td) if they have not been administered during childhood or the history is uncertain; boosters are needed every 10 years. Young adults need to have documentation of two doses of MMR. Offer varicella vaccine to those who are susceptible. Assess risk factors that indicate the need for other vaccines: hepatitis A, hepatitis B, influenza, or pneumococcal vaccines.

B. **Adults 25–64 years of age**

1. Adults 25–64 years of age should complete a primary series of Td if they have not done so during childhood or the history is uncertain; boosters are needed every 10 years.

2. All adults who were born in 1957 or later should receive measles vaccine (preferably MMR) unless they have a dated record of vaccination with at least one dose of live measles vaccine on or after the first birthday, documentation of physician-diagnosed disease, or serologic evidence of immunity. The killed measles vaccine, which was used for some vaccinations in the 1960s, did not confer adequate protection, and those persons must be revaccinated. Most persons born before 1957 are immune and do not need to be vaccinated, except health care workers, who need to have immunity verified.

3. All adults, especially women of childbearing age, should receive rubella vaccine unless there is documentation of previous vaccination or serologic evidence of immunity.

4. All adults aged 50 and older should receive annual influenza vaccination, even if healthy [*MMWR Morb Mortal Wkly Rep* 2000;49(RR-3):1–38].

5. The age of 50 years is an appropriate time to review preventive health measures, especially vaccinations. More than one-third of persons aged 50–64 have risk factors that are indications for pneumococcal immunization, and many need tetanus boosters (or even a primary series).

C. **Adults age 65 years and older**

1. One-third of tetanus cases occur after age 60 years. All older adults should complete a primary series of Td if they have not done so during childhood or the history is uncertain (the vaccine was first widely used during World War II).

2. All older adults should receive influenza vaccine annually and should receive a single dose of pneumococcal vaccine.

D. **Persons who lack documentation of vaccinations.** If records cannot be located, the age-appropriate schedule of primary immunizations should be started. Persons who have served in the military have been vaccinated against measles, rubella, tetanus, diphtheria, and polio.

E. **Vaccines received outside the United States** are usually of adequate potency; foreign records are acceptable if they include written documentation of the date of vaccination and the schedule (age and interval) was comparable with that recommended in the United States.

F. **Breast-feeding is not a contraindication** for any vaccine for infant or mother.

G. **Pregnancy.** Risk from vaccination during pregnancy is largely theoretical. Pregnant women who are not fully immunized against **tetanus** should begin the primary series. **Influenza vaccine** is now recommended for women who will be in the second or third trimester of pregnancy during influenza season [*MMWR Morb Mortal Wkly Rep* 1999;48(RR-4):1–28]. **Vaccines for hepatitis B, hepatitis A, and pneumococcus** are indicated for pregnant women who are at high risk for these infections or their complications. **Pregnancy is a contraindication for live virus vaccines, such as MMR, varicella, or oral polio vaccine (OPV)**, but these vaccines can safely be administered to the children of a pregnant woman. All pregnant women **should be tested for rubella antibodies**; women who are susceptible to rubella should be vaccinated immediately after delivery.

H. Immunosuppressed patients
1. **Live vaccines are generally contraindicated** in immunosuppressed patients, such as those with congenital immunodeficiency, HIV infection, leukemia, lymphoma, generalized malignancy or therapy with alkylating agents, antimetabolites, radiation, or supraphysiologic doses of corticosteroids.
2. **Killed (inactivated) vaccines can be safely administered**, but the response may be suboptimal. Vaccination during (or within 2 weeks before) chemotherapy or radiation therapy results in a poor antibody response and therefore should be delayed or repeated 3 months after therapy is discontinued.
3. Because measles infection may cause serious illness in persons with HIV infection, the CDC recommends **MMR vaccination for asymptomatic HIV-infected persons**. Because of the theoretical risk, and one reported fatal case of vaccine-type measles pneumonitis 1 year after vaccination (*Ann Intern Med* 1998;129:104–106), the CDC believes it prudent to **withhold MMR in severely immunocompromised HIV-infected patients**.
4. **Symptomatic or severely immunocompromised HIV-infected patients who are exposed to measles should receive immune globulin** (0.25 ml/kg; maximum dose 15 ml), regardless of prior vaccination status.

I. Hemophilia and bleeding disorders. Many patients tolerate IM injections well if a fine (23-gauge) needle is used and firm pressure is applied to the site for at least 2 minutes without rubbing. If the patient receives factor replacement therapy, IM vaccination can be scheduled shortly after such therapy.

J. Persons with liver disease are at increased risk of suffering complications from many vaccine-preventable diseases. One should ensure immunity to hepatitis A, hepatitis B, pneumococcus, influenza, tetanus, MMR, and varicella.

K. Persons with chronic renal disease and transplant recipients should receive influenza and pneumococcal vaccines. Hemodialysis patients should be screened for hepatitis B, and susceptible patients should receive a primary series of hepatitis B virus (HBV) vaccine (see sec. III.G for special schedules and precautions).

L. Persons with splenic dysfunction, including sickle cell disease, or anatomic asplenia are at increased risk of contracting fatal pneumococcal and meningococcal bacteremia and should receive the vaccines. The *Haemophilus* vaccine should be considered. Persons who are scheduled for elective splenectomy should receive these vaccines at least 2 weeks before the operation.

M. Health care workers and public safety workers are at risk for exposure to and possible transmission of vaccine-preventable diseases. **Hepatitis B** is an occupational hazard for any worker with possible exposure to blood or bloody fluids. **Influenza vaccine** is recommended annually for all health care workers and can also be considered for those who provide essential community services. All health care workers should document **immunity to measles and rubella**. Additional vaccines are indicated for veterinarians, laboratory technicians, animal handlers, and others who may have occupational exposure to rabies, poliovirus, smallpox virus, *Yersinia pestis* (plague), or *Bacillus anthracis* (anthrax).

N. Travelers. The risk of acquiring illness during international travel depends on the areas to be visited and the extent to which the traveler is likely to be exposed to diseases. Influenza is present in the Southern Hemisphere from April through September and year-round in the tropics. Travelers should be counseled about safe sex practices. Selected travelers may need immunization against yellow fever, cholera, typhoid, plague, meningococcus, rabies, hepatitis B, or hepatitis A. Resources for up-to-date information for travelers include the **CDC website (http://www.cdc.gov)**, which has detailed information about worldwide destinations, and the **CDC's toll-free 24-hour Travelers' Health Hotline, 877-394-8747 (877-FYI-TRIP)**.

III. **Specific immunobiological agents**
   A. **MMR**
      1. **Indications**
         a. Adequate evidence of immunity to measles can include
            (1) A dated record of vaccination with at least one dose of live measles vaccine on or after the first birthday, or
            (2) Documentation of physician-diagnosed disease, or
            (3) Serologic evidence of immunity (presence of measles antibodies)
         b. Persons born before 1957 can be considered to be immune.
         c. All adults born in 1957 or later should receive one dose of MMR unless they have evidence of immunity to measles, mumps, and rubella.
         d. **Health care workers** should have documentation of having received **two doses** of live MMR, at least a month apart, on or after their first birthday, or serologic evidence of immunity.
         e. **All students** should have documentation of having received **two doses** of live MMR, at least a month apart, on or after their first birthday, or serologic evidence of immunity.
         f. **Prior recipients of killed measles vaccine** or an unknown type in the period 1963–1967 should be revaccinated with live measles vaccine.
      2. **Contraindications, side effects, precautions**
         a. MMR is a live attenuated virus; it is **contraindicated in pregnancy and is generally contraindicated in immunocompromised hosts** (see sec. II.H).
         b. Persons with a history of **anaphylactic hypersensitivity to eggs or neomycin** should be given MMR only with extreme caution and under special protocols by an allergist.
         c. In a minority of vaccine recipients, fever (5–15%), rash (5%), or arthralgias (up to 25% of adult females) may develop.
         d. Because **blood products** can interfere with the antibody response, MMR administration should be delayed (consult manufacturer's information for exact intervals). However, rubella-susceptible women should be vaccinated immediately postpartum even if anti-Rho(D) or other blood products were administered in pregnancy or at delivery. Antibody levels should be measured 3 months later to assess response.
         e. **Tuberculin test response** can be inhibited by live virus vaccines; tuberculosis skin testing can be done on the same day as the vaccination or 4–6 weeks later.
   B. **Polio.** Because wild-type polio has been eradicated from the Western Hemisphere, adults do not need polio vaccination unless they travel to endemic areas or have occupational exposure to poliovirus. The OPV is a live attenuated virus and can cause vaccine-associated paralytic poliomyelitis (approximate rate: 1 in 6 million). It is now recommended that OPV not be used for routine vaccination, even in healthy children; **only inactivated polio vaccine (IPV) should be used** [*MMWR Morb Mortal Wkly Rep* 1999:48(27);590]. **Anaphylactic hypersensitivity to streptomycin, polymyxin B, or neomycin is a contraindication to inactivated polio vaccine.**
   C. **Tetanus**
      1. **Indications.** In the United States, tetanus is a rare disease (<100 cases/year); one-third of cases occur after age 60 years. Because infection does not confer complete immunity, the patient should be immunized after recovery.

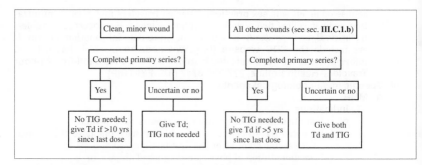

Fig. 1-1. Guidelines for postexposure prophylaxis to prevent tetanus. Td, tetanus and diphtheria toxoids, adsorbed; TIG, tetanus immune globulin.

   a. All adults of any age should complete a primary series of three doses of Td if they have not done so during childhood or the history is uncertain. Doses that are given as part of wound management may count toward the three doses needed.
   b. Tetanus-producing wounds are often not the classic puncture wounds but can include minor wounds, burns, frostbite, bullet wounds, crush injuries, and chronic wounds such as abscesses and chronic ulcers (14% of cases). Approximately 4% of patients with tetanus can recall no antecedent wound.
   c. The CDC recommends a Td booster every 10 years throughout life, whereas the ACP recommends a single booster at age 50 years (assuming a full childhood series, including the adolescent booster); either schedule is acceptable in immunocompetent adults.
   d. See Fig. 1-1 for guidelines for postexposure prophylaxis.
 2. Contraindications, side effects, precautions. Local reactions are common and consist of erythema, induration, or tenderness. Too frequent administration can produce increased rates of local or systemic reactions due to antigen-antibody complexes (Arthus-type reaction). Td can rarely cause urticarial or anaphylactic reactions. If such a history exists, then serologic testing to determine immunity to tetanus can be performed to evaluate the need for a booster dose. If additional doses are needed to ensure immunity, referral to an allergist is indicated.
D. Influenza. Annually, many deaths occur among the elderly and chronically ill, who are at high risk for complications of influenza infection (more than 10,000 excess deaths in the United States in many years). Antibodies from previous infections or vaccinations are not fully protective against new strains because the virus undergoes constant antigenic drift (point mutations) and occasional antigenic shift (change in subtype). Those who are at highest risk of the disease and its complications are also the least able to respond to vaccination. Overall the vaccine is approximately 70–80% effective against vaccine type viruses.
 1. Indications. Annual influenza vaccination is recommended for the following target groups [*MMWR Morb Mortal Wkly Rep* 2000;49(RR-3):1–38]:
   a. All healthy persons 50 years or older
   b. Women who will be in the second or third trimester of pregnancy during flu season
   c. Residents of nursing homes
   d. Adults or children with chronic cardiovascular or pulmonary disorders (including asthma), chronic metabolic diseases [including DM],

renal dysfunction, nephrotic syndrome, alcoholism, cirrhosis, asplenia, hemoglobinopathies (including sickle cell anemia), or immunosuppression (including organ transplantation, HIV infection, hematologic malignancies, or corticosteroid use)

    e. Health care personnel, caregivers, and household contacts of high-risk patients (to reduce transmission to patients)

    f. Anyone in the general public (especially those who provide essential community services) who wishes to reduce the chance of influenza infection

  2. Contraindications, side effects, precautions. A history of **anaphylactic hypersensitivity to eggs is a contraindication** to the influenza vaccine. Side effects are usually limited to mild arm soreness; placebo-controlled trials have demonstrated no increase in systemic symptoms (*Arch Intern Med* 1996;156:1546–1550, and *JAMA* 1990;264:1139–1141). The vaccine is **not a live virus and cannot cause the flu.** Guillain-Barré syndrome has not been associated with the influenza vaccine since the 1976–1977 swine flu vaccine (which was associated with approximately 5–10 excess cases of Guillain-Barré syndrome/million vaccinees).

E. Pneumococcal vaccine. Pneumococcal disease causes approximately 40,000 deaths annually in the United States. The vaccine contains purified capsular materials of 23 serotypes; efficacy is controversial and is estimated at 40–70%. Because polysaccharide vaccines do not induce T-cell–dependent responses associated with immunologic memory, there is no anamnestic response to additional doses of vaccine (although antibody levels will rise).

  1. Indications

    a. All healthy persons age 65 years or older who were not previously vaccinated or with unknown vaccination status

    b. All healthy persons age 65 years or older who were vaccinated 5 or more years ago and were younger than 65 years old at first vaccination

    c. Persons aged 2–64 years with chronic health conditions, including chronic cardiovascular or pulmonary disease, DM, alcoholism, chronic liver disease or cirrhosis, cerebrospinal fluid leaks, and functional or anatomic asplenia, including sickle cell disease

    d. Nursing home residents

    e. Alaskan natives and certain American Indian populations

    f. Immunocompromised persons, including those with HIV infection; leukemia, lymphoma, Hodgkin's disease, multiple myeloma, or generalized malignancy; chronic renal failure or nephrotic syndrome; organ or bone marrow transplant; immunosuppressive chemotherapy, including corticosteroids (the interval between vaccination and initiation of immunosuppressive therapy should be at least 2 weeks; do not vaccinate during chemotherapy or radiation therapy)

  2. Revaccination is not routinely recommended and is contraindicated if the patient had a severe reaction to the first dose (Arthus or anaphylactic). **A single revaccination should be considered after 5 years** for those who are at highest risk for serious pneumococcal infection or those who are likely to have a rapid decline in antibody levels, or both; those with anatomic or functional asplenia (sickle cell disease); and immunocompromised patients (i.e., all in sec. **III.E.1.f.**).

  3. Contraindications, side effects, precautions. Approximately half of patients experience injection site soreness, redness, or swelling; systemic symptoms are rare. Pneumococcal vaccine is contraindicated in those with a severe reaction to a previous dose (anaphylaxis or local Arthus-type reaction).

F. Hepatitis A vaccine (HAV) and immune globulin (Ig). The levels of antibody following HAV vaccine or Ig are much lower than those following natural infection and are usually below the level of detection of most commercial assays but are protective against infection (>90% effective by 1 month).

1. **Indications for vaccination for pre-exposure prophylaxis.** In high-prevalence populations it may be reasonable (but not necessary) to check serology before offering HAV vaccine. Target groups include persons traveling to/working in countries in which HAV is endemic; homosexual men; illicit drug users; persons with chronic liver disease or liver transplant recipients (no increased risk of acquiring infection, but complications would be more likely); persons with an occupational risk (e.g., laboratory workers); and persons who receive clotting factor concentrates. Vaccination can also be considered for food handlers to reduce potential transmission and to control outbreaks, according to local health authorities.

2. **Contraindications, side effects, and precautions.** Contraindications include hypersensitivity to alum or the preservative 2-phenoxyethanol. The most frequent side effects are injection site soreness (up to one-half) and headache (approximately 15%). The vaccine and Ig can be given at the same time at separate anatomic sites.

3. **Travelers** (see also sec. II.N)
   a. Travelers to Canada, western Europe, Australia, New Zealand, and Japan are at no greater risk for infection than in the United States. Elsewhere, there is increased risk even if travelers observe precautions against enteric infection or stay in urban areas or luxury hotels.
   b. Ideally, travelers should receive HAV at least 4 weeks before travel (a second dose 6–12 months later is necessary for long-term protection). Persons who travel to a high-risk area less than 4 weeks after the initial dose also should receive Ig (0.02 ml/kg) at a different anatomic site.
   c. Travelers who do not receive the vaccine should be administered a single dose of Ig (0.02 ml/kg), which will provide protection for up to 3 months. For travel periods that exceed 2 months, the dose should be 0.06 ml/kg; administration must be repeated if the travel period exceeds 5 months.

4. **Postexposure prophylaxis.** In high-prevalence populations it may be reasonable (but not necessary) to check serology before offering Ig. The Ig (0.02 ml/kg) should be given as soon as possible, but no later than 10 days to 2 weeks after exposure. Persons who received HAV vaccine at least 1 month before exposure do not need Ig. Postexposure prophylaxis is indicated for household and sexual contacts of confirmed cases (but not casual contacts). Day care center staff and attendees need prophylaxis if one or more cases are confirmed. If a food handler is diagnosed with hepatitis A, other food handlers at the same location need Ig (and should consider vaccine). Transmission to patrons is unlikely, but prophylaxis can be considered if an infectious worker directly handled uncooked or previously cooked foods *and* had diarrhea or poor hygienic practices *and* patrons can be contacted and treated within 2 weeks.

G. **Hepatitis B**
   1. **Efficacy and postvaccination testing**
      a. **In immunocompetent adults** the vaccine is 80–95% effective in preventing disease. Protection is essentially complete for those with an adequate antibody response (≥10 mIU/ml measured 1–6 months after immunization). Antibody levels decline over time, but protection against disease appears to persist despite undetectable antibody. Routine booster doses of vaccine are not recommended for immunocompetent children or adults.
      b. **Efficacy is lower in hemodialysis patients.** Antibody levels should be tested annually and a booster dose administered when antibody levels decline to less than 10 mIU/ml.

   c. Postvaccination testing for serologic response (1–6 months after completion of the vaccine series) is advised only for persons whose subsequent clinical management depends on knowledge of their immune status [e.g., infants born to hepatitis B surface antigen (HBsAg)-positive mothers, dialysis patients and staff, and persons with HIV infection] or those who are expected to have a suboptimal response (age >50, renal disease, HIV infection). Postvaccination testing should also be considered for persons at occupational risk.

   d. When nonresponders are revaccinated, 15–25% produce an adequate antibody response after one additional dose and 30–50% after three additional doses.

  2. Indications. The vaccine is indicated for susceptible persons in the following groups (serologic testing may be reasonable, but there is no harm in vaccinating persons who are already immune):

   a. All newborns and all previously unimmunized adolescents

   b. Those at occupational risk: health care workers, morticians

   c. Residents and staff of institutions for the developmentally disabled

   d. Hemodialysis patients, hemophiliacs, and other recipients of blood products

   e. High-risk lifestyles: homosexual men; men and women with multiple sex partners who are seen for STDs; intravenous drug users

   f. Household and sexual contacts of known hepatitis B carriers

   g. Immigrants from eastern Asia or sub-Saharan Africa; native Alaskans, native Pacific Islanders

   h. Travelers to endemic areas who will have close contact with the local population

  3. Patients on hemodialysis require larger or increased number of doses, or both, to achieve adequate antibody levels (measure titers 1–6 months after immunization). For adult dialysis patients use the special 40-μg/ml formulation of Recombivax-B, 1.0 ml IM at 0, 1, and 6 months, *or* use the regular 20-μg/ml formulation of Engerix-B, 2.0 ml IM at 0, 1, 2, and 6 months. Booster doses should be given when annual testing shows antibody levels of less than 10 mIU/ml.

  4. Contraindications and side effects. The vaccine is well tolerated; pregnancy is not a contraindication.

  5. Postexposure prophylaxis. Hepatitis B immune globulin (HBIG) is used for postexposure prophylaxis in susceptible individuals (no vaccine or known nonresponder). Vaccine and HBIG can be administered at the same time, but at separate sites.

   a. Sexual partners of patients with acute HBV infection or who are HBsAg positive should begin prophylaxis within 14 days of the last sexual contact or if ongoing sexual contact will occur. Administer a single dose of HBIG (0.06 ml/kg) and begin the vaccine series.

   b. Household contacts of patients with acute HBV infection do not need prophylaxis except infants and those with identifiable blood exposure (shared toothbrush or razor). Administer a single dose of HBIG (0.06 ml/kg) and begin the vaccine series. If the index patient becomes a chronic carrier, all household contacts should be given the hepatitis B vaccine.

   c. After any percutaneous exposure to blood, the source patient and the exposed person should be checked for HBsAg status. See Table 1-2 for treatment algorithm.

H. Varicella. Approximately 10% of U.S. adults are susceptible to the varicella-zoster virus and its complications. Approximately 100 deaths occur annually, over half in adults; even healthy young adults can succumb to acute respiratory distress syndrome after varicella infection. A reliable history of varicella is considered a valid measure of immunity; most adults with negative or uncertain histories are actually immune.

Table 1-2. Hepatitis B prophylaxis following percutaneous exposure to blood

Exposed person is	Treatment when source patient is		
	HBsAg positive	HBsAg negative	Status unknown
Unvaccinated	HBIG × 1; initiate HB vaccine	Initiate HB vaccine	Initiate HB vaccine
Previously vaccinated, known responder	Recheck anti-HBs level; if adequate, no treatment; if inadequate, HB vaccine booster dose[a]	No treatment	No treatment
Previously vaccinated, known nonresponder	HBIG × 2 (1 mo apart) *or* HBIG × 1 + 1 HB vaccine	No treatment	If known high-risk source patient, can treat as if HBsAg positive
Previously vaccinated, response unknown	Check anti-HBs level; if adequate, no treatment; if inadequate, HBIG plus HB vaccine booster dose	No treatment	Check anti-HBs level; if adequate, no treatment; if inadequate, HB vaccine booster dose

HB, hepatitis B; HBIG, hepatitis B immune globulin; HBsAg, hepatitis B surface antigen.
[a]Adequate anti-HBsAg level is 10 SRU by radioimmunoassay or positive by enzyme immunoassay.

1. **Indications.** The varicella vaccine is a live attenuated virus vaccine. It is indicated for all susceptible adolescents and adults, with emphasis on the following groups: health care workers, household contacts of immunocompromised persons, workers in schools and day care centers, those who live in closed populations such as colleges or the military, all nonpregnant women of childbearing age, international travelers, and susceptible adolescents and adults who live with young children [varicella deaths in young mothers reported in *MMWR Morb Mortal Wkly Rep* 1997;46(19):409–412].

2. **Contraindications, side effects, precautions.** Approximately 25–33% of recipients had injection site soreness, swelling, erythema, or rash. In fewer than 1%, a diffuse rash developed with a median of five lesions, most caused by wild-type virus. Vaccine-type virus from the varicella-like rash after immunization can infrequently be transmitted to susceptible contacts, but the secondary cases are subclinical or mild. Varicella vaccine is contraindicated in pregnancy (defer pregnancy 1 month after vaccination), in individuals with compromised cellular immune function, or in adults who receive more than 20 mg/day prednisone.

3. **Efficacy.** In adolescents and adults, the seroconversion rate is 99% after two doses. Pediatric studies show an efficacy of 70–90% in preventing infection and 95% protection against severe disease for 7–10 years. Cases that occur in vaccinated persons were usually mild with fewer than 50 lesions. It is unknown whether booster doses will be needed in the future. The incidence of herpes zoster may be less after vaccination than after the natural disease (*N Engl J Med* 1991;325:1545–1550, and *Pediatrics* 1997;99:35–39).

I. *Haemophilus influenzae* type B (Hib). Most invasive Hib disease occurs in very young children but can also occur in adults with chronic pulmonary disease and conditions that predispose to infections with encapsulated organisms (splenic dysfunction, hematologic malignancies). Most *H. influ-*

enzae disease in adults is due to nontypable strains. Hib-conjugated vaccine can be considered for adults with functional or anatomic asplenia or HIV infection (although of unproven benefit). Side effects of injection site swelling, redness, and/or pain have been reported in 5–30% of children; systemic reactions are infrequent.

J. Meningococcus. The quadrivalent meningococcal polysaccharide vaccine includes serogroups A, C, Y, and W135, but not serogroup B, which causes half of U.S. cases. Serogroup A is the most common cause of epidemics worldwide. **Indications** include travelers to endemic areas (e.g., pilgrimage to Mecca), for controlling outbreaks, and for individuals with terminal complement deficiencies or anatomic or functional asplenia. Vaccine-induced immunity is of unknown duration, and the need for revaccination is unknown. Adverse reactions are mild and infrequent. Meningococcal vaccine is **contraindicated in cases of sensitivity to thimerosal or other vaccine component**. Safety in pregnancy is unknown.

K. Rabies. Most reported cases of animal rabies in the United States are in wild raccoons, skunks, foxes, and bats. Worldwide, wild dogs account for most cases; some U.S. cases of rabies originate from dog bites sustained abroad, even years earlier. Rabies prophylaxis in foreign countries may be inadequate. **Vaccine side effects** include injection site soreness and erythema; mild systemic symptoms (such as headache, nausea, myalgias) are common.

1. **Pre-exposure prophylaxis is indicated in** persons whose jobs or hobbies bring them into contact with potentially rabid animals. Those at continuing risk should have a booster (or check serology) every 2 years.

2. **Postexposure prophylaxis**

   a. **The most important element of postexposure prophylaxis is immediate and thorough washing of all wounds with copious soap and water**, not just antiseptics. Tetanus prophylaxis should be considered.

   b. Previously immunized patients should receive two doses of vaccine: 1.0 ml IM in the deltoid on days 0 and 3.

   c. Persons not previously immunized should be treated with a single 20-IU/kg dose of human rabies immune globulin (HRIG; up to one-half infiltrated in the area of the wound and one-half IM) as well as five doses of vaccine (1.0 ml IM in the deltoid on days 0, 3, 7, 14, and 28). HRIG should be given immediately but can be administered up to the eighth day after vaccine was started.

   d. Immunocompromised persons should be tested for adequacy of antibody response.

   e. The decision to initiate postexposure prophylaxis should include the following considerations. The local department of health should be notified.

      (1) Bats and wild carnivores should be regarded as rabid unless proved negative by laboratory tests. Contact with a bat may have occurred if a bat is found in a room with a sleeping person. Airborne rabies can be acquired in bat-infested caves. Rabbits, hares, and rodents are rarely rabid.

      (2) Healthy domestic dogs and cats should be held for observation for 10 days; if signs of rabies develop in the animal, the human contact should be immediately treated with HRIG and vaccine while the animal is tested. Bites from a suspected rabid dog or cat require immediate prophylaxis. Casual contact (petting) does not require prophylaxis.

      (3) Because **bites to the head or neck can result in rabies in less than 1 week**, immediate prophylaxis is indicated.

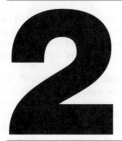

Care of the Surgical Patient

Thomas M. DeFer

General Considerations

I. **Elective versus emergent surgery.** Elective surgery carries less risk of perioperative complications than does emergent surgery, as the patient's general medical condition may be improved by treating cardiovascular and pulmonary conditions, malnutrition, metabolic and electrolyte abnormalities, and anemia. Further, emergency surgeries are often associated with serious medical comorbidities. However, in emergency situations, the disadvantages of delaying surgery may offset the benefits of stabilizing the patient.

II. **Routine preoperative laboratory testing** of all patients before elective surgery is generally unnecessary. The frequency of unanticipated abnormalities or abnormalities that ultimately change patient management is too low to justify "routine labs" for all patients (*Med Clin North Am* 1993;77:289). A very large randomized study of preoperative medical testing before cataract surgery failed to show a significant difference in the rates of intraoperative and postoperative events between the testing group and the no-testing group (*N Engl J Med* 2000;342:168).

   A. **Preoperative hemostatic screening tests** need not be performed routinely unless suggestive historical or physical examination findings are present (*Am J Surg* 1995;170:19).

   B. **Preoperative CBCs** are not warranted unless more than minimal blood loss is expected or the history or physical examination indicates them.

   C. **Multiphasic biochemical testing** may reveal abnormalities in a significant number of patients. Such results, however, rarely alter the outcome of surgery and are frequently not acted on (*Am J Surg* 1992;163:565). Multiphasic biochemical testing should be ordered when a thorough history and physical examination dictate.

   D. **Routine preoperative chest radiography** is not indicated. Testing should be performed only on those patients in whom an abnormality is expected and for whom the course of perioperative care may be changed based on the results (*Can J Anaesth* 1993;40:1022).

   E. **Preoperative ECGs** are useful in patients older than the age of 40 years who are undergoing more than minor surgery, for patients with a history of heart disease, and when the history and physical examination dictate.

III. **The modality of anesthesia** (i.e., general vs. regional) is an often-debated aspect of preoperative assessment. No absolute consensus on this issue has been reached. The basal rate of morbidity and mortality related to anesthesia is very low and requires large sample sizes to demonstrate differences between regional and general anesthesia. Furthermore, there are countless types of surgeries and medical conditions that may confound the results. Several studies have failed to show a difference in perioperative cardiopulmonary complications or mortality between regional and general anesthesia (*Anesthesiology* 1992;77:1095). A careful assessment before anesthesia is always necessary to uncover comorbidities that may increase the risk of anesthesia.

IV. Surgery in the elderly. Studies regarding the effect of age on perioperative complications have been variable. A large, prospective cohort study found that elderly patients (≥ 70 years) who underwent nonemergent major surgery were at higher risk for perioperative complications (cardiac and noncardiac) and death, after adjustment for clinical data, including functional status and type of surgery (*Ann Intern Med* 2001;134:637). However, the rate of complications does not appear to be prohibitive, and age alone should not be used to withhold clinically necessary surgery.

   A. Preoperative assessment. Older patients have more pre-existing comorbidities, particularly cardiopulmonary diseases and declining functional status. Therefore, they require an especially careful preoperative evaluation. As with all patients, the medical problems of the elderly should be optimally treated to reduce perioperative morbidity and mortality. Poor exercise capacity has been associated with perioperative cardiopulmonary complications (*JAMA* 1989;261:1909). Age seems to be associated with surgery on an emergent basis, which carries a substantially greater risk of cardiac complications (*J Am Coll Cardiol* 1996;27:910).

   B. Postoperative delirium. Older patients, especially those with dementia, are at increased risk for postoperative agitation and delirium. Preoperative mental status examination is vital for comparison postoperatively. Careful attention must be paid to the medical factors that may be contributing, such as pre-existing alcohol and sedative dependency, medications, infection, cardiopulmonary complications, cerebral ischemia, metabolic abnormalities, and pain.

      1. Supportive measures include a quiet well-lit environment, reassurance, reorientation, and the presence of family members. Physical restraints must be avoided whenever possible, as they may worsen agitation and the potential for self-harm.

      2. Pharmacologic treatments are appropriate for postoperative agitation, but great care must be taken to avoid oversedation. When necessary, low doses of antipsychotics (haloperidol, 1 mg PO or IM) or benzodiazepines (e.g., lorazepam, 0.5–1.0 mg PO, IM, or IV) can be used.

 V. Obesity and surgery. Obesity is associated with a wide variety of comorbidities, including type II diabetes, dyslipidemia, hypertension, cardiovascular disease, and sleep apnea (*J Am Diet Assoc* 1998;98:S9). These problems should be the focus of preoperative assessment in obese patients. Multiple elective procedures have been studied. Although most are associated with a modest increase in perioperative complications, particularly wound problems, the preponderance of data suggest that obesity, even severe obesity, does not result in an increase in mortality or unacceptable operative results (*Annu Rev Med* 1998;49:215). It is important to recall that obesity is a risk factor for the development of venous thromboembolism, and appropriate prophylaxis should be used (see Prophylaxis).

VI. Alcohol dependency and alcoholic liver disease can pose special problems in the perioperative period.

   A. The **CAGE** questionnaire is an effective screening tool for alcoholism (*Am J Psychiatry* 1974;131:1121, and see Chap. 1, sec. **VIII.B**).

   B. The **history, physical, and laboratory evaluation of patients with known alcohol dependency** should be aimed at uncovering the consequences of chronic alcohol use, including hypertension, alcoholic cardiomyopathy, malnutrition, GI bleeding, hepatitis, cirrhosis, ascites, anemia, thrombocytopenia, coagulopathy, and encephalopathy. The presence of comorbid conditions (e.g., seizure disorder, chronic obstructive pulmonary disease, coronary artery disease, and diabetes mellitus), prior perioperative complications, concomitant drug use, and previous episodes of alcohol withdrawal are clearly important as well. Patients with active withdrawal should not have elective surgery.

   C. The **Child-Pugh classification** (see Chap. 14, Table 14-7) can be used to predict risk in alcohol-dependent patients who are undergoing surgery (*Ann Surg* 1984;199:648). The operative mortality of abdominal surgeries in class A, B, and C patients is 5–10%, 10–30%, and 50–70%, respectively.

D. Confusion and alcohol withdrawal are major challenges in the perioperative period. Supportive care and pharmacologic treatment of agitation and other signs of withdrawal are indicated. Benzodiazepines are effective for reducing the symptoms of alcohol withdrawal and the risk of withdrawal seizures and delirium tremens (*JAMA* 1997;278:144). Chlordiazepoxide (25–100 mg q6h), diazepam (5–20 mg q6h), and lorazepam (1–4 mg q6h) are similarly efficacious. Dosages must be carefully adjusted depending on patient response.

Cardiovascular Considerations

I. **General considerations.** Preoperative evaluation and intraoperative management should be aimed at eliminating or treating risk factors to reduce the risk of cardiac events [myocardial infarction (MI), unstable angina, CHF, arrhythmia, and death]. A thorough preoperative history and physical examination and an ECG are important components. The risk of the surgery to be done and the functional status of the patient may also be important considerations. Elective surgery carries less risk than emergent surgery because the patient's general medical condition can be improved by treating malnutrition, metabolic and electrolyte abnormalities, hypoxemia, and anemia. In emergency situations, however, the disadvantages of delaying surgery may offset the benefit of stabilizing the patient. Very young patients and persons who are undergoing very minor surgery can generally proceed directly to surgery. Patients who have previous angiography results indicating mild coronary artery disease or successful coronary revascularization (and have no new clinical symptoms) have a risk for perioperative cardiac events that is probably similar to that of patients without coronary artery disease.

II. **Two rational strategies for preoperative cardiovascular risk assessment** have been suggested. Both stress the importance of a thorough clinical assessment of the patient with minimal diagnostic testing.

A. **American College of Cardiology (ACC)/American Heart Association (AHA) Task Force** (*J Am Coll Cardiol* 1996;27:910). Clinical markers that predict perioperative risk of cardiac events are grouped into major, intermediate, and minor predictors (Table 2-1). **Major clinical predictors** mandate aggressive management that may delay or cancel elective surgery; **intermediate clinical predictors** identify patients who have increased risk for cardiac events and may require further evaluation; **minor clinical predictors** alone are not associated with increased perioperative risk. Preoperative risk is also influenced by functional capacity (Table 2-2) and the risk associated with the type of surgery (Table 2-3). Table 2-4 summarizes recommendations for preoperative management based on clinical predictors, functional capacity, and surgery-specific risk. If the patient has undergone complete coronary revascularization within the past 5 years or percutaneous transluminal coronary angioplasty (PTCA) within 6 months to 5 years and there are no recurrent symptoms or signs of ischemia, further cardiac testing is generally unnecessary. If the patient has undergone thorough invasive or noninvasive cardiac testing with favorable results during the past 2 years and there has been no change in symptoms or the development of symptoms compatible with ischemia, **repeat testing is generally unnecessary**. When the surgery is truly emergent, a detailed cardiac assessment is usually not possible. In such situations, the medical consultant should provide clear recommendations for perioperative medical management and surveillance. Subsequent postoperative risk stratification and treatment are often appropriate for such patients.

B. **American College of Physicians (ACP)–American Society of Internal Medicine clinical guideline (ASIM)** (*Ann Intern Med* 1997;127:309). As with the ACC/AHA Task Force strategy, the ACP-ASIM clinical guideline concen-

Table 2-1. Clinical predictors of increased perioperative cardiovascular risk (myocardial infarction, CHF, death)

Major

    Unstable coronary syndromes

    Recent MI (>1 wk, <1 mo) with evidence of important ischemic risk by clinical symptoms or noninvasive study

    Unstable or severe angina (Canadian class III or IV)

    Decompensated CHF

    Significant arrhythmias

    High-grade atrioventricular block

    Symptomatic ventricular arrhythmias in the presence of underlying heart disease

    Supraventricular arrhythmias with uncontrolled ventricular rate

    Severe valvular disease

Intermediate

    Mild angina (Canadian class I or II)

    Prior MI by history or pathologic Q waves

    Compensated or prior CHF

    Diabetes mellitus

Minor

    Advanced age

    Abnormal ECG (LVH, LBBB, ST-T abnormalities)

    Rhythm other than sinus

    Low functional capacity

    History of stroke

    Uncontrolled systemic hypertension

LBBB, left bundle branch block; LVH, left ventricular hypertrophy; MI, myocardial infarction. Modified with permission from KA Eagle, BH Brundage, BR Chaitman, et al. Guidelines for perioperative cardiovascular evaluation for noncardiac surgery. Report of the American College of Cardiology/American Heart Association Task Force on Practice Guidelines (Committee on Perioperative Cardiovascular Evaluation for Noncardiac Surgery). *J Am Coll Cardiol* 1996;27:910.

trates on variables that enable the clinician to classify the patient as low risk, intermediate risk, or high risk. The modified **cardiac risk index** (*J Gen Intern Med* 1986;1:211) should be performed on all patients (Table 2-5). **Class II or III** predicts a **high risk** (>10%) for irreversible perioperative cardiac events (MI or cardiac death). **Class I** on the index does not reliably identify those at low risk for perioperative events. The presence of **"low-risk" variables** (*Ann Intern Med* 1989;110:859, and *Am J Cardiol* 1996;77:143) should be determined in these patients (Table 2-6). The presence of only 0 or 1 "low-risk" variables is predictive of low risk (<3%) of irreversible perioperative cardiac events. Low-risk patients do not require further testing before surgery. A substantial number of patients are at intermediate risk for irreversible perioperative cardiac events (3–10%). Such patients may benefit from further diagnostic testing, particularly those who undergo vascular surgery. Functional status is not considered in this strategy. Other than nonvascular or vascular surgery, the type of surgery is not specifically considered. Fig. 2-1 summarizes the ACP-ASIM guideline. Further characterization of high-risk patients and management guidelines are presented in Fig. 2-2.

Table 2-2. Estimated energy requirements for various activities

1 MET	Light ADLs	4 METs	Climb a flight of stairs or walk up a hill
	Eat, dress, or use the toilet		Walk on level ground at 4 mph
	Walk indoors around the house		Run a short distance
	Walk a block or two on level ground at 2–3 mph		Do heavy work around the house such as scrubbing the floor or lifting or moving heavy furniture
	Do light work around the house such as dusting or washing dishes		Moderate sports such as golf, bowling, dancing, doubles tennis
		>10 METs	Strenuous sports such as swimming, singles tennis, football, basketball, skiing

ADLs, activities of daily living; MET, metabolic equivalent.
Modified with permission from KA Eagle, BH Brundage, BR Chaitman, et al. Guidelines for perioperative cardiovascular evaluation for noncardiac surgery. Report of the American College of Cardiology/American Heart Association Task Force on Practice Guidelines (Committee on Perioperative Cardiovascular Evaluation for Noncardiac Surgery). *J Am Coll Cardiol* 1996;27:910.

Table 2-3. Cardiac risk[a] for noncardiac surgery

High (reported cardiac risk often >5%)

   Emergent major operations, particularly in the elderly

   Aortic and other major vascular

   Peripheral vascular

   Anticipated prolonged surgical procedures associated with large fluid shifts and/or blood loss

Intermediate (reported cardiac risk generally <5%)

   Carotid endarterectomy

   Head and neck

   Intraperitoneal and intrathoracic

   Orthopedic

   Prostate

Low (reported cardiac risk generally <1%)

   Endoscopic procedures

   Dermatologic procedures

   Cataract surgery

   Breast surgery

[a]Combined incidence of cardiac death and nonfatal myocardial infarction.
Modified with permission from KA Eagle, BH Brundage, BR Chaitman, et al. Guidelines for perioperative cardiovascular evaluation for noncardiac surgery. Report of the American College of Cardiology/American Heart Association Task Force on Practice Guidelines (Committee on Perioperative Cardiovascular Evaluation for Noncardiac Surgery). *J Am Coll Cardiol* 1996;27:910.

Table 2-4. Recommendations for preoperative management before elective noncardiac surgery

Clinical predictor group	Functional capacity	Surgery-specific risk	Recommendations
Minor			
	>4 METs	Low	Generally safe to undergo surgery
		Moderate	
		High	
	<4 METs	Low	Generally safe to undergo surgery
		Moderate	
		High	Consider further noninvasive testing
Intermediate			
	>4 METs	Low	Generally safe to undergo surgery
		Moderate	
		High	Consider further noninvasive testing
	<4 METs[a]	Low	Generally safe to undergo surgery
		Moderate	Consider further noninvasive testing
		High	
High			
	Not relevant	Low	Consider invasive evaluation and intensive management
		Moderate	
		High	

MET, metabolic equivalent.
[a]Or two or more intermediate predictors regardless of functional capacity.
Modified with permission from KA Eagle, BH Brundage, BR Chaitman, et al. Guidelines for perioperative cardiovascular evaluation for noncardiac surgery. Report of the American College of Cardiology/American Heart Association Task Force on Practice Guidelines (Committee on Perioperative Cardiovascular Evaluation for Noncardiac Surgery). *J Am Coll Cardiol* 1996;27:910.

   C. **Noninvasive cardiac testing.** Dipyridamole thallium imaging and dobutamine stress echocardiography may be useful when the presence, type, or severity of coronary artery disease is unknown.
      1. **The ACC/AHA Task Force** recommends noninvasive testing for patients with intermediate clinical risk who have poor functional capacity or multiple intermediate clinical predictors or are undergoing a high-risk surgical procedure (including major vascular procedures).
      2. **The ACP-ASIM guideline** recommends either dipyridamole thallium imaging or dobutamine stress echocardiography for further risk stratification in intermediate-risk patients who are having vascular surgery. Noninvasive testing is not recommended for low-risk patients undergoing vascular surgery or low- and intermediate-risk patients undergoing nonvascular surgery. If used indiscriminately, noninvasive testing may lead to potentially harmful subsequent interventions and unnecessary costs.
   D. **Preoperative cardiac catheterization** should be performed in patients with markedly positive stress tests and individuals with high clinical risk who

Table 2-5. Modified cardiac risk index

Variable	Points[a]
Coronary artery disease	
MI <6 mos earlier	10
MI >6 mos earlier	5
Canadian Cardiovascular Society angina classification[b]	
Class III	10
Class IV	20
Pulmonary edema	
Within 1 wk	10
Ever	5
Suspected critical aortic stenosis	20
Arrhythmias	
Rhythm other than NSR or NSR with APCs	5
>5 PVCs on ECG	5
Poor general medical condition, defined as any of the following:	
PO_2 <60 mm Hg, PCO_2 >50 mm Hg	
K^+ <3 mmol/L, BUN >140 mg/dl	
Creatinine >3 mg/dl	
Bedridden	5
Age >70	5
Emergency surgery	10

APC, atrial premature contraction; MI, myocardial infarction; NSR, normal sinus rhythm; PCO_2, carbon dioxide pressure; PO_2, oxygen pressure; PVC, premature ventricular contraction.
[a]Class I = 0–15 points; class II = 20–30 points; class III >30 points.
[b]Canadian Cardiovascular Society classification of angina: 0 = asymptomatic; I = angina with strenuous exercise; II = angina with moderate exercise; III = angina with walking 1–2 blocks or climbing one flight of stairs or less at a normal pace; IV = inability to perform any physical activity without development of angina.
Modified with permission from VA Palda, AS Detsky. Guidelines for assessing and managing the perioperative risk from coronary artery disease associated with major noncardiac surgery. *Ann Intern Med* 1997;127:309.

would be considered for revascularization independent of the scheduled noncardiac surgery.
   - **E. Preoperative echocardiography** does not add to the assessment of perioperative cardiac risk in patients who are undergoing noncardiac surgery (*Ann Intern Med* 1996;125:433).
   - **F. Referral to a cardiologist** should be considered in all high-risk patients and when noninvasive testing is being considered for intermediate-risk patients.
   - **G. Hemodynamic monitoring.** Intraoperative and postoperative use of a pulmonary artery catheter may be beneficial in patients with signs and symptoms of CHF preoperatively and in patients at risk for major hemodynamic disturbances who are undergoing a procedure that is likely to result in these hemodynamic changes (e.g., when major fluid shifts are expected) (*Anesthesiology* 1993;78:380). **Referral to a cardiologist** is appropriate in all such patients.
   - **H. Medical therapies**
     1. **β-Adrenergic antagonists** are recommended for all patients without major contraindications and at intermediate or high risk of cardiac

Table 2-6. Low-risk variables

Criteria of Eagle et al.[a]	Criteria of Vanzetto et al.[b]
Age >70 yrs	Age >70 yrs
History of angina	History of angina
Diabetes mellitus	Diabetes mellitus
Q wave on ECG	Q wave on ECG
History of ventricular ectopy	History of myocardial infarction
	ST-segment ischemic abnormalities on resting ECG
	Hypertension with severe LVH
	History of CHF

LVH, left ventricular hypertrophy.
[a]*Ann Intern Med* 1989;110:859.
[b]*Am J Cardiol* 1996;77:143.
Modified with permission from VA Palda, AS Detsky. Guidelines for assessing and managing the perioperative risk from coronary artery disease associated with major noncardiac surgery. *Ann Intern Med* 1997;127:309.

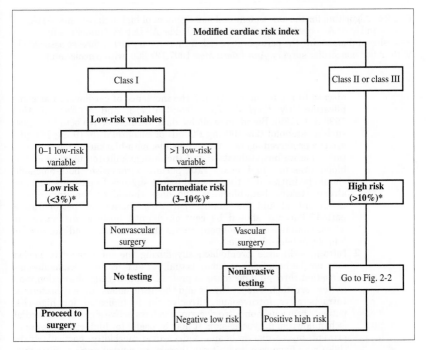

Fig. 2-1. Suggested algorithm for the risk assessment and management of patients at low or intermediate risk for perioperative cardiac events.
*Risk of irreversible perioperative cardiac events (myocardial infarction and cardiac death). (Modified from VA Palda, AS Detsky. Guidelines for assessing and managing the perioperative risk from coronary artery disease associated with major noncardiac surgery. *Ann Intern Med* 1997;127:309, with permission.)

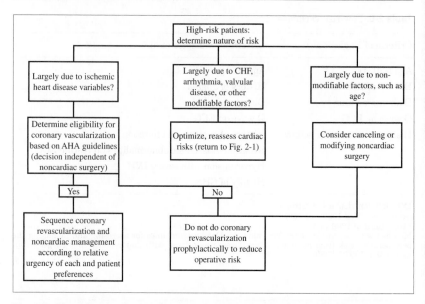

Fig. 2-2. Algorithm for the assessment and management of high-risk patients. AHA, American Heart Association. (Modified from VA Palda, AS Detsky. Guidelines for assessing and managing the perioperative risk from coronary artery disease associated with major noncardiac surgery. *Ann Intern Med* 1997;127:309, with permission.)

disease to reduce mortality and the incidence of cardiovascular complications (*N Engl J Med* 1996;335:1713, and *N Engl J Med* 1999;341:1789). Based on available data, cardioselective beta-blockers, such as atenolol (25–100 mg PO qd) or bisoprolol (5–10 mg PO qd), are the preferred agents. When feasible, beta-blockade should be initiated before hospitalization and the dosage adjusted upward as the blood pressure and heart rate permit. Otherwise, beta-blockade should be initiated in the hospital before surgery. In patients who are already taking beta-blockers, the dose should be maximized and treatment should be maintained throughout the perioperative period. Therapy should be continued until hospital discharge, at which time it can be stopped, unless there are other indications for long-term beta-blockade.

2. **Nitroglycerin** used prophylactically during the intraoperative period may not be beneficial and may actually lead to cardiovascular decompensation through a decrease in preload. Transdermal absorption may be very erratic intraoperatively, and the intravenous route is preferred. Intraoperative intravenous nitroglycerin is indicated for high-risk patients previously on nitroglycerin who have active signs of myocardial ischemia without hypotension. It may be useful for high-risk patients to prevent myocardial ischemia and cardiac morbidity, particularly in those who have required nitrate therapy to control angina. Nitroglycerin should not be initiated in patients with signs of hypovolemia or hypotension.

3. **Angiotensin-converting enzyme inhibitors and digoxin** should be considered in the preoperative treatment of patients with signs and symptoms of systolic heart failure.

4. Patients who are chronically taking a **calcium channel blocker** should continue this medication in the perioperative period.

I. Specific conditions

1. **Atrial fibrillation (AF)** that is controlled is only a minor clinical predictor for perioperative cardiovascular complications. Additional risk may come from the cardiac conditions associated with the AF. Antiarrhythmic and rate-control agents should be continued in the perioperative period. Anticoagulation should be discontinued before surgery (see Medication Adjustments in the Perioperative Period, sec. **III**). Loss of rate control in the postoperative period is not uncommon and should be treated aggressively (see Chap. 8, Mechanisms of Arrhythmia, sec. **III.B**).

2. **Ventricular arrhythmias**, including premature ventricular contractions, complex ventricular ectopy, and nonsustained ventricular tachycardia, usually do not require specific treatment. When these arrhythmias occur in the setting of myocardial ischemia or moderate to severe left ventricular dysfunction, however, they represent a significant risk factor, and elective noncardiac surgery should be postponed so that a thorough evaluation and treatment can take place. These and more serious ventricular arrhythmias are discussed in Chap. 8.

3. **Conduction disorders.** Temporary transvenous pacemakers or transthoracic pacing units should be used preoperatively in patients who have indications for a permanent pacemaker and in whom this cannot be done safely before surgery. Patients with intraventricular conduction delays, bifascicular block, or left bundle branch block do not require temporary pacemaker implantation in the absence of history of syncope or more advanced atrioventricular block.

4. **Valvular heart disease. Aortic stenosis** presents the greatest risk in noncardiac surgery. Elective noncardiac surgery should usually be postponed or canceled if the aortic stenosis is severe and symptomatic. These patients require aortic valve replacement before elective surgery. Patients with **severe mitral regurgitation** benefit from afterload reduction and diuretics to optimize hemodynamic stability before surgery. Endocarditis prophylaxis is discussed in Appendix H.

5. **Patients with prosthetic valves** are at risk for complications of anticoagulation and bacterial endocarditis.

6. **Stable hypertension** with a diastolic blood pressure of less than 110 mm Hg is not an independent risk factor for perioperative cardiovascular complications (*Med Clin North Am* 1993;77:349). More severe hypertension should be controlled before surgery. Antihypertensive medication, particularly β-adrenergic antagonists, should be continued through the surgery.

7. **Congestive heart failure** is an important clinical predictor of increased risk when noncardiac surgery is performed. Decompensated CHF is a marker of patients at very high risk. The preoperative history and physical examination should be directed at detecting unsuspected heart failure. CHF should be thoroughly evaluated and stabilized before any elective surgery (see Chap. 7).

8. **Cardiomyopathies** should be thoroughly evaluated before elective noncardiac surgery (see Chap. 7). Patients with hypertrophic obstructive cardiomyopathy may have special problems with reduced blood volume, decreased systemic vascular resistance, increased venous capacitance, and reduced filling pressures. All may potentially increase the tendency to outflow obstruction and potentially disastrous results.

9. **History of prior stroke** is a minor clinical predictor of perioperative cardiovascular complications. For patients who have recently had a stroke or transient ischemic attack (TIA) or who are having recurrent TIAs, a neurologic consultation should be obtained. Patients with asymptomatic carotid bruits do not have a significantly increased risk of postoper-

ative stroke unless they are undergoing coronary artery bypass surgery. It should be remembered that there is a strong correlation between carotid and coronary artery disease.

Pulmonary Considerations

I. **Patient-related risk factors** that may increase the risk of pulmonary complications in the perioperative period include chronic obstructive airways disease, chronic bronchitis, asthma, smoking, and poor general health status. When controlled for coexisting conditions, age is not a strong predictor of pulmonary complications. Obesity itself probably does not significantly increase the risk, but this is somewhat controversial (*N Engl J Med* 1999;340:937).

II. **Procedure-related risk factors** include abdominal or thoracic surgery and duration of surgery longer than 3 hours. Some studies have shown fewer pulmonary complications with spinal/epidural than with general anesthesia, but this difference has not been convincingly demonstrated in others. Regional nerve blockade does carry less risk of pulmonary complications. Laparoscopic procedures may have less risk of pulmonary complications in relatively low-risk patients. In patients with poor gas exchange, however, intraperitoneal carbon dioxide may be absorbed and significantly increase the carbon dioxide pressure (PCO_2) and cause pulmonary decompensation.

III. **Preoperative evaluation** begins with a thorough history and physical examination. If no risk factors are uncovered, further preoperative evaluation is unnecessary.
   A. **Spirometry** (forced vital capacity maneuver and lung volumes) should be done if risk factors are present (e.g., patients with pulmonary symptoms or a history of smoking who are undergoing thoracic or upper-abdominal surgery and when the adequacy of control of existing obstructive lung disease is unclear). Abnormal forced vital capacity or forced expiratory volume in 1 second may be predictive of more frequent and severe perioperative pulmonary complications. It should be noted that spirometry results alone should not be used to deny surgery.
   B. **Arterial blood gases** should be performed in patients with abnormal spirometry. A PCO_2 of greater than 45 mm Hg may identify patients at high risk for perioperative pulmonary complications (*BMJ* 1975;3:670). Blood gas results alone should not be used to deny surgery.

IV. **Perioperative management**
   A. **Smoking cessation** should be advised at least 8 weeks before an elective surgery (see Chap. 1). Smoking cessation hours to days before the procedure may have no beneficial effect.
   B. **Obstructive pulmonary disease** (emphysema, chronic bronchitis, and asthma) should be aggressively treated, including inhaled bronchodilators, inhaled or systemic corticosteroids, and antibiotics when indicated. Elective surgery should be postponed in the face of an acute exacerbation.
   C. **Postoperative management** should include therapeutic maneuvers that increase lung volume and reduce the risk of pulmonary complications, including **deep-breathing exercises**, **incentive spirometry**, and perhaps **continuous positive airway pressure** (for patients who cannot perform the other methods or for those who use it at home). Deep-breathing exercises and incentive spirometry should be taught to patients preoperatively. Patients at increased risk for pulmonary complications should have frequent monitoring of oxygen saturation and arterial blood gases. Bronchodilators and antibiotics should be used when indicated for bronchospasm and infection.

V. **Referral to a pulmonologist** should be considered for patients with serious chronic lung disease and those who are being considered for lung resection.

Table 2-7. Classification of level of risk for deep venous thrombosis and pulmonary embolism

Level of risk	Low	Moderate	High	Highest
Clinical characteristics	Uncomplicated minor surgery in patients <40 yrs with no clinical risk factors	Any surgery (minor or major) in patients 40–60 yrs but no additional risk factors; major surgery in patients <40 yrs but no additional risk factors; minor surgery in patients with risk factors	Major surgery in patients >60 yrs without additional risk factors; major surgery in patients 40–60 yrs with additional risk factors, patients with MI and medical patients with risk factors	Major surgery in patients >40 yrs with prior DVT/PE or cancer or hypercoagulable state; patients with elective major lower-extremity orthopedic surgery, hip fracture, stroke, multiple trauma, or spinal cord injury
Calf vein thrombosis (%)	2	10–20	20–40	40–80
Proximal vein thrombosis (%)	0.4	2–4	4–8	10–20
Clinical PE (%)	0.2	1–2	2–4	4–10
Fatal PE (%)	0.002	0.1–0.4	0.4–1.0	1.0–5.0

DVT, deep venous thrombosis; MI, myocardial infarction; PE, pulmonary embolism.
Modified from GP Clagett, FA Anderson, W Geerts, et al. Prevention of venous thromboembolism. *Chest* 1998;114:531S.

Prophylaxis

I. **Deep venous thrombosis (DVT) and pulmonary embolism (PE) prophylaxis.** Risk factors for the development of DVT include age greater than 40 years (risk progressively increases with age); prolonged immobility or paralysis; prior DVT or PE; cancer; major surgery (particularly those involving the abdomen, pelvis, and lower extremities); obesity; varicose veins; CHF; MI; cerebrovascular accident; leg, hip, or pelvis fractures; indwelling femoral vein catheter; inflammatory bowel disease; nephrotic syndrome; estrogen use; and congenital or acquired hypercoagulable states (*Chest* 1998;114:531S). In many patients multiple risk factors are present, and the risks are cumulative. Based on these risk factors, patients can be classified as **low risk, moderate risk, high risk, or highest risk** (Table 2-7). Perioperative anticoagulation is effective in decreasing the incidence of DVT and PE. Early ambulation reduces the risk of thromboembolism but is not a substitute for anticoagulation in higher-risk patients.
   A. **Low-risk general surgery patients** require no specific prophylaxis other than early ambulation.
   B. **Moderate-risk general surgery patients** should receive prophylaxis with elastic compression stockings; **intermittent pneumatic compression (IPC);**

low-dose unfractionated heparin (LDUH), 5000 units q12h; **or low-molecular-weight heparin (LMWH)**. Either dalteparin, 2500 units, or enoxaparin, 40 mg, 1–2 hours before surgery and qd after surgery can be used. Elastic compression stockings and IPC are appropriate adjuvants for higher-risk patients.

C. **High-risk general surgery patients** should receive LDUH (5000 units q8h) or LMWH (dalteparin, 5000 units, or enoxaparin, 40 mg, 10–12 hours before surgery and qd after surgery). IPC is an acceptable alternative when bleeding complications are of major concern.

D. Like high-risk patients, **highest-risk general surgery patients** should be treated with LDUH or LMWH, **with** the addition of IPC. Perioperative warfarin [international normalized ratio (INR) 2.0–3.0] may also be an appropriate prophylactic strategy for selected very high-risk general surgery patients.

E. Patients who are undergoing **orthopedic surgery** (e.g., total hip and knee replacements, hip fracture surgery) are at especially high risk. Either oral anticoagulation (INR 2.0–3.0) or LMWH can be used (ardeparin, 50 units/kg q12h starting 12–24 hours after surgery; dalteparin, 5000 units 8–12 hours before surgery and qd after surgery; enoxaparin, 30 mg q12h starting 12–24 hours after surgery; or enoxaparin, 40 mg qd starting 10–12 hours before surgery). IPC is probably as effective as LMWH or warfarin in patients with total knee replacement but must be used consistently and properly.

F. Reductions in LMWH doses may be necessary in the setting of chronic renal failure and could potentially be guided by anti–factor Xa levels. In the morbidly obese, doses may need to be increased.

G. The optimum duration of prophylaxis in hip and knee replacement patients is unclear. At least 7–10 days of warfarin or LMWH is recommended, but newer data suggest that a longer duration may offer further benefit.

H. IPC, with or without elastic compression stockings, is recommended for patients who are undergoing elective intracranial neurosurgery. LMWH and LDUH may also be acceptable alternatives.

II. **Antibiotic prophylaxis of surgical wounds.**

A. In general, antibiotic prophylaxis is indicated only for procedures that are associated with a high rate of infection and the implantation of prosthetic material and in situations in which the consequences of infection are especially serious (*Med Lett Drugs Ther* 1999;41:75).

1. **Patient characteristics** that may be associated with surgical wound infections include diabetes, nicotine use, steroid use, severe malnutrition, preoperative nares colonization with *Staphylococcus aureus*, advanced age, obesity, and infection at a remote body site.

2. **Operative and local factors** may also influence the risk of surgical site infection. Preoperative shaving the night before an operation, prolonged duration, abdominal procedures, foreign body in the surgical site, and surgical drains have all been associated with an increased risk of infection (*Infect Control Hosp Epidemiol* 1999;20:247).

3. **The classification of the surgical procedure** strongly influences the likelihood of infection.

a. **Clean (class I) procedures** [nonemergent, do not involve acutely inflamed tissue, not associated with a break in sterile technique, do not involve entering the respiratory, GI, or genitourinary (GU) tract] have the lowest risk. Antimicrobial prophylaxis is recommended for clean operations that involve the implantation of any prosthetic material (e.g., pacemaker placement, prosthetic arterial grafts, or joint replacement) or when the consequences of a surgical wound infection would be particularly serious (e.g., cardiac and neurosurgical procedures).

b. Antimicrobial prophylaxis is indicated for many **clean-contaminated (class II) procedures** (opening of the respiratory, GI, or GU tract under controlled conditions without unusual contamination/spillage).

c. Antibiotic usage in **contaminated (class III) procedures** (open, accidental wounds, major breaks in sterile technique, gross spillage from the GI tract, incision of acutely inflamed but nonpurulent tissue, or entry into an infected biliary or GU tract) is generally more therapeutic than prophylactic.

d. Wound infection rates in **dirty-infected (class IV) procedures** are high, up to 40%. In these situations, antibiotic usage is clearly therapeutic rather than prophylactic. The clinical situation dictates appropriate antibiotic selection and duration.

4. **The timing of antibiotic administration** is crucial. Parenteral prophylactic antibiotics should be given within 30 minutes of the actual skin incision rather than "on call" to the operating room. A second administration should be given at intervals of one to two times the half-life of the selected antibiotic. For cefazolin, redosing at 3–4 hours is appropriate. Routine administration of prophylactic antibiotics after the surgery is not indicated unless gross contamination has occurred during the procedure.

5. **Selection of prophylactic antibiotics** should be directed against the most likely organism. For the majority of procedures, **cefazolin** is effective. Routine prophylactic use of vancomycin is not indicated unless methicillin-resistant *S. aureus* or methicillin-resistant coagulase-negative staphylococci are significant causes of surgical site infections in a particular institution. For improved anaerobic coverage, **cefotetan** or **cefoxitin** is recommended for colorectal procedures and appendectomy. Catharsis and oral neomycin and erythromycin base should precede elective colorectal surgery.

Medication Adjustments in the Perioperative Period

I. **Diabetes mellitus in surgical patients.** Diabetes is an important predictor of increased perioperative cardiovascular risk. It is associated with important comorbidities that also impart increased risk. Surgery is a significant stress on diabetic control, and it usually interferes with oral intake. Surgeries that require general anesthesia also put more stress on glycemic control. Renal transplantation and coronary artery bypass surgery, obesity, and steroid use are associated with increased insulin requirements during surgery. Reasonable glycemic control (120–200 mg/dl) should be maintained to help avoid dehydration, electrolyte abnormalities, ketoacidosis, impaired wound healing, and wound infection. If possible, minor surgeries should be scheduled early in the morning to minimize disruption of the patient's usual regimen. Elective surgery should be postponed if the patient's diabetic control is poor (*Endocrinol Metab Clin North Am* 1997;26:631).

A. Patients managed with **diet alone** generally require no additional measures, although their blood glucose should be monitored.

B. **Oral hypoglycemics** should be withheld on the day of surgery and resumed when reliable oral intake has returned. Hyperglycemia can be controlled with insulin as necessary. Because of its long half-life, chlorpropamide should be stopped 2–3 days before surgery.

C. **Metformin** should be temporarily stopped before surgery because of the possibility of lactic acidosis. It can be resumed once the patient is reliably taking PO and renal function has been evaluated as normal. Insulin can be given as necessary for hyperglycemia.

D. **Insulin-treated patients** require careful management with adjustments of insulin dosage and frequent glucose monitoring in the perioperative period.

1. **Type I diabetics** require uninterrupted insulin to prevent ketoacidosis.

a. The most reliable way to accomplish this is with simultaneous administration of **intravenous insulin** and 5% glucose in 0.45%

sodium chloride with supplemental potassium. The dextrose and insulin infusions should be controlled by separate volumetric pumps, but they can be piggybacked through a single intravenous line. Blood glucose should be monitored hourly. The rate of infusion can be based on half of the patient's usual total daily dose prescribed in units/hour. For most patients, a conservative insulin infusion rate is between 0.5 and 1.0 units/hour.

   b. Alternatively, **subcutaneous insulin** can be used in well-controlled type I diabetics who are scheduled for early-morning procedures. Half the usual total morning insulin dosage is given as neutral protamine Hagedorn insulin (NPH) on the morning of surgery. Regular insulin is given as needed every 4 hours guided by frequent blood glucose monitoring. Although this is a seemingly simpler regimen, it is much less physiologic and can result in wider swings in blood glucose and the development of ketosis. It also does not allow for unforeseen occurrences in the operating room.

   2. Type II diabetics who are taking insulin require dosage alterations that reflect the anticipated extent of insulin deficiency, stress of the surgery, and disruption of oral intake.

   a. In patients with well-controlled type II diabetes who are taking modest insulin doses (<50 units/day) and are undergoing minor surgical procedures in the early morning, it may be appropriate to withhold a.m. insulin and give modified therapy based on blood glucose and anticipated postoperative diet.

   b. Well-controlled type II diabetics who are undergoing more than minor procedures and those taking insulin doses greater than 50 units/day should continue to receive insulin in the perioperative period. Half of the usual total morning insulin dosage is given as NPH preoperatively, plus as-needed regular insulin every 4–6 hours until PO intake resumes. When this technique is used, at least some dextrose should be given.

   c. IV insulin is appropriate for some type II diabetics with more than modest insulin requirements (>50 units/day) or those who are undergoing particularly stressful surgery.

II. In general, **antiplatelet therapy** should be stopped before elective surgery if possible. **Aspirin** irreversibly acetylates cyclooxygenase (COX), resulting in dysfunction of exposed platelets for their remaining lifetimes (7–10 days). It should be stopped at least 1 week before surgery. Other **nonsteroidal anti-inflammatory agents** (e.g., ibuprofen, diclofenac, oxaprozin, nabumetone, etc.) also inhibit COX, but this effect is more reversible and generally lasts less than 24 hours. These agents should be stopped 1–2 days before surgery. The thienopyridine derivatives, **ticlopidine** and **clopidogrel**, also irreversibly inhibit platelet activity. Both should be stopped at least a week before elective surgery. **Dipyridamole** does not prolong the bleeding time or inhibit platelet aggregation and does not appear to increase bleeding risk. Because platelets contain only COX-1, the selective COX-2 inhibitors, **celecoxib** and **rofecoxib**, have no effect on platelet function and are safe from this standpoint during the perioperative period (*Lancet* 1999;353:307).

III. The determination of when and how to discontinue **long-term oral anticoagulation** before surgery involves careful consideration of the opposing risks of thrombosis and bleeding. It is prudent for the medical consultant to discuss the anticoagulation management in detail with the surgeon. No absolute consensus has been reached, and decisions must be individualized. In patients who are maintained at an INR between 2.0 and 3.0, it takes 4 days after warfarin is stopped for the INR to fall to 1.5 or less in almost all patients. Surgery is generally believed to be safe when the INR is 1.5 or below (*N Engl J Med* 1995;122:40).

   A. When chronic anticoagulation is stopped, there will be some increased **risk of thrombosis**, and the degree of risk depends in large measure on the indication for anticoagulation. The greatest risk of recurrent thromboembolism occurs in the first month after an acute episode of venous thromboembolism or cardioembolic stroke (*Lancet* 1993;342:1255). The risk declines during the following 2 months. If possible, elective surgery should be postponed until after this time period. Patients who are receiving long-term warfarin for recurrent venous thromboembolism are at a lesser but still increased risk. Although the conglomerate risk of thromboembolism in patients with nonvalvular AF is 4.5%/year, the risk is clearly variable. Clinical factors that are associated with an increased risk of thromboembolism include history of cerebrovascular accident or TIA, hypertension, diabetes mellitus, heart disease (e.g., CHF and mitral stenosis), and increasing age. Patients younger than 65 years of age who do not have any of these risk factors are at very low risk of stroke (*Arch Intern Med* 1994;154:1449). The estimated rate of thromboembolism in patients with mechanical heart valves is 8%/year. The risk is higher with mitral versus aortic valve replacements and caged-ball versus tilting-disk prostheses (*N Engl J Med* 1996;335:407). The increased risk of thrombosis that is associated with the surgery itself must also be considered.

B. The **risk of bleeding** must also be taken into account. The typical replacement for chronic oral warfarin is full-dose intravenous heparin. The absolute increased bleeding risk with this therapy in the perioperative setting is uncertain but becomes more important as the risk of recurrent thrombosis decreases. Depending on the surgery, the consequences of bleeding may be catastrophic. LDUH and prophylactic-dose LMWH are alternatives and offer a degree of protection with a reduced risk of major bleeding.

C. Therapeutic recommendations are based on an overall appraisal of these opposing risks in specific clinical situations.

   1. In patients with a **lesser risk** of thrombosis (e.g., AF in an individual without risk factors or dilated cardiomyopathy alone), warfarin should be stopped 4–5 days before invasive surgery without the addition of full-dose heparin. Warfarin should be resumed immediately postoperatively. Such patients should receive the appropriate DVT prophylactic regimen until they are ambulatory.

   2. Patients at **higher risk** (e.g., prosthetic valves, AF with risk factors, and recurrent DVT/PE) should also have warfarin stopped 4–5 days preoperatively, but it should be replaced with full-dose IV heparin or LMWH before and after surgery. IV heparin must be stopped 6 hours before surgery and LMWH 12–24 hours before surgery. Heparin should be resumed postoperatively along with warfarin. Some authorities recommend a less aggressive approach with the use of IV heparin or LMWH in only the highest-risk patients (*N Engl J Med* 1997;336:1506). In higher-risk patients, some minor procedures can be safely performed even while the patient is receiving oral warfarin with a therapeutic INR (2.0–3.0), including most dental extractions and cleaning, endoscopy without polypectomy, and most skin biopsies.

   3. For patients who are undergoing **dental procedures**, locally applied ε–aminocaproic acid solution has been used successfully without stopping warfarin (*J Oral Maxillofac Surg* 1996;54:27).

IV. Antihypertensive medications, particularly β-adrenergic antagonists, should be continued throughout the perioperative period. If the patient is to be NPO for more than a short period, intravenous alternatives can be given. Clonidine can be administered via the transdermal route. Abrupt withdrawal of beta-blocker and clonidine can result in rebound hypertension and tachycardia. Although not commonly used, reserpine and guanethidine should be stopped before surgery, as they can cause markedly fluctuating blood pressure during anesthesia.

V. Medications to control chronic CHF, including stable doses of diuretics, should be continued during the perioperative period.

VI. In patients with **AF**, antiarrhythmic and rate-control agents should be continued in the perioperative period.

VII. Antiarrhythmic drugs in usual doses should be given on the morning of surgery to patients with a history of arrhythmias and those who are chronically taking such medications.

VIII. 3-Hydroxy-3-methylglutaryl coenzyme A reductase inhibitors can be stopped the day before surgery because of the small risk of rhabdomyolysis.

Special Considerations in the Perioperative and Postoperative Period

I. Preoperative

A. Patients who receive **chronic glucocorticoid therapy** require stress doses of hydrocortisone, 50–100 mg IV every 8 hours perioperatively (the first dose is given preoperatively). The dose can be reduced to maintenance therapy 3–4 days after uncomplicated surgery. Doses of prednisone as low 7.5 mg/day can cause clinically significant adrenal suppression. Partial adrenal insufficiency can persist for up to a year after a prolonged course of steroids has been stopped.

B. Patients with **hypothyroidism** who are clinically euthyroid and receiving chronic **levothyroxine** replacement can safely skip this medication for several days given its long half-life. It can be resumed as soon as the patient is able to take PO. If the patient is NPO for a prolonged period of time, intravenous levothyroxine can be given, usually at half the oral dose.

C. Patients who are taking **anticonvulsants** for generalized **seizures** should continue to receive this medication perioperatively, parenterally if needed. Phenytoin has a fairly long half-life and a single dose can be withheld safely. When IV or IM preparations are not available, phenytoin IV or phenobarbital IV/IM can be substituted if this is believed to be warranted. Patients with a poorly controlled seizure disorder should not undergo elective surgery.

D. Elective surgery should be postponed in patients with unstable **psychiatric conditions**, and the use of any psychotropic drugs should be clearly communicated to the anesthesiologist. Because of the possibility of withdrawal, **benzodiazepines** should be continued postoperatively in those who take them chronically. **Tricyclic antidepressants** can have significant anticholinergic and α-adrenergic blocking properties, and the potential for drug interactions exists. Tricyclics should preferably be stopped several days before elective surgery. **Monoamine oxidase inhibitors** have the potential for severe drug interactions and must be stopped at least 2 weeks before elective surgery. If emergency surgery is necessary, the anesthesiologist must be notified so that sympathomimetic drugs and meperidine can be avoided. **Selective serotonin reuptake inhibitors** have relatively long half-lives and can generally be given safely in the perioperative period. A single missed dose is of no clinical importance. The concomitant use of other serotonergic medications should be carefully avoided to minimize the risk of the serotonin syndrome. **Antipsychotics** can also generally be continued perioperatively without adverse effects. Phenothiazines may potentiate the action of other CNS depressants, and when they are used concomitantly, care should be used to avoid excess sedation. The use of **lithium** is complex because of its narrow margin of safety and its serious side effects when overdosed. It can result in fluid and electrolyte abnormalities and may prolong the effects of anesthetic and neuromuscular blocking agents. Lithium should usually be stopped 1–2 days preoperatively and can be resumed once the patient is reliably taking PO. However, the physician should be aware that stopping lithium may precipitate mania. The mood stabilizer **valproic acid** can be safely continued in the perioperative period. Since it can cause thrombocytopenia and reduced platelet aggregation, a platelet count and bleeding time should be done before surgery.

   E. Many patients take **herbal preparations** but may not report this when asked for a medication list. They should be specifically questioned about the use of alternative or herbal preparations (*N Engl J Med* 1993;328:246). Certain herbal preparations should be stopped before elective surgery. Feverfew (*Tanacetum parthenium*), ginger (*Zingiber officinale*), and ginkgo (Ginkgo biloba) may all potentially increase the risk of bleeding and should be discontinued preoperatively. Because of its ability to potentiate the effects of sedatives and anxiolytics, valerian root (*Valeriana officinalis*) should not be given perioperatively. St. John's wort (*Hypericum perforatum*) is believed to have monoamine oxidase inhibitor activity and should be stopped before surgery. In combination with other serotonergic medication, it may precipitate the serotonin syndrome. Ma huang's (*Ephedra sinica*) toxic effects include hypertension, arrhythmias, palpitations, and myocardial ischemia. It, too, should be discontinued before elective surgery (*Arch Intern Med* 1998;158:2192, and *Arch Intern Med* 1998;158:2200). "Herbal phen-fen" is actually a combination of St. John's wort and ma huang and should be stopped before surgery.

 II. Postoperative. Patients frequently have questions about wound care, suture/ staple removal, incisional pain, lifting and activity restriction, returning to work, and sexual functioning following surgery. These questions are best adressed by the surgeon.

   A. Early ambulation should be stressed preoperatively, not only to reduce the risk of DVT/PE but also to prevent the generalized weakness that can occur with prolonged bed rest. The potential for incisional pain and orthostasis should also be explained to the patient before surgery so that it can be anticipated. These issues are particularly important for elderly patients.

   B. Physical and occupational therapies are important adjuvants and should be started as soon as possible after surgery for appropriate patients. The goals of rehabilitation may include pain control, prevention of medical complications, maintenance of range of motion and muscle strength, and early ambulation. Physical therapy is especially important after orthopedic procedures. Issues of weightbearing are best determined by the surgeon. More prolonged rehabilitation or nursing home placement may be necessary.

   C. Postoperative fatigue is a common occurrence and can last for more than a month. Drugs, hypovolemia, anemia, poor PO intake, depression, and other medical conditions may all contribute. Patients should be carefully assessed for these potential causes, and they should be corrected if possible. Patients should be encouraged to be out of bed and as active as their condition allows. Gradually increasing physical therapy may be appropriate for such patients.

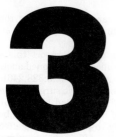

Nutrition

Mary F. Chan and
Arlyn Pittler

I. **Introduction. Malnutrition** refers to either deficiency or excess of one or more nutrients. Thus, the term refers to both undernutrition and overnutrition. For simplification, the terms **undernutrition** and **malnutrition** and the terms **obesity** and **overnutrition** are used interchangeably in this chapter.

II. **Undernutrition** causes significant morbidity and mortality. The 90-day mortality for undernourished patients admitted to a geriatric ward is 50%, in contrast to 16% for the well-nourished control group. Furthermore, the cost of treating medical complications in malnourished inpatients is four times greater than the cost of treating the same complications in a well-nourished control population. Thus, it is important to identify persons in the community at risk for malnutrition who might benefit from early intervention. Risk factors for undernutrition include advanced age, chronic medical illnesses, drug-nutrient interactions, low socioeconomic status, and social isolation.

A. **Pathophysiology.** Malnutrition occurs when intake or absorption of nutrients fails to meet metabolic requirements, leading to impairment of physiologic functions. It results in loss of skeletal and cardiac muscle function, impairment of immune function, apathy, and depression. Death often results when weight falls to 65% of ideal body weight (IBW).

B. **Wasting syndromes** may result from inadequate nutrient intake, malabsorption, increased metabolic demands, ineffective substrate use, or any combination of these. Systemic illnesses and depression may negatively affect appetite. Pulmonary diseases, oropharyngeal disorders, and upper GI lesions may result in decreased oral intake. Intestinal, pancreatic, and biliary diseases can lead to malabsorption of macro- and micronutrients. Chronic febrile illnesses and cancer may cause cachexia, despite what should otherwise be adequate nutritional intake, since fever increases metabolic demands and cancer is associated with ineffective metabolism. Detailed medical history and physical examination are mandatory in assessing nutritional risk. A thoughtful approach to the patient with weight loss results in an efficient and cost-effective evaluation and treatment plan. Causes for wasting syndromes are listed in Table 3-1.

III. **Overnutrition.** More than 30% of Americans are overweight, and another 15% are obese. Medical conditions that are associated with obesity include diabetes mellitus, hypertension, hyperlipidemia, atherosclerosis, gout, and sleep apnea. Risk factors for obesity include genetic factors, increased food intake, increased proportion of fat calories, sedentary lifestyle, and physical inactivity. Although weight loss programs to treat obesity are designed to maintain weight loss over time, it is estimated that only 5–10% of people can maintain a weight loss over 5 years. A combination of diet, exercise, and behavioral modification is the best approach to treat obesity.

IV. **Office assessment.** All methods of nutritional assessment attempt to identify individuals who have or who are at risk for significant malnutrition. A general office assessment of nutritional status needs to include a medical history, a nutritional history, and a physical examination. Ancillary tests and anthropometry may be indicated to complete the evaluation. **Anthropometrics** means measurement of the human body.

Table 3-1. Causes of wasting syndromes

Inadequate oral intake	Malabsorption	Altered metabolism
Limited finances	Pancreatic insufficiency	Fever
Ill-fitting dentures	Regional enteritis	Sepsis
Oral ulcers	Gluten sensitivity	Cancer cachexia
Dysphagia	Whipple's disease	AIDS wasting syndrome
Gastric ulcer	Gastrectomy	
Depression	Small-bowel resection	
Anorexia nervosa	Bariatric surgery	

A. **Nutritional history.** The nutritional history needs to elicit a weight history, especially a recent change in weight. It should also elicit other contributory factors, including medical illnesses, access to food, and psychosocial environment.
   1. **Weight loss.** The clinician must note how weight has changed over a period of time. The **rate** of weight loss has important prognostic implications and is the single best indicator of nutritional risk. Rapid weight loss usually indicates an acute aggressive illness and a need for a more aggressive evaluation and treatment plan. Slow weight loss is usually associated with a more chronic illness, allowing the clinician the relative luxury of time when evaluating and treating such a patient.
   2. **Additional symptoms and psychosocial factors.** Other questions to be asked as part of the nutritional history are: Is taste or smell altered? If so, is there an apparent cause? Are gingival or dental problems present? Who does the grocery shopping and who prepares the meals? Can patients afford adequate nutrition or are financial constraints present? Are risk factors for micronutrient deficiencies, such as alcoholism (thiamine, folate), lactose intolerance (calcium, vitamin D), or ileal disease (vitamin B_{12}) present? Are meals social events or does the patient eat alone? Is the patient depressed? Is the patient taking medications that may have drug-nutrient interactions (i.e., sulfasalazine and folate, tetracycline and divalent cations, and cholestyramine and fat-soluble vitamins)?
B. **Physical examination.** The physical examination needs to include height and weight, vital signs, and an assessment of fat and muscle stores. A subjective assessment of skeletal muscle mass can be made visually by the examiner. Extremity, thenar, and temporal muscle wasting all indicate severe protein depletion. Objective measurements of muscle mass can be made with anthropometrics. Trained dietitians, nurses, and physicians use standard measures of skin folds, midarm circumference, height, and weight to estimate lean body mass. It should be noted, though, that technical measures of nutritional status, such as anthropometrics, are not superior to bedside examination. The skin, hair, and oral cavity may hold additional clues to micronutrient deficiencies. Table 3-2 lists important physical findings that are associated with malnutrition.
V. **Macronutrient deficiency.** Protein, carbohydrate, and fat deficiencies can be identified by medical and dietary histories and by physical examination. Macronutrient deficiencies lead to weight loss because of the discrepancy between energy and protein requirements and energy and protein intake. Weight loss occurs with a decrease in oral intake, malabsorption of nutrients, or an uncompensated increase in energy needs. **Weight loss over time is probably the most useful single indicator of significant undernutrition.** The medical history must identify the medical and socioeconomic conditions that lead to undernutrition. The physical examination should identify signs of

Table 3-2. Symptoms and signs of nutrient deficiencies

Symptom or sign	Associated nutrient deficiency
General	
Muscle wasting	Protein-calorie
Skin	
Pallor	Iron, folate, vitamin B_{12}
Perifolliculitis	Vitamins C, A
Dermatitis	Protein, zinc, essential fatty acids, niacin, riboflavin, vitamin A
Bruising, purpura	Vitamin K, vitamin C
Hair	
Sparse and thin	Protein, zinc, biotin
Easy pluckability	Protein
Corkscrew hairs	Vitamin C
Nails	
Spoon nails	Iron
Transverse lines	Protein
Eyes	
Night blindness, keratitis	Vitamin A
Mouth	
Glossitis, burning tongue, fissuring	Vitamin B_{12}, folate, iron, protein, riboflavin, niacin
Gingiva-bleeding, -receding	Vitamins C, A, and K, folate, niacin
Cheilosis, stomatitis	Riboflavin, pyridoxine, niacin
Hypogeusia (loss of taste)	Zinc
Neck	
Goiter	Iodine
Abdomen	
Distention	Protein-calorie
Hepatomegaly	Protein-calorie
Cardiac	
High-output failure	Thiamine
Low-output failure	Protein-calorie
Neurologic	
Tetany	Calcium, magnesium
Peripheral neuropathy	Vitamins B_{12} and E, thiamine, pyridoxine
Mental status changes	Thiamine, niacin, vitamin B_{12}
Depression	Protein-calorie, vitamin B_{12}, folate, biotin
Bone	
Osteomalacia, rickets	Vitamin D, calcium, phosphorus
Osteoporosis	Vitamin D, calcium

Source: Position of the American Dietetic Association: functional foods. *J Am Diet Assoc* 1999;99:1278–1285.

macronutrient and micronutrient deficiency. Height and weight are easily measured. Temporal wasting, thenar atrophy, skeletal muscle mass, and distribution of body fat should all be noted. Percentage of IBW and percentage of usual body weight should be calculated. Percentage usual body weight is more reliable than percentage IBW as an indicator of individual risk. IBW is associated with longevity. Historically, serum protein levels and immune competence have been used as measurements of nutritional status. Serum protein levels are not markers of malnutrition per se, however, as negative acute-phase reactants they are markers of severity of illness, and do have negative prognostic implications. Like depressed serum protein levels, anergy is more often an indicator of disease severity than of malnutrition.

VI. Micronutrient deficiencies. Multiple vitamin and mineral deficiencies may be found in the severely malnourished patient. An isolated micronutrient deficiency is usually a manifestation of a specific disease or drug effect. Circulating levels and functional tests provide information about micronutrient stores.

VII. Obesity. Weight gain results when energy intake exceeds energy expenditure. More than 30% of Americans are overweight, and another 15% are obese as defined in terms of **body mass index (BMI)** or weight (kg) divided by height^2 (m^2). Obesity-associated morbidity increases proportionately with BMI.

Underweight: BMI <18.5 kg/m^2
Normal weight: BMI 18.5–25.0 kg/m^2
Overweight: BMI >25 kg/m^2
Obesity: BMI >30 kg/m^2
Morbid obesity: BMI >40 kg/m^2

VIII. Professional and consumer nutrient guidelines
  A. Recommended dietary allowances (RDAs). The RDAs, first established in 1941, are levels of intake of essential nutrients that are adequate to meet the known nutritional needs of practically all (97–98%) healthy persons. Traditionally, RDAs have focused on preventing nutritional deficiencies and not preventing disease.
  B. Dietary reference intakes (DRIs). To improve on the concept of RDAs, the Food and Nutrition Board in 1997 adopted a new approach to quantifying nutrient needs called the **dietary reference intakes** that incorporates the RDAs. Where RDAs have focused on nutrient deficiency, DRIs focus on the relationship of nutrients and food components to health and chronic disease. DRIs represent a change from a primary concern for the prevention of deficiency to an emphasis on the beneficial effects of healthy eating. DRIs are quantitative estimates of nutrient intakes that can be used for planning and assessing diets for healthy individuals. The DRIs consist of four reference intakes: the RDA, the tolerable upper limit (UL), estimated average requirement (EAR), and adequate intake (AI). DRIs have been published for calcium, phosphorus, magnesium, vitamin D, and fluoride (Institute of Medicine. *Dietary Reference Intakes for Calcium, Phosphorus, Magnesium, Vitamin D and Fluoride*. Washington, DC: National Academy Press, 1997) and for thiamine, riboflavin, niacin, vitamin B$_6$, folate, vitamin B$_{12}$, pantothenic acid, biotin, and choline (Institute of Medicine. *Dietary Reference Intakes for Calcium, Phosphorus, Magnesium, Vitamin D and Fluoride*. Washington, DC: National Academy Press, 1998). A report for vitamins C and E and for beta-carotene is due soon. Additional nutrients and food components will be published over the next few years. Tables 3-3 and 3-4 contain the most current recommendations of the Food and Nutrition Board.
    1. Recommended dietary allowances (RDAs). The RDA in the framework of DRI takes on a new role, serving only as a goal for intake for individuals. RDA is the intake that meets the nutrient needs of almost all healthy individuals in a specific age and gender group. Its values are based on estimating an **average requirement plus an increase** to

Table 3-3. Food and Nutrition Board, Institute of Medicine: National Academy of Sciences dietary reference intakes: recommended intakes for individuals

Life-stage group	Calcium (mg/day)	Phosphorus (mg/day)	Magnesium (mg/day)	Vitamin D (mg/day)[a,b]	Fluoride (mg/day)	Thiamin (mg/day)	Riboflavin (mg/day)	Niacin (mg/day)[c]	Vitamin B6 (mg/day)	Folate (μg/day)[d]	Vitamin B12 (μg/day)	Pantothenic acid (mg/day)	Biotin (μg/day)	Choline (mg/day)[e]
Infants														
0–6 mos	210*	100*	30*	5*	0.01*	0.2*	0.3*	2*	0.1*	65*	0.4*	1.7*	5*	125*
7–12 mos	270*	275*	75*	5*	0.5*	0.3*	0.4*	4*	0.3*	80*	0.5*	1.8*	6*	150*
Children														
1–3 yrs	500*	460	80	5*	0.7*	0.5	0.5	6	0.5	150	0.9	2*	8*	200*
4–8 yrs	800*	500	130	5*	1*	0.6	0.6	8	0.6	200	1.2	3*	12*	250*
Males														
9–13 yrs	1300*	1250	240	5*	2*	0.9	0.9	12	1.0	300	1.8	4*	20*	375*
14–18 yrs	1300*	1250	410	5*	3*	1.2	1.3	16	1.3	400	2.4	5*	25*	550*
19–30 yrs	1000*	700	400	5*	4*	1.2	1.3	16	1.3	400	2.4	5*	30*	550*
31–50 yrs	1000*	700	420	5*	4*	1.2	1.3	16	1.3	400	2.4	5*	30*	550*
51–70 yrs	1200*	700	420	10*	4*	1.2	1.3	16	1.7	400	2.4[f]	5*	30*	550*
>70 yrs	1200*	700	420	15*	4*	1.2	1.3	16	1.7	400	2.4[f]	5*	30*	550*
Females														
9–13 yrs	1300*	1250	240	5*	2*	0.9	0.9	12	1.0	300	1.8	4*	20*	375*
14–18 yrs	1300*	1250	360	5*	3*	1.0	1.0	14	1.2	400[g]	2.4	5*	25*	400*
19–30 yrs	1000*	700	310	5*	3*	1.1	1.1	14	1.3	400[g]	2.4	5*	30*	425
31–50 yrs	1000*	700	320	5*	3*	1.1	1.1	14	1.3	400[g]	2.4	5*	30*	425*
51–70 yrs	1200*	700	320	10*	3*	1.1	1.1	14	1.5	400	2.4[f]	5*	30*	425*
>70 yrs	1200*	700	320	15*	3*	1.1	1.1	14	1.5	400	2.4[f]	5*	30*	425*

Pregnancy														
≤18 yrs	1300*	1250	400	5*	3*	1.4	1.4	18	1.9	600[h]	2.6	6*	30*	450*
19–30 yrs	1000*	700	350	5*	3*	1.4	1.4	18	1.9	600[h]	2.6	6*	30*	450*
31–50 yrs	1000*	700	360	5*	3*	1.4	1.4	18	1.9	600[h]	2.6	6*	30*	450*
Lactation														
≤18 yrs	1300*	1250	360	5*	3*	1.6	1.6	17	2.0	500	2.8	7*	35*	550*
19–30 yrs	1000*	700	310	5*	3*	1.6	1.6	17	2.0	500	2.8	7*	35*	550*
31–50 yrs	1000*	700	320	5*	3*	1.6	1.6	17	2.0	500	2.8	7*	35*	550*

Note: This table presents recommended dietary allowances (RDAs) in **bold** type and adequate intakes (AIs) in ordinary type followed by an asterisk (*). RDAs and AIs can both be used as goals for individual intake. RDAs are set to meet the needs of almost all (97–98%) individuals in a group. For healthy breast-fed infants, the AI is the mean intake. The AI for other life-stage and gender groups is believed to cover the needs of all individuals in the group, but lack of data or uncertainty in the data prevent the ability to specify with confidence the percentage of individuals who are covered by this intake.

[a]As cholecalciferol, 1 μg cholecalciferol = 40 IU vitamin D.

[b]In the absence of adequate exposure to sunlight.

[c]As niacin equivalents (NE). 1 mg niacin = 60 mg tryptophan; 0–6 mos = preformed niacin (not NE).

[d]As dietary folate equivalents (DFE). 1 DFE = 1 μg food folate = 0.6 μg folic acid from fortified food or as a supplement consumed with food = 0.5 μg of a supplement taken on an empty stomach.

[e]Although AIs have been set for choline, there are few data to assess whether a dietary supply of choline is needed at all stages of the life cycle, and the choline requirement may be able to be met by endogenous synthesis at some of these stages.

[f]Because 10–30% of older people may malabsorb food-bound B_{12}, it is advisable for those older than 50 years to meet their RDA mainly by consuming foods that are fortified with B_{12} or a supplement containing B_{12}.

[g]In view of evidence linking folate intake with neural tube defects in the fetus, it is recommended that all women who are capable of becoming pregnant consume 400 μg from supplements or fortified foods in addition to intake of food folate from a varied diet.

[h]It is assumed that women will continue to consume 400 μg from supplements or fortified food until their pregnancy is confirmed and they enter prenatal care, which ordinarily occurs after the end of the periconceptional period—the critical time for formation of the neural tube.

Institute of Medicine. *Dietary Reference Intakes for Calcium, Phosphorus, Magnesium, Vitamin D, and Fluoride.* A Report of the Standing Committee on the Scientific Evaluation of Dietary Reference Intakes and Its Panel on Calcium and Related Nutrients and Subcommittee on Upper Reference Levels of Nutrients, Food and Nutrition Board. Washington, DC: National Academy Press, 1997.

Institute of Medicine. *Dietary Reference Intakes for Thiamin, Riboflavin, Niacin, Vitamin B_6, Folate, Vitamin B_{12}, Pantothenic Acid, Biotin, and Choline.* A Report of the Standing Committee on the Scientific Evaluation of Dietary Reference Intakes and Its Panel on Folate, Other B Vitamins, and Choline and Subcommittee on Upper Reference Levels of Nutrients, Food and Nutrition Board. Washington, DC: National Academy Press, 1998.

Table 3-4. Food and Nutrition Board, National Academy of Sciences: National Research Council recommended dietary allowances,[a] revised 1989 (abridged)

Category	Age (yrs) or condition	Weight[b] (kg)	(lb)	Height[b] (cm)	(in.)	Protein (g)	Vitamin A (µg RE)[c]	Vitamin E (mg α-TE)[d]	Vitamin K (µg)	Vitamin C (mg)	Iron (mg)	Zinc (mg)	Iodine (µg)	Selenium (µg)
Infants	0.0–0.5	6	13	60	24	13	375	3	5	30	6	5	40	10
	0.5–1.0	9	20	71	28	14	375	4	10	35	10	5	50	15
Children	1–3	13	29	90	35	16	400	6	15	40	10	10	70	20
	4–6	20	44	112	44	24	500	7	20	45	10	10	90	20
	7–10	28	62	132	52	28	700	7	30	45	10	10	120	30
Males	11–14	45	99	157	62	45	1000	10	45	50	12	15	150	40
	15–18	66	145	176	69	59	1000	10	65	60	12	15	150	50
	19–24	72	160	177	70	58	1000	10	70	60	10	15	150	70
	25–50	79	174	176	70	63	1000	10	80	60	10	15	150	70
	51+	77	170	173	68	63	1000	10	80	60	10	15	150	70
Females	11–14	46	101	157	62	46	800	8	45	50	15	12	150	45
	15–18	55	120	163	64	44	800	8	55	60	15	12	150	50
	19–24	58	128	164	65	46	800	8	60	60	15	12	150	55
	25–50	63	138	163	64	50	800	8	65	60	15	12	150	55
	51+	65	143	160	63	50	800	8	65	60	10	12	150	55

Pregnant	—	—	—	60	800	10	65	70	30	15	175	65
Lactating	1st 6 mos	—	—	—	65	1300	12	65	95	15	19	200	75
	2nd 6 mos	—	—	—	62	1200	11	65	90	15	16	200	75

RE, retinol equivalents; α-TE, α-tocopherol equivalents.

Note: This table does not include nutrients for which dietary reference intakes have recently been established [see *Dietary Reference Intakes for Calcium, Phosphorus, Magnesium, Vitamin D, and Fluoride* (1997) and *Dietary Reference Intakes for Thiamin, Riboflavin, Niacin, Vitamin B₆, Folate, Vitamin B₁₂, Pantothenic Acid, Biotin, and Choline* (1998)].

[a] The allowances, expressed as average daily intakes over time, are intended to provide for individual variations among most normal persons as they live in the United States under usual environmental stresses. Diets should be based on a variety of common foods to provide other nutrients for which human requirements have been less well defined.

[b] Weights and heights of reference adults are actual medians for the U.S. population of the designated age, as reported by National Health and Nutrition Examination Survey (NHANES II). The use of these figures does not imply that the height-weight ratios are ideal.

[c] 1 retinol equivalent = 1 μg retinol or 6 μg beta-carotene.

[d] 1 mg/day α-tocopherol = 1 α-TE.

©Copyright 1998 by the National Academy of Sciences. All rights reserved.

Institute of Medicine. *Dietary Reference Intakes for Calcium, Phosphorus, Magnesium, Vitamin D, Folate, and Fluoride.* A Report of the Standing Committee on the Scientific Evaluation of Dietary Reference Intakes and Its Panel on Calcium and Related Nutrients and Subcommittee on Upper Reference Levels of Nutrients, Food and Nutrition Board. Washington, DC: National Academy Press, 1997.

Institute of Medicine. *Dietary Reference Intakes for Thiamin, Riboflavin, Niacin, Vitamin B₆, Vitamin B₁₂, Pantothenic Acid, Biotin, and Choline.* A Report of the Standing Committee on the Scientific Evaluation of Dietary Reference Intakes and Its Panel on Folate, Other B Vitamins, and Choline and Subcommittee on Upper Reference Levels of Nutrients, Food and Nutrition Board. Washington, DC: National Academy Press, 1998.

45

Table 3-5. 2000 Dietary Guidelines for Americans from the U.S. Department of Agriculture and the Department of Health and Human Services

Aim for fitness
    Aim for a healthy weight
    Be physically active each day
Build a healthy base
    Let the pyramid guide your food choices
    Choose a variety of grains daily, especially whole grains
    Choose a variety of fruits and vegetables daily
    Keep food safe to eat
Choose sensibly
    Choose a diet that is low in saturated fat and cholesterol and moderate in total fat
    Choose beverages and foods to moderate your intake of sugars
    Choose and prepare foods with less salt
    If you drink alcoholic beverages, do so in moderation

account for the variation within a particular group. The RDA should be used in guiding individuals to achieve adequate nutrient intake aimed at decreasing the risk of chronic disease.

2. **Estimated average requirement (EAR).** EAR is the intake that meets the estimated nutrient need of half the individuals in a specific group. This figure is used for developing the RDA. If the EAR for a given nutrient cannot be established through sufficient scientific data, the RDA for that nutrient cannot be established. When the RDA cannot be established, the AI is used instead.

3. **Adequate index (AI).** When sufficient data are not available to estimate an average requirement, an AI is set. AI is a goal for intake where no RDA exists. As with the RDA, the AI is used as a goal for the nutrient intake of individuals. It is based on observed or experimental calculations.

4. **Tolerable upper limit (UL).** The UL is the upper limit of intake that is safe to most individuals. Increasing consumption above the upper limit also increased the chance of adverse effects. The UL of a nutrient assumes daily use.

C. **Dietary guidelines.** The U.S. Department of Agriculture (USDA) and the Department of Health and Human Services developed guidelines for healthy eating called **Dietary Guidelines for Americans**. The latest edition from 2000 is summarized in Table 3-5. These guidelines are based on current scientific knowledge and are an attempt to promote health and to reduce the risk of major chronic diseases. They are revised every 5 years. The USDA and Department of Health and Human Services also developed a graphic depiction (**food guide pyramid**), shown in Fig. 3-1, to convey the message of moderation, proportionality, and variety, using the five major food groups (USDA, Home and Garden Bulletin 252, U.S. Government Printing Office, 1992). Other pyramids have also evolved.

D. **Alternate food plans.** Other organizations have created additional graphics to represent the nutrient needs of diverse populations. The Mediterranean diet pyramid received much attention for its potential for protecting against cancer and cardiovascular disease. Researchers at Tufts University developed the Food Guide Pyramid for People over 70 Years Old, with special emphasis on nutrient-dense foods, high-fiber foods, and water. Various cultural food habits and vegetarian diets have been displayed on other pyramids. The Asian

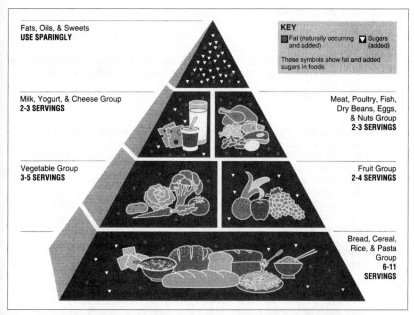

Fig. 3-1. U.S. Department of Agriculture and Department of Health and Human Services food guide pyramid.

Diet Pyramid developed by Cornell and Harvard universities and Oldways Preservation and Exchange Trust stress the traditional plant-based rural diets. These and other food guide pyramids can be found at http://www.nal.usda.gov/fnic/etext/000023.html.

IX. Energy

A. Requirements. Total energy expenditure (TEE) is equal to basal energy expenditure (BEE) or basal metabolic rate (BMR) and the energy expenditure of activity plus the thermic effect of food. The thermic effect of food is a small percentage of TEE and is largely ignored when energy requirements are estimated. Thus, energy needs are calculated from an estimate of BMR with an activity factor that adjusts for the stress of various medical conditions and for the level of activity. Rarely is BMR or TEE measured. Many methods are available for estimating energy requirements. The easiest method in a healthy individual is to provide 25 kcal/kg body weight for weight loss, 30 kcal/kg body weight for weight maintenance, and 35 kcal/kg body weight for weight gain.

B. Harris-Benedict equations estimate BMR based on gender, height, age, and weight. BMR is multiplied by an activity and stress factor ranging between 0.8 and 1.8 to yield an estimate of TEE. The Harris-Benedict equations are

Male: BMR (kcal) $= 66.5 + (13.8 \times \text{wt in kg}) + (5 \times \text{ht in cm}) - 6.8 \times \text{age in yrs}$

Female: BMR (kcal) $= 655 + (9.6 \times \text{wt in kg}) + (1.9 \times \text{ht in cm}) - 4.7 \times \text{age}$

Multiply BMR by an activity factor to estimate daily caloric needs. The activity factors that are most often used are 1.2 for sedentary lifestyle, 1.3 for little activity, and 1.5 for regular activity.

C. **Indirect calorimetry** measures oxygen consumption and carbon dioxide production. Energy expenditure is calculated using the respiratory quotient. This method is expensive, requires special equipment, trained personnel, and is not readily available.

D. **An easy method** for estimating BMR uses the formula 1 kcal/kg/hour for men and 0.9 kcal/kg/hour for women. The estimated BMR for a 70-kg man is

$$\text{BMR} = 1 \text{ kcal} \times 70 \text{ kg} \times 24 \text{ hours} = 1680 \text{ kcal/day}.$$

X. **Protein**
   A. **Assessment.** Extremity, thenar, and temporal muscle wasting indicates chronic protein-calorie malnutrition. Although serum proteins have traditionally been used to assess total body protein status, these **protein levels rarely reflect protein homeostasis and are not recommended as part of a nutritional assessment**. Serum proteins that are manufactured within the liver are often acute-phase reactants and better reflect overall health status, not nutritional status. For example, serum albumin is often depressed in chronic illness despite normal nutritional status. Nonetheless, a low serum albumin level may have negative prognostic value and can be very important in the overall assessment of the patient.
   B. **Food sources.** Dietary sources of protein include animal products, such as meat, poultry, fish, and dairy products (excluding butter, sour cream, and cream cheese), and plant products, such as grains, legumes, and vegetables. Complete proteins contain all nine indispensable (essential) amino acids in the approximate amounts needed by humans. Sources of complete proteins are foods of animal origin, with the exception of gelatin, which does not have tryptophan. Incomplete proteins or low-quality proteins are derived from plant foods. These foods tend to have too little of one or more indispensable amino acid. To ensure that the body receives all the indispensable amino acids, plant proteins can be ingested in combination so that their amino acid patterns become complementary. For example, legumes complement grains. The lacto-ova vegetarian should have no problem with protein adequacy, because when milk and eggs are combined with plant foods, the indispensable amino acids are supplied in adequate amounts. The formula for **vegan** protein balance is 60% of protein from grains, 35% from legumes, and 5% from leafy greens.
   C. **Recommended protein intake.** Protein and amino acid requirements of humans are influenced by age, body size, physiologic state, and level of energy intake. The RDA for protein intake in young healthy adults of both sexes is 0.8 g/kg body weight/day. No evidence has been shown that protein intakes above the RDA are beneficial, and they may in fact be detrimental. Nonetheless, the average American's daily protein intake far exceeds the RDA.

XI. **Carbohydrate**
   A. **Types of carbohydrate**
      1. **Polysaccharides.** Roughly half of dietary carbohydrates are in the form of complex carbohydrates that are derived largely from cereal grains and vegetables. Starch is the most common digestible polysaccharide. Cellulose, the major component of cell walls in plants, is resistant to digestion and is therefore defined as a dietary fiber.
      2. **Sugars.** The remaining half of dietary carbohydrate intake is supplied as oligo- or monosaccharides, also known as sugars. The disaccharides, sucrose and lactose, are the predominant dietary sugars. Fructose is commonly used as an additive in foods. Maltose and glucose are less common sugars. Maltose is a disaccharide; glucose and fructose are monosaccharides, also known as **simple sugars**.
   B. **Requirements.** In general, it is recommended that Americans increase their intake of complex carbohydrates and fiber. Once daily energy requirements

have been estimated, the proportion of calories provided as carbohydrates and as fat can be calculated, and diets and menus can be planned. It is recommended that **fat intake** should be limited to 30% or less of total calories, with the balance of the energy requirements being met by carbohydrates and protein intakes. **Carbohydrates** should comprise 55–65% total daily calories. **Fiber intake** should range between 25 and 35 g/day. Daily recommendations are for five or more servings of vegetables and fruits and for six or more servings of breads, cereals, and legumes.

C. **High- and low-fiber diets.** Dietary fiber is not a single entity. It is best defined as plant polysaccharides, which are resistant to hydrolysis by the digestive enzymes of humans. Fibers are often categorized by their solubility in water, water-holding capacity and viscosity, ability to bind organic and inorganic compounds, and fermentability by intestinal bacteria. Pectin, gum, mucilages, and some hemicelluloses are considered soluble fibers. Cellulose, lignin, and some hemicelluloses are considered insoluble fibers.

   1. **Benefits of soluble fiber.** Soluble fibers delay gastric emptying, slow intestinal transit, and decrease glucose absorption. These properties can improve glycemic control in a diabetic patient because complex carbohydrates are absorbed more slowly than simple sugars. Water-soluble fibers in general have high water-holding capacity and can form viscous solutions in the gut. This decreases luminal wall tension (pain and cramps) and diarrhea in irritable bowel syndrome. Soluble fibers and lignin (an insoluble fiber) adsorb fatty acids, cholesterol, and bile acids, and have the beneficial effects of lowering serum lipid levels and preventing atherosclerosis. Legumes are a good source of soluble fiber. Psyllium (Metamucil) and methylcellulose (Citrucel) are soluble fibers that are marketed as laxatives. These same fiber supplements are often beneficial for patients with chronic diarrhea.

   2. **Benefits of insoluble fiber.** Insoluble fibers increase intestinal transit and increase fecal bulk, providing a laxative effect. This may translate into lower rates of diverticulosis and colonic neoplasms. Wheat bran is a good source of insoluble fiber.

   3. **Recommended daily intake of fiber.** Several governmental and private agencies have recommended increasing the amount of dietary fiber in the American diet. The recommended daily intake of fiber is 25–35 g/day. The minimum recommended fiber intake is 20 g/day. To achieve these recommendations, individuals should consume fiber-rich legumes, at least 5 servings of fruits and vegetables/day, and at least 2–3 servings/day of whole grains as part of the 6–11 recommended servings by the food guide pyramid depicted in Fig. 3-1.

   4. **Low-fiber diet.** Patients with acute GI disorders, such as a flare of inflammatory bowel disease, diverticulitis, or infectious diarrhea, may benefit temporarily from a low-fiber diet. The **BRAT diet** is an example of a low-fiber diet and consists of **b**ananas, white **r**ice, **a**pples or applesauce, and **t**oast made with white bread. Other low-fiber foods include canned fruits, canned vegetables, pasta made with processed wheat, and meats. Dairy products are without fiber but may not be tolerated in acute GI disorders because of the lactose (see below) they contain.

D. **Lactose.** Lactose is a disaccharide of glucose and galactose that is cleaved by the brush border enzyme, lactase. The disaccharidase activity occurs in the microvilli of the intestinal mucosa. Diminished or absent lactase activity leads to maldigestion of lactose.

   1. **Lactose intolerance** is the symptomatic response to lactase deficiency. The undigested sugar causes an osmotic diarrhea. Distention, bloating, abdominal pain, and flatulence are caused by bacterial fermentation of lactose within the colon. Individuals generally develop symptoms with the ingestion of 12–18 g lactose, which is roughly the equivalent of 1–1 1/2 glasses of milk (see Chap. 13).

2. Causes of lactose intolerance

a. Congenital lactase deficiency is rare, but acquired deficiency is common (>50%) in adults.

b. Primary delayed-onset lactase deficiency is a genetically predetermined reduction of enzyme activity during childhood or adolescence. Lactase deficiency is the norm (>90%) in several populations in Africa and Asia. Northern Europeans have the lowest incidence (5–15%) of lactose intolerance in the world.

c. Secondary lactase deficiency occurs in response to diffuse intestinal insult, such as giardiasis, rotavirus, regional enteritis (Crohn's disease), celiac disease, or bacterial overgrowth.

3. Diagnosis. Simply withholding dietary lactose can serve as the diagnostic test in most cases, especially in a patient from a high prevalence population with a history compatible with lactase deficiency syndrome.

a. Lactose tolerance test. The diagnosis of lactose intolerance can be established, if necessary, with this test. Following a 50-g dose of lactose, blood glucose levels are determined at serial time points for 2 hours. Adequate hydrolysis of the disaccharide and subsequent absorption of the component sugars are reflected by a greater than 20-mg/dl rise in blood glucose and the lack of symptoms. Gastric dysmotility syndromes and diabetes mellitus may affect test results. Diabetes may increase blood glucose levels to this degree because of faulty glucose metabolism. Blood glucose response may be higher with rapid gastric emptying and lower with delayed gastric emptying.

b. Breath hydrogen testing is an alternative, noninvasive method for diagnosing lactose intolerance. Hydrogen is liberated during colonic fermentation of the unabsorbed carbohydrate. Detection of a rise in breath hydrogen greater than 20 ppm following the administration of oral lactose is considered diagnostic.

E. Sweeteners and sugar substitutes. Sweeteners come with calories (nutritive) and without calories (nonnutritive). The demand for sweeteners, especially without added energy, has exponentially grown over the years and resulted in the development of new products.

1. Nutritive sweeteners are sugars (sucrose, fructose, glucose, dextrose, high fructose corn syrup, honey, maple sugar) and sugar alcohols (sorbitol, mannitol, xylitol). They have 4 "empty" calories/gram. Some sugar alcohols are not fully absorbed, leading to diarrhea with increasing consumption.

2. Nonnutritive sweeteners provide sweetness without calories. Four sweeteners have been approved by the U.S. Food and Drug Administration (FDA): saccharin, aspartame, acesulfame, and sucralose. Saccharin (Sweet 'N Low) is 300 times sweeter than sucrose. It still comes with a warning label for possible cancer risk. Aspartame (NutraSweet and Equal) is made from two amino acids, aspartic acid and phenylalanine. It is 160–220% sweeter than sucrose. Cooking tends to decrease its sweetness. Acesulfame K (Sunette) is an organic salt. It is used in soft drinks and is 200 times sweeter than sucrose. Sucralose (Splenda) is a sucrose derivative but is not absorbed by the body. It is 600 times sweeter than sucrose and is heat stable.

F. Alcohol. Ethanol has a structure that resembles carbohydrates. It is readily absorbed by the GI tract, and each gram of ethanol yields 7 kcal. Thus, it can be a significant source of empty calories, and is devoid of other beneficial nutrients. The alcohol content in one jigger of distilled liquor, one 12-oz beer, and one 3.5-oz glass of wine are roughly equivalent. One serving of an alcoholic beverage provides 10–13 g ethanol (70–90 kcal). Beer or distilled alcohol mixed with soda may provide even more calories. Alcohol consumption must be factored into weight loss programs. Ethanol is known to increase high-density lipoprotein (HDL) in serum; thus, moderate ethanol use may convey a cardioprotective effect.

XII. Fat

A. **Fatty acids** are the simplest forms of lipids and are components of complex dietary lipids. The length of the fatty acid chain may vary from 4 to 24 carbon atoms, and the terms **short-chain**, **medium-chain**, and **long-chain fatty acids** are applied to categorize these molecules into classes with distinct physiologic properties. Fatty acids may be saturated, monounsaturated, or polyunsaturated, and the degree of saturation also has health implications. Essential fatty acids are plant-derived unsaturated fatty acids that are required to prevent a clinical syndrome characterized by growth retardation, dermatitis, kidney disease, and death. **Omega-3 fatty acids** (N-3 polyunsaturated fatty acids) are found in fish oils and are thought to have hypolipidemic and antithrombotic effects. The risk for cardiovascular disease increases with hypercholesterolemia or an unfavorable shift in low-density lipoprotein (LDL)–HDL ratio. Increased consumption of total fat, saturated fatty acids, and cholesterol correlates with increased risk for cardiovascular disease. Monounsaturated and polyunsaturated fatty acids, including N-3 polyunsaturated fatty acid, have cardioprotective properties via hypocholesterolemic effects or a favorable shift in LDL-HDL ratio.

B. **Trans fatty acids and cholesterol.** Trans fatty acids, also known as **trans fat**, are made through the process of hydrogenation that solidifies vegetable oils. Hydrogenation increases the shelf life and flavor of oils and the foods that contain them. Trans fat is found in vegetable shortening, stick margarine, crackers, cookies, and snack foods. Trans fatty acids contribute to increased blood LDL cholesterol, which increases the risk of coronary artery disease. The FDA now proposes to amend its regulations on nutrition labeling to require that the amount of trans fatty acids in a food be included in the nutrition facts panel. Included in this proposal is a new nutrient content claim defining "trans fat free" and a limit on trans fatty acids wherever there are limits on saturated fat in nutrient content claims or health claims.

C. **Requirements.** Fat should comprise no more than 30% total daily calories. Saturated fatty acid intake should be restricted to less than 10% total calories. Intake of cholesterol should be restricted to 300 mg daily.

XIII. Approaches to weight loss (Fig. 3-2)

A. **Low-calorie diets.** A number of major weight loss programs are based on the calorie-controlled meal plan. If clients maintain a regular exercise program, weight loss may still be achieved at calorie levels above 1200 kcal for women and 1500 kcal for men. Such a plan provides flexibility and individualization.

B. **Fat gram monitoring.** Monitoring fat grams instead of calories, or reducing dietary fat without severe calorie restriction, is another approach to weight reduction. Clients make lower-fat food choices. A food diary and a fat gram counter are required. Fat gram allowances are determined by the individual's daily energy requirement.

$$\text{Daily kcal requirement} \times \frac{\text{desired \% of total kcal from fat}}{100}$$

(9 kcal/g fat = recommended number of fat grams/day)

This system works best when fresh foods are consumed, as it is difficult to consume excess calories on a low-fat diet. Weight loss experts have backed away from this strategy. Food technology has allowed low-fat but high-calorie foods to be labeled as low-fat food. Consumers who choose such products may not lose weight, because their caloric intake has not been reduced.

C. **Fad and novelty diets.** Fad diets are notorious for promising miracle weight losses with minimal effort. Some promote high-protein and low-carbohydrate intake to induce ketosis, which can result in electrolyte imbalances and cardiac arrhythmias. Most fad diets lack balance. "Gimmicks" are usually inef-

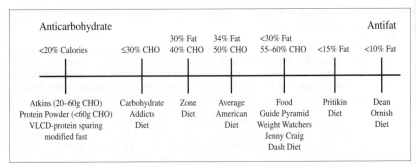

Fig. 3-2. The continuum of popularly known self-help diets ranging from anticarbohydrate to antifat. CHO, carbohydrate; VLCD, very low-calorie diet.

fective. Weight loss through fad dieting is primarily due to energy restriction or water loss (diuresis), which is quickly regained with cessation of the diet. Fad diets often lead to binge eating of prohibited foods, which may contribute to further weight gain.

D. **Very low-calorie diets (VLCDs).** VLCDs were designed to produce rapid, maximum weight loss while minimizing the protein losses of starvation. VLCDs should never be used as first-line therapy for obesity.
   1. Calories. VLCDs commonly supply only 400–800 kcal/day, usually in liquid form.
   2. Criteria. Candidates for VLCDs should meet the following criteria:
      a. Weight $\geq 30\%$ of IBW or BMI 30–40 kg/m^2
      b. Willing to make a lifelong commitment to changes in lifestyle
      c. Commitment to completion of treatment and maintenance programs
      d. No medical contraindications, including renal or hepatic disease, cardiac arrhythmias, insulin-dependent diabetes, cerebrovascular accidents, cancer, cholecystitis, alcoholism, and psychiatric disease
      e. Support. These comprehensive weight loss programs combine dietary and behavioral modification with an exercise routine and have staff with expertise in behavioral psychology, nutrition, and exercise physiology.

E. **Surgery.** Morbidly obese individuals (BMI >40 kg/m^2) who have tried and failed medical treatment can be considered for bariatric surgery. Candidates for surgery should be chosen by a team of medical, surgical, psychiatric, and nutrition experts who determine that the risk-benefit ratio is favorable for the given individual.

F. **Drug therapy.** Pharmacologic treatments for obesity are becoming available, but they have not been shown to induce long-term results for most people. The beneficial results are maintained only as long as the drug is taken. Dexfenfluramine (Redux) was approved in 1996 by the FDA, but dexfenfluramine and fenfluramine (Pondimin) were withdrawn in 1997 because of postmarketing reports of valvular heart disease associated with these medications. The combination of fenfluramine and phentermine (Fen-Phen) had been used to treat obesity for several years before. Phentermine was not withdrawn from the market. The FDA has approved orlistat, which interferes with fat absorption (see below). The protein-products of the so-called obesity genes hold promise for novel treatments of obesity in the near future.

G. **Fat replacements**
   1. **Olestra** was developed as a fat replacement to impart palatability to a diet without the consequences of high-calorie fat. It is a mixture of

hexa-, hepta-, and octaesters of sucrose with long-chain fatty acids. It imparts taste that is indistinguishable from fat, yet it is not hydrolyzable by pancreatic lipase, and therefore it has no caloric value. It is debated whether or not olestra, as an undigestible food, causes abdominal discomfort, flatulence, and diarrhea.

  2. Orlistat interferes with the absorption of fat. This compound inhibits pancreatic lipase and reduces the absorption of fat. At therapeutic doses (300–400 mg/day), orlistat inhibits fat absorption by 30%, resulting in a calorie deficit of approximately 200 calories. At recommended doses, orlistat does not have significant GI side effects.

XIV. Vitamins

A. Requirements.
Vitamins are essential organic compounds that are required to maintain growth, metabolism, and overall health. Tables 3-3 and 3-4 contain the DRIs for vitamins and minerals. Unlike fat-soluble vitamins, water-soluble vitamins (with the exception of cyanocobalamin–vitamin B_{12}) cannot be retained for long periods by the body.

B. Fat-soluble vitamins

1. Vitamin A
  a. Functions: visual pigments, cell differentiation, gene regulation
  b. Sources: Preformed retinol: liver, whole and fortified milk, eggs; carotenoids: yellow-orange vegetables and fruits (sweet potato, carrot, squash, cantaloupe, apricot), dark-green leafy vegetables (spinach, broccoli)
  c. Deficiency: Adults: night blindness, xeroderma
  d. Toxicity: Hepatomegaly and abnormal liver tests, bone pain, anorexia, fatigue
  e. Replacement dose: 100,000 IU IM once
  f. Maintenance dose: 100,000 IU IM monthly or 5000–30,000 IU PO qd

2. Vitamin D
  a. Functions: Calcium homeostasis, bone metabolism
  b. Sources: Fortified cow's milk, herring, salmon, sardines, liver
  c. Deficiency: Adults: osteomalacia
  d. Toxicity: Hypercalcification of bone, kidney stones, metastatic calcification of soft tissues, hypercalcemia, headache, weakness, nausea, vomiting, constipation, polyuria, polydipsia
  e. Replacement dose: Vitamin D_2 (ergocalciferol, Calciferol), 500,000 IU in sesame oil IM once
  f. Maintenance dose: Vitamin D_2 (Calciferol), 100,000 IU IM monthly or 25,000–50,000 IU PO 3 times weekly for malabsorption; 25-hydroxyvitamin D_3 (Calderol), 50 µg PO daily for osteopenia or renal disease; 1,25-dihydroxyvitamin D_3 (Rocaltrol), 0.5–1.0 µg PO daily for chronic renal failure or vitamin D–dependent rickets

3. Vitamin E
  a. Functions: Membrane antioxidant. Vitamin E is currently under investigation to determine if it has a role in preventing cardiovascular disease or prostate cancer.
  b. Sources: Vegetable oils, wheat germ, rice bran, nuts, and seeds.
  c. Deficiency: Adults: neuropathy, myopathy.
  d. Toxicity: Postsurgical bleeding, bleeding in patients who receive anticoagulation.
  e. Maintenance dose: 30–200 IU PO qd.

4. Vitamin K
  a. Functions: Blood clotting, calcium metabolism. Dietary and pharmaceutical supplements should be avoided in patients who are anticoagulated with warfarin.
  b. Sources: Seaweed (kelp), green leafy vegetables (kale, turnip greens, spinach, broccoli, cabbage, lettuce), green beans, peas.

    c. Deficiency: Coagulopathy (hypoprothrombinemia), bleeding dyscrasia.

    d. Toxicity: None.

    e. Replacement dose: 10 mg SC or IM daily for 3 days or until pro-thrombin time corrects.

    f. Maintenance dose: 10 mg PO qd.

C. Water-soluble vitamins

  1. Vitamin C (ascorbic acid)

    a. Functions: Reductant in hydroxylations in biosynthesis of collagen and carnitine and in the metabolism of drugs and steroids.

    b. Sources: Fruits (especially citrus, kiwi, cantaloupe, strawberries), juices (especially orange, grapefruit, tomato), vegetables (especially broccoli, bell pepper, potato, asparagus, cabbage, greens, peas, carrots).

    c. Deficiency: Scurvy: loss of appetite, fatigue, retarded wound healing, bleeding gums, spontaneous rupture of capillaries, perifolliculitis, corkscrew hairs.

    d. Toxicity: Vitamin C is considered safe in doses up to 1 g/day. Osmotic diarrhea from unabsorbed vitamin C is the main side effect of large doses. A hypothetical concern is that large doses of vitamin C can cause oxalate and uric acid kidney stones. Vitamin C may also give false-positive fecal occult blood tests. Increased iron absorption associated with vitamin C ingestion may lead to iron overload in susceptible patients with hemochromatosis, thalassemia, or sideroblastic anemia.

  2. Vitamin B$_1$ (thiamine)

    a. Functions: Coenzyme for oxidative decarboxylations of 2-keto acids and transketolations.

    b. Sources: Brewer's yeast, meats (especially pork), sunflower seeds, wheat germ, enriched grain products, nuts, legumes.

    c. Deficiency (beriberi): Muscle weakness, anorexia, tachycardia, cardiomegaly, edema.

    d. Toxicity: Excessive (100 times recommendations) thiamine, administered parenterally (IV or IM), has been associated with headache, convulsion, cardiac arrhythmias, and anaphylactic shock. Little or no danger of thiamine toxicity appears to be associated with oral ingestion of large amounts of thiamine (500 mg/day for 1 month).

  3. Vitamin B$_2$ (riboflavin)

    a. Functions: Coenzyme in redox reactions of fatty acids and the tricarboxylic acid (TCA) cycle

    b. Sources: Liver, meats, brewer's yeast, milk, cheese, egg, fortified cereals, broccoli, spinach, mushrooms

    c. Deficiency: Cheilosis, glossitis, hyperemia and edema of pharyngeal and oral mucous membranes, angular stomatitis, photophobia

    d. Toxicity: None

  4. Niacin

    a. Functions: Coenzyme for dehydrogenases. **Niacin** is a term that is used for both nicotinic acid and nicotinamide.

    b. Sources: Meat, poultry, fish, fortified cereals, wheat flour, corn, potato, noncitrus fruits and juices.

    c. Deficiency (pellagra): Diarrhea, dermatitis, confusion or dementia.

    d. Toxicity: Nicotinic acid is used in high doses to treat hypercholesterolemia. Side effects are frequent at doses of 1 g/day or more of nicotinic acid. At doses as low as 10 mg/day, nicotinic acid can cause flushing via release of histamine, which may also aggravate asthma and peptic ulcer disease. Other side effects include elevated liver enzymes, elevated serum uric acid levels, pruritus, hyperglycemia, heartburn, nausea, and vomiting.

  5. Vitamin B$_6$ (pyridoxine)

    a. Functions: Coenzyme in amino acid metabolism.

    b. Sources: Liver, oatmeal, banana, chicken, potato, wheat germ, rice.

c. Deficiency: Dermatitis, glossitis, convulsions.

d. Toxicity: Excessive ingestion (>500 mg/day) of pyridoxine can cause degeneration of the dorsal root ganglia, demyelination, and peripheral neuropathy.

6. Folic acid

a. Functions: Coenzyme in single carbon metabolism.

b. Sources: Fortified cereals, brewer's yeast, legumes, spinach, broccoli, citrus fruit and juices, meat, poultry, fish.

c. Deficiency: Megaloblastic anemia, diarrhea, fatigue, depression, confusion, glossitis.

d. Toxicity: None. Folate replacement, however, may mask the bone marrow effect of vitamin B_{12} deficiency without correcting the neurologic manifestations of vitamin B_{12} deficiency.

7. Biotin

a. Functions: Coenzyme for carboxylations.

b. Sources: Cereals, eggs, liver, meat, fish, shellfish, brewer's yeast, nuts, legumes, peanut butter.

c. Deficiency: Very rare; usually induced by ingestion of large amounts of raw egg whites containing avidin. Anorexia, nausea, glossitis, depression, dry-scaly dermatitis, hair loss. Sufficient quantities are needed for the maintenance of healthy hair and skin.

d. Toxicity: None.

8. Pantothenic acid

a. Functions: Coenzyme for fatty acid metabolism

b. Sources: Meat (especially liver), fish, poultry, milk, yogurt, legumes, whole grain cereals, wheat germ

c. Deficiency: Very rare; numbness and tingling of hands and feet, vomiting, fatigue

d. Toxicity: None; intakes up to 20 g/day may cause intestinal distress and diarrhea

9. Vitamin B_{12} (cobalamin)

a. Functions: Coenzyme in metabolism of propionate, amino acids, and single carbon fragments

b. Sources: Clams, liver, oysters, crab, tuna, beef, halibut

c. Deficiency: Megaloblastic anemia, depression, neuropathy, psychosis, glossitis

d. Toxicity: None

XV. Minerals

A. Calcium

1. Function: Structural component of bones and teeth; role in cellular processes, including signal transduction, muscle contraction, blood clotting

2. Sources: Milk, milk products, sardines, clams, oysters, turnip, mustard greens, broccoli, legumes

3. Deficiency: Rickets, osteomalacia, osteoporosis, dental caries, tetany

4. Toxicity: Kidney stones, constipation

B. Phosphorus

1. Function: Structural component of bones, teeth, cell membranes, phospholipids, adenosine triphosphate; regulation of pH

2. Sources: Meat, poultry, fish, eggs, milk, milk products, legumes, nuts, grains, chocolate

3. Deficiency: Rickets, osteomalacia, anorexia, tetany, cardiac arrhythmias

4. Toxicity: Hypocalcemia, tetany

C. Magnesium

1. Function: Component of bones; role in nerve conduction, protein synthesis, enzyme activation.

2. Sources: Nuts, legumes, grains, corn, peas, carrots, seafood, brown rice.

3. Deficiency: Depression, muscle weakness, tetany, abnormal behavior, convulsions, growth failure.

   4. Toxicity: Osmotic diarrhea, nausea, flushing, double vision, slurred speech, weakness, paralysis, cardiac failure, respiratory failure. Magnesium-containing antacids and laxatives can cause inadvertent toxicity in patients with renal failure.

D. Potassium
   1. Function: Water, electrolyte, and pH balances; cell membrane transfer
   2. Sources: Fruits, potato, beans, wheat bran, dairy products, eggs
   3. Deficiency: Muscular weakness, apathy, cardiac arrhythmias, paralysis
   4. Toxicity: Cardiac arrhythmia, cardiac arrest

E. Iron
   1. Function: Oxygen transport
   2. Sources: Organ meats, meat, molasses, clams, oysters, nuts, legumes, seeds, green leafy vegetables, and enriched whole grains, breads, and cereals
   3. Deficiency: Microcytic anemia, listlessness, fatigue, sore tongue, angular stomatitis
   4. Toxicity: Hemochromatosis, hemosiderosis

F. Zinc
   1. Function: Cofactor in energy metabolism, protein synthesis, collagen formation, alcohol detoxification, taste, smell
   2. Sources: Oysters, wheat germ, beef, liver, poultry, whole grains
   3. Deficiency: Poor wound healing, abnormal growth, anorexia, abnormal taste and smell; changes in skin, hair, and nails
   4. Toxicity: Metallic taste, nausea, vomiting, epigastric pain, abdominal cramps, diarrhea; copper deficiency (competitive absorption)

G. Copper
   1. Function: Utilization of iron stores, lipids, collagen, pigment, neurotransmitter synthesis
   2. Sources: Liver, shellfish, whole grains, legumes, eggs, meat, fish
   3. Deficiency: Anemia, neutropenia, bone abnormalities
   4. Toxicity: Nausea, vomiting, diarrhea, hematuria, jaundice, oliguria, or anuria

H. Selenium
   1. Function: Protects against free radicals and hydrogen peroxide
   2. Sources: Grains, meats, poultry, fish, dairy products
   3. Deficiency: Myalgia, cardiomyopathy, pancreatic degeneration
   4. Toxicity: Nausea, vomiting, fatigue, hair and nail loss, changes in nail beds

I. Chromium
   1. Function: Regulation of blood glucose level
   2. Sources: Mushrooms, prunes, asparagus, organ meats, whole grains, breads, cereals
   3. Deficiency: Glucose intolerance, lipid abnormalities
   4. Toxicity: Respiratory disease, skin ulcerations, liver injury

J. Iodine
   1. Function: Thyroid hormone synthesis
   2. Sources: Iodized table salt, saltwater seafood, sunflower seeds, mushrooms, liver, eggs
   3. Deficiency: Goiter, hypothyroidism
   4. Toxicity: None

K. Manganese
   1. Function: Brain, collagen, bone function.
   2. Sources: Wheat bran, legumes, nuts, lettuce, blueberries, pineapple, seafood, poultry, meat.
   3. Deficiency: Impaired growth, skeletal abnormalities, impaired CNS function.
   4. Toxicity: In liver failure and cholestatic liver diseases, manganese can cause neurotoxicity. Miners may experience parkinsonian-like syndrome and memory loss.

L. Molybdenum
  1. Function: Metabolism of purines and pyrimidines
  2. Sources: Soybeans, lentils, buckwheat, oats, rice, bread
  3. Deficiency: Hypermethioninemia, increased urinary xanthine, decreased urinary sulfate and urate excretion
  4. Toxicity: Gout
M. Fluorine
  1. Function: Maintenance of teeth and bone
  2. Sources: Fluorinated drinking water, fish, meat, legumes, grains
  3. Deficiency: Dental caries, bone disorders
  4. Toxicity: Chronic toxicity (fluorosis): bone, kidney, nerve, and muscle dysfunction and mottled teeth; acute toxicity: nausea, vomiting, acidosis, cardiac arrhythmias, death (5–10 g sodium fluoride or 32–64 mg fluoride/kg body weight
XVI. Drug-nutrient interactions. It is well known that mixing food and medications is not always a benign action. Food can delay or negate a drug's activity and efficacy. It can also enhance drug effects. Medication can influence food and nutrient intake, absorption, metabolism, and excretion. Many reported interactions are of questionable clinical significance however, either due to short duration of drug therapy or insufficient research. It is beyond the scope of this chapter to list all of the possible drug-nutrient interactions. Table 3-6 lists some important food/nutrient-drug interactions.
XVII. Dietary supplements. Americans spend billions of dollars annually on supplements. The estimate of herb sales alone topped $1.2 billion in 1996.
  A. Dietary Supplement Health and Education Act of 1994 (DSHEA). In 1994, the U.S. Congress passed DSHEA. The law provides a new definition for a dietary supplement, describes labeling requirements, and requires the establishment of a commission and Office of Dietary Supplements within the National Institutes of Health.
  B. Definition. A dietary supplement is a "product (other than tobacco) that is intended to supplement the diet that bears or contains one or more of the

Table 3-6. Important food/nutrient-drug interactions

Food/nutrient	Medication	Interaction
Grapefruit juice	Carbamazepine	Increases concentration of medication. This effect is mediated by cytochrome P-450 enzyme CYP3A4 in the small intestine. The effect of grapefruit juice can last 24 hrs. Drugs with high presystemic metabolism are affected the most.
	Calcium channel blockers	
	Cyclosporin	
	Saquinavir	
	Terfenadine	
	Astemizole	
	Lovastatin	
	Simvastatin	
	Atorvastatin	
	Cisapride	
	Buspirone	
	Clomipramine	
	Midazolam	
	Diazepam	
	Tacrolimus	(continued)

Table 3-6. (continued)

Food/nutrient	Medication	Interaction
Tyramine-containing foods: aged cheese, overripe fruit, spoiled foods, fermented/dry salami or sausage, soy sauce, marmite concentrated yeast extract, sauerkraut, fava and broad beans, banana peel, tap beer	Furazolidone Isocarboxazid Phenelzine Tranylcypromine Isoniazid Procarbazine Toloxatone[a] Moclobemide[a] Selegiline[a]	Tyramine foods enhance the release of norepinephrine, resulting in vasoconstriction and hypertension. MAOIs increase levels of norepinephrine and serotonin. The combination can lead to hypertensive crisis. Food restrictions have been re-evaluated. Suggested upper limit of tyramine is 6 mg/day. Caution should be taken with selective MAOIs and higher doses of tyramine.
Potassium supplements	Amiloride Triamterene Spironolactone	Risk of hyperkalemia.
Vitamin K–rich foods: dark leafy green vegetables; soybean, canola, cottonseed, olive oils	Warfarin Phenindione	Antagonist to effect of warfarin. Intake needs to be consistent.
Vitamin B$_6$	Hydralazine Isoniazid Chloramphenicol Cycloserine	Antipyridoxine effect.
Fat-soluble vitamins	Cholestyramine Colestipol Mineral oil	Inhibits absorption of fat-soluble vitamins.
Folic acid	Sulfasalazine Phenytoin Primidone Colestipol Cholestyramine Methotrexate Pyrimethamine Nitrofurantoin Trimethoprim	Decreased absorption; folic acid antagonists.
Vitamin B$_{12}$	Histamine-2 receptor antagonists Proton pump inhibitors Chloramphenicol Cycloserine	Decreased absorption.

MAOIs, monoamine oxidase inhibitors.
[a]Selective monoamine oxidase inhibitors.

following dietary ingredients: a vitamin, a mineral, an herb or other botanical, an amino acid, a dietary substance for use by man to supplement the diet by increasing the total daily intake, or a concentrate, metabolite, constituent, extract, or combinations of these ingredients."

C. Regulations. The law requires the product label to include ingredient labeling (name, part of plant for herbs, quantity of each ingredient and strength), the words **dietary supplement**, and nutritional labeling. The law restricts the authority of the FDA and allows the products to be sold without the proof of safety and efficacy that is required for drugs and food additives. It is the burden of the FDA to show that a product is not safe. DSHEA prohibits labeling that indicates the treatment or prevention of disease. Manufacturers must state on the labels of supplements, "This product is not intended to diagnose, treat, cure or prevent disease." They can, however, state "structure-function" claims; for example, "Calcium builds strong bones."

D. Adverse events. For reporting adverse events, health care providers can contact the FDA at FDA MedWatch, 1-800-FDA-1088, or http://www.fda.gov/medwatch/report/hcp.htm. Consumers can report events to the MedWatch telephone number or http://www.fda.gov/medwatch/report/consumer/consumer.htm.

XVIII. Herbals and botanicals. Herbal products have been used for centuries, but many herbs have little research to back their claims. Some argue that long-term use implies safety and efficacy. Other industrialized nations have clearer guidelines and regulations for herbals and phytomedicines.

A. Regulations. The World Health Organization published *Guidelines for the Assessment of Herbal Medicines*, and the European Scientific Cooperative on Phytotherapies published a set of monographs. Because quality assurance is lacking in the United States at this time, consumers must be aware that biochemical analyses of products have shown great variability in strength, potency, and purity. Some products contain no active ingredient.

B. Safety. Botanicals have also been contaminated with pesticides, drugs, heavy metals, and other inactive herbs. It is important to buy products from a reputable manufacturer. The Office of Dietary Supplements and the National Center for Complementary and Alternative Medicine are currently facilitating and conducting research in the area of safety and efficacy of herbs and botanicals. Consult Table 3-7 for a description of popular botanicals that are being consumed.

XIX. Functional foods and other popular supplements. A surge of interest, popular and research, has been shown in food and food components that might prevent disease or provide for a healthy longevity, or both. Terms such as **nutriceutical**, **medicinal foods**, and **functional foods** have appeared in the literature.

A. Functional foods. Functional foods are foods or substances found in foods that have health and medical benefits beyond traditional nutrients. Table 3-8 reviews some functional foods, level of intake, and disease association.

1. Creatine is an amino acid involved in the transfer of phosphate to adenosine diphosphate that provides energy for muscle activity. It is used as an ergogenic aid and can be found in food (meat, milk, and fish) or supplement form (powder, tablets, capsules, energy bars, and drink mixes). Increased intake can increase skeletal muscle stores by 20–50% and has been shown to help in high-intensity, brief, repetitive activity (*Am J Clin Nutr* 2000;72:607S). Creatine taken with a carbohydrate drink increases muscle accretion. Caffeine intake negates the advantage of supplementation. Recommended intake of creatine monohydrate for athletes is 15–30 g/day in divided doses with food or a carbohydrate drink for 1 week, then 2–5 g/day. The usual supplementation period is 3 months, then off 1 month. It is usually well tolerated and safe but should be avoided in people with impaired renal function (*Clin Sports Med* 1999;8:651). Creatine supplementation holds promise in patients with muscle weakness and atrophy from a neurologic cause.

Table 3-7. Popular herbal and botanical supplements

Name	Reported uses/actions	Adverse side effects	Doses	Potential interactions	Other
Echinacea	Cold, flu, or other infections—used as treatment, not prevention	No toxic effects	1–2 g dried root	May interfere with effectiveness of immunosuppressive medications	Has been adulterated with other members of the Compositae family with no pharmacologic activity
Echinacea pallida	Immune stimulant	Avoid if allergic to plants in daisy family	Liquid extract (1:1 in 45% alcohol), 0.25–1.0 ml tid		Part used: active constituents have not been confirmed; a few controlled trials favor the root of *E. pallida* and above-ground parts of *E. purpurea* for effectiveness
Echinacea purpurea	Applied topically to healing wound		Tincture (1:5) 50% ethanol 1–2 ml tid		Do not use longer than 6–8 wks; may cause immune suppression
Echinacea angustifolia	Stimulates phagocytosis and mobility of leukocytes		Capsules: 0.9–1.0 g qd		
Family: Compositae Common: **Echinacea**, black susans, comb flower, snakeroot, purple cone flower			*E. purpurea* herb, 6–9 ml (expressed juice)		
Valeriana officinalis	Sedative and sleep aid	Mild GI upset	As sleep aid: 400–900 mg extract, 30 mins before bedtime; daily dose 100–1800 mg/day extract	Avoid use with other sedatives and anxiolytics	Part used: fresh underground plant parts

Herb	Uses	Side Effects	Dosage	Interactions	Comments
Family: Valerianaceae Common: **Valerian**, All-heal, Amantilla, Capon's tail, heliotrope	Reduces nervous tension, stress, anxiety, and restlessness	Increased dose: headache, nausea, grogginess, and blurred vision	Tea, 1 cup 3–4 × day and qhs (1 tsp dry–150 ml water) Takes 2–4 wks to see effects No abuse potential	Not synergistic with alcohol	
Tanacetum parthenium Family: Asteraceae/Compositae Common: **Feverfew**, bachelor button, nosebleed, Santa Maria, wild quinine	Most known for migraine prophylaxis—may work like methysergide, menstrual pain, headaches, arthritis Traditionally: antipyretic	Allergic reactions Mouth ulcers Rebound headache if discontinued abruptly	1–3 fresh leaves or 25–50 mg crushed dried leaves or 125 mg dried leaf preparation with standardized product with at least 0.2% parthenolide—1–2 × day.	Possible interaction with anticoagulants May inhibit prostaglandin production	Parts used: leaf and aerial parts May take wks to mos before benefit is realized; does not relieve acute pain

(continued)

Table 3-7. (continued)

Name	Reported uses/actions	Adverse side effects	Doses	Potential interactions	Other
Ginkgo biloba	Antioxidant	Increased bleeding, headache, and nausea	Most popular form: extract (GBE)-leaf extract standardized to contain 24% ginkgoflavone glycosides and 6% terpene lactones, 40–60 mg tid-qid	Ginkgolides competitively inhibit binding of PAF to membrane receptor	One of the most researched herbs
Family: Ginkgoaceae	Improve cerebral and peripheral blood circulation, improve memory, intermittent claudication, vertigo, and tinnitus	Rare: headache, dizziness, palpitations, and mild GI distress	Tincture (1:5), 2–4 ml tid	Reduce platelet aggregation; does not interfere with clotting cascade; avoid concurrent use with anticoagulants and antiplatelet drugs	Approved for peripheral arterial vascular disease, vertigo, tinnitus, and dementia in Germany
Common: **Ginkgo**, maidenhair tree, knew tree, yingsing	Antioxidant properties	Allergenic: ginkgo pollen Seed ingestion: loss of consciousness and seizures Patients with known risk factors of intracranial hemorrhage should avoid	Fluid extract: (1:1), 1–3 ml tid		Part used: leaf See improvement in 4-6 wks, can take for 6 mos

Herb	Uses	Dosage	Side effects	Comments
Hypericum perforatum Family: Hypericaceae Common: **St. John's wort**, goatweed, rosin rose, klamath weed	Internal: mild depression and anxiety Topically: relieve inflammation and promote healing burns and wounds	200–1000 mg/day Recommended product standardized to 0.3% hypericin extract (1:1), 2–4 ml tid Tincture (1:10), 2–4 ml tid Tea, 2–4 g dried herb in 1–2 cups water daily	Fatigue Mild GI distress: lessened with food Photosensitivity Allergic reaction	Do not combine with other psychoactive mediations Possible slight MAO activity Induces the P-450 enzyme system leading to drug interactions	Dried above ground parts and flowers Meta-analysis showed herb more effective than placebo for mild depression Recommend to take for 4–6 wks; if no improvement, discontinue May cause serotonin syndrome when taken with SSRI antidepressants
Serenoa repens Family: Arecaceae Common: **saw palmetto**, cabbage palm, American dwarf palm tree	Antiandrogen for BPH May ↑ urinary flow, reduce residual urine volume, and ↓ frequency of urination Used as mild diuretic Reduces symptoms of BPH without reducing size	Recommended standardized product that contains 85–95% fatty acids or sterols 1–2 g berry or 320 mg lipophilic extract (160 mg bid)	Mild: headache, GI upset	Concern that herb can cause false-positive PSA level	Use berries (fat-soluble components), not leaves Studies show *S. repens* to be superior to placebo and has similar efficacy to finasteride

(continued)

Table 3-7. (continued)

Name	Reported uses/actions	Adverse side effects	Doses	Potential interactions	Other
Piper methysticum Family: Piper-aceae	Reduce stress Anxiolytic	May affect motor reflexes With chronic use: temporary yellow discoloration of skin, hair, and nails; scaly rash; puffy face	50–240 kavalactones/pyrones/day Recommend standardized product with 70% kavalactones content	Potentiation of CNS depressants Alcohol ↑ kava toxicity	Part used: dried rhizome and roots Studies show the herb to be more effective than placebo for anxiety
Common: **Kava-Kava**, awa, knew, tonga	Sedative Tranquilizer	↑ GGT and acute hepatitis with high doses have been reported	Root extract, 150–300 mg bid Tincture, 30 gtts tid May take 4 wks to see improvement	Not recommended for people with endogenous depression Antagonistic effect with dopamine Kava used with alprazolam resulted in coma	Not recommended for long periods of time (>3 mos) without medical supervision
Panax ginseng: Asian, Chinese, Korean	Reduction of fatigue	Generally safe: mild diarrhea, insomnia, nervousness, headache, breast tenderness	Extract, 100–300 mg tid (1.5–7.0% ginsenodides)	Caffeine may potentiate	Quality root very expensive; concentrations of ginsenosides vary among preparations; some have no ginseng at all
Panax quinquefolius: American	Energy enhancement		0.5–3.0 g crude herb	Avoid with MAOIs	Approved by Commission E for lack of stamina

Herb	Actions/Effects	Side effects	Dose	Interactions/Cautions	Notes
	"Cure all"			Watch blood sugar levels if given with diabetic agents Antiplatelet effect	Part used: root
Eleutherococcus senticosus: Siberian	T-lymphocyte increase Hypoglycemic effect Binds to estrogen receptors		Average daily dose: 2–3 g/day root	Increased amounts may increase excretion of vitamins B_1, B_2, and C	From root and root bark
Ginseng	Hypoglycemic effect Possible immunomodulatory activities: T lymphocytes ↑ in healthy volunteers	Occasional gastric discomfort		Digoxin: monitor levels closely	Clinical studies do not substantiate claims
Cimicifuga racemosa	Estrogenic activity: binds to estrogen receptors; suppress LH secretion		In studies doses range from 8 to 2400 mg/day	Avoid if taking BCPs or hormone replacement	Part used: rhizomes and roots
Family: Ranunculaceae	Relief of premenstrual and menopausal symptoms (hot flashes, night sweats, vaginal dryness, and anxiety)	Large dose: dizziness, nausea, headache, stiffness, trembling	No standardized doses	May potentiate antihypertensives	Do not confuse with blue cohosh Take for no longer than 6 mos

(continued)

Table 3-7. (continued)

Name	Reported uses/actions	Adverse side effects	Doses	Potential interactions	Other
Common: **Black cohosh**, black snake root, rattle weed, bug wort, squaw root Roots **Not recommended**	Vascular: hypotensive activity				Studies show it to be effective in reducing menopausal symptoms at 8 mg/day Remifemin, 40 gtts bid
Ephedra: more than 40 species	Most activity from ephedrine component	Tachycardia, high BP	FDA wants limited amount of ephedrine alkaloid to <24 mg/daily dose (prohibits sale >8 mg/dose)	Coffee potentiates	Ephedrine content varies widely in products
Family: Ephedraceae	CNS stimulant	>1000 adverse reactions		Avoid concomitant use with beta-blockers, ephedra alkaloids, MAOIs, phenothiazines, theophylline	Found in Metabolife
Common: **Ma huang**, sea grape, yellow horse, mormon tea, squaw tea	Decongestant Bronchodilator and peripheral vasoconstrictor Weight loss: appetite suppressant	>54 deaths High doses associated with MI, sudden death, strokes, seizures Insomnia, dizziness, anxiety			

Symphytum officinale Family: Boraginaceae Common: **Comfrey** knitbone, blackwort, slippery root	Historical use: internal—GI and pulmonary disorders External: wound healing	Internal use—linked to cancer and cirrhosis Potentially fatal External use not to exceed 1 μg pyrrolizidine alkaloids calculated with 5–7% drug External use limit to 10 days or less	Oral use not recommended; however, it can be found as tea, tablets, capsules, and tincture		Comfrey root is approved by Commission E for *external* use only on intact skin
Pausinystalia yohimbe Family: Rubiaceae Common: **yohimbe**	Men's aphrodisiac Found in body-building products Orthostatic hypotension Investigated for organic impotence	High doses associated with weakness, paralysis, and death Seizures and kidney failure Orthostatic hypotension	Impotence studies: 2.7–5.4 PO tid Orthostatic hypotension: 12.5 mg/day	Tyramine foods may increase blood pressure Not recommended with tricyclics, SSRIs, or OTC stimulants	Declared unsafe by FDA Studies of efficacy are contradictory

BCPs, birth control pills; BPH, benign prostatic hypertrophy; FDA, U.S. Food and Drug Administration; GGT, γ-glutamyltransferase; LH, luteinizing hormone; MAO, monoamine oxidase; MAOIs, monoamine oxidase inhibitors; MI, myocardial infarction; OTC, over-the-counter; PAF, platelet-activating factor; PSA, prostate-specific antigen; SSRIs, selective serotonin reuptake inhibitors.

Table 3-8. Approximate intake levels for select functional foods or food components to promote optimal health status

Food/food component	Level of intake	Disease association	References
Green or black tea	4–6 cups/day	Reduced gastric and esophageal cancer risk	*Crit Rev Food Sci Nutr* 1997;36:691 *Proc Soc Exp Biol Med* 1999;220:271
Soy protein	25 g/day	Reduced low-density lipoprotein cholesterol, non–high-density lipoprotein Reduced menopausal symptoms	*N Engl J Med* 1995;333:276 *Obstet Gynecol* 1998;91:6
Garlic	600–900 mg/ day (approximately 1 fresh clove/ day)	Reduced BP Reduced serum cholesterol	*Hypertension* 1994;12:463 *Am J Clin Nutr* 1996;64:866 *Ann Intern Med* 1993;119:599
Vegetables and fruits	5–9 servings/ day	Reduced risk of cancer (colon, breast, prostate) BP reduction Reduced risk of cardiovascular disease	*J Am Diet Assoc* 1996;96:1027 *N Engl J Med* 1997;336:1117 *Am J Clin Nutr* 2000;72:922
Fructo-oligosaccharides	3–10 g/day	Blood pressure reduction Beneficial effect on lipid metabolism, improved GI health, and serum cholesterol reduction	*Br J Nutr* 1998;80:S197 *J Nutr* 1999;129:113
Fish rich in omega-3 fatty acids	>180 g (6 oz)/ wk	Reduced risk of heart disease	*Ann Intern Med* 1999;130:554
Grape juice or red wine	8–16 oz/day 8 oz/day	Platelet aggregation reduction	*Pharmacol Biol* 1998;36:21 *Circulation* 1999;100:1050 *J Nutr* 2000;130:53

Source: Adapted from Position of the American Dietetic Association: functional foods. *J Am Diet Assoc* 1999;99:1278–1285. Used with permission.

2. **Coenzyme Q10** (CoQ10) has been demonstrated to be an antioxidant and possibly an immunomodulating agent. Supplements have been shown to be effective in cardiomyopathy and CHF. It has been suggested that limited synthesis might be a problem in the etiology of heart disease. Foods that are high in CoQ10 are fish oils, nuts, fish, and meats. Supplemental doses for CHF are 90–150 mg/day. The most common side effects of CoQ10 are nausea, diarrhea, and cardiac arrhythmias.

3. **Glucosamine** is an amino sugar that is synthesized by the body from glucose and glutamine. It is found in almost all human tissue including cartilage, where it is the principal component of glycosaminoglycans. Supplements of glucosamine are sold as sulfate, hydrochloride (HCl), and N-acetyl- and chlorhydrate salts. Most research has been done using the sulfate form. On a weight basis, glucosamine HCl has more bioactive glucosamine than the sulfate form (2608 mg sulfate = 1500 mg HCl). However, it is suggested that the sulfate moiety may have therapeutic benefit. Research has demonstrated improvement in pain and inflammation and in range of motion associated with osteoarthritis. Glucosamine appears to be safe in short-term studies (*Rheum Dis Clin North Am* 1999;25:379). It can be given PO, IM, IV, and intra-articularly. The effective dose is 500 mg PO tid (1000–2000 mg/day glucosamine). **Chondroitin** is the most abundant glycosaminoglycan in cartilage. It has demonstrated similar anti-inflammatory properties in people with osteoarthritis. It is usually given with glucosamine. The usual dose is 400 mg PO tid (800–1600 mg/day chondroitin), however, oral absorption of chondroitin sulfates is poor.

4. **Alpha-lipoic acid** is an antioxidant and a cofactor in glucose metabolism. It is fat and water soluble, and therefore it has a greater ability to work as a free-radical scavenger. It has been used in Germany for years for the complications of diabetes. It appears to improve intracellular glucose utilization and diabetic neuropathy, and it may be effective in other neurodegenerative disorders. Doses for diabetic neuropathy are 600–1200 mg/day PO. An antioxidant dose is not recommended, although some suggest one or two 50-mg capsules daily. Good food sources are organ meats, beef, yeast, broccoli, and spinach.

XX. Internet nutrition resources

American Dietetic Association, http://www.eatright.org

Tufts University Nutrition Navigator, http://www.navigator.tufts.edu

National Center for Complementary and Alternative Medicine, http://nccam.nih.gov

American Botanical Council, http://www.herbalgram.org

Office of Dietary Supplements, http://odp.od.nih.gov/ods/

Food and Nutrition Information Center, http://www.nal.usda.gov/fnic

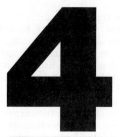

Hypertension

Tammy L. Lin and
Scott W. Rypkema

Definitions and Diagnostic Evaluation

Hypertension is defined as the presence of BP elevation to a level that places patients at increased risk for target organ damage in several vascular beds, including the retina, brain, heart, kidneys, and large conduit arteries (Table 4-1). Hypertension characterized by a BP of greater than 140/90 mm Hg is a common condition that affects an estimated 50 million Americans and imposes significant financial and social burdens on all Americans. Of these patients, 90% have essential hypertension; the remainder have secondary hypertension caused by renal parenchymal disease, renovascular disease, pheochromocytoma, Cushing's syndrome, primary hyperaldosteronism, coarctation of the aorta, and uncommon autosomal dominant or recessive diseases of the adrenal-renal axis that result in salt retention. Disease-associated morbidity and mortality, including atherosclerotic cardiovascular disease, stroke, heart failure (HF), and renal insufficiency, increase with higher levels of systolic and diastolic BP. Isolated systolic hypertension of the elderly is also associated with increased cardiovascular and cerebrovascular complications (*JAMA* 1991;265:3255). Patients with a recent substantial increase in BP above their baseline value that is sufficient to cause acute damage to retinal vessels (hemorrhage, exudates, papilledema) are considered to have accelerated malignant hypertension, regardless of the absolute level of BP.

I. **Detection and classification.** BP measurements should be performed on **multiple** occasions under nonstressful circumstances (e.g., rest, sitting, empty bladder, comfortable temperature, no tobacco or caffeine within 30 minutes) to obtain an accurate assessment of BP in a given patient. Hypertension should not be diagnosed on the basis of one measurement alone unless it is greater than 210/120 mm Hg or accompanied by target organ damage. Three or more abnormal readings should be obtained, preferably over a period of several weeks, before therapy is considered. Care should also be used to exclude pseudohypertension, which usually occurs in elderly individuals with stiff noncompressible vessels. A palpable artery that persists after cuff inflation (Osler's sign) should alert the physician to this possibility. Home and ambulatory BP monitoring can be used to assess a patient's true average BP, which correlates better with target organ damage. Circumstances in which ambulatory BP monitoring might be of value include (1) suspected "white-coat hypertension" (increases in BP associated with the stress of physician office visits), (2) evaluation of possible drug resistance, (3) high-normal BP (130–139 mm Hg systolic, 85–89 mm Hg diastolic), (4) episodic hypertension, and (5) hypotensive symptoms associated with medication or autonomic dysfunction. Hypertension is present if a patient's average BP is greater than 140 mm Hg systolic or greater than 90 mm Hg diastolic (Table 4-2).

II. **Initial clinical evaluation.** BP elevation is usually discovered in asymptomatic individuals during screening. Optimal detection and evaluation of hypertension

Table 4-1. Manifestations of target organ disease

Organ system	Manifestations
Large vessels	Aneurysmal dilatation
	Accelerated atherosclerosis
	Aortic dissection
Cardiac	
Acute	Pulmonary edema, myocardial infarction
Chronic	Clinical or ECG evidence of CAD; LVH by ECG or echocardiogram
Cerebrovascular	
Acute	Intracerebral bleeding, coma, seizures, mental status changes, TIA, stroke
Chronic	TIA, stroke
Renal	
Acute	Hematuria, azotemia
Chronic	Serum creatinine >1.5 mg/dl, proteinuria >1+ on dipstick
Retinopathy	
Acute	Papilledema, hemorrhages
Chronic	Hemorrhages, exudates, arterial nicking

CAD, coronary artery disease; LVH, left ventricular hypertrophy; TIA, transient ischemic attack.

require accurate noninvasive BP measurement, which should be obtained in a seated patient with the arm level with the heart. A calibrated, appropriately fitting BP cuff should be used because falsely high readings may be obtained if the cuff is too small. Two readings should be taken, separated by at least 2 minutes. Systolic BP should be noted with the appearance of Korotkov's sounds (phase I) and diastolic BP with the disappearance of sounds (phase V). In certain patients, the Korotkov's sounds do not disappear but are present to 0 mm Hg. In this case, the initial muffling of Korotkov's sounds (phase IV) should be taken as the diastolic BP (*Hypertension* 1988;11:211A). One should be careful to avoid spuriously low BP readings due to an auscultatory gap, which is caused by the disappearance and reappearance of Korotkov's sounds in hypertensive patients and may account for up to a 25-mm Hg gap between true and measured BP. Hypertension should be confirmed in both arms and the higher reading used. The history should seek to discover secondary causes of hypertension and note the presence of medications that may affect BP (e.g., decongestants, oral contraceptives, appetite suppressants, nonsteroidal anti-inflammatory agents, exogenous thyroid hormone, recent alcohol consumption, and illicit stimulants). A diagnosis of secondary hypertension should be considered in the following situations: (1) age at onset younger than 30 years or older than 60 years, (2) hypertension that is difficult to control after therapy has been initiated, (3) stable hypertension that becomes difficult to control, (4) clinical occurrence of a hypertensive crisis, (5) the presence of signs or symptoms of a secondary cause such as hypokalemia or metabolic alkalosis that is not explained by diuretic therapy, and (6) stage 3 hypertension. The **physical examination** should include investigation for target organ damage or a secondary cause of hypertension by noting the presence of carotid bruits, a third or fourth heart sound, cardiac murmurs, neurologic deficits, elevated jugular venous pressure, rales, retinopathy, unequal pulses, enlarged or small kidneys, cushingoid features, and abdominal bruits.

Table 4-2. Classification of blood pressure for adults aged 18 years and older[a]

Category	Systolic pressure (mm Hg)	Diastolic pressure (mm Hg)
Optimal[b]	<120	<80
Normal	<130	<85
High normal	130–139	85–89
Hypertensive[c]		
Stage 1	140–159	90–99
Stage 2	160–179	100–109
Stage 3	≥ 180	≥ 110

[a]Not taking antihypertensive drugs and not acutely ill. When systolic and diastolic pressures fall into different categories, the higher category should be selected to classify the individual's BP status. Isolated systolic hypertension is defined as a systolic BP of 140 mm Hg or more and a diastolic BP of less than 90 mm Hg and should be staged appropriately (e.g., 170/85 mm Hg is defined as stage 2 isolated systolic hypertension). In addition to classifying stages of hypertension on the basis of average BP levels, the clinician should specify the presence or absence of target organ disease and additional risk factors. This specificity is important for risk classification and management.
[b]Optimal BP with respect to cardiovascular risk is <120 mm Hg systolic and <80 mm Hg diastolic. However, unusually low readings should be evaluated for clinical significance.
[c]Based on the average of two or more readings taken at each of two or more visits after an initial screening.
Source: Sixth Report of the Joint National Committee on Detection, Evaluation, and Treatment of High Blood Pressure. *Arch Intern Med* 1997;157:2413–2446, with permission.

III. Laboratory evaluation. All newly diagnosed hypertensive patients should have a laboratory assessment to evaluate for target organ damage (Table 4-1) and other risk factors. Routine tests include a urinalysis, CBC, fasting plasma glucose, serum sodium, serum potassium, serum creatinine, and ECG. Fasting cholesterol levels should be obtained to screen for hyperlipidemia (see Chap. 5). This battery of tests helps to identify patients with possible target organ damage and provides a baseline for assessing adverse effects of therapy. Other tests to consider include a chest x-ray, creatinine clearance, 24-hour urine protein, serum calcium, uric acid, thyroid-stimulating hormone, and hemoglobin A_{1C}. Assessment of cardiac function or left ventricular hypertrophy (LVH) by echocardiography may be of value for certain patients.

Therapeutic Considerations

I. General considerations and goals (Fig. 4-1). The goal of treatment for hypertension is to prevent long-term sequelae (i.e., target organ damage). Barring an overt need for immediate pharmacologic therapy, most nondiabetic patients with stage 1 hypertension should be given the opportunity to achieve a reduction in BP over an interval of 3–6 months by applying nonpharmacologic modifications. The primary goal is to reduce BP to less than 140/90 mm Hg while concurrently controlling other modifiable cardiovascular risk factors. As isolated systolic hypertension is also associated with increased cerebrovascular and cardiac events, the therapeutic goal in this subset of patients should be to lower BP to less than 140 mm Hg systolic. Treatment should be more aggressive for those patients in whom target organ damage or other cardiovascular risk factors are present (*Ann Intern Med* 1993;119:329). In the absence of hypertensive crisis, BP should be reduced gradually to avoid end-organ (e.g., cerebral) ischemia. Patient education is an essential component of the treatment plan and promotes patient compliance. Physicians should

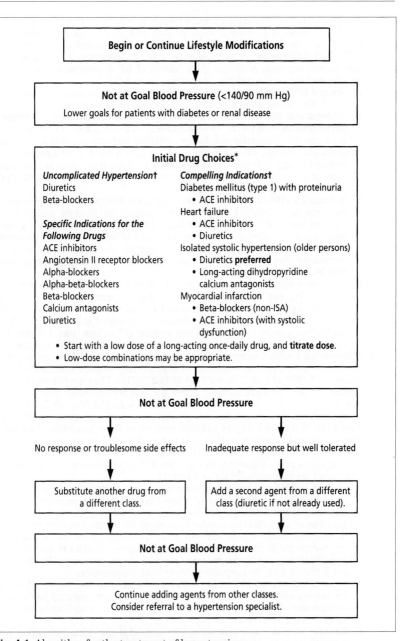

Fig. 4-1. Algorithm for the treatment of hypertension.
*Unless contraindicated. †Based on randomized controlled trials.
ACE, angiotensin-converting enzyme; ISA, intrinsic sympathomimetic activity. (From the National Institutes of Health).

emphasize that (1) lifelong treatment usually is required, (2) symptoms are an unreliable gauge of severity of hypertension, and (3) prognosis improves with proper management. Cultural factors that affect compliance and other individual differences among patients must be considered in planning a therapeutic regimen. Although classification of BP is somewhat arbitrary, it may be useful in making clinical decisions (Table 4-2).

A. **Normal BP is defined as <130/85**; pharmacologic intervention is not indicated. For cardiovascular risk factors, optimal BP is <120/80.

B. **High-normal BP is defined as a BP of 130–139/85–89**, whereas **stage 1 hypertension is a BP of 140–159/90–99**. In these patients with no more than one cardiovascular risk factor excluding diabetes mellitus and no target organ damage, BP can be followed for up to 6 months with nonpharmacologic therapy. If treatment is ineffective or there is evidence of end-organ damage or diabetes, or both, with or without additional risk factors, pharmacologic therapy should be initiated.

C. **In stages 2 (160–179/100–109) and 3 (>180/110) hypertension**, pharmacologic therapy should be initiated in addition to lifestyle modification. Patients with BP levels of greater than 180/110 mm Hg often require more than one medication and frequent intervals of follow-up before adequate control is achieved. Patients with an average BP of 200/120 or greater need immediate therapy and, if symptomatic end-organ damage is present, require hospitalization.

D. **Isolated systolic hypertension** is defined as a systolic BP of greater than 140 mm Hg and a diastolic BP of less than 90 mm Hg. This occurs frequently in the elderly, beginning after the fifth decade and increasing with age. Nonpharmacologic therapy should be attempted initially. If this fails, medication should be used to lower systolic BP to less than 140 mm Hg. Patient tolerance of antihypertensive therapy should be assessed frequently.

II. **Nonpharmacologic therapy.** Lifestyle modifications should be encouraged in all hypertensive patients regardless of whether they require medication (*Arch Intern Med* 1997;157:2412, and *JAMA* 1993;270:713). They are potential opportunities to prevent hypertension, lower BP, and reduce other cardiovascular risk factors at little cost and with minimal risk (*N Engl J Med* 1997;336:1117–1124). Even modest weight loss can produce long-term reductions in BP (*Ann Intern Med* 2001;134:1–11). In addition, even when lifestyle modifications alone cannot control hypertension, they may reduce the number and dosage of medications needed (*JAMA* 1993;270:713–724). Physicians should advise every patient who smokes cigarettes that cessation is an effective measure in reducing overall cardiovascular risk (see Chap. 1).

A. **Weight reduction** should be encouraged strongly in patients whose body mass index is 27 (kg/m^2) or greater (see Chap. 3). Reduction in body weight, especially truncal obesity, may obviate the need for drug therapy or decrease the amount of medication required to control BP. Weight loss of as little as 10 lb may reduce BP significantly in many overweight patients. Additionally, improvements in cholesterol, diabetes, and regression of LVH may occur in hypertensive patients who are managed with weight reduction. Weight loss is not recommended for pregnant patients with hypertension.

B. **Alcohol consumption** should be decreased to 1 oz or less/day or 0.5 oz/day for women and lighter-weight people. In large amounts, ethanol has a direct vasopressor effect and can exacerbate hypertension as well as cause resistance to antihypertensive therapy.

C. **Regular dynamic exercise** should be advised if the clinical situation permits. Repeated periods of exercise result in a significant reduction in BP independent of weight loss or altered sodium excretion (*Lancet* 1986;2:473) and decrease all-cause risk and cardiovascular morbidity and mortality (*JAMA* 1989;262:2395). Exercise should be performed at least three times/ week for at least 30 minutes and should achieve approximately 60–70% of a patient's maximum predicted heart rate (220 – age). Patients with known or suspected coronary artery disease and those older than age 40 years with coronary risk factors should undergo exercise stress testing before beginning an exercise program (see Chap. 6).

D. Dietary modifications include sodium restriction, which modestly reduces BP in hypertensive patients (*JAMA* 1996;275:1590). Sodium restriction may also decrease drug resistance and enhance efficacy, especially in African-Americans, diabetics, and the elderly. Total sodium chloride intake should be limited to less than 6 g/day (2.4 g sodium). The use of potassium as a therapeutic agent is controversial but may be of some benefit (*Hypertension* 1994;23:485). Normal serum potassium levels should be maintained in patients with spontaneous or drug-induced hypokalemia. Adequate intake of calcium and magnesium should be maintained as well. Dietary intake of cholesterol and saturated fat should be reduced to lessen hyperlipidemia and facilitate weight loss. The combination of decreased sodium intake and a diet with reduced total and saturated fat that is rich in fruits, vegetables, and low-fat dairy foods has been shown to substantially decrease BP (*N Engl J Med* 1997;336:1117–1124).

III. Pharmacologic therapy

A. Diuretics (Table 4-3) are effective agents in the therapy of hypertension, and data have accumulated to demonstrate their safety and benefit in reducing the incidence of stroke and cardiovascular events. Chlorthalidone, a thiazide diuretic, may be more effective than α-adrenergic antagonists (doxazosin) in the treatment of hypertension and may also carry less risk of cardiovascular disease and stroke in patients with hypertension and at least one risk factor for coronary heart disease (*JAMA* 2000;283:1967). However, diuretics have shown a less consistent decrease in ischemic cardiac events at higher doses (e.g., >50 mg hydrochlorothiazide) and may increase ventricular arrhythmias.

1. **The mechanism of action** is to initiate a natriuresis and subsequently to decrease intravascular volume. Diuretics may initially cause an increase in peripheral resistance and a decrease in cardiac output, but with chronic administration, these parameters return to normal. Diuretics may also produce mild vasodilation by inhibiting sodium entry into vascular smooth-muscle cells. Indapamide in particular has a pronounced vasodilating effect.

2. **Several classes of diuretics** are available, generally categorized by their site of action in the kidney. Thiazide and thiazide-like diuretics (e.g., hydrochlorothiazide, chlorthalidone) block sodium reabsorption predominantly in the distal convoluted tubule. Loop diuretics (e.g., furosemide, bumetanide, ethacrynic acid, and torsemide) block sodium reabsorption in the thick ascending loop of Henle and are effective agents in patients with renal insufficiency (creatinine >2.5 mg/dl). Spironolactone, a potassium-sparing agent, acts by competitively inhibiting the actions of aldosterone on the kidney. Triamterene and amiloride are potassium-sparing drugs that act on the distal convoluted tubule to inhibit the secretion of potassium ions. Potassium-sparing diuretics are weak agents when used alone; thus, they are often combined with a thiazide for added potency.

3. **Side effects** of diuretics vary by class. Thiazide diuretics can produce weakness, muscle cramps, and impotence. Metabolic side effects include hypokalemia, hypomagnesemia, hyperlipidemia (with increases in low-density lipoproteins and triglyceride levels), hypercalcemia, hyperglycemia, hyperuricemia, hyponatremia, and, rarely, azotemia. Thiazide-induced pancreatitis also has been reported. Metabolic side effects may be limited when thiazides are used in low doses (e.g., hydrochlorothiazide, 12.5–25.0 mg/day). Loop diuretics can cause electrolyte abnormalities, such as hypomagnesemia, hypocalcemia, and hypokalemia, and also can produce irreversible ototoxicity (usually dose related and more common with parenteral therapy). Spironolactone can produce hyperkalemia; gynecomastia may occur in men, and breast tender-

Table 4-3. Commonly used antihypertensive agents by functional class

Drugs by class	Properties	Initial dose	Usual dosage range
β-Adrenergic antagonists			
Atenolol[a,b]	Selective	50 mg PO qd	25–100 mg
Betaxolol	Selective	10 mg PO qd	5–40 mg
Bisoprolol[a]	Selective	5 mg PO qd	2.5–20 mg
Metoprolol	Selective	50 mg PO bid	50–450 mg
Metoprolol XL	Selective	50–100 mg PO qd	50–400 mg
Nadolol[a]	Nonselective	40 mg PO qd	20–240 mg
Propranolol[b]	Nonselective	40 mg PO bid	40–240 mg
Propranolol LA	Nonselective	80 mg PO qd	60–240 mg
Timolol[b]	Nonselective	10 mg PO bid	20–40 mg
Acebutolol[a]	ISA, selective	200 mg PO bid, 400 mg PO qd	200–1200 mg
Carteolol[a]	ISA	2.5 mg PO qd	2.5–10.0 mg
Penbutolol	ISA	20 mg PO qd	20–80 mg
Pindolol	ISA	5 mg PO bid	10–60 mg
Labetalol	α- and β-antagonist properties	100 mg PO bid	200–2400 mg
Carvedilol	α- and β-antagonist properties	6.25 mg PO bid	12.5–50.0 mg
Calcium channel antagonists			
Amlodipine	DHP	5 mg PO qd	2.5–10.0 mg
Diltiazem	—	30 mg PO qid	90–360 mg
Diltiazem SR	—	60–120 mg PO bid	120–360 mg
Diltiazem CD	—	180 mg PO qd	180–360 mg
Diltiazem XR	—	180 mg PO qd	180–480 mg
Isradipine	DHP	2.5 mg PO bid	2.5–20.0 mg
Nicardipine[b]	DHP	20 mg PO tid	60–120 mg
Nicardipine SR	DHP	30 mg PO bid	60–120 mg
Nifedipine	DHP	10 mg PO tid	30–120 mg
Nifedipine XL (or CC)	DHP	30 mg PO qd	30–90 mg
Nisoldipine	DHP	20 mg PO qd	20–40 mg
Verapamil[b]	—	80 mg PO tid	80–480 mg
Verapamil HS	—	180 mg PO qd	180–480 mg
Verapamil SR	—	120–180 mg PO qd	120–480 mg
Angiotensin-converting enzyme inhibitors			
Benazepril[a]	—	10 mg PO bid	10–40 mg
Captopril[a]	—	25 mg PO bid–tid	50–450 mg
Enalapril[a]	—	5 mg PO qd	2.5–40.0 mg

(continued)

Drugs by class	Properties	Initial dose	Usual dosage range
Fosinopril	—	10 mg PO qd	10–40 mg
Lisinopril[a]	—	10 mg PO qd	5–40 mg
Moexipril	—	7.5 mg PO qd	7.5–30.0 mg
Quinapril[a]	—	10 mg PO qd	5–80 mg
Ramipril[a]	—	2.5 mg PO qd	1.25–20.00 mg
Trandolapril	—	1–2 mg PO qd	1–4 mg
Angiotensin II–receptor blocker			
Candesartan	—	8 mg PO qd	4–32 mg
Irbesartan	—	150 mg PO qd	150–300 mg
Losartan	—	25 mg PO qd	25–100 mg
Telmisartan	—	20 mg PO qd	20–80 mg
Valsartan	—	80 mg PO qd	80–160 mg
Diuretics			
Bendroflumethiazide	Thiazide diuretic	5 mg PO qd	2.5–15.0 mg
Chlorothiazide	Thiazide diuretic	500 mg PO qd (or IV)	125–1000 mg
Chlorthalidone	Thiazide diuretic	25 mg PO qd	12.5–50.0 mg
Hydrochlorothiazide	Thiazide diuretic	25 mg PO qd	12.5–50.0 mg
Hydroflumethiazide	Thiazide diuretic	50 mg PO qd	50–100 mg
Indapamide	Thiazide diuretic	1.25 mg PO qd	2.5–5.0 mg
Methyclothiazide	Thiazide diuretic	2.5 mg PO qd	2.5–5.0 mg
Metolazone	Thiazide diuretic	2.5 mg PO qd	1.25–5.00 mg
Polythiazide	Thiazide diuretic	2.0 mg PO qd	1–4 mg
Quinethazone	Thiazide diuretic	50 mg PO qd	25–100 mg
Trichlormethiazide	Thiazide diuretic	2.0 mg PO qd	1–4 mg
Bumetanide	Loop diuretic	0.5 mg PO qd (or IV)	0.5–5.0 mg
Ethacrynic acid	Loop diuretic	50 mg PO qd (or IV)	25–100 mg
Furosemide	Loop diuretic	20 mg PO qd (or IV)	20–320 mg
Torsemide	Loop diuretic	5 mg PO qd (or IV)	5–10 mg
Amiloride	Potassium-sparing diuretic	5 mg PO qd	5–10 mg
Spironolactone	Potassium-sparing diuretic	50 mg PO qd	25–100 mg
Triamterene	Potassium-sparing diuretic	50 mg PO bid	50–200 mg
α-Adrenergic antagonists			
Doxazosin	—	1 mg PO qd	1–16 mg

(continued)

Table 4-3. (continued)

Drugs by class	Properties	Initial dose	Usual dosage range
Prazosin	—	1 mg PO bid–tid	1–20 mg
Terazosin	—	1 mg PO qhs	1–20 mg
Centrally acting adrenergic agents			
Clonidine[b]	—	0.1 mg PO bid	0.1–1.2 mg
Clonidine patch	—	TTS 1/weekly (equivalent to 0.1 mg/day release)	0.1–0.3 mg
Guanfacine	—	1 mg PO qd	1–3 mg
Guanabenz	—	4 mg PO bid	4–64 mg
Methyldopa[b]	—	250 mg PO bid–tid	250–2000 mg
Direct-acting vasodilators			
Hydralazine	—	10 mg PO qid	50–300 mg
Minoxidil	—	5 mg PO qd	2.5–100 mg
Miscellaneous			
Reserpine[b]	—	0.05 mg PO qd	0.01–0.25 mg

DHP, dihydropyridine; ISA, intrinsic sympathomimetic activity.
[a]Adjusted in renal failure.
[b]Available in generic form.

ness has been noted in women. Triamterene (usually in combination with hydrochlorothiazide) can cause renal tubular damage and renal calculi. Unlike thiazides, potassium-sparing and loop diuretics do not cause adverse lipid effects.

B. Sympatholytic agents

1. **β-Adrenergic antagonists** (Table 4-3) are effective antihypertensive agents and are part of medical regimens that have been proven to decrease the incidence of stroke, myocardial infarction (MI), and HF. These agents may offer advantages in selected populations, including patients with increased adrenergic drive (i.e., those with a wide pulse pressure and tachycardia), LVH, and a previous MI. β-Adrenergic antagonists have been shown to improve survival in patients with mild to moderate HF (see Chap. 7, Heart Failure, sec. II.C.5).

   a. The **mechanism of action** of β-adrenergic antagonists is competitive inhibition of the effects of catecholamines at β-adrenergic receptors, which decreases heart rate and cardiac output. These agents also decrease plasma renin and cause a resetting of baroreceptors to accept a lower level of BP. β-Adrenergic antagonists cause release of vasodilatory prostaglandins, decrease plasma volume, and also may have a CNS-mediated antihypertensive effect.

   b. **Classes of β-adrenergic antagonists** can be subdivided into those that are cardioselective, with primarily β_1-blocking effects, and those that are nonselective, with β_1- and β_2-blocking effects. At low doses, the cardioselective agents can be given with caution to patients with mild chronic obstructive pulmonary disease, diabetes mellitus, or peripheral vascular disease. At higher doses, these agents lose their β_1 selectivity and may cause unwanted effects in these patients. β-Adrenergic antagonists also can be categorized according to the presence or absence of partial agonist or intrinsic sympathomimetic activity (ISA). β-Adrenergic antagonists with ISA cause less bradycardia than do those without it.

   c. Side effects include high-degree atrioventricular block, HF, Raynaud's phenomenon, and impotence. Lipophilic β-adrenergic antagonists, such as propranolol, have a higher incidence of CNS side effects, such as insomnia and depression, than do the more hydrophilic agents. Propranolol also can cause nasal congestion. β-Adrenergic antagonists can cause adverse effects on the lipid profile; increased triglyceride and decreased high-density lipoprotein (HDL) levels occur mainly with nonselective β-adrenergic antagonists but generally do not occur when β-adrenergic antagonists with ISA are used. Because β-receptor density is increased with chronic antagonism, abrupt withdrawal of these agents can precipitate angina pectoris, increases in BP, and other effects that are attributable to an increase in adrenergic tone (*Br Heart J* 1981;45:637). Therefore, the dose should be tapered on discontinuation.

2. **Selective α-adrenergic antagonists,** such as prazosin, terazosin, and doxazosin, have replaced nonselective α-adrenergic antagonists, such as phenoxybenzamine (Table 4-3), in the treatment of essential hypertension.

   a. The **mechanism of action** of selective α_1-adrenergic antagonists is to block postsynaptic α-receptors, producing arterial and venous vasodilation.

   b. Side effects of these agents include a "first-dose effect," which results from a greater decrease in BP with the first dose than with subsequent doses. Selective α_1-adrenergic antagonists can cause syncope, orthostatic hypotension, dizziness, headache, and drowsiness. In most cases, side effects are self-limited and do not recur with continued therapy. Selective α_1-adrenergic antagonists may improve lipid profiles by decreasing total cholesterol and triglyceride levels and increasing HDL levels (*Am Heart J* 1991;121:251). Additionally, these agents can improve the negative effects on lipids that are induced by thiazide diuretics and β-adrenergic antagonists (*Am Heart J* 1991;121:1307). However, doxazosin specifically may be less effective in lowering systolic BP than thiazide diuretics and may additionally be associated with a higher risk of cardiovascular disease, particularly CHF, and stroke in patients with hypertension and at least one risk factor for coronary heart disease (*JAMA* 2000;283:1967).

3. **Agents with mixed properties** (labetalol, carvedilol) have α- and β-adrenergic antagonist actions (Table 4-3). In addition, carvedilol may have antioxidant properties. These agents are effective in Caucasian and in African-American hypertensive patients.

   a. The **mechanism of action** of these drugs is to antagonize the effects of catecholamines at β-receptors and peripheral α_1-receptors. The effects of labetalol on α-receptors decrease with chronic administration and are essentially gone within a few months.

   b. Side effects of labetalol include hepatocellular damage, postural hypotension, a positive antinuclear antibody test (ANA), a lupuslike syndrome, tremors, and potential hypotension in the setting of halothane anesthesia. Reflex tachycardia rarely occurs because of the initial vasodilatory effect. Labetalol has negligible effects on lipids. Carvedilol appears to have a similar side effect profile as other β-adrenergic antagonists.

4. **Centrally acting adrenergic agents** (Table 4-3) are potent antihypertensive drugs. In addition to oral dosage forms, clonidine is available as a transdermal patch that is applied weekly.

   a. The **mechanism of action** of centrally acting adrenergic agents is to stimulate the presynaptic α_2-adrenergic receptors in the CNS. This stimulation leads to a decrease in peripheral sympathetic tone, which reduces systemic vascular resistance. Also, it causes a modest decrease in cardiac output and heart rate. Renal blood flow is not compromised by centrally acting adrenergic agents, but fluid retention may occur.

   b. **Side effects** may include bradycardia, drowsiness, dry mouth, orthostatic hypotension, galactorrhea, and sexual dysfunction. Transdermal clonidine may cause a rash in up to 20% of patients. These agents can precipitate HF in individuals with decreased left ventricular function, and abrupt cessation can precipitate an acute withdrawal syndrome (AWS) of elevated BP, tachycardia, and diaphoresis. Methyldopa produces a positive direct antibody (Coombs') test in up to 25% of patients, but significant hemolytic anemia is much less common. The drug should be withdrawn if hemolytic anemia develops, and severe cases of hemolytic anemia may require treatment with glucocorticoids. Methyldopa also causes positive ANA test results in approximately 10% of patients and can cause an inflammatory reaction in the liver that is indistinguishable from viral hepatitis; fatal hepatitis has been reported. Guanabenz and guanfacine decrease total cholesterol levels, and guanfacine also can decrease serum triglyceride levels.

5. **Other sympatholytics** (reserpine, guanethidine, guanadrel). These agents (Table 4-3) were among the first effective antihypertensive agents to be available. Currently, these drugs are not regarded as first- or second-line therapy because of their significant side effects.

   a. The **mechanism of action** of these agents is to inhibit the release of norepinephrine from peripheral neurons. Reserpine, which is more lipophilic than are other drugs in this class, also affects the CNS. Reserpine depletes biogenic amines from being packaged into storage vesicles within neurons, thereby allowing norepinephrine to be degraded by cytoplasmic monoamine oxidase. Guanethidine and guanadrel directly inhibit the release of norepinephrine from peripheral nerve terminals.

   b. **Side effects** of reserpine include severe depression in approximately 2% of patients. Sedation and nasal stuffiness also are potential side effects. Guanethidine can cause severe postural hypotension by effecting a decrease in cardiac output, a decrease in peripheral resistance, and venous pooling in the extremities. Patients who are receiving guanethidine with orthostatic hypotension should be cautioned to arise slowly and to wear support hose. Guanethidine also can cause ejaculatory failure and diarrhea.

C. **Calcium channel antagonists** (Table 4-3) are effective agents in the treatment of hypertension. Generally, they are effective in African-American and in Caucasian hypertensive patients, have no significant CNS side effects, and can be used to treat diseases, such as angina pectoris, that can coexist with hypertension. Concern has risen that the use of short-acting dihydropyridine calcium channel antagonists may increase the number of ischemic cardiac events (*JAMA* 1995;274:620); however, long-acting agents are safe in the management of hypertension (*Am J Cardiol* 1996;77:81).

   1. **The mechanism of action** is to cause arteriolar vasodilation by selective blockade of the slow inward calcium channels in vascular smooth-muscle cells. These agents also cause an initial natriuresis, which may dissipate with time.

   2. **Classes of calcium channel antagonists** include diphenylalkylamines (e.g., verapamil), benzothiazepines (e.g., diltiazem), and dihydropyridines (e.g., nifedipine). The dihydropyridines include many newer second-generation drugs (e.g., amlodipine, felodipine, isradipine, and nicardipine) that are more vasoselective and have longer plasma half-lives than nife-

dipine. Verapamil and diltiazem have negative cardiac inotropic and chronotropic effects. Nifedipine also has a negative inotropic effect, but, in clinical use, it is much less pronounced than verapamil or diltiazem because of peripheral vasodilatation and reflex tachycardia. Less negative inotropic effects have been observed with the second-generation dihydropyridines. All calcium channel antagonists are metabolized in the liver; thus, in patients with cirrhosis, the dosing interval should be adjusted accordingly. Some of these drugs also inhibit the metabolism of other hepatically cleared medications (e.g., cyclosporine). Verapamil and diltiazem should be used with caution in patients with cardiac conduction abnormalities and are contraindicated in patients with decreased left ventricular function. Amlodipine and felodipine appear to be safe in HF, but they do not improve survival (*N Engl J Med* 1996;335:1107).

   3. **Side effects** of verapamil include constipation, nausea, headache, and orthostatic hypotension. Diltiazem can cause nausea, headache, and rash. Dihydropyridines can cause lower-extremity edema, flushing, headache, and rash; only the long-acting preparations should be used. Calcium channel antagonists have no significant effects on glucose tolerance, electrolytes, or lipid profiles. In general, calcium channel antagonists should not be initiated in patients immediately after MI because of increased mortality in all but the most stable patients without evidence of HF. Additionally, in patients with hypertension and non–insulin-dependent diabetes mellitus dihydropyridines (nisoldipine) may be associated with a higher incidence of fatal and nonfatal MIs (*N Engl J Med* 1998;338:645).

D. Inhibitors of the renin-angiotensin system (Table 4-3) are effective antihypertensive agents in a broad array of patients.

   1. **Angiotensin-converting enzyme (ACE) inhibitors** have beneficial effects in patients with concomitant HF or kidney disease. One study has also suggested that ACE inhibitors (ramipril) may significantly reduce the rate of death, MI, and stroke in patients without HF or low ejection fraction (*N Engl J Med* 2000;342:145). Additionally, they can reduce hypokalemia, hypercholesterolemia, hyperglycemia, and hyperuricemia caused by diuretic therapy and are particularly effective in states of hypertension that are associated with a high renin state (e.g., scleroderma renal crisis) (*Med Clin North Am* 1987;71:979). Fosinopril is unique in that 50% of the drug is eliminated by the liver under normal conditions, but this percentage increases in the presence of renal insufficiency.

      a. **Mechanism of action.** ACE inhibitors block the production of angiotensin II, a vasoconstrictor, by inhibiting ACE competitively, thereby leading to arterial and venous vasodilation and to natriuresis. Furthermore, ACE inhibitors, by inhibiting the formation of angiotensin II, reduce aldosterone secretion, thus producing a mild natriuresis and a decrease in K^+ secretion. Additionally, ACE inhibitors increase levels of vasodilating bradykinins. Some agents (i.e., captopril) directly stimulate production of renal and endothelial vasodilatory prostaglandins. Despite these vasodilating effects, ACE inhibitors do not cause significant reflex tachycardia, perhaps because of a resetting of the baroreceptor reflex.

      b. **Side effects** associated with the use of ACE inhibitors are infrequent. They do not cause levels of lipids, glucose, or uric acid to increase. ACE inhibitors can cause a dry cough (up to 20% of patients), angioneurotic edema, and hypotension. ACE inhibitors that contain a sulfhydryl group (e.g., captopril) may cause a glomerulopathy with proteinuria, taste disturbance, and leukopenia. Because ACE inhibitors cause preferential vasodilation of the efferent arteriole in the kidney, worsening of renal function may occur in patients who have decreased renal perfusion or who have pre-existing severe renal insufficiency. ACE inhibitors can cause hyperkalemia and should be used with caution in patients with a decreased glomerular filtration rate, in those who are taking potassium supplements, or in those who are receiving potassium-sparing diuretics.

2. **Angiotensin-receptor antagonists (ARBs)** are a class of antihypertensive drugs that are effective in diverse patient populations (*N Engl J Med* 1996;334:1649). Several of these agents are now approved for the management of mild to moderate hypertension (Table 4-3). Additionally, ARBs may be a useful alternative in patients with HF who are unable to tolerate ACE inhibitors (*Lancet* 2000;355:1582).

   a. **The main mechanisms of action** of these drugs are to antagonize the vasoconstrictor effects on smooth muscle and the secretory effects on the zona glomerulosa of angiotensin II at the angiotensin II type 1 receptor. These actions result in decreased peripheral vascular resistance.

   b. **Side effects** of losartan occur rarely but include angioedema, allergic reaction, and rash. The cough seen with ACE inhibitors occurs much less frequently with losartan. The side effect profile is otherwise similar to that of the ACE inhibitors. Losartan specifically is uricosuric. These agents do not appear to affect lipids.

E. **Direct-acting vasodilators,** potent antihypertensive agents (Table 4-3), now are reserved for refractory hypertension or specific circumstances, such as the use of hydralazine in pregnancy. Hydralazine in combination with nitrates is useful in treating patients with hypertension and HF.

   1. **The mechanism of action** of these agents (e.g., minoxidil and hydralazine) is to produce direct arterial vasodilation. Minoxidil hyperpolarizes and relaxes smooth muscle by stimulating an adenosine triphosphate–dependent K^+ channel. The mechanism of action of hydralazine is unknown. Although these drugs lower BP when used alone, their sustained antihypertensive action is limited because of reflex sodium and fluid retention and sympathetic hyperactivity that produces tachycardia. Often, concomitant diuretic or β-adrenergic antagonist use is required to ameliorate these unwanted effects. These agents should be used with caution or avoided in patients with ischemic heart disease because of the reflex sympathetic hyperactivity that they induce.

   2. **Side effects** of hydralazine therapy may include headache, nausea, emesis, tachycardia, and postural hypotension. Asymptomatic patients may have a positive ANA test result, and a hydralazine-induced systemic lupus–like syndrome may develop in approximately 10% of patients. Individuals who may be at increased risk for this latter complication include (1) those treated with excessive doses (e.g., >400 mg/day), (2) those with impaired renal or cardiac function, and (3) those with the slow acetylation phenotype. Hydralazine should be discontinued if clinical evidence of a lupus-like syndrome develops and a positive ANA test result is present. The syndrome usually resolves with discontinuation of the drug, leaving no adverse long-term effects. Side effects of minoxidil include weight gain, hypertrichosis, hirsutism, ECG abnormalities, and pericardial effusions.

F. **Oral loading of antihypertensive agents** has been used successfully in patients with hypertensive crisis when urgent but not immediate reduction of BP is indicated.

   1. **Oral clonidine loading** is achieved by using an initial dose of 0.2 mg PO followed by 0.1 mg PO q1h to a total dose of 0.7 mg or a reduction in diastolic pressure of 20 mm Hg or more. BP should be checked at 15-minute intervals over the first hour, 30-minute intervals over the second hour, and then hourly. After 6 hours, a diuretic can be added, and an 8-hour clonidine dosing interval can be initiated. Sedative side effects are significant.

2. **Sublingual nifedipine** has an onset of action within 30 minutes but can produce wide fluctuations and excessive reductions in BP. **Because of the potential for adverse cardiovascular events (stroke/ MI), the use of sublingual nifedipine is contraindicated** (*Ann Intern Med* 1987;107:185). Side effects include facial flushing and postural hypotension.

IV. **Individual patient considerations.** A vast array of effective antihypertensive agents is available. Logical therapeutic choices require consideration of a patient's pathogenic derangement of renin secretion, sympathetic tone, and renal sodium excretion and the attendant changes in cardiac output, peripheral vascular resistance, and volume status.

A. **Hypertension in the elderly patient** (older than 60 years) generally is characterized by increased vascular resistance, decreased plasma renin activity, and greater LVH than in younger patients. Systolic BP is a better predictor of events than diastolic BP in the elderly (*Hypertension* 1994;23:275), and an elevated pulse pressure signals an increased risk for cardiovascular events (*Hypertension* 1994;23:395). Lifestyle modifications such as salt reduction and weight loss should be attempted first. Often, elderly hypertensive patients have coexisting medical problems that must be considered in initiating antihypertensive therapy. Drug doses should be initiated at low doses and increased slowly to avoid adverse effects and hypotension. Diuretics alone as initial therapy have been shown to decrease the incidence of stroke, fatal MI, and overall mortality in this age group (*JAMA* 2000;283:1967; *JAMA* 1991;265:3255; and *Lancet* 1985;1: 1349). Calcium channel antagonists decrease vascular resistance, have no adverse effects on lipid levels, and are good choices for elderly patients. Even though elderly patients tend to have low plasma renin activity, ACE inhibitors and ARBs may be effective agents in this population (*N Engl J Med* 1993;328:914). Long-term studies have documented the safety and efficacy of β-adrenergic antagonists, especially after acute MI; however, they may increase peripheral resistance, decrease cardiac output, and decrease HDL cholesterol. Combining beta-blockers with thiazide diuretics has also been shown to reduce morbidity and mortality in multiple trials (*Clin Exp Hypertens* 1993;15:967). Agents that produce postural hypotension (i.e., prazosin, guanethidine, guanadrel) should be avoided. Central α-adrenergic agents generally are effective in elderly patients but commonly cause sedation. In elderly patients with isolated systolic hypertension, the same approach to initiating therapy should be used, but smaller doses should be given, and adjustments should be made less frequently.

B. **African-American hypertensive patients** generally have a lower plasma renin level, higher plasma volume, and higher vascular resistance than do Caucasian patients. Given the demonstrated reduction in morbidity and mortality and good response to diuretic use, diuretics should be the agent of choice in African-American patients without any contraindications, alone or in combination with calcium channel antagonists. ACE inhibitors, ARBs, and labetalol (an α- and β-adrenergic antagonist) are also effective agents in this population, and addition of a diuretic to these drugs often increases the response.

C. **The obese hypertensive patient** is characterized by more modest elevations in vascular resistance, higher cardiac output, expanded intravascular volume, and lower plasma renin activity at any given level of arterial pressure. Weight reduction is the primary goal of therapy and is effective in reducing BP and causing regression of LVH. Weight reduction should be part of any therapeutic regimen. In addition, obese patients are at higher risk for obstructive sleep apnea, which may result in hypertension that is more difficult to control.

D. **The diabetic patient** with nephropathy may have significant proteinuria and renal insufficiency, which can complicate management (see Chap. 18). Control of BP (especially diastolic BP) to below 130/85 is the most important intervention that has been shown to slow the loss of renal function. Tight BP control better protects against stroke, CHF, MI, sudden death, and retinopathy in diabetic patients (*BMJ* 1998;317:703–713). Lifestyle modifications including weight reduction are essential. ACE inhibitors should be used as first-line therapy, as they have been shown to decrease proteinuria and to slow progressive loss of renal function independent of their antihypertensive effects (*N Engl J Med* 1993;329:1456). ACE inhibitors may be beneficial in reducing the rates of death, MI, and stroke in diabetics who have cardiovascular risk factors but lack left ventricular dysfunction (*N Engl J Med* 2000;342:145). Furthermore, ACE inhibitors may have a lower incidence of MI than the dihydropyridine class of calcium channel antagonists (*N Engl J Med* 1998;338:645). Hyperkalemia is a common side effect in diabetic patients who are treated with ACE inhibitors, especially in those with moderate to severe impairment of their glomerular filtration rate. ARBs also are effective antihypertensive agents and have been shown to slow the rate of progression to end-stage renal disease, thus supporting a renal protective effect. Calcium channel antagonists are also effective in diabetic patients; diltiazem and verapamil may have a selective beneficial effect in decreasing proteinuria in diabetic patients with renal disease (*Ann Intern Med* 1990;113:987). In patients with evidence of nephropathy, a β-adrenergic antagonist and diuretic may be considered if ACE inhibitors or ARBs are not tolerated.

E. **The hypertensive patient with chronic renal insufficiency** has hypertension that usually is partially volume dependent. Retention of sodium and water exacerbates the existing hypertensive state, and diuretics are important in the management of this problem. With a serum creatinine greater than 2.5 mg/dl, loop diuretics are the most effective class. BP control in this patient group decreases progression to end-stage renal disease (*N Engl J Med* 1996;334:13). Other causes of renal insufficiency such as renovascular disease must be excluded before the initiation of ACE inhibitors.

F. **The hypertensive patient with LVH** is at increased risk for sudden death, MI, and all-cause mortality. Although there is no direct evidence, regression of LVH could be expected to reduce the risk for subsequent complications. Sodium restriction, weight loss, and all drugs except direct-acting vasodilators can decrease left ventricular mass and wall thickness. ACE inhibitors appear to have the greatest effect on regression (*JAMA* 1996;275:1507).

G. **The hypertensive patient with coronary artery disease** is at increased risk for unstable angina and MI. β-Adrenergic antagonists can be used as first-line agents in these patients, as they can decrease cardiac mortality and subsequent reinfarction in the setting of acute MI and can decrease progression to MI in those who present with unstable angina. β-Adrenergic antagonists also have a role in secondary prevention of cardiac events and in increasing long-term survival after MI (*Arch Intern Med* 1996;156:1267). Care should be exercised in those with cardiac conduction system disease; reflex tachycardia and sympathetic activation avoided by lowering the BP too quickly or excessively. Calcium channel antagonists should be used with caution in the setting of acute MI, as studies have shown conflicting results from their use. They have modest benefit after a non–Q-wave MI or following an MI with preserved left ventricular function (*J Am Coll Cardiol* 1996;28:1328). ACE inhibitors are also useful in patients with coronary artery disease and decrease mortality in individuals who present with acute MI, especially those with left ventricular dysfunction; more recently they have been shown to decrease mortality in patients without left ventricular dysfunction (*N Engl J Med* 2000;342:145).

H. **The hypertensive patient with CHF** is at risk for progressive left ventricular dilatation and sudden death. In this population, ACE inhibitors decrease mortality (*N Engl J Med* 1992;327:685), and in the setting of acute MI, they decrease the risk of recurrent MI, hospitalization for HF, and mortality (*N Engl J Med* 1992;327:669, and *Lancet* 1995;345:669). It would also be anticipated that, based on this mechanism of action, the angiotensin-receptor blockers would have similar beneficial effects, and they appear to be an effective alternative in patients who are unable to tolerate an ACE inhibitor (*Lancet* 2000;355:1582). Carvedilol (an alpha-beta–blocker) has been shown to decrease morbidity and mortality when added to ACE inhibitors (*N Engl J Med* 1996;334:1349). Nitrates and hydralazine also decrease mortality in patients with HF irrespective of hypertension, but hydralazine can cause reflex tachycardia and worsening ischemia in patients with unstable coronary syndromes and should be used with caution. Calcium channel antagonists should generally be avoided in patients in whom negative inotropic effects will affect their status adversely.

I. Hypertension in women increases with age. Studies demonstrate that treatment of elderly women is effective and should be initiated (see sec. **IV.A**) along with lifestyle modifications. In patients in whom osteoporosis is also a concern, diuretics decrease urinary calcium excretion. No therapeutic trials have shown clinically significant sex differences in BP response and outcomes; treatment of hypertension lowers the risk of cardiovascular morbidity and mortality in women older than 55 years of age and benefits African-American women of all ages [*J Gen Intern Med* 1999;14(12):718–729]. Although trials are in progress, treatment of mild to moderate hypertension in young to middle-aged women with no other risk factors should be conservative, with particular emphasis on lifestyle modifications. Individual treatment thresholds may decrease for women at increased risk of stroke or cardiovascular disease. Gender-specific considerations include (1) hypertension associated with use of oral contraceptives, (2) hormone replacement therapy, (3) pregnancy, and (4) the increased incidence of fibromuscular dysplasia causing renovascular hypertension. With close monitoring, hormone replacement therapy is safe for women with hypertension [*JAMA* 1995;273(3):199–208], as are oral contraceptives in nonsmokers whose hypertension is well controlled.

V. Initial drug therapy. Currently, diuretics, β-adrenergic antagonists, calcium channel antagonists, ACE inhibitors, ARBs, and α-adrenergic antagonists are regarded as first-line agents. Data from long-term trials have shown decreased cardiovascular and cerebrovascular morbidity and mortality with the use of thiazide diuretics and β-adrenergic antagonists; thus, these drugs may be favored as first-line agents in the absence of a contraindication to their use (hyperlipidemia, glucose intolerance, or an elevated uric acid) or if characteristics of a patient's profile (concomitant disease, age, race) mandate institution of a different agent. Calcium channel antagonists and ACE inhibitors have been shown to decrease BP to degrees similar to those observed with diuretics and β-adrenergic antagonists and also are good initial agents because of their low side effect profile. The majority of patients with stage 1 or stage 2 hypertension can attain adequate BP control with single-drug therapy. Initial drug choice may be affected by coexistent factors, such as age, race, angina, CHF, renal insufficiency, LVH, obesity, hyperlipidemia, gout, and bronchospasm. Cost and drug interactions also should be considered. The BP response usually is consistent within a given class of agents; therefore, if a drug fails to control BP, another agent from the same class is unlikely to be effective. At times, however, a change within drug class may be useful in reducing adverse effects. The lowest possible effective dosage should be used to control BP, adjusted every 1–3 months as needed.

VI. Additional therapy. When a second drug is needed, it can generally be chosen from among the other first-line agents. A diuretic should be added first, as doing so may enhance effectiveness of the first drug, yielding more than a simple additive effect. Several combination preparations of first-line agents are available.

VII. Adjustments of a therapeutic regimen. In considering a modification of therapy because of inadequate response to the current regimen, the physician should investigate other possible contributing factors. Poor patient compliance, use of antagonistic drugs (i.e., sympathomimetics, antidepressants, steroids, nonsteroidal anti-inflammatory drugs, cyclosporine, caffeine, thyroid hormones, cocaine, erythropoietin), inappropriately high sodium intake, or increased alcohol consumption should be considered before antihypertensive drug therapy is modified. Unacceptable side effects from a particular agent may contribute to poor patient compliance. Excessive fluid retention should be evaluated and treated. Secondary causes of hypertension must be considered when a previously effective regimen becomes inadequate and other confounding factors are absent. If hypertension has been well controlled for 1 year, gradual efforts to streamline the therapeutic regimen may be considered. Close follow-up is needed as hypertension can recur months or years after cessation of therapy.

Special Considerations

I. **Hypertension associated with withdrawal syndromes.** Hypertension may be part of several important syndromes of withdrawal from drugs, including alcohol, cocaine, and opioid analgesics. Rebound increases in BP also may be seen in patients who abruptly discontinue antihypertensive therapy.
   A. **Cocaine and other sympathomimetic drugs** (e.g., amphetamines, phencyclidine hydrochloride) can produce hypertension in the setting of acute intoxication and when the agents are discontinued abruptly after chronic use. No evidence has been found that chronic hypertension is caused by continued cocaine abuse (*J Am Soc Nephrol* 1996;7:1547). Hypertension often is complicated by other end-organ insults, such as ischemic heart disease, stroke, and seizures. Management of acute cocaine-induced hypertension should be done in an inpatient setting. β-Adrenergic antagonists should be avoided due to the risk of unopposed α-adrenergic activity, which can exacerbate hypertension.
   B. **Monoamine oxidase inhibitors** used in association with certain drugs or foods can produce a catecholamine excess state and accelerated hypertension. Interactions are common with tricyclic antidepressants, meperidine, methyldopa, levodopa, sympathomimetic agents, and antihistamines. Tyramine-containing foods that can lead to this syndrome include certain cheeses, red wine, beer, chocolate, chicken liver, processed meat, herring, broad beans, canned figs, and yeast. Nitroprusside, labetalol, and phentolamine have been used effectively in the treatment of accelerated hypertension that is associated with monoamine oxidase inhibitor use.
II. **Withdrawal syndrome associated with discontinuation of antihypertensive therapy.** In substituting therapy for patients with moderate to severe hypertension, it is reasonable to increase doses of the new medication in small increments while tapering the previous medication to avoid excessive BP fluctuations. On occasion, an acute withdrawl syndrome (AWS) develops (usually within the first 24–72 hours), and BP rises to a level that is much greater than baseline. The most severe complications of AWS include encephalopathy, stroke, MI, and sudden death. The AWS is associated most commonly with centrally acting adrenergic agents (particularly clonidine) and β-adrenergic antagonists, but has been reported with other agents, including diuretics. Rarely should BP medications be withdrawn, but in discontinuing therapy, these drugs should be tapered over several days to weeks unless other medications are used to substitute in the interim. Discontinuation of antihypertensive medications should be done with caution in patients with pre-existing cerebrovascular or cardiac disease. Management of AWS by reinstitution of the previously administered drug is generally effective and may be best done in an inpatient setting. In the AWS caused by clonidine, β-adrenergic antagonists should not be used because unopposed α-adrenergic activity will be augmented and may exacerbate hypertension. However, labetalol (Table 4-3) may be useful in this situation.

III. Hypertensive crisis. Hypertensive emergencies include accelerated hypertension (systolic BP >210 mm Hg and diastolic BP >130 mm Hg) that presents with headaches, blurred vision, or focal neurologic symptoms and malignant hypertension (includes above and papilledema). In hypertensive emergency, control of acute or ongoing end-organ damage is more important than is the absolute level of BP. BP control with a rapidly acting parenteral agent should be accomplished as soon as possible (within 1 hour) to reduce permanent organ dysfunction and death (Table 4-1). A reasonable goal is a 20–25% reduction of mean arterial pressure or a reduction of the diastolic pressure to 100–110 mm Hg over a period of minutes to hours. This should be managed in an inpatient setting. BP control in **hypertensive urgencies** (defined as a substantial increase in BP, with distolic BP >120–130 mm Hg) can be accomplished more slowly. The initial goal of therapy in urgency should be to achieve a diastolic BP of 100–110 mm Hg. Excessive or rapid decreases in BP should be avoided to minimize the risk of cerebral hypoperfusion or coronary insufficiency. Normal BP can be attained gradually over several days as tolerated by the individual patient.

IV. Aortic dissection. Acute, proximal aortic dissection (type A) is a surgical emergency, whereas uncomplicated distal dissection (type B) can be treated successfully with medical therapy alone. Sodium nitroprusside is considered the initial drug of choice along with the simultaneous addition of a β-adrenergic antagonist. IV labetalol has also been successfully used as a single agent (*JAMA* 1987;258:78). All patients, including those treated surgically, require acute and chronic antihypertensive therapy to provide initial stabilization and to prevent complications (e.g., aortic rupture, continued dissection). Medical therapy of chronic stable aortic dissection should seek to maintain systolic BP at or below 130–140 mm Hg if tolerated. Antihypertensive agents with negative inotropic properties, including non-DHP calcium channel antagonists, β-adrenergic antagonists, methyldopa, clonidine, and reserpine, are preferred for management in the postacute phase.

V. Pregnancy and hypertension (see Appendix A). Hypertension in the setting of pregnancy is a special situation because of the potential for maternal and fetal morbidity and mortality associated with elevated BP and the clinical syndromes of preeclampsia and eclampsia. The possibility of teratogenic or other adverse effects of antihypertensive medications on fetal development also should be considered. ACE inhibitors and angiotensin II–receptor blockers have been associated with renal failure and death and should not be used in pregnant women (*N Engl J Med* 1996;335:257). β-Adrenergic blockers are effective but should be used only in the latter part of pregnancy, because their earlier use may be associated with growth retardation (*N Engl J Med* 1996;335:257).

Lipid Disorders

Anne Carol Goldberg

The relationship between the risk of atherosclerotic heart disease and serum lipoproteins is well established. Elevated levels of total cholesterol and low-density lipoprotein cholesterol (LDL-C) and low levels of high-density lipoprotein cholesterol (HDL-C) are associated with increased risk. Elevated triglycerides are associated with an increased risk of cardiovascular disease in some situations, such as familial combined hyperlipoproteinemia (FCHL), dysbetalipoproteinemia, diabetes mellitus (DM), and the polymetabolic syndrome. Severely elevated triglycerides confer an increased risk of pancreatitis. Lowering LDL-C levels has been shown to decrease the risk of coronary events and procedures in patients with and without coronary artery disease. Guidelines to help physicians detect, evaluate, and treat patients with dyslipidemia have been issued by the National Cholesterol Education Program Adult Treatment Panel III (*JAMA* 2001;285:2486–2497; http://www.nhlbi.nih.gov).

Detection and Evaluation

All adults older than age 20 should have a fasting lipoprotein profile and evaluation of cardiac risk factors every 5 years (Table 5-1). An HDL-C level of less than 40 mg/dl is considered low. High HDL-C, greater than 60 mg/dl, is treated as a negative risk factor. Total cholesterol and HDL-C can be measured in a nonfasting state, but triglycerides and calculated LDL-C must be performed fasting. Fasting lipoprotein analysis should be obtained in all patients with coronary heart disease (CHD) and in patients with a total cholesterol of greater than 200 mg/dl and an HDL-C of less than 40 mg/dl.

I. **Lipoprotein analysis** is performed on serum obtained after a **12-hour fast**. Total cholesterol, triglycerides, and HDL-C are measured, and LDL-C is calculated using the following formula:

$$LDL\text{-}C = \text{total cholesterol} - HDL\text{-}C - (\text{triglyceride}/5)$$

where triglyceride/5 represents the cholesterol contained in very low-density lipoprotein (VLDL). This formula is not valid when triglyceride levels are greater than 400 mg/dl. In such patients, direct measurement of LDL-C using ultracentrifugation is the most reliable way of ascertaining LDL-C. Cholesterol should be measured while patients are on their usual diet. In patients who are losing weight, are pregnant, have had major surgery, or are seriously ill (e.g., myocardial infarction), cholesterol levels may not be representative, and analysis should be deferred for at least 6 weeks. In patients who have had an acute myocardial infarction, lipoprotein levels measured within the first 24 hours provide an approximation of their usual levels; otherwise levels will not be stable for up to 6 weeks.

II. **Risk assessment is the first step in the evaluation of patients for management of elevated lipid levels.** Risk is determined based on the lipoprotein profile, the presence or absence of CHD, and other major risk factors (Table 5-1).

Table 5-1. Major risk factors [exclusive of low-density lipoprotein cholesterol (LDL-C)] that modify LDL goals

Cigarette smoking

Hypertension (BP ≥ 140/90 mm Hg or on antihypertensive medication)

Family history of premature CHD (CHD in male first-degree relative <55 yrs; CHD in female first-degree relative <65 yrs)

Low HDL-C (<40 mg/dl)[a]

Age: men ≥ 45 yrs
women ≥ 55 yrs

CHD, coronary heart disease; HDL-C, high-density lipoprotein cholesterol.
[a]HDL-C level ≥ 60 mg/dl counts as a "negative" risk factor; its presence removes one risk factor from the total count.
Source: Executive summary of the third report of the National Cholesterol Education Program (NCEP) Expert Panel on Detection, Evaluation, and Treatment of High Blood Cholesterol in Adults (Adult Treatment Panel III). *JAMA* 2001;285:2487.

A. **Initial classification is based on LDL-C level**, which is the primary target of therapy.
   1. **Optimal LDL-C** is less than 100 mg/dl.
   2. **Near or above optimal LDL-C** is 100–129 mg/dl.
   3. **Borderline-high LDL-C** is 130–159 mg/dl.
   4. **High LDL-C** is 160–189 mg/dl.
   5. **Very high LDL-C** is greater than or equal to 190 mg/dl.
B. **Total cholesterol and HDL-C are classified.**
   1. **Desirable total cholesterol** is less than 200 mg/dl.
   2. **Borderline-high blood cholesterol** is from 200–239 mg/dl.
   3. **High blood cholesterol** is greater than or equal to 240 mg/dl.
   4. **Low HDL-C** is less than 40 mg/dl and is counted as a risk factor.
   5. **High HDL-C** is greater than or equal to 60 mg/dl and is a negative risk factor; its presence removes one risk factor from the total count.
C. **Risk categories modify LDL-C goals.**
   1. **Patients in the category of highest risk are those with CHD and CHD risk equivalents.** CHD risk equivalents include clinical CHD, symptomatic carotid artery disease, peripheral vascular disease, and abdominal aortic aneurysm. Other CHD risk equivalents include DM and the presence of multiple risk factors that confer a 10-year risk for CHD greater than 20% (see Table 6-1). Patients in this category have an LDL goal of less than 100 mg/dl.
   2. **The next category consists of patients with multiple (2+) risk factors** (Table 5-1). Goal LDL for these patients is less than 130 mg/dl.
   3. **The third category consists of people with no or one risk factor.** The goal LDL for this group is less than 160 mg/dl.
D. **The estimation of 10-year risk of CHD** is performed in patients with two or more risk factors using Framingham scoring (see Table 6-1).
   1. **A 10-year risk of greater than 20%** is considered a CHD risk equivalent, and the goal LDL is less than 100 mg/dl.
   2. **A 10-year risk of 10–20%** qualifies patients for a more aggressive approach than a 10-year risk of less than 10%, even though the goal LDL is less than 130 mg/dl for both groups.
   3. **A 10-year risk of less than 10%** usually corresponds to fewer than 2 risk factors.
III. **Classification of patients with CHD.** Patients with CHD or CHD risk equivalents need aggressive therapy to lower LDL-C.

A. **Optimal LDL-C** is less than or equal to 100 mg/dl. These patients should have instruction on diet and physical activity. Other lipid and nonlipid risk factors should be treated.

B. **Higher than optimal LDL-C** is above 100 mg/dl. Patients with baseline LDL above 130 mg/dl require intensive lifestyle therapy and maximal control of other risk factors. Drug therapy can be started simultaneously with lifestyle therapy. The goal of therapy is less than 100 mg/dl. Patients with LDL-C levels between 100 and 129 mg/dl should have lifestyle therapy started or intensified and should also be considered for initial or intensified drug therapy.

IV. **Elevated serum triglyceride levels** are an independent risk factor for atherosclerotic disease. They may be associated with increased concentrations of atherogenic particles such as chylomicron remnants, VLDL remnants, and small, dense LDL particles. Patients with hypertriglyceridemia frequently have low levels of HDL-C.

A. **Normal triglycerides** are less than 150 mg/dl.

B. **Borderline-high hypertriglyceridemia** levels are between 150 and 199 mg/dl. Nonpharmacologic therapy, including diet, exercise, and weight loss, is the initial form of therapy in these patients. Drug therapy is considered for patients who are not at goal level of LDL, which is the first target of therapy in this group.

C. **High triglycerides** are defined as triglyceride levels between 200 and 499 mg/dl. Nonpharmacologic treatment with diet, exercise, and weight loss is initial therapy. LDL-C remains the primary target of therapy, but non–HDL-C is a secondary target of therapy. Non–HDL-C is equal to total cholesterol minus HDL-C.

D. **Very high triglycerides** are over 500 mg/dl. These patients are at increased risk for pancreatitis. Nonpharmacologic measures and a search for secondary causes are needed. These patients must be treated aggressively. Once triglyceride levels are lowered to less than 500 mg/dl, LDL is again the primary target of therapy.

V. **Screening for other risk factors.** In addition to the risk factors listed in Table 5-1, measurement of other risk factors may be useful in some patients in whom the decision to treat with medication is uncertain.

A. **Elevated levels of lipoprotein (a)** above 30 mg/dl are associated with increased risk of atherosclerotic cardiovascular disease. Measurement of lipoprotein (a) may be useful in assessing risk, particularly in patients with few risk factors but with a strong family history of premature atherosclerosis.

B. **Elevated levels of homocysteine** have been associated with increased rates of atherosclerotic events. Measurement of homocysteine may be useful in assessing risk, particularly in patients with few risk factors but with a strong family history of premature atherosclerosis.

Diagnosis of
Specific Disorders

I. **Primary causes of hypercholesterolemia**

A. **Familial hypercholesterolemia (FH)** is an autosomal dominant disorder involving the LDL receptor.

1. **Heterozygotes** for FH have 50% of the normal number of LDL receptors, elevated LDL-C levels, and cholesterol levels of 250–500 mg/dl. The incidence is approximately one in 500 persons. Affected patients often have premature vascular disease and may have tendinous xanthomas. Treatment usually requires drug as well as diet therapy. More severe cases may require the combination of two or more medications. Patients with insufficient response to tolerated doses of lipid-lowering medications may be candidates for LDL-apheresis.

2. **Homozygotes** for FH have few or no LDL receptors and thus have markedly elevated LDL-C levels and blood cholesterol levels of 600–1000 mg/dl. The incidence is one in one million. Heart disease often begins in early childhood, and many patients die of heart disease in their 20s and 30s. Affected children may have planar and tuberous as well as tendinous xanthomas. They respond poorly to diet and to drug therapy, although they may have some response to higher doses of potent statins. LDL-apheresis is the preferred therapy. Liver transplantation has been performed in a few patients.

3. **Familial defective apolipoprotein B-100** is an autosomal dominant disorder caused by an abnormality in the LDL receptor-binding region of apoprotein B-100, the major protein on the surface of LDL particles. It appears to have frequency, clinical features, and lipoprotein levels that are similar to those of the FH heterozygous form.

B. **Familial combined hyperlipoproteinemia (FCHL)** is associated with an increased risk of vascular disease. Patients may have elevated cholesterol, triglycerides, or both. The molecular basis of this disorder is unknown; many patients overproduce VLDL. FCHL appears to be an autosomal dominant disorder and occurs in 1–2% of the population. The diagnosis is made by the presence of multiple lipoprotein phenotypes within one family. Family members may have elevated VLDL (type IV), elevated LDL-C (type IIa), or increased levels of VLDL and LDL-C (type IIb). Diet therapy, weight loss, and exercise are useful initial therapies, but many patients require drug therapy that is aimed at correcting specific lipoprotein abnormalities.

C. **Severe polygenic hypercholesterolemia** is found in adults whose LDL-C is above 220 mg/dl and who do not clearly demonstrate a monogenic inheritance of hypercholesterolemia. These patients are usually at increased risk for premature CHD. Many require medication to achieve LDL-C goals.

II. **Hypertriglyceridemia** may be secondary to diet, obesity, excess alcohol intake, DM, hypothyroidism, uremia, dysproteinemias, β-adrenergic antagonists, estrogen, oral contraceptive drugs, and retinoids. Triglyceride levels greater than 400 mg/dl are often associated with an underlying primary disorder. Primary hypertriglyceridemia can be due to FCHL or familial hypertriglyceridemia (FHTG). Families with FHTG have multiple members with elevated triglyceride levels due to increased VLDL levels. FHTG appears to be an autosomal dominant disorder without a clearly defined molecular basis. Families may show less pronounced risk of CHD than those with FCHL.

III. **Dysbetalipoproteinemia** (type III hyperlipoproteinemia) is a rare (approximately 1 in 5000) disorder caused by an abnormality of apoprotein E, a protein on the surface of VLDL and other lipoproteins, that is important in the uptake of remnant particles by cell surface receptors. Cholesterol-enriched VLDL (β-VLDL), an atherogenic particle, accumulates. Cholesterol and triglycerides are elevated. Isoelectric focusing shows an abnormal apoprotein E pattern, which can be confirmed by specific genotyping. Patients may have palmar or tuberoeruptive xanthomas, and there is increased risk of vascular disease. Patients with this disorder may respond well to diet and weight loss.

IV. **Hyperchylomicronemia** is diagnosed by the presence of a chylomicron layer when plasma is centrifuged or when chylomicrons float to the top of plasma that has been refrigerated overnight. Chylomicrons can be seen when triglyceride levels are in excess of 1000 mg/dl. The patient may have rare syndromes that involve absence of lipoprotein lipase activity or absent apoprotein CII (a cofactor of lipoprotein lipase). Chylomicrons alone may be increased, as in lipoprotein lipase deficiency, or VLDL and chylomicrons may be elevated. Total cholesterol levels are often markedly elevated because of the presence of large numbers of VLDL particles that contain cholesterol as well as triglycerides. In patients with primary hypertriglyceridemia, FCHL, or dysbetalipoproteinemia, hyperchylomicronemia may develop in the presence of excessive dietary fat intake, uncontrolled diabetes, alcohol excess, obesity, or other secondary causes of hyperlipidemia. The chylomicronemia syndrome may include abdominal pain, hepatomegaly, splenomegaly, eruptive xanthomas, lipemia retinalis, and pancreatitis. Memory loss, paresthesias, and peripheral neuropathy can also occur.

V. **Low HDL-C levels (<40 mg/dl)** may be due to a genetic disorder or to secondary causes.

   A. **Primary disorders** include familial hypoalphalipoproteinemia, primary hypertriglyceridemias, and rare disorders such as fish-eye disease, Tangier disease, and lecithin-cholesterol-acyltransferase deficiency.

   B. **Secondary causes** of low HDL-C levels include cigarette smoking, obesity, lack of exercise, androgens, some progestational agents, anabolic steroids, β-adrenergic antagonists, and hypertriglyceridemia.

VI. **Family members** of patients with hyperlipidemia should be screened to facilitate diagnosis of primary hyperlipidemias as well as to identify other patients who are in need of treatment.

Therapy of Hyperlipidemia

I. **The rationale for therapy** of hyperlipidemia is to reduce the risk of atherosclerotic cardiovascular disease. For patients with severe hypertriglyceridemia, the aim is to prevent pancreatitis.

   A. **Reduction of cholesterol and LDL-C levels** is associated with a reduction of risk of cardiovascular disease. This has been demonstrated by a number of clinical trials that involve primary and secondary prevention (*Lancet* 1994;344:1383–1389, *N Engl J Med* 1996;335:1001–1009, and *N Engl J Med* 1995;333:1301–1307) as well as angiographic studies of plaque regression (*Circulation* 1993;87:1781).

   B. **Hypertriglyceridemia** is less clearly associated with cardiovascular disease, but risk is believed to be increased in FCHL, in diabetic dyslipidemia, or when other risk factors are present. Triglyceride levels above 500 mg/dl should be treated to prevent hyperchylomicronemia and pancreatitis.

II. **Therapeutic lifestyle changes (TLCs) including dietary changes, increased physical activity, and weight reduction are the first-line therapy** for hyperlipidemia and may be sufficient for mild to moderate hypercholesterolemia and hypertriglyceridemia. Most patients have a 10–15% decrease in LDL levels with diet; this may be enough to reach goal levels in some patients and is important in patients in whom the ultimate drop in LDL needs to be 30–60%. Hypertriglyceridemia often responds quite well to decreased intakes of fat, sugar, alcohol, and calories (where necessary). Response to lipid-lowering drugs may be disappointing in patients who continue to consume high-fat diets. The physician and the entire health team should stress the benefits of TLCs.

   A. **Goals** of therapy of hypercholesterolemia should be set. These are minimal goals, and lower levels of LDL should be attained whenever possible (Table 5-2).

      1. **In the absence of risk factors,** a target goal LDL-C is less than 160 mg/dl.

      2. **The presence of two or more risk factors** calls for a target goal LDL-C of less than 130 mg/dl.

      3. **In patients with CHD or CHD risk equivalents (including diabetes),** the goal LDL-C is less than 100 mg/dl.

   B. **Diet therapy** calls for reduction in saturated fat and cholesterol.

      1. **Saturated fat should be reduced to less than 7% of total calories and cholesterol intake to less than 200 mg/day.** Total fat should be 25–35% of calories.

         a. **Saturated fat** intake is reduced by cutting portion sizes of beef, pork, chicken, and fish and limiting total meat consumption to 6 oz/day. Lean cuts of beef and pork should be well trimmed, skin should be removed from chicken and turkey, and fried foods should be avoided. Vegetable oils that are highly saturated, such as coconut oil and palm oil, should

Table 5-2. National Cholesterol Education Program 2001 Adult Treatment Panel
guidelines: treatment decisions based on low-density lipoprotein (LDL) cholesterol

Risk category	LDL goal	LDL level at which to initiate therapeutic lifestyle changes	LDL level at which to consider drug therapy
CHD or CHD risk equivalents (10-yr risk >20%)	<100 mg/dl	≥100 mg/dl	≥130 mg/dl (100–129 mg/dl: drug optional)
2+ risk factors (10-yr risk ≤20%)	<130 mg/dl	≥130 mg/dl	10-year risk 10–20%: ≥130 mg/dl 10-year risk <10%: ≥160 mg/dl
0–1 risk factor	<160 mg/dl	≥160 mg/dl	≥190 mg/dl (160–189 mg/dl: LDL-lowering drug optional)

CHD, coronary heart disease.
Source: Executive summary of the third report of the National Cholesterol Education Program (NCEP) Expert Panel on Detection, Evaluation, and Treatment of High Blood Cholesterol in Adults (Adult Treatment Panel III). *JAMA* 2001;285:2487.

be avoided. Low-fat dairy products can be substituted for whole-milk products. Soft margarine, liquid vegetable oils, and low-fat cheese should replace butter, solid vegetable shortening, and high-fat cheese. **Trans fatty acids**, produced during hydrogenation of liquid oils to make solid fats, raise LDL-C and lower HDL-C (*N Engl J Med* 1990;323:439). Avoidance of fried foods, use of low-fat baked goods, and soft margarine will decrease dietary intake of trans fatty acids.
  b. **Polyunsaturated fats** can be obtained from vegetable oils and margarine. Intake of polyunsaturated fat should not exceed 10% of total calories.
  c. **Monounsaturated fat** should be 10–20% of total calories. These fats are found in vegetable oils, especially olive and canola oil.
  d. **Cholesterol intake** can be reduced by restricting egg yolks and organ meats, such as liver, kidney, brains, and sweetbreads, as well as by keeping portions of beef, poultry, and fish to 5–6 oz/day. A maximum of one egg yolk/week (including those used in prepared foods) can be used.
  e. **Fresh fruits, vegetables, and whole-grain products** should be used to increase variety and provide nutrients and fiber. Carbohydrates, especially complex carbohydrate, should make up 50–60% of total calories. A minimum of two to three servings of vegetables, two to three servings of fruits, and six servings of bread, cereal, or other grain products should be included daily.
  f. **Dietary fiber** intake should be 20–30 g/day.
  g. **Total calories** should be adjusted to maintain desirable body weight and to prevent weight gain.
2. **If goal LDL-C is not met** after 6 weeks, plant stanols and soluble fiber can be added. After 12 weeks, referral to a **registered dietitian** may be helpful.
3. **Addition of drug therapy can be considered after 3 months** for patients who do not have CHD and who have not reached LDL goal.

Diet instruction and drug therapy may be started at the time of diagnosis of CHD or an acute event. Cholesterol levels should be monitored at 6-week intervals to provide incentive for change. Gradual initiation of diet changes often works better than drastic alterations.

4. **Adjustments in dietary therapy** need to be made for the elderly, who may have poor nutritional intake, and in pregnant women, who have increased requirements for a number of nutrients. Severely restrictive diets should not be used in young children with the exception of those with primary lipoprotein lipase deficiency, in whom dietary fat restriction is necessary to prevent hyperchylomicronemia.

5. **Improved compliance can be achieved** by setting realistic goals with an emphasis on gradual change; involving the patient, food preparers, and family in making and implementing decisions; and referring patients to registered dietitians who can offer endorsement and encouragement of diet as a major therapy. It is important to pay attention to the individual patient's needs and habits.

C. **Increased physical activity** is an important part of the overall management of patients with hyperlipidemia. It is helpful in lowering triglyceride and cholesterol levels and in raising HDL-C. It can also contribute to weight loss. Regular exercise will also help patients who have lost weight to maintain their weight. An exercise program must be designed for the individual, depending on his or her state of health, fitness, and cardiac status.

D. **Weight loss** is beneficial in patients who are overweight or have the metabolic syndrome. Total calories should be adjusted for gradual weight loss. Elevated triglycerides often respond well. HDL-C may increase with weight loss, and LDL-C may decrease. A general approach is to lower caloric intake by 250–500 calories/day. Very low-calorie diets are not recommended in most cases.

E. **Hypertriglyceridemic patients** usually respond to restriction of dietary fat and may also require decreased intake of simple sugars and alcohol. Some patients who markedly increase their carbohydrate intake have increases in triglyceride levels. Hypertriglyceridemic patients should generally not be on diets with fat content less than 25% of calories, except for patients with the chylomicronemia syndrome. The response to very low-fat diets (i.e., 10% of calories from fat) may be disappointing in patients with impaired glucose tolerance unless the diet is sufficiently hypocaloric. Very high-carbohydrate diets that are isocaloric can lead to poor glycemic control and increased triglyceride levels. A particular problem is a high intake of nonfat desserts, which leads to increased calories in an otherwise low-fat diet.

F. **The chylomicronemia syndrome** requires a diet that is very low in total fat. Patients with triglycerides above 2000 mg/dl should initiate a diet with less than 10% of total calories as fat. It may be possible to increase the fat content gradually as the triglyceride level falls to less than 500 mg/dl. Primary lipoprotein lipase deficiency is treated with fat restriction and does not respond to drug therapy.

G. **Adjuncts to dietary therapy** include food-derived substances that may help lower lipid levels.

1. **Soluble fiber** may produce modest decreases in LDL-C. **Psyllium** in doses of 5 g twice a day can produce a 5–10% decrease in LDL-C. Oat bran, pectin, and guar gum may produce similar effects (*Curr Opin Lipidol* 1995;6:14–19).

2. **Plant sterols and stanols** are compounds that can affect the absorption of cholesterol in the intestine. These are available in the form of margarine that can be used in spreads or cooking. Use of two to three servings/day can produce LDL reductions of 10–14%.

3. **Soy protein** has been shown to decrease LDL-C. The effects vary depending on the type and amount of soy protein used and on the baseline LDL levels. At 20–50 g/day soy protein in the diet, LDL levels may decrease by approximately 10–15% (*N Engl J Med* 1995;333:276–282).

4. **Omega-3 fatty acids,** found in fish oils, can reduce triglyceride levels. Fish oil capsules that contain the long-chain fatty acids, **eicosapentaenoic acid and docosahexaenoic acid**, can be used as an adjunct to other therapies in patients with hypertriglyceridemia. At doses of 3–6 g/day eicosapentaenoic acid plus docosahexaenoic acid, triglycerides may decrease by up to 30%. The major drawbacks to high doses of these fatty acids are the large number of pills to be taken, eructation, and occasional diarrhea. A mild antiplatelet effect occurs, which may be of concern in patients who are receiving warfarin or antiplatelet drugs.

III. **Discontinuation of thiazide diuretics and β-adrenergic antagonists,** if possible, sometimes leads to reduction of triglycerides, cholesterol, and LDL-C and to increased HDL-C. Substitution of a selective β-adrenergic antagonist for a nonselective one may be helpful. In postmenopausal women who have triglycerides over 500 mg/dl on estrogen replacement therapy, switching from an oral estrogen preparation to transdermal estrogen often leads to improvement in triglyceride levels.

IV. **Secondary causes of hyperlipidemia** should be treated. Patients who are hypothyroid should be on adequate replacement dosages of L-thyroxine. Control of hyperglycemia is critical if diabetic dyslipidemia is to be adequately managed.

V. **The metabolic syndrome is a secondary target of risk reduction therapy.** It is a constellation of factors, including abdominal obesity, insulin resistance or diabetes, hypertension, and atherogenic lipid profile (elevated triglyceride levels, small dense LDL, low HDL).

A. **Patients are considered to have the metabolic syndrome** if they have three of the following:

1. **Abdominal obesity:** waist circumference greater than 102 cm in men and 88 cm in women.
2. **Triglycerides** greater than or equal to 150 mg/dl.
3. **HDL-C** less than 40 mg/dl in men and 50 mg/dl in women.
4. **BP** greater than or equal to 130/85 mm Hg.
5. **Fasting glucose** greater than or equal to 110 mg/dl.

B. **Weight control and increased physical activity** are important in the treatment of the metabolic syndrome. Other risk factors such as hypertension should also be treated.

C. **Elevated triglycerides** and/or low HDL should be treated once LDL goal has been reached.

VI. **Drug therapy** is considered if maximal diet, weight reduction, and exercise efforts do not reduce serum lipids to goal levels after an adequate trial.

A. **Initiation of drug therapy** of hypercholesterolemia should be considered if LDL-C remains greater than 190 mg/dl in patients without CHD or two or more cardiac risk factors. For those with LDL of 160–189 mg/dl, drug therapy is optional. In patients with two or more risk factors, the cutoff point is LDL-C greater than 160 mg/dl in patients with a 10-year risk of less than 10% and greater than 130 mg/dl in patients with a 10-year risk of 10–20% (see Table 6-1). In patients with CHD or CHD risk equivalents, one should initiate drug therapy if the LDL-C remains above 130 mg/dl in spite of diet. For patients with CHD who have LDL-C levels between 100 and 130 mg/dl, use of drug therapy depends on the physician's clinical judgment about the benefits of adding medication. Many CHD patients require medication to reach the LDL goal of less than 100 mg/dl.

B. **Goals of therapy** are the reduction of LDL-C to less than 100 mg/dl in patients with CHD or CHD risk equivalents, less than 130 mg/dl in those with two or more risk factors, and less than 160 mg/dl in patients without CHD or two or more risk factors. Diabetes is a CHD risk equivalent, and adult patients with diabetes have a goal LDL of less than 100 mg/dl.

C. **TLCs** are continued even if drug therapy is used.

D. Drugs that lower LDL-C are the 3-hydroxy-3-methylglutaryl coenzyme A (HMG CoA) reductase inhibitors (statins), bile acid sequestrant resins, and nicotinic acid. The statins, resins, and nicotinic acid have been shown to have safety and efficacy in reduction of cholesterol and risk of CHD.

E. Triglyceride-lowering drugs include niacin, gemfibrozil, and fenofibrate.

F. Patients with triglycerides of 500 mg/dl or less and elevated LDL-C levels may respond adequately to a statin added to nonpharmacologic measures. If the triglycerides remain elevated after LDL goal is reached, a secondary goal is the non–HDL-C. For patients with CHD or CHD risk equivalents, the non–HDL-C goal is less than 130 mg/dl. For patients with multiple risk factors, non–HDL-C goal is less than 160 mg/dl and for patients with 0–1 risk factor, the non–HDL-C goal is less than 190 mg/dl. If the triglycerides are above 500 mg/dl and diet and exercise are reasonable, the choice of medication could include a statin at higher doses, gemfibrozil, fenofibrate, or niacin. When triglycerides are over 1000 mg/dl, fibrates and niacin are initial drugs. If LDL-C levels remain high after the triglycerides are lowered, combination therapy may be considered.

G. Dysbetalipoproteinemia responds well to diet and weight loss. When drugs are needed, nicotinic acid, gemfibrozil, or fenofibrate can be used. Some patients with this disorder also respond well to statins.

H. Low HDL-C levels are associated with an increased risk of cardiovascular disease. Attention should be given to factors that lower HDL, such as cigarette smoking and certain medications, such as β-adrenergic blocking agents, androgenic compounds, and progestins. Nonpharmacologic therapy, such as exercise, weight loss, and smoking cessation, should be stressed. Niacin is the most effective agent for increasing HDL. Some increase can occur with fibrates, approximately 10–20%.

I. Drug combinations may be useful in certain situations.

    1. In severe hypercholesterolemia, it is often necessary to use a combination of diet and two or more drugs to reduce LDL-C to desired levels. Useful combinations include statin plus resin, statin plus nicotinic acid, or the combination of all three. Triple-drug therapy with statin, resin, and niacin may be needed in some patients with the heterozygous form of FH to reach goal LDL-C levels.

    2. Combined LDL-C and triglyceride elevations may respond to nicotinic acid or statin as single-drug therapy. A few patients may have adequate control with a fibric acid derivative alone. Combinations of nicotinic acid plus statin or fibric acid plus statin are used but carry an increased risk of severe myopathy or rhabdomyolysis.

    3. Low doses of two drugs can be combined if higher doses of a single agent are not tolerated by the patient. Combination of statin and resin or nicotinic acid and a resin may be quite effective.

J. Response to therapy should be monitored by checking cholesterol and triglyceride levels after 6–8 weeks of therapy. If the patient has no response to a drug in spite of dosage adjustments, or if unacceptable side effects occur, the drug should be discontinued. If the initial drug produces only a partial response at tolerated dosage, addition of a second drug with a different mechanism of action may be useful.

VII. LDL-apheresis and liver transplantation have been used to treat patients with the homozygous form of FH because these patients respond poorly to drug therapy. LDL-apheresis can be used for some patients with severe heterozygous FH who do not have an adequate response to tolerated doses of medications.

Drugs

I. The HMG CoA reductase inhibitors (statins) inhibit the rate-limiting step in cholesterol biosynthesis. Drugs in this class are lovastatin, pravastatin, simvastatin, fluvastatin, and atorvastatin. All have the same mechanism of action and similar side effects. Inhibition of enzyme activity leads to a decrease in intracellular cholesterol pools and consequently an increase in LDL receptors. The statins lower LDL-C well in most patients. These drugs are the drugs of choice for lowering LDL for secondary prevention. LDL-C can drop by 20–60% depending on the drug and dosage. HDL may increase by up to 15%, and triglycerides decrease by up to 30%. Atorvastatin has a longer half-life, approximately 13 hours, than the other reductase inhibitors, which have half-lives of about 2–3 hours.

A. **Dosages** for lovastatin are 10–80 mg/day, for pravastatin 10–40 mg/day, for simvastatin 5–80 mg/day, for fluvastatin 20–80 mg/day, and for atorvastatin 10–80 mg/day. Lovastatin is best given with food, usually with the evening meal, but pravastatin, simvastatin, and fluvastatin can be given without food, preferably in the evening. Atorvastatin can be given at any time during the day.

B. **Side effects** occur infrequently (approximately 5% of patients), are usually mild and transient, and most commonly include bloating, gassiness, nausea, and indigestion. Myopathy is an infrequent side effect but has been reported more often when the reductase inhibitors are combined with cyclosporine, gemfibrozil, niacin, or erythromycin. Liver function tests should be followed, preferably at 6-week intervals for the first 3 months, then at 3-month intervals during the first year of therapy, and thereafter every 6 months. Mild elevations of transaminases may occur after starting therapy; these usually decrease with continued therapy. Approximately 1% of patients have transaminase elevations to greater than three times the upper limit of normal, and the medication must be discontinued. The HMG CoA reductase inhibitors should be avoided in the presence of active liver disease. It may be useful to check creatine kinase in the presence of myalgias, but in many cases, it is not elevated. Rhabdomyolysis is a rare side effect, which has been reported particularly when statins have been combined with fibric acid derivatives, cyclosporine, niacin, or erythromycin. Such combination should be used with caution and with note of the manufacturer's package inserts.

II. **Bile acid sequestrant resins** (cholestyramine and colestipol) are insoluble, nonabsorbable, anion-exchange resins that bind bile acids within the intestine, preventing their reabsorption. Because more cholesterol must be used to synthesize bile acids, there is an increase in cell surface receptors for LDL, producing a fall in circulating LDL-C levels. Reduction of LDL-C is dose dependent; up to a 35% reduction can be seen. HDL-C may increase, and VLDL sometimes increases, usually transiently. The use of resins as single-drug therapy is contraindicated in the presence of elevated triglyceride levels greater than 300 mg/dl.

A. **Dosages** are 4–30 g cholestyramine or colestipol daily. The initial dosage of cholestyramine is 4 g (1 scoop or packet) PO daily with a meal and one scoop or packet (5 g) of colestipol PO daily with a meal. Up to 24 g cholestyramine or 30 g colestipol can be used. Cholestyramine and colestipol are available in powder form; a single dose of cholestyramine is 4 g resin and of colestipol 5 g. Colestipol is also available in 1-g tablets, with typical dosing schedules of 4–16 tablets/day.

B. **Compliance** is enhanced and side effects minimized by starting therapy with low dosages and carefully educating the patient about these drugs. The granule form of cholestyramine and colestipol must be mixed with a liquid. Increasing by one scoop or packet every few weeks may decrease GI side effects. The drug can be mixed in almost any liquid or semiliquid food. Timing close to meals is important. It should be taken within 1 hour of a meal, especially the evening meal if once-a-day dosing is used. For colestipol tablets (1 g), once- or twice-daily dosing close to meals is desirable. A single daily dose of up to 8–12 g may be useful to fit the resin into a medication schedule. Side effects and efficacy of colestipol tablets are comparable to those of powdered resin. Tablets may be more convenient or palatable for patients who dislike the powder.

C. Side effects include constipation, abdominal pain, nausea, vomiting, bloating, heartburn, belching, and flatulence. These effects often diminish with continued use of the drug. Use of stool softeners or psyllium can decrease constipation. Patients with severe constipation and very complicated drug regimens are not usually good candidates for resin therapy. The resins can interfere with absorption of thiazides, digoxin, warfarin, thyroxine, and cyclosporine; other medications should be given at least 1 hour before or 4 hours after the resins.

D. Colesevelam is a recently approved bile acid–binding drug. It is available in 625-mg tablets, with a recommended dose of six tablets/day and a maximum dose of seven tablets/day. LDL-C reduction is 15–18%. Less of a problem may occur with certain drug interactions. Side effects are similar to those of the other resins.

III. Nicotinic acid (niacin) is a water-soluble vitamin that lowers triglycerides by 20–50%, raises HDL-C by 10–40%, and can lower LDL-C by 15–30%. Niacin is particularly useful in combined hyperlipidemia and in patients with low levels of HDL. Niacin has been used in several secondary and angiographic trials of lipid lowering (*J Am Coll Cardiol* 1986;8:1245, *JAMA* 1987;257:3233, and *N Engl J Med* 1990;323:1289).

A. Dosage should be low initially with a gradual increase. Initial dosage is 100 mg PO one to three times/day **with meals**, increasing slowly (e.g., by 300 mg/day each week), to 2–4 g/day. The highest dose that is conventionally used is 3000 mg/day crystalline niacin, although higher doses have been used.

B. Side effects tend to be dose dependent, but cutaneous flushing occurs in most patients. Patient education and attention to how niacin is taken are important for compliance. Tolerance to flushing usually develops. Niacin should be taken with food to help decrease flushing. Aspirin, 81 mg PO 30 minutes before each dose, can decrease flushing. Niacinamide does not cause flushing but has no significant effect on lipid levels. Other side effects include pruritus, rash, nausea, dyspepsia, anorexia, dizziness, and hypotension. Hyperuricemia, liver function abnormalities, and worsening of glucose intolerance may occur. Baseline liver profiles and uric acid and fasting blood glucose levels should be obtained, and these should be monitored every 6–8 weeks while the dosage is being titrated and thereafter every 3–4 months. Queasiness, nausea, or increased fatigue may be signs of toxicity; liver function tests should be checked and the dose decreased if these are elevated. Use of **nicotinic acid is contraindicated in patients with gout, peptic ulcer disease, inflammatory bowel disease, and significant arrhythmias**. Niacin can be used in patients with DM who have well-controlled blood glucose levels, but blood sugar levels must be monitored carefully. Use of **over-the-counter sustained-release preparations should be avoided** due to an associated increased toxicity, including severe hepatotoxicity (*Ann Intern Med* 1989;111:253). Severe toxicity is more likely to occur when patients switch abruptly from a non–sustained-release to a sustained-release preparation without reducing the total dosage. A **prescription-only, extended-release formulation** can be given once a day at bedtime; significant liver toxicity was not reported at doses up to 2000 mg/day in clinical trials. The maximum dose is 2000 mg/day.

IV. Fibric acid derivatives include gemfibrozil and fenofibrate. They lower levels of triglycerides by 30–50% and raise HDL-C by 10–20%. LDL-C may decrease by 10–20% in some patients with combined hyperlipidemia but increase in others, especially patients with markedly elevated triglyceride levels.

A. Dosage of gemfibrozil is 600 mg PO bid before meals. The dose should be reduced in patients with renal insufficiency. Fenofibrate is given once a day with a meal. The full dose is 160 mg/day, but lower doses may also be useful. Fenofibrate is available in 54- and 160-mg tablets. Lower doses should be used in patients with renal insufficiency.

B. Side effects include bloating, abdominal pain, diarrhea, nausea, headaches, occasional rashes, and pruritus. Liver enzymes and creatinine should be checked at baseline and 8–12 weeks after the drug is started, after another 3 months, and then yearly. Increased transaminases occur in approximately 5% of patients on fenofibrate and return to normal when the drug is discontinued. Infrequently, myalgias and increased creatine kinase have been reported. Gemfibrozil potentiates the effects of warfarin and may be associated with an increased risk of gallstones.

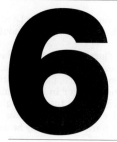

Cardiovascular I: Ischemic Heart Disease

Charles F. Carey

Ischemic heart disease is the leading cause of mortality in adults in North America and most other developed countries. Primary care physicians have an important role in preventing, diagnosing, and treating coronary artery disease (CAD). The initial clinical presentation of CAD is usually either stable angina pectoris or acute coronary syndromes such as myocardial infarction (MI) or unstable angina (USA), but it may also present as CHF or sudden death or can be clinically silent. More than 1 million patients in the United States have an MI each year, with up to one-half of these individuals not surviving to hospitalization. CAD is usually secondary to a lipid-rich plaque with a fibrous cap that, if it ruptures or erodes, results in thrombus formation that typically presents as an acute coronary syndrome. Interventions that prevent atherosclerosis, stabilize the lipid-rich plaque, and decrease the risk of plaque rupture or reduce the physiologic significance of a plaque are important aspects of ambulatory adult medicine.

Ischemic Heart Disease Risk Factors

I. **Major risk factors are additive in predicting CAD risk and include advancing age (male age >45 years or female age >55 years or premature menopause without estrogen replacement), cigarette smoking, diabetes, hypertension, elevated low-density lipoprotein cholesterol (LDL-C), low high-density lipoprotein cholesterol (HDL-C) (<40 mg/dl), and premature family history of CAD (<55 years old for male or 65 years old in female first-degree relatives).** A HDL-C greater than 60 mg/dl reduces the risk of CAD. Table 6-1 provides a method for predicting the risk of clinically developing coronary heart disease based on the major risk factors.

II. Other risk factors that contribute to the risk for CAD that should be evaluated in clinical practice include obesity (particularly truncal obesity), physical inactivity, elevated triglycerides, and psychosocial factors. An elevated sensitive C-reactive protein is a risk factor for future events, but its role in clinical practice is currently not defined.

Prevention

Primary and secondary prevention have the greatest potential for decreasing the mortality and morbidity of CAD.

I. **Cholesterol** is an important modifiable risk factor for primary and secondary prevention (see Chap. 5). It should be evaluated at least every 5 years in asymptomatic patients starting at age 20 years. In patients with no major risk factors, two or more major risk factors (see Ischemic Heart Disease Risk Factors, sec. I), or CAD or CAD risk equivalent, the goal for LDL-C should be less than 160, 130, and 100 mg/dl, respectively. Diet and lifestyle changes should be prescribed to all patients. If after 4–6 months the patient's LDL-C remains 30 mg/dl over goal, pharmacologic therapy should be considered. For secondary prevention if the initial LDL is greater than 130 mg/dl, it is reasonable to start pharmacologic therapy initially, usually with a statin, along with diet and lifestyle changes. The ideal triglyceride level is less than 150 mg/dl. The HDL-C goal is greater than 40 mg/dl, with the CAD risk inversely proportional to the level.

II. **Hypertension** should be treated if the BP is greater than 140/90 mm Hg after lifestyle modifications. A direct relationship is found between risk of CAD and BP. ECG evidence of left ventricular (LV) hypertrophy has also been shown to be a powerful predictor of cardiovascular (CV) risk. In patients with CHF or renal disease, the BP should be less than 130/85 mm Hg and in diabetic patients less than 130/80 mm Hg. In patients with CAD, beta-blockers should be used to manage hypertension [see Chap. 4 and *JNC VI* (NIH Publication No. 98-4080, 1997; http://www.nhlbi.nih.gov/guidelines) for further details].

III. **Diabetes** greatly increases the risk of CAD, and there is a disproportionate CV mortality in diabetics, especially in women. Prevention and risk modification must be aggressive in this population, with particular attention to cholesterol (LDL <100) and BP control (*BMJ* 1998;317:703). An angiotensin-converting enzyme (ACE) inhibitor should be strongly considered as part of the regimen (*N Engl J Med* 2000;342:145). It is recommended that glycemic control be tightly regulated with target hemoglobin A_{1c} of less than 7. This intervention has been extremely effective in decreasing microvascular complications. An effect probably also occurs in reducing macrovascular disease, with a modest reduction (16% over 10 years, p = .052) in MI compared to a nonintensive strategy (*Lancet* 1998;352:837). Insulin sensitizers, such as metformin, potentially result in further reduction of macrovascular risk, particularly in an obese patient, but further study is needed (see Chap. 18 and *Lancet* 1998;352:854).

IV. **Smoking cessation** decreases the risk of cardiac events by 25–50% for primary and for secondary prevention. A linear relationship exists between the risk of CAD and number of cigarettes smoked. Smoking is estimated as being the number one leading cause of preventable death in North America (*JAMA* 1995;273:1047). Three years after smoking cessation, a patient's risk of CAD returns to normal. It is important to emphasize smoking cessation at every opportunity. The addition of bupropion hydrochloride or nicotine replacement, or both, to a counseling and smoking cessation program increases the success rate (see Chap. 1). Secondhand smoke from a person in the same household results in an increased risk of CV mortality.

V. **Lifestyle modification** with changes in physical activity, nutrition, weight management, and psychosocial factors requires frequent discussion and reinforcement. Patients who have CAD benefit from a structured cardiac rehabilitation program, which has been associated with a one-fourth reduction in CV mortality and reinforces the following lifestyle changes.

   A. **Physical activity** consisting of at least 30 minutes of aerobic activity a day is important for primary and for secondary prevention. A history and physical examination should be performed in patients who plan an exercise program. Walking at a regular pace is safe in most patients, starting at 5–10 minutes at a time and increasing the duration of walking up to 30–60 minutes over several weeks. A symptom-limited stress test should be performed to exclude ischemia at the planned levels of activity in patients with suspected CAD, age over 40 years, or two or more major risk factors who are planning to participate in an exercise program that is more strenuous than walking (*Circulation* 1990;82:2286). A general guide in patients without CAD who want to participate in a more intense aerobic exercise program would be to start at an exercise intensity that achieves 50–60% of maximal predicted

Table 6-1. Ten-year risk for developing coronary artery disease

Men

Age (yrs)	Points	Age (yrs)	Points	Age (yrs)	Points
20–34	–9	50–54	6	65–69	11
35–39	–4	55–59	8	70–74	12
40–44	0	60–64	10	75–79	13
45–49	3				

Total choles-terol (mg/dl)	Points				
	Age 20–39 yrs	Age 40–49 yrs	Age 50–59 yrs	Age 60–69 yrs	Age 70–79 yrs
<160	0	0	0	0	0
160–199	4	3	2	1	0
200–239	7	5	3	1	0
240–279	9	6	4	2	1
≥280	11	8	5	3	1

	Points				
	Age 20–39 yrs	Age 40–49 yrs	Age 50–59 yrs	Age 60–69 yrs	Age 70–79 yrs
Nonsmoker	0	0	0	0	0
Smoker	8	5	3	1	1

High-density lipoprotein (mg/dl)	Points
≥60	–1
50–59	0
40–49	1
<40	2

Systolic BP (mm Hg)	If untreated	If treated
<120	0	0
120–129	0	1
130–139	1	2
140–159	1	2
≥160	2	3

Point total	10-year risk (%)	Point total	10-year risk (%)
<0	<1	9	5
0	1	10	6
1	1	11	8
2	1	12	10
3	1	13	12
4	1	14	16
5	2	15	20
6	2	16	25
7	3	≥17	≥30
8	4		

Women

Age (yrs)	Points	Age (yrs)	Points	Age (yrs)	Points
20–34	–7	50–54	6	65–69	12
35–39	–3	55–59	8	70–74	14
40–44	0	60–64	10	75–79	16
45–49	3				

Total choles-	Points				
terol (mg/dl)	Age 20–39 yrs	Age 40–49 yrs	Age 50–59 yrs	Age 60–69 yrs	Age 70–79 yrs
<160	0	0	0	0	0
160–199	4	3	2	1	1
200–239	8	6	4	2	1
240–279	11	8	5	3	2
≥280	13	10	7	4	2

	Points				
	Age 20–39 yrs	Age 40–49 yrs	Age 50–59 yrs	Age 60–69 yrs	Age 70–79 yrs
Nonsmoker	0	0	0	0	0
Smoker	9	7	4	2	1

High-density lipoprotein (mg/dl)	Points
≥60	–1
50–59	0
40–49	1
<40	2

Systolic BP (mm Hg)	If untreated	If treated
<120	0	0
120–129	1	3
130–139	2	4
140–159	3	5
≥160	4	6

Point total	10-year risk (%)	Point total	10-year risk (%)
<9	<1	17	5
9	1	18	6
10	1	19	8
11	1	20	11
12	1	21	14
13	2	22	17
14	2	23	22
15	3	24	27
16	4	≥25	≥30

Note: Add points in each category (age, total cholesterol, smoking status, high-density lipoprotein cholesterol, systolic BP) to determine point total. Use this number in determining 10-year risk.
Source: Executive summary of the third report of the National Cholesterol Education Program (NCEP) expert panel on detection, evaluation, and treatment of high blood cholesterol in adults (Adult Treatment Panel III). *JAMA* 2001;285:2497.

heart rate (MPHR = 220 – age) and gradually increase the intensity and duration over several months to a target heart rate of 70–80% of MPHR. A warm-up period and a cool-down period of 5–15 minutes with vigorous activity should be included (see also Cardiac Rehabilitation).

B. Nutrition counseling should recommend a diet that is rich in fruits, vegetables, and dietary fiber. Most patients should have less than 30% of total calories from fat, less than 10% of calories from saturated fat, and less than 300 mg cholesterol/day. Patients with established CAD or other major risk factors should follow the American Heart Association Step II diet, with less than 7% of calories from saturated fat and less than 200 mg cholesterol/day. N-3 polyunsaturated fatty acids (fish oil) have been shown to decrease CV death in secondary prevention by 2% over 3.5 years (see Chap. 3, http://www.americanheart.org, and *Lancet* 1999;354:447).

C. Weight management continues to be a growing problem in the United States. Obtaining a desirable body mass index is important in achieving other goals for prevention, particularly regarding diabetes, hyperlipidemia, and hypertension. Proper diet and exercise are the cornerstones of weight reduction.

D. Stress reduction or management particularly in patients with CAD has been shown to reduce the risk of future cardiac events. Psychological stress has been associated with increased risk for CAD.

VI. Hormone replacement therapy (HRT) in postmenopausal women has been associated with decreased risk of CAD in multiple large observational studies. However, in a large randomized study in women with CAD using estrogen and medroxyprogesterone, there was an increased 1-year risk of MI and CV death with HRT, with no significant difference at 4 years. An increased incidence of thromboembolisms (0.4% annual increased risk) and gallbladder disease was also found in the patients treated with HRT (*JAMA* 1998;280:605). HRT should not be initiated for secondary prevention of CAD. A clear answer regarding the use of HRT for primary prevention of CAD will await the results of ongoing randomized studies. Currently, the decision to initiate HRT should be based more on other potential benefits such as for osteoporosis than on CAD prevention. It is currently recommended that most patients who are already receiving HRT should remain on this regimen (see Chap. 24).

VII. Aspirin [acetylsalicylic acid (ASA)], 81–325 mg/day, should be given to all patients with suspected or proven CAD. No benefit has been found in giving patients higher doses of ASA, and potential side effects, such as GI bleeding, are dose related (*Am Heart J* 1999;137:S9). ASA for primary prevention reduces the incidence of nonfatal MI in men older than 40 years of age, but the overall vascular and total mortality is not significantly different (*BMJ* 1994;308:81, and *N Engl J Med* 1989;321:129). The decision to prescribe ASA for primary prevention should be based on the clinical assessment of CAD risk and potential side effects, using a low dose of ASA once a day or every other day.

VIII. Antioxidants and decreasing homocysteine levels conceptually should decrease cardiac events. However, currently no convincing clinical benefit has been shown in large randomized studies either for treatment with antioxidants, such as vitamin C, vitamin E, or beta-carotene, or treatment of elevated homocysteine. **Beta-carotene** in multiple large randomized studies has not been shown to reduce CAD and may increase overall mortality (*N Engl J Med* 1994;330:1029, and *N Engl J Med* 1996;334:1145 and 1150). The use of **vitamin E**, 400–800 IU qd, except in one smaller study (*Lancet* 1996;347:781), has shown no clinical benefit in large randomized studies (*N Engl J Med* 2000;342:154, and *Lancet* 1999;354:447). Homocysteine is associated with CAD, and levels can be decreased with folic acid and vitamins B_6 or B_{12}, or both. However, currently there are no large studies that demonstrate a decrease in CV events by treating an elevated homocysteine level (>10 µmol/L) (*Circulation* 1999;99:178). A reasonable approach until more definitive studies are available is to encourage a well-balanced diet that is high in fruits and vegetables and, particularly in the elderly, a daily complete multivitamin containing folic acid.

IX. Alcohol in moderate consumption (1–2 drinks qd) in observational studies has been associated with a decreased risk of CV events. Alcohol consumption can raise triglyceride and HDL-C levels. The recommendation to consume alcohol for prevention of CAD with its many other potential complications, including myocardial toxicity at high levels, has not been studied in randomized controlled studies.

Stable Angina

The most common manifestation of atherosclerotic CAD is stable angina (*J Am Coll Cardiol* 1999;33:2092). Other causes of angina include valvular heart disease, hypertrophic cardiomyopathy, coronary spasm, myocardial bridging, arrhythmia, endothelial dysfunction, drugs, hypoxemia, severe hypertension, or anemia. Noncardiac conditions related to esopageal, pulmonary, or chest wall disorders may present with symptoms that mimic angina. When one assesses a patient with chest pain, the goals should be an expedient diagnosis and risk stratification in the patient. The **five most important predictors** of CAD during the initial examination, in order, are angina description, prior MI, sex, age, and number of other major risk factors such as diabetes, smoking, dyslipidemia, and hypertension.

I. **The Canadian Cardiovascular Society Classification** of angina is helpful in risk stratifying and following patients. USA is usually defined as class III or IV angina that starts or progresses within the past 2 months. See Table 6-2 for the prevalence of CAD based on gender, age, and symptoms.

   A. Class I: Angina occurs only with strenuous activity.

   B. Class II: Angina occurs with moderate activity such as walking quickly or climbing stairs, walking uphill, or walking at a normal pace more than two blocks or more than one flight of stairs.

   C. Class III: Angina occurs with mild activity such as climbing one flight of stairs or walking level for one to two blocks.

   D. Class IV: Angina occurs with any physical activity and may be present at rest.

II. **Clinical characteristics** and risk factors help predict the likelihood of CAD as the etiology of chest discomfort.

   A. The history in typical angina is usually described as (1) "pressure," "heavy," or "suffocating" **discomfort or ache (often not "pain") in the substernal region** that may radiate to the neck, jaw, epigastric region, or arms; (2) **usually lasting for minutes** (not seconds and usually not hours); and (3) **provoked by physical or emotional stress and relieved by rest or nitroglycerin**. Atypical angina does not have all three of these characteristics. Sometimes there is only neck, jaw, or arm discomfort without chest discomfort, and frequently exertional dyspnea is an anginal equivalent. Associated symptoms include dyspnea, diaphoresis, and nausea. The patient often has a difficult time describing the discomfort, and it may be difficult to separate from an upper gastrointestinal etiology. **Symptoms that are not suggestive of angina** include pain lasting for days or a few seconds, pain localized with one finger, pain mainly in the umbilical region or lower in the abdomen, pain radiating to the lower extremities, or pain that is exactly or only reproduced with movement of the chest or arms.

   B. The physical examination and ECG may provide further clues, particularly during ongoing angina, but frequently are unremarkable when the patient is seen with chronic stable angina. On auscultation with ongoing chest pain, a new gallop, a new mitral regurgitation murmur, or pulmonary crackles are predictive of CAD. With ongoing chest pain, 50% of patients with CAD have a new ECG abnormality such as ST- or T-wave changes. During the examination, evidence of previous MI, LV dysfunction, peripheral vascular dis-

Table 6-2. Percentage with coronary artery disease based on age, symptoms, and gender

Age (yrs)	Typical angina		Atypical angina		Nonanginal pain	
	Men	Women	Men	Women	Men	Women
30–39	70	26	22	4	5	1
40–49	87	55	46	13	14	3
50–59	92	79	59	32	22	8
60–69	94	91	67	54	28	19

Adapted from *N Engl J Med* 1979;300:1350.

ease, or other CV risk factors may be identified, along with noncardiac etiologies of chest pain such as musculoskeletal or pulmonary disease. A hemoglobin, fasting glucose, and fasting lipid profile should also be ordered at the time of initial examination. A chest radiograph should be obtained in patients with evidence of CHF, valvular disease, or aortic abnormalities.

III. Stress testing to establish the diagnosis is recommended for patients with an intermediate suspicion of CAD and further allows for risk stratification in all patients with CAD (*J Am Coll Cardiol* 1997;30:260).

   A. Exercise ECG stress testing has an average sensitivity of 70% and a specificity of 75%. In studies without work-up bias, which more likely reflects a population seen by primary care physicians, the sensitivity and specificity are 50% and 90%, respectively. Exercise stress tests should be performed to confirm the diagnosis of CAD in patients with an intermediate (15–85%) probability of CAD and also allow for risk stratification. In patients with a very low or high probability of CAD, the sensitivity and specificity are sufficiently low that the predictive value is poor. Therefore, in patients with a very low likelihood of CAD, the positive predictive value is decreased, resulting in more false positives than true positives. Very high-likelihood patients will have a low negative predictive value. For the diagnosis of CAD, beta-blockers are typically held for several half-lives before an exercise stress test to increase the sensitivity. Patients with ECG evidence of pre-excitation (Wolff-Parkinson-White), LV hypertrophy, left bundle branch block, digoxin effects, paced ventricular rhythm, or resting ST-segment and T-wave changes should also have an imaging study because the ECG has significantly decreased accuracy in this setting. Exercise stress testing has been proven to predict future risk of complications from CAD and should be considered for risk stratification in all patients with suspected CAD, including those with a high likelihood of CAD. A stress test should not be terminated just because the patient reaches the target heart rate, because important prognostic information will not be obtained.

   1. A positive exercise test is based on greater than –1 mm (0.1 mV) of new ST-segment deviation 60–80 msec from the J point compared to the PR segment in three consecutive beats. Horizontal or downsloping ST depression does not localize the area of ischemia but is the most common change with a positive stress test. ST elevation in a lead without a Q wave localizes the area of ischemia and is suggestive of high-grade stenosis or spasm. An upsloping ST segment that has 1 mm ST depression or greater 60–80 msec from the J point should be considered nondiagnostic, as should a "negative" submaximal stress test (<85% of

MPHR). Patients with a nondiagnostic stress test should be considered for an imaging stress test.

2. **Risk stratification** on an exercise treadmill test is related to the workload, symptoms, and degree of ischemia (associated with degree of ST depression) and is important in patients with suspected CAD. LV function also is an important factor in further risk stratification. The Duke treadmill score is one of many formulas that are used to help predict future CV events. The score is equal to exercise time in minutes on the Bruce protocol – (5 × ST deviation in mm) – [4 × exercise angina score (0 for no angina, 1 for angina with the test, and 2 for angina that causes the patient to stop exercising)] (*N Engl J Med* 1991;325:849).

   a. **High-risk** patients have an exercise score of –11 or less and have at least a 5% annual mortality from CAD. Other markers of high risk include evidence of ischemia at less than 4 metabolic equivalents (METs) or stage I of the Bruce protocol, new ST depression greater than 2 mm, or new ST elevation greater than 1 mm; decrease in systolic pressure by 10 mm Hg from baseline; ST changes greater than 1 mm that persist greater than 5 minutes into recovery, or sustained ventricular tachycardia. High-risk patients should be referred for angiography.

   b. **Intermediate-risk** patients (Duke score –10 to 4) have a 1.25% annual mortality from CAD. In this population further risk stratification should be performed either with angiography or with an imaging stress test that allows assessment of LV function and area of myocardium at risk.

   c. **Low-risk** patients have a score of 5 or more and have an annual CV mortality of 0.25% in stable angina. An ability to exercise for greater than 10 METs indicates low risk.

B. **Imaging studies** with echocardiography or radionuclide perfusion imaging are indicated when the ECG would have decreased accuracy (see sec. **A**) or when a pharmacologic stress test is performed because the patient is unable to exercise. **High-risk characteristics** include severe LV dysfunction [ejection fraction (EF) <35%], large or multiple areas of ischemia particularly involving the anterior wall, LV dilation or a decrease in EF with stress, or thallium uptake in the lungs with stress. Intermediate risk characteristics include mild to moderate LV dysfunction or one moderate-sized (two segments with echocardiography) area of ischemia not including the anterior wall. Exercise echocardiography has a sensitivity of 85% and a specificity of 77%, whereas exercise radionuclide single photon emission computed tomography has a similar sensitivity of 87% but a decreased specificity of 64% (*JAMA* 1998;280:913). Generally, in patients with a lower suspicion of CAD, stress echocardiography is preferred because of the better specificity. However, the most important aspect of **deciding which imaging study to use depends greatly on the expertise at the individual institution**.

   1. **Echocardiography** should be used in all patients with suspected valvular disease. Accuracy is marginally increased compared with nuclear perfusion in women and in patients with left bundle branch block. Stress echocardiography can be very useful in evaluating patients with unexplained dyspnea on exertion because it can evaluate for ischemia, valvular disease, LV function, and diastolic function and estimate pulmonary artery pressures in most patients. Stress echocardiography costs less than nuclear perfusion studies.

   2. **Nuclear perfusion** with thallium or technetium allows for assessment of regional LV function with the advent of single photon emission computed tomographic imaging. These tests have better prognostic value and have been studied longer than stress echocardiography. A normal test has less than 1% per year risk of MI or death. Patients with a positive ECG portion but a normal imaging study still have an excellent

prognosis. The rate of false-positive nuclear perfusion tests is increased in the first 2 months after angioplasty.

IV. **Angiography** can be used for diagnosis and risk stratification and determines the suitability for revascularization either percutaneously or surgically. Angiography should be considered in patients with class III or IV angina despite medical treatment, high-risk criteria on stress testing, clinical evidence of CHF, moderate LV dysfunction with intermediate-risk criteria, or indeterminate diagnostic or prognostic information with stress testing (*J Am Coll Cardiol* 1999;331:756). The mortality of diagnostic angiography is 0.11% with a morbidity of 1–2% mainly consisting of vascular complications.

V. **Hospitalization** is initially prudent in patients with a significant suspicion of CAD with greater than 20 minutes of rest pain, associated CHF, ST- or T-wave changes, or USA in patients over 65 years of age or starting in the preceding 2 weeks.

VI. **Treatment** is aimed at reducing symptoms and preventing MI and death.

A. **Pharmacologic treatment** is important for all patients with angina. The usual initial drug regimen consists of aspirin, a beta-blocker, and immediate-release nitroglycerin prn. Calcium channel blockers (CCBs) or long-acting nitrates, or both, are often added, depending on whether the angina symptoms are not controlled with beta-blockers or because of contraindications to beta-blockers.

1. **Aspirin**, 81–325 mg PO qd, decreases the risk of MI and death by one-third and is standard therapy. Clopidogrel, 75 mg PO qd, should be used if aspirin is contraindicated (*Lancet* 1996;348:1329).

2. **Beta-blockers**, by decreasing myocardial oxygen demand, decrease angina episodes and decrease CV complications in patients with stable angina. These agents have negative inotropic and chronotropic effects, decrease BP, and decrease myocardial oxygen consumption with activity. A reasonable goal for the resting heart rate is between 55 and 60 beats/minute. Absolute contraindications for beta-blockers include severe bradycardia and high-degree atrioventricular block. In patients with relative contraindications, such as peripheral vascular disease, bronchospastic disease, insulin-dependent diabetes mellitus, or CHF, a trial with β_1-selective agents starting at a low dose should be attempted, particularly if they have a previous MI history (Table 6-3).

a. **Classification** of beta-blockers depends on their selectivity for cardiac β_1-receptors, hydrophilic or lipophilic properties, and whether they possess intrinsic sympathomimetic activity (ISA). No difference is found in antianginal effects between the different groups of beta-blockers except that agents with ISA are less efficacious in patients with rest angina or class III–IV angina. β_1-selective agents at low doses may decrease side effects in patients with reactive airway disease, peripheral vascular disease, or diabetes. Hydrophilic beta-blockers have less central nervous system penetration, may have decreased central nervous system side effects compared to lipophilic agents, and are usually excreted by the kidneys. Agents with ISA result in less bradycardia and would be selected in patients with pre-existing bradycardia with exertional angina (Table 6-3).

b. **Side effects** include bronchospasm, claudication, depression, insomnia, fatigue, impaired intellectual capacity, impotence, nightmares, decreased libido, and masking of symptoms of hypoglycemia. In patients with mild or moderate CHF (New York Heart Association class I–III), the initial dose should be low and slowly increased, observing for worsening CHF symptoms. Beta-blockers should not be discontinued for asymptomatic resting bradycardia. Abrupt discontinuation of beta-blockers should be avoided to prevent rebound, which may worsen CAD signs and symptoms.

3. **CCBs** should be initiated when beta-blockers are contraindicated or in combination with beta-blockers if treatment with beta-blockers alone

Table 6-3. Common medicines in angina

Medication	Total daily dose	Frequency
Beta-blockers		
Atenolol[a,b]	25–200 mg	qd
Propranolol[c]	40–640 mg	bid–tid[d]
Metoprolol[a,c]	50–400 mg	bid[d]
Bisoprolol[a]	2.5–20.0 mg	qd
Nadolol[b]	20–320 mg	qd
Timolol	20–60 mg	bid
Betaxolol[a]	10–20 mg	qd
Acebutolol[a,e]	200–1200 mg	qd–bid
Pindolol[e]	10–60 mg	bid
Labetalol[f]	200–2400 mg	bid
Carvedilol[f]	6.25–50.0 mg	bid
Calcium channel blockers		
Diltiazem	120–480 mg	qid[d]
Verapamil	120–480 mg	tid[d]
Dihydropyridines		
Amlodipine	2.5–10.0 mg	qd
Felodipine	2.5–20.0 mg	qd
Isradipine	5–20 mg	bid[d]
Nicardipine	60–120 mg	tid[d,h]
Nifedipine (XL or CC)	30–120 mg	qd[d,h]
Nisoldipine	10–60 mg	qd
Nitrates		
2% nitroglycerin ointment	0.5–2.0 in. tid	tid[g]
Transdermal patch	0.1–0.8 mg/hr for 12 hrs	qd[g]
Nitroglycerin sustained release	5–18 mg	bid[g]
Isosorbide dinitrate	30–120 mg	tid[d,g]
Isosorbide mononitrate	30–240 mg	qd[g]
Sublingual nitroglycerin	0.3, 0.4, 0.6 mg	prn q5min
Aerosol nitroglycerin	0.4 mg	prn q5min

[a]β_1 selective.
[b]Hydrophilic, mostly excreted by kidneys and decreased CNS penetration.
[c]Lipophilic, mostly metabolized by liver and increased CNS penetration.
[d]Long-acting forms available usually qd.
[e]Intrinsic sympathomimetic activity.
[f]Combination α and β antagonist.
[g]8- to 12-hr nitrate-free period should be provided to avoid tolerance.
[h]Short-acting form contraindicated in coronary artery disease.

does not control symptoms. CCBs are as effective as beta-blockers in decreasing angina symptoms and have an important role in coronary vasospasm. The mechanism of action is by coronary artery and peripheral artery vasodilatation, resulting in decreased afterload and increased coronary flow. The negative inotropic and chronotropic effects, which vary with specific agents, further decrease myocardial oxygen consumption. In patients with moderate or severe LV dysfunction or bradycardia, amlodipine or felodipine should be used instead of verapamil or diltiazem. **Short-acting dihydropyridines (e.g., nifedipine tid) are contraindicated in patients with CAD** (Table 6-3).

   a. **Classification** is usually broken into dihydropyridines, verapamil (a papaverine derivative), and diltiazem (a benzothiazepine). The dihydropyridines include the second-generation CCB-like amlodipine, felodipine, isradipine, and nicardipine. Amlodipine and felodipine have been shown to be safe in patients with LV dysfunction (*Circulation* 1997;96:856, and *N Engl J Med* 1996;335:1107). All the dihydropyridines cause marked arteriolar vasodilatation and minimal negative inotropic and chronotropic effects in the clinical setting. Verapamil and diltiazem have negative chronotropic and inotropic effects. The negative chronotropic effects may be particularly useful in patients who are unable to take beta-blockers or who have atrial arrhythmias.

   b. **Side effects** from all CCBs include peripheral edema, constipation, headaches, and flushing. Nifedipine can cause reflex tachycardia. Verapamil or diltiazem can worsen conduction abnormalities or CHF, and this is additive to the effects of beta-blockers.

4. **Nitroglycerin** mainly reduces preload by venodilation but also vasodilates large epicardial coronary arteries independent of endothelial function. Patients should be warned about headaches, hypotension, and the contraindication of taking sildenafil while on nitroglycerin. Sildenafil should not be prescribed to patients who use nitrates in any form, as it can cause severe hypotension even 24 hours after the last dose (see Chap. 25) (*J Am Coll Cardiol* 1999;33:273). Headaches are not unusual with the initiation of nitrates but usually resolve in several days, and acetaminophen is usually effective for relief of this side effect. Other side effects include hypotension, flushing, and reflex tachycardia.

   a. **Immediate-release** sublingual nitroglycerin (SLNTG) tablets (0.3–0.6 mg) or spray (0.4 mg) is useful for immediate relief of angina symptoms and should be prescribed for all patients with angina along with an explanation of proper use. When angina starts, the patient should immediately sit down and rest. If the patient still has chest discomfort after several minutes, he or she should take one SLNTG and repeat this every 5 minutes until the symptoms disappear or a total of three SLNTG have been administered. If the chest pain is still present after three SLNTG, the patient should be taken by ambulance immediately to the emergency room. If a patient has increasing requirement of SLNTG, he or she should be reassessed (see Acute Coronary Syndromes and Indications for Hospitalization), and possibly other long-acting antianginal regimens should be increased. Patients can take nitroglycerin prophylactically if they are involved in an activity that is known to cause angina. The peak effect occurs in the first 2 minutes and continues for approximately 30 minutes. The patient may initially experience tingling under the tongue with SLNTG. The tablets should be replaced every 6 months and must be stored in the original bottle.

   b. **Long-acting** nitrates with an appropriate nitrate-free period of 8–12 hours are indicated for reducing symptoms when beta-blockers with or without CCBs are ineffective in controlling symptoms. These are usually prescribed in an oral or transdermal form. The transdermal forms have variable absorption and generally are less effective than the oral forms (Table 6-3).

B. **Predisposing medical problems**, which can provoke angina and require treatment, include severe anemia, thyrotoxicosis, arrhythmias, marked hypertension, and severe valvular disease.

C. Risk modification can greatly decrease cardiac events (**see Prevention**). Lipid-lowering therapy, particularly with statins, has been effective in decreasing the risk of MI or death by one-third and along with diet should be initiated in all patients with elevated LDL-C (see Chap. 5). Smoking cessation is important to decreasing the risk of future CV events. ACE inhibitors also decrease the risk of secondary ischemic events and are appropriate in addition to the standard antianginal regimen if BP permits (*N Engl J Med* 2000;342:145).

D. Revascularization is indicated to improve survival or in patients with persistent symptoms despite maximal medical treatment. Improved survival is conferred by revascularization of (1) significant (>50%) left main disease or (2) an EF of less than 50% with significant (>70%) three-vessel disease or two-vessel disease that involves the proximal left anterior descending (LAD) coronary artery. Patients with chronic stable angina with high-risk factors on stress testing or continued class III or IV angina despite medical therapy should also be evaluated for revascularization. Other situations in which revascularization is generally considered warranted include proximal LAD stenosis, a moderate to large area of hibernating myocardium or ischemia, or sustained ventricular tachycardia or sudden cardiac death. Overall, there has been no significant mortality difference between angioplasty and coronary artery bypass grafting (CABG) in nondiabetics (*J Am Coll Cardiol* 2000;35:1116 and 1123), but certain clinical situations favor CABG over angioplasty, and certain lesions may not be amenable to revascularization by angioplasty or CABG, or both. Consultation with a cardiologist is appropriate when considering revascularization. In asymptomatic patients after revascularization, there is no indication for routine follow-up stress tests or angiography. A stress imaging test may be useful at 3–6 months after angioplasty to screen for clinically silent restenosis in patients with high-risk characteristics such as LV dysfunction, diabetes, multivessel disease, proximal LAD disease, or suboptimal revascularization results. Risk modification, particularly smoking cessation, lifestyle changes, and treating hyperlipidemia, is critical because **revascularization is not a cure for the underlying disease process**.

   1. **CABG** is the preferred method for revascularization for left main disease, left main equivalent (proximal LAD and circumflex), or three-vessel disease with moderate LV dysfunction. Diabetics and high-risk patients (CHF or proximal LAD disease) with multivessel disease also benefit from this type of revascularization compared with angioplasty (*J Am Coll Cardiol* 1999;34:1261). An important aspect of improved survival with CABG is a mammary artery bypass to the LAD with a 10-year patency rate of 90% compared to a 50% patency rate of saphenous vein grafts at 10 years.

   2. **Percutaneous coronary intervention (PCI)** using angioplasty with or without stent deployment has become widely prevalent. PCI is usually favored over CABG for patients with approachable lesions with class III–IV angina with one-vessel disease that does not involve the proximal LAD. Typical antithrombotic therapy after stent placement is usually indefinite ASA and a several-week course of clopidogrel, 75 mg PO qd, or ticlopidine, 250 mg PO bid. In the first 6 months after PCI, there is a 10–40% clinical risk of restenosis at the site of intervention, which is usually heralded by recurrent angina. This generally occurs progressively and rarely results in abrupt vessel closure. The risk of restenosis is increased in patients with diabetes or end-stage renal disease or in those who smoke, and possibly in patients with USA or proximal LAD revascularization. Routine angioplasty for CAD with class I or II stable angina is not indicated. Angioplasty in a low-risk population is associated with initial improvement in symptoms and exercise performance but has a small but significantly increased incidence of MI or death in the intervention group compared with standard medical treatment (*Lancet* 1997;350:461). Medical treatment including aggressive lipid-lowering treatment (atorvasta-

tin, 80 mg qd) resulted in a decreased time to an ischemic event compared with angioplasty in a low-risk population (*N Engl J Med* 1999;341:70). In high-risk patients (see Stable Angina, sec. **III**), however, there was improved mortality and symptoms in the revascularization group as opposed to medical treatment alone (*Circulation* 1997;95:2037). Nuclear perfusion studies have an increased false-positive rate in the revascularized territory during the first 2 months after PCI.

   E. **Long-term treatment goals** are secondary prevention with risk factor modification (see Prevention) and reduction of symptoms to class I angina. If there is change in the patient's stable angina pattern, predisposing factors should be sought out and the antianginal regimen increased, and the patient should be reassessed with angiography or stress testing (see Stable Angina, sec. **III**).

VII. **Unusual causes of angina in adults.** CAD is usually manifested as atherosclerosis, but other unusual diseases of the coronary arteries may result in ischemia. These causes include vasospasm; congenital coronary artery anomalies; myocardial bridges; coronary artery aneurysm, fistulas, emboli, or dissection; or trauma.

   A. **Vasospastic, variant, or Prinzmetal's angina is uncommon.** It is caused by endothelial dysfunction resulting in coronary artery spasm usually at a site of atherosclerosis but can occur in angiographically normal-appearing coronary arteries. Characteristically, the chest pain is associated with ST-segment elevation on the ECG.

   1. **Diagnosis** is made by the characteristic symptoms with associated ST-segment elevation at the time of chest discomfort. Patients with this manifestation of CAD frequently have angina symptoms at rest, at night, or early in the morning and are often smokers. An ECG at the time of angina usually reveals ST-segment elevation, but generally a longer recording device such as a 24-hour ambulatory electrocardiographic monitor is required to capture an episode. Pharmacologically induced coronary spasm at the time of angiography with agents such as ergonovine or acetylcholine is sometimes required to make the diagnosis correctly.

   2. **Treatment** goals should be aimed at preventing spasm and improving endothelial function. CCBs and nitrates in combination are usually effective at preventing spasm. Sometimes a dihydropyridine CCB and verapamil or diltiazem can be used in combination. Patients should also be prescribed ASA, 81 mg/day. Endothelial function should be improved by secondary prevention. Smoking cessation and treatment of hyperlipidemia are critical. ACE inhibitors also may play a role in improving endothelial dysfunction and decreasing spasm (*Circulation* 1996;94:258). Beta-blockers should be avoided in patients with vasospasm and hemodynamically insignificant CAD. Revascularization should be considered in patients with significant CAD. The long-term prognosis of vasospastic angina is related to the extent of underlying CAD.

   B. **Myocardial bridging** or tunneling of the coronary artery into the myocardium usually involves the LAD and angiographically is seen in approximately 5% of the population. However, this **is usually a clinically benign condition** and rarely causes angina or MI. In the symptomatic patient, treatment with a beta-blocker is usually effective by increasing diastolic coronary flow. Nitrates may worsen the condition. In refractory patients with proven hemodynamically significant systolic compression, stenting or surgical myotomy can be considered.

   C. **Cocaine** can cause tachycardia, hypertension, vasoconstriction, and coronary artery thrombosis that can lead to angina or MI. Risk of atherosclerosis may also be increased. Patients with ongoing chest pain should be directed immediately to the emergency room for evaluation and frequently have repolarization abnormalities on the ECG that may be confused with ischemia. However, the majority of patients with chest pain after cocaine use do not have enzymatic evidence of MI (*Ann Intern Med* 1991;115:282). Beta-blockers alone should be avoided in patients with cocaine exposure because of the risk of worsening spasm and unopposed α-adrenergic activation. A key goal is cessation of cocaine use. In patients with suspected CAD or coronary spasm and a high likelihood of future cocaine abuse, ASA should be used along with nitrates, CCBs, and/or labetalol.

VIII. Silent ischemia
   A. Silent or asymptomatic ischemia is evidence of ischemia without symptoms of angina or an angina equivalent. It is usually detected during exercise stress testing or ambulatory ECG monitoring with ST-segment depression. Patients who have silent ischemia at low levels of exertion, similar to patients who have angina symptoms at low levels of exertion, are at increased risk of complications of CAD. Currently, there is a much larger body of evidence using stress testing for predicting CAD complications, and the additional use of ambulatory electrocardiographic monitoring to detect silent ischemia is generally not warranted.
   B. Treatment for silent ischemia is similar to that of symptomatic angina. Patients with evidence of ischemia at low levels of activity despite medical treatment (like class III–IV angina) should be considered for revascularization. A pilot study in high-risk patients with angina detected on stress tests and silent ischemia on a 48-hour ambulatory ECG suggests an improved mortality in patients who receive revascularization (*Circulation* 1997;95:2037).

Acute Coronary Syndromes and Indications for Hospitalization

Acute coronary syndromes usually result from thrombus formation on a ruptured or ulcerated plaque and manifest as USA or MI with or without ST elevation (historically Q-wave or non–Q-wave MI). Typically, the thrombus with ST-elevation MI is fibrin rich, whereas the thrombus in USA or non-ST elevation MI is a platelet-rich plaque. USA and non–ST-elevation MI do not respond to thrombolytics, and the treatment strategies in the hospital are usually similar (*Circulation* 1998;97:1195).
   I. USA is defined as chest pain at rest for greater than 20 minutes or new class III or IV angina that has progressed or started within the past 2 months (*J Am Coll Cardiol* 2000;36:970).
   A. Initial risk stratification is based on patient characteristics, the frequency and severity of angina, evidence of CHF or ischemic mitral regurgitation, and ischemic ECG changes such as ST-segment depression or elevation or T-wave inversions, or both. Patients who call the office with ongoing prolonged (usually greater than 20 minutes) chest discomfort that is consistent with ischemia should be directed immediately to the emergency room by ambulance for evaluation. Patients who are not having ongoing chest pain and do not have intermediate- or high-risk characteristics can be initially evaluated in the office in an expedient fashion.
      1. Hospitalization is initially prudent in patients with a moderate to high suspicion of CAD with any of the following: (1) greater than 20 minutes of rest pain, (2) nocturnal angina, (3) CHF, (4) ST- or T-wave changes, (5) known atherosclerosis, (6) an elevated troponin, or (7) USA either in patients who are 65 years of age or older or starting in the last 2 weeks (*J Am Coll Cardiol* 2000;36:970). Patients who are admitted to the hospital are usually treated with ASA, therapeutic heparin (unfractionated or low-molecular-weight heparin), beta-blockers, nitrates, and possible use of a IIB/IIIA antagonist (*J Am Coll Cardiol* 2000;35:1699). Stabilized

patients should undergo a stress test for risk stratification and diagnosis. **Angiography** is usually indicated instead of a stress test in patients with persistent (>1 hour despite aggressive medical therapy) or recurrent angina, prior revascularization, associated CHF, LV dysfunction, more than 1 mm ST depression at rest with angina, or malignant ventricular arrhythmias. **Angiography** is also indicated after a high-risk stress test and in the majority of patients at experienced centers with an elevated troponin I or T (*Lancet* 1999;354:708, and *N Engl J Med* 2001;344:1879).

2. **Outpatient evaluation** is reasonable in patients who do not have any of the above indications for hospitalization, with low suspicion of CAD, and no prolonged rest pain in the preceding 2 weeks. If there are no contraindications, patients should be instructed to take an aspirin immediately. Patients who are deemed low risk do not require immediate hospitalization but should have further CV evaluation in the following 72 hours if not done initially. Treatment strategies in this population are similar to those of stable angina.

   a. **Stress testing** for diagnosis and risk stratification is indicated in the majority of patients. In patients with a very low suspicion of CAD and low risk, empiric treatment or further testing of suspected noncardiac etiologies may be initially warranted because of the high rate of false-positive stress tests in this population. Risk stratification is similar to stable angina (see Stable Angina).

   b. **Treatment** is similar to that of stable angina, with use of ASA, betablockers, immediate-release nitrates, and potentially long-acting nitrates or CCBs (see Stable Angina).

   c. **Angiography** is typically indicated in patients who have continued symptoms despite medical treatment, high-risk criteria on stress testing, recurrent USA, exclusion or diagnosis of CAD in patients with multiple episodes of chest pain without documentation of ischemia, or a prior revascularization procedure.

B. **Follow-up** in patients who return after their initial evaluation should include an assessment for any change in intensity or frequency of symptoms. If a change is noted, possible exacerbating factors should be screened for, such as anemia, noncompliance, changes in lifestyle, concurrent illnesses, hyperthyroidism, illicit drug use, or arrhythmias. Patients with class II or greater angina should have their antianginal regimen increased. In all patients risk modification is critical and should be reviewed periodically (see Prevention). If there is no change in the patient's clinical status, routine follow-up stress testing is not indicated in all patients. A stress imaging test may be useful at 3–6 months after angioplasty to screen for clinically silent restenosis in patients with high-risk characteristics such as LV dysfunction, diabetes, multivessel disease, proximal LAD disease, or suboptimal revascularization results.

II. **Acute MI** requires immediate hospitalization with a goal of opening the closed artery as soon as possible. Up to one-fourth of MIs may not be recognized at the time of infarction. Patients who have had evidence of an MI several weeks to months previously and have not had any recent chest pain or significant CHF do not require hospitalization but should have a stress test and assessment of LV function (see Post–Myocardial Infarction Care).

Post–Myocardial Infarction Care

I. **Risk stratification** should initially be performed in the hospital before discharge (*Ann Intern Med* 1997;126:556 and 561). Assessment of LV function should be obtained in all MI patients. Patients with uncomplicated MIs and

Table 6-4. Contraindications to exercise testing

Relative contraindications	Absolute contraindications
Moderate valvular stenosis	MI in past 48 hrs
SBP >200 mm Hg or DBP >110 mm Hg	Unstable angina, not stabilized
Electrolyte abnormalities	Symptomatic severe aortic stenosis
Hypertrophic cardiomyopathy	Uncontrolled CHF
Left main CAD	Uncontrolled arrhythmias
Significant arrhythmias or AV block	Acute pulmonary embolism
Disabling mental or physical impairment	Acute aortic dissection
	Acute myocarditis or pericarditis

AV, atrioventricular; CAD, coronary artery disease; DBP, diastolic BP; MI, myocardial infarction; SBP, systolic BP.
Source: Modified from *J Am Coll Cardiol* 1997;30:260.

without LV dysfunction (EF <40%) should undergo a stress test. If LV function has not been assessed, it is usually practical to obtain a stress imaging test that also evaluates LV function, increases the sensitivity and specificity of the stress test, and quantifies the degree and territory of ischemia. Patients who have high-risk predictors on the stress test, are clinically unstable, or have LV dysfunction (EF <40%) should undergo angiography before hospital discharge. Stress testing is not routinely required after angioplasty except to determine the clinical significance of an intermediate lesion that has not received intervention.

A. **Stress testing** can be done 4 days after an MI (Table 6-4). Traditionally, a submaximal (<70% of MPHR or 5 METs) exercise test was done during the first week after an MI and a symptom-limited stress test was performed at least 10 days after an MI. Evidence is growing that stable ambulating patients without angina can undergo a symptom-limited stress test safely 4–7 days after an MI (*J Am Coll Cardiol* 2000;35:1212). A stress test, preferably symptom limited, should be performed before discharge in patients who have not had angiography. If a patient has a submaximal stress test in the hospital, a follow-up symptom-limited stress test should be performed 3–6 weeks after the MI (*Circulation* 1997;96:345). Patients who are unable to exercise should have pharmacologic stress tests in the first week after an MI. Stress tests that use vasodilators such as dipyridamole or adenosine can be performed after the first 48–72 hours, and dobutamine stress echocardiography can be used starting 72–96 hours after an MI.

B. **LV function** is the most important prognostic indicator of survival after MI and should be assessed in all patients. This can be done using clinical characteristics, echocardiography, angiography, or radionuclide ventriculography. Patients with a normal EF have a 1-year mortality of less than 5%, whereas patients with severe LV dysfunction (EF <30%) have a 10-fold increase in mortality (*Arch Intern Med* 1997;157:273).

C. **Arrhythmia screening** is currently not indicated after hospital discharge in asymptomatic patients. Patients who have nonsustained ventricular tachycardia and an EF of less than 40% should be evaluated for possible use of an implantable cardiac defibrillator. If an antiarrhythmic agent is indicated after an MI, amiodarone or dofetilide has been shown to be safe in this setting (see Chap. 8).

II. **Pharmacologic therapy** can greatly improve the quality and quantity of life. The following medicines should strongly be considered in every patient after an

MI: ASA, beta-blocker, ACE inhibitor, lipid-lowering therapy, and immediate-release nitrates. Anticoagulation, long-acting nitrates, or CCBs are indicated in some patients.

A. Aspirin (81–325 mg) is standard of care. In patients who cannot take ASA, clopidogrel, 75 mg PO qd, is an effective substitute and, compared to ASA, resulted in a small reduction in atherosclerotic events (*Lancet* 1996;348:1329).

B. Beta-blockers should be considered in all patients and decrease mortality by up to 40%. Because of beta-blockers' significant benefits, they should be tried even in patients with relative contraindications by starting at low doses of β_1-selective beta-blockers.

C. ACE inhibitors can greatly improve the quality and quantity of life. The benefit obtained from ACE inhibitors increases as the LV function decreases. However, even patients with normal LV function benefit from these agents, with a significant decreased risk for MI, death, and stroke (see Chap. 7 and *N Engl J Med* 2000;342:145).

D. Lipid-lowering therapy, particularly with statins, should be considered in every patient. If a patient has an LDL-C of greater than 125 mg/dl, it is reasonable to start a statin along with lifestyle changes, with an LDL-C goal of less than 100 mg/dl (*J Am Coll Cardiol* 1999;33:125). Lifestyle changes should be initiated first for patients with a low HDL-C (<40 mg/dl) or high triglycerides (>150 mg/dl). Drug therapy can be considered in patients who do not reach their goal with lifestyle changes. Patients who did not have a fasting lipid profile collected on the first day of hospitalization and have a normal cholesterol should have a repeat lipid profile 8–12 weeks after discharge because the lipid level declines rapidly in hospitalized patients (see Chap. 5).

E. Immediate-release nitrates should be prescribed for every patient for symptom relief, as needed (see Stable Angina).

F. Warfarin therapy with an international normalized ratio goal of 2–3 should be considered in patients with atrial fibrillation, LV thrombus, LV aneurysm, or a large akinetic region, particularly associated with anterior MI. In patients with an akinetic region or LV thrombus, unless otherwise indicated, anticoagulation can be discontinued 3–6 months after the MI.

G. Long-acting nitrates are useful in patients who continue to have angina despite treatment with a beta-blocker (see Stable Angina, sec. **VI.A.4.b**).

H. CCBs are second-line agents. They should be reserved for people who are unable to take a beta-blocker or when beta-blockers and ACE inhibitors are inadequate to control hypertension or angina. Diltiazem or verapamil should not be used in patients with an EF of less than 40% or CHF.

III. Physical activity and limitations should be discussed, and an inpatient cardiac rehabilitation program should be initiated before discharge. Patients can start walking for 5–10 minutes at a time at home. Outpatient cardiac rehabilitation should be prescribed for everyone. **Sexual activity** usually can be resumed a week after an MI. Each state has its own regulations, but generally **driving** can be initiated in the first week after an uncomplicated MI. In the stable patient without complications, **commercial air travel** is reasonable, with the caveat that in the first 2 weeks the patient has a companion and uses ground transportation to limit strenuous activity in the terminal. It is important that the patient has immediate-release nitroglycerin available during all these activities.

IV. Return to work in most asymptomatic patients can occur 2 weeks after an MI but must be individualized. Patients whose job requires a high physical demand should wait until a symptom-limited stress test is performed to make sure that there is no ischemia at the level of their work activity.

V. Secondary prevention is a continuous process and should focus on modifying lifestyle habits, including smoking, exercise, and diet, while treating hyperlipidemia, hypertension, and diabetes (see Prevention). The utility of treating potentially inflammatory biologic agents, such as *Chlamydia pneu-*

moniae, Helicobacter pylori, cytomegalovirus, or herpesvirus, is currently being investigated.

Cardiac Rehabilitation

Cardiac rehabilitation should be considered in all patients after an acute coronary syndrome or revascularization procedure and in patients with stable angina (*Circulation* 1994;90:1602). A cardiac rehabilitation program is not simply an aerobic exercise program but a structured program that incorporates lifestyle modification, which should be reinforced lifelong at every follow-up visit. Cardiac rehabilitation reduces mortality by one-fourth and is safe. Furthermore, it results in decreased cigarette use while improving symptoms (e.g., effort angina), exercise tolerance, plasma lipids, and psychosocial well-being (AHCPR Publication No. 96-00672 clinical guideline No. 17, 1997; http://www.ahcpr.gov/clinic/cpgonline.htm).

I. **An exercise test** is needed to develop an exercise prescription. A common initial exercise prescription is a constant work level (e.g., walking, cycling, etc.) for 10–30 minutes, which attains 50–60% of the maximal work load or MPHR achieved during the stress test (MPHR = 220 – age). The duration of the exercise is increased by 5 minutes every week up to 30–60 minutes. The minimum recommended frequency is three times a week. Later, in selected patients who are clinically stable, the exercise intensity can be increased, with a goal of 70–85% of the maximal workload or MPHR achieved during the stress test. Generally, patients should not engage in high-intensity endurance exercise without supervision. After 6 months or a year, another stress test can be performed to reassess the patient's status and modify the exercise program. The exercise prescription should include a warm-up and cool-down period of 5–15 minutes.

II. **Home exercise programs** should be considered in low-risk patients who will not or cannot participate in a formal cardiac rehabilitation program. Patients should still undergo a treadmill stress test to determine risk and the exercise prescription. Low-risk characteristics include class I–II angina, exercise capacity over 6 METs without evidence of ischemia by 6 METs, no evidence of CHF, no sequential premature ventricular contractions, and an appropriate rise in BP with exercise (*Circulation* 1990;82:2286). The initial exercise prescription is similar to a supervised regimen with a warm-up and cool-down period and an initial workload of 50–60% of that achieved with the stress test for 5–10 minutes. The duration should be increased every week until a minimum of 30 minutes is achieved with each session. The intensity can then be gradually increased every few weeks to a goal of 70% of the maximal workload or MPHR attained on the exercise stress test. A less strenuous program of walking at a slow or regular pace starting at 5–10 minutes and progressing over weeks to 30–60 minutes can also be prescribed as an outpatient regimen and can be initiated immediately after discharge from the hospital.

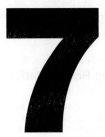

Cardiovascular II: Heart Failure, Cardiomyopathy, and Valvular Heart Disease

Michael W. Rich

Heart Failure

I. Introduction

A. Definition. Heart failure (HF) is a condition in which an abnormality in cardiac function leads to an inability of the heart to provide sufficient cardiac output to meet the metabolic needs of the body while maintaining normal intracardiac pressures.

B. Epidemiology. Despite recent declines in age-adjusted mortality from coronary heart disease and stroke, the population prevalence of HF has been increasing for more than 2 decades, primarily due to the aging of the population. HF affects approximately 5 million Americans, and 550,000 new cases are diagnosed each year. HF is the most costly cardiovascular illness in the United States, with annual expenditures in excess of $20 billion, and it is the leading indication for hospitalization in persons over 65 years of age. HF also accounts for up to 12 million physician office visits each year, ranking second only to hypertension among cardiovascular indications for outpatient physician contacts. HF is a highly lethal condition, with 5-year survival rates of less than 50% in men and in women. HF is listed as the primary cause of death in more than 45,000 cases each year and as a contributory cause in an additional 238,000 cases. Nearly 80% of HF hospitalizations and more than 85% of HF deaths occur in individuals over 65 years of age.

C. Pathophysiology. HF occurs when reduced cardiac output results in tissue hypoperfusion and inadequate oxygen delivery or when elevated cardiac filling pressures lead to pulmonary and systemic venous congestion. Compensatory mechanisms for augmenting cardiac output, restoring tissue perfusion, and normalizing filling pressures include (1) an increase in heart rate, (2) ventricular dilatation and hypertrophy, and (3) activation of multiple neuroendocrine pathways, including the adrenergic nervous system, renin-angiotensin system, and vasopressin system. Although these mechanisms are often effective in acutely stabilizing hemodynamics, chronic activation is deleterious and contributes to the progressive decline in cardiac function that is observed in persons with chronic HF. Classically, HF has been viewed primarily as a disorder of contractile function. More recently, the syndrome of HF with preserved left ventricular (LV) systolic function (i.e., normal LV ejection fraction) has become increasingly recognized. This disorder accounts for 30–50% of all HF cases, with the majority occurring in individuals over 65 years of age (*Arch Intern Med* 1996;156:146). HF with normal LV systolic function is often attributable to abnormal diastolic relaxation and increased myocardial stiffness, resulting in increased intraventricular pressures despite normal (or reduced) intraventricular volumes.

D. Etiology and precipitants. HF is not a disease but rather a syndrome that represents the final common pathway for a wide range of cardiac disorders. In the United States, 70–80% of HF cases are attributable to hypertension or coronary heart disease. Other common etiologies are listed in Table 7-1. Frequently,

Table 7-1. Common etiologies of heart failure in the United States

Hypertension
Coronary heart disease
  Myocardial infarction
Cardiomyopathy
  Dilated
    Idiopathic
    Toxic (ethanol, cocaine, anthracyclines)
    Infectious (viral, parasitic)
    Peripartum
    Inflammatory (myocarditis, sarcoid)
  Hypertrophic
  Restrictive/infiltrative
    Amyloid
    Hemochromatosis
    Endocardial fibroelastosis
Valvular heart disease
  Aortic stenosis or regurgitation
  Mitral stenosis or regurgitation
  Infective endocarditis
Pericardial disease
  Pericardial tamponade
  Constrictive pericarditis
Congenital heart disease
  Cyanotic
  Acyanotic
Cardiac neoplasms
  Primary
    Benign (myxoma)
    Malignant (rhabdomyosarcoma)
  Metastatic
Pulmonary disease
  Chronic lung disease
  Pulmonary hypertension
High-output states
  Chronic anemia
  Thyrotoxicosis
  Arteriovenous malformations
  Thiamine deficiency
Age-associated diastolic dysfunction

Table 7-2. Common precipitants of heart failure

Myocardial ischemia or infarction
Uncontrolled hypertension
Arrhythmias
   Supraventricular (especially atrial fibrillation)
   Ventricular
   Bradyarrhythmias (e.g., sick sinus syndrome)
Noncompliance with diet, medications
Excess fluid intake (including iatrogenic volume overload)
Medications
   Nonsteroidal anti-inflammatory drugs
   Corticosteroids
   β-Adrenergic blockers (including ophthalmologicals)
   Calcium channel antagonists
   Antiarrhythmic agents
   Antihypertensives (e.g., minoxidil)
Drugs
   Ethanol
   Cocaine
Systemic illness
   Anemia
   Thyroid dysfunction
   Infection (especially pneumonia, sepsis)
   Pulmonary disease (including pulmonary embolism)
Pregnancy

multiple potential etiologies can be identified, especially in older patients. Acute HF exacerbations are often precipitated by factors that are discrete from the primary or secondary etiologies (Table 7-2). The most common cause of repetitive HF episodes is noncompliance with diet or medications.

E. Clinical manifestations. The cardinal symptoms of HF are exertional dyspnea and fatigue, exercise intolerance, orthopnea, paroxysmal nocturnal dyspnea, nocturia, and swelling of the feet and ankles. Atypical symptoms occur with increasing frequency at older age and include confusion, irritability, lethargy, lassitude, anorexia, and GI disturbances. The classic signs of HF are jugular venous engorgement, hepatojugular reflux, moist pulmonary rales, pleural effusions, an S_3 gallop, hepatic congestion, ascites, and dependent pitting edema. In more advanced cases, hypotension, impaired sensorium, cyanosis, diminished carotid pulses, and pulsus alternans may be present.

F. Diagnostic evaluation. No single diagnostic test is specific for HF, although studies indicate that plasma levels of brain natriuretic peptide hold promise as a diagnostic tool (*Lancet* 1997;350:1349). At present, HF remains a **clinical diagnosis** that is based on a constellation of symptoms, signs, laboratory findings, and response to treatment. In advanced cases, the diagnosis is usually straightforward, but in patients with nonspecific symptoms and signs, the diagnosis may be subtle, and a high index of suspicion must be maintained. In persons with new-onset HF, the diagnostic assessment should include a chest radiograph, ECG, CBC, serum electrolytes and standard chemistries (glucose, creatinine, BUN, hepatic enzymes), urinalysis, and assessment of cardiac function with echocardiography, radionuclide ventriculography, MRI, or contrast ventriculography (*J Am Coll Cardiol* 1995;26:1376). If coronary heart disease is suspected, serial cardiac enzymes or biomarkers (e.g., troponin) should be obtained, and a stress test or cardiac catheterization with coronary angiography should be performed. A fasting lipid profile and an assessment of thyroid function may be appropriate in selected cases.

II. Management of heart failure

A. General principles. The initial assessment should include a detailed history and physical examination to establish the presence of HF, determine the primary and secondary etiologies, and identify any precipitating factors or events. The clinical examination should be supplemented by appropriate laboratory studies as indicated above, recognizing that persons with recurrent HF exacerbations do not require comprehensive evaluations with each episode. Ambulatory patients with new-onset or worsening HF of mild to moderate severity can often be evaluated and treated in the outpatient setting, but patients with more severe symptoms or acute pulmonary edema require hospitalization (see secs. **II.E** and **F**). The principal goals of HF therapy are to reduce disability, improve quality of life and functional capacity, decrease hospitalization rates, and extend survival. These goals can be accomplished through the judicious use of lifestyle modifications, pharmacologic agents, and invasive therapies (e.g., percutaneous or surgical coronary revascularization, cardiac valve repair or replacement, heart transplantation). Whenever possible, the underlying etiology should be corrected [e.g., valve replacement for aortic stenosis (AS), revascularization for severe multivessel coronary artery disease], and precipitating factors should be identified and managed accordingly. Management of acute HF includes correcting volume overload and relieving congestion and edema through the use of diuretics, preload and afterload reducing agents, and, if indicated, inotropic drugs. Long-term management includes maintenance of euvolemia; optimization of preload, afterload, and myocardial contractile function; and amelioration of the adverse effects of chronic neurohumoral activation. A multidisciplinary approach to HF disease management, involving nurses, dietitians, pharmacists, social workers, therapists, home health representatives, and physicians may be more efficacious in improving clinical outcomes than conventional physician-directed care, particularly in patients with more advanced disease (*N Engl J Med* 1995;333:1190).

B. Nonpharmacologic therapy. Nonpharmacologic measures are an important adjunct to drug therapy and can contribute significantly to improving quality of life and reducing HF exacerbations.

    1. Patient education and self-management. HF is a chronic illness frequently characterized by periods of clinical stability that are interrupted, often abruptly, by episodes of acute decompensation. Behavioral factors, particularly noncompliance, play a pivotal role in repetitive HF exacerbations, thus providing the rationale for implementing behavioral interventions to improve HF outcomes. Patients with newly diagnosed HF should be provided with educational materials that discuss HF as a chronic illness, including specific information about how it is diagnosed and treated, what the clinical manifestations and prognosis are, and, most important, what the patient can do to minimize symptoms and improve quality of life. The importance of specific self-management tasks, such as compliance with diet and medications, daily weights, regular exercise, and smoking cessation, should be emphasized, and the patient should understand that all of these aspects of disease management are under his or her direct control. Reinforcement of these points should be provided during subsequent office visits. (Note: Patient education materials are available in English and in Spanish at http://www.heartfailure.org).

2. **Diet.** A no-added-salt diet coupled with avoidance of high-salt foods (i.e., most snack foods and "fast foods," canned soups and vegetables not specifically labeled as low salt, many lunch meats and frozen entrees, tomato juice and tomato-based sauces, pickles) is appropriate for most HF patients. Patients with more severe HF and those with diastolic HF, who tend to be particularly salt sensitive, may require more aggressive sodium restriction (e.g., <1.5 g Na$^+$/day). The availability of salt substitutes and other salt-free seasonings allows patients to enjoy their meals while maintaining compliance with sodium restrictions. In addition to salt restriction, patients with coronary heart disease or diabetes should receive dietary instruction on lipid and glucose control. Weight loss is also appropriate in patients who are more than 20 lb (9 kg) over ideal body weight.

3. **Fluid intake.** In patients with mild to moderate HF, fluid restriction is usually unnecessary, but excessive fluid intake (>3 L/day) should be discouraged. In patients with more advanced HF, fluid intake should be limited to 2 L/day. In patients with hyponatremia (<130 mEq/L), fluid intake should be restricted to less than 1.5 L/day.

4. **Daily weights.** Patients should be instructed to weigh themselves each morning after urinating but before eating and to maintain a record of their weights. A baseline "dry" weight should be established, and patients should be instructed to contact their physician or other health care provider if their weight increases or declines by more than 3–5 lb (1.5–2.5 kg) from baseline, as such changes may require an adjustment in diuretic dosage.

5. **Physical activity.** Although strenuous activity should be avoided, most HF patients should be encouraged to participate in some form of low-impact, low-intensity physical activity (e.g., walking or pedaling a stationary cycle) on a daily basis. Such activity helps to preserve physical function, avoid chronic muscular deconditioning, and maintain quality of life. Specific activity recommendations vary from patient to patient, but a general guideline is that patients should exercise for a comfortable period of time at a comfortable pace, then gradually increase the duration (not the intensity) until they are able to exercise continuously for 20–30 minutes without chest pain, lightheadedness, undue shortness of breath, or severe palpitations.

6. **Oxygen.** Supplemental oxygen is appropriate for patients with a resting oxygen tension of less than 60 mm Hg and for those whose oxygen saturation declines to less than 90% during activity.

7. **Home care.** Patients with advanced HF and home-bound patients with significant disability may benefit from regular home visits by a qualified home health professional.

8. **Immunizations.** A pneumococcal vaccination and annual influenza vaccination are indicated in all patients with HF.

C. **Pharmacotherapy of HF due to LV systolic dysfunction**

1. **General principles.** Although there is substantial overlap between systolic and diastolic HF, for practical purposes patients with a left ventricular ejection fraction (LVEF) of less than 0.40 can be defined as having predominantly systolic HF, those with an LVEF of 0.50 or greater can be defined as having predominantly diastolic HF, and those with an LVEF of 0.40–0.49 can be considered as having mixed systolic and diastolic HF.

2. **Angiotensin-converting enzyme inhibitors (ACE inhibitors) are the cornerstone of therapy for patients with systolic HF** based on clinical trials involving more than 100,000 patients that demonstrate significant improvements in survival, functional capacity, and quality of life (*JAMA* 1995;273:1450). Importantly, ACE inhibitors improve outcomes in

patients with LV systolic dysfunction even in the absence of clinical HF (*N Engl J Med* 1992;327:685). ACE inhibitors block the conversion of angiotensin I to angiotensin II and also inhibit the breakdown of bradykinins. Clinically, ACE inhibitors are mixed arterial and venodilators that reduce ventricular filling pressures (preload), decrease vasoconstriction and lower vascular resistance (afterload), and attenuate fluid retention, hyponatremia, and hypokalemia caused by the compensatory activation of the renin-angiotensin system. Cardiac output and tissue perfusion are increased with little or no effect on heart rate and only a modest effect on BP. Significant hypotension (>15 mm Hg decline in systolic BP) or worsening renal function in response to an ACE inhibitor suggests decreased filling pressures or volume contraction and should prompt a reduction in diuretic dosage. Less commonly, hypotension and renal insufficiency may be due to bilateral renal artery stenosis. Dry cough occurs in 10–20% of patients who take an ACE inhibitor, but fewer than 5% require discontinuation of therapy. Worsening HF, chronic pulmonary disease, and sinus drainage should be considered as potential causes of cough before stopping ACE inhibitor therapy. Other adverse effects include rash, angioedema, dysgeusia and other GI disturbances (especially with captopril), mild increases in serum creatinine, hyperkalemia, and, rarely, blood dyscrasias. Renal function and serum electrolytes should be monitored periodically in patients who take ACE inhibitors, particularly on initiation of therapy and following an increase in dosage. Potassium supplements, potassium-based salt substitutes, and potassium-sparing diuretics should be used with caution in patients who take ACE inhibitors because of an increased risk of hyperkalemia. Most ACE inhibitors are renally excreted, and careful dosage titration is required in patients with renal insufficiency.

   a. **Captopril** is often used when initiating ACE inhibitor therapy in HF patients because its short half-life (2–3 hours) permits more rapid dosage titration and may minimize the risk of hypotension and worsening renal function. In ambulatory patients younger than 70 years of age with resting systolic BP of 120 mm Hg or greater and normal renal function (serum creatinine <1.5 mg/dl), the initial dose of captopril is 12.5 mg q8h. In the absence of adverse effects, the dosage should be doubled at 1- to 2-week intervals until a target dosage of 50 mg q8h is achieved. In patients older than 70 years of age or with systolic BP of less than 120 mm Hg or pre-existing renal dysfunction (serum creatinine ≥1.5 mg/dl), a starting dose of 6.25 mg q8h is recommended. Upward titration should be more gradual, and BP, electrolytes, and renal function should be monitored more closely, but the target dosage remains 50 mg q8h in the absence of adverse effects. Because captopril contains a sulfhydryl group (unlike other ACE inhibitors), angioedema and agranulocytosis may be more common with this agent.

   b. **Enalapril** is hydrolyzed by the liver to enalaprilat, the active moiety. The duration of action (12–24 hours) is longer than with captopril, permitting once- or twice-daily dosing, but the potential for hypotension or renal insufficiency is slightly higher. The initial dose in ambulatory patients is 5 mg once a day (2.5 mg/day in patients >70 years, with systolic BP <120 mm Hg, or with serum creatine ≥1.5 mg/dl), and the dose should be doubled at 1- to 2-week intervals to achieve a target dosage of 20 mg once a day or 10 mg bid. Further increases in dosage, up to 20 mg bid, may be beneficial in patients with more advanced symptoms or more severe LV dysfunction (LVEF <0.25).

   c. **Lisinopril** is a long-acting ACE inhibitor that is suitable for once-daily administration. The initial dosage is 5 mg (2.5 mg in patients

>70 years, with systolic BP <120 mm Hg, or serum creatinine ≥1.5 mg/dl). The dose should be increased at 1- to 2-week intervals to achieve a target dosage of 20 mg/day. As with enalapril, additional increases in dosage, up to 40 mg/day, may be beneficial in selected patients (*Circulation* 1999;100:2312).

   d. **Ramipril** and **trandolapril** have been shown to improve survival in patients with HF following acute myocardial infarction (*Lancet* 1993;342:821, and *N Engl J Med* 1995;333:1670). The initial dose of ramipril is 2.5 mg bid, increasing to 5 mg bid after 1–2 weeks. The initial dose of trandolapril is 1–2 mg once daily, increasing to 4 mg/day over 2–4 weeks. As with other ACE inhibitors, the initial dosage of these agents should be reduced in patients who are at increased risk for adverse renal and hemodynamic effects.

   e. **Quinapril** is approved for use in HF, with an initial dose of 10 mg/day and a maximum dose of 40 mg/day or 20 mg bid. **Fosinopril, moexipril, perindopril** and **benazepril** are approved to treat hypertension and may be effective in HF, but there is less experience with these agents compared to other ACE inhibitors.

3. **Angiotensin II receptor blockers** (ARBs) inhibit the actions of angiotensin II by selectively binding to the cell surface receptor for angiotensin II, subtype 1. ARBs provide more complete blockade of angiotensin II than ACE inhibitors, and because they do not increase bradykinin levels, cough, angioedema, and possibly hyperkalemia occur less frequently. The hemodynamic effects of ARBs are similar to those of ACE inhibitors, and although ARBs appear to be better tolerated than ACE inhibitors, their relative value in improving clinical outcomes in HF patients has not yet been established. As a result, **ACE inhibitors remain first-choice therapy for systolic HF**; however, ARBs are a suitable alternative in those patients who are intolerant to ACE inhibitors. None of the ARBs have been approved for use in HF.

   a. **Losartan** reduced mortality compared to captopril in a single small trial (*Lancet* 1997;349:747), but no survival advantage was demonstrated in a larger trial with longer follow-up (*Lancet* 2000;355:1582). Losartan undergoes extensive first-pass hepatic metabolism, and the parent compound and its major metabolite are pharmacologically active. Losartan is also mildly uricosuric. The starting dose of losartan is 12.5 to 25.0 mg once a day, and the maintenance dose is 50 mg once a day or bid. Renal function and serum electrolytes should be monitored periodically.

   b. In the Valsartan Heart Failure trial, **valsartan** added to an ACE inhibitor had no effect on mortality but had a favorable impact on morbidity, hospitalizations for HF, and quality of life. Importantly, this benefit was limited to patients who did not receive a betablocker. The initial dose of valsartan in the Valsartan Heart Failure trial was 40 mg bid, and the target dose was 160 mg bid.

   c. **Candesartan** is currently under investigation for the treatment of HF. The starting dose is 4 mg once a day, and the maximum dose is 32 mg qd.

   d. **Irbesartan** and **telmisartan** are approved for use in hypertension, but there is limited experience with these agents in HF.

4. **Hydralazine** in combination with **isosorbide dinitrate** improves exercise tolerance and reduces mortality in patients with systolic HF (*N Engl J Med* 1986;314:1547), but the effect on survival is less pronounced than with an ACE inhibitor (*N Engl J Med* 1991;325:303). Nonetheless, this combination is a suitable alternative in ACE inhibitor–intolerant patients, and it can be used as an adjunct to ACE inhibitors in patients with severe HF who remain symptomatic despite intensive therapy. Hydralazine is a direct arterial vasodilator, and its afterload-

reducing effects may be particularly useful in the treatment of mitral or aortic regurgitation. The initial dose of hydralazine is 25 mg tid, and the dosage should be gradually increased over a period of several weeks to 75 mg qid or 100 mg tid–qid. Hydralazine can cause reflex tachycardia and should be used with caution in patients with active coronary heart disease. As with other vasodilators, BP should be monitored in patients who are treated with hydralazine, particularly during the dose titration phase. Hydralazine has been associated with the drug-lupus syndrome in approximately 10% of patients who receive daily dosages in excess of 300 mg. Other adverse effects include headache, nausea, and postural hypotension. Nitrates act by transiently increasing the production of nitric oxide, an endogenous vasodilator. At lower dosages, venodilation predominates, but arterial vasodilation also occurs at higher dosages. Nitrates reduce preload, decrease symptoms of pulmonary congestion, and diminish myocardial ischemia. For chronic use, nitrates can be administered orally or transdermally. A daily nitrate-free period of 6–12 hours is recommended to avoid nitrate tolerance. In HF trials, isosorbide dinitrate (in combination with hydralazine) was initiated at a dose of 10 mg qid, and the dosage was increased to 40 mg qid over a period of several weeks. Other nitrate formulations may also be efficacious. Aside from tolerance, the most common adverse effects of nitrates are headache, hypotension, and flushing.

5. β-**Adrenergic receptor antagonists** (beta-blockers) inhibit the deleterious effects of sympathetic nervous system activation and have been shown to improve survival and left ventricular function in patients with mild to moderate HF (New York Heart Association class I–III) (*N Engl J Med* 1996;334:1349, *Lancet* 1999;353:9, and *Lancet* 1999;353:2001). Data from the Carvedilol Prospective Cumulative Survival (COPERNICUS) trial indicate that beta-blockers also improve outcomes in stable New York Heart Association class IV patients (*N Engl J Med* 2001;344:1651). The beneficial effects include reductions in deaths due to pump failure and arrhythmias and a decrease in the need for heart transplantation. Based on these studies, **beta-blockers should be considered standard therapy in the treatment of all appropriately selected patients with systolic HF** in the absence of contraindications. Before beta-blocker therapy is initiated, the dosages of ACE inhibitors, diuretics, and digoxin (if used) should be optimized. In addition, although initiation of beta-blockers in the ambulatory setting is appropriate and desirable, the patient's HF should be clinically stable before initiation of treatment. In addition to decompensated HF, other contraindications to beta-blockade include bradycardia (heart rate <50/min), relative hypotension (systolic BP <90–100 mm Hg), heart block [PR interval ≥240 msec or higher-degree atrioventricular (AV) block], active bronchospastic lung disease, and severe chronic obstructive pulmonary disease. The presence of mild lung disease, diabetes mellitus, or peripheral arterial disease does not preclude the use of beta-blockers. Potential adverse effects of beta-blockers include bradycardia, hypotension, worsening dyspnea, bronchospasm, claudication, fatigue or low energy level, and sexual dysfunction. Importantly, beta-blockers should be initiated at a very low dose in all HF patients to minimize the risk of worsening HF due to the negative inotropic and chronotropic effects of these agents.

a. **Metoprolol** at low to moderate doses (<200 mg/day) is relatively selective for β_1-adrenergic receptors and is less likely to induce bronchospasm or worsen claudication than are nonselective agents. The starting dose of metoprolol is 12.5 mg bid in patients with class I–II HF and 6.25 mg bid in class III–IV patients. The dose should be doubled at approximately 2-week intervals as tolerated to achieve a maintenance dose of 50–100 mg bid. If there is an increase in HF symptoms during titration, a dosage reduction may be required. Once a stable dosage has been reached, changing to a long-acting, once-daily formulation at an equivalent daily dosage should be considered.

   b. Carvedilol is a nonselective antagonist of β_1-, β_2-, and α_1-adrenergic receptors; it also has antioxidant properties. Carvedilol is initiated at a dose of 3.125 to 6.25 mg bid, and the dose is doubled at 2-week intervals as tolerated to achieve a maintenance dose of 25–50 mg bid.

   c. Bisoprolol is a once-daily β_1-selective agent with an initial dose of 1.25 mg/day and a maintenance dose of 5–10 mg/day.

6. **Diuretics** are effective in relieving pulmonary congestion and peripheral edema but have not been shown to influence the natural history of HF. Diuretics are particularly useful for the management of acute HF; in chronic HF diuretics should be used in conjunction with dietary sodium and fluid restriction (see secs. **II.B.2** and **II.B.3**), and the minimum effective dose that is required to maintain euvolemia should be used. Diuretics are usually well tolerated but may be associated with serious electrolyte disturbances, including hypokalemia, hyponatremia, and hypomagnesemia. Other common adverse effects include intravascular volume contraction, metabolic alkalosis, worsening renal function (especially prerenal azotemia), impaired glucose metabolism, hyperuricemia, rash, and allergic reactions. Serum electrolytes and renal function should be monitored closely during diuretic therapy, and potassium supplementation or the use of a potassium-sparing diuretic should be considered for the prevention or treatment of hypokalemia.

   a. Thiazide diuretics (hydrochlorothiazide, chlorthalidone) can be used in patients with mild HF and normal renal function, but most patients with moderate to severe HF require a loop diuretic. The initial dose of hydrochlorothiazide and chlorthalidone is 12.5–25.0 mg/day, and the maximum recommended dose is 50 mg/day. Thiazides are ineffective when the serum creatinine level is 3 mg/dl or greater.

   b. Loop diuretics (furosemide, bumetanide, torsemide) are more potent than thiazides and are effective in the management of acute and chronic HF, as well as in patients with renal insufficiency. The initial doses of these agents are furosemide, 10–20 mg/day; bumetanide, 0.5–1.0 mg/day; and torsemide, 5–10 mg/day. Subsequent dosing should be based on the clinical response and severity of HF. All three agents can be administered intravenously at equivalent dosages for the treatment of acute HF. Higher dosages may be required to promote diuresis in the setting of renal insufficiency.

   c. Metolazone acts at the proximal and the distal tubules and is useful in the management of HF that is resistant to conventional doses of loop diuretics and in patients with low glomerular filtration rates. Metolazone should be administered 30–60 minutes before giving a loop diuretic and initiated at a dose of 2.5 mg/day with a maximum dose of 10 mg/day. Metolazone can induce profound electrolyte disturbances even during short-term administration, and careful monitoring of electrolytes and renal function is essential.

   d. Spironolactone is a relatively weak potassium-sparing diuretic that acts as a competitive aldosterone antagonist. It has been shown to improve outcomes in patients with class III or IV HF when used in combination with an ACE inhibitor (*N Engl J Med* 1999;341:709). The starting dose of spironolactone is 12.5–25.0 mg/day, and the maximum recommended dose in patients with HF is 50 mg/day. Spironolactone may cause significant hyperkalemia, particularly in diabetics and in patients who use ACE inhibitors or nonsteroidal anti-inflammatory drugs. Gynecomastia and breast tenderness occur in up to 10% of patients.

7. **Digoxin** and other digitalis glycosides increase myocardial contractility by inhibiting the sarcolemmal Na-K exchange mechanism, thereby facilitating Na-Ca exchange and increasing intracellular calcium. Digoxin improves symptoms and reduces hospitalizations for HF but has no effect on survival when used in combination with ACE inhibitors and diuretics (*N Engl J Med* 1997;336:525). Digoxin is indicated in the management of patients with severe LV dysfunction (LV ejection fraction <0.25) and in those who remain symptomatic despite appropriate therapy with an ACE inhibitor, diuretic, and beta-blocker. In addition to its inotropic effect, digoxin slows conduction through the AV node, and it is useful in the management of HF patients with supraventricular arrhythmias, especially atrial fibrillation.

   a. **Pharmacokinetics and dosing.** When taken orally, digoxin has an onset of action of 30–120 minutes, and the peak effect is reached 2–5 hours after administration. The half-life is 36–48 hours in patients with normal renal function, and it may be substantially prolonged in patients with renal insufficiency. In ambulatory patients, a loading dose of digoxin is not recommended. The starting dose is 0.25 mg/day in persons less than 70 years of age with normal renal function (serum creatinine <1.5 mg/dl) and a body weight of 60 kg or greater. In persons who do not meet these criteria, the starting dose should be 0.125 mg/day. Very elderly patients and those with more advanced renal insufficiency (serum creatinine ≥3.0 mg/dl) may require lower dosages or longer dosing intervals. Conversely, younger patients and those who weigh 90 kg or more may require higher dosages, for example, 0.375 mg/day. When in doubt, a lower dose of digoxin should be administered because the toxic-therapeutic index is narrow.

   b. **Monitoring.** Although the value of monitoring serum digoxin levels in stable patients without evidence of toxicity is unproven, most experts recommend obtaining a digoxin level approximately 1 month after initiating therapy. The therapeutic range for digoxin in our laboratory is 0.8–2.0 µg/L (1.0–2.6 nmol/L), but levels above 1.5 µg/L provide little additional inotropic effect and are associated with increased toxicity (*J Am Coll Cardiol* 1997;29:1206). In addition, patients older than 70 years of age may be more susceptible to the therapeutic and the toxic effects of digoxin, and a suggested therapeutic digoxin range for this age group is 0.6–1.2 µg/L. Once a stable dose of digoxin has been achieved, routine monitoring of digoxin levels is not recommended. However, it is appropriate to obtain a digoxin level whenever toxicity is suspected or when there is concern about worsening renal function or drug interactions.

   c. **Drug interactions** with digoxin are common, and include impaired absorption with cholestyramine, antacids, and kaolin-pectin, which may reduce bioavailability by 25%. Oral antibiotics such as erythromycin and tetracycline may increase digoxin levels by 10–40%. Quinidine, verapamil, flecainide, and amiodarone may increase digoxin levels by up to 100%.

   d. **Digoxin toxicity** occurs in 5–15% of patients during chronic therapy. Risk factors for digoxin toxicity include older age, renal insufficiency, volume contraction, chronic lung disease, hypothyroidism, drug interactions, and electrolyte abnormalities. Cardiac arrhythmias are the most important manifestation of digitalis intoxication and frequently occur in the absence of other signs or symptoms. Common arrhythmias include frequent ventricular premature depolarizations (often in a bigeminal pattern), junctional tachycardia, and varying degrees of AV block, ranging from first-degree to complete heart block. Paroxysmal atrial tachycardia with block, atrial fibrillation with regular ventricular response, and bidirectional ventricular tachycardia are hallmarks of digitalis toxicity. In severe cases, sustained ventricular tachycardia, ventricular fibrillation, and asystole may occur. Noncardiac manifestations of digoxin toxicity include neuropsychiatric symptoms (altered mental status, agitation, lethargy, and visual disturbances, especially scotomas and changes in color perception) and GI disorders (anorexia, nausea, vomiting, and diarrhea).

e. **Treatment of digoxin toxicity** includes discontinuation of digoxin and any other agents that may increase digoxin levels, maintaining serum potassium in the range of 4.0–5.0 mEq/L and serum magnesium in the range of 1.6–2.2 mEq/L and correction of other precipitating factors. Patients with digoxin-induced arrhythmias require continuous ECG monitoring in a hospital setting, but mild digitalis intoxication (digoxin level <3 µg/L) in the absence of arrhythmias or electrolyte abnormalities does not usually require hospitalization. Management of serious digoxin toxicity is beyond the scope of this manual but may include atropine or temporary pacing for bradyarrhythmias and lidocaine or phenytoin for supraventricular or ventricular tachyarrhythmias. Life-threatening arrhythmias and massive digitalis overdoses should be treated with digoxin-specific Fab antibody fragments (*Circulation* 1999;99:1265).

8. **Calcium channel antagonists** have not been shown to improve clinical outcomes in patients with HF, and first-generation calcium channel antagonists (nifedipine, diltiazem, verapamil) are contraindicated in patients with LV systolic dysfunction because they may increase HF exacerbations and decrease survival. Newer agents, such as amlodipine and felodipine, appear to be safe in HF patients, but they do not improve survival (*N Engl J Med* 1996;335:1107, and *Circulation* 1997;96:856).

9. **Antithrombotic therapy.** Aspirin, 81–325 mg/day, is indicated in all patients with documented coronary heart disease, but aspirin may inhibit the beneficial effects of ACE inhibitors and should probably be avoided in the absence of atherosclerotic vascular disease. Warfarin titrated to an international normalized ratio (INR) of 2.0–3.0 is indicated in HF patients with atrial fibrillation or flutter (chronic or paroxysmal), mechanical prosthetic heart valves (INR, 2.5–3.5), prior arterial thromboembolism, or anterior myocardial infarction within 3–6 months. The value of warfarin in other situations is unproven. Similarly, the role of newer antithrombotic agents, such as ticlopidine, clopidogrel, and glycoprotein IIb/IIIa inhibitors, in the management of HF remains to be established.

10. **Inotropic agents** such as intravenous dobutamine and milrinone may improve symptoms and quality of life in patients with severe HF that is refractory to conventional pharmacologic and nonpharmacologic therapies. The effect of intravenous inotropic therapy on survival is unknown, and such agents should generally be used only under the supervision of a HF specialist.

D. **Management of diastolic HF.** Up to 50% of HF patients have preserved LV systolic function, and the proportion of patients with diastolic HF increases progressively with advancing age. With the exception of digoxin, there has been no major clinical trials evaluating specific pharmacologic agents for the treatment of diastolic HF; as a result, treatment of this disorder remains largely empiric. General measures include appropriate BP control, management of other cardiac risk factors, and treatment of ischemia. The nonpharmacologic measures outlined in sec. **II.B** are equally appropriate in patients with systolic or diastolic HF. Diuretics are indicated for relief of congestion and edema but must be used cautiously in patients with diastolic HF, who are often "volume sensitive" and require elevated filling pressures to maintain cardiac output. Clinical features that are indicative of overdiuresis include relative hypotension (especially orthostatic hypotension), increased fatigue, reduced exercise tolerance, and worsening prerenal azotemia. By lowering preload, nitrates may reduce exertional dyspnea, thereby improving exercise tolerance. Administration of nitrates at bedtime may be effective in reducing orthopnea. ACE inhibitors, beta-blockers, calcium channel antagonists, and angiotensin receptor blockers have all been shown to provide symptomatic palliation in selected patients with diastolic HF, but the effect of these agents on major clinical outcomes is unknown. Use of these agents should therefore be individualized, based on comorbid conditions (e.g., diabetes, asthma, coronary heart disease, atrial fibrillation), heart rate, tolerability, convenience, and cost. Patients who remain symptomatic on monotherapy should be switched to an alternative agent, or a second agent from another class should be added. Based on data from the Digitalis Investigation Group study, digoxin should be considered in patients with persistent class III–IV diastolic HF without evidence for LV outflow tract obstruction (*N Engl J Med* 1997;336:525).

E. **Ambulatory management of HF exacerbations.** In many cases, mild to moderate HF exacerbations can be managed in the outpatient setting. A detailed history should be obtained, focusing on issues of compliance with diet and medications, as well as on other potential factors that contribute to worsening symptoms (Table 7-2). An ECG should be obtained if ischemia is suspected, and a chest radiograph is appropriate if the diagnosis is in doubt. Serum electrolytes and creatinine should be assessed in most situations; additional chemistries and a CBC may be appropriate in selected cases. In patients with mild HF exacerbations, increasing the doses of oral diuretics and vasodilators is appropriate. In patients who are already on high doses of loop diuretics (furosemide, 160 mg/day or equivalent), the addition of metolazone, 2.5 mg/day, should be considered. The dose of beta-blockers should **not** be increased and may need to be temporarily reduced. The importance of sodium restriction and of monitoring daily weights should be emphasized, and a target weight loss should be specified (e.g., 5 lb in 3 days). Failure to achieve this goal should prompt a follow-up call to the physician or HF manager. In patients who experience significant symptomatic improvement in response to the above measures, telephone follow-up after 1 week is appropriate, with a follow-up office visit in 2–4 weeks. Patients with more severe HF exacerbations require more aggressive therapy. In addition to the above measures, intravenous diuretic therapy (e.g., furosemide) is indicated, either in the office or at home, with the latter option requiring the assistance of a home health nurse. The addition of metolazone, 2.5–5.0 mg/day, should be considered, and the beta-blocker dose should be reduced by 50%. As with mild HF exacerbations, a target weight reduction should be specified, and telephone follow-up should be arranged within 3–5 days, with subsequent follow-up contingent on the initial response to therapy. In patients who respond to the above interventions with symptomatic improvement, satisfactory diuresis, and significant weight loss, renal function and electrolytes should be reassessed, and maintenance therapy should be resumed, perhaps with more frequent follow-up.

F. **Indications for hospitalization or referral.** Hospitalization is indicated for the treatment of severe HF exacerbations, acute pulmonary edema, and moderate exacerbations that fail to respond to intensified therapy as outlined above. Hospitalization is also warranted if significant myocardial ischemia or infarction is suspected or if new or worsening ventricular or supraventricular arrhythmias (including new-onset or recurrent atrial fibrillation or flutter) are identified. In addition, hospitalization is appropriate in patients with other high-risk features, including relative hypotension (systolic BP <90–100 mm Hg), marked tachycardia or bradycardia, significant renal insufficiency (serum creatinine >1.5–2.0 mg/dl), or suspected severe AS, infective endocarditis, pericardial disease, or drug toxicity. In the

United States, up to 80% of HF patients are managed by primary care physicians. However, referral to a cardiologist or HF specialist should be considered for patients with persistent New York Heart Association class III or IV symptoms despite appropriate medical therapy. Inability to titrate medical therapy to optimal levels (e.g., due to low BP or renal dysfunction) is also an indication for referral. Patients with significant ventricular arrhythmias (e.g., frequent ventricular premature depolarizations, nonsustained or sustained ventricular tachycardia) or unexplained syncope should be evaluated by a cardiologist or cardiac electrophysiologist, and patients with potentially correctable lesions, including severe coronary artery disease, valvular lesions, and pericardial disease, should also be referred for further evaluation and therapy. In addition, patients with HF of obscure origin, frequent HF exacerbations (≥3 hospitalizations within a 12-month period), or heart failure that is difficult to manage due to comorbidities, drug intolerance, or noncompliance should be seen in consultation by a cardiologist with expertise in HF. Finally, patients with advanced HF who may be suitable candidates for heart transplantation, ventricular assist devices, intravenous inotropic therapy, or other novel HF treatments should undergo a comprehensive evaluation by an HF specialist.

Cardiomyopathy

I. **Cardiomyopathy** refers to any process that results in substantial injury or damage to the myocardium or that causes significant abnormalities in myocardial function. Broadly, this includes most causes of HF (Table 7-1), but certain disease processes appear to affect the myocardium primarily, and the management of these disorders is discussed in this section. In general, primary cardiomyopathies account for 10–20% of all HF cases, with dilated cardiomyopathy being the most common form, followed by hypertrophic cardiomyopathy (HCM) and restrictive cardiomyopathy.

II. **Dilated cardiomyopathy** is characterized by dilatation of all four cardiac chambers and by impaired ventricular contractility. It is a common cause of systolic HF, particularly in persons younger than 55 years of age, and accounts for approximately 40% of referrals for heart transplantation. The majority of cases are idiopathic, and the putative role of viral myocarditis in this syndrome remains speculative. Chronic ethanol abuse, anthracycline toxicity, and cocaine are other common causes of dilated cardiomyopathy.

A. **Clinical features.** Symptomatic HF is the most frequent mode of presentation, but nonspecific symptoms, often simulating a viral upper respiratory infection, are also a common reason for patients to seek medical attention. Chest pain and arrhythmias, including sudden cardiac death, are less common presentations but are not rare. The ECG often reveals nonspecific ST-segment and T-wave abnormalities; LV hypertrophy and conduction abnormalities are also common. The chest radiograph reveals diffuse cardiomegaly, and pulmonary congestion may be present. Other laboratory findings are nonspecific. The echocardiogram reveals four-chamber dilatation and reduced LV systolic function, which may be severe. Mitral and tricuspid regurgitation are often present, varying from mild to severe. Pulmonary hypertension may also be noted. Stress testing and coronary angiography, if performed, are useful in excluding coronary heart disease as the cause of LV dysfunction. In most cases, endomyocardial biopsy is of little value in the diagnosis or management of dilated cardiomyopathy.

B. **Management.** Medical therapy is similar to that for systolic HF of any cause. In particular, maximally tolerated doses of ACE inhibitors and beta-blockers should be administered, diuretics should be given to maintain euvolemia, and other therapies should be considered based on symptom severity. Nonpharmacologic measures as discussed above are an important adjunct to pharmacologic treatment.

III. HCM is characterized by ventricular hypertrophy, myocyte disarray, reduced LV cavity dimensions, normal or increased LV contractility, and markedly impaired ventricular relaxation. Approximately 50% of cases are inherited with an autosomal dominant transmission pattern, and more than a dozen single gene mutations that can cause the HCM phenotype have been identified. The age at onset, clinical course, and prognosis are highly variable, with the most severe forms presenting in childhood and being associated with a high risk of sudden cardiac death. Conversely, up to 30% of cases are initially diagnosed in persons older than 65 years of age, and the prognosis in these cases is more favorable. A pathophysiologically similar disorder, **hypertensive HCM**, occurs in older individuals, especially women, with long-standing hypertension or chronic renal disease (*N Engl J Med* 1985;312:277).

A. Clinical features. Many patients with HCM are asymptomatic, and the diagnosis may be occult. Common symptoms include exertional dyspnea, chest pain, arrhythmias (supraventricular and ventricular), and syncope. Sudden cardiac death may occur, most commonly in patients younger than 30 years of age with a family history of premature sudden death; other risk factors for sudden death include syncope and ventricular tachycardia. Physical findings may include pulsus bisferiens (if LV outflow obstruction is present; see below), an S_4 gallop, an LV heave, and a coarse ejection systolic murmur that is best heard along the left sternal border and accentuated by standing or the Valsalva maneuver. An apical murmur of mitral regurgitation (MR) may also be present. Chest radiography demonstrates LV prominence, and ECG often reveals LV hypertrophy with ST-segment and T-wave abnormalities. Echocardiography is usually diagnostic, and classic features of HCM include asymmetric septal hypertrophy and systolic anterior motion of the mitral valve (SAM), with or without obstruction of the LV outflow tract. Alternatively, LV hypertrophy may be concentric, especially in older persons with hypertensive HCM, and provocative maneuvers, such as Valsalva or amyl nitrite, may be necessary to induce SAM of the mitral valve. LV outflow tract obstruction results from the combination of asymmetric septal hypertrophy and SAM of the mitral apparatus and may occur at rest or with provocation; when present, the outflow gradient can be quantified with Doppler flow studies. Although markedly increased LV outflow gradients (≥ 80 mm Hg) are often associated with severe symptoms, the prognosis is similar whether or not LV outflow obstruction is present.

B. Management. Therapy for HCM is directed at symptom relief and the prevention of endocarditis and life-threatening arrhythmias. Treatment of asymptomatic individuals, especially those at low risk for serious arrhythmias, is controversial, because there is no conclusive evidence that medical therapy is beneficial in such patients.

1. General measures. All individuals with HCM should receive bacterial endocarditis prophylaxis before dental work and other procedures (see Appendix H). Strenuous physical activity, including most competitive sports, should be avoided, especially when there is a family history of premature sudden cardiac death. First-degree relatives of patients with familial HCM should undergo a screening echocardiogram, even in the absence of symptoms.

2. Medical therapy. β-**Adrenergic antagonists** may reduce symptoms by decreasing myocardial contractility and slowing heart rate. Propranolol, 40–80 mg/day can be initiated in the ambulatory setting, and the dose should be gradually increased to 160–320 mg/day based on clinical response and tolerability. Some patients may require higher dosages to achieve maximum symptomatic improvement. Equivalent dosages of other beta-blockers are also effective. **Calcium channel antagonists**, especially diltiazem and verapamil, may be effective in relieving symptoms, but the dihydropyridines should be avoided in patients with LV outflow obstruction due to their vasodilatory properties. **Disopyramide** is a type I antiarrhythmic agent with negative inotropic effects that may be useful in managing patients with refractory symptoms. The starting dose of disopyramide is 200–300 mg/day, and the usual maintenance dose is 400–600 mg/day. Disopyramide may prolong the QT interval and induce torsades de pointes ventricular tachycardia; an ECG should be obtained after each dose titration. Disopyramide also has significant anticholinergic effects, and it should be avoided in persons who are at risk for developing urinary retention, for example, men with prostatic hypertrophy. **Diuretics** may be useful in relieving congestive symptoms, but overdiuresis should be avoided because LV outflow obstruction may be worsened. Nitrates and other vasodilators are relatively contraindicated in patients with significant LV outflow obstruction.

3. **Atrial and ventricular arrhythmias** occur commonly in patients with HCM. **Supraventricular arrhythmias**, including atrial fibrillation, are often poorly tolerated and require aggressive treatment. Beta-blockers, diltiazem, and verapamil are effective in slowing heart rate, but digoxin should be avoided due to its inotropic effect and potential for increasing LV outflow obstruction. For long-term suppression of supraventricular arrhythmias, **amiodarone** and **disopyramide** are often effective, although neither has been approved for this indication. In stable patients without active HF or ventricular arrhythmias, many clinicians initiate amiodarone in the ambulatory setting at a dosage of 200–400 mg bid for 2–4 weeks, with a subsequent maintenance dose of 100–200 mg/day (see Chap. 8 for additional details on the use of amiodarone). Patients with chronic atrial fibrillation or flutter and those with frequent episodes of paroxysmal atrial fibrillation or flutter should be treated with warfarin to maintain an INR of 2.0–3.0. Patients with HCM and symptomatic **ventricular arrhythmias**, nonsustained ventricular tachycardia, or unexplained syncope should be referred to a cardiologist or electrophysiologist for further evaluation, because empiric antiarrhythmic therapy has not been shown to improve clinical outcomes in these patients.

4. **Dual-chamber pacing, percutaneous transcoronary septal ablation with ethanol, and surgical therapies,** including septal myectomy and mitral valve replacement, may provide effective palliation in patients with HCM that is refractory to other therapies, but the impact of these interventions on long-term clinical outcomes is unknown.

IV. **Restrictive cardiomyopathy** is a relatively rare cause of HF that results from infiltration of the myocardium by various processes. Amyloidosis and sarcoidosis are the two most common causes of restrictive cardiomyopathy in the United States. Less common causes include hemochromatosis (primary or secondary), hypereosinophilic syndromes, endomyocardial fibrosis, tumor infiltration, and glycogen storage diseases.

A. **Pathophysiology and diagnosis.** The hallmark of restrictive cardiomyopathy is markedly impaired ventricular diastolic filling due to myocardial infiltration. Varying degrees of systolic dysfunction may also be present. The ECG often demonstrates a low-voltage QRS and AV and intraventricular conduction abnormalities. Echocardiography usually demonstrates generalized or focal myocardial hypertrophy, reduced ventricular cavity dimensions, and biatrial enlargement. A characteristic "sparkling" appearance of the myocardium may be seen in patients with advanced amyloid infiltration. Doppler studies reveal a restrictive pattern of ventricular filling. Restrictive cardiomyopathy may be difficult to differentiate from constrictive pericarditis, the latter of which can be successfully treated with pericardiectomy;

computed tomography, MRI, or endomyocardial biopsy may be required to make this distinction.

B. Management. The prognosis for restrictive cardiomyopathy is poor unless the underlying disease process can be successfully treated. Diuretics and vasodilators may be beneficial in some cases, but excessive preload reduction should be avoided. Digoxin is contraindicated in patients with cardiac amyloidosis due to enhanced susceptibility to digoxin toxicity.

Valvular Heart Disease

I. **Valvular heart disease (VHD)** is common in the adult population, and the prevalence increases with advancing age. VHD may be congenital (e.g., bicuspid aortic valve) or acquired (e.g., rheumatic heart disease, calcific AS), and its clinical spectrum ranges from very mild to severe and life threatening. VHD should be considered in all patients with cardiac symptoms or a heart murmur on physical examination. In most cases, echocardiography provides a definitive diagnosis and can reliably estimate disease severity. Treatment is based on the specific lesion and its severity, as well as the potential risks associated with invasive interventions.

II. **Aortic stenosis (AS)**

    A. AS is the most common valvular lesion requiring surgical intervention in the United States. Congenital bicuspid aortic valve is the most common cause of severe AS in patients younger than 60 years of age, and calcific degeneration of a normal trileaflet valve is the most common cause of AS in patients older than 60 years of age. Rheumatic AS occurs infrequently, principally in men.

    B. Clinical manifestations. AS is associated with a prolonged latency period, and patients often remain asymptomatic for years or even decades following the detection of an aortic valvular murmur. Classic symptoms of AS include the triad of anginal chest pain, HF, and syncope, but few patients manifest all three. Once any of these symptoms occurs, the prognosis is poor, with median survival rates of 1–3 years in the absence of aortic valve replacement. The cardinal physical finding of AS is a harsh, mid- to late-peaking ejection systolic murmur that radiates to the carotids. Additional findings may include a delayed carotid upstroke, LV heave, S_4 gallop, and low-intensity or absent A_2 component of the second heart sound. ECG often reveals increased QRS voltage and ST-segment and T-wave abnormalities, but these findings are nonspecific and not invariably present. Echocardiography demonstrates a thickened or calcified aortic valve with restricted opening. Doppler echocardiography provides information regarding the peak and mean pressure gradients across the aortic valve, and the effective aortic valve area can be estimated by means of the continuity equation. In adults of average size, the normal aortic valve area is 2.5 cm^2 or greater. A calculated aortic valve area of less than 0.7–0.8 cm^2 is indicative of severe AS (*J Am Coll Cardiol* 1998;32:1486). In addition to echocardiography, most persons over age 40 with severe AS should undergo cardiac catheterization with coronary angiography before valve surgery, because coronary artery disease coexists in up to 50% of cases.

    C. Management. Endocarditis prophylaxis is indicated in all cases (see Appendix H), and vigorous physical activity should be avoided in patients with moderate to severe AS by echocardiography. Digoxin, diuretics, nitrates, and vasodilators may provide symptomatic palliation in patients with mild to moderate AS, but caution is needed to avoid overdiuresis and excessive reduction of preload and afterload. Sublingual nitroglycerin and other vasodilators should be avoided in patients with severe AS, particularly if the systolic BP is less than 110–120 mm Hg. In the absence of symptoms, patients with mild to moderate AS can be followed closely at 3- to 6-month intervals. Patients with symptomatic severe AS should be referred for aortic valve replacement, which represents definitive therapy for this condition. Percutaneous balloon aortic valvuloplasty, once considered an alternative to surgery, has been associated with a high rate of restenosis and poor long-term clinical results.

III. **Aortic insufficiency (AI)**

    A. AI that is severe enough to warrant surgical intervention is relatively uncommon except in selected patient populations (e.g., Marfan's syndrome). AI may result from a primary valvular abnormality or from dilatation or distortion of the aortic root. Common causes of valvular AI include rheumatic heart disease, trauma, endocarditis, and deformities due to bicuspid or calcific AS. Aortic root dilatation may be due to hypertension, aortic dissection, hereditary and acquired connective tissue diseases (Marfan's syndrome, ankylosing spondylitis), and luetic aortitis. Acute AI often presents with severe HF and pulmonary edema, whereas chronic AI usually has an insidious onset.

    B. Clinical manifestations. Chest pain, fatigue, exercise intolerance, palpitations, and HF are the most common symptoms associated with AI. Physical findings include bounding pulses, a wide pulse pressure, and a diastolic murmur of variable intensity. The chest x-ray usually demonstrates cardiomegaly, and the ECG often reveals LV hypertrophy. Echocardiography with Doppler can reliably confirm the diagnosis, estimate AI severity, and provide insight into potential etiology. In most cases, cardiac catheterization is not required before valve surgery unless coronary artery disease is suspected.

    C. Management. Patients with chronic AI should receive prophylaxis for bacterial endocarditis (see Appendix H). If LV dysfunction is present, strenuous physical activity (especially isometric activity) should be avoided. Whenever possible, the underlying condition should be treated (e.g., antibiotics for endocarditis or syphilis, anti-inflammatory agents for ankylosing spondylitis). Afterload reduction delays the need for surgery and is appropriate for patients with moderate or severe AI. In individuals with preserved LV systolic function, nifedipine is effective (*N Engl J Med* 1994;331:689), whereas ACE inhibitors should be used if LV function is impaired (*J Am Coll Cardiol* 1994;24:1046). Diuretics and digoxin are useful for the treatment of congestive symptoms. In patients with acute severe AI, urgent surgery is usually required. Patients with mild to moderate chronic AI often remain stable for prolonged periods of time, and conservative medical management is appropriate (see also sec. **VII.A**). Patients with severe chronic AI should be considered for surgical intervention when New York Heart Association class II–III symptoms develop or when the echocardiogram demonstrates LV systolic dysfunction or evidence for progressive LV dilatation (*J Am Coll Cardiol* 1998;32:1512).

IV. **Mitral stenosis (MS)**

    A. MS is usually due to rheumatic heart disease, with other causes (congenital malformations, severe mitral annular calcification, atrial myxoma) occurring much less frequently.

    B. Clinical manifestations. MS in adults usually runs an indolent course, with significant symptoms occurring many years after an episode of acute rheumatic fever. Typical symptoms include fatigue and a gradual reduction in exercise tolerance. Cough, hemoptysis, exertional dyspnea, and peripheral edema tend to occur later in the course. Often the presenting manifestation is atrial fibrillation that is associated with pulmonary congestion. Physical findings include signs of left and right HF as well as evidence for pulmonary hypertension [right ventricular (RV) heave, accentuated P_2]. Cardiac auscultation reveals a loud first heart sound, an opening snap, and a rumbling diastolic murmur that is heard best at the apex. The chest x-ray often shows left atrial enlargement and evidence for chronic pulmonary congestion. ECG may reveal left atrial enlargement or atrial fibrillation and signs of RV hypertrophy (right axis deviation, increased right precordial R-wave voltage). Echocardiography is diagnostic in almost all cases and is useful in assessing the severity of MS and pulmonary hypertension, as well as for identifying associated valvular lesions. Cardiac catheterization with coronary angiography is indicated in older persons who are being considered for mitral valve surgery.

C. **Management.** Endocarditis prophylaxis is recommended (see Appendix H), and vigorous physical activity should be avoided in patients with moderate or severe MS. Daily antibiotic prophylaxis (e.g., with penicillin) against recurrent rheumatic fever is indicated for patients with a recent episode of rheumatic fever (within 5 years) and for those at high risk for streptococcal infection (school teachers, military personnel) (*J Am Coll Cardiol* 1998;32:1498). Warfarin is indicated in all patients with MS and intermittent or chronic atrial fibrillation, as well as in those with marked left atrial enlargement ($\geq$ 5.5–6.0 cm by echocardiography), demonstrated atrial thrombus, or a prior embolic event. Because atrial fibrillation is often poorly tolerated, consideration should be given to maintaining sinus rhythm with an antiarrhythmic agent such as flecainide, sotalol, or amiodarone. Diuretics are the mainstay of therapy for pulmonary and systemic venous congestion, and nitrates may provide additional symptomatic relief. Digoxin, β-adrenergic blockers, diltiazem, and verapamil are useful for controlling heart rate in patients with chronic atrial fibrillation. ACE inhibitors are indicated if there is LV systolic dysfunction or valvular insufficiency (MR or AI). Indications for percutaneous or surgical intervention include severe symptoms (New York Heart Association class III–IV) that are not responsive to medical therapy, severe pulmonary hypertension, and recurrent thromboembolic events. Percutaneous balloon mitral valvuloplasty and open mitral commissurotomy provide effective treatment for patients with severe MS in the absence of significant MR or advanced calcification of the mitral valve apparatus. Mitral valve replacement is appropriate for patients with severe MS who are not candidates for less invasive interventions.

V. **Mitral regurgitation (MR)**
A. **MR** is the most common clinically significant valvular lesion in adults. Common etiologies include myxomatous degeneration, ischemic heart disease with papillary muscle dysfunction, mitral valve annular calcification, rheumatic heart disease, endocarditis, and connective tissue disorders (e.g., Marfan's syndrome). MR may also occur as a consequence of LV dilatation, resulting in the inability of the mitral valve leaflets to coapt properly.

B. **Clinical manifestations.** MR may be acute, subacute, or chronic. Acute severe MR is usually due to ischemia, endocarditis, or rupture of a chordae tendineae. Patients with acute severe MR often present with pulmonary edema and incipient cardiogenic shock. The prognosis is poor unless the patient can be rapidly stabilized for prompt surgical intervention. Subacute MR usually occurs when an acute event, such as a ruptured chordae tendineae, is superimposed on chronic MR, resulting in symptomatic deterioration but with a less fulminant presentation than acute severe MR. Chronic MR is usually asymptomatic in mild to moderate cases with preserved LV systolic function. In more severe cases and in patients with impaired LV function, chronic MR presents with typical symptoms of HF, including orthopnea, edema, and exertional dyspnea and fatigue. In addition to signs of HF, physical examination reveals a holosystolic or mid to late systolic murmur that is best heard at the apex with radiation to the axilla. An S_3 gallop is often present in patients with LV systolic dysfunction and active HF. The chest x-ray reveals cardiomegaly, left atrial enlargement, and signs of volume overload. ECG findings are nonspecific but may include left atrial enlargement or atrial fibrillation, as well as evidence for LV or RV hypertrophy. Echocardiography with Doppler and color flow studies confirms the presence of MR and may provide information about the etiology. MR severity can be estimated and LV function quantified. Transesophageal echocardiography is particularly useful in elucidating mitral valve pathology.

C. **Management.** Prophylaxis against bacterial endocarditis is indicated for all patients with significant mitral valve pathology (see Appendix H). In patients with mild to moderate MR, vasodilators (ACE inhibitors, hydralazine, and nitrates), diuretics, and digoxin often provide effective symptom control. In addition, afterload reduction may slow disease progression and delay the need for surgery (*Am J Cardiol* 1998;82:242). Anticoagulation is indicated if atrial fibrillation is present. Patients with mild to moderate MR and preserved LV systolic function can be managed medically with close follow-up at 3- to 6-month intervals. Indications for surgery in patients with severe MR include New York Heart Association class II–III symptoms, mild to moderate LV dysfunction (even in the absence of symptoms), and progressive LV dilatation with an LV end-systolic dimension of 4.5 cm or greater (*J Am Coll Cardiol* 1998;32:1532). Patients with severe LV dysfunction tolerate mitral valve surgery poorly, and surgical intervention is contraindicated. When feasible, mitral valve repair is associated with more favorable hemodynamics and superior long-term clinical outcomes compared with valve replacement (*Circulation* 1995;91:1022).

VI. **Mitral valve prolapse (MVP)**

A. **MVP** occurs in 1–5% of the adult population and is approximately twice as common in women as in men, although men are more likely to require surgery for severe MR. The most common pathologic finding is myxomatous degeneration of the mitral valve apparatus, with elongation and redundancy of the chordae tendineae. MVP is the most common antecedent valvular abnormality in persons in whom infective endocarditis develops, and it is also the most common cause of chronic MR. In addition, MVP is an important cause of palpitations and nonspecific chest pain, and it may be associated with an increased risk of stroke and sudden cardiac death.

B. **Clinical manifestations.** Many individuals with MVP are asymptomatic, whereas others experience palpitations or nonspecific chest pain that may resemble angina pectoris. Less frequently, lightheadedness, syncope, embolic phenomena, or HF may occur. Physical findings include a midsystolic click and late systolic or holosystolic murmur. Chest radiography and ECG are often normal, but 24-hour ambulatory monitoring may reveal frequent atrial and ventricular premature depolarizations. Echocardiography demonstrates redundant mitral valve tissue with systolic prolapse of the mitral valve leaflets into the left atrium. In severe cases, ruptured chordae tendineae may be seen. MR, when present, ranges from minimal to severe. In persons with chest pain, stress testing may be necessary to evaluate for coronary artery disease.

C. **Management.** Endocarditis prophylaxis is recommended for persons with MVP that is associated with MR by physical examination or echocardiography, whether or not symptoms are present (see Appendix H). Mild symptoms should be treated with reassurance that MVP is rarely life threatening. For patients with moderate symptoms, beta-blockers are the treatment of choice. Verapamil or diltiazem may be beneficial in patients who are unable to tolerate beta-blockers. Infrequently, antiarrhythmic agents are necessary to control symptomatic arrhythmias. MR should be managed similarly to MR due to other causes (see sec. **V.C**).

VII. **Long-term surveillance**

A. Patients with mild to moderate VHD and stable symptoms and exercise tolerance should have routine follow-up physical examinations at 6- to 12-month intervals. Patients with severe symptoms or evidence for clinical deterioration should be evaluated more frequently. Echocardiography should be performed annually in patients with moderate or severe AI or MR to identify early signs of LV dysfunction or dilatation. Echocardiography is also appropriate in all patients with worsening symptoms, but routine serial echocardiograms are not indicated in patients with mild to moderate AS or MS, stable symptoms, and normal LV function. Similarly, serial echocardiograms are not necessary in patients with stable symptoms and physical findings following valve repair or replacement.

B. Anticoagulation. Patients with mechanical prosthetic heart valves require long-term anticoagulation with warfarin to maintain an INR of 2.5–3.5 (*Chest* 1998;114:602S). The addition of aspirin, 80–100 mg/day, reduces the risk of valve thrombosis and embolization at the expense of a small increase in bleeding risk (*Am Heart J* 1995;130:547). Most patients with mechanical prosthetic valves do not require heparin before elective surgery. Aspirin should be stopped 1 week before surgery and resumed as soon as possible after surgery. Warfarin should be stopped 72 hours before surgery and restarted on the day of surgery. Patients with mechanical valves and atrial fibrillation, prior thromboembolism, or both, are at increased risk for thromboembolic events when warfarin is discontinued. In such cases, warfarin should be stopped 72 hours before surgery, and intravenous heparin should be initiated to maintain an activated partial thromboplastin time of 1.5–2.5 times control until the day of operation. Following surgery, heparin and warfarin should be resumed as soon as possible, and heparin should be continued until the INR is 2.0 or greater. The use of low-molecular-weight heparins in the perioperative management of patients with prosthetic valves has not been evaluated and is not currently recommended. In most cases, it is not necessary to withhold warfarin before routine dental work or minor ophthalmologic procedures (e.g., cataract surgery).

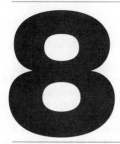

Cardiovascular III: Cardiac Arrhythmias

Benigno F. Decena and
Joseph M. Smith

I. **Role of the primary care physician (PCP).** With regard to the management of patients with cardiac arrhythmias, the emergence of radiofrequency catheter ablation and the development of nonthoracotomy transvenous pacemakers and internal cardioverter-defibrillators (ICDs) have shifted much of the emphasis of treatment to invasive procedures. However, the outpatient evaluation and treatment of arrhythmias remain critically important, and the PCP should continue to play an integral role in the management of those disorders. The PCP is often the first clinician to identify a rhythm abnormality. He or she then needs to determine the significance of the finding and decide what course of action to take. Perhaps most important, the PCP can help outline a long-term treatment strategy that incorporates a more intimate knowledge of the patient's overall condition and the patient's wishes. This chapter reviews cardiac arrhythmias, paying particular attention to aspects that are applicable to outpatient management.

II. **Recognition and diagnosis**
   A. **History and physical.** The patient history remains an important tool in the evaluation of patients with suspected cardiac arrhythmias. Although certain rhythm disorders are identified only as incidental findings, patients with clinically significant arrhythmias are typically symptomatic. Tachyarrhythmias may produce symptoms of palpitations, lightheadedness, dyspnea, angina, or syncope. Bradyarrhythmias are generally associated with exercise intolerance, fatigue, lightheadedness, or syncope. A history of familial or congenital causes of arrhythmias (e.g., Wolff-Parkinson-White syndrome, long QT syndrome, Brugada syndrome), a history of noncardiac diseases that potentiate rhythm abnormalities (e.g., endocrinopathies or inflammatory, infiltrative, or infectious processes), and symptoms of organic heart disease (e.g., ischemic, valvular) should be sought. A detailed history of the patient's medications (prescription, over-the-counter, and illicit drugs) must be obtained. Physical examination should emphasize pulse rate and regularity, BP, orthostatic changes, signs of organic heart disease (e.g., midsystolic click of mitral valve prolapse), or evidence of relevant systemic diseases. Serum electrolytes, CBC, serum levels of electrophysiologically active drugs, thyroid function tests, and toxicology studies should be considered in all patients under investigation for a suspected arrhythmia.
   B. **Available tests.** None of the symptoms described above are specific for rhythm disorders. Thus, with the exception of life-threatening arrhythmias, for which primary prevention in certain patient populations plays a clear role, therapy for suspected cardiac arrhythmias should not be initiated unless symptoms have been directly correlated with a rhythm disturbance. Depending on the frequency of symptoms, the clinician has several options to document temporally related arrhythmias.
      1. **A 12-lead ECG** should be obtained in all patients with suspected arrhythmias. When an ECG is obtained while the patient is having symptoms, the diagnosis is easily made. However, the patient's symptoms are frequently not present. In those instances, abnormalities on a

baseline ECG may offer important clues as to the etiology of the patient's symptoms. For example, a short PR interval and delta wave suggest ventricular pre-excitation, the substrate for Wolff-Parkinson-White syndrome. Left atrial abnormalities suggest a possible substrate for atrial fibrillation (AF). Q waves that are characteristic of myocardial infarction raise the question of ventricular tachycardia (VT). First-degree atrioventricular (AV) block or interventricular conduction delays may suggest possible causes of complete heart block.

2. **A continuous rhythm strip** is another simple, bedside test that can provide further insight regarding suspected arrhythmias. This type of monitoring can document (1) spontaneous changes in rhythm, rate, or morphology and (2) the response to interventions (e.g., vagal maneuvers, antiarrhythmic drug therapy).

3. **Holter monitoring** for 24–48 hours allows capture of symptomatic and asymptomatic arrhythmias. Holter monitoring is most useful when symptoms occur relatively frequently (i.e., daily). However, correlation of symptoms to rhythm disturbances requires the patient to keep an accurate diary during the recording.

4. **Transtelephonic electronic monitors** can be used for weeks to months in patients with relatively infrequent symptoms. These devices require manual activation by the patient (or witness) to record data. Most commonly, a **continuous-loop event recorder** is worn for extended periods and can record and save data that occurred before and after patient activation. Alternatively, smaller devices can be applied and activated at the time of symptoms but cannot record the onset of the arrhythmia. Lastly, an implantable, continuous-loop event recorder has become commercially available for patients with very infrequent symptoms.

5. **Head-up tilt-table testing** may be helpful in establishing a neurocardiogenic mechanism for syncope. After the patient is secured to a tilt table, the table is raised to an upright position (60–90 degrees) for periods ranging from 5 to 60 minutes. If passive testing alone is unsuccessful in eliciting a positive response, defined as reproduction of the patient's symptoms associated with a **cardioinhibitory** response (abrupt decrease in heart rate), a **vasodepressor** response (marked decrease in systolic BP), or both, chemical agents (isoproterenol or nitroglycerin) can be used to increase the likelihood of a positive response.

6. **Electrophysiologic studies** involve the placement of percutaneous, endocardial catheters to record intracardiac electrograms and to provide programmed electrical stimulation for the provocation and evaluation of tachyarrhythmias and bradyarrhythmias. Despite the invasive nature of this examination, it is often performed as an outpatient procedure with discharge the same day.

7. **Miscellaneous tests** that are designed to noninvasively assess the risk of sudden cardiac death from ventricular arrhythmias include (1) signal-averaged ECGs, (2) heart rate variability, (3) T-wave alternans, (4) QT dispersion, (5) body surface mapping, and (6) baroreceptor sensitivity. The exact role of these tests remains to be determined.

Mechanisms of Arrhythmia

I. **Premature complexes**, resulting from the depolarization of cardiac tissue earlier than would be predicted by the baseline rhythm, represent the most common disturbances of normal sinus rhythm. They may originate from any location in the heart, but **premature ventricular complexes (PVCs)** are more frequently seen than either **premature atrial complexes** or **premature junctional complexes**. Potential triggers include infection, inflammation, myocardial ischemia, drug toxicity, catecholamine excess, electrolyte imbalance, and excessive use of tobacco, alcohol, or caffeine. Patients may be asymptomatic or may complain of "skipped" beats that reflect the postextrasystolic beat rather than the premature beat. On ECG recordings, PVCs are manifest as premature and wide (i.e., >120 msec) QRS complexes with bizarre morphologies. Premature atrial complexes are recognized by early P waves with morphologies that are different than the sinus P wave. Premature junctional complexes result in premature, normally conducted QRS complexes without preceding P waves. A retrograde P wave may be seen just after the QRS. Asymptomatic premature complexes require no treatment, and initial therapy for symptomatic patients should be directed toward correction or removal of provocative stimuli. Regarding long-term prognosis, only PVCs have been correlated with future morbidity and mortality and only in a subset of patients who have survived acute myocardial infarction. Thus, treatment should be undertaken with great care. β-Adrenergic antagonists (beta-blockers) or calcium channel blockers (CCBs) may be useful, with a low incidence of side effects. However, treatment with antiarrhythmic agents to suppress premature complexes may be associated with significant adverse effects and should be reserved for severely symptomatic patients.

II. **Bradyarrhythmias** are defined as rhythms that result in a ventricular rate of less than 60 beats/minute (bpm). This definition does not distinguish between physiologic (e.g., endurance training) and pathologic etiologies of slow rhythms. It is important to remember that symptoms that are directly attributable to bradyarrhythmias or signs of hemodynamic compromise, or both, determine the need for treatment rather than the heart rate itself, because bradyarrhythmias are frequently asymptomatic. Two key points regarding the treatment of bradyarrhythmias are (1) no oral medication is currently available that can reliably increase the heart rate and (2) the only effective, long-term treatment for symptomatic bradycardia is permanent pacing. Additionally, acutely symptomatic patients and patients with hemodynamically unstable bradyarrhythmias should be considered critically ill and treated as recommended by current advanced cardiac life support (ACLS) protocols. Bradyarrhythmias can be divided into those due to sinus node dysfunction and those secondary to disturbances in AV conduction.

A. **Sinus node dysfunction**

1. **Sinus bradycardia** describes a bradyarrhythmia in which electrical activity originates from the sinus node region, the intrinsic pacemaker during normal conduction. ECGs demonstrate an atrial rate of less than 60 bpm with a normal P-wave configuration and axis. Primary sinus node disease (common with aging), increased vagal tone, antiarrhythmic drug therapy, hypothyroidism, and ischemia are typical etiologies. Asymptomatic sinus bradycardia is a common finding and in most cases requires no treatment. However, some patients experience excessive fatigue or CHF symptoms due to chronic sinus bradycardia or **chronotropic incompetence**, the inability to increase the sinus rate appropriately with increases in myocardial oxygen demand (e.g., exercise). In the absence of a reversible cause, symptomatic patients require permanent pacing.

2. **Sinus arrest (or pause) and sinoatrial (SA) exit block** are conditions that are recognized by a pause in the sinus rate. With sinus arrest, sinus node automaticity slows or ceases. SA exit block is due to conduction disturbances between the sinus node and atrial tissue. Transient sinus arrest or SA block may be asymptomatic if a stable escape rhythm is present. (Prolonged ventricular asystole reflects the lack of a reliable escape rhythm and implies conduction system disease distal to the sinus node.) Permanent pacing is recommended for symptomatic patients.

3. **Bradycardia-tachycardia (tachy-brady) syndrome**, characterized by the presence of supraventricular tachyarrhythmias and bradyarrhythmias, is the form of sinus node dysfunction that is most frequently associated with symptoms. Symptoms of bradycardia, including syncope, generally occur

with the marked pauses following termination of the tachycardia. Sinus node dysfunction and related symptoms are often exacerbated by medications prescribed for the associated tachyarrhythmia. Once again, treatment for symptomatic patients involves permanent pacing.

B. AV block occurs when an atrial impulse is conducted with delay or fails to conduct to the ventricle at a time when the ventricle should not be refractory. Delay or block can occur at any level of the AV conduction system (i.e., atria, AV node, His bundle, or His-Purkinje system).

1. **First-degree AV block**, or prolonged AV conduction, is defined as a PR interval greater than 200 msec. It usually results from delay within the AV node and can be due to intrinsic conduction system disease, increased vagal tone, antiarrhythmic drug therapy, electrolyte imbalances, ischemia, or infarction. It is usually asymptomatic, but may exacerbate CHF symptoms if marked delay affects AV synchrony. Symptomatic patients are treated with permanent pacing.

2. **Second-degree AV block**, or intermittent AV conduction, occurs when some atrial impulses are not conducted to the ventricle at a time when the ventricle should not be refractory. Two types of second-degree AV block are recognized.

   a. **Mobitz type I (Wenckebach) block** is characterized by progressive delay in AV conduction (and PR prolongation on ECG) before block. The site of block is almost always within the AV node. Etiologies include increased vagal tone, intrinsic conduction system disease, antiarrhythmic drug therapy, electrolyte abnormalities, and myocardial ischemia (typically in an inferior or posterior distribution). Mobitz I block, especially with a normal QRS, is benign and usually does not portend development of complete heart block. For persistent symptoms, permanent pacing is recommended.

   b. **Mobitz type II block** is characterized by AV conduction block without preceding conduction delay. The ECG reveals no change in the PR interval preceding a nonconducted P wave. The site of block is localized most often to the His-Purkinje system. Etiologies include intrinsic conduction system disease, antiarrhythmic drug therapy, myocardial ischemia (typically in an anterior distribution), and increased vagal tone. Mobitz II block, especially in the setting of bundle branch block, often precedes the development of complete heart block. Permanent pacing is recommended if symptoms are present.

   c. **2:1 AV block** may be either type I or type II. The concomitant presence of bundle branch block suggests a type II mechanism, and various maneuvers (e.g., carotid massage; atropine, 1 mg IV) may help distinguish the two. However, a precise diagnosis can only be made by intracardiac recordings during invasive electrophysiologic studies.

3. **Third-degree AV block (complete heart block)** is the failure of all conduction from the atria to the ventricles. This pattern is distinct from competitive **AV dissociation**, which is present when the ventricular rate exceeds the atrial rate. The site of block in complete AV block may be the AV node or within the His-Purkinje system. Etiologies of acquired complete AV block include ischemia or infarction, drug toxicity, idiopathic degeneration of the conduction system, infiltrative diseases (amyloidosis, sarcoidosis, metastatic disease), rheumatologic disorders (polymyositis, scleroderma, rheumatoid nodules), infectious diseases (Chagas' disease, Lyme disease), calcific aortic stenosis, or endocarditis. Symptoms depend on the presence and adequacy of the underlying escape rhythm. In the absence of a reversible cause, permanent pacing is indicated for acquired complete heart block. Asymptomatic patients with congenital complete heart block and significant bradycardia (i.e., <45 bpm) can be treated with permanent pacemaker implantation to prevent a malignant ventricular arrhythmia.

III. Tachyarrhythmias are defined as rhythms that result in a ventricular rate greater than 100 bpm. Symptoms may include palpitations, lightheadedness, angina, and syncope. Tachyarrhythmias can be classified by mechanism (i.e., re-entry, increased automaticity, or triggered activity), site of origin (i.e., supraventricular vs. ventricular), regularity (vs. irregularity), or width of the QRS complex (i.e., narrow complex or wide complex).

A. Regular narrow-complex tachycardias are almost exclusively supraventricular in origin. They encompass a diverse group of disorders, all of which typically have a 1:1 association between atrial and ventricular activation. A differential diagnosis can be generated on the basis of the **R-P interval**, the time interval between the peak of an R wave and the subsequent P wave during tachycardia.

1. **Short R-P tachycardias** have an R-P interval less than 50% of the R-R interval.

    a. **Typical AV nodal re-entrant tachycardia (AVNRT)** is the most common paroxysmal supraventricular tachycardia (PSVT). It is believed to be due to re-entry involving two distinct pathways (slow and fast) through the AV node. The ECG reveals a ventricular rate between 150 and 250 bpm with a retrograde P wave that is either obscured by or occurs at the end of the QRS complex. Vagal maneuvers alone (e.g., carotid massage, Valsalva) are often effective in terminating acute episodes. If unsuccessful, administration of adenosine (6–12 mg IV push) or diltiazem (15–20 mg IV over 2 minutes) can be used, although adenosine is preferred given its shorter half-life. Hospital admission is not required in the absence of persistent or associated symptoms. Chronic drug therapy with CCB or beta-blockers may be effective in decreasing the frequency of episodes, but radiofrequency catheter ablation can now obviate the need for such therapy.

    b. **Orthodromic AV reciprocating tachycardia (AVRT)**, the second most commonly observed PSVT, results from re-entry using an accessory pathway as the retrograde limb. In most instances, the accessory pathway is concealed (i.e., conducts only in the retrograde direction). Orthodromic AVRT typically occurs with ventricular rates of 150–250 bpm. A retrograde P wave may be seen at the end of the QRS complex (indistinguishable from AVNRT) or in the early part of the ST segment. Symptoms and therapy are similar to those outlined for AVNRT.

    c. **AV junctional tachycardia** is an uncommon rhythm in outpatient settings. It is likely due to increased automaticity within the AV node. On ECG, normal (baseline) QRS complexes are seen with a ventricular rate between 60 and 130 bpm. Retrograde P waves may be present; otherwise, AV dissociation may be seen. Therapy consists of correcting the underlying pathophysiologic process. Beta-blockers, phenytoin, or lidocaine may be effective, as may atrial overdrive pacing in patients with hemodynamic compromise.

2. **Long R-P tachycardias** have an R-P interval greater than 50% of the RR interval.

    a. **Sinus tachycardia** occurs when the sinus mechanism is accelerated and atrial activation is otherwise normal. Increased sympathetic or diminished vagal tone, catecholamine excess, pain, hypovolemia, hypoxemia, myocardial ischemia or infarction, pulmonary embolism, fever, and inflammation are common etiologies. The ECG is characterized by an atrial rate that is typically between 100 and 160 bpm, with normal P waves and a normal (baseline) QRS pattern. Therapy should be targeted at the underlying pathophysiologic process. Otherwise, beta-blockers can be used to slow the sinus rate, particularly in the setting of myocardial ischemia.

    b. **Atrial tachycardia** occurs when an ectopic focus, distinct from the sinus node, drives the atrial rate greater than 100 bpm. Uncommon in patients with structurally normal hearts, it is seen in patients with pulmonary disease, coronary artery disease, acute alcohol ingestion, or digitalis intoxication. The ECG typically reveals an atrial rate between 100 and 200 bpm with abnormal P waves. Therapy is targeted at the underlying pathophysiologic process. With the notable exception of suspected digitalis toxicity, CCBs, beta-blockers, or digitalis can be used to slow the ventricular rate. In refractory cases, antiarrhythmic drug therapy or radiofrequency catheter ablation can be considered. However, the success rate of radiofrequency ablation for atrial tachycardia is lower than that seen with either AVNRT or AVRT.

   c. **Atypical AVNRT** is an uncommon cause of PSVT. Symptoms and therapy are similar to those for typical AVNRT. However, unlike the situation seen in typical AVNRT, antegrade conduction occurs over the fast pathway and retrograde conduction occurs over the slow pathway.

   d. **AVRT using a slowly conducting accessory pathway** is another uncommon type of long R-P, narrow-complex tachycardia. Unlike most accessory pathways, which conduct in an all-or-none fashion, slowly conducting accessory pathways behave similarly to the AV node, exhibiting decremental conduction as the rate of activation increases. Clinically, this is typically manifest as an incessant tachycardia, **permanent junctional reciprocating tachycardia**, in young patients. Pharmacologic therapy is often ineffective, but radiofrequency ablation provides a potential cure.

B. **Irregular, narrow-complex tachycardias** include AF, atrial flutter, and multifocal tachycardia.

   1. **AF** is the most common sustained tachyarrhythmia. It is often associated with structural heart disease (e.g., valvular, hypertensive, and ischemic) but can occur in patients with structurally normal hearts ("lone AF"). Transient or reversible etiologies include hypertension, acute alcohol ingestion, theophylline or other stimulant toxicity, endocrinopathies (hypothyroidism, hyperthyroidism, pheochromocytoma), pericarditis, and myocardial infarction. Patients may or may not be symptomatic, but importantly, symptoms generally reflect the heart rate rather than the irregularity of the rhythm, and most patients with paroxysmal AF cannot reliably distinguish AF from sinus rhythm. On the ECG, a fluctuating baseline with indistinguishable atrial activity and an irregular ventricular response are hallmarks of AF. AF may occur and resolve spontaneously (paroxysmal), it may require intervention for termination (persistent), or it may frustrate all attempts at management (permanent or chronic). Regardless of the pattern, thromboembolic phenomena, including strokes, are potential complications. The optimal treatment strategy for AF has not yet been determined, but management must emphasize reducing the risk of thromboembolism and the frequency and severity of symptoms. Once again, acutely ill patients should be treated as outlined by ACLS protocols.

      a. **Anticoagulation.** With the exception of patients who are successfully converted to normal sinus rhythm from their first episode of AF, therapy to reduce the risk of thromboembolism is indicated in all patients with AF. Factors that are associated with an increased risk of cerebrovascular accident include (1) prior transient ischemic attack, (2) valvular heart disease, (3) CHF, (4) hypertension, (5) diabetes, (6) age greater than 75 years, and (7) coronary artery disease. Patients with any of these risk factors should be treated with chronic warfarin anticoagulation, with the goal of maintaining an international normalized ratio (INR) level between 2.0 and 3.0. If warfarin is contraindicated, aspirin (325 mg qd) should be given. If the patient is aspirin intolerant, clopidogrel (75 mg qd) or ticlopidine (250 mg bid) can be used. The need for anticoagulation and the role of aspirin are controversial in patients who are younger than 65 years without risk factors because of the low rate of strokes in this population. In patients with newly diagnosed AF, anticoagulation can be safely initiated on an outpatient basis provided that careful follow-up of INR levels is available.

b. **Rate control** in AF can be achieved with CCBs, beta-blockers, or digoxin. Diltiazem (30 mg qid) and metoprolol (25 mg bid) are equally reasonable options for initial therapy depending on comorbid conditions. Although digoxin is generally less efficacious and may predispose to recurrence of AF, it may be the only agent that is tolerated in patients with left ventricular systolic dysfunction.

c. **Cardioversion.** Restoration of sinus rhythm can be accomplished either electrically (DC current) or pharmacologically, but chemical cardioversion with class IA (quinidine or procainamide), class IC (i.e., propafenone or flecainide) or class III (amiodarone, sotalol, ibutilide, or dofetilide) antiarrhythmic agents is clearly less effective than DC cardioversion. Before proceeding with either method, one must consider the potential for a thromboembolic event. If AF has persisted longer than 48 hours, patients should be anticoagulated, with documentation of therapeutic INRs for at least 3 weeks before any attempt is made. The use of transesophageal echocardiography to shorten the duration of anticoagulation therapy is discussed in Related Topics, sec. **I.A.** Regardless, therapeutic warfarin should be continued for at least 3 weeks after the cardioversion.

d. **Maintenance of sinus rhythm.** The use of long-term antiarrhythmic therapy to prevent the recurrence of AF is controversial. Antiarrhythmic agents (classes IA, IC, and III) are modestly effective but have not been shown to reduce stroke risk or to reduce overall mortality. In addition, each is associated with potential side effects, some of which may be life threatening (i.e., proarrhythmia). As a result, the use of antiarrhythmic drugs should be reserved for patients with highly symptomatic AF, and these patients should be admitted for initiation or adjustment of therapy.

e. **Refractory AF.** Despite repeated attempts to convert AF or maintain sinus rhythm, or both, some patients continue to experience frequent paroxysms of AF or remain in chronic AF. If the patient is asymptomatic, it is reasonable to treat only with anticoagulation and rate control. However, patients with poorly tolerated refractory AF should be referred to specialists for consideration of more invasive treatment options, which include catheter ablation of the AV node with pacemaker implantation, the Maze surgical procedure, and, in a subset of patients with frequent episodes of AF, catheter ablation.

2. **Atrial flutter** results from re-entrant circuits around functional or structural barriers within the atria. It is seen more commonly in patients with structural heart disease. In typical (type I) flutter, the 12-lead ECG has a characteristic "sawtooth" pattern that is apparent in the inferior leads (II, III, avF), with an effective atrial rate of 280–350 bpm. Atypical (type II) flutter lacks the characteristic sawtooth pattern of typical flutter and may reach atrial rates of up to 420 bpm. In either case, the ventricular response may be regular (e.g., 2:1 AV block) or variable. The goals of therapy for atrial flutter are identical to those for AF. However, because of the differences in mechanisms between the disorders, two important distinctions with regard to management must be made.

a. **Overdrive atrial pace-termination** of atrial flutter can be attempted as a substitute for DC or chemical cardioversion, particularly in patients with temporary or permanent pacemakers.

b. **Radiofrequency catheter ablation** is another alternative to restore and maintain sinus rhythm. It is particularly effective for patients with typical atrial flutter. A successful ablation is considered a cure and obviates the need for further antiarrhythmic therapy.

3. **Multifocal atrial tachycardia** is an irregular supraventricular tachycardia (SVT) associated with hypoxemic states (i.e., chronic obstructive pulmonary disease and CHF) and can be potentiated by concomitant therapy with theophylline. It is diagnosed when three or more distinct P-wave morphologies are recorded on a single ECG. Therapy is targeted at treatment of the underlying pathophysiologic process.

C. **Wide-complex tachycardias** may be either supraventricular or ventricular in origin, and correct diagnosis is critical to the selection of appropriate treatment. Given the high risk of sudden death with ventricular arrhythmias, **all wide-complex tachycardias should be considered life threatening and treated accordingly,** as per ACLS protocols, until proven otherwise.

1. **SVT with aberration.** Any typically "narrow-complex" tachycardia can present with wide QRS complexes as a result of fixed intraventricular conduction defects (right bundle branch block, left bundle branch block) or rate-dependent conduction block.

2. **SVT with ventricular pre-excitation.** Although most accessory pathways are concealed, some may conduct in the antegrade direction. These accessory pathways provide alternate, typically more rapid routes for atrial activity to reach the ventricles. The resultant ventricular pre-excitation is manifest on the ECG as a delta wave and a short PR interval. **Wolff-Parkinson-White syndrome** describes tachycardias using an accessory pathway for antegrade conduction.

   a. **Pre-excited AF**, though uncommon, is important to recognize because of its association with malignant ventricular arrhythmias. Although AF is not, in general, a life-threatening rhythm, it may, in combination with a manifest accessory pathway, predispose toward ventricular fibrillation (VF). The ECG of pre-excited AF is characterized by an irregularly undulating baseline without recognizable P waves, an irregular rapid ventricular rate (180–300 bpm), and varying QRS complex morphologies. Pre-excited AF should be treated emergently with intravenous procainamide or electrical cardioversion as soon as is feasible. AV nodal-blocking agents, particularly CCBs and digoxin, must be avoided, as they can increase the ventricular rate and initiate VF. Options for chronic treatment include radiofrequency ablation or antiarrhythmic drug therapy with class IA, IC, or III agents.

   b. **Antidromic AVRT** descibes a re-entrant rhythm in which antegrade conduction occurs over the accessory pathway and retrograde conduction occurs through the specialized conduction system. Clinically, it is similar to orthodromic AVRT, except that the ECG reveals a regular, wide-complex tachycardia, which may be difficult to distinguish from VT. Once a correct diagnosis is made, acute therapy is the same as that for orthodromic AVRT (i.e., vagal maneuvers, adenosine). The choice of chronic therapy, on the other hand, depends on the perceived risk of developing AF and sudden death. If the risk is believed to be low, beta-blockers or diltiazem can be used. Otherwise, antidromic AVRT should be treated similarly to pre-excited AF.

3. **Accelerated idioventricular rhythm** is an uncommon arrhythmia in the outpatient setting. It is generally associated with myocardial infarction or digitalis toxicity. The ECG reveals a ventricular rate of 60–110 bpm, usually exceeding the spontaneous atrial rate. The QRS complex is wide and bizarre. Accelerated idioventricular rhythm is usually transient and asymptomatic but can cause hemodynamic deterioration in patients who require AV synchrony. In symptomatic patients, therapy is directed at increasing the sinus rate (e.g., atropine, isoproterenol, atrial pacing).

4. **VT** is defined as a series of three or more ventricular complexes that occur at a rate greater than 100 bpm. VT can be characterized as sus-

tained (i.e., longer than 30 seconds) versus nonsustained or monomorphic (a single QRS morphology throughout the arrhythmia) versus polymorphic (characterized by an ever-changing QRS morphology).

  a. **Sustained VT** requires prompt recognition and acute treatment as outlined by ACLS protocols due to the risk of hemodynamic collapse and cardiac arrest. Further evaluation should be performed in a hospital setting. A small subset of patients with sustained VT has a structurally normal heart (idiopathic VT). This condition is associated with a benign course, and treatment options include beta-blockers, CCBs, and radiofrequency ablation.

  b. **Nonsustained VT**, although commonly asymptomatic, warrants further investigation in certain patient populations. More specifically, patients with coronary artery disease and an ischemic cardiomyopathy (i.e., ejection fraction <40%), who have documented nonsustained VT, should undergo electrophysiologic studies to determine their risk of sudden cardiac death (*N Engl J Med* 1996;335:1933).

  5. **VF** is invariably associated with cardiac arrest and requires immediate defibrillation for survival. It is not addressed in this chapter.

IV. **Miscellaneous electrocardiographic abnormalities.** Several findings on the ECG of an asymptomatic patient should raise a clinician's suspicion and warrant further investigation.

  A. **Ventricular pre-excitation** has been discussed in detail with respect to its role in **Wolff-Parkinson-White syndrome**. However, evidence of pre-excitation (i.e., a delta wave and a short PR interval) may be found incidentally in asymptomatic individuals. In these patients, observation alone is a reasonable approach. However, the ability of the pathway to conduct 1:1 to the ventricles at very rapid rates (i.e., >240 bpm) suggests a higher risk of VF in patients who are already at risk of AF. An exercise stress test to evaluate accessory pathway conduction at increased rates has been advocated to distinguish high-risk from low-risk patients.

  B. **Long QT syndrome** describes two broad groups of disorders characterized by the ECG finding of a prolonged corrected QT interval (QTc) and an association with torsades de pointes (TdP), a form of polymorphic VT. TdP is recognized by QRS complexes of changing amplitude and axis that appear to twist around the isoelectric line at rates of 200–250 bpm. Therapy for sustained TdP is immediate DC cardioversion.

  1. **Congenital long QT syndromes** comprise a group of inherited genetic disorders that affect cell membrane ion channels. A family history of sudden cardiac death and a prolonged QTc (i.e., >440 msec) on a 12-lead ECG are suggestive of congenital long QT syndrome. No consensus has been reached regarding the optimal treatment for these patients, but beta-blocker therapy and surgical unilateral sympathectomy have been shown to decrease the mortality in this syndrome. Permanent pacemakers or ICDs, or both, may also be effective in selected patients.

  2. **Acquired long QT syndrome.** A variety of influences can prolong the QT interval in patients who do not have the congenital long QT syndrome and, thereby, promote TdP. Factors that have been associated with aquired long QT syndrome include electrolyte abnormalities (hypokalemia, hypomagnesemia, and, rarely, hypocalcemia), drugs (Table 8-1), cardiac disease (ischemia or myocarditis), bradycardia, CNS disease (intracranial trauma, subarachnoid hemorrhage, or cerebrovascular accident), or toxic exposures (organophosphate poisoning, cesium). Once a prolonged QTc is identified, a cause should be sought immediately. Patients who have had an episode of TdP or in whom the QTc is greater than 500 msec should be admitted for evaluation and treatment.

  3. **Brugada syndrome** is a clinical entity that is characterized by a typical ECG pattern (ST-segment elevation in lead V1 and V2, often with a

Table 8-1. Drugs associated with torsades de pointes

Amiodarone	Encainide	Pentamidine
Amitriptyline	Erythromycin	Perhexiline
Arsenic	FK506	Prenylamine
Astemizole	Flecainide	Probucol
Bepridil	Haloperidol	Procainamide
Bretylium	Ibutilide	Propafenone
Chlorpromazine	Imipramine	Quinidine
Cisapride	Indapamide	Quinine
Cocaine	Itraconazole	Sotalol
Disopyramide	Ketanserin	Sparfloxacin
Dofetilide	Ketoconazole	Sultopride
Doxepin	Maprotiline	Terfenadine
Droperidol	Moricizine	Terodiline
		Thioridazine

right bundle branch block pattern) and sudden cardiac death. The syndrome, which has been linked to a genetic defect, is associated with a very poor prognosis. Recognition of this ECG finding should warrant immediate evaluation by a specialist for the need for an ICD.

Antiarrhythmic Drug Therapy

 I. Many pharmacologic agents are commercially available for the treatment of cardiac arrhythmias.
 II. The **Vaughan-Williams classification** describes four classes, based on the drugs' mechanism of action. Class I agents inhibit the fast sodium channel, class II agents are beta-blockers, class III agents primarily block potassium channels, and class IV agents are CCBs, but specific drugs may have actions that span multiple classes. Class II and IV agents are commonly used medications for the treatment of hypertension, angina pectoris, and, in the case of β-adrenergic antagonists, myocardial infarction. As previously mentioned, drugs in these two classes can be used to suppress premature complexes, control the ventricular rate of AF and atrial flutter, or terminate and prevent recurrences of re-entrant forms of SVT. However, in general practice, the term **antiarrhythmic drugs** more often refers to class I and III agents that are used solely for the treatment of recurrent symptomatic ventricular arrhythmias or refractory SVTs, or both. They are associated with significant side effect profiles, including a risk, with certain agents, of proarrhythmia, defined as the exacerbation of a rhythm disturbance or the initiation of a potentially life-threatening arrhythmia. Because of these side effects, patients should be admitted for continuous ECG monitoring during the initiation and titration of class I and III agents. PCPs will have some patients taking antiarrhythmic drugs, and they should be familiar with their indications, usual doses, side effects, and important drug interactions. These are listed in Table 8-2.

Table 8-2. Antiarrhythmic drugs commonly used in the outpatient setting

Drug	Indications	Maintenance doses (oral)	Common side effects	Drug interactions
IA				
Quinidine	PACs, PVCs, AF, PSVT, VT, VF	Sulfate, 200–400 mg q6h Polygalacturonate, 275–550 mg q8–12h Gluconate, 324–648 mg q8–12h	Nausea, vomiting, diarrhea, rash, cinchonism (↓ hearing, tinnitus, blurred vision), ↓ platelets, hemolytic anemia, proarrhythmia (VT/VF)	Digoxin, warfarin, propranolol, metoprolol, propafenone, heparin, verapamil, cimetidine, amiodarone, phenobarbital, phenytoin, rifampin, nifedipine
Procainamide	PACs, PVCs, AF, PSVT, VT, VF	2–4 g/day in divided doses	Nausea, vomiting, diarrhea, rash, fever, Raynaud's phenomenon, agranulocytosis, depression, psychosis, lupus syndrome, proarrhythmia	Cimetidine, aminoglycosides, alcohol, amiodarone, trimethoprim
Disopyramide	PACs, PVCs, AF, PSVT, VT, VF; neurocardiogenic syncope	100–300 mg q6–8h	Anticholinergic effects (dry mouth, blurred vision, constipation, urinary retention), hypoglycemia, nausea, vomiting, rash, jaundice, agranulocytosis, proarrhythmia	Phenobarbital, phenytoin, rifampin, β-adrenergic antagonists, erythromycin
IB				
Mexiletine	VT, VF, congenital long QT syndrome	200 mg q8h	Nausea, vomiting, tremor, dizziness, blurred vision, proarrhythmia	Phenytoin, phenobarbital, rifampin, cimetidine, chloramphenicol, isoniazid, theophylline
IC				
Flecainide	AF, A-Flutter, PSVT	100–200 mg q12h	Conduction abnormalities, proarrhythmia, CHF exacerbation, confusion, irritability, blurred vision, dizziness, nausea, headache	Digoxin, amiodarone, cimetidine, propranolol, quinidine

148

Propafenone	AF, A-Flutter, PSVT	150–300 mg q8h	Nausea, dizziness, metallic taste, blurred vision, paresthesias, constipation, increased LFTs, asthma exacerbations, conduction abnormalities, proarrhythmia	Digoxin, warfarin, propranolol, metoprolol, theophylline, cyclosporine, desipramine, phenytoin, phenobarbital, rifampin, quinidine, cimetidine
III				
Amiodarone	VT, VF, AF, A-Flutter	200–400 mg/day	Dry cough, dyspnea, photosensitivity (blue-gray skin discoloration), hypo- and hyperthyroidism, corneal deposits, nausea, anorexia, ↑ LFTs, proarrhythmia	Digoxin, warfarin, cyclosporine
Sotalol	VT, VF, AF, A-Flutter	80–240 mg q12h	Fatigue, proarrhythmia, bradyarrhythmias, bronchospasm, CHF exacerbation	β-Adrenergic antagonists
Dofetilide	AF, A-Flutter	125–500 μg q12h	Proarrhythmia	Verapamil, cimetidine, ketoconazole, trimethoprim-sulfamethoxazole, megesterol, prochlorperazine

AF, atrial fibrillation; A-Flutter, atrial flutter; LFTs, liver function tests; PACs, premature atrial complexes; PSVT, paroxysmal supraventricular tachycardia; PVCs, premature ventricular complexes; VF, ventricular fibrillation; VT, ventricular tachycardia.

Related Topics

I. **Electrocardioversion.** Synchronized DC cardioversion is successful in restoring sinus rhythm in more than 90% of patients with recent-onset atrial flutter, AF, re-entrant SVTs, and VT. Although symptomatic or hemodynamically unstable tachyarrhythmias require immediate treatment, DC cardioversion can be performed electively on an outpatient basis in patients with well-tolerated dysrhythmias, particularly AF and atrial flutter. Indeed, DC cardioversion is often the initial therapy. However, it must be made clear that cardioversion is capable only of restoring but **not maintaining** sinus rhythm. Failure to convert to sinus or early/immediate recurrence of the dysrhythmia indicates a need for antiarrhythmic drug therapy depending on the clinical scenario.

   A. **Technique.** Elective cardioversions are performed in a hospital setting. Patients with either AF or flutter of greater than 48 hours' duration should be anticoagulated with warfarin (INR 2.0–3.0) for at least 3 weeks. An alternative, although still controversial, approach involves the use of transesophageal echocardiography to exclude the presence of left atrial thrombus or spontaneous echo contrast (i.e., "smoke") to minimize the duration of anticoagulation preceding the cardioversion (*N Engl J Med* 2001;344:1411–1420). In patients who are successfully cardioverted from AF or flutter, anticoagulation should be continued for 3–4 weeks after the procedure.

   B. **Contraindications.** Cardioversion is relatively contraindicated in certain circumstances.

      1. **Digoxin toxicity.** If digoxin toxicity is known or suspected, elective cardioversion should be deferred.

      2. **Repetitive, short-lived tachycardias.** These disorders should not be treated with cardioversion, as their recurrence demonstrates an abnormal substrate that requires pharmacologic manipulation.

      3. **Multifocal atrial tachycardia** or other automatic arrhythmias.

      4. **Hyperthyroidism.** Patients should be functionally euthyroid before elective cardioversion to limit the likelihood of recurrence.

   C. **Adverse effects.** DC cardioversion rarely produces adverse effects. Sinus pauses and atrial, junctional, or ventricular ectopic beats may occur transiently after restoration of sinus rhythm, especially in patients with longstanding AF and a slow ventricular response. Serious arrhythmias, such as VT, VF, or asystole, are rare. Thromboembolic events are uncommon if appropriate anticoagulation has been achieved. Muscle pain and irritation of the skin at the paddle site may occur.

II. **Permanent pacemakers** are the only reliable, long-term treatment option for patients with symptomatic bradycardia or those at high risk of progression to complete heart block. Although patients with pacemakers should be followed by specialists, at times such follow-up is not available. Additionally, questions regarding permanent pacing often arise when patients are being evaluated for unrelated problems. Thus, it is important that the PCP have some understanding of pacemaker function. Unfortunately, as technology improves and pacemakers more closely mimic normal cardiac physiology, it becomes more difficult to differentiate normal and abnormal function. Adding to the difficulty is the lack of a uniform standard between the various pacemaker manufacturers. Accordingly, the single most important pieces of historical information that a clinician can obtain from a patient with a permanent pacemaker is the name of the manufacturer of the pacemaker. Once this is known, the device can be interrogated using the appropriate programmer, and an assessment of device function can be readily made.

   A. **Pacing modalities.** On a basic level, pacemakers do only two things, sense intrinsic electrical activity or discharge pulses of electrical current to stimulate the myocardium. Both of these functions can be performed in the right atrium or the right ventricle, or both. (Protocols are currently evaluating the role of left ventricular pacing via the coronary sinus.) Based on the number of implanted leads, various configurations are possible. A five-letter alphabetic code has been used to identify the various ways in which a permanent pacemaker can be programmed. The first initial defines which chambers can be paced (**V**entricular, **A**trial, or **D**ual). The second initial identifies the chambers in which electrograms are sensed (**V**, **A**, or **D**). The third indicates the pacemaker's response to a sensed event [**I**nhibition of electrical stimulus, **T**riggering of electrical stimulus (typically used to assess sensing function), or **D**ual (allows AV sequential pacing)]. The fourth initial is used primarily to denote rate-responsive mode and is represented by the letter **R** when present. The fifth initial applies only to devices with anti-tachycardia functions (i.e., ICDs) and includes antitachycardia **P**acing, **S**hocks, or **D**ual functions. The most commonly used modes are DDD/DDDR and VVI/VVIR. DDD pacemakers sense and pace in the atrium and the ventricle. A sensed atrial event inhibits the atrial stimulus and triggers a ventricular response after a programmed AV interval. A sensed ventricular event inhibits ventricular and atrial stimuli and resets the atrial timer. This mode allows maintenance of normal AV sequential activation with either sinus or paced atrial rhythms. VVI pacemakers sense and pace only in the ventricle. A sensed ventricular event inhibits the ventricular stimulus. This mode is preferred in patients in whom AV synchrony is not required or is contraindicated (i.e., chronic AF). Newer dual-chamber models have a mode-switching feature, in which the pacing mode can be changed automatically when the atrial rate increases abruptly (e.g., DDD to DDI with paroxysmal AF). Rate responsiveness allows the pacemaker to adjust its lower rate limit, depending on input from various sensors (e.g., acceleration, QT interval, ventricular impedance, thoracic impedance, and temperature).

B. Assessing pacemaker function. It is difficult to confirm pacemaker malfunction without knowing what type of device is implanted and how it is programmed. It therefore behooves any clinician who is managing a patient with a pacemaker to keep records of the patient's device, including, at a minimum, the manufacturer, the programmed mode, and the lower rate limit. In the absence of this information, some useful data can still be derived from an ECG provided that the patient is being paced at least occasionally (i.e., if the patient's intrinsic rate is greater than the programmed lower rate limit, neither sensing nor pacing functioning can be assessed). One can determine if the pacemaker is a single- or dual-chamber device by the presence of atrial or ventricular pacing signals, or both. The lower rate limit can be determined by measuring the interval between consecutive ventricular pacing signals (in VVI mode) or between atrial pacing signals (in dual-chamber or AAI modes). Failure to capture is characterized by the presence of a pacing spike that is not associated with an appropriate P-wave or QRS complex at a time when the respective chamber should not be refractory. For example, a ventricular pacing spike that occurs simultaneously or shortly after the QRS complex (i.e., with a PVC) would not be expected to activate the ventricle. Failure to sense is characterized by a pacing spike that occurs earlier than would be expected based on the programmed, lower rate limit. In addition to a lower rate limit, dual-chamber devices have upper tracking rate limits above which the ventricle will not pace 1:1 with intrinsic atrial rates. Further discussion of normal and abnormal pacemaker function is beyond the scope of this chapter, and more specific questions should be referred to a specialist. However, if the ability to capture must be known, a magnet placed over the device itself results in a transient mode switch to asynchronous pacing (i.e., no inhibition by sensed activity).

C. Complications associated with permanent pacing
   1. **Pacemaker syndrome** is the name given to a variety of symptomatic manifestations (e.g., fatigue, dizziness, syncope), referable most often to the loss of AV synchrony during single-chamber ventricular pacing or, less

commonly, alterations in AV timing or contractility during dual-chamber pacing. The mainstays of therapy are revision of the existing system into a dual-chamber system or optimization of the existing device's timing.

2. **Pacemaker-mediated tachycardia (PMT)** occurs in dual-chamber pacemakers that are programmed to DDD mode when a ventricular depolarization (usually a PVC) results in retrograde atrial activation that is sensed by the atrial lead, resulting in a subsequent paced ventricular depolarization. The paced ventricular beat then reinitiates the same sequence, resulting in an incessant A-sensed, V-paced rhythm at or near the programmed upper rate limit of the pacemaker. Although vagal maneuvers (transient interruption of retrograde AV nodal conduction) occasionally terminate PMT, application of a pacemaker magnet is always successful. PMT can be prevented in newer devices by specific programming algorithms.

3. **Infection** of the pacing system hardware is an uncommon complication of implanted pacemakers with potentially devastating consequences (i.e., endocarditis). Although prophylactic antibiotics are not routinely recommended before high-risk procedures (e.g., dental procedures), a high degree of suspicion must be maintained when evaluating patients with pacemakers (see Appendix H). Persistent or recurrent bacteremia should raise the question of an infected lead or generator pocket. When infection is diagnosed, explantation of the pacing system is usually required.

4. **Electromagnetic interference (EMI)** can affect pacemaker functioning, resulting in either inhibition of pacing or reprogramming of the parameters. If sources of EMI cannot be avoided, it is often necessary to make adjustments before the time of exposure. Examples of EMI that are commonly encountered in hospitals include electrocautery, magnetic resonance imaging, radiofrequency catheter ablation, electroshock therapy, and lithotripsy. Nonhospital sources of EMI include heavy motors, arc welding, digital cellular phones (in very close proximity to the generator), and antitheft devices.

III. **ICDs** are implantable devices similar to permanent pacemakers that are also able to recognize and treat life-threatening ventricular arrhythmias. They are capable of tiered therapy, including (1) bradycardia pacing, (2) antitachycardia pacing, (3) low-energy cardioversion for stable VT, and (4) high-energy cardioversion for VT or VF. Studies have confirmed the efficacy of ICDs for primary and secondary prevention of sudden cardiac death. Accordingly, ICDs are becoming increasingly prevalent in the general population and patients with ICDs are seen in practice by PCPs. However, even more so than patients with pacemakers, patients with ICDs must be closely followed by physicians who are specially trained to do so. All questions regarding normal or abnormal functioning of an ICD should be immediately referred directly to a specialist, particularly when a patient is shocked by the device. Inappropriate shocks (in response to SVTs or ICD malfunction) in some series account for up to 30% of shocks and cannot be differentiated from appropriate therapy without analyzing electrograms recorded during the episode. Various programmable features have been developed to minimize inappropriate shocks. These mechanisms are beyond the scope of this chapter, but the generalist should be aware that patients with ICDs should avoid sources of EMI, such as those described previously for patients with pacemakers (see sec. **II.C.4**).

Syncope

I. **Syncope**, defined as the transient loss of consiousness and postural tone, is a very common clinical problem. Although syncopal spells may be benign, they may also indicate otherwise unsuspected, potentially lethal, cardiac conditions. Therefore, a careful evaluation to exclude life-threatening causes must be undertaken, particularly after unheralded syncope and syncope associated with significant injury to the patient.

II. **Etiologies** of syncope are myriad and can be divided into primary cardiac and noncardiac mechanisms. Primary cardiac syncope is caused either by mechanical obstruction of cardiac output (e.g., hypertrophic cardiomyopathy, valvular stenosis, aortic dissection, myxomas, pulmonary embolism) or by arrhythmias, including bradyarrhythmias (e.g., sinus node disease, AV node disease, conduction system disease, pacemaker malfunction) or tachyarrhythmias, including VT or, rarely, SVT. Noncardiac mechanisms include **neurocardiogenic syncope**, orthostatic hypotension, toxic or metabolic influences (e.g., drug toxicities, hypoglycemia, hypoxia, etc.), neurologic etiologies (e.g., seizures or cerebrovascular events), and psychiatric etiologies (e.g., conversion disorders and anxiety disorders). Neurocardiogenic syncope, also called **vasovagal syncope**, is the most common cause of syncope, particularly in patients without underlying heart disease. Stimulation of a variety of afferent neural pathways results in peripheral vasodilatation or bradycardia, or both, leading to hypotension and syncope. Specific stimuli may evoke the neurocardiogenic mechanism, leading to a situational syncope (e.g., associated with micturition, defecation, coughing, swallowing).

III. **History and physical examination.** The clinical history and physical examination have the highest utility for identifying a potential mechanism of syncope. In addition to a careful interview of the patient, historical details should be obtained from witnesses and emergency medical services personnel. Special attention should focus on the events or symptoms preceding and following the syncopal event, the time course of loss and resumption of consciousness (abrupt vs. gradual), and any description of vital signs before, during, and after the event. A characteristic prodrome of nausea, diaphoresis, or flushing preceding loss of consciousness suggests neurocardiogenic syncope, as does the identification of a particular emotional or situational trigger or a postsyncopal sensation of fatigue that lasts for many minutes to hours. Alternatively, an unusual sensory prodrome, incontinence, or a decreased level of consciousness that gradually clears suggests a seizure as a likely etiology. With transient ventricular arrhythmias, an abrupt loss of consciousness may occur with a rapid recovery. A clear history of palpitations is elicited infrequently. Physical examination should include assessment of orthostatic vital signs and careful neurologic, pulmonary, and cardiovascular assessment. Bedside manipulations may be useful, including Valsalva maneuvers and squatting, with attention to cardiac auscultatory findings to detect valvular and subvalvular lesions. In patients with a clinical history that is suggestive of carotid sinus hypersensitivity (e.g., syncope with turning the head), carotid sinus massage can be performed.

IV. **Diagnostic testing.** A 12-lead ECG and ECG monitoring (Holter or transtelephonic, or both) lead to a diagnosis in fewer than 10% of cases. Routine laboratory tests typically are generally unhelpful, but toxicology screening should be performed if illicit drug use or inadvertent drug exposure is suspected. Echocardiograms should be performed in patients in whom history or physical examination suggests structural heart disease. Invasive electrophysiologic studies are most useful in patients with structural heart disease or with documented tachyarrhythmias. Head-up tilt-table testing may be helpful in confirming a clinical diagnosis of neurocardiogenic syncope in patients with structurally normal hearts. Routine CT scans or EEGs, or both, in unselected patients with syncope are not supported by available data. A psychiatric evaluation should be considered in patients with frequent unexplained episodes.

V. **Therapy.** Appropriate therapy for patients with syncope is determined by the underlying etiology. In cases of suspected neurocardiogenic syncope, empiric therapy can be targeted at various aspects of the physiologic response.

Treatment can be targeted at minimizing the impact of peripheral vasodilatation by the use of support stockings or volume expansion with fludrocortisone. Beta-blockers may be useful to block peripheral adrenergic-mediated vasodilatation and to decrease cardiac inotropy. Disopyramide may be useful, probably through its strong negative inotropic action, reducing stimulation of ventricular mechanoreceptors, to prevent neurocardiogenic syncope. Centrally acting agents such as serotonin-reuptake inhibitors or yohimbine may be useful in attenuating central reflex centers that are involved in neurocardiogenic mechanisms. Permanent dual-chamber pacemakers with a hysteresis function (high rate pacing in response to a detected sudden drop in pulse rate) have been shown to be useful in highly selected patients with recurrent neurocardiogenic syncope who have a prominent cardioinhibitory component.

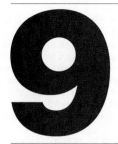

Vascular Disease and Antithrombotic Therapy

Brian S. Gage and
Roger D. Yusen

I. Arterial disease and arterial embolism
A. Atrial fibrillation (AF) and stroke prophylaxis

1. **Pathophysiology. AF is characterized by disorganized electrical and mechanical atrial activity.** The loss of atrial contraction results in impaired ventricular filling, thereby favoring the formation of atrial thrombi. Because these thrombi can embolize to the brain, AF is associated with a fivefold increase in the risk of stroke. The most common causes of AF are mitral valve disease, advanced age, hypertension, ischemic heart disease, and congestive heart failure (*Annu Rev Med* 1988;39:41). Other causes of AF include myocardial infarction (MI), atrial septal defect, alcohol intoxication, pulmonary embolism (PE), and genetic predisposition.

2. **Sign/symptoms.** At presentation, half of patients with AF have **palpitations**. Chest pain, heart failure, fatigue, dyspnea, dizziness, presyncope, and syncope also occur, but many episodes of AF are asymptomatic. On physical examination, the peripheral pulse and cardiac rhythm are irregularly **irregular**.

3. **Diagnosis. ECG** typically shows an irregular cardiac rhythm without defined P waves, often with rapid ventricular response (i.e., a heart rate >100 beats/minute).

4. **Therapy**
   a. **Hospital admission** is not required for all patients with new-onset AF; indications for admission include hemodynamic compromise, severe symptoms, and the desire for immediate cardioversion. AF patients with unstable angina or ECG findings that are suggestive of myocardial ischemia should be hospitalized. In contrast, the most asymptomatic patients can be managed in the outpatient setting, including the initiation of warfarin therapy (see sec. **III.B.3**).

   b. **Electrical or pharmacologic cardioversion** of acute AF to normal sinus rhythm (NSR) is often attempted to improve cardiac function, to relieve symptoms, and to decrease the potential risk for thromboembolism. The hypothesis that cardioversion of AF will decrease the long-term risk for thromboembolism is being tested in a National Institutes of Health trial (the AFFIRM trial). That trial also will evaluate the risks and benefits of prescribing antiarrhythmic agents to help maintain NSR.

   (1) **Emergent** cardioversion should be performed for patients with AF who have symptoms of cardiac ischemia, hypotension, or pulmonary edema.

   (2) **Elective** cardioversion has approximately a 1% risk of thromboembolism. Elective cardioversion of AF should be preceded by 3 weeks of anticoagulation [international normalized ratio (INR) approximately 2.5] unless the AF is acute (duration <48 hours) or a high-quality transesophageal echocardiogram (TEE) has documented the absence of atrial and ventricular thrombi (*N Engl J Med* 2001; 344:1411). IV unfractionated heparin (UFH) or SC low-molecular-

weight heparin (LMWH), prescribed at the time of TEE and continued for at least 24 hours after the cardioversion, may reduce the risk of stroke from this strategy. After any cardioversion (with or without a prior TEE), warfarin therapy (INR goal of 2.5) should be initiated and continued for 4–6 weeks. If the patient remains in NSR throughout this period, the warfarin therapy can be stopped and aspirin can be substituted in most patients. Warfarin should be prescribed for at least 4 weeks after successful cardioversion because it may require this long for the atria to recover their normal mechanical function.

   c. **Ventricular rate control** can be achieved by prescribing atrioventricular nodal blocking agents (see Chap. 8). In outpatients without left ventricular systolic dysfunction, verapamil, diltiazem, or β-adrenergic antagonists are preferred over digoxin because they provide more reliable rate control during exertion (*J Fam Pract* 2000;49:47).

   d. **Antithrombotic therapy for stroke prophylaxis**
      (1) **Warfarin is the preferred therapy for most patients who have chronic or paroxysmal AF because it reduces the risk of stroke by 62%** (*Ann Intern Med* 1999;131:492). In general, warfarin should be initiated with a daily dose of 5 mg or less (see sec. **III.B.3**). In patients with AF who cannot or who choose not to take warfarin or who lack risk factors for stroke (in addition to the AF), **aspirin should be prescribed because it reduces stroke by approximately 22%**.
      (2) **Risk factors for stroke.** Patients with AF and valvular disease (mitral valve stenosis or a prosthetic heart valve) require warfarin therapy; they are likely to have ≥10 strokes/100 patient years without anticoagulant therapy. The stroke rate in patients with nonvalvular AF depends on other risk factors for stroke. One clinical prediction rule that estimates the stroke rate in these patients is $CHADS_2$. Patients with a $CHADS_2$ score of 0 have a low rate of stroke with aspirin therapy (Table 9-1); they do not need warfarin therapy. Patients with a $CHADS_2$ score of 1 have a moderate rate of stroke with aspirin therapy; they generally benefit from adjusted-dose warfarin therapy, depending on their risk of hemorrhage and personal preferences. Anticoagula-

Table 9-1. Risk of stroke in nonvalvular atrial fibrillation

$CHADS_2$ score	Estimated rate[a] (strokes/100 patient yrs)
0	1.9
1	2.8
2	4.0
3	5.9
4	8.5
5	12.5
6	18.2

Note: $CHADS_2$ score = +1 point each for the following conditions: CHF, hypertension, age >75 years, or diabetes mellitus; +2 points for a prior stroke or transient ischemic attack.
[a]Estimated rates are for aspirin therapy. The rate without any antithrombotic therapy will be approximately one-fourth greater; rates with warfarin will be approximately one-half those shown.
Source: JAMA 2001;285:2864.

tion candidates with a CHADS$_2$ score of 2–6 should take warfarin because of their high risk of stroke with aspirin therapy.

(3) Trials and guidelines support a **target INR of 2.5** (range, 2.0–3.0) for most patients with AF, except that higher INRs (target of 3.0) are advocated for patients with AF and a mechanical heart valve. An INR of 3.0 also can be used in patients with AF and a recent stroke or TIA (*N Engl J Med* 1995;333:5).

B. Use of aspirin for primary prophylaxis of MI (see Chap. 6 for secondary prophylaxis). Aspirin [acetylsalicylic acid (ASA)] is the most widely used drug in the world. By inhibiting the enzyme cyclooxygenase (especially COX-1), ASA decreases platelet production of thromboxane A$_2$ and leads to inhibition of platelet aggregation and decreased vasoconstriction. Although a rectal suppository is available, ASA is usually given by mouth, preferably with food. The oral dose of ASA to achieve an antithrombotic effect should be 75–325 mg/day or 160–325 mg every other day; higher doses of ASA are not more effective at preventing thrombosis (although they do have greater analgesic, anti-inflammatory, and antipyretic effects).

1. **Risks. GI side effects, including hemorrhage**, occur with ASA. However, the absolute risk of GI hemorrhage is low with daily doses of 325 mg or less. Although enteric-coated ASA can decrease gastric irritation, neither buffered nor enteric-coated ASA appears to lower the risk of major upper-GI bleeding substantially (*Lancet* 1996;348:1413). The absolute increase in the rate of **hemorrhagic stroke** from ASA is less than 1/1000 patient years of therapy (*JAMA* 1998;280:1930).

2. **Benefits. ASA reduces the relative risk of a first MI** by approximately 20%. Five major trials have randomized more than 50,000 participants to either ASA or placebo. Although the relative risk reduction in MI was statistically significant in only two of these trials (*N Engl J Med* 1989;321:129, and *Lancet* 1998;351:233), when all five trials are taken together, they provide significant evidence of aspirin's effectiveness. How this 20% relative risk reduction translates into absolute terms depends on the patient's underlying risk of MI. For example, there is little to be gained by prescribing ASA in healthy patients who are younger than age 40 years. In contrast, the benefits of ASA generally outweigh the risks in older patients who have coronary risk factor(s) [including peripheral arterial occlusive disease (PAOD), see sec. **I.E**], coronary artery disease (see Chap. 6), or cerebral ischemia (see sec. **I.C**).

C. Internal carotid artery disease and prevention of ischemic stroke

1. **Pathophysiology. Atherothrombotic** strokes arise from atherosclerotic plaques on large arteries that limit flow from in situ stenosis or that shower plaque or fibrin clots distally. **Lacunar** infarcts typically occur in the deep white matter of the hemisphere or brain stem (often in the basal ganglia) because of hypertension-induced lipohyalinosis or arteriosclerosis of small arteries. **Embolic** strokes generally arise from the heart, but paradoxical emboli may occur in patients who have a patent foramen ovale and a deep venous thrombosis (DVT).

2. **Signs/symptoms.** Cerebral infarction resulting in a neurologic deficit that persists for greater than 24 hours is designated as a stroke, whereas a deficit of shorter duration is referred to as a **TIA**.

3. **Diagnosis and evaluation. Carotid duplex ultrasound** is the primary screening test for carotid stenosis because it is noninvasive and less expensive than other noninvasive tests, such as magnetic resonance angiography. However, routine ultrasound screening of asymptomatic patients is not recommended. If stenosis is seen on ultrasound, conventional angiography may be required to clarify the anatomy before carotid endarterectomy (CEA) or other procedure can be recommended. In younger patients with a stroke or TIA, some experts advocate a search for thrombophilia (sec. **II.F.7**).

4. **Prognosis and therapy.** Surgical therapy for carotid artery stenosis includes CEA or angioplasty (often with stent placement). Medical therapy for prevention of an ischemic stroke includes treatment of risk factors and antithrombotic therapy (http://circ.ahajournals.org/cgi/content/full/103/1/163).

   a. **Treatment of risk factors** consists of the following: maintenance of systolic BP at less than 140 mm Hg and diastolic BP at less than 90 mm Hg [lower targets are appropriate in certain settings, such as DM (*Lancet* 1998;351:1755)]; reduction of low-density lipoprotein cholesterol (LDL-C) with 3-hydroxy-3-methylglutaryl coenzyme A reductase inhibitors ("statins") if diet and exercise fail to lower the LDL-C level to less than 130 mg/dl [with statin therapy, the target LDL is less than 100mg/L (2.59 mmol/L)]; avoidance of smoking and heavy alcohol intake; control of diabetes; and engagement in regular exercise (*Stroke* 1999;30:1991).

   b. **Antiplatelet therapy** should be prescribed after cerebral ischemia, unless the ischemia was of embolic origin (*N Engl J Med* 2001;345:1444) or there is a separate indication for anticoagulant therapy.

      (1) **ASA** reduces the relative risk of a subsequent stroke by 25% (*BMJ* 1994;308:81). Although other antiplatelet therapies (see below) are slightly more effective than ASA, many experts prescribe ASA after a first-time ischemic stroke because it is inexpensive, widely available, and well tolerated (http://www.americanheart.org/Scientific/statements). **ASA doses that exceed 325 mg qd (e.g., 650 mg bid) are no more effective, and they cause more bleeding** (*Lancet* 1999;353:2179). Thus, the dose of ASA after stroke should be 50–325 mg taken once/day. In patients who are undergoing CEA, ASA can be started preoperatively.

      (2) **Dipyridamole (Persantine)** is a vasodilator that interferes with platelet function by increasing the cellular concentration of cyclic adenosine monophosphate. When used alone, it offers no benefit over ASA, but the combination of ASA, 25 mg, plus dipyridamole, 200 mg, taken bid together (e.g., **Aggrenox**), may be more effective than either agent alone in preventing stroke recurrence (*J Neurol Sci* 1996;143:1). This combination has not been compared to either ticlopidine or clopidogrel for the prevention of stroke. Dipyridamole also has been used in combination with warfarin in high-risk patients with prosthetic heart valves, but combination therapy consisting of warfarin (INR target, 3.0) plus low-dose ASA may be more effective for this population (*J Am Coll Cardiol* 2000;35:739). Dipyridamole's pregnancy category is B.

      (3) **Ticlopidine** is a thienopyridine that inhibits platelet aggregation. Two randomized, controlled trials that compared ticlopidine, 250 mg PO bid, to ASA in patients with stroke or TIA found that ticlopidine reduced the relative risk of stroke recurrence by 20% more than did ASA. Ticlopidine can cause diarrhea, nausea, skin rash, hyperlipidemia, and hematologic complications. Because of a 1–2% risk of **neutropenia or thrombotic thrombocytopenic purpura**, CBC monitoring (with platelet count) must be done every 2 weeks for the first 3 months of ticlopidine therapy. If hematologic complications develop, the ticlopidine must be stopped immediately and appropriate therapy undertaken. Ticlopidine should be taken with food. It is contraindicated in the presence of advanced liver or renal disease. Because of its long half-life, ticlopidine should be stopped 10–14 days before invasive procedures. The drug is pregnancy category B.

      (4) **Clopidogrel** also is a thienopyridine that inhibits adenosine diphosphate–induced platelet aggregation. A single large trial (CAPRIE) compared clopidogrel, 75 mg PO qd, to ASA, 325 mg, and found that clopidogrel reduced the relative risk of the combined end point

(recurrent stroke, MI, or vascular death) by 9% more than ASA did, with an absolute risk reduction of 0.5%. As compared to ticlopidine, clopidogrel is well tolerated and has fewer hematologic adverse events. Although rare cases of thrombotic thrombocytopenic purpura have been reported within 2 weeks of starting clopidogrel, routine CBC monitoring is not recommended by the manufacturer. Thus, although ticlopidine may be the more effective thienopyridine, clopidogrel is safer. No dose reduction is necessary with renal disease, as the liver metabolizes clopidogrel. The drug is pregnancy category B.

   c. Surgical therapy and evaluation
   (1) Carotid artery disease causing recent symptoms (i.e., stroke, TIA, transient monocular blindness, or retinal ischemia) carries a substantial risk of stroke.
      (a) The risk of stroke increases with the degree of stenosis (*N Engl J Med* 1998;339:1415). For example, a moderate (i.e., 50–69%) stenosis that was recently symptomatic has a 20–25% incidence of ipsilateral stroke over the next 5 years, but this risk would drop to 8–16% with **CEA**. In symptomatic patients with high-grade (i.e., 70–99%) carotid artery stenosis, the absolute benefits of CEA are even greater. In contrast, in patients whose stenosis is less than 50%, CEA offers no advantage over medical therapy.
      (b) Referral to a surgeon for CEA is recommended for symptomatic surgical candidates who have a stenosis that is 50% or greater: CEA can lower their long-term risk of ipsilateral stroke (*N Engl J Med* 1998;339:1415). However, the benefit of CEA is lower in patients who have a stenosis that is less than 70%, are female, or have a high risk of perioperative complications. CEA is not indicated for patients who have a complete (100%) carotid occlusion. Patients who undergo CEA also should receive medical therapy, including antiplatelet therapy (*Lancet* 1999;353:2179). Trials now in progress are comparing angioplasty and stent placement to CEA (*Lancet* 2001;357:1722).
   (2) Asymptomatic carotid artery disease. CEA may lower the long-term risk of ipsilateral stroke in asymptomatic patients who meet all of the following criteria: (1) stenosis of 60% or greater, (2) a perioperative complication rate (of death and stroke combined) of less than 3%, and (3) life expectancy of 5 years or greater (http://www.americanheart.org/Scientific/statements). CEA may also be beneficial for asymptomatic patients in special circumstances, such as patients who are undergoing simultaneous coronary artery bypass graft. Some experts reserve CEA for asymptomatic patients whose stenosis is 80% or greater, because this population has a higher risk of stroke than patients with less stenosis, and because ultrasound may tend to exaggerate the rate of stenosis as compared to angiography.

D. Aortic disease
   1. Aneurysm is a pathologic enlargement of a segment of a blood vessel. In a true aneurysm all three walls of the artery (intima, media, adventitia) are involved; a pseudoaneurysm spares the adventitia. The most common cause of aneurysm is **atherosclerosis**. Other causes include cystic medial necrosis (often caused by Marfan's or Ehlers-Danlos syndrome), syphilis, tuberculosis, Takayasu's arteritis, giant cell arteritis, rheumatoid arthritis, human leukocyte antigen B27–associated spondyloarthropathies, bicuspid aortic valve, trauma, and genetic predisposition.
      a. Thoracic aortic aneurysms can be asymptomatic or they can cause dysphagia from compression of the esophagus, hoarseness due to compression of the recurrent laryngeal nerve, or pain that radiates to the

back or chest. Physical examination may reveal aortic regurgitation. Although the diagnosis may be suspected based on chest radiographic findings (widened mediastinum, left-sided pleural effusion, or calcified aorta), it requires confirmation with CT, MRI, angiogram, or echocardiogram (with transesophageal being better than transthoracic echocardiogram). **Referral to a surgeon** is recommended for surgical candidates who have symptoms or an aortic aneurysm diameter of greater than 5–6 cm (>5 cm with **Marfan's**). Patients who are undergoing aortic aneurysm repair require careful preoperative cardiac evaluation because of their high risk for perioperative cardiac complications.

b. **Acute aortic dissection** results from an intimal tear. Independent predictors of the presence of an acute aortic dissection are the **acute onset of tearing or ripping pain in the chest, back, and/or neck; pulse deficit and/or BP differential** (i.e., >20 mm Hg difference in systolic pressure) between left and right arm; and **widening of the mediastinum or aorta** on the chest radiograph (*Arch Intern Med* 2000;160:2977). Migratory pain, focal neurologic signs, acute renal failure, aortic regurgitation, and hypertension also may occur.

c. **Treatment** of acute aortic dissection includes hospitalization for parenteral therapy (i.e., beta-blockers) that reduces systemic BP, left ventricular contractility, and heart rate and urgent surgical consultation. Ascending aortic dissection (type A) requires emergency surgical repair, whereas uncomplicated descending (type B) dissections are treated medically.

d. **Abdominal aortic aneurysm (AAA)** may be detected on physical examination as a **pulsatile nontender mass**. Abdominal palpation to detect abnormal widening of the aortic pulsation has a sensitivity of 0.76 in detecting AAA of 5 cm or greater, but the sensitivity is lower in patients with abdominal obesity (*JAMA* 1999;281:77). Although some experts advocate screening of high-risk patients (e.g., older male smokers) for AAA by physical examination or ultrasound, whether this strategy prevents mortality from AAA rupture is unknown. **Referral to a surgeon** is recommended for surgical candidates who have an AAA that is rapidly expanding, symptomatic, or **5.5 cm or greater** (*Lancet* 1998;352:1649). Either open surgical or percutaneous grafting can be used to repair an AAA. Patients who are undergoing AAA repair require careful preoperative cardiac evaluation because of their high risk for perioperative cardiac complications (http://www.americanheart.org/Scientific/statements1996/039607.html).

2. **Aortitis** is inflammation of the aorta that usually affects the aortic arch, but the process may extend proximally to the sinuses of Valsalva, as in **rheumatic aortitis**, or extend distally into branches of the aorta, as in **Takayasu's arteritis**. Takayasu's arteritis typically affects young Asian women. Because of the risk of arterial occlusions, especially the left subclavian artery, it is labeled **pulseless disease**. Takayasu's disease can be treated with warfarin, glucocorticoids, immunosuppressive therapy, or surgical bypass of critical stenoses. **Syphilitic** aortitis presents one or more decades after initial infection and typically results in calcification and dilatation of the aortic root (often leading to aortic insufficiency), but it may involve the entire aorta or cause coronary artery ostial disease. Treatment includes penicillin and surgical repair.

3. **Giant cell arteritis** is a disease of the elderly. Because of its predilection for the temporal artery, it also is called **temporal arteritis**. When the temporal artery is affected, symptoms may include headache, jaw claudication, and loss of vision. The diagnosis of temporal arteries may be suggested based on the clinical presentation and laboratory abnormalities (anemia and erythrocyte sedimentation rate elevation), but the diagnosis should be made by temporal artery biopsy. When the diagnosis

is suspected, urgent treatment with glucocorticoids (e.g., prednisone, 1 mg/kg/day) can prevent blindness. To prevent relapses, the glucocorticoid should be tapered gradually over the ensuring months, and concomitant therapy with methotrexate (10 mg PO/week) may be considered (*Ann Intern Med* 2001;124:106).

   4. Aortic occlusive disease from atherosclerosis presents similarly to bilateral PAOD (see sec. **I.E.2**) except that aortic disease may cause bilateral claudication that extends to the buttocks or back and impotence (Leriche syndrome). Chronic aortic occlusive disease is treated similarly to PAOD. In contrast, acute occlusion requires immediate thrombectomy or revascularization to salvage the affected limb, which is usually painful, pulseless, pale, and cool.

E. Peripheral arterial occlusive disease

   1. Pathophysiology. The most common cause of PAOD is atherosclerosis leading to inadequate perfusion of an exercising muscle. Other causes include arteritis, fibrosis, and thromboangiitis obliterans (Buerger's disease). In **thromboangiitis obliterans**, inflammatory thrombi occlude the small- and medium-sized arteries and veins in the distal extremities of younger smokers (*N Engl J Med* 2000;343:864). Although **pseudoclaudication** may mimic PAOD, it arises from compression of the distal spinal cord (typically from lumbar spine stenosis) or when intrinsic muscle disease is present.

   2. Signs/symptoms. The classic symptom of PAOD is **claudication**, the exercise-induced pain or cramping that occurs in muscle groups and is relieved with a few minutes of rest. Claudication is reproducible, often occurring after walking a specific distance. As PAOD progresses, rest pain can develop, and infarction, ulceration, and gangrene in the periphery may occur. The usual site of claudication is the limb just distal to the occluded artery. Common signs of claudication are **diminished pulses, arterial bruits, hair loss, dystrophic nails, and skin changes** (hairless, cool, thin, shiny, pallor on elevation, dependent rubor, or livedo reticularis), but many of these signs are absent in patients who have mild disease or vasospastic claudication. PAOD should be distinguished from acute arterial occlusion of an extremity, an emergency that is treated with vascular surgery (e.g., thrombectomy or bypass surgery) or thrombolytic therapy (*J Vasc Surg* 1996;23:64). Acute arterial occlusion, which is caused by either embolism or in situ thrombus, presents with some or all of the 5 Ps: **p**ain, **p**allor, **p**ulselessness, **p**oikilothermia, and **p**aresthesias.

   3. Differential diagnosis and evaluation. The **ankle-arm index (AAI)** is the ratio of the systolic BP in the posterior tibial (or dorsalis pedis) artery divided by the systolic BP in the brachial artery. A continuous-wave Doppler device applied distal to multiple BP cuffs can measure the index at rest and after walking. An AAI of less than 0.95 at rest or after exertion is abnormal, but symptomatic patients typically have an index of less than 0.80. The AAI is not useful in some patients, especially those with diabetes, who have small-vessel disease or noncompressible arteries. Patients with low AAIs should undergo further evaluation. Noninvasive tests for these patients include pulse-volume recordings, transcutaneous oximetry, magnetic resonance angiography, and two-dimensional real-time ultrasound.

   4. Therapy and management

   a. Medical management

   (1) Cessation of smoking and other forms of tobacco use decrease symptoms. Even minimal use of products that contain nicotine can be deleterious, especially for patients who have thromboangiitis obliterans.

   (2) Exercise that is done regularly up to the point of claudication (and then resumed once symptoms subside) increases the pain-free walking distance by more than 100% (*JAMA* 1995;274:975).

        (3) Hyperlipidemia should be treated aggressively, with a target LDL of less than 100.

        (4) Pharmacologic therapy

           (a) Aspirin, ticlopidine, or clopidogrel (see sec. **I.C.4.b**) should be prescribed to reduce the risk of a major vascular event and possibly to lessen the need for peripheral arterial surgery (*Lancet* 1992;340:143).

           (b) Cilostazol (Pletal), 100 mg PO bid, is a phosphodiesterase inhibitor that increases the pain-free walking distance by 40–50% (*Arch Intern Med* 1999;159:2041). The dosage should be reduced to 50 mg bid in patients who have end-stage renal disease or who are taking drugs that inhibit CYP3A4 (e.g., ketoconazole) or CYP2C19 (e.g., omeprazole). Cilostazol inhibits platelet aggregation, but it can be taken with aspirin. Cilostazol causes arterial vasodilation, but how it decreases claudication is unknown. Side effects include headache, diarrhea, palpitations, and dizziness. Cilostazol should **not** be taken with food or grapefruit juice. It is contraindicated in patients with congestive heart failure. The drug is pregnancy class C.

           (c) Pentoxifylline (Trental), 400 mg PO tid, is a phosphodiesterase inhibitor that increases erythrocyte flexibility, but it has inconsistent benefit for patients with PAOD; on average, it increases the pain-free walking distance by 30% or less.

           (d) Although not approved by the U.S. Food and Drug Administration, the following agents increased pain-free walking distance in trial participants who had claudication: **beraprost sodium** (an oral prostaglandin I_2 analogue with antiplatelet and vasodilating properties), **calcium-heparin** (administered SC), **propionyl-L-carnitine**, and possibly **ginkgo biloba** extract.

        (5) Referral for revascularization is indicated for advanced PAOD as indicated by rest claudication, debilitating symptoms that fail to respond to medical management, infarction, ulceration, or gangrene. The perioperative risk of a cardiac complication is high in patients who undergo vascular surgery. This high-risk population should undergo preoperative cardiac evaluation if they have poor functional capacity (i.e., <4 metabolic equivalents), heart disease, or DM (http://www.americanheart.org/Scientific/statements/1996/039607.html).

II. Venous thromboembolism (VTE) and other venous diseases

  A. Introduction. VTE represents **DVT** and **PE**. VTE is often unsuspected, leading to diagnostic and therapeutic delays that can increase morbidity and mortality. DVTs that arise from the proximal veins of the lower extremities (popliteal vein or above) and pelvis are the primary source of PE. Calf vein DVTs rarely cause significant emboli unless they propagate proximally first: 0–30% of calf vein DVTs extend into the proximal leg, and, if not treated, some of these will cause PE. DVTs that arise from abdominal veins or upper-extremity veins can also cause PE. DVT of the upper extremity is often secondary to an indwelling catheter.

  B. Pathophysiology of VTE. Blood stasis, blood vessel wall abnormalities, and changes in the soluble and formed elements of the blood are the major contributors to thrombosis. Blood vessel wall injuries typically occur with trauma and surgery. Hypercoagulable states may be inherited or acquired, such as those seen in cancer patients (see sec. **II.F.7**).

  C. DVT. Venous thrombosis is typically described by anatomic location. Thrombosis in the lower extremity can be classified as **deep** or **superficial** and as **proximal** or **distal**. The **superficial femoral vein** is actually a deep vein, and its preferred term is **femoral vein**. Because superficial venous thrombosis can be a sign of DVT, objective assessment for DVT is recommended when superficial venous thrombosis is present. A DVT that is found in the popliteal vein or more proximal is considered **proximal,** whereas a DVT found inferior to the popliteal vein is termed **distal.**

D. The **differential diagnosis** for unilateral lower-extremity edema includes Baker's cyst, hematoma, venous insufficiency, lymphedema, sarcoma, arterial aneurysm, myositis, cellulitis, rupture of the medial head of the gastrocnemius, and abscess. Compression ultrasound, MRI, and CT are useful for detecting DVT and other pathology.

    1. History and physical examination are neither sensitive nor specific for DVT. Thus, the presence of symptoms or signs, such as pain or edema, implies the need for objective diagnostic testing. Clinical suspicion may dictate the speed and type of evaluation.

    2. Diagnostic testing

        a. The initial diagnostic test for symptomatic acute DVT should be a **noninvasive test,** either **compression ultrasound** (called **duplex examination** when performed with Doppler testing) or impedance plethysmography (*Am J Respir Crit Care Med* 1999;160:1043). Although validated protocols and experienced technicians improve the accuracy of these tests, their accuracy is diminished in special circumstances. Compression ultrasound is not sensitive at detecting calf DVT and may fail to visualize other veins as well, especially parts of the deep femoral vein and the upper-extremity venous system. Noninvasive testing also is difficult to interpret in the setting of an old DVT, unless the original thrombus is known to have resolved. Finally, noninvasive testing has a low sensitivity in asymptomatic patients.

        Serial noninvasive testing can improve the diagnostic yield of noninvasive tests. If the initial noninvasive test is negative in patients with a clinically suspected calf DVT, anticoagulant therapy can be withheld provided that an objective test is repeated 3–14 days later. The repeat study may detect extension of a previously nonvisualized calf DVT to the proximal veins.

        A **simplified compression ultrasound** procedure that is limited to the common femoral vein in the groin and the popliteal vein down to the trifurcation of the calf veins is not as sensitive as a complete examination, but one or two repeated simplified noninvasive tests within 2 weeks improve sensitivity. When patient follow-up is unreliable, either full noninvasive testing or venography should be used.

        b. Venography is the gold standard technique for diagnosing DVT. It is used for diagnosing calf DVT and DVT in the asymptomatic patient. Venography requires placement of a pedal IV catheter, administration of iodinated contrast, and exposure to radiation. Thus, noninvasive tests are the preferred initial tests in symptomatic patients with suspected DVT. Contraindications to venography include renal dysfunction and dye allergy.

        c. D-dimer is a specific degradation product that is released into the circulation when cross-linked fibrin undergoes fibrinolysis. Rapid bedside assays are now available, and these are read as negative or positive. D-dimer testing has a low positive predictive value, and thus **patients with a positive test require further evaluation.** In contrast, the negative predictive value of a negative D-dimer is high enough to exclude a DVT when a noninvasive test is negative (*Arch Intern Med* 1997;157:1077) or the clinical probability is low, or both (http://med.mssm.edu/ebm/cpr/dvt2.html). In settings in which the pretest probability is moderate or high, including patients with cancer, a D-dimer test is not useful because it is not sufficiently accurate to rule out a DVT (*Ann Intern Med* 1999;131:17).

        d. MRI has had high sensitivity for acute, symptomatic proximal DVT in small studies. Although expensive, MRI is noninvasive.

e. **CT venography** is being used to diagnose DVT in conjunction with a contrast-enhanced spiral CT for diagnosis of PE (see sec. **II.D.2.b**). Although CT venography allows for visualization of the veins in the abdomen, pelvis, and proximal lower extremities, data supporting the use of spiral CT for DVT evaluation are preliminary (*Ann Intern Med* 2000;132:227).

E. **PE.** PEs are classified as proximal or distal (subsegmental or smaller) based on their location within the pulmonary arteries. In the absence of contraindications, any PE warrants anticoagulant therapy (see below). Smaller PEs are more difficult to diagnose, but the clinical significance of PEs that are too small to be detected by conventional testing remains unclear. The differential diagnosis of PE includes dissecting aortic aneurysm (see sec. **I.D.1**), pneumonia, bronchitis, lung cancer, pericardial or pleural disease, heart failure, costochondritis, and myocardial ischemia. Contrast-enhanced spiral CT and MRI are useful for detecting pathology other than PE. Electrocardiography, blood gases, and chest radiography, may help to focus the differential diagnosis and assess cardiopulmonary reserve, but they cannot rule in or rule out PE.

1. **History and physical examination. Symptoms and signs of PE** are neither sensitive nor specific. However, predictors of PE are shortness of breath; chest pain, especially pleuritic chest pain; hypoxemia or oxyhemoglobin; hemoptysis; a pleural rub; new right-sided heart failure; and tachycardia (*Ann Intern Med* 1998;129:997). Validated **clinical risk factors** for PE are a prior or family history of VTE, immobilization, surgery, fracture, cancer, and recent obstetric delivery (*Ann Intern Med* 1998;129:997). Clinical **suspicion of PE should lead to objective diagnostic evaluation**.

2. **Diagnostic testing** (*Am J Respir Crit Care Med* 1999;160:1043)

   a. **Ventilation-perfusion (V̇/Q̇) scanning** requires placement of an IV catheter and administration of radioactive material (via inhaled and IV routes). V̇/Q̇ scanning is most useful in patients with normal chest radiographs, because nondiagnostic scans are extremely common in the setting of an abnormal chest radiograph. V̇/Q̇ scans can be classified as normal, nondiagnostic (i.e., very low probability, low probability, intermediate probability), or high probability for PE. Clinical suspicion improves the accuracy of V̇/Q̇ scanning: In patients with normal- or high-probability V̇/Q̇ scans that agree with the pretest clinical suspicion, PE is absent or present, respectively, in 96% of patients (*JAMA* 1990;263:2753). When the V̇/Q̇ findings and the pretest probability conflict, further testing should be performed.

   b. **Contrast-enhanced spiral (helical) chest CT** requires placement of an IV catheter, administration of iodinated contrast, and exposure to radiation. Used according to standardized protocols in conjunction with expert interpretation, spiral CT appears accurate for large (proximal) PEs but is less than 75% sensitive for small (distal) emboli. Based on the current evidence, spiral CT alone is not adequate to confidently rule out PE. Similar to V̇/Q̇, spiral CT ought to be used in conjunction with other noninvasive diagnostic test information. A clinical trial that is now in progress is further evaluating the accuracy of spiral CT (PIOPED II). In contrast to V̇/Q̇ scans, most spiral CT scans produce a diagnostic result (positive or negative), with few (<10%) indeterminate or inadequate studies. CT has the benefit of suggesting alternative diagnoses, such as dissecting aortic aneurysm, pneumonia, malignancy, pleural disease, etc. Contraindications to spiral CT include renal dysfunction and dye allergy.

   c. **MRI**, in small studies, is sensitive for diagnosing acute PE. Similar to spiral CT, MRI may detect alternative diagnoses. The role of MRI in the diagnosis of PE is not clearly defined.

   d. **D-dimer** testing is sensitive but not specific for diagnosing PE. Consequently, **patients with a positive test require further evaluation**.

However, a negative D-dimer in combination with low pretest probability can exclude almost all PE (*Ann Intern Med* 1998;129:1006). Thus, some experts reserve the use of D-dimer for patients who have a low pretest probability for PE (*Arch Intern Med* 2001;161:567).

    e. Pulmonary **angiography** is the gold standard for diagnosing PE, although noninvasive tests are preferred for the initial evaluation. Even though angiography is the gold standard, it can be inadequate or inaccurate in some situations. Angiography requires placement of a pulmonary artery catheter, infusion of IV contrast, and exposure to radiation. Contraindications to angiography include renal dysfunction and dye allergy.

    f. **Noninvasive testing of the legs** may be useful for patients with suspected PE who have nondiagnostic V̇/Q̇ scans, serving as an alternative means to diagnose PE in the patient with a clinical scenario highly suggestive of PE. However, further evaluation is required if the noninvasive test is negative and the suspicion of PE is present.

F. Treatment and management of DVT and PE

    1. The goal of VTE therapy is to prevent clot extension, recurrent VTE, embolism, and death. In addition, therapy should minimize postthrombotic complications, including postphlebitic syndrome and pulmonary hypertension. Treatment of DVT and of PE is similar because these two conditions are manifestations of the same disease process, although the duration of treatment may vary. Approximately half of patients with proximal DVT have asymptomatic PE, and the majority of PEs are thought to arise from DVTs of the legs or pelvis. Clinical trials have validated similar treatment regimens for DVT and PE. Anticoagulants are recommended for patients with proximal DVT, any PE, or symptomatic calf DVT. Treatment is usually recommended for asymptomatic calf DVT as well.

        a. **Primary prevention** (prophylaxis) is mostly an issue for inpatients whereas **secondary prevention** occurs in the inpatient and outpatient setting (see below).

        b. **In addition to anticoagulants, treatment** of VTE may include breakdown or removal of a clot with thrombolysis or embolectomy (see below).

    2. Treatment of VTE should begin with **heparin**, either unfractionated (UFH) or LMW (see sec. **III.A** for dosing), and with a vitamin K antagonist (see sec. **III.B** for dosing). Heparin can be discontinued after 4–5 days once the INR is 2 or greater for 2 consecutive days. Patients with **massive thromboembolism** should possibly undergo more than 4–5 days of heparin therapy.

        a. **UFH** is an inexpensive, safe, and effective way to treat acute DVT or PE. Initial treatment with UFH (combined with long-term warfarin) decreases the recurrence rate of VTE to less than 5% over 3 months and helps prevent pain and swelling at the site of a DVT. The administration of UFH is discussed in sec. **III.A.1**.

        b. **LMWHs** are made from UFH and are as safe and effective as UFH for the treatment of DVT or PE (*Ann Intern Med* 1999;130:800). In addition, LMWHs are used subcutaneously, once or twice/day, at a constant dose and do not require monitoring except in special populations (see sec. **III.A.2**). Given these advantages, LMWHs are the preferred initial antithrombotic therapy for **stable outpatients** who have an acute DVT (*N Engl J Med* 1996;334:677, and *N Engl J Med* 1996;334:682). Ideally, outpatients who receive LMWH have none of the following **relative contraindications to outpatient therapy**: signs or symptoms of PE, high risk for recurrent clotting (ongoing risk factor) or for bleeding (e.g., age >80 years), limited cardiopulmonary reserve, or need for hospitalization due to another illness (*Chest* 1999;115:972). The administration of LMWH is discussed in sec. **III.A.2** and in Table 9-2. Given the

Table 9-2. Disease-specific antithrombotic therapy

Indication	First-line Rx	Alternate Rx	Comment and duration
AF			
Low risk (i.e., no risk factors)[b]	ASA	INR 2.5	Duration: lifelong[a]
Typical patient	INR 2.5	ASA	
DVT/PE	INR 2.5[c] and UFH or LMWH	INR 2–5[c] and pentasaccharide	LMWH options: dalteparin, 100 units/kg SC q12h; dalteparin, 200 units/kg SC qd; enoxaparin, 1.0 mg/kg SC q12h; enoxaparin, 1.5 mg/kg SC qd; nadroparin, 90 units/kg q12h; tinzaparin, 175 units/kg SC qd
			Duration for warfarin: 6 mos typically, but shorter for postoperative DVT and longer for multiple events or ongoing risk factors
Ischemic stroke (secondary prophylaxis)			
Noncardioembolic stroke	ASA 81–325 mg	Ticlopidine, 250 mg bid; clopidogrel, 75 mg qd; or ASA, 25 mg, + dipyridamole, 200 mg bid	In patients taking ticlopidine, check CBC q2wk for 3 mos
Cardioembolic stroke, MS, or history of AF	INR 2.5	—	Use warfarin in patients with AF, MS, or acute cardioembolic stroke (rule out hemorrhage with CT first)
			Duration: lifelong
Post-MI			
Typical patient	ASA 81–325 mg	INR 2.5	Duration for ASA: lifelong
High risk for embolism (e.g., anterior MI, severe LV dysfunction, AF, mural thrombosis, or history of embolism)	INR 2.5 or 3.0	ASA ± warfarin	Except for chronic embolic risk factors (e.g., AF), warfarin duration: 3 mos; then substitute ASA

Heart valve replacement			
Tissue	INR 2.5	ASA 325 mg	Duration, tissue: 3 mos for warfarin; subsequently, ASA can be used lifelong
Mechanical			Duration, mechanical: lifelong warfarin
Low risk (i.e., aortic St. Jude valve)	INR 2.5	INR 3.0	Can add ASA or use INR >3 for patients with CAD, caged-ball, or caged-disk valves (e.g., Bjork-Shiley), or prior embolism
Typical patient	INR 3.0	INR 3.0 + ASA 81 mg	—

AF, atrial fibrillation; ASA, acetylsalicylic acid; CAD, coronary artery disease; DVT, deep venous thrombosis; INR, international normalized ratio from warfarin therapy; LMWH, low-molecular-weight heparin; LV, left ventricular; MI, myocardial infarction; MS, mitral stenosis; PE, pulmonary embolus; UFH, unfractionated heparin.

[a]Warfarin for cardioversion should begin 3 wks before cardioversion and can be stopped once rhythm has been maintained for >4 wks.

[b]Risk factors for stroke: history of stroke, transient ischemic attack, hypertension, diabetes mellitus, CHF, MS, or age >75 yrs.

[c]Higher INR may be needed for patients who had a DVT or PE with an INR of 2–3 or who have the antiphospholipid antibody syndrome.

Adapted from J Hirsh, J Dalen, DR Anderson, et al. Oral anticoagulants: mechanism of action, clinical effectiveness, and optimal therapeutic range. *Chest* 2001;119:8S–21S.

long half-life of LMWH, IV UFH is preferred in inpatients who plan to undergo an invasive procedure.

3. Systemic or IV **thrombolytic therapy** may be appropriate for patients with PE and systemic hypotension (*Chest* 2001;119:176S). For patients with DVT, thrombolytic therapy can help to decrease the postphlebitic syndrome, but it should only be considered in patients with massive DVT because of its risk of intracranial hemorrhage (*N Engl J Med* 1994;330:1864).

4. An **inferior vena cava (IVC) filter** should be placed in patients who have an acute DVT or PE and an absolute contraindication to anticoagulation (*N Engl J Med* 1998;338:409). IVC filters are also indicated for patients who have had a recurrent VTE during adequate anticoagulant therapy. Although IVC filters prevent PEs, they can increase the incidence of DVT. Thus, patients who have an IVC filter placed because of a recurrence while receiving adequate anticoagulation should continue to receive anticoagulant therapy, unless contraindicated. IVC filters can also be used in select populations (e.g., trauma patients) without VTE who are at high risk for VTE and for hemorrhage, especially those patients with a limited cardiopulmonary reserve.

5. As with heparin, **warfarin** appears to have a threshold that is necessary to achieve an antithrombotic state.
   a. An **INR of 2.0–3.0 is the usual intensity of treatment**, with a target of 2.5. At least 4–5 days of heparin therapy is recommended for VTE, overlapping with warfarin therapy for at least 4 days (*Arch Intern Med* 1998;158:1005).
   b. The **duration of anticoagulation** depends on the etiology of the thrombosis, the ongoing risk for recurrence, the patient's preferences, and the risk of hemorrhage. The following guidelines apply to patients who do not have an excessive risk of hemorrhage:
      (1) Patients with a **PE or an idiopathic proximal DVT** should receive at least 6 months of therapy.
      (2) Patients who have a single **proximal DVT associated with a transient reversible risk factor**, such as surgery or trauma, should receive at least 3 months of anticoagulation for DVT (*Chest* 2001;119:176S–193S).
      (3) Patients with **isolated symptomatic calf vein DVT** should undergo at least 6–12 weeks of anticoagulation.
      (4) Patients with one-time proximal **DVT or PE and ongoing risk factors**, such as cancer, antithrombin deficiency, or anticardiolipin antibody syndrome, should be treated for at least 12 months. Anticoagulant treatment for 12 months also is appropriate for patients who have VTE and deficiency of protein C or protein S, homocysteinemia, homozygous factor V Leiden (activated protein C resistance), or multiple thrombophilic states (see sec. **II.F.7**).
      (5) Patients with **recurrent idiopathic VTEs** should usually receive anticoagulants for life or until a contraindication develops.
      (6) When stopping anticoagulant therapy after a VTE, the clinician should consider prescribing aspirin. Aspirin can prevent MI (see sec. **I.B**). Aspirin may also prevent VTE: In the PEP study of orthopedic patients, patients randomized to aspirin, 160 mg, had a one-third reduction in perioperative VTE (*Lancet* 2000; 355:1295).

6. Patients with an apparently **idiopathic** DVT or PE may have an **underlying malignancy** (*N Engl J Med* 1992;327:1128). Thus, once an idiopathic DVT or PE is found, the clinician should search for malignancy. No special cancer screening is recommended; instead, the patient should undergo a careful history and physical examination, chest radio-

graph, and routine cancer screening (e.g., flexible sigmoidoscopy with barium enema or colonoscopy, prostate examination or Papanicolaou smear and mammography). Further evaluation (e.g., CT scan) should be done if indicated by the initial workup. By definition, patients who have a visceral malignancy and migratory thrombophlebitis have **Trousseau's syndrome**. Patients with Trousseau's syndrome may fail treatment with warfarin. If so, they should receive long-term heparin therapy instead (*West J Med* 1993;158:364).

7. **Thrombophilia**, acquired or genetic, is commonly associated with VTE.

   a. **Acquired thrombophilias** include those associated with malignancy, pregnancy, estrogen use, nephrotic syndrome, myeloproliferative disorders, paroxysmal nocturnal hemoglobinuria, heparin-induced thrombocytopenia (HIT), vasculitis, and thrombotic thrombocytopenic purpura. Treatment of VTE associated with these disorders generally should occur in the usual fashion, except that the duration of therapy can be prolonged if the risk factor is ongoing. Patients with **antiphospholipid antibody syndrome** may require a target INR of 3.0 or greater (*N Engl J Med* 1995;332:993). If these patients have a lupus anticoagulant, INR monitoring may be inaccurate, especially if the baseline INR was prolonged (*Ann Intern Med* 1997;127:177). Heparin (UFH or LMW) should be avoided in patients with a history of HIT.

   b. The classic **heritable deficiencies** of endogenous anticoagulants protein C, protein S, and antithrombin III are rare. In Caucasians, hereditary resistance to activated protein C (the factor V Leiden mutation) is more common. A variant in the prothrombin gene (the 20210A allele) is another newly discovered genetic cause of thrombophilia. Hyperhomocystinemia, influenced by genetics and diet, also is associated with thrombosis. More than half of patients with familial thrombosis have one or more genetic abnormalities associated with thrombosis. However, many patients with a genetic abnormality never experience a symptomatic VTE or stroke. Searching for these hypercoagulable states in an older patient with a single VTE or stroke is not necessary, because they are unlikely to affect management (*Stroke* 2001;32:1793). Screening is often recommended in populations with a high prevalence of genetic thrombophilias: younger patients (age <40 years) with a VTE or stroke, patients with a personal and family history of VTE, and patients with recurrent VTE. The intensity and duration of anticoagulation prophylaxis in the setting of other risk factors (surgery, pregnancy, or estrogen therapy) may be affected by genetic test results. Proteins C and S depend on vitamin K levels; they should not be assayed while the patient is receiving warfarin therapy. Protein S levels also should not be checked during pregnancy, when they are depressed. Functional assays of activated protein C resistance and antithrombin III levels should not be checked while the patient is receiving heparin or LMWH therapy. Anticoagulation does not interfere with genetic tests, lupus anticoagulant and antiphospholipid antibody testing, or assessment of homocysteine levels (measured while fasting).

8. The **postthrombotic syndrome** consists of pain, swelling, and possibly ulceration after a DVT and is often related to recurrent thrombosis (*Ann Intern Med* 1996;125:1). Elevation of the affected leg and use of fitted graduated compression stockings help to prevent postthrombotic syndrome and decrease its symptoms if it occurs.

G. **Treatment and management of distal DVT and superficial thrombophlebitis.** Anticoagulant therapy is recommended for all patients with symptomatic calf DVT and some patients with asymptomatic calf DVT. If relative but not absolute contraindications to anticoagulation are present, an alternative approach is to follow the patient with serial noninvasive testing over 3–14 days, watching for proximal extension. Patients with DVT that is confined to the calf are at low risk for clinically important PE, and anticoagulant therapy should be withheld in patients for whom the risks outweigh the benefits. If the DVT does propagate proximally, heparin and an oral anticoagulant should be prescribed. Once objective testing has excluded the diagnosis of DVT, patients with superficial thrombophlebitis can be treated with nonsteroidal anti-inflammatory drugs (NSAIDs) rather than anticoagulants.

III. Antithrombotic therapy
A. Heparins
1. The anticoagulant action of **UFH** is mediated largely by its interaction with antithrombin, resulting in the inhibition of factors II (thrombin), factor Xa, and other activated coagulation factors.
   a. **UFH can be begun with an IV bolus of 60–80 units/kg, followed by an infusion of 14–18 units/kg/hr**, with subsequent doses determined by nomogram (*Ann Intern Med* 1993;119:874). UFH is cleared and degraded primarily by the reticuloendothelial system; dose adjustment is not required in the setting of renal dysfunction.
   b. Because the response to systemic doses of IV UFH is unpredictable, **activated partial thromboplastin time (aPTT) monitoring is required** (q6h initially) to titrate the dose to a therapeutic level.
   c. **UFH can also be administered by SC injection** given q8h or q12h, with the dose depending on the purpose: 5000 units is used for **prophylaxis** of thromboembolism, whereas larger doses that are sufficient to prolong the aPTT to at least 1.5 times control are used for **systemic anticoagulation**. If an immediate anticoagulant effect is required, the initial SC dose should be accompanied by an initial IV bolus injection because the SC anticoagulant effect does not peak until approximately 2 hours after SC injection. Large doses of SC heparin are used for systemic anticoagulation, such as 12,000 IU SC q8h or 16,000 IU SC q12h. With SC heparin the aPTT should be drawn 6 or more hours after the injection.
   d. **Side effects** include hemorrhage and HIT, and therefore a CBC with platelet count should be monitored routinely (e.g., every other day initially and less frequently subsequently). Other side effects of heparin include allergy, skin necrosis, priapism, heparin-induced hypoaldosteronism (leading to hyperkalemia), and osteoporosis (with long-term use). Mild asymptomatic elevation of hepatic transaminases is common and does not require cessation of therapy.
      (1) **Hemorrhage.** An unexplained drop in hematocrit requires a search for a source of bleeding. Patients who require immediate reversal of their UFH therapy, because of overdose or significant bleeding, should be hospitalized for IV administration of fresh frozen plasma, protamine sulfate, or both.
      (2) **HIT** should be suspected when thrombocytopenia occurs after 3–10 days of heparin therapy, but it can occur earlier in patients who have been exposed to heparin previously. Despite the presence of thrombocytopenia, HIT can cause venous or arterial thrombosis as well as hemorrhage. It also can result in adrenal insufficiency from thrombosis or hemorrhage into the adrenal glands. If HIT is suspected, all heparin must be stopped and the diagnosis should be confirmed by an assay for antibodies that react with the heparin–platelet factor 4 complex or detection of heparin-dependent platelet activation. Warfarin may paradoxically increase the risk of thrombosis and should therefore be withheld until the platelet count has risen to above $100 \times 10^3/L$ or

until therapeutic anticoagulation has been achieved with recombinant hirudin (lepirudin), danaparoid (if cross reactivity is not present), or argatroban. LMWH should not be substituted for UFH in the setting of HIT.

e. Although its **pregnancy category is C**, heparin is safer than warfarin during pregnancy, especially during the first trimester. Heparin does not cross the placenta and is not excreted in breast milk. Full-dose heparin is recommended during pregnancy for patients who would otherwise take warfarin. For pregnant women with a single remote DVT or PE, a strategy of either prophylactic SC heparin or watchful waiting can be used, but heparin therapy is advocated if the initial event was idiopathic or if there is a laboratory diagnosis of thrombophilia (*N Engl J Med* 2000;343:1439). Heparin should be stopped at the onset of labor and resumed 12–24 hours after birth. If warfarin is initiated postpartum, the heparin can be stopped after the INR is therapeutic.

2. **LMWHs** are chemically or enzymatically prepared from UFH, and they have relatively high anti-Xa activity. LMWHs are as safe and effective as UFH in patients with VTE (*Ann Intern Med* 1999;130:800) or an acute coronary syndrome.

a. **LMWH is administered by SC injection** adjusted for the patient's weight (Table 9-2). The dose of LMWHs used for VTE treatment is significantly greater than the doses used for prophylaxis.

b. **Monitoring** for LMWHs is required only in special situations: renal insufficiency, pregnancy, or morbid obesity. For these populations, monitoring of plasma **anti-Xa activity is recommended**; the aPTT typically becomes only minimally elevated and is not used to guide LMWH therapy. As with UFH, regular **monitoring of CBC (with platelet count)** is advisable.

c. **Side effects** of LMWHs are similar to those seen with UFH (see above), although HIT and osteoporosis may be less common. Bleeding from LMWH is handled similarly to bleeding induced by UFH, but LMWH has a longer half-life than UFH, and protamine sulfate may not reverse LMWH as well as it reverses UFH.

d. **Patients who are self-injecting LMWH should be educated** about the risks and benefits of anticoagulant therapy and about the mechanics of self-injection. They should receive instructions regarding symptoms or signs of bleeding (including pink urine or black stool) and recurrent VTE (pain, swelling, shortness of breath, hemoptysis, fainting) and how to notify their clinician if any of these occur. Patients should be taught about the administration of LMWH, including the expectation that a small hematoma will form at the site of injection. The injection should be SC, not IM, and the site of LMWH injection should be rotated, primarily using the anterolateral abdominal wall and thighs. Patients should also be taught about the storage of medications and equipment as well as the appropriate way to dispose of needles.

B. **Warfarin (Coumadin and others)**

1. **Warfarin** is the most commonly prescribed antagonist of vitamin K. It is completely absorbed after oral administration and then is highly bound to albumin in the plasma. Commercially available warfarin is a racemic mixture, and both enantiomers interfere with the vitamin K–dependent carboxylation of glutamic acid residues on the procoagulant forms of the clotting factors (factors II, VII, IX, and X).

2. The effect of warfarin is measured using the prothrombin time (PT) or the **INR**. The INR is calculated by dividing the patient's PT by the mean of the normal PT and then raising this ratio to an exponent, the international sensitivity index (ISI). The ISI reflects the sensitivity of the

thromboplastin reagent to warfarin-induced changes in the levels of the clotting factors. The INR should be used to adjust dosing of warfarin, and the target INR is typically 2.5 or 3.0, depending on the indication and comorbid condition (Table 9-2). Because the INR may be spuriously elevated in patients who have the lupus anticoagulant (see sec. **II.F.7**), alternative methods of monitoring warfarin therapy may be required in this setting.

3. **Warfarin initiation**
   a. **Most stable outpatients with disorders such as AF can begin warfarin therapy without concomitant heparin therapy.** In contrast, patients with an acute thrombosis should have overlapping heparin therapy. In patients with an acute DVT or PE, the heparin and warfarin should be overlapped for at least 4–5 days (*Arch Intern Med* 1998;158:1005) even if the INR is therapeutic sooner, because the early INR rise primarily reflects depletion in factor VII, with relatively little depletion of factor II.
   b. Loading warfarin doses (e.g., >10 mg on the first day of therapy) can cause a supratherapeutic INR; they should be used cautiously or avoided altogether (*Arch Intern Med* 1999;159:46). Most patients should begin their warfarin therapy by taking **approximately 5 mg warfarin PO**. However, individuals who have liver disease, advanced age, poor nutrition, low body mass, or an elevated INR at baseline should begin with a 2- to 5-mg dose.
   c. After an initial 5-mg dose, **warfarin induction can be guided by an algorithm** (Table 9-3).
   d. **Patients who are starting warfarin for the first time should be educated** about the risks and benefits of anticoagulation (Table 9-4).

Table 9-3. Warfarin nomogram

Day	INR	Dosage (mg)
2	<1.5	5.0
	1.5–1.9	2.5
	2.0–2.5	1.0–2.5
	>2.5	0
3	<1.5	5.0–10.0
	1.5–1.9	2.5–5.0
	2.0–3.0	0–2.5
	>3.0	0
4	<1.5	10.0
	1.5–1.9	5.0–7.5
	2.0–3.0	0–5.0
	>3.0	0
5	<1.5	10.0
	1.5–1.9	7.5–10.0
	2.0–3.0	0–5.0
	>3.0	0

INR, international normalized ratio.
Adapted from MA Crowther, L Harrison, J Hirsh. Warfarin: less may be better—in response. *Ann Intern Med* 1997;127:333.

Table 9-4. Information for patients who are using warfarin

√ Warfarin can cause bleeding and bruising. If excessive bruising or any bleeding (e.g., pink urine or a black bowel movement) develops, call your health care provider.

√ The amount of vitamin K in your diet should be consistent. Bingeing on foods that are rich in vitamin K (e.g., green leafy vegetables) counteracts the effect of warfarin.

√ Because alcohol interacts with warfarin and can cause stomach ulcers, you should minimize alcohol consumption (i.e., no more than two drinks/day).

√ While you are taking warfarin, you will require regular monitoring by a blood test (international normalized ratio).

√ If you miss one warfarin dose, take it as soon as possible. If you miss more than one warfarin dose, call your health care provider for instructions.

√ Many drugs interact with warfarin. When starting any new medication, including aspirin and herbal remedies, check with your doctor or pharmacist to find out whether it is safe for you to take.

√ Women who take warfarin must avoid pregnancy; if you want to bear children, a different blood thinner can be prescribed.

Adapted from BF Gage, SD Fihn, RH White. Warfarin therapy for an octogenarian who has atrial fibrillation. *Ann Intern Med* 2001;134:465–474.

4. The **target INR** depends on the indication for anticoagulation (Table 9-2). The target INR is 2.5 (range, 2.0–3.0) for most indications, except for most types of metallic valves. Patients who have a **St. Jude valve in the aortic position** have a target INR of 2.5, whereas other patients who have metallic valves have a target INR of 3.0 (range, 2.5–3.5). The target INRs may have to be adjusted downward for patients at high risk of hemorrhage, including those who recently have had a hemorrhage. Likewise, they may have to be adjusted upward for patients at high risk of thrombosis (e.g., individuals who have the **antiphospholipid antibody syndrome**) or for those patients who have had a thrombotic event while their INR was therapeutic.

5. **Warfarin dose adjustments**
   a. Once an appropriate warfarin dose has been determined, the frequency of INR monitoring can be decreased to once weekly and then to once every other week. Eventually, most compliant patients can be managed with INR monitoring every 4 weeks. Even in stable compliant patients, INR monitoring should be done at least every 4–6 weeks (*J Gen Intern Med* 1994;9:131).
   b. Most dose **adjustments should raise or lower the weekly dose by 20% or less** (*Am J Med* 2000;109:481). In addition to adjusting the dose and rechecking the INR within approximately 1 week (Table 9-5), the clinician should **search for the cause of an aberrant INR**. These causes include laboratory error, nonadherence, a warfarin-drug interaction (Table 9-6), a change in the intake of vitamin K, or a change in health status.
   c. **When to increase the warfarin dose** depends on the clinical scenario; the dose need not be raised just because a single INR is 0.1 or 0.2 (e.g., INR = 1.8 or 1.9 for a target INR of 2–3) lower than the target range. Lower INRs generally should prompt a dose increase (*Clin Lab Haematol* 1995;17:339), except that INRs that appear to be erroneous should be repeated before one acts on them.
   d. **When to decrease the warfarin dose** also depends on the clinical scenario: In a nonbleeding patient, the dose need not be lowered just because a single INR is a few tenths too high (e.g., INR = 3.3 for a

Table 9-5. Dosage adjustment guidelines for warfarin maintenance therapy with target international normalized ratio of 2.5 (range, 2–3)

INR	Therapeutic intervention	Recheck INR in approximately
<1.8	↑ Weekly dose by 5–20%	≤1 wk
1.8–1.9	None	1–2 wks
2.0–3.0	None	2–6 wks
3.1–3.3	None	1–2 wks
3.4–4.0	↓ Weekly dose by 5–20%	1 wk
4.1–6.0	Hold 1–2 daily dose(s) and	≤1 wk
	↓ Weekly dose by 10–25%	
6.0–9.0	Hold warfarin until INR has fallen	1–5 days
	↓ Weekly dose by 10–40%	
	Vitamin K_1 (1.0–2.5 mg) PO if at increased risk of bleeding or INR rising	
>9.0	Hold warfarin until INR has fallen	1 day
	↓ Weekly dose by 15–50%, and	
	Vitamin K_1 (3–10 mg) PO, SC, or slow IV	

INR, international normalized ratio.
Note: Warfarin dosage adjustments depend on the clinical scenario; recommendations in this table are not appropriate for some clinical scenarios, including bleeding (see sec. **III.B.11**).
Adapted from JD Horton, BM Bushwick. Warfarin therapy: evolving strategies in anticoagulation. *Am Fam Physician* 1999;59:635–646.

   target INR of 2–3). On the other hand, lowering the warfarin dose would be prudent if the patient is feeling ill, eating poorly, or starting a drug that is known to elevate the INR.
   e. **Warfarin-drug interactions** should be considered when making dose adjustment (Table 9-6). For example, a patient who is beginning a drug that is known to increase the INR significantly (e.g., amiodarone) should have his or her warfarin dose reduced prophylactically. In contrast, when minimal warfarin-drug interaction is expected, the usual warfarin dose can be maintained (and the INR checked as appropriate).
6. **Anticoagulation clinics** provide systematic monitoring of outpatient anticoagulant therapy: They monitor the INR, dose the warfarin, and educate patients. One trial found lower rates of bleeding in elderly participants who were randomized to have access to a multidisciplinary anticoagulation clinic that used patient self-testing (*Ann Intern Med* 2000;133:687). Several manufacturers (Avocet Medical, San Jose, CA; Dade Behring, Inc., Deerfield, IL; International Technidyne, Edison, NJ; and Roche Diagnostics, Indianapolis, IN) have developed hand-held instruments that measure the INR, thereby allowing patients to monitor their INR values at home, with remote supervision by a physician or anticoagulation service. Use of **patient self-testing** requires outpatient teaching, supervised practice, and quality assurance testing. In randomized trials, self-testing has improved the quality of anticoagulation control (*JAMA* 1999;281:145).
7. **Side effects include hemorrhage**, GI symptoms, and alopecia. Warfarin also can cause rashes: Coumarin-induced skin necrosis occurs

Table 9-6. Common drugs known to increase the effect of warfarin

Antibiotic/ antifungal	Anti-inflammatory drugs and analgesics	Antiarrhythmics	Miscellaneous
Azoles (e.g., fluconazole)	Acetaminophen[a]	Amiodarone	Alcohol
	Aspirin	Quinidine	Anabolic steroids
Carbenicillin	Allopurinol		Chloral hydrate
Cephalosporins	Methylprednisolone[a]		Cimetidine
Clarithromycin	NSAIDs[b]		Clofibrate
Erythromycin	Propoxyphene		Disulfiram
Isoniazid	Sulfinpyrazone[c]		Heparins
Metronidazole	Zafirlukast		Omeprazole
Quinolones (e.g., ciprofloxacin)			Simvastatin
Tetracycline			Phenytoin (diphenylhydantoin)[c]
Trimethoprim-sulfamethoxazole			Tamoxifen
			Thyroxine

NSAIDs, nonsteroidal anti-inflammatory drugs.
[a]Low doses may not increase the effect of warfarin.
[b]Many NSAIDs, including celecoxib (Celebrex) and rofecoxib (Vioxx), can raise the international normalized ratio (INR).
[c]This drug raises the INR initially, but later it may lower it. The INR also rises when a patient discontinues a drug that lowers the INR (e.g., rifampin, barbiturates, or anticonvulsants).
Adapted from PS Wells, AM Holbrook, NR Crowther, J Hirsh. Interactions of warfarin with drugs and food. *Ann Intern Med* 1994;121:676–683, and BF Gage, SD Fihn, RH White. Management and dosing of warfarin therapy. *Am J Med* 2000;109:481–488.

after 3–10 days of therapy, and the purple toe syndrome typically develops 3–8 weeks after warfarin initiation or after an endovascular procedure. Warfarin is a **pregnancy category D** drug, because it can impair development of the fetal central nervous system and cause other birth defects. Although their side effects and mechanism of action are similar to that of warfarin, other vitamin K antagonists (e.g., **acenocoumarol** and anisindione) have different half-lives and dosing recommendations. The risks for thrombosis and for hemorrhage both increase **with advanced age**, and therefore careful monitoring and avoidance of warfarin interactions are especially important in the elderly.

8. Because **simultaneous use of aspirin and warfarin increases the risk of hemorrhage**, the combination should be used only in special circumstances. Aspirin does **not** need to be added to warfarin therapy in patients who have stable coronary artery disease and a separate indication for warfarin therapy. Warfarin adjusted to an INR of greater than 2 is as effective as aspirin in preventing MI (*JAMA* 1999;282:2058). In contrast, combination therapy with aspirin and warfarin (INR >2) may be justified in patients taking warfarin for another indication who then develop an acute coronary syndrome or in other patients at risk of a thrombotic event.

9. **Very high INRs in the nonbleeding patient** should be treated with vitamin K$_1$. Experts recommend administering vitamin K when the INR is >9 or when the INR is >5 and the patient is at high risk of hemorrhage (*Chest* 2001;119:33S). Patients who have a defect in platelet function (e.g., from concomitant use of ASA or NSAID) or in platelet number (platelet count <100,000) are at high risk of hemorrhage. Patients with

alcoholic binge drinking, liver disease, renal disease, prior bleeding, recent stroke, and advanced age also have an increased risk of hemorrhage (*Am J Med* 1999;107:414). When vitamin K is given, **only vitamin K₁ (phytonadione) should be given**, as other formulations of vitamin K may not reverse the warfarin effect.

   a. For nonbleeding patients at high risk of hemorrhage whose **INR is 5–9, oral administration of vitamin K₁** is recommended because of its ease of administration, greater safety, and lower cost as compared to parenteral vitamin K. An oral vitamin K dose of 1.0–2.5 mg usually is sufficient to lower an INR that is 5–9 to a safe range within 24 hours (*Ann Intern Med* 1997;125:959). Because the smallest available vitamin K tablet is 5 mg, one can administer half of a 5-mg tablet or have the patient drink the appropriate quantity of parental phytonadione diluted in a flavored beverage.

   b. **For INRs of greater than 9**, either oral or parental vitamin K₁ is appropriate and moderate doses of vitamin K (e.g., 3–10 mg) are recommended. If administering vitamin K₁ by the IV route, one should dilute it in 50 ml 5% dextrose solution and then give it slowly to minimize the risk of anaphylactoid reaction. As compared to IV administration, SC administration has less risk of anaphylactoid reaction, but it does not lower the INR as reliably in the subsequent 24 hours.

10. **Treating the bleeding patient**
   a. **Minor bleeds** often can be treated in the outpatient setting, but the INR should be checked and local measures should be instituted. If bleeding is easily controlled and the INR is therapeutic, the warfarin dose can be left unchanged or slightly lowered. For example, minor **anterior epistaxis** often can be controlled with digital pressure to the alae of the nose and a cold compress applied to the bridge of the nose while the patient is sitting upright. If the epistaxis is readily controlled and the INR is not elevated above the recommended range, warfarin can be continued (*Clin Otolaryngol* 1997;22:542), but ASA and other NSAIDs should be avoided and hypertension should be controlled. In contrast to patients who have a single episode of self-resolving anterior epistaxis, individuals who have posterior epistaxis, hematuria, or a stool with occult blood should be thoroughly evaluated; warfarin-induced bleeding may unmask a serious underlying disorder.

   b. **Major bleeds** require hospitalization and correction of the elevated INR.
      (1) **Functional clotting factors** should be given in sufficient quantity to lower the INR to approximately 1.3 or less (i.e., 2–4 units of fresh frozen plasma (FFP), depending on the patient's size and the degree of INR elevation). Because warfarin has a longer half-life than the effect of FFP, vitamin K should be given with the **FFP**, and both treatments may require frequent administration to prevent bleeding recurrence. If available, prothrombin complex concentrate can lower the INR more rapidly than FFP can.
      (2) **Vitamin K₁** should be given in sufficient quantity (e.g., 10 mg phytonadione diluted in 50 ml 5% dextrose solution, given IV over 20 minutes) to overcome the warfarin effect. Because the warfarin effect lasts longer than the vitamin K, vitamin K often has to be administered every 12–24 hours to maintain the INR at less than 1.3.

11. **Perioperative antithrombotic therapy** (see Chap. 2 for details). Holding warfarin for 4–5 days before surgery allows the INR to drift below 1.5 (*Ann Intern Med* 1995;122:40), and holding aspirin for 7 days preoperatively allows enough time for unaffected platelets to enter the circulation. If anticoagulation is needed until just before surgery, LMWH or

UFH can be given, with discontinuation of LMWH at least 24–48 hours before operation and discontinuation of UFH at least 6 hours before surgery.

12. Formulations of **generic warfarin** that are available in the United States are bioequivalent to Coumadin. Some generic formulations (e.g., Barr Warfarin) share a common color scheme with Coumadin; for example, the 2-mg tablets are violet, the 2.5-mg tablets are lime, and the 5-mg tablets are peach.

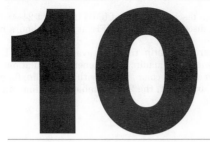

**Pulmonary I:
Common
Symptoms and
Complaints**

Daniel M. Goodenberger

I. Cough

A. Definition. A cough is considered chronic if it persists for 3 or more weeks. Acute cough, lasting for less than 3 weeks, is most often due to the common cold.

B. Significance. Cough is the most common complaint that results in medical attention and is the second most common reason for a general medical examination. It results in more than 30 million office visits annually and accounts for 10–38% of a pulmonologist's office practice. More than 1 billion dollars is spent on cough and cold products each year [*Chest* 1998;114(2 Suppl):133S–181S]. Complications include exhaustion and insomnia, social isolation due to self-consciousness, musculoskeletal chest and abdominal pain, and urinary incontinence. Spouses may also be affected.

C. Causes

1. **Chronic bronchitis** is defined as 3 or more months of cough with sputum production for 2 or more consecutive years. Chronic bronchitis due to cigarette smoking is the **most common cause** of chronic cough in the United States. Of smokers who consume one-half pack/day, 25% have cough, and more than 50% who smoke more than two packs/day are affected. However, in most studies, chronic bronchitis due to cigarette smoking accounts for only approximately 5% of cases of chronic cough, presumably because cigarette smokers are aware that the cough is secondary to smoking and rarely present solely for evaluation of cough. Smokers are more likely to be seen when they are afflicted by a superimposed infectious bronchitis or if chronic bronchitis results in disabling dyspnea.

2. **Chronic cough among nonsmokers** is predominantly due to three causes: postnasal drip, asthma, and gastroesophageal reflux. More than one etiology may be present: 38–82% have a single etiology, and 18–62% have two or more. Asthma and reflux may occur simultaneously, with the gastroesophageal reflux sometimes triggering the asthma. Similarly, postnasal drip or sinusitis, or both, may occur simultaneously with asthma; successful treatment of the asthma is difficult without clearing the postnasal drip or sinusitis, or both.

   a. Postnasal drip is responsible in 8–60% of cases (average, 34%) and is therefore the most common cause of cough. Symptoms other than cough may not be present. Favorable response to treatment is the best evidence to support the diagnosis and its frequency.

   b. Asthma may account for another 7–39% of cases (average, 28%). In some, the asthma has been previously diagnosed or is clinically apparent. In others, cough may be the only manifestation.

   c. Gastroesophageal reflux may cause 3–40% of chronic cough (average, 18%). As many as two-fifths of these, with etiology confirmed by esophageal pH monitoring, may lack symptoms that are referable to reflux other than cough. Cough due to actual aspiration is probably infrequent but is rather most often due to a vagally mediated reflex from acid stimulation of the lower esophagus. This assertion is supported by the observation that acid infused into the lower esophagus of individuals with reflux and cough increased cough frequency and duration as compared with saline (*Am J Respir Crit Care Med* 1994;149:160–167).

d. The remaining etiologies occur less frequently than the three above but still should be considered. **Postviral bronchial hyperreactivity** is responsible for approximately one-sixth of cases of chronic cough (range, 7–25%). Symptoms persist after resolution of an upper or lower respiratory tract infection for up to 12 weeks. Pulmonary function tests are normal. **Bronchiectasis** accounts for 4–5% of cases. It may be localized, as a result of prior severe pulmonary infection, or diffuse, as the result of humoral immunodeficiency, cystic fibrosis, or ciliary dyskinesia. The cough is typically productive. **Lung cancer** is often thought of first by the physician but is a relatively unusual cause (0–2%) of isolated chronic cough. It is extremely unlikely to occur in a nonsmoker. Exposure to asbestos, radioactive materials, and certain metals and organic chemicals may increase the likelihood.

e. **Medications** may also be responsible. Beta-blockers may induce cough via bronchospasm or otherwise subclinical left ventricular dysfunction. Angiotensin-converting enzyme inhibitors (ACE inhibitors) are all capable of causing a chronic cough, which may begin 1 week to 6 months after initiation of therapy. Occasionally, the cough begins almost immediately. ACE inhibitors may account for 0–3% of cases, with the incidence decreasing as clinicians have become more aware of the complication, which occurs in 0.2–33.0% (average, approximately 10%) of those exposed. The pathophysiology remains unclear but may be due to accumulation of bradykinins.

f. **Miscellaneous causes** are responsible for the remainder of cases. Interstitial lung diseases (including sarcoid) occasionally present in this way. Chronic infection is more common in other parts of the world than the United States, with tuberculosis among the most frequent causes. Foreign bodies are unusual in adults but should be remembered in the mentally and neurologically impaired and in those with an episodic altered level of consciousness (alcoholics, drug abusers, epileptics, and diabetics). Pulmonary venous hypertension due to left ventricular dysfunction or mitral valvular disease may cause chronic cough. Psychogenic cough and habit cough are diagnoses of exclusion. Other rare causes include occult cystic fibrosis; recurrent aspiration; ear irritation by hair, cerumen, or foreign body; hyperthyroidism; carcinoid syndrome; lymphangitic carcinomatosis; retained suture; and Zenker's diverticulum.

D. Evaluation and diagnosis

1. History of present illness. Obtain information regarding onset, frequency, severity, and associated symptoms (hemoptysis, dyspnea, weight loss, fever). Ascertain cigarette use. Ascertain whether a respiratory tract infection has occurred within the last 3 months. Ask about tuberculosis exposure and prior purified protein derivative skin testing. Inquire about halitosis, which may be present in lung abscess. Take a careful history of medication use—ACE inhibitors, beta-blockers, inhalants, amiodarone, and nitrofurantoin.

a. **Sputum production.** Inquire about sputum production of significant amounts, which is essentially limited to chronic bronchitis, bronchiectasis, and, rarely, lung abscess. The cough of chronic bronchitis is typically productive of white to grayish sputum and is most prominent in the morning. Cigarette smokers are aware of this and rarely present solely for evaluation of cough; they are more likely to be seen when they are afflicted by a superimposed infectious bronchitis or if chronic bronchitis results in disabling dyspnea. The sputum of bronchiectasis is typically purulent and may be associated with hemoptysis. The sputum associated with lung abscess is typically putrid.

b. **Sinus complaints.** Ask about symptoms that suggest postnasal drip: nasal discharge or congestion, throat clearing, a sensation of pharyngeal tickle or of "dripping" down the back of the throat, and prior sinusitis. Those who are affected may report symptoms that are worse when they are recumbent and are most prominent in the early mornings. Sinusitis may be associated with fever and facial pain.

c. **Reflux.** Ask about heartburn, nocturnal water brash, and exacerbation by recumbency. Unfortunately, more than 40% of patients with reflux have cough as the sole symptom.

d. **Asthma.** Determine if they have a history of asthma, now or in childhood, or a history of allergic rhinitis. Inquire about wheezing (although 28% of patients with asthma may not wheeze) and whether cough worsens with exposure to cold or with exercise. Cough may also be most prominent at night. If the cough worsens at work, that may indicate an occupational cause. Take a careful occupational history—not just job title but what is actually done.

2. **Medical history.** Are any autoimmune diseases associated with interstitial lung disease (polymyositis, rheumatoid arthritis, scleroderma, Sjögren's syndrome)? Is there underlying neurologic disease (prior stroke, motor neuron disease, epilepsy, myasthenia) that may promote aspiration? Is there a history of CHF? Has the patient had laryngeal or thoracic surgery (stitch granuloma)? Is the patient diabetic and given to hypoglycemia? Does the patient abuse alcohol or narcotics?

3. **Family history** should include inquiries about cystic fibrosis, asthma, and tuberculosis.

4. **Social history** should include information regarding tobacco and alcohol use as well as a history of exposure to industrial respiratory toxins (asbestos, silica, coal dust, cotton, isocyanates, fumes) in the past as well as the present.

5. **Physical examination.** Obtain the patient's weight. Examine the ears for wax, foreign material that is touching the tympanic membrane, and otitis (rare causes of cough). Evaluate the eyes for signs of allergic disease, such as allergic conjunctivitis, as well as for iritis, which may suggest an underlying systemic disease. Examine the nose for evidence of mucopurulent secretions, sinus tenderness, boggy turbinates, or polyps, all of which suggest postnasal drip and perhaps a predisposition to asthma. Postnasal drip may also cause a cobblestone appearance of the pharyngeal mucosa as well as erythematous vertical bands along the tonsillar pillars. The throat should also be examined for signs of bulbar neurologic dysfunction. Examine the chest carefully for generalized or localized wheezes and crackles. Auscultate the heart to evaluate ventricular function and valvular abnormalities. Inspect the extremities for edema and the clubbing that may accompany interstitial lung disease and bronchiectasis as well as carcinoma and for signs of autoimmune disease (sclerodactyly, telangiectasia).

6. **Laboratory and radiologic evaluation** should be directed by the history and physical examination and by knowledge of the relative frequency of etiologies. Chronic bronchitis due to cigarette smoking is the most common cause of chronic cough in the United States. Among nonsmokers, three causes (postnasal drip, asthma, and gastroesophageal reflux) account for most chronic cough (see sec. **I.C.2**).

a. **Obtain a chest x-ray first.** If the chest x-ray is abnormal, focus on directed evaluation of the abnormality. If it is normal, obtaining sputum cytology, microbiological stains, and cultures is neither warranted nor cost-effective. If the chest x-ray is normal, the patient is a smoker, and there are no other systemic symptoms, he or she should stop smoking for 4–6 weeks, using whatever assistance is necessary (see Chap. 1, Tobacco Use and Cessation), with further evaluation only if the cough persists.

b. Characteristic symptoms of postnasal drip without signs or symptoms that suggest an alternate diagnosis should prompt 1 week of empiric therapy for postnasal drip without further evaluation. Firm diagnosis requires a positive response to therapy. Response usually occurs within 1 week, and failure to respond suggests an alternative diagnosis or coexistent sinusitis. Imaging of the sinuses should be done if coexistent sinusitis is suspected.

c. **Sinus CT scan** provides superior imaging and is no more expensive than plain radiography, but there is no validation of its predictive value. Nevertheless, it has become the imaging modality of choice in many centers. Sinus x-rays are reported to have a positive predictive value of 81% and a negative predictive value of 95% for sinusitis.

d. **Pulmonary function tests (PFTs).** If empiric therapy for postnasal drip is unsuccessful and no signs or symptoms point to an alternative diagnosis, obtain **PFTs**. If they show reversible obstruction, treat the patient for asthma. **Methacholine challenge.** If pulmonary function tests are normal when the patient is asymptomatic, perform a **methacholine inhalation challenge**. If the methacholine challenge is positive, treat the patient for asthma and evaluate for response. If the methacholine challenge is negative, cough-variant asthma is essentially ruled out (*Arch Intern Med* 1997;157:1981–1987). Because methacholine challenge is more sensitive than either exercise or cold exposure for detection of bronchial hyperreactivity in cold- or exercise-induced asthma, it is rarely necessary to perform postexercise or post–cold air exposure pulmonary function tests for these diagnoses. Because methacholine administration, particularly at higher doses, may have a nearly 20% false-positive rate, failure to alleviate the cough should prompt further workup.

e. **Further management.** If other evaluations, including chest x-ray, pulmonary function tests, and methacholine inhalation challenge, are nondiagnostic, 4 weeks of empiric therapy with a **proton pump inhibitor** for esophageal reflux is recommended, with monitoring of pH performed only if the response to proton pump inhibition is inadequate. **Barium swallow** is insensitive (48%) but inexpensive and not uncomfortable. If it is positive for reflux, treat the patient as a therapeutic trial. However, many experts would skip this step. **Twenty-four–hour esophageal pH monitoring** has been reported to have a sensitivity of 92%; evaluation is most useful if pH drop is correlated with cough (*Chest* 1993;104:1511–1517). Because only approximately one-third of individuals with cough that is not due to postnasal drip or asthma who had a positive pH study responded to proton pump inhibition (*Am J Gastroenterol* 1999;94:3131–3138), expert gastroenterologists recommend evaluation by pH monitoring only after 4 weeks of proton pump inhibitor therapy (*Gastroenterology* 1996;110:1981). The study should be done while the patient is taking the drug to document adequacy of therapy. High-dose proton pump inhibitor therapy (omeprazole, 80 mg/day) is reported to be 83–90% sensitive for the diagnosis of reflux-induced cough; however, because some patients require therapy for up to 6 months, a positive study in a patient with no other apparent cause warrants a longer therapeutic trial.

7. Referral and further evaluation

a. If all other evaluation continues to be negative, consultation with a pulmonologist and a **high-resolution spiral CT** scan of the chest for detection of bronchiectasis and the rare cases of occult interstitial lung disease should be considered. High-resolution CT has been reported to have a sensitivity of 60–100% and a specificity of 92–100% for bronchiectasis. Endobronchial disease (tumor, broncholith) may also be detected.

(1) If the high-resolution spiral CT scan is negative, **laryngoscopy** and **fiberoptic bronchoscopy** may then be indicated. Broncholiths, tumors, stitch granulomas, and so forth almost always call attention to themselves via the history or symptoms.

(2) **Echocardiography** may detect otherwise occult left ventricular failure or occult mitral valvular disease.

(3) Relatively low-yield tests in otherwise asymptomatic patients include **sweat test** for cystic fibrosis, **quantitative immunoglobulins**, and **HIV** testing.

b. If all of the above evaluation is negative, **history and physical examination should be repeated**, and the presence of two or more simultaneous causes should be considered. If cough onset followed a viral infection, **postviral cough** is likely because postviral bronchial hyperreactivity is responsible for approximately one-sixth the cases of chronic cough (range, 7–25%). Symptoms persist for up to 12 weeks after resolution of an upper or lower respiratory tract infection.

c. If all other evaluation is negative, consider psychogenic or habit cough.

E. Treatment. When possible, therapy should be directed by diagnosis. Some studies suggest resolution in as many as 97% with specific therapy.

1. **Chronic bronchitis.** Smoking cessation is crucial, and the patient should be offered nicotine replacement (gum, patch, or nasal spray). Smoking cessation reduces cough in 94–100% of patients, an effect that occurs in 4 weeks or less in over one-half of patients. Ipratropium bromide (2 puffs qid) reduces cough and may help associated bronchospasm. A meta-analysis of 15 studies suggests that mucolytics reduce the frequency of exacerbations, disability days, and antibiotic use in chronic bronchitis (*ACP J Club* 1999;131:14).

2. **Postnasal drip.** In the absence of infectious symptoms, begin therapy with a first-generation oral antihistamine (dexbrompheniramine maleate, 6 mg bid, or azatadine maleate, 1 mg bid) and a sustained-release decongestant (pseudoephedrine sulfate, 120 mg bid). **Nonsedating antihistamines do not appear to be effective** (*Drugs* 1993;46:80–91). Response usually occurs within 1 week and is confirmatory of the diagnosis. If there are symptoms suggestive of allergic rhinitis (see Chap. 12, Rhinitis and Rhinoconjunctivitis, sec. **IV**), initiate a regimen of inhaled nasal steroids (fluticasone nasal spray, 2 sprays in each nostril daily). Nonsedating antihistamines (loratadine) may be effective in allergic rhinitis. Ipratropium nasal spray may be useful in vasomotor rhinitis. If therapy is unsuccessful in relieving symptoms in 2 weeks, consider obtaining a sinus CT scan.

3. **Sinusitis** [see Chap. 19, Specific Infectious Diseases, sec. **I.A.2.d.(4)**]. Select an appropriate antibiotic (e.g., amoxicillin-clavulanate, 500 mg tid, or clarithromycin, 500 mg bid) for a minimum of 3 and up to 6 weeks. Maintain the patient on inhaled steroids (fluticasone, 1 spray each nostril qd). If therapy is unsuccessful, refer to an otolaryngologist to evaluate for endoscopic sinus surgery.

4. **Asthma.** Treat as you would other patients with asthma (see Chap. 12, Asthma, sec. **IV**). Steroids are effective in reducing cough due to asthma, with or without β agonists. Initiate inhaled steroids (fluticasone, 88–220 mg bid). Oral steroids (prednisone, 40 mg/day) may be necessary initially. Steroid therapy may be needed for 6–8 weeks. It can be discontinued when resolution occurs, although recurrence may necessitate resumption of therapy. Use β agonists (albuterol MDI, 2 puffs prn, with longer-acting

salmeterol, 2 puffs bid, as maintenance). **Zafirleukast does not help asthmatic cough. Nedocromil**, however, is effective in reducing asthmatic cough (*Chest* 1990;97;299–306). Exercise- or cold air–induced asthma may be ameliorated by cromolyn (2 puffs qid) or nedocromil (2 puffs qid). For nocturnal cough due to asthma, **long-acting theophylline**, 400 mg qhs, or **albuterol**, 2–4 mg qhs, taken orally may prevent sleep disruption. Once it is controlled, maintenance with **inhaled steroid or cromolyn** may be all that is necessary, with or without prophylactic inhaled albuterol before exercise or cold exposure. Inhaled steroids are ineffective in chronic cough that is not due to asthma (*Can Respir J* 1999;6:323–330, and *Allergy* 1989;44:510–514).

5. **Gastroesophageal reflux** (see Chap. 14, Esophageal Diseases, sec. I). Standard antireflux measures should be used. Gastroenterologists overestimate compliance with head-of-bed elevation using 20-cm blocks. Compliance is more likely with a foam wedge or, if economic circumstances allow, a mechanical bed (double beds that allow one partner to remain flat while the other has the head elevated). The patient should be advised to **avoid eating for 3 hours before bedtime** and to **avoid chocolate, caffeine, and alcohol. Weight loss** may be helpful. High-protein, low-fat diets are recommended. **Smoking** should be curtailed. **Medications that promote reflux** should be avoided (theophylline, anticholinergics, calcium channel blockers). **Omeprazole** (40 mg bid) should be prescribed. Therapy may need to continue for up to 6 months to achieve optimal response. Because of tachyphylaxis and frequent side effects, metoclopramide should be reserved for resistant cases. Failure to respond should prompt consideration of other or additional etiologies. **Antireflux surgery** should be considered only after intensive medical therapy has failed, although laparoscopic fundoplication makes this a more attractive option.

6. **Postviral bronchial hyperreactivity.** This tends to be resistant to therapy but fortunately is self-limited. Ipratropium bromide (two puffs q4–6h) is significantly more effective than placebo in reducing cough in this entity; in one study, ipratropium improved cough in 12 of 14 patients, with resolution in 5 patients (*Respir Med* 1992;86:425–429). Evidence for efficacy of inhaled steroids and oral steroids is weaker, but they can be given if cough persists despite ipratropium use. Resistant cough should be treated with antitussives (see below) and reassurance.

7. **ACE inhibitors.** Discontinuing ACE inhibitors often results in relief of symptoms in less than a week, and virtually all patients are better in 4 weeks. **Changing ACE inhibitors is unlikely to be effective**, as this is a class effect. For those who need these drugs for severe disease, such as refractory CHF or scleroderma with previous renal crisis, treatment with sulindac, indomethacin, nifedipine, and inhaled sodium cromoglycate may provide some relief (anecdotal reports). Alternatives, such as angiotensin receptor antagonists (CHF) or strong antitussives (scleroderma), can be used. Coordination and consultation with involved subspecialists are crucial. On occasion, nebulized lidocaine [200–400 mg q6h (5–10 ml 4% solution)] may be useful if no other drug can be substituted.

8. **Bronchiectasis.** Antibiotics that are effective against *Haemophilus influenzae*, *Staphylococcus aureus*, or *Pseudomonas aeruginosa* reduce cough and sputum production. Improvement may require more than 2 weeks of therapy. Physical therapy, postural drainage, and drugs that enhance mucociliary clearance may provide benefit.

9. **Interstitial lung disease.** Therapy is directed at the underlying disease. Nonspecific antitussive therapy may be required.

10. **Lung cancer.** Treatment for non–small-cell lung cancer is resection and, for small-cell lung cancer, chemotherapy. Nonresectable cancer may require nonspecific antitussive therapy.

11. **CHF.** Therapy is directed at the underlying disorder.
12. **Psychogenic cough.** Modest evidence supports biofeedback and psychotherapy, supported by short-term use of nonspecific antitussive therapy.
13. **Nonspecific therapy. Expectorants** (guaifenesin, iodinated glycerol) are useful only for those with significant, and tenacious, sputum production. **Antitussives** may allow rest and sleep. Dextromethorphan, 30–60 mg every 4 hours, is effective for mild cough, lowers cough intensity to a greater extent, and is rated better as an antitussive by patients than codeine, although both lowered cough frequency (*J Int Med Res* 1983;11:92–100). Codeine can also be used. If the dose of 10–20 mg in cough elixirs is ineffective, codeine given alone in doses of 30–60 mg every 4 hours may increase efficacy. The patient should be counseled regarding anticonstipation measures, and a stool softener or bulk-forming agent should be considered. Hydrocodone (5 mg q4h) and similar potent narcotics should be used judiciously. They are rarely necessary for treatable or self-limited causes of chronic cough. However, they should not be withheld because of inappropriate fear of addiction (i.e., chronic racking cough due to otherwise untreatable disease). They may provide the only available relief for a patient with unresectable lung cancer or severe scleroderma lung disease.

F. **Prognosis.** Overall prognosis is excellent. Diagnosis is successful in 87–100% of patients and specific therapy in 87–98%.

II. **Hemoptysis**

A. **Definition.** Coughing up blood from a pulmonary source is called **hemoptysis**. On occasion, it is confused with hematemesis or the expectoration of blood from a nasopharyngeal source. Blood originates from the bronchial circulation in most cases but has a pulmonary arterial source in pulmonary arteriovenous malformations, Rasmussen's aneurysms in tuberculous cavities, and the diffuse alveolar hemorrhage syndromes of autoimmune origin.

Massive hemoptysis is a poorly defined entity. Definitions are widely varied, ranging from 200 ml/24 hours to 600 ml/16 hours. It is probably more useful to think of hemoptysis as either small volume (<50 ml) or large volume. Large-volume hemoptysis is more likely to be due to tuberculosis, bronchiectasis, and cryptogenic causes. Other causes include aspergilloma, lung abscess, aortobronchial fistula, lung cancer, and pulmonary artery rupture due to pulmonary artery catheter. Bland or septic pulmonary embolism occasionally causes massive hemoptysis.

B. **Significance.** Hemoptysis is an infrequent complaint for those who seek primary care but is of great concern to the patient. When present in small amounts, the greatest concern is about lung cancer. When there is a large amount, the event itself is frightening to the patient and physician.

C. **Causes.** The causes of hemoptysis vary significantly in reported frequency, depending on the patient population, frequency of smoking, amount of hemoptysis, and time period studied. Bronchitis (5% to 37%), tuberculosis (6% to 16%), and lung cancer (12% to 29%) are all common causes. Bronchiectasis appears to be declining in frequency, from as much as 25% to current figures closer to 1%. Aspergilloma is usually found in patients with advanced sarcoid. It is common in city hospital surveys but rare in other settings. Other less frequent causes include trauma, necrotizing pneumonia, lung abscess, mitral stenosis, CHF, pulmonary embolism, foreign body, broncholith, arteriovenous malformation, bronchovascular fistula, pulmonary sequestration, metastasis from extrapulmonary cancer, and pseudohemoptysis (factitious illness). The cause remains elusive in 4–22% of cases.

D. **Evaluation**

1. **History**

a. **Acute hemoptysis.** Obtain an estimate of the volume of hemoptysis. If the history suggests acute hemoptysis of 2 oz or more, refer the patient immediately to a hospital emergency service and arrange for pulmonary and thoracic surgical consultation. Carefully evaluate whether the complaint represents true hemoptysis or is due to expectoration from a nasopharyngeal source. Establish the duration and tempo of the complaint. A long history of episodic hemoptysis is more likely to be due to a benign cause such as chronic bronchitis or bronchiectasis.

   b. **Sputum production.** Ask about the appearance of the sputum. Frothy pink sputum suggests CHF or mitral stenosis. Fever, shaking chills, purulent sputum, and hemoptysis suggest pneumonia. Chronic sputum production is common in chronic bronchitis, bronchiectasis, tuberculosis, and lung abscess. Purulent sputum with streaks of blood suggests bronchitis. Chronic large-volume purulent sputum punctuated by episodes of frank blood suggests bronchiectasis.

   c. **Chest pain.** Inquire about chest pain, which may accompany pulmonary embolism, lung cancer involving the parietal pleura, and pneumonia.

2. **Medical history.** Inquire about severe childhood respiratory infections and previous pneumonias, which may have resulted in bronchiectasis. Obtain a history of any prior malignancy or chest surgery. Inquire about past rheumatic fever. Ascertain whether there is any other known cardiac disease. Inquire about any known respiratory diagnoses, such as sarcoid or cystic fibrosis. Determine whether there are any diseases that would result in episodes of altered consciousness and consequent aspiration, such as diabetes, epilepsy, and alcoholism. Inquire about a prior diagnosis of or exposure to tuberculosis.

3. **Social history.** Determine whether the patient has ever smoked cigarettes and quantify the amount. Obtain an occupational history, with particular attention to asbestos exposure. Obtain a history of alcohol or drug use, with particular attention to whether consciousness has been lost as a result.

4. **Family history.** Inquire about a family history of cystic fibrosis or hereditary hemorrhagic telangiectasia.

5. **Review of systems.** Weight loss and anorexia imply a chronic illness, particularly lung cancer, although tuberculosis and lung abscess can cause similar symptoms. Tuberculosis in particular may cause night sweats. Chronic exertional dyspnea may accompany chronic bronchitis, bronchiectasis, heart failure, and mitral stenosis, as well as cystic fibrosis. Inquire about symptoms of rash, pleurisy, arthralgias, arthritis, and Raynaud's phenomenon, and other rheumatologic symptoms that may implicate systemic lupus erythematosus.

6. **Physical examination.** Fever suggests an infectious cause. Examine the nasopharynx carefully (indirect laryngoscopy may be helpful) to rule out an upper-airway source of bleeding. Halitosis may accompany lung abscess. Auscultate the chest for signs of consolidation (pneumonia), a pleural rub (pulmonary infarction, pneumonia), or a localized wheeze (bronchial obstruction by a neoplasm). Examine the heart carefully for signs of heart failure and the murmur of mitral stenosis. Clubbing may be present in severe bronchiectasis, cystic fibrosis, and lung cancer. Synovitis and rash may suggest vasculitis. Telangiectasia on face, lips, tongue, and fingers may indicate hereditary hemorrhagic telangiectasia and coexistent pulmonary arteriovenous malformation.

7. **Laboratory evaluation.** Obtain CBC, prothrombin time, partial thromboplastin time, and platelet count. Examine the urine for microscopic hematuria and red-cell casts that may suggest a vasculitic pulmonary-renal syndrome and obtain a serum creatinine. Arterial blood gases are unreliable in the diagnosis of pulmonary embolism, but an assessment

of oxygenation is important. Send sputum for Gram stain, acid-fast stain, culture, and cytologic examination. In cases in which pulmonary vasculitis is a consideration, obtain antinuclear antibodies and antineutrophil cytoplasmic antibodies. An echocardiogram may be obtained if there is concern for a cardiac source of hemoptysis.

8. **Radiography.** The **chest x-ray** should be evaluated for a localizing infiltrate or mass. Volume loss or atelectasis suggests bronchial obstruction. Pulmonary cavitation may occur with lung abscess, tuberculosis, or cavitary cancer. The "crescent sign" suggests aspergilloma. **High-resolution CT** with contrast is the best method for diagnosis of bronchiectasis. It is also excellent for the diagnosis of aspergilloma and may detect a broncholith or arteriovenous malformation. If pulmonary embolism is suspected, **ventilation-perfusion lung scan** has been the standard examination. However, **helical CT** with thin sections provides so much more information that it should become the standard.

9. **Bronchoscopy.** Fiberoptic bronchoscopy should be performed in all patients with an abnormal chest x-ray and less than massive hemoptysis. The diagnostic sensitivity varies from study to study depending on the population evaluated but at best is localizing or diagnostic in approximately half (*Arch Intern Med* 1991;151:221–225, and *Chest* 1994;105:1155–1162). Identification of the bleeding site is three times as likely if bronchoscopy is done within 48 hours as when done later (*Am Rev Respir Dis* 1981;124:221–225). Use in patients with normal or nonsuspicious chest x-ray depends on risk factors for bronchogenic carcinoma. Up to 6% of patients may have an occult carcinoma, with male sex, age over 50 years, and significant smoking history being predictors (*Chest* 1989;95:1043–1047, and *Chest* 1988;92:70–76). If the patient is younger than 40 and has never smoked, it is safe to conclude the evaluation without bronchoscopy (*Chest* 1985;87:142–144).

E. **Treatment.** Massive hemoptysis is a medical emergency that requires rapid evaluation and treatment by medical and surgical thoracic specialists and is not further discussed here. The treatment of small-volume hemoptysis is directed at the underlying disease process. Hemoptysis that is associated with chronic bronchitis and bronchiectasis should be treated with antibiotics and antitussives (see Chap. 11). Lung cancer is resected when possible and treated with radiation or chemotherapy, or both, when surgery is not an option. Pulmonary embolism is treated with anticoagulation. The treatment of the other diagnoses listed is beyond the scope of this discussion.

III. **Dyspnea**

A. **Definition.** Dyspnea is, at its most severe, disabling shortness of breath. At the other end of the spectrum, it may simply be an uncomfortable awareness of the effort of breathing.

B. **Significance.** Dyspnea is a common complaint in an office-based practice. Not life-threatening in and of itself, its importance is in the underlying pathophysiologic process.

C. **Causes**

1. **Acute dyspnea** is caused most often by diseases of the heart and lungs.

   a. **Cardiac causes** are most often related to acute pulmonary edema. CHF may occur acutely as a result of myocardial infarction. It may also be the result of acute decompensation of chronic CHF related to ischemic heart disease, long-standing hypertension, and nonischemic cardiomyopathy occurring as a result of a wide variety of diseases (see Chap. 7). Acute pulmonary edema may also be due to diseases of the left-sided cardiac valves (see Chap. 7).

   b. **Pulmonary causes** of acute dyspnea include acute severe bronchospasm, which may be due to asthma or anaphylaxis, or decompensation of chronic obstructive pulmonary disease (COPD). Pulmonary embolism may have acute dyspnea as its major manifestation, with little or no chest pain. Pneumothorax is another cause of acute dyspnea.

c. **Psychogenic dyspnea** may present acutely. Usually a manifestation of an anxiety disorder or panic disorder, it is recognized as acute hyperventilation syndrome.

d. **Evaluation** of acute dyspnea is rarely appropriate in an office setting. When one is alerted to its onset, usually by phone from the patient or a relative, the patient is best referred to an emergency room; transport should be by emergency medical service.

2. **Chronic dyspnea** is usually due to disorders of the heart, lungs, or blood.

  a. **Cardiac causes** include left ventricular dysfunction, valvular abnormalities, and pericardial disease.

  (1) **Left ventricular dysfunction** results in increased left ventricular end-diastolic pressure, which causes interstitial fluid accumulation. The resultant reduction in pulmonary compliance causes increased work of breathing. Exercise worsens the situation, leading to exertional dyspnea. The recumbent position of sleep promotes reabsorption of peripheral edema, and the resultant volume overload may cause orthopnea and, occasionally, paroxysmal nocturnal dyspnea. Causes include coronary disease, hypertensive heart disease, and nonischemic cardiomyopathies (see Chap. 7).

  (2) **Valvular heart disease** is usually left sided. Severe aortic stenosis results in left ventricular dysfunction, manifested by the symptoms listed above. Critical aortic stenosis may also be accompanied by angina, syncope, and atrial fibrillation. Aortic insufficiency may cause progressive left ventricular dilatation and dysfunction. Mitral stenosis results in pulmonary venous hypertension. In addition to dyspnea on exertion, orthopnea, and nocturnal dyspnea, hemoptysis may occur. Mitral insufficiency may cause similar symptoms. Left atrial myxoma, by obstructing the mitral valve, may mimic mitral stenosis.

  (3) **Constrictive pericarditis** may result in exertional dyspnea and peripheral edema.

  b. **Pulmonary diseases** that cause chronic dyspnea extend from the larynx to the alveoli.

  (1) **Vocal cord dysfunction** may result in symptoms that may be difficult to distinguish from those of asthma. Indeed, many patients are treated aggressively (including the use of chronic systemic corticosteroids) before a diagnosis is reached. An accompanying anxiety disorder may occur. The cause is inappropriate vocal cord apposition. Clues include central wheezing, which occurs on inspiration and on expiration.

  (2) **Tracheal stenosis** may have a similar presentation and may also be mistaken for asthma. It may occur as a result of tracheal injury from prior endotracheal intubation or tracheostomy. It may also result from inflammation due to Wegener's granulomatosis or relapsing polychondritis. Rare causes include fibrosing mediastinitis that compresses the trachea, amyloid, and tracheopathia osteoplastica. Tracheal tumors present in a similar fashion.

  (3) **Asthma** (Chap. 12, sec. I–IV) causes episodic or waxing and waning dyspnea. When a cause of dyspnea, it is nearly always associated with wheezing.

  (4) **COPD** is a common cause of dyspnea. Chronic bronchitis is accompanied by cough and sputum production. Emphysema may produce severe dyspnea with few other symptoms. COPD is typically preceded by an extensive cigarette smoking history. Presentation is more fully described in Chap. 11. **Bronchiectasis** is also often accompanied by sputum production and intermittent

hemoptysis. It is often due to prior significant pulmonary infection. In recent years, *Mycobacterium avium-intracellulare* has been recognized as an increasing cause, particularly among middle-aged women. Other associated diseases include cystic fibrosis, common variable immunodeficiency, disorders of ciliary function including Kartagener's syndrome, and Young's syndrome.

   (5) A wide variety of **interstitial lung diseases** may result in dyspnea and progressive pulmonary disability (see Chap. 11). Pulmonary fibrosis may be idiopathic. It may also be secondary to rheumatologic diseases (scleroderma, polymyositis, rheumatoid arthritis), occupational exposures (asbestosis, silicosis, coal worker's pneumoconiosis), or systemic granulomatous disease (sarcoidosis, eosinophilic granuloma), or it may be drug induced (bleomycin). Dyspnea may be due to diminished lung compliance, airways disease, or hypoxemia (typically worsened with exercise), alone or in combination.

   (6) **Chest wall deformities** may also cause pulmonary restrictive disease. Severe kyphoscoliosis may result in dyspnea and, ultimately, respiratory failure, due to mechanical reduction of lung volumes, diminished respiratory compliance, and mechanical muscle disadvantage. Ultimately, hypercarbic respiratory failure and cor pulmonale may result. Very occasionally, severe pectus excavatum may result in exertional dyspnea, likely due to impairment of cardiac filling.

   (7) **Neuromuscular disease** may cause dyspnea. Muscular dystrophies, including Duchenne's, Becker's, limb-girdle dystrophy, and myotonic dystrophy, cause progressive dyspnea and respiratory failure due to muscular weakness. Later in life, respiratory difficulties may develop in polio survivors, particularly those who had respiratory paralysis during the acute illness. Primary neurologic disease, such as amyotrophic lateral sclerosis, hereditary motor neuropathies (Charcot-Marie-Tooth, Dejerine-Sottas), and spinal muscular atrophy, have a similar pathophysiology and symptomatology. Bilateral phrenic nerve paralysis may result from cardiac surgery, trauma, amyotrophic lateral sclerosis, or neuralgic amyotrophy after viral infection or serum administration. Diaphragm paralysis is marked by chronic dyspnea and orthopnea, as well as increased symptoms caused by submersion.

   (8) **Pleural effusion** frequently has dyspnea as a primary symptom. Depending on the cause, pain may accompany dyspnea.

   (9) **Pulmonary vascular disease** results in pulmonary hypertension. Primary pulmonary hypertension (Chap. 11) causes dyspnea on exertion and may cause exertional chest pain and syncope. Right heart failure supervenes, accompanied by edema. Pulmonary hypertension may be **secondary**, due to drugs (anorexiants, amphetamines, and intravenous drug use) and to HIV infection. It may also result from chronic pulmonary thromboembolism, chronic hypoxemia (right-to-left shunts, intrinsic lung disease), lung fibrosis or destruction (idiopathic pulmonary fibrosis, emphysema), left-sided heart failure, chronic liver disease (portopulmonary hypertension), and obstructive sleep apnea with obesity-hypoventilation syndrome. Tumor microemboli may result in lymphangitic carcinomatosis and hypoxemia.

   (10) **Extrapulmonary causes** include massive ascites (pulmonary restriction and hepatopulmonary syndrome–related hypoxemia) and obesity (from restriction and from deconditioning).

   c. **Severe anemia** may cause marked dyspnea, probably from reduced oxygen-carrying capacity and from a high-output cardiac state that may result in elevated left ventricular end-diastolic pressure and pulmonary congestion.

d. **Anxiety disorders** may be accompanied by a chronic sense of dyspnea. Physical signs and symptoms that accompany organic causes of dyspnea are generally absent.

D. Evaluation

1. **History.** Assess the degree of disability; inquire whether dyspnea is present at rest or only with activity. If the latter, ask about the degree of exercise that is necessary to provoke symptoms. Distance walked at a normal pace on level ground and ability to climb stairs provide an approximation of function and are a way to follow symptoms over time. Determine whether dyspnea is constant or episodic. Ask about edema, orthopnea, or paroxysmal nocturnal dyspnea.

   a. **Cardiac etiologies.** Inquire about a history of angina, myocardial infarction, or known coronary artery disease. Ask about cardiac risk factors, including cigarette smoking, hypertension, family history, and hyperlipidemia. Consider causes of nonischemic cardiomyopathy, including alcohol use, hemochromatosis, and amyloid, and inquire about related symptoms. Ask about a history of rheumatic fever or known valvular heart disease. Inquire about medication use, particularly with respect to medicines recently prescribed that might worsen ventricular function or cardiac medicines with which the patient has not been compliant. Determine whether there have been recent dietary changes or indiscretion.

   b. **Pulmonary etiologies.** Elicit a smoking history. Ask about chronic cough and sputum production, which might suggest chronic bronchitis. Determine if there is episodic wheezing; a personal or family history of asthma or atopy; symptom provocation by specific exposures, cold, or exercise; and relief of symptoms with β agonists, any or all of which suggest asthma. Inquire about prior severe respiratory infection, chronic sputum production, intermittent hemoptysis, and recurrent pneumonia, which may suggest bronchiectasis. When bronchiectasis is present, recurrent sinusitis may suggest cystic fibrosis or immune globulin deficiency, as may diarrhea and malabsorption (villous atrophy and *Giardia* in the latter, pancreatic insufficiency in the former). Male infertility may result from cystic fibrosis, ciliary dyskinesia, and Young's syndrome. Obtain a thorough occupational exposure history. Inquire about current and prior medication and drug use. Ask about rheumatologic symptoms, including arthritis, Raynaud's phenomenon, rash, and dysphagia. Obtain a history of any known neurologic disease and neurologic symptoms including weakness. Determine whether there are any HIV risk factors. Ask about prior deep venous thrombosis, pulmonary embolism, and current risk factors.

   c. **Other etiologies.** Inquire whether there is any history of blood loss or known hematologic disease. Ask about symptoms of anxiety or known prior psychiatric diagnosis.

2. **Medical history**

   a. **General.** Inquire about prior myocardial infarction or cardiac surgery. Determine if there is a past history of rheumatic fever. Determine whether the patient has had tuberculosis or radiation therapy in the past, either of which might lead to constrictive pericarditis. Ask about prior serious or recurrent respiratory infections, or both, or previous diagnosis of known pulmonary disease. Ask about known rheumatologic or neurologic disease. Inquire about prior deep venous thrombosis, pulmonary embolism, cancer, hematologic disease, or bleeding disorder. Obtain a history of psychiatric disease or treatment.

   b. **Medications.** Take a history of current and prior medication and drug use. β-Adrenergic blockers, some calcium channel antagonists, and some antidysrhythmics may worsen left ventricular dysfunction. β-Adrenergic antagonists and tartrazine-containing medications may worsen asthma and COPD. Bleomycin may cause pulmonary fibrosis; the onset may be delayed for long periods and be precipitated by oxygen administration. A wide variety of other drugs may induce interstitial lung disease; if in question, review relevant literature to ascertain whether a current or past drug may be responsible. Intravenous drug use may lead to HIV infection; it may also result in pulmonary hypertension due to talc contamination. Anorexiants may induce pulmonary hypertension, as may prior use of contaminated L-tryptophan.

3. **Social history.** Take a careful occupational history. Inquire about symptoms and exposure that suggest occupational asthma. Symptoms may improve over the weekend and worsen at work. Agents may be sensitizers (e.g., isocyanates used in paints) or nonspecific irritants. Ask particularly about exposures to asbestos and silica. Determine and quantify cigarette use. Ask about alcohol use. Inquire about past and present drug use. Inquire about sexual behaviors and HIV risk factors.

4. **Family history.** Inquire about premature coronary disease. Ask about a family history of atopy or asthma. Determine if the patient has a history of early emphysema (α_1-antitrypsin deficiency) or cystic fibrosis. Ask about family history of neurologic or muscular disease.

5. **Review of systems.** Ask about symptoms of allergic rhinitis and recurrent sinus infections. Inquire about symptoms of pain and swelling of the ear and nasal cartilage. Determine presence, frequency, and precipitants of chest pain and discomfort. Note if pleurisy is present. Ask about cough, sputum production, hemoptysis, and wheezing. Inquire about orthopnea, nocturnal dyspnea, nocturia, and edema. Determine if there are GI symptoms, particularly diarrhea and GI blood loss and if there has been weight loss. Ask about genitourinary symptoms, including hematuria. Inquire about rheumatologic symptoms, including arthritis, Raynaud's phenomenon, rash, photosensitivity, pleuritic chest pain, and dysphagia. Ask about syncope or weakness. Determine if the patient has symptoms of anxiety or panic attacks.

6. **Physical examination**
   a. **General appearance and vital signs.** Elevated pulse and respiratory rate are nonspecific but suggest organic disease. Hypertension may have led to diastolic dysfunction or frank heart failure. Excessive obesity and sleepiness during the interview raise the possibility of obstructive sleep apnea and obesity-hypoventilation syndrome. Posture (leaning forward with the arms tripoding), accessory muscle use, and pursed lip breathing suggest COPD. Pallor suggests anemia, jaundice liver disease, and cyanosis hypoxemia. The skin should be examined for rashes that may accompany dermatomyositis, vasculitides, and the purpura of amyloid, and for telangiectasia.
   b. **Ear, nose, and throat examination.** Look for nasal polyps and purulent nasal discharge. Signs of current or past ear or nasal cartilage inflammation may suggest tracheal involvement from relapsing polychondritis or Wegener's granulomatosis. An enlarged tongue may accompany amyloid. Cigarette use may be suggested by the odor of the breath and finger nicotine stains. Lip and tongue telangiectasia are manifestations of hereditary hemorrhagic telangiectasia and may lead to blood loss anemia. Auscultate over the trachea; a prominent central wheeze suggests a laryngeal or tracheal etiology. Adenopathy may be due to infection, sarcoid, or malignancy. Jugular venous distention and hepatojugular reflux suggest right ventricular failure. Examine the carotids for a delayed upstroke and transmitted systolic murmur consistent with aortic stenosis.

c. **Chest examination.** Inspection of the chest reveals relevant chest wall deformities. Dullness to percussion and diminished breath sounds at the chest base(s) indicate pleural effusion. Hyperresonance, hyperexpansion, prolonged expiratory phase, and Hoover's sign (lower chest wall retraction with inspiration) are signs of emphysema. Expiratory wheezes indicate airway obstruction; auscultation during forced expiration may be necessary to detect them. Listen carefully to determine whether the wheezing is most marked peripherally or centrally; inspiratory wheeze also suggests a central lesion. Rales occur with pulmonary fluid accumulation and with pulmonary fibrosis. Those that are associated with fibrosis are characteristically dry and begin in mid- or late inspiration; they are often characterized as sounding like strips of Velcro being pulled apart.

d. **Cardiac examination.** Pay attention to all aspects of the cardiac examination. Palpation may reveal a right ventricular heave or palpable P_2 (pulmonic second sound) associated with pulmonary hypertension, a thrill associated with aortic stenosis, or a dyskinetic left ventricular impulse associated with left ventricular dysfunction. Cardiac auscultation may reveal a dysrhythmia that is suggestive of organic heart disease. S_1 (first heart sound) is accentuated in mitral stenosis and has fixed splitting in atrial septal defect. S_2 may be muffled or absent in the aortic area with severe aortic stenosis or aortic insufficiency and increased in the pulmonic area with pulmonary hypertension. An S_3 may be present in CHF. An opening snap and diastolic rumble indicate mitral stenosis, whereas the murmur without the snap may be present in aortic insufficiency (Austin Flint murmur), even when the characteristic diastolic blowing murmur is difficult to hear. Listen also for the murmurs of aortic stenosis and mitral insufficiency.

e. **Abdominal examination.** Observe the abdomen for inappropriate inward movement with inspiration in the supine position (abdominal paradox), which indicates bilateral diaphragm paralysis or severe weakness or fatigue. The presence of ascites suggests chronic liver disease, as does a firm nodular liver. Enlargement of the liver may be due to primary disease or engorgement from right ventricular failure or impaired filling due to pericardial constriction.

f. **Extremities.** Examine the extremities for edema that suggests right heart failure. Clubbing may accompany pulmonary malignancy, as well as right-to-left shunts and pulmonary fibrosis that is either idiopathic or due to asbestosis. Signs of thrombophlebitis include swelling, pain, and palpable cords but are often absent, particularly in chronic pulmonary thromboembolism. Diminished pulses and signs of vascular insufficiency may indicate significant atherosclerosis. Active synovitis, chronic joint deformity, subcutaneous nodules, muscle tenderness, sclerodactyly, and digital telangiectasia may indicate one of the rheumatologic disorders. The presence of fasciculations may indicate a case of amyotrophic lateral sclerosis with early respiratory involvement. The muscle weakness and atrophy that are associated with hereditary neuromuscular disorders are usually obvious.

7. **Laboratory studies.** CBC detects anemia. Other laboratory tests are not often useful before assessment of pathophysiology by imaging and pulmonary function testing as described below. Restrictive and dilated cardiomyopathies without other obvious cause should prompt transferrin saturation and ferritin measurement (hemochromatosis) and serum and urine electrophoresis (amyloid). Specific patterns of positive antinuclear antibodies may suggest specific rheumatologic syndromes, and a positive antineutrophil cytoplasmic antibody suggests Wegener's granulomatosis. Sputum culture may detect atypical mycobacteria, and

mucoid *P. aeruginosa* suggests cystic fibrosis. The recognition that less severe forms of cystic fibrosis may present in adulthood should prompt sweat testing in those with diffuse bronchiectasis and, if the results are borderline, genetic testing. Diffuse bronchiectasis should also prompt measurement of immune globulin levels and, on occasion, electron microscopy of cilia. Angiotensin-converting enzyme levels are neither sensitive nor specific for sarcoidosis. If lower lobe–predominant emphysema is present, α_1-antitrypsin level should be obtained.

8. **Electrocardiography** may show evidence of previous myocardial infarction. Rhythm disturbances, changes that are characteristic of left ventricular hypertrophy and right ventricular strain, and conduction blocks suggesting infiltrating cardiomyopathies may also be detected.

9. **Radiography and other imaging studies**
   a. **Posteroanterior and lateral chest x-ray** should be one of the initial diagnostic evaluations. Severe kyphoscoliosis is easily apparent. Cardiomegaly and pleural effusion, associated with upward vascular redistribution and, on occasion, interstitial edema, suggest CHF. Filling of the retrosternal space and enlarged pulmonary arteries indicate pulmonary hypertension. Peripherally, the vessels may be pruned, suggesting severe pulmonary hypertension, or plethoric, as may be seen in left-to-right shunt. Occasionally, valvular calcification or pericardial calcification is visible. Increased lung volumes, increased retrosternal air space, and flattened diaphragms are consistent with emphysema. Diminished lung volumes may be due to decreased compliance, as in fibrosis, or weak musculature. The lung parenchyma should be inspected. Bullae and hyperlucency suggest emphysema. Bilateral lower-lobe bullous disease may be particularly suggestive of panacinar emphysema due to antitrypsin deficiency. Signs of bronchiectasis include tram tracking and, in more severe cases, cystic changes, sometimes with air fluid levels. Diffuse involvement, particularly of the upper lobes, suggests an underlying systemic disease such as cystic fibrosis, immune globulin deficiency, or ciliary dyskinesia.
      (1) **Distribution of findings.** Interstitial disease may be categorized by lung volumes and location. Small lung volumes are associated with fibrosis, idiopathic or secondary to rheumatologic diseases, and drugs. Normal or large lung volumes occur with granulomatous disease (sarcoid, eosinophilic granuloma, and hypersensitivity pneumonitis), lymphangioleiomyomatosis, and advanced cystic fibrosis. Lower-lobe involvement is characteristic of idiopathic fibrosis, rheumatologic disease, and asbestosis. Mid- and upper-lung zone development is associated with the granulomatous diseases and silicosis.
      (2) **Additional signs.** Kerley B lines are seen in heart failure and mitral stenosis but may also be present in lymphangitic carcinomatosis and lymphangioleiomyomatosis. Hilar and mediastinal lymphadenopathy may be due to sarcoid, infection, and malignancy. Peripheral calcification of lymph nodes ("eggshell") is characteristic of silicosis but may occur in sarcoidosis.
   b. **Further imaging studies.** If the diagnosis remains obscure after standard radiography and pulmonary function tests, **high-resolution CT** may be helpful. It detects the approximately 10% of cases of idiopathic fibrosis that are not visible on x-ray and is the best method for the diagnosis of bronchiectasis. It may be definitive as well for constrictive pericarditis, lymphangioleiomyomatosis, and lymphangitic carcinomatosis. It may reveal chronic thromboembolic disease when performed with contrast administration and is preferable to ventilation-perfusion scan for this purpose. When pulmonary hypertension is present, the radio-

nuclide dose should be reduced. **Pulmonary angiography** is the most definitive examination for diagnosis of chronic thromboemboli. **Diaphragmatic fluoroscopy** in the supine position is preferable to the "sniff test" for diagnosis of bilateral diaphragm paralysis.

  c. If pulmonary disease is not evident, **echocardiography** can reveal left ventricular dysfunction, detect and estimate the severity of valvular disease, and reveal and quantify the degree of pulmonary hypertension. Administration of saline contrast reveals the presence of intracardiac or intrapulmonary shunt. It is useful for revealing pericardial effusion and thickening. When performed during exercise or dobutamine infusion, it may reveal otherwise inapparent cardiac ischemia.

10. **Pulmonary function testing** should also be used early in the diagnostic evaluation.

  a. **Obstructive physiology** is marked by a reduced ratio of forced expiratory volume in 1 second (FEV_1) to forced vital capacity (FVC) ratio and is common to emphysema, chronic bronchitis, bronchiectasis, and asthma. When interstitial disease is present, obstruction is associated with eosinophilic granuloma, lymphangioleiomyomatosis, and sometimes sarcoid. Increased lung volumes are associated with emphysema and asthma; the latter typically shows improvement when bronchodilators are administered. Methacholine administration may cause a fall in FEV_1 when asthma is in remission. Diminished diffusing capacity accompanying obstruction suggests emphysema.

  b. **Restrictive physiology** is marked by a reduction in total lung capacity. The FEV_1/FVC ratio is usually normal or increased. Fibrotic disease is generally accompanied by symmetric reduction in all lung volumes. Neuromuscular disease is associated with reduction in the vital capacity, with relative preservation of the functional residual capacity and residual volume, and is accompanied by reduced maximal inspiratory and expiratory pressures. Reduction in diffusing capacity is characteristic of pulmonary fibrosis.

  c. When central airway obstruction is present, **flow-volume loops** may show characteristic flattening of the inspiratory or expiratory limbs, or both, depending on the location of the lesion and pliability of the central airway. A characteristic sawtooth abnormality may be seen in obstructive sleep apnea.

11. **Assessment of gas exchange.** Arterial blood gases should be obtained as part of pulmonary function testing. An increased alveolar-arterial gradient or frank hypoxemia is nonspecific and common to many cardiac and pulmonary diseases. Hypercapnia is likewise nonspecific but implies severe pulmonary disease. It is also characteristic of the obesity-hypoventilation syndrome. If resting oxygen pressure is normal, a decrease with exercise may be seen in emphysema, interstitial lung disease, and pulmonary vascular disease. Such testing can be used to guide oxygen therapy.

12. **Exercise testing.** When diagnosis is not obvious, cardiopulmonary exercise testing may be useful. In addition to detecting cardiac ischemia, specific patterns of response are seen in heart disease, lung disease, pulmonary vascular disease, and deconditioning. It may also give strong evidence that chronic dyspnea is not due to disease of the cardiopulmonary axis. Further, it is useful in determining degree of disability.

13. **Lung biopsy** may be required to establish a definitive diagnosis of interstitial lung disease. This is further discussed in Chap. 11.

14. **Overall approach.** History and physical examination result in a high likelihood of the correct diagnosis in the majority of cases, with subsequent testing done for confirmation and to guide therapy. If initial history and physical do not suggest heart disease, chest x-ray and pulmonary function tests, including arterial blood gases, should be ordered first. The hemoglobin concentration determined as part of the blood gas test rap-

idly detects or rules out anemia. If lung disease is confirmed as the cause, further evaluation may include specialized radiography, laboratory testing, oxygen needs assessment, and, when indicated, lung biopsy. If a cardiac cause is suspected, echocardiography should be performed early in the evaluation to aid in determination of etiology and severity. When the diagnosis remains obscure, exercise testing may be helpful, particularly in ruling out significant cardiac or pulmonary disease.

E. **Treatment.** Treatment is aimed at the disease process that is responsible for the patient's dyspnea. Specifics are covered in the portions of this book that address each.

IV. **Noncardiac chest pain**

A. **Definition.** Noncardiac chest pain is that due to causes other than heart disease. Often referred to as **atypical chest pain**, it is generally used to include all chest pain that is not caused by coronary disease.

B. **Significance.** Noncardiac chest discomfort is quite common in ambulatory practice. Its greatest importance lies in the concern it causes to patient and physician alike that significant heart disease underlies the symptom. Given the frequency with which chest discomfort caused by coronary disease is not classic angina pectoris, particularly in women and diabetics, this concern is warranted.

C. **Causes.** This discussion assumes that the presence of coronary disease has been evaluated and ruled out (Chap. 6). Evaluation of valvular heart disease, aortic dissection, and pericarditis is discussed in Chap. 7. The remaining common causes involve the chest wall, pleura, and esophagus. Diseases of the gallbladder, pancreas, and large and small bowel, and psychiatric disorders, account for the majority of the remainder.

1. **Chest wall disorders.** Musculoskeletal is more common than neurogenic pain. Costochondral and chondrosternal pain is frequently the result of exercise, injury, or inflammation of obscure cause (costochondritis). Rib fracture may occur from direct trauma, cough, or malignancy. Intercostal or pectoral muscle strain may occur from exercise. Nerve pain may be a result of pre-eruption herpes zoster, postviral or idiopathic neuritis, or referred nerve root pain from compression or irritation of cervical or thoracic nerve roots.

2. **Pleural pain** results from inflammation of the pleura. It is frequently due to infection. Viral pleuritis may follow Coxsackie B infection (pleurodynia). Pneumonia is often accompanied by pleural inflammation, sometimes accompanied by pain. This is particularly characteristic of pneumococcal disease. Pleural involvement with tuberculosis is sometimes associated with pain. Pulmonary infarction occurs in a minority of cases of pulmonary embolism and is often accompanied by pain. Rheumatoid arthritis and systemic lupus erythematosus are often complicated by pleural involvement; pain is much more common in lupus. Carcinomatous involvement of the pleura is usually accompanied by effusion; the associated sensation is more often described as heavy or dragging than painful. The pain associated with pneumothorax is probably due to disruption of adhesions of the parietal to the visceral pleura.

3. **Esophageal pain** can easily be confused with coronary ischemia. It is most often due to reflux or spasm.

4. **Gallbladder pain** may radiate to the chest. It is most often due to cystic duct obstruction but may be caused by frank cholecystitis.

5. **Uncommon causes**, such as gastric and duodenal ulcer, bowel distention secondary to gas or obstruction, and pancreatic inflammation, may result in chest pain.

D. **Evaluation**

1. **History**

a. Any **significant chest pain** should prompt consideration of coronary artery disease. If one is notified of acute severe pain by phone, **refer**

the patient to an emergency room via emergency medical service for initial evaluation of coronary insufficiency, aortic dissection, and pulmonary embolism, any of which may be rapidly fatal; office evaluation is not appropriate.

b. Initiate the history by establishing the **character and quality of the pain**, assuming that the pain is not suggestive of an acute coronary syndrome or another serious emergency, or that coronary disease has been ruled out. Determine the location, nature, and duration of the pain. Ascertain whether the pain is precipitated by exercise, emotion, eating, or posture. Inquire whether the pain is worsened by cough or deep breath. Ask whether the pain is relieved or improved by rest, nitrates, antacids, or histamine-2 (H_2) blockers or by changes in posture. Ask about accompanying symptoms, including nausea, vomiting, heartburn, sweating, fever, dyspnea, cough, sputum production, or hemoptysis. Inquire about recent viral infection, unaccustomed exercise, or chest trauma. **Musculoskeletal pain** is of widely varying duration, from a few seconds to days. It is typically aggravated by movement, deep inspiration, and cough. The patient may notice that it hurts to touch. Systemic symptoms are absent. **Neurologic pain** is less likely to be increased by thoracic movement, but neck, arm, and shoulder movement may worsen nerve root irritation or thoracic outlet compression. **Pleuritic pain** is typically sharp and aggravated by inspiration and cough, but less so by movement. An exception is the pleural pain component that may accompany pericarditis; the pericardial component may be improved by sitting up and leaning forward. The patient may have had recent or current infectious symptoms, including fever, chills, coryza, cough, and sputum production. **Pulmonary infarction** due to thromboembolism may be accompanied by dyspnea and hemoptysis. Its likelihood is increased by the presence of predisposing factors, such as prolonged immobilization, heart failure, previous venous thrombosis, extended travel, cancer, and recent surgery. **Pleurisy** due to lupus erythematosus is often accompanied by other systemic signs of the disease, including arthralgias, arthritis, rash, photosensitivity, and Raynaud's phenomenon. Often the diagnosis has been made previously. Pleural involvement with **cancer** often follows a known prior diagnosis. **Pneumothorax** is characterized by abrupt onset, often accompanied by dyspnea.

Esophageal pain may be difficult to differentiate from that of a cardiac etiology. Classic heartburn, occurring after a large meal and worsened by the supine position, presents little diagnostic confusion. Typically, it is improved or relieved with antacids or H_2 blockers. The duration is typically longer than that caused by angina. However, it may be dull or heavy rather than burning and may radiate to the neck or arm. It may improve with nitrates or calcium channel blockers and may even occasionally worsen with exercise. **Peptic ulcer disease** is typically epigastric but may be perceived as originating in the chest. It is typically relieved by antacids and H_2 blockers. **Gallbladder** pain is usually of acute onset, associated with nausea and vomiting, and felt in the right upper quadrant or epigastrium. However, it may radiate substernally or more typically to the right infrascapular area and may improve with nitroglycerin. It may last for hours. **Pancreatitis** usually presents as severe epigastric pain with radiation to the back, nausea, and vomiting, but on occasion it is mistaken for cardiac pain.

2. **Medical history.** Ask about a history of past deep venous thrombosis, cancer, or rheumatologic disease. Determine whether there has been interstitial lung disease that may predispose to pneumothorax. Inquire whether there has been prior pancreatitis or ulcer disease. Determine whether med-

icines are being taken that may cause drug-induced lupus (procainamide, hydralazine, isoniazid, among others) or that reduce lower esophageal sphincter pressure (theophylline, calcium channel blockers). Oral contraceptives may increase the risk of thromboembolism.

3. **Social history.** Obtain a history of cigarette smoking (which may predispose to esophageal reflux, ulcer disease, and pneumothorax, in addition to cancer) and alcohol use (reflux and pancreatitis).

4. **Physical examination.** Most patients with noncardiac chest pain who present to an office look well. Exceptions include those with acute infection, who may be febrile and dyspneic; those with pulmonary embolism, who may be dyspneic; those with acute biliary colic, who may be diaphoretic and vomiting; those with pancreatitis, who may be acutely ill and have emesis; and those with malignancy, who may appear chronically ill. Tachycardia may accompany any of the acute illnesses and is characteristic of pulmonary embolism and infarction. Tachypnea may accompany embolism and pneumothorax. Fever suggests infection but may be a manifestation of pulmonary embolism, malignancy, or lupus. Examine the fundi for signs of vascular disease. Palpate the chest wall for tenderness; although characteristic of musculoskeletal pain, it may also be present in empyema, pleurodynia, and, rarely, pulmonary infarction. Percuss and auscultate for dullness or hyperresonance; the former may herald pleural effusion or consolidation, the latter pneumothorax. Listen for consolidation or rales, suggesting pneumonia, and a pleural rub, suggesting pleural inflammation. Diminished breath sounds, when accompanied by dullness, may suggest effusion. When accompanied by hyperresonance and sometimes tracheal deviation, they may indicate pneumothorax. Examine the heart for signs of heart failure or pericardial friction rub. Inspect the skin for the eruption of herpes zoster. Palpate the abdomen for right upper quadrant tenderness and a Murphy's sign, suggestive of gallbladder disease. Pancreatitis and peptic ulcer disease may have associated epigastric tenderness. Palpate for any abdominal masses. Examine the cervical and thoracic spine for any signs of tenderness and determine if pain is worsened by cervical spine motion or vertical compression. Examine the extremities for swelling, tenderness, or cords that are suggestive of venous thrombosis.

5. **Laboratory evaluation and radiography** are guided by history and physical examination. The patient who has a **benign history**, appears well, has normal vital signs, and whose physical examination is entirely negative except for localized chest wall tenderness that reproduces the symptoms complained of may require nothing other than reassurance. In practice, however, obtaining a normal ECG may be worth its cost in providing that reassurance. Similarly, definite diagnosis of a benign process such as herpes zoster requires no further evaluation as to cause. If chest wall tenderness follows **trauma** or is accompanied by systemic symptoms, rib films may show evidence of fracture or malignancy. Pain that is **radicular** and unremitting may warrant MRI of the cervical or thoracic spine. If the symptoms suggest **pleuropulmonary infection**, obtain a chest x-ray, and if pneumonia is present, sputum Gram stain and culture and blood cultures. If a pleural effusion is present, it should be evaluated as described in sec. **V.** Appropriate systemic symptoms should prompt one to obtain an antinuclear antibody and rheumatoid factor. Suspicion of **pulmonary embolism and infarction** requires the workup outlined in Chap. 9. **Nonpleuritic pain** without an obvious origin should prompt evaluation for a GI source. Barium swallow is neither sensitive nor specific for pain caused by reflux, and the invasiveness and expense of esophageal pH monitoring and endoscopy make a trial of H_2 blocker a reasonable first alternative. If there is inadequate response or the diagnosis remains in doubt, those studies and esophageal manometry can be considered, with gastroenterologic consultation. Perform right upper

quadrant ultrasound for suspected biliary colic. Obtain a serum amylase or lipase as a screen for pancreatitis.

E. Treatment is directed at the specific diagnosis that is responsible for the chest pain. Treat musculoskeletal pain with nonsteroidal anti-inflammatory medication, which may also be helpful for nonspecific neuritis. Please refer to the appropriate sections for treatment of the other diagnoses listed.

V. Pleural effusion*

A. Transudative pleural effusions are formed when the normal hydrostatic or oncotic pressures are perturbed [e.g., increased mean capillary pressure (heart failure) or decreased oncotic pressure (cirrhosis or nephrotic syndrome)]. **Exudative pleural effusions** occur when damage or disruption of the normal pleural membranes or vasculature occurs and leads to increased capillary permeability or decreased lymphatic drainage (e.g., tumor involvement of the pleural space, infection, inflammatory conditions, or trauma).

B. Diagnosis. Most pleural effusions require further evaluation unless their origin is clear (e.g., heart failure) and the patient is responding well to therapy (*Am Rev Respir Dis* 1989;140:257).

1. **Thoracentesis** can be performed safely in the absence of disorders of hemostasis on effusions that demonstrate a thickness of greater than 10 mm on lateral decubitus films. Loculated effusions can be localized with ultrasonography or CT scan. Proper technique and sonographic guidance minimize the risk of pneumothorax and other complications.

   a. **The etiology** of an effusion frequently can be deduced from the clinical circumstances (e.g., CHF or hepatic failure with ascites). Exudates have at least one (and transudates none) of the following: (1) a pleural fluid protein–serum protein ratio of greater than 0.5, (2) a pleural fluid–serum lactate dehydrogenase (LDH) ratio of greater than 0.6, or (3) a pleural fluid LDH of more than two-thirds of the upper limit of normal for serum LDH. Proposed additional criteria for an exudative pleural effusion include (1) a cholesterol level of greater than 45 mg/dl, (2) a serum–pleural albumin gradient of less than 1.2 g/dl, or (3) a pleural–serum bilirubin ratio of greater than 0.6 (*Chest* 1997;111:970). Parapneumonic effusions are exudates that develop secondary to pulmonary infections. An empyema is pus in the pleural space. The pleural fluid glucose, pH, and LDH are helpful in differentiating complicated parapneumonic effusions and are useful to identify the patients who usually will require chest tube drainage.

   b. **Other studies** involving pleural fluid that may be useful in specific clinical settings include cell count and differential, amylase, triglycerides, microbiologic stains, cultures, and cytology. Some useful observations have been obtained from the results of studies on pleural fluid.

      (1) Gross blood is seen with tumor, pulmonary infarction, or trauma; a pleural fluid–blood hematocrit ratio of more than 0.5 establishes the diagnosis of a **hemothorax**.

      (2) A **pH of less than 7.3** is seen with empyema, tuberculosis, malignancy, collagen vascular disease, or esophageal rupture.

      (3) **Glucose** concentration of less than 40 mg/dl is associated with an empyema, rheumatoid arthritis, tuberculosis, or malignancy.

      (4) An **elevation of eosinophil count** (>10% of total nucleated cell count) may occur with bloody effusions, pneumothorax (or previous thoracentesis), fungal and parasitic infection, drug-induced disease, and malignancy.

      (5) An **elevation of amylase** may occur with pancreatitis, pancreatic pseudocyst, renal failure, malignancy, esophageal rupture, or ruptured ectopic pregnancy.

*Dan Schuller and Subramanian Paranjothi contributed to this section.

    (6) Elevation of triglycerides (>110 mg/dl) indicates chylous effusions, which are caused by thoracic duct rupture from trauma, surgery, or malignancy (usually lymphoma).

    (7) Cytology is positive in approximately 60% of malignant effusions. Priming the fluid collection bag with 300–1000 IU heparin and submitting a large pleural fluid volume maximize the diagnostic yield for cytologic diagnosis.

  2. Closed pleural biopsy should be performed when the cause of an exudative pleural effusion cannot be determined by thoracentesis. For tuberculous effusions, pleural fluid cultures alone are positive in only 20–25% of cases; however, the combination of pleural fluid studies and pleural biopsy (demonstrating granulomas or organisms) is 90% sensitive in establishing tuberculosis as the etiology of the effusion. For malignant effusions, pleural biopsies add a small but significant diagnostic yield to fluid cytology alone.

  3. Other diagnostic procedures that are useful in establishing the etiology of a pleural effusion when the foregoing tests are normal include biopsy of other abnormal sites (e.g., a mediastinal or lung mass), diagnostic thoracoscopy, and evaluation for pulmonary emboli.

C. Treatment

  1. Symptomatic pleural effusions may require removal of large amounts of pleural fluid. The rapid removal of more than 1 L of pleural fluid may result (rarely) in re-expansion pulmonary edema. When frequent or repeated thoracentesis is required for effusions that reaccumulate, early consideration should be given to tube drainage and pleurosclerosis.

  2. Parapneumonic effusions and empyema. Appropriate management is instituted according to a classification based on the size of the effusions, the gross characteristics of the pleural fluid, the biochemical analysis, and the presence of loculations (*Chest* 1995;108:299). Insignificant parapneumonic effusions (small, <10 mm thick on decubitus film) almost always resolve with antibiotic therapy alone. Performing a thoracentesis is unnecessary unless the effusion becomes symptomatic or increases in size. Pleural effusions greater than 10 mm thick require a thoracentesis, and management depends on the pleural fluid characteristics.

  3. Malignant pleural effusions arise from tumor involvement of the pleura or mediastinum. Patients with malignancy are also at increased risk for pleural effusions from postobstructive pneumonia, pulmonary emboli, chylothorax, and drug or radiation reactions. If pleural tissue or cytology is positive for malignancy or if other causes of effusion are reasonably excluded in a patient with malignancy, several therapeutic options exist (*Clin Chest Med* 1993;14:189).

    a. Therapeutic thoracentesis may improve patient comfort and relieve dyspnea. The subjective response to drainage and the rate of fluid reaccumulation should be monitored. Repeated thoracenteses are reasonable if they achieve symptomatic relief and if fluid reaccumulation is slow. This may be done in the outpatient setting.

    b. Chemical pleurodesis is an effective therapy for recurrent effusions. This treatment is recommended in patients whose symptoms are relieved with initial drainage but who have rapid reaccumulation of fluid. Talc pleurodesis appears to be the most effective and least expensive agent, particularly in malignant pleural effusions with a pH of less than 7.30 (*Chest* 1998;113:1007). Doxycycline or minocycline can be instilled in the pleural space at the bedside without thoracoscopy or general anesthesia. Bleomycin appears to be less effective and more expensive than other drugs. All require admission and referral as appropriate.

    c. **Pleurectomy or pleural abrasion** requires thoracotomy and should be reserved for patients with a good prognosis when pleurodesis has been ineffective.

    d. **Chemotherapy and mediastinal radiotherapy** may control effusions in responsive tumors such as lymphoma or small-cell bronchogenic carcinoma but are seldom useful in metastatic carcinoma.

    e. **Observation** without invasive interventions may be appropriate for some patients.

VI. Solitary pulmonary nodule

A. Definition. A solitary pulmonary nodule is defined as an asymptomatic round lesion less than 3 cm in diameter, completely surrounded by lung, and unaccompanied by atelectasis or intrathoracic adenopathy.

B. Significance. Solitary nodules are usually found on routine screening x-rays or those taken as part of the evaluation of another process. It is estimated that they occur on 0.09–0.20% of such films, for a total incidence of approximately 150,000 yearly in the United States. Although most are benign, a significant minority represent lung cancer in a potentially curable state (stage I). Thus, the goal is to separate those that are malignant from those that are benign, resecting all the malignant lesions and avoiding resection of as many as possible of those that are benign.

C. Causes. Approximately 50% are granulomas, and another 5% are benign tumors, most often hamartomas. Another 5% are due to miscellaneous benign causes, including arteriovenous malformations, healed pulmonary infarction, vasculitides such as Wegener's granulomatosis, rheumatoid nodules, and bronchogenic cysts. The remaining 40% are malignant. Four of five malignancies are primary bronchogenic carcinomas, a small number are other primary nonbronchogenic pulmonary malignancies, and the remainder are solitary metastases of nonpulmonary origin. It is important to recognize that even when there has been a prior nonpulmonary malignancy, the majority of malignant solitary nodules are bronchogenic carcinomas.

D. Evaluation

    1. **History.** Patients often have few symptoms. The age of the patient is important, as fewer than 2% of nodules in those under the age of 30 years are malignant, as opposed to more than 50% in patients older than 60 years. Determine whether cough, hemoptysis, weight loss, or bone pain is present. Obtain a smoking history. Inquire as to residence in an area with endemic mycoses (histoplasmosis, coccidioidomycosis), and whether the patient has had exposure to individuals with tuberculosis.

    2. **Medical history.** Inquire about previous malignancies.

    3. **Social history.** Determine whether the patient has ever smoked cigarettes, as the risk of lung cancer after a significant smoking history never returns to baseline. Take a careful occupational history. Significant asbestos exposure, even many years earlier, increases the risk of lung cancer, particularly in smokers. Miners may have increased radon exposure.

    4. **Family history.** Hereditary hemorrhagic telangiectasia dramatically increases the incidence of pulmonary arteriovenous malformations.

    5. **Physical examination.** Note evidence of wasting or weight loss. Look for adenopathy, which may provide a convenient site for biopsy. In women, examine the breasts carefully for masses. Palpate the abdomen for hepatomegaly or abdominal masses. Palpate a man's testicles for masses, particularly if he is young. Do a rectal examination and test the stool for occult blood. Look for clubbing. The presence of telangiectasia may be a clue to hereditary hemorrhagic telangiectasia.

    6. **Radiography**

        a. **Chest x-ray.** The most important radiograph is a previous chest x-ray. If a prior film demonstrates that the nodule is unchanged for 2 years or more, the lesion is almost certainly benign. If the lesion has increased in size, the doubling time is useful in estimating the likelihood of malignancy. This refers to increase in the volume, which doubles when the diameter increases 1.26 times. If the doubling time is more than 400 days (which may occur with hamartomas or granulomas) or less than 30 days (which is typically due to infection), malignancy is unlikely. The **presence of calcification** is also a useful predictor of benign status, as fewer than 2% of cancers are calcified. Lesions that have laminated, central, diffuse, or popcorn calcification are invariably benign. Those with stippled or eccentric calcification may be benign or malignant. Lesions with spiculated or irregular lesions are more likely to be malignant, whereas those with smooth borders are more likely to be benign. Size has a rough correlation, with larger lesions more likely to be malignant.

b. **Chest CT** has proved a valuable adjunct, increasing to 60–80% the percentage of nodules that are malignant when resected. Lesion diameter can be measured precisely, allowing more accurate estimation of doubling time. Thin cuts through the lesion are more sensitive for presence and pattern of calcification, and the nature of the lesion's margins may be seen more easily. It was previously observed that lesions with a density greater than 185 Hounsfield units were usually benign and those with lower density more likely to be malignant. However, the use of phantoms for densitometry proved insufficiently accurate for diagnosis and is no longer recommended. Contrast enhancement with evidence of feeding and draining vessels may suggest an arteriovenous malformation. Enlarged mediastinal nodes may represent metastasis. Location is important in planning for biopsy by transbronchial needle aspiration or mediastinoscopy. CT may also reveal asymptomatic metastases in liver, adrenal, or bones.

c. **Positron emission tomographic scans** are based on the fact that radioactive fluorodeoxyglucose[18] is taken up by metabolically active lesions but not metabolized. Thus, malignant lesions are more likely to be "hot" than are benign ones. Sensitivity of 89–100% and specificity of 79–100% have been reported in populations with generally high pretest probabilities of cancer. Metastases are demonstrated in up to 14% of cases of lung cancer. False negatives occur in slowly growing tumors such as bronchoalveolar carcinoma and carcinoids, and false positives may occur in active infections. Insufficient data exist at present to recommend the use of positron emission tomography as a routine decision-making tool.

d. **Routine bone scan** and **brain CT scan** are not recommended in the absence of symptoms that suggest involvement of those organ systems.

7. **Laboratory evaluation** is of limited use. The serum calcium level may be increased in epidermoid cancers. Serum sodium may be reduced as part of the syndrome of inappropriate antidiuretic hormone secretion associated with small-cell cancer, although this rarely presents as a solitary nodule. Alkaline phosphatase may be elevated when bone metastases are present. Sputum acid-fast bacteria stain (AFB stain) is unlikely to be productive when there is no other parenchymal disease. Sputum cytology is unlikely to be positive with peripheral nodules. A tuberculin skin test does not add useful decision-making information.

8. **Bronchoscopy** is unlikely to result in diagnosis of small peripheral nodules. Sensitivity is less than 20% for lesions smaller than 2 cm and 40–60% for those that are 2–3 cm in size.

9. **General diagnostic approach and decision-making process.** The reasonable desire is that all primary lung cancers be resected while the unnecessary resection of benign lesions is avoided. This is tempered by a desire not to mistake a malignant lesion for a benign one when it is at

its most resectable stage; resected stage I lesions have a 5-year survival of approximately 70%.

a. **Observation.** In general, three strategies are available. The first is observation with serial CT. This is favored when there is a low risk of cancer, the patient has a strong aversion to surgery, or there is serious comorbid disease or pulmonary dysfunction, which substantially increases the 2–4% mortality associated with resection in otherwise healthy individuals. This approach is supported by the observation that average life expectancy is similar whether surgery is performed immediately, biopsy is performed before surgery, or a strategy of serial observation is followed.

b. **Biopsy.** A second strategy is transthoracic needle aspiration biopsy followed by resection of demonstrated malignancy and avoidance of resection for a confirmed benign diagnosis. This approach is favored for lesions with an intermediate risk of malignancy, for patients who decline surgery absent a firm diagnosis of malignancy, and for those with significant surgical risk. It is supported by a sensitivity of more than 90% for the diagnosis of malignancy. Limitations are that a specific diagnosis is made in fewer than 50% of benign lesions and that pneumothorax occurs in 15–30% of biopsies, approximately half of which require treatment. Failure to make a specific diagnosis does not resolve the dilemma of whether to operate or to continue observation.

c. **Surgery.** The third approach is to resect the lesion immediately. This is favored in patients with a high risk of malignancy and no contraindications to surgery.

d. **Risk of malignancy.** A formal prediction model has been developed to estimate risk of malignancy (*Arch Intern Med* 1997;157:849–855). Risk is estimated based on age (younger than 40 years vs. older than 50 years), smoking history (never smoked or quit more than 4 years before vs. moderate to heavy smoking or quit less than 4 years before), growth rate (sec. **VI.D.6**), diameter (<1.5 cm vs. >2 cm), location (upper lobe favoring malignancy), edge (smooth vs. spiculated), and calcification (specific patterns favoring benign lesion). However, prospective evaluation of this instrument as compared to the decisions made by experienced physicians failed to demonstrate an advantage (*Mayo Clin Proc* 1999;74:319–329). Thus, patients with indeterminate lesions are probably best managed by referral to a physician who is experienced in their management.

E. **Treatment.** Treatment of lung cancer is as described in Chap. 11. Specific benign diagnoses and healed granulomas seldom require treatment.

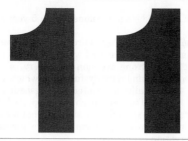

Pulmonary II: Diseases

Roger D. Yusen and
Stephen S. Lefrak

Chronic Obstructive Lung Disease

I. **Introduction.** Chronic obstructive pulmonary disease (COPD) describes a pattern of disease that is **c**hronic (time scale is measured in years), **o**bstructive (characterized by a fully or partially irreversible decrease in maximal expiratory airflow at any lung volume), **p**ulmonary (involving the lungs, airways, or pulmonary parenchyma), and a **d**isease (a pathophysiologic entity with defining symptoms and signs). Approximately 14 million Americans have COPD; although most have chronic bronchitis, 2 million have emphysema. COPD is the fourth leading cause of death in the United States, with higher death rates associated with the more severe airflow obstruction as measured by the forced expiratory volume in 1 second (FEV_1). The major diseases that produce chronic airway obstruction are chronic bronchitis and emphysema. Although bronchiectasis (see Cystic Fibrosis) and asthma (see Chap. 12) can both produce chronic airflow obstruction, they are usually not categorized as COPD.

II. **Etiology and pathophysiology** Emphysema is defined as dilatation of the terminal air passages with alveolar wall destruction and the absence of fibrosis. **Chronic bronchitis** is defined clinically as cough that is productive of at least two tablespoons of sputum on most days, for 3 consecutive months in 2 consecutive years, in the absence of any other lung disease. The etiology of emphysema and chronic bronchitis is almost always tobacco smoking (cigarettes). Even those patients with α_1-antitrypsin deficiency in whom clinically significant disease develops are often smokers. In the 15–20% of smokers in whom airflow obstruction develops, the only treatment modality that has been demonstrated to stop the excessive decline in pulmonary function and decrease mortality is the halting of cigarette use. This cannot be overemphasized. Physicians should work with all patients to help stop tobacco smoking.

COPD is particularly insidious, as dyspnea usually does not develop until the FEV_1 is 60% or less than the predicted normal value, and once developed it is hard to alleviate. The pathways to dyspnea are complex but include (1) airflow obstruction, (2) hyperinflation that produces abnormalities in chest wall and respiratory muscle function, (3) increased respiratory drive, and (4) maldistribution of ventilation that produces frequency dependence and abnormalities in alveolar gas exchange. These four mechanisms are important to understand, as therapy is directed toward correcting them so that dyspnea can be alleviated. As dyspnea becomes severe, there is a particularly unfortunate tendency to do less physical activity. This leads to deconditioning of the cardiovascular system and peripheral muscles, further impairing the ability to exercise. As a result, the patient is unable to perform even basic activities of daily living (ADLs) without difficulty.

III. **Evaluation**
   A. **History and physical examination.** The symptoms of COPD include dyspnea, cough, sputum production, and occasionally wheezing. It is useful to quantitate

a patient's dyspnea either by using a readily available scale, such as the Modified Medical Research Council Dyspnea Scale, or a simple self-devised one, which is useful to compare the patient's level of function from visit to visit. The physical signs of COPD are present only with far-advanced disease and relate predominantly to the complications of the disease. Wheezing may be audible with the stethoscope. The apparent "barrel chest," accessory muscle use, and inward movement of the lower costal margin (Hoover's sign) with inspiration are all reflections of hyperinflation. Pursed lip breathing may be present. Ankle edema from right heart failure is a sign of far-advanced disease. Clubbing is not a sign of chronic bronchitis or emphysema. If clubbing is present, a search for another cause is indicated, especially lung cancer. Attention must be paid to the patient's weight and nutrition, as **weight loss** is a particularly ominous sign in severe emphysema. Weight loss due to COPD, however, should be a diagnosis of exclusion, and other causes of weight loss should be investigated.

B. **Pulmonary function testing**, especially spirometry, should be included in the initial examination of every patient who is or was a cigarette smoker for the detection of COPD. Spirometry is the only reliable means for diagnosing COPD, and that measurement and understanding of FEV_1 and forced vital capacity are critical in office practice. Spirometry is not only valuable for diagnosis, but also can be used to classify the disease by the severity of impairment of the FEV_1 and to plan treatment. Patients with mild disease (FEV_1 <80%, but ≥50% predicted) require office management by a primary care physician, whereas those patients with severe disease (FEV_1 <35% predicted) may well require office management by a pulmonologist if one is available. Those with moderate (FEV_1 <49%, but ≥35% predicted) disease should probably have at least a consultation by a pulmonologist, and their continuous management can be carried out by their primary care physician.

C. **Arterial blood gases** should be obtained in patients with moderate and severe impairment. A measurement of oxyhemoglobin saturation obtained with a pulse oximeter is insufficient, as it provides no information about alveolar ventilation ($PaCO_2$).

D. **Supplemental oxygen requirements** should be assessed at rest and during exercise in patients with moderate to severe disease. Many patients with COPD have an adequate arterial oxygen pressure (PaO_2) at rest but experience oxyhemoglobin desaturation with exercise. A simple test can be performed by having the patient, wearing a pulse oximeter, walk as rapidly as possible for 6 minutes accompanied by a therapist, who monitors the pulse oximeter. Supplemental oxygen flow is increased as needed to keep the measured saturation at 89% or greater. This provides an assessment of oxygen needs with exercise and quantitates the distance that the patient can actually walk, both of which are important in planning the exercise regimen. **Sleep desaturation** is common in COPD. Supplemental oxygen requirements during sleep can be determined with nighttime recording pulse oximetry. If the patient manifests signs of daytime sleepiness or a nocturnal history that is compatible with sleep apnea, polysomnography should be performed (see Obstructive Sleep Apnea–Hypopnea Syndrome).

E. **Imaging studies** such as chest radiographs are helpful in excluding concomitant disease (e.g., lung cancer) and evaluating for hyperinflation, but they are not very sensitive for diagnosing emphysema. CT scans may be diagnostic of emphysema but are not usually indicated except in unusual circumstances. Both chest radiographs and CT scans often appear normal in patients with chronic bronchitis.

F. **α$_1$-Antitrypsin levels** are indicated in patients with (1) premature onset of COPD or severe impairment before the age of 50, (2) predominance of basilar emphysema, (3) a family history of α$_1$-antitrypsin deficiency or early COPD, (4) chronic bronchitis with airflow obstruction in a patient who never smoked, or (5) unexplained bronchiectasis or cirrhosis. Genetic phenotyping should be performed if α$_1$-antitrypsin levels are low.

IV. General management
   A. All patients should **cease smoking tobacco**. Nicotine addiction, however, is extremely tenacious, and efforts to end tobacco use must be vigorous. The use of nicotine in chewing gum, transdermal patches, nasal spray, or inhaled devices is very helpful and provides benefit when compared to placebo (see Chap. 1). Bupropion hydrochloride (Zyban or Wellbutrin) is another mode of tobacco cessation therapy. Support groups and even hypnosis can be tried. However, only 20% of those who enter such "cease smoking" programs are successful for more than a year. The poor long-term outcome for giving up nicotine is ample demonstration of its addictive power. Physicians must be encouraging and supportive rather than threatening or punitive in their approach to patients and their families.
   B. **Educational materials** should be made available for patients so that they can understand their disease, its treatment, and its prognosis. Such information can be obtained from the local American Lung Association or its Web site (http://www.ALA.org). It is important to stress to the patient that emphysema is not a rapidly progressive disease but rather a chronic problem that can be managed successfully.
   C. **Health maintenance** should include polyvalent (Pneumovax) inoculation every 5 years and the yearly influenza vaccine. All patients should receive a chest radiograph on at least a yearly basis.
V. Pharmacologic therapy
   A. **Inhaled bronchodilators** are the mainstays of therapy in metered-dose inhalers (MDI) that contain either a β agonist, an anticholinergic agent, or both. Albuterol may be found combined with ipratropium (Combivent). Patients with severe disease should be instructed to use at least 2–4 puffs every 4–6 hours. This dose can be increased two (or even, rarely, three) times to achieve maximum bronchodilation. Patients must be instructed in the proper use of the MDI, and if they have difficulty, a spacer may prove of benefit. The predominant advantage to a nebulizer is a larger dose administered, but most patients are adequately treated by MDIs. Nebulizers are also helpful for those with poor MDI technique. The addition of a long-acting β agonist, salmeterol (Serevent), 2 puffs bid, may produce further symptomatic improvement, especially if the patient is awakening at night to use the inhaler. A new longer-acting anticholinergic agent (Tiotropium) has shown promise in preliminary reports (*Chest* 2000;118:1294).
   B. **Systemic bronchodilators** can be tried if the patient's condition does not improve. A trial can be given of theophylline, in sustained-release form, 600–800 mg total/day. Although theophylline use has declined in view of its potential toxicity, it is particularly helpful in patients who cannot use inhaled drugs appropriately or regularly. Theophylline and a number of other drugs interact, leading to a change in the dosage requirements and possible toxicity. Thus, changes in drug levels should be anticipated and monitored when certain medications are changed in a patient's regimen. Continued inhalation of tobacco smoke lowers theophylline levels, which should be maintained at between 6 and 12 mg/L. Theophylline produces anxiety and tremor, which many patients cannot tolerate. Nausea, vomiting, tachycardia, and tachyarrhythmias are signs of theophylline toxicity; levels should be obtained and the drug stopped immediately. Seizures and death can occur in seriously toxic patients. Oral β agonist therapy is usually not recommended because inhaled agents provide similar benefits with fewer side effects.
   C. **Anti-inflammatory drugs** such as corticosteroids may benefit as many as 30% of patients with COPD. A trial of oral prednisone may be indicated in patients with wheezing, frequent exacerbations, or severe impairment. An objective improvement in measured FEV_1 must be demonstrated for maintaining corticosteroid therapy. Subjective feelings of improvement by themselves are insufficient criteria for maintenance of these drugs. A reasonable starting dose is 40 mg prednisone for 10–14 days,

then gradually tapering to the minimal required for objective improvement. In patients who respond to oral therapy, inhaled corticosteroids offer the ability to maintain the improvement with less risk of systemic effects. Inhaled steroids can be administered by MDI, for example, fluticasone (Flovent), in doses ranging from 44 to 220 µg/puff. Inhaled steroids should be administered at 2 puffs bid (patient may use a spacer), following bronchodilator treatment, and the patient should thoroughly wash the mouth and throat out after each use to avoid thrush and hoarseness. Caution should be used when substituting inhaled steroids for oral steroids due to the risk of adrenal insufficiency.

D. **Oxygen therapy** has been shown to decrease mortality and improve physical and mental function in patients who are hypoxemic. An arterial blood gas should be obtained to document whether hypoxemia is present when breathing room air. Pulse oximetry may be useful for routine checks after a baseline oxyhemoglobin saturation is determined. Oxygen therapy is indicated for any patient with a PaO_2 of 55 mm Hg or less or oxyhemoglobin saturation (SaO_2) of 88% or less. If a patient has evidence of cor pulmonale, pulmonary hypertension, or a hematocrit of greater than 55%, oxygen therapy is indicated, with a PaO_2 of ≤ 59 mm Hg or SaO_2 of $\leq 89\%$. If patients require oxygen either at rest or with exercise, then they need supplemental oxygen during sleep. Although the exact amount required nocturnally might be measured with pulse oximetry, it is not unreasonable to set the oxygen to be delivered during sleep as 1 L greater than that required during rest when awake. If patients do not require oxygen at rest or with exercise, it is unlikely that they need it with sleep. Desaturation is more common during sleep in patients with COPD. Therefore, unexplained pulmonary hypertension or polycythemia is an indication for measuring oxyhemoglobin saturation during sleep. Supplemental oxygen requirements may decrease after treatment of an acute exacerbation. Therefore, an oxygen reassessment can be made 1–3 months after initiation of therapy. One should be cautious in removing oxygen therapy from a patient who has benefited from the initiation of pharmacologic and oxygen therapy, as this is usually a lifetime commitment.

E. **Oxygen delivery systems** should be prescribed to ensure the most active lifestyle for the patient, as exercise should be encouraged. Essentially, there are three systems for delivering long-term oxygen therapy: compressed gas, liquid oxygen, or oxygen concentrators. The highest cost and greatest mobility occur with the liquid system, whereas the lowest cost and least mobility result from the concentrators. If patients use a concentrator, they must have another source for ambulation outside the home. Most frequently, oxygen is delivered via continuous-flow, dual-prong nasal cannula. This serves virtually all patients regardless of activity level. Patients rarely require high concentrations of oxygen (e.g., exercise), and the use of a reservoir system with an Oxymizer may be the most cost effective in these cases. Also, demand pulse systems are available in which oxygen is only delivered during inspiration. Transtracheal oxygen is rarely needed in COPD, although it may be necessary in some patients with other problems who require high concentrations of oxygen to maintain an adequate oxyhemoglobin saturation. It is also occasionally useful in patients who prefer a cosmetic alternative to nasal prongs. The physician, when writing an oxygen prescription, should state the delivery system required as well as the required oxygen dose (L/min) for rest, exercise, and sleep.

F. **Antibiotics** are useful only in patients with an acute exacerbation of their disease.

VI. **Pulmonary rehabilitation**

  A. **General.** Patients with severe COPD frequently find their enjoyment of life curtailed by respiratory symptoms, especially dyspnea. Pulmonary rehabilitation comprises a multidimensional continuum of services aimed at providing improvement in functioning and quality of life. Rehabilitation should be a central element of the treatment program for virtually all patients with severe COPD and has been shown to decrease frequency of hospitalization (*Ann Intern Med* 1969;70:1109). Patients with COPD who should be referred to a comprehensive rehabilitation program include those who (1) continue to demonstrate severe dyspnea after maximum pharmacologic therapy, (2) who have had several emergency department visits or hospital admissions in the past year, or (3) exhibit impaired quality of life, limited functional status, or restricted ADLs as a result of dyspnea or other respiratory symptoms.

B. Graded exercise. The initiation and maintenance of a graded exercise program are a mainstay of rehabilitation of the patient with severe COPD. Although the use of oxygen and pharmacologic therapy may produce symptomatic improvement, exercise rehabilitation may further improve the patient's quality of life and performance of ADLs. A graded exercise program may return a patient to a more functional and satisfactory life. To initiate an exercise program for the markedly impaired patient, an evaluation of exercise capability and need for supplemental oxygen should first be undertaken. The patient then should enter a graded exercise program a minimum of three times/week with a goal of 30 minutes of continuous aerobic activity. Oxygen should be worn if required and the patient monitored with pulse oximetry to ensure an adequate oxyhemoglobin saturation. The workload should be gradually increased at weekly intervals until patients reach 80% of their maximum heart rate ($220 - \text{age} \times 0.8$) or breathlessness. A treadmill is preferred for exercise, although a stationary bicycle can be used as well. An arm ergometer can be used along with lifting of light weights to increase upper-extremity strength. Flexibility exercise should be included, especially in elderly patients. Noninvasive cardiac stress testing or cardiopulmonary testing is recommended prior to initiation of exercise rehabilitation in patients at higher risk for coronary artery disease.

C. Nutrition and psychosocial support. Malnutrition, especially undernutrition, commonly occurs in patients with marked COPD and is associated with increased mortality. Patients may benefit from nutritional counseling and the use of nutritional supplements. Unless the carbohydrate intake is excessively high, excess carbon dioxide production is not a problem. As part of the initial comprehensive rehabilitation evaluation, counseling can be offered to address coping with anger, depression, and fear related to the chronic illness and to provide encouragement and support. Referral to a support group that is composed of patients with similar pulmonary problems may be beneficial.

VII. Surgery offers three options for carefully selected patients with severe COPD. Referral to the appropriate centers with the most experience should be considered in any patient with severe dyspnea. **Lung transplantation** is an alternative for patients with marked airflow obstruction (FEV_1 <25% predicted), hypercapnia, marked hypoxemia, pulmonary hypertension, and marked limitation in the ADLs. In general, this is an option for younger patients without significant comorbidity. **Bullectomy** is a procedure that has been in use for decades. It is used in patients with airway obstruction and dyspnea in whom a bulla or bullae occupy at least 50% of the hemithorax. **Lung volume reduction surgery** has had excellent results in highly selected patients with severe emphysema (FEV_1 <35%). Target areas consist of volume-occupying and poorly functioning lung, which are accessible to surgical resection.

VIII. Replacement therapy with α_1-antitrypsin (Prolastin) is available for patients with emphysema and α_1-antitrypsin deficiency. Although the benefits of replacement therapy have not been well defined, this extremely expensive therapy may be useful in these patients. Therapy should be instituted before disease is severe and after smoking has been discontinued. Hepatitis B vaccination is recommended before initiation of replacement therapy.

IX. Monitoring of disease progression is important. Patients should be followed at regular intervals (every 3–4 months). At these visits, information concerning severity of dyspnea with certain activities should be obtained using a simple quantitative dyspnea scale. A directed physical examination should be performed with the intent of detecting complications (e.g., ankle swelling indicating right heart failure), as well as maintaining general health. Proper use of MDIs should be reviewed, abstinence from smoking should be encouraged, and rehabilitation and graded exercise goals reviewed. Spirometry and chest radiography should be performed at least once a year. FEV_1 typically declines <60 cc/yr if the patient continues to smoke and <30 cc/yr if the patient is not smoking.

Obstructive Sleep Apnea–Hypopnea Syndrome

I. **Introduction. Obstructive sleep apnea–hypopnea syndrome (OSAHS)** is a disorder of symptomatic sleep-disordered breathing. OSAHS is characterized by repetitive episodes of upper-airway narrowing or collapse during sleep, often associated with sleep fragmentation and oxyhemoglobin desaturation. OSAHS frequently causes excessive daytime sleepiness (hypersomnolence) and other sequelae that adversely affect the daily functioning of the patient. The sequelae of OSAHS may include motor vehicle accidents (*Sleep* 1997;20:608), systemic hypertension (*N Engl J Med* 2000;342:1378, and *JAMA* 2000;283:1829), pulmonary hypertension (*Eur Respir J* 1996;9:787), polycythemia, and increased morbidity and mortality, typically due to cardiovascular disease (*Eur Respir J* 1999;13:179). OSAHS is a major public health concern, present in an estimated 2–4% of middle-aged adults (*N Engl J Med* 1993;328:1230). The National Commission on Sleep Disorders Research estimated that OSAHS causes 38,000 cardiovascular deaths/year at a cost of $42 million annually for related hospitalizations. The cumulative 8-year mortality of untreated OSAHS has been estimated to be as high as 37% for patients with moderate-severe disease compared to 4% for patients with less severe disease (*Chest* 1988;94:9). The most significant problem is **recognition** and **diagnosis** of OSAHS.

II. **Pathophysiology.** Sleep apnea may be central, obstructive, or a combination of both. Some patients have a combination of central and obstructive sleep apnea. **Obstructive** sleep apnea results from decreased or absent respiratory airflow due to narrowing or collapse of the upper airway. In **central** sleep apnea, the airway patency is adequate, the central drive to breathe is absent, there is no respiratory effort, and airflow is absent. Most cases of sleep apnea are **obstructive** and are grouped under the heading **OSAHS.**

The patency of the pharynx depends on the surrounding musculature. While awake, patients with OSAHS typically prevent pharyngeal collapse with upper-airway dilatory muscles. During sleep, the upper-airway muscles relax and the pharynx narrows or collapses. Decreased or absent respiratory airflow and oxyhemoglobin desaturation occur. Pulmonary vascular hypoxic vasoconstriction leads to elevation of the pulmonary arterial pressures. As attempts to inspire against the obstructed airway continue, the intrathoracic pressure becomes increasingly negative. Reflexes then cause the brain to arouse the patient from sleep. An increased sympathetic nervous system response leads to variations in heart rate and BP. As the patient arouses, the airway patency is restored and the oxyhemoglobin saturation, heart rate, and BP normalize. As the patient returns to sleep, the cycle may repeat.

III. **Diagnosis of OSAHS. OSAHS** is a disorder of sleep characterized by recurrent apneic and hypopneic episodes (*Sleep* 1999;22:667). Patients with risk factors and symptoms or sequelae of OSAHS should be referred to a sleep specialist and sleep laboratory for further evaluation.

A. **Symptoms of OSAHS** (Table 11-1). Habitual loud snoring is the most common symptom of OSAHS, and patients most often seek medical attention

Table 11-1. Symptoms associated with obstructive sleep apnea–hypopnea syndrome

Excessive daytime sleepiness

Snoring

Nocturnal arousals

Apneas

Nocturnal gasping, grunting, and choking

Nocturia

Awakening unrefreshed

Morning headaches

Impaired memory and concentration

Irritability and depression

Impotence

because of the complaints of their bed partner. Not all people who snore have OSAHS. The partner's description of the sleep-related events can provide very important information. Excessive daytime sleepiness (daytime hypersomnolence) is a classic symptom of OSAHS. Patients may describe falling asleep while driving or having difficulty in concentrating at work. Subjective sleepiness can be assessed by a validated scale such as the **Epworth sleepiness scale** (*Sleep* 1991;14:40). With this scale, patients estimate their likelihood of falling asleep on a four-point scale during eight normal daily situations (Table 11-2). An Epworth score of greater than 10

Table 11-2. Epworth sleepiness scale

How likely are you to doze off or fall asleep in the following situations, in contrast to just feeling tired? This refers to your usual way of life in recent times. Even if you have not done some of these things recently, try to work out how they would have affected you. Use the following scale to choose the most appropriate number for each situation.

0 = would never doze	2 = moderate chance of dozing
1 = slight chance of dozing	3 = high chance of dozing

Situation	Chance of dozing
Sitting and reading	_____
Watching TV	_____
Sitting, inactive, in a public place	_____
As a passenger in a car for an hour	_____
Lying down in the afternoon	_____
Sitting and talking to someone	_____
Sitting quietly after a lunch without alcohol	_____
In a car, while stopped for a few minutes in traffic	_____

Adapted from MW Johns. Reliability and factor analysis of the Epworth sleepiness scale. *Sleep* 1992;15:376–381.

suggests that significant daytime sleepiness is present, although an elevated Epworth score is not specific for OSAHS.

B. Testing

  1. The gold standard for the diagnosis of OSAHS is overnight **polysomnography** ("sleep study"), with direct observation by a qualified technician. Sleep studies are typically done in the outpatient setting. A standard sleep study consists of an EEG to determine the stages of sleep, electromyography to monitor muscle activity, and electro-oculography to monitor eye movements. Respiratory airflow, respiratory effort, oxyhemoglobin saturation, heart electrical activity (ECG), and body position are monitored.

  a. The sleep study is analyzed for sleep staging and for the frequency of respiratory events. Events are categorized as

   (1) Obstructive: Airflow is absent or reduced despite continuous respiratory efforts.

   (2) Central: Airflow and respiratory effort are absent.

  b. The **respiratory disturbance index (RDI) or the apnea-hypopnea index (AHI)** is used to diagnose sleep-disordered breathing and to quantify its severity. **Apnea** is defined as complete cessation of airflow that lasts for at least 10 seconds. **Hypopnea** is defined as a significant reduction in airflow or thoracoabdominal movement for at least 10 seconds that is associated with at least a 4% drop in the arterial oxyhemoglobin saturation. The RDI or AHI is the sum of apneic and hypopneic episodes/hour of sleep. **OSAHS** exists when clinical features are present and a sleep study shows an AHI of at least five events/hour. Mild-severity OSAHS has an AHI of 5–15, moderate severity has an AHI of 16–30, and severe OSAHS has an AHI of more than 30 (*Sleep* 1999;22:667). Symptoms and sequelae should also define the severity of OSAHS. The risk of death, hypertension, and poor neuropsychological functioning rise as the AHI increases.

  c. A single sleep study is usually sufficient to diagnose OSAHS. A second night study should be performed for treatment titration (see sec. **V**). However, if classic symptoms of OSAHS are present and if the diagnosis of severe OSAHS is made early in the study, a "split-night" study can be performed. The first half is done to make the diagnosis of OSAHS, and the second half is used to titrate positive airway pressure treatment.

IV. Therapeutics and management of OSAHS. Once a diagnosis of OSAHS is made, therapy should be instituted.

A. Weight loss, even small amounts, may lead to a marked improvement in overweight patients (*Chest* 1987;92:631). Successful sustained weight loss is difficult, and education, psychological support, and close follow-up may be beneficial.

B. Positive airway pressure

  1. Continuous positive airway pressure (CPAP) is used to deliver air via a nasal or oral mask. **Nasal continuous positive airway pressure (nCPAP)** is the current **treatment of choice** for most patients with OSAHS. nCPAP pneumatically splints open the upper airway and prevents collapse. The airway pressure that is required to optimize airflow is determined during the sleep study. The nCPAP pressure (cm H_2O) is gradually increased until obstructive events, snoring, and oxygen desaturations are most improved. Some patients require supplemental oxygen to maintain adequate oxygen saturations ($Sao_2 \geq 89\%$). CPAP leads to consolidated sleep and decreased daytime hypersomnolence in almost all patients. BP, nocturia, polycythemia, and pulmonary hypertension may also improve.

  2. Efforts to improve **compliance** with therapy are a key to the successful treatment of patients. Unfortunately, the mechanical treatment of

OSAHS has been associated with compliance problems in 50% of patients. Compliance may be improved with education, instruction, follow-up, adjustment of the mask for fit and comfort, heated humidification of the air to decrease dryness, and treatment of nasal or sinus symptoms. Use of a full mask (oronasal) has not improved compliance compared to the use of nasal masks.

   3. Bilevel positive airway pressure (BiPAP) can be used to treat patients with OSAHS. It is more expensive than CPAP and does not improve patient compliance. BiPAP is reserved for patients who are intolerant of very high levels of CPAP or do not have a good response to CPAP. These individuals may respond well to noninvasive mechanical ventilation with BiPAP or volume ventilation. **AutoPap** ("smart" CPAP) machines use flow and pressure transducers to sense airflow patterns and then automatically adjust the CPAP. The effectiveness of AutoPap has not been well studied.

   4. Adverse effects of CPAP or BiPAP. All noninvasive positive pressure or mechanical ventilation devices may induce dryness of the airway, nasal congestion, rhinorrhea, epistaxis, skin reactions to the mask, nasal bridge abrasions, and aerophagia.

C. Oral appliances, such as the mandibular repositioning device, are used to increase airway size to improve airflow. The devices can be fixed or adjustable, and most require customized fitting. Many devices have not been well studied.

D. Surgical treatment

   1. For patients with OSAHS, **tracheostomy** has been consistently effective, but it is rarely used given the advent of positive airway pressure therapy. Tracheostomy should be performed in patients with life-threatening disease (cor pulmonale, arrhythmias, or severe hypoxemia) that cannot be controlled with nonsurgical therapy. Patients can plug the tracheostomy tube during the day. Tracheostomy has the usual risks associated with anesthesia, and the procedure causes disfigurement of the neck and may result in psychological distress. Granulation tissue may develop, and patients may rarely experience life-threatening hemoptysis and airway obstruction.

   2. Uvulopalatopharyngoplasty (UPPP) is the most common surgical treatment of **obstructive sleep apnea** in patients who do not respond to medical therapy. UPPP enlarges the airway by removing tissue from the tonsils, tonsillar pillars, uvula, and posterior palate. UPPP may be complicated by change in voice, nasopharyngeal stenosis, foreign body sensation, and velopharyngeal insufficiency. UPPP's success rate is only 50%, and improvements related to it may diminish over time. Thus, it is considered a second-line treatment for patients with moderate to severe OSAHS who cannot successfully use CPAP and who have retropalatal obstruction. Laser-assisted uveoplasty has not been as well studied. Other surgical procedures have been used separately or in conjunction with UPPP, but the efficacy of most has not been proven. The most promising other procedure is maxillomandibular advancement, which may be best for patients with retroglossal obstruction.

E. Pharmacologic treatment. At this time, medications have a minimal role in the treatment of OSAHS. Patients should be assessed and treated for hypothyroidism. Patients with OSAHS should **avoid use of alcohol, tobacco, and sedatives**.

V. Return evaluation. Initially, frequent visits to the home by respiratory technicians to assist in mask and machine setting adjustments may be necessary. After a period of stability, patients should be monitored at least once a year to assess symptoms (Table 11-1) and the adequacy of therapy. Weight loss recommendations should be reinforced, and counseling should continue as needed. Symptoms of rhinorrhea and nasal congestion should be sought, and appropriate treatment should be instituted if problems are noted. Causes of noncompliance should be addressed. Patients should also undergo repeat polysomnography for **CPAP titration** if symptoms or sequelae worsen or return.

Cystic Fibrosis

I. **Cystic fibrosis (CF)** is the most common lethal genetic disease in Caucasians, with an incidence of 1 in 3200 live births in the United States (*J Pediatr* 1998;132:255). Although it is less common in non-Caucasians, the diagnosis needs to be considered in patients of diverse backgrounds. The diagnosis of CF is typically made during childhood, but 8% of patients are diagnosed during adolescence or adulthood (*J Pediatr* 1993;122:1). With improved therapy, the median survival has been extended to approximately 30 years (*J Pediatr* 1993;122:1).

II. **Pathophysiology.** CF is an autosomal recessive disorder that is caused by mutations of a gene located on chromosome 7. All patients with the clinical syndrome of CF have mutations in both gene copies, although all mutations do not necessarily produce the clinical syndrome. CF-related gene mutations lead to abnormal production of a **CF transmembrane conductance regulator** protein that normally regulates and participates in the transport of electrolytes across epithelial cell and probably intracellular membranes (*Science* 1989;245:1073). Although the primary manifestations of disease are thought to be related to abnormal electrolyte transport, the pathophysiology is not completely understood.

III. The **diagnosis** of CF is based on clinical and family history in combination with persistently elevated concentrations of sweat chloride, two known disease-causing CF mutations, or nasal transepithelial potential difference measurements that are typical of CF. Atypical patients may lack classic symptoms and signs or have normal sweat tests. Although genotyping may assist in the diagnosis, it alone cannot establish or rule out the diagnosis of CF.

A. **Clinical manifestations**

1. **Pulmonary symptoms** lead to the consideration of the diagnosis of CF in 50% of cases (*J Pediatr* 1993;122:1). Almost all patients eventually develop chronic sinopulmonary disease, most notable for bronchiectasis and chronic airflow obstruction. Symptoms typically include cough and purulent sputum production, and dyspnea ensues as the disease progresses. Acute pulmonary disease exacerbations may lead to significant deterioration and subsequent hospitalization. Isolation of a mucoid variant of *Pseudomonas aeruginosa* from the respiratory tract occurs frequently in patients with CF. Other pulmonary problems may include allergic bronchopulmonary aspergillosis, hemoptysis, and pneumothorax.

2. **Extrapulmonary manifestations** of CF include exocrine pancreatic insufficiency, seen in 90% of patients, leading to fat malabsorption and malnutrition. CF affects the GI tract (steatorrhea, constipation, impaction, distal intestinal obstruction, volvulus, intussusception, and rectal prolapse). Constipation must be distinguished from the other complications that may present with similar symptoms. CF also affects the endocrine pancreas (diabetes mellitus and pancreatitis), hepatobiliary (fatty liver, cirrhosis, portal hypertension, cholelithiasis, and cholecystitis), genitourinary (male infertility and epididymitis), and skeletal (retardation of growth, demineralization, and osteoarthropathy) systems. Digital clubbing appears in childhood in virtually all symptomatic patients.

B. **Differential diagnosis.** Primary ciliary dyskinesia or immunoglobulin deficiency may lead to bronchiectasis, sinusitis, and infertility, but few GI symptoms and no sweat electrolyte abnormalities are present. Shwachman syndrome, consisting of pancreatic insufficiency and cyclic neutropenia, may also lead to lung disease, but sweat chloride concentrations are normal and the neutropenia is distinguishing. Men with Young's syndrome have bronchiectasis, sinusitis, and azoospermia, but the respiratory disease is usually mild, and GI symptoms or sweat manifestations are not present.

C. Testing

1. **Skin sweat testing** using a standardized quantitative pilocarpine iontophoresis method remains the gold standard for the diagnosis of CF. A **sweat chloride concentration of greater than 60 mmol/L** is consistent with the diagnosis of CF. The diagnosis should be made only if there is an elevated sweat chloride concentration on two separate occasions in a patient with a typical phenotype or with a history of CF in a sibling. Borderline sweat test results (40–60 mmol/L sweat chloride) or nondiagnostic results in the setting of high clinical suspicion should also lead to repeat sweat testing, nasal potential difference testing, or genetic testing. Abnormal sweat chloride concentrations are rarely detected in non-CF patients (e.g., Addison's disease and untreated hypothyroidism).

2. **Genetic tests** have detected more than 900 putative CF mutations (*Hum Mutat* 1994;4:167). The most common CF transmembrane conductance regulator mutation in patients with CF is ΔF508. Commercially available probes are quite sensitive but test for only a minority of the known CF genes, although they identify more than 90% of the abnormal genes in a Caucasian Northern European population. Two of these recessive genes must be abnormal to cause CF.

3. **Other tests** may be supportive of the diagnosis of CF and clinically useful, although they are not absolutely diagnostic. **Chest radiography** eventually typically shows enlarged lung volumes, with cystic lung disease and bronchiectasis, especially in the upper lobes. **Pulmonary function tests** eventually typically show expiratory airflow obstruction with increased residual volume and total lung capacity. Impairment of alveolar gas exchange may be present as well, progressing to hypercapnia and hypoxemia. **Sputum cultures** typically identify *P. aeruginosa* and *Staphylococcus aureus*, or both, and **sputum sensitivity testing** is useful for directing therapy. **Testing for malabsorption** is often not formally performed, because clinical evidence [the presence of foul-smelling, bulky, and loose stools; **low fat-soluble vitamin levels (vitamins A, D, and E)**; and a **prolonged prothrombin time** (vitamin K dependent)] and a clear response to pancreatic enzyme treatment are usually considered sufficient for diagnosing exocrine insufficiency. Tests that identify sinusitis or infertility, especially obstructive azoospermia in men, would also be supportive of the diagnosis of CF.

IV. Therapeutics and management.
The goals of CF therapy include improving quality of life and functioning, decreasing the number of exacerbations and hospitalizations, avoiding complications associated with therapy, and decreasing mortality. A large portion of therapy is focused on clearing pulmonary mucus and controlling infections. A comprehensive program that addresses multiple organ/system derangements, as provided at CF core centers, is recommended. Because most adults with CF have significant lung disease, pulmonologists often manage or comanage the care of these patients.

A. Pulmonary disease

1. **Nonpharmacologic treatment**

   a. **Mucus mobilization** can be accomplished by various airway clearance techniques, including postural drainage with chest percussion and vibration, with or without mechanical devices (flutter valves, high-frequency chest oscillation vests, low- and high-pressure positive expiratory pressure devices, etc.), and breathing and coughing exercises.

   b. **Pulmonary rehabilitation** is recommended, and exercise rehabilitation may improve functional status.

2. **Pharmacologic treatment**

   a. **Bronchodilators** (see Chronic Obstructive Lung Disease, sec. **V.A**, and Chap. 12) such as β-adrenergic agonists (albuterol MDI, 2–4 puffs bid–qid; salmeterol MDI, 2 puffs bid) are used to treat the reversible components of airflow obstruction and facilitate mucus clearance. These agents are contraindicated in the rare patient with associated paradoxical deterioration of airflow after their use.

b. **Recombinant human deoxyribonuclease (DNase; Dornase alpha; Pulmozyme)** digests extracellular DNA, decreasing the viscoelasticity of the sputum. DNase improves pulmonary function and decreases the incidence of respiratory tract infections that require parenteral antibiotics (*N Engl J Med* 1992;326:812, and *Am Rev Respir Dis* 1993;148:145). The recommended dose of Pulmozyme is 2.5 mg (1 ampule)/day inhaled using a jet nebulizer. Adverse effects may include pharyngitis, laryngitis, rash, chest pain, and conjunctivitis.

c. **Antibiotics.** *P. aeruginosa* is the most frequent pulmonary pathogen. A combination of an intravenous semisynthetic penicillin, a third- or fourth-generation cephalosporin, or a quinolone and an aminoglycoside is typically recommended during acute exacerbations. Sputum culture sensitivities are used to guide therapy. The duration of antibiotic therapy is dictated by the clinical response. At least 10–14 days of antibiotics are typically given to treat an exacerbation. Home IV antibiotic therapy is common, but hospitalization may allow better access to comprehensive therapy and diagnostic testing. Oral antibiotics are recommended only for mild exacerbations. The use of chronic or intermittent prophylactic antibiotics can be considered, especially in patients with frequent recurrent exacerbations, but antimicrobial resistance may develop. Inhaled aerosolized tobramycin [300 mg nebulized bid (28 days on alternating with 28 days off) using appropriate nebulizer and compressor] improves pulmonary function, decreases the density of *P. aeruginosa*, and decreases the risk of hospitalization (*N Engl J Med* 1999;340:23).

d. **Oxygen therapy** is indicated based on standard recommendations (see Chronic Obstructive Lung Disease, sec. **V.D**). Rest and exercise oxygen assessments should be performed as clinically indicated.

e. **Glucocorticoids** are only indicated for refractory lung disease that has demonstrated subjective (less dyspnea) and objective (decreased airflow obstruction or improved exercise tolerance, or both) benefit during a trial period. Short courses of glucocorticoid therapy may be helpful to some patients, but long-term therapy should be avoided to minimize the side effects, which include glucose intolerance, osteopenia, and growth retardation.

f. **Vaccinations.** Yearly influenza vaccinations (0.5 ml IM) decrease the incidence of infection and subsequent deterioration (*N Engl J Med* 1984;311:1653). Pneumovax, 0.5 ml IM every 5 years, may also provide benefit.

3. **Other treatments**

a. **Lung transplantation.** The majority of patients with CF die from pulmonary disease. FEV_1 has been the best predictor of mortality (*N Engl J Med* 1992;326:1187), and it is helpful in deciding when to refer patients for lung transplantation. An FEV_1 of less than 30% of the predicted normal value, marked alveolar gas exchange abnormalities (resting hypoxemia or hypercapnia), evidence of pulmonary hypertension, or increased frequency or severity of pulmonary exacerbations should lead to consideration of lung transplantation as a treatment option (*Am J Respir Crit Care Med* 1997;155:789).

b. **Noninvasive ventilation** for chronic respiratory failure due to CF has not been clearly demonstrated to be effective.

c. **Avoidance of irritating fumes, dusts, or chemicals** is recommended.

B. Extrapulmonary disease
1. **Pancreatic enzyme supplementation** should be instituted after pancreatic insufficiency and malabsorption have been demonstrated. Enzyme dose is titrated to achieve one to two semisolid stools/day. Enzymes are taken immediately before meals and snacks. Dosing of pancreatic enzymes should be initiated at 500 units lipase/kg/meal and should not exceed 2500 units lipase/kg/meal. High doses (6000 units lipase/kg/meal) have been associated with chronic intestinal strictures (*N Engl J Med* 1997;336:1283). **Generic** enzyme substitutes may not provide adequate lipase needs for absorption and should be avoided.
2. **Vitamin supplementation** is recommended, especially the fat-soluble vitamins that are not well absorbed in the setting of pancreatic insufficiency. Vitamins A, D, E, and K can all be taken orally on a regular basis. Iron deficiency anemia requires iron supplementation. Osteopenia from chronic steroid use should be treated (see Chap. 17).
3. **Sinusitis regimens** are used in the typical fashion (see Chap. 18).
4. **Treatment of pancreatic endocrine dysfunction**, specifically diabetes mellitus, is done with insulin in the standard fashion (see Chap. 18), but typical diabetic dietary restrictions are liberalized (high-calorie diet with unrestricted fat) to encourage appropriate growth and weight maintenance.

V. Return evaluation
A. Changes in therapeutics. Spirometry is the best objective measurement of lung function in CF, and routine spirometry monitoring is recommended. A significant decline in spirometry, even in the absence of increased symptoms, is an indication for intensification of therapy. Sputum culture and sensitivity testing can be used to guide antimicrobial therapy. Quantity and quality of stool, as well as laboratory evidence of malabsorption (see sec. **III.C.3**) can be used to guide pancreatic enzyme replacement.
B. Laboratory monitoring. Patients with CF have atypical pharmacokinetics and often require higher drug doses at more frequent intervals. Monitoring levels (peaks and troughs) of drugs such as aminoglycosides helps to assure therapeutic levels and decrease the risk of toxicity. In patients with CF, for example, cefepime is often dosed at 2 g IV q8h, and gentamicin or tobramycin is often dosed at 3 mg/kg IV q8h (aiming for peak levels of 9–10 mg/ml and trough levels of <2 mg/ml). Monitoring of electrolytes is indicated in patients with a history of electrolyte abnormalities or renal insufficiency.
C. Complications from therapy. Resistant bacterial organisms in the sputum may develop based on exposure to antibiotics. Use of multiple drugs against *P. aeruginosa* and rotation of antibiotics have been proposed as modes of protection against resistance. Patients with CF should be observed for complications of antibiotics, such as ototoxicity, renal dysfunction, and so forth, and these are managed in the standard fashion.

Diffuse Interstitial Lung Disease

I. Introduction. The patient with bilateral or diffuse pulmonary infiltrates presents the physician with many challenges. **Diffuse parenchymal lung disease (DLD)** occurs less commonly than obstructive lung disease but nevertheless represents a significant clinical problem. Approximately 30% of patients with DLD have idiopathic pulmonary fibrosis (IPF), a primary lung disease.
II. Pathophysiology. Regardless of etiology, DLD produces dyspnea primarily by decreasing the distensibility of the lung. As the lungs become stiffer, the vital capacity and total lung capacity decrease, producing a restrictive pattern on

pulmonary function testing. To various degrees, restriction is accompanied by a decrease in the diffusing capacity for carbon monoxide, a widening of the alveolar-arterial difference for oxygen at rest, and at times a dramatic fall in oxygenation with exercise. Most patients present with a respiratory alkalosis. Carbon dioxide retention occurs only in very severe and terminal disease. Distortion of the small airways may produce concomitant airway obstruction with long-standing or far-advanced DLD. Pulmonary hypertension usually occurs late in the course and, unlike COPD, may not be fully treatable with supplemental oxygen. Correlation among the patient's symptoms, radiographic findings, and physiologic abnormalities is poor.

III. **Approach to the patient.** With DLD the physician must consider these questions: Is the disease **acute or chronic**? Does the patient have an **underlying systemic disease** or exposure that is likely to give rise to DLD, or is this is a **primary lung** problem? Is the patient **immunosuppressed**? A careful and detailed history is necessary to help answer these questions. Patients present either with the onset of symptoms, especially cough and dyspnea, or with an incidental finding on chest radiograph of diffuse infiltrates. Most of the patients demonstrate audible inspiratory crackles, often at the lung bases. Clubbing of the digits may occur in up to 40% of the patients. Other signs are rarely present on physical examination unless the DLD is a manifestation of a systemic disease. A chest radiograph is imperative, as is obtaining previous radiographic examinations.

IV. **Evaluation**

A. If the patient is known to be **immunosuppressed**, urgent consultation with a pulmonologist is imperative and immediate hospitalization is frequently required, especially if the patient has rapidly advancing symptoms or fever (see Chap. 18). The most common etiologies are **infection**, either with community-acquired or opportunistic organisms; **drug toxicity or hypersensitivity**; and complications of lung or bone marrow **transplantation**. Regardless of the state of the immune system, it is imperative to consider disorders that may mimic DLD. The appearance of DLD can be caused by inflammation (infectious or not), increased lung water, alveolar blood, or infiltrative material. A careful history, physical examination, and obtaining old chest radiographs and medical records are necessary for evaluation. Differential diagnosis includes congestive heart failure, noncardiogenic pulmonary edema, lymphangitic spread of malignancy, acute (usually viral) pneumonia, alveolar hemorrhage, and alveolar proteinosis, among others. The differential diagnosis list can be narrowed with history and imaging but occasionally requires bronchoscopy or other testing. Occasionally, bilateral pleural effusions or scarring may be misinterpreted as parenchymal disease.

B. If the patient is **not** known to be immunosuppressed, the first question is whether he or she is ill enough to be admitted to the hospital or requires urgent consultation with a pulmonologist. This is best answered by an analysis of the patient's vital signs. If the patient is **febrile**, or if the **respiratory rate exceeds 35 breaths/minute**, hospitalization may well be in order. An arterial blood gas that demonstrates a PaO_2 of less than **60 mm Hg or an SaO_2 of less than 90%** while the patient is breathing room air also indicates the need for immediate hospitalization. Outpatient evaluation should be commenced if the patient is not hospitalized.

C. All stable patients who present with DLD should undergo pulmonary function testing with measurement of lung volumes, flow rates, diffusing capacity, a resting arterial blood gas, and an assessment of arterial oxygenation with exercise. The diseases that produce DLD can only be broadly categorized, as shown in Table 11-3. The evaluation must proceed in an orderly manner to either implicate or acquit these categories as the cause for the pulmonary problem. The treatment depends on either eliminating an offending agent, treating the underlying disease, or use of an immunosuppressant drug.

Table 11-3. Classification of diffuse parenchymal lung disease

Category	Examples
Granulomatous disease	Sarcoidosis
	Berylliosis
	Hypersensitivity pneumonitis
Collagen vascular disease	Scleroderma
	Rheumatoid arthritis
	Polymyositis
Iatrogenic	Drug induced
	Nitrofurantoin
	Bleomycin
	Amiodarone
	Radiation
Familial	Tuberous sclerosis
Bronchiolitis obliterans	With or without organizing pneumonia
Occupational	Inorganic dusts
	Asbestosis
	Silicosis
	Organic dusts
	Farmer's lung (hypersensitivity pneumonitis)
Infections	*Pneumocystis carinii*
	Mycobacteriosis
Chronic eosinophilic pneumonia	—
Idiopathic	Idiopathic pulmonary fibrosis (IPF)
	Eosinophilic granuloma (EG)
	Lymphangioleiomatosis (LAM)

Adapted from G Raghu. Interstitial lung disease: a diagnostic approach. Are CT scan and lung biopsy indicated in every patient? *Am J Respir Crit Care Med* 1995;151:909–914, with permission.

V. Laboratory evaluation
  A. Routine blood testing is **rarely** helpful, although the following abnormalities may help to guide the evaluation: iron deficiency anemia–alveolar hemorrhage, eosinophilia–eosinophilic pneumonia or drug reaction, thrombocytopenia–collagen vascular disease, and hypercalcemia–sarcoid. Targeted blood testing for the following markers may sometimes be helpful. Rheumatoid factor and antinuclear antigen are present in high titer in rheumatoid arthritis and scleroderma. Unfortunately, they are present in lower titers nonspecifically in IPF as well as silicosis. The presence of antineutrophil cytoplasmic antibody provides evidence for Wegener's granulomatosis, necrotizing vasculitis, and pulmonary capillaritis. A positive assay for anti–Jo 1 is helpful in diagnosing polymyositis. Hypersensitivity antigen/antibody testing is suggestive of farmer's lung, pigeon breeder's disease, and so forth. Less specific is an increased level of angiotensin-converting enzyme, which is present in sarcoid, berylliosis, and other granulomatous diseases.
  B. Distribution patterns on **chest radiographs** (Table 11-4) are not specific but can be suggestive of certain etiologies and direct further inquiry.

Table 11-4. Chest radiograph patterns in diffuse parenchymal lung disease

Pattern	Examples
Lower-lobe predominance	Idiopathic pulmonary fibrosis
	Collagen vascular disease (scleroderma)
	Asbestosis
Upper-lobe predominance	Pneumoconiosis (silicosis)
	Ankylosing spondylitis
	Eosinophilic granuloma (Langerhans cell granulomatosis)
	Chronic hypersensitivity pneumonitis
Hilar adenopathy	Sarcoid
	Hypersensitivity pneumonitis (including some drugs, e.g., methotrexate)
Associated pneumothorax	Eosinophilic granuloma
	Lymphangioleiomatosis
	Tuberous sclerosis

   C. Imaging studies. The CT scan, including high-resolution CT (HRCT), although more sensitive than chest radiographs, has not proved to provide specific diagnostic information or information that obviates the need for invasive diagnostic studies except in rare situations such as lymphangioleiomatosis. Perhaps the strongest reason for obtaining an HRCT is to provide guidance for obtaining tissue from the most active sites of parenchymal disease and to detect associated findings such as mediastinal lymphadenopathy.
 VI. Invasive diagnostic studies. Samples can be obtained for diagnosis through three major routes.
   A. Bronchoalveolar lavage (BAL) can be used to obtain cells and material from the periphery of the lung during bronchoscopy. This is most useful in patients with infections, particularly those who are immunosuppressed or those with alveolar hemorrhage. The role of BAL as a diagnostic tool in other patients with DLD is so limited as to almost never be worthwhile as a sole procedure.
   B. Transbronchial lung biopsy obtains small pieces of lung tissue through the bronchoscope close to the perivascular-bronchiolar areas. It therefore is most useful in diseases that follow that distribution (e.g., sarcoid or lymphangitic carcinoma). With the exception of infection, it is much less useful and may be inadequate if a large amount of tissue is needed to make a diagnosis of other types of DLD.
   C. Surgical lung biopsy. Either video-assisted thoracoscopic surgery or **thoracotomy** is probably the procedure of choice to obtain lung tissue that is sufficient for diagnosis. The surgical biopsy should be directed toward the most active sites of inflammation as determined by HRCT, not a routine biopsy of the easily accessible right middle lobe or lingula.
      Younger patients with rapidly advancing disease, suspicion of vasculitis, marked systemic symptoms, or atypical imaging findings should receive strong consideration for surgical biopsy. The decision as to whether video-assisted thoracoscopic surgery or a thoracotomy procedure is performed is best left to the surgeon, although the HRCT should be used to delineate the area from which lung should be sampled. In some patients with DLD, the risks of a biopsy may exceed the benefits of a tissue-based diagnosis, particularly in the elderly (>age 75) or those with (1) severe comorbidity, (2) sta-

ble or very slowly progressive disease, (3) known collagen vascular disease, and (4) typical imaging and functional abnormalities.

VII. Treatment

A. General. Treatment of DLD depends on the underlying etiology. Exposures to offending agents should be avoided, appropriate antibiotics begun, or specific immunosuppressant therapy instituted. In many cases, particularly those of sarcoid, bronchiolitis obliterans–organizing pneumonia, and chronic eosinophilic pneumonia, various regimens of corticosteroids can be used effectively. Before embarking on a course of treatment, the physician likely needs to obtain lung tissue and exclude infection for as accurate a diagnosis as possible.

B. Sarcoidosis is a syndrome of multiorgan involvement characterized by noncaseating granuloma without known cause. The lungs and thoracic lymph nodes are the organs most commonly affected, with skin and eyes involved in approximately 20% of the cases. The diagnosis is most often made by demonstrating the characteristic noncaseating granuloma in the affected organs, and this is usually accomplished by transbronchial lung biopsy. If skin lesions or enlarged lymph nodes are present, they are a productive site for biopsy, as are lymph nodes.

   1. Corticosteroids are the mainstay of treatment and are indicated in the face of vital organ dysfunction (eye, CNS, heart), hypercalcemia, or progressive impairment of pulmonary function.

      a. Lung involvement. Patients with bilateral hilar adenopathy alone have an 85% chance of obtaining resolution without therapy. Those with pulmonary infiltrates alone have an approximately 50% chance of improvement without therapy within 2 years. After 2 years, hyalinization and fibrosis appear in increasing frequency, so that treatment should begin before 2 years have elapsed with objective demonstration of worsening pulmonary function. Although there is still debate as to their long-term effectiveness, corticosteroids do appear to reverse the early changes of pulmonary parenchymal involvement. The decision to begin corticosteroid therapy is a long-term commitment, as the patient will likely require them for approximately 1 year, if not longer, to prevent relapse. The usual initial dose regimen of oral prednisone is 40 mg/day, with plans to taper over weeks to approximately 20 mg/day. The lowest dose that will continue to suppress the patient's symptoms should be maintained, while monitoring for toxicity. The efficacy of other immunosuppressant drugs in sarcoid has not been clearly defined.

   2. Other organ involvement. All patients with sarcoid should receive an ophthalmologic evaluation with a slit lamp, because untreated posterior uveitis leads to blindness. Central nervous system and cardiac involvement are poorly responsive to therapy. Hypercalcemia is treatable with corticosteroids, but hyperparathyroidism should first be excluded. Patients should be cautioned to avoid ultraviolet exposure.

C. IPF is a relatively uncommon chronic disease that is limited to the lung and associated with the histologic appearance of usual interstitial pneumonitis on lung biopsy. IPF is more frequent in men than in women, with onset occurring in middle age and a mean age at time of diagnosis of 66 years. The approach to evaluation is similar to that of other patients with DLD (see sec. **III**). HRCT shows lower lobe–predominant patchy peripheral and subpleural basal reticular abnormalities. Traction bronchiectasis and honeycombing may be present. Although HRCT increases the accuracy of diagnosis compared to chest radiography, there is a large interobserver variation depending on experience. The specific diagnosis frequently relies on obtaining lung tissue (see sec. **VI**). In general, transbronchial lung biopsy does not obtain sufficient lung tissue to define the disease process adequately, and a surgical approach is generally justified (see sec. **VI.B**).

1. IPF does not respond well to **therapy** and has a relatively poor outcome, with mean survival of 2–4 years. Treatment options include corticosteroids, immunosuppressives, and antifibrotic agents, either alone or in combination. At best, only 30% of patients demonstrate objective response to corticosteroid therapy alone. No large randomized placebo-controlled trials are available as to the effectiveness of this therapy. Because of this and the complications of such treatment, the American Thoracic Society (*Am J Respir Crit Care Med* 2000;161:646–664) recommends that undertaking treatment in the following categories of patients be done with circumspection: those older than age 70 years, those with extreme obesity, patients with concomitant severe comorbidity (e.g., diabetes mellitus, cardiac disease, osteoporosis), and those with end-stage honeycomb lung on HRCT examination. For those patients who are made aware of the risks of therapy, the American Thoracic Society recommends combined therapy with corticosteroids and either azathioprine or cyclophosphamide. The efficacy of interferon-gamma is being evaluated. Supplemental oxygen (see Chronic Obstructive Lung Disease, sec. **V.D.**) requirements should be tested and met.

   Treatment should be continued for at least 6 months, and then studies should be performed to evaluate response (see Monitoring, below). If the patient's condition is worse, as is frequently the case, the drugs can be tapered and stopped or switched to an alternative. If the patient is improved or stable, the drugs should be maintained at the same dose. After 18 months, therapy should be individualized.

2. **Monitoring** the clinical course is difficult, but the use of clinical, radiographic, and physiologic parameters may be useful, especially if the patient is being treated with corticosteroids alone or in combination with immunosuppressants. A battery of information should be obtained at baseline and at 3- to 6-month intervals in patients who are being treated for IPF to assess progression or remission. Dyspnea and functional status should be assessed using established scales. HRCT scans are useful to evaluate change in the distribution or anatomy of the disease process. Lung volumes, spirometry, diffusing capacity, resting arterial blood gases, and an oxygen and exercise assessment help quantify severity of illness and changes in physiology.

   If the patient is being treated, **evaluation of side effects** of corticosteroids and azathioprine or cyclophosphamide (Cytoxan) should be undertaken carefully. The major adverse effects of corticosteroids include increases in blood sugar and BP as well as production of cataracts and glaucoma. Azathioprine places patients at increased risk for leukopenia, thrombocytopenia, hepatotoxicity, cancer, and pancreatitis. Cyclophosphamide may cause hemorrhagic cystitis, leukopenia, thrombocytopenia, and cardiomyopathy. Infection with community-acquired or opportunistic organisms is a concern for all three agents. For the patient who is younger than 65 years of age, **lung transplantation** evaluation should be considered at the time of diagnosis, because IPF may progress quickly.

Pulmonary Hypertension

I. **Pulmonary hypertension** is defined as sustained elevation of the mean pulmonary artery pressure (>25 mm Hg at rest or 30 mm Hg during exertion) or of the systolic pulmonary artery pressure (>40 mm Hg). The World Symposium on Primary Pulmonary Hypertension 1998 (World Health Organization, 1999, and http://www.who.int/ncd/cvd/pph.html) suggested the classification schema in Table 11-5, based on the clinical features of pulmonary hypertension.

Table 11-5. Diagnostic classification of pulmonary hypertension

Pulmonary arterial hypertension

Primary pulmonary hypertension

  Sporadic

  Familial

Related to

  Collagen vascular disease

  Congenital systemic to pulmonary shunts

  Portal hypertension

  HIV infection

  Drugs/toxins

    Anorexigens

    Other

  Persistent pulmonary hypertension of the newborn

  Other

Pulmonary venous hypertension

Left-sided atrial or ventricular heart disease

Left-sided valvular heart disease

Extrinsic compression of central pulmonary veins

  Fibrosing mediastinitis

  Adenopathy/tumors

Pulmonary veno-occlusive disease

Other

Pulmonary hypertension associated with disorders of the respiratory system or hypoxemia, or both

Chronic obstructive pulmonary disease

Interstitial lung disease

Sleep-disordered breathing

Alveolar hypoventilation disorders

Chronic exposure to high altitude

Neonatal lung disease

Alveolar-capillary dysplasia

Other

Pulmonary hypertension due to chronic thrombotic and/or embolic disease

Thromboembolic obstruction of proximal arteries

Obstruction of distal pulmonary arteries

  Pulmonary embolism (thrombus, tumor, ova and/or parasites, foreign material)

  In situ thrombosis

  Sickle cell disease

(continued)

Table 11-5. (continued)

Pulmonary hypertension due to disorders directly affecting the pulmonary vasculature

Inflammatory

Schistosomiasis

Sarcoidosis

Other

Pulmonary capillary hemangiomatosis

Adapted from 1999 World Health Organization.

Pulmonary hypertension is commonly caused by **pulmonary venous hypertension**, defined by the presence of a pulmonary capillary wedge pressure of greater than 15 mm Hg. Increased intravascular pressures distal to the pulmonary arterioles, either in the pulmonary veins or in the left heart (i.e., left heart failure), produce increased pressure in the pulmonary veins and arteries. The other etiologies of pulmonary hypertension are listed in Table 11-5.

Primary (arterial) pulmonary hypertension (PPH) is an uncommon disease of unclear etiology. A number of risk factors or possible triggers for the development of PPH have been identified, such as use of diet pills, including fenfluramine and dexfenfluramine. The main cause of death in patients with PPH is right heart failure. The median survival in a U.S. registry was 2.8 years (*Ann Intern Med* 1987;107:216), but therapies have been improving over time.

II. **The diagnosis** of pulmonary hypertension is usually based on symptoms of dyspnea (especially on exertion), fatigue, palpitations, presyncope, syncope, chest pain, hemoptysis, and cough. **Signs** of pulmonary hypertension are most notable from the cardiovascular examination, typically including a right ventricular heave, a prominent P_2 (second heart sound), a right ventricular S_4, and a tricuspid regurgitation murmur. A pulmonic insufficiency murmur may also be present. With **right heart failure**, elevated jugular venous pressure, a right ventricular S_3, a pulsatile liver, pedal edema, and sometimes ascites develop.

The diagnosis of PPH **requires the exclusion of other causes** of pulmonary hypertension, especially chronic thromboembolic disease, collagen vascular disease, and left-sided and congenital heart disease. Raynaud's phenomenon is associated with PPH, but it is also associated with scleroderma and other collagen vascular diseases. Telangiectasias and sclerodactyly suggest the presence of other underlying illnesses such as scleroderma. Clubbing is not associated with PPH.

A **modified New York Heart Association (NYHA) classification** is often used to define the clinical severity of disease (Table 11-6).

III. **Testing.** Once signs and symptoms that are suggestive of pulmonary hypertension are present, diagnostic testing should be undertaken. Acute illnesses with reversible pulmonary hypertension (pneumonia, pulmonary edema, etc.) should be treated before a thorough evaluation for chronic etiologies is performed.

A. A **transthoracic echocardiogram** is the preferred test for the initial evaluation of suspected pulmonary hypertension because noninvasive Doppler techniques can be used to estimate the pulmonary artery systolic pressure. Patients with pulmonary arterial hypertension should be evaluated for the presence of a **right-to-left shunt** (i.e., patent foramen ovale, atrial septal defect, etc.) with an echocardiogram bubble or contrast study (or a radionuclide lung perfusion scan that looks for abnormal accumulation of tracer in the brain or kidneys). Transthoracic echocardiography usually demon-

Table 11-6. Functional assessment

Class	Description
I	No limitation of physical activity. Ordinary physical activity does not cause undue dyspnea or fatigue, chest pain, or near syncope.
II	Slight limitation of physical activity. Comfortable at rest. Ordinary physical activity causes undue dyspnea or fatigue, chest pain, or near syncope.
III	Marked limitation of physical activity. Comfortable at rest. Less than ordinary activity causes undue dyspnea or fatigue, chest pain, or near syncope.
IV	Unable to carry out any physical activity without symptoms. Dyspnea and/or fatigue may be present at rest. Discomfort is increased by any physical activity. Signs of right heart failure are present.

Modified from the New York Heart Association Functional Classification; 1999 World Health Organization.

strates the presence of left ventricular dysfunction or valvular heart disease in patients with pulmonary venous hypertension secondary to cardiac disease, a common cause of pulmonary hypertension.

B. Once pulmonary hypertension is diagnosed, a thorough evaluation for causes should be performed. The type of pulmonary hypertension (Table 11-5) assists in directing the evaluation. If not already done in the initial evaluation, further testing should include the following.

1. **Chest radiography** may show enlarged pulmonary arteries, right ventricular enlargement, and signs of secondary causes of pulmonary hypertension.

2. **Pulmonary function tests** often show a mild to moderate reduction in diffusing capacity for carbon monoxide (DLCO). A decrease in the DLCO is often the sole abnormality seen on pulmonary function testing of patients with PPH. Additional abnormalities of airflow, lung volumes, or alveolar gas exchange often suggest the presence of secondary causes of pulmonary hypertension.

3. **Arterial blood gas measurement** may show hypoxemia and oxyhemoglobin desaturation that worsen with exertion.

4. **Six-minute walk distance** achieved may be lower than expected.

5. **Electrocardiography** may demonstrate signs of right ventricular and right atrial hypertrophy. Other findings suggestive of cardiovascular disease may be present.

6. **A cardiopulmonary exercise test should be performed with caution** and only if necessary. Exercise is usually limited by cardiovascular function, especially if oxyhemoglobin saturation is maintained with oxygen supplementation.

7. **Ventilation-perfusion (V̇/Q̇) lung scanning** should be performed to evaluate for the presence of chronic thromboembolic disease. In the presence of thromboembolic pulmonary hypertension, the V̇/Q̇ scan is usually interpreted as high probability for pulmonary embolism. If the perfusion is in any way abnormal, a pulmonary angiogram should be performed to assess for the presence and extent of disease.

8. **Contrast-enhanced helical chest CT/high-resolution CT (pulmonary embolism protocol).** In addition to the assessment for thromboembolic disease, the CT can be used to look for signs of secondary causes of pulmonary hypertension. The spiral CT is not yet considered specific enough to exclude definitively the presence of chronic thromboembolic disease.

9. **Pulmonary arteriography.** If the perfusion portion of the V̇/Q̇ scan is abnormal, pulmonary arteriography is used in conjunction with CT to

assess for the presence (and extent) of thromboembolic disease. Patients with chronic thromboemboli should be referred for a thromboendarterectomy evaluation at an experienced center.

10. **Lung biopsy** is indicated only when a lung disease that requires a tissue diagnosis for confirmation, such as pulmonary vasculitis, is suspected.

11. **Radionuclide ventriculography** is used to assess function of the right and left heart, including ejection fraction and wall motion.

12. **Sleep study.** A sleep study is indicated in patients with signs or symptoms of sleep apnea (see Obstructive Sleep Apnea–Hypopnea Syndrome, sec. **III.B**).

13. Screening **laboratory tests** are used to assess for **underlying** liver disease, collagen vascular disease, and HIV infection, as well as **secondary** polycythemia, anemia, or thrombocytopenia. **Other signs of systemic diseases** may include anemia, thrombocytopenia, leukopenia, renal dysfunction, hematuria, and proteinuria.

14. **Right heart catheterization** should be performed for further evaluation of echocardiographic findings of pulmonary arterial hypertension or for evaluation of patients who have clinical signs of pulmonary hypertension that are not confirmed by echocardiogram, because echocardiographic estimates of pulmonary artery pressures can be significantly lower than those found with right heart catheterization (*Circulation* 1997;95:1479). If the catheterization does not reveal pulmonary arterial hypertension, pulmonary hemodynamics should be measured during exercise. Right heart catheterization may also help to determine the cause of the pulmonary hypertension and can be used to assess for the presence of a **left-to-right shunt**.

15. If pulmonary arterial hypertension is confirmed, all patients should undergo **vasodilator testing** with short-acting intravenous adenosine, intravenous epoprostenol sodium (Flolan), or inhaled nitric oxide (NO). Calcium channel blockers (CCBs) are no longer recommended for use in determination of vasoreactivity, because they may induce prolonged systemic hypotension, syncope, and cardiovascular collapse. Patients with severe right heart failure may be at higher risk for circulatory collapse during vasodilator testing. One definition of vasodilator responsiveness is a reduction in the mean pulmonary artery pressure of at least 10 mm Hg with either no change or an increase in the cardiac output (World Symposium on Primary Pulmonary Hypertension, 1998). Patients with an acute vasodilator response of more than a 20% decrease in mean pulmonary artery pressure and more than a 20% decrease in pulmonary vascular resistance were found to have a favorable response to treatment with oral CCBs (*N Engl J Med* 1992;327:76).

16. Patients with pulmonary arterial hypertension, especially those with PPH, should be **referred to a specialist** with expertise in the evaluation and care of such patients.

IV. **Therapeutics and management.** The underlying cause of pulmonary hypertension determines the appropriate treatment. For example, pulmonary hypertension in patients with COPD and untreated hypoxemia is often due to hypoxic vasoconstriction, and treatment should include oxygen supplementation. Pulmonary hypertension secondary to left heart failure requires treatment of the left heart failure and its causes. This section focuses on the treatment of pulmonary arterial hypertension, including PPH and other diseases.

A. **Pharmacologic treatment**

1. **Vasodilator therapy** has been demonstrated to be most useful in the treatment of PPH, leading to improved pulmonary hemodynamics, right ventricular function, cardiac output, oxygen delivery, symptoms, functioning, and survival (*N Engl J Med* 1992;327:76, and *N Engl J Med* 1996;334:296). Individual responses to vasodilator therapy are variable and often difficult to predict. Systemic hypotension is the most common complication of therapy, and other adverse effects include

lower arterial oxygen tensions. **After chronic use of vasodilator therapy, abrupt discontinuation can result in rebound pulmonary hypertension and death.**

a. **CCBs** vasodilate the pulmonary and systemic vascular smooth muscle. Caution should be exercised, because they also possess negative inotropic properties and cause reflex β-adrenergic tone. Patients who respond to vasodilator therapy during the acute challenge should receive a trial of a CCB. Only 20% of patients with PPH respond to oral CCB therapy, with improved symptoms, exercise tolerance, hemodynamics (decreased pulmonary artery pressure and increased cardiac output), and survival. **Vasodilator responders** should be treated with CCB therapy titrated according to a protocol (*N Engl J Med* 1996;334:296), typically guided by right heart catheterization. Nifedipine is commonly used, and diltiazem may be more appropriate for patients with resting tachycardia. Vasodilator responders are started with low-dose CCB therapy, and doses are cautiously advanced until a significant improvement in hemodynamic parameters is reached, as tolerated by BP. Over time, dosing is regulated based on symptoms, as tolerated by BP. The optimal dosing of CCB therapy in patients with PPH is uncertain. Patients who have **no evidence of a hemodynamic response** to CCBs are unlikely to benefit from chronic therapy. In addition, these nonresponders may experience such adverse events as systemic hypotension, pulmonary edema, right ventricular failure, and death if treated with CCBs. Patients who do not respond to vasodilator therapy during the acute challenge should be considered for prostaglandin therapy.

b. **Prostaglandins.** Continuous intravenous **prostacyclin (epoprostenol, PGE$_2$ Flolan)** therapy is indicated for patients with **pulmonary arterial hypertension.** Prostacyclin has been demonstrated in prospective randomized clinical trials of **PPH** to improve exercise tolerance, hemodynamics, and survival in patients who are NYHA (Table 11-6) functional class III or IV (*N Engl J Med* 1996;334:296). Studies have also demonstrated that lack of an acute response to prostacyclin does not preclude a chronic beneficial response. Prostacyclin therapy should be instituted in the hospital, and initial dosing is typically limited by side effects such as jaw pain, headache, diarrhea, and musculoskeletal pain. The development of tolerance to the effects of intravenous prostacyclin is common, and appears to respond to dose escalation. However, overmedication with prostacyclin can occur, requiring gradual dose reduction. Sudden discontinuation of therapy can be dangerous, and this may be due to accidental kinking or disconnection of the infusion catheter. Catheter-related infections can be problematic as well. The optimal dosing of intravenous prostacyclin for PPH remains uncertain. **Analogue molecules of prostacyclin** that can be inhaled [e.g., iloprost (*N Engl J Med* 2000;342:1866)] or taken orally [e.g., beraprost (*Lancet* 1997;349:1365)] have been studied, but their efficacy remains to be demonstrated in adequately sized, randomized, placebo-controlled trials. In a 12-week study, treprostinil sodium (Remodulin) led to statistically significant but small improvements in dyspnea, exercise capacity, and hemodynamics in patients with primary and secondary pulmonary hypertension who were NYHA functional class II–IV (*Am J Resp Crit Care Med* 2002;165:800). A survival benefit was not demonstrated. Treprostinil was administered subcutaneously via an infusion device, and 85% of patients experienced infusion site pain, leading to discontinuation of treprostinil in 8% of patients.

c. An **oral endothelin receptor antagonist**, bosentan (Tracleer), was studied in patients with symptomatic severe pulmonary arterial hypertension who were NYHA functional class III or IV (*N Engl J Med* 2002;346:896). Patients had PPH or pulmonary hypertension due to scleroderma or systemic lupus erythematosus. Bosentan significantly improved exercise capacity and time to clinical worsening as compared to placebo over a 3-month period, although a survival benefit was not demonstrated. Drug side effects were similar to placebo.

d. **NO** is a potent and selective pulmonary vasodilator when administered by inhalation. The rapid combination of inhaled NO with hemoglobin inactivates any NO diffusing into the blood, thereby preventing systemic vasodilation. The role of NO for PPH remains investigational.

2. **Inotropic therapy** may improve right heart function, cardiac output, and symptoms (*Chest* 1998;114:792), but data are lacking in terms of effect on survival.

3. **Anticoagulation** with oral warfarin therapy may improve survival (*N Engl J Med* 1992;327:76–81), and may prevent strokes in patients with intracardiac shunts, although a large definitive randomized controlled trial has not been performed. Warfarin is dosed (see Chap. 9) with a goal international normalized ratio of 1.5–2.5, lower than that typically used for treatment of venous thromboembolism. Patients with recurrent syncope or hemoptysis may not be good candidates for anticoagulation therapy.

4. **Diuretic therapy** is indicated for the treatment of peripheral edema and ascites.

5. **Other medications** can be used to treat problems that may lead to increased intrathoracic pressure, decreased cardiac output, and syncope. Stool softeners can be used to prevent constipation and straining.

6. **Avoidance of causal drugs, vasoactive substances, and exacerbating activities is advised.** Due to their vasoactive properties, nasal decongestants should be avoided. Sedatives that can lower BP should be cautiously administered. Narcotics, nitrates, and other agents that decrease preload and right ventricular filling should be avoided, as should barbiturates and other drugs that depress cardiac output. Platelet and fresh frozen plasma transfusions should be cautiously administered because of their volume load and presence of vasoactive compounds. Vigorous exercise should be avoided because of the risk of developing cardiovascular collapse. High altitudes should be avoided because of the low inspired concentration of oxygen. Patients should not smoke cigarettes. Pregnancy should usually be avoided, but the use of oral contraceptives is normally not recommended because they may exacerbate the symptoms or increase the risk of thrombosis.

7. An **intravenous filter** should be put in line with all intravenous lines in patients with documented right-to-left shunt to prevent air embolism.

B. **Supplemental oxygen therapy** is indicated based on standard **recommendations** (see Chronic Obstructive Lung Disease, sec. **V.D**). Rest, exertion, and sleep oxygen assessments should be performed as clinically indicated.

C. **Vaccinations** with the influenza vaccine and the Pneumovax may provide benefit.

D. **Surgical therapy**

1. **Lung transplantation** (or heart-lung transplantation) was the treatment for PPH in patients who did not remain improved on CCB vasodilator therapy until the mid-1990s. Since the inception of intravenous epoprostenol therapy, the need for early transplantation for patients with PPH has decreased. If interested, all patients with a diagnosis of PPH should be referred for lung transplant evaluation in case medical therapy does not produce satisfactory results. Patients should be referred early for

transplantation because of the long wait list time and the fast rate of deterioration of PPH, especially individuals with NYHA functional class III–IV, mean right atrial pressure greater than 15 mm Hg, mean pulmonary artery pressure greater than 55 mm Hg, or a cardiac index of less than 2 L/min/m^2 (*Am J Respir Crit Care Med* 1998;158:335). A randomized trial of medical versus transplant therapy has not been conducted, but lung transplant is thought to prolong survival in select patients with PPH. Single lung and bilateral lung transplantation have been successful for patients with PPH, and simultaneous heart transplantation is usually not necessary. The 5-year survival of patients with PPH has been 40–45%, slightly lower than the survival of other patients who undergo lung transplantation.

2. **Atrial septostomy** allows decompression of the right heart by creating a hole between the right and left atrium, leading to improved left ventricular filling and cardiac output. Currently, atrial septostomy is considered an investigational palliative procedure. Indications for this procedure include severe PPH that is refractory to maximal medical therapy with recurrent syncope or ascites. Atrial septostomy may also serve as a last effort bridge to transplantation in patients whose conditions are deteriorating despite all medical efforts. Because of the procedure-induced right-to-left shunt, hypoxemia will likely worsen. The procedure-related mortality is high, and only highly experienced centers should perform this procedure.

V. **Return evaluation**

A. **Changes in therapeutics.** Adjustments to vasodilator, diuretic, anticoagulation, and oxygen therapy are made as needed. Echocardiographic assessment and oxygen assessments should be performed on an intermittent but regular basis.

B. **Laboratory monitoring.** Asymptomatic individuals with pulmonary hypertension should have repeat testing with transthoracic echocardiogram 6 months after the initial diagnosis. International normalized ratio monitoring should occur at least monthly.

C. **Screening.** The World Symposium on Primary Pulmonary Hypertension 1998 has recommended echocardiographic screening of asymptomatic individuals with scleroderma or first-degree relatives of patients with pulmonary hypertension.

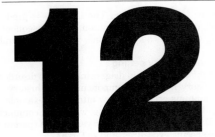

Allergy and Asthma

Mitchell H. Grayson,
H. James Wedner, and
Phillip E. Korenblat

Allergy

I. **Pathophysiology.** For an **allergic reaction** to occur, allergen-**specific immunoglobulin E (IgE)** must be cross-linked on the surface of mast cells and basophils. This event leads to the release of a number of mediators that are responsible for the subsequent allergic response. The initial mediators are released from mast cells and basophils within minutes of exposure to the allergen, a response that is known as the **early phase**. Lymphocytes and eosinophils arrive at the site 4–72 hours after the initial event, the so-called **late-phase** response. Often symptoms subside or disappear completely after the early phase only to reappear with the late phase.

A. **Mediators**

 1. **Early phase. Mast cells** release histamine, various cytokines, leukotrienes, prostaglandins, and tryptase. Because mast cells are the only cells in the body that release **tryptase**, the serum level of this enzyme is increased after a systemic allergic reaction. **Basophils** also release histamine and various cytokines. Histamine mainly binds to the H_1 receptor, leading to increased vascular permeability and edema. In addition, perturbation of nerve endings leads to increased mucus production and the sensation of itch.

 2. **Late phase. Lymphocytes** are recruited to the site of the reaction by the cytokines that are released in the early-phase response. These cells further exacerbate the reaction through the release of additional cytokines. The presence of certain cytokines and leukotrienes attracts **eosinophils**. These cells release additional leukotrienes, which can lead to bronchoconstriction. They also release several toxic proteins, including major basic protein, which leads to disruption of the airway epithelium.

B. **Allergens**

 1. An **allergen** is a protein or carbohydrate moiety against which the body can produce IgE. Allergens may be inhaled, ingested, or injected into the body, where they encounter IgE bound to mast cells or basophils and an allergic reaction occurs. The first time that a person is exposed to a specific allergen, no allergic response can occur because this initial exposure is required for the immune system to make IgE against the allergen. Certain airborne allergens are more prevalent at certain times of the year. These **seasonal** allergens include tree, grass, and weed pollens (most often seen in the spring, early summer, and early fall, respectively). Other allergens are present year-round. The **perennial** allergens include dust mites, cockroaches, and molds (although some molds have a seasonal increase in midsummer). Other allergens are encountered only through specific exposures. These include medications, stinging insect venoms, animal danders, and foods.

 2. **Most medications** are too small to elicit an IgE response; however, through a process called **haptenation**, the drug may bind to serum pro-

teins, which then allow for sensitization. The IgE that is produced in this manner is directed against the medication, and subsequent exposure leads to binding of IgE to the drug alone, without any binding to serum proteins.

II. Approach to allergies in the ambulatory setting

A. History.
The most important component in diagnosing allergic disorders is to take a full and complete history. Important components of the history include

1. **Symptoms.** What symptoms occur and how often? For example, is the patient complaining of a runny nose, sneezing, wheezing, conjunctivitis, rashes, or swelling? Do these symptoms occur year-round (perennial) or are they restricted to specific exposures, and so forth?

2. **Exacerbating/alleviating factors.** Does exposure to pets, smoke, perfume, or a change in air temperature affect the patient's symptoms? Are certain seasons better or worse?

3. **Environmental history.** Where does the patient work, live, and play? What exposures are present in each of these environments? Does the patient have a pet?

4. **Family history.** Are there other members of the family with allergic diseases (including asthma)? A child with one parent with allergic disorders has a 40% chance of having allergies (and/or allergic asthma). Two parents increase the risk to 60–80%.

5. **Psychosocial issues.** It is important to determine if any psychosocial issues exist that may interfere with the patient's care. For example, one should determine if the patient has appropriate social support. It is also helpful to determine the patient's goals for the visit.

B. Diagnostic tests.
All testing modalities may have false positives, and therefore, correlation with the patient's symptoms and exposures is necessary.

1. **Skin testing.** This is the most rapid and specific testing modality. Results are obtained within 20 minutes of starting the test. These tests evaluate for mast cell degranulation when the patient's skin is exposed to allergen. Antihistamines block the effects of skin testing and, therefore, must be discontinued before testing (Table 12-1). Skin tests are of two types.

   a. **Epicutaneous.** This is the most specific test available and identifies most clinically significant allergens. Although sensitivity to most allergens can be evaluated using epicutaneous and intradermal skin tests, food allergens should only be evaluated using epicutaneous methods.

   b. **Intradermal.** This type of skin test is more sensitive than epicutaneous testing but less specific. Irritant effects may cause many more false positives with this test. The risk of a systemic reaction is also increased with intradermal testing.

2. **In vitro tests [radioallergosorbent test (RAST) or PRIST test].** These tests evaluate for the presence of IgE in the patient's serum against specific allergens, which are usually immobilized on a disk or plastic plate. They only determine if specific IgE exists in the blood and have the potential to give positives to allergens to which the patient is not being exposed or to allergens to which the patient is not clinically allergic. In general, the sensitivity and specificity of in vitro tests are similar to those of intradermal skin testing alone.

C. Physical examination

1. **Appearance**

   a. **Mouth breathing** due to nasal congestion may be present.

   b. Due to edema in the nasal tissues, the draining veins under the eyes may be compressed, leading to pooling of blood and darkening of the region under the eyes. This is known as **allergic shiner**.

   c. Patients may also have infraorbital folds or **Dennie's lines**, as well as a **nasal crease**, a transverse line across the lower portion of the nose.

Table 12-1. Commonly used outpatient medications in allergy and immunology

Medication	Class	Usual adult dosage	Indications	Major side effects	Other
Chlorpheniramine	CA	4 mg q12h	AR, UR, ANA	Fatigue/drowsiness/impaired mental performance	72 hrs[a]
Diphenhydramine	CA	25–50 mg q6-8h	AR, UR, ANA	Fatigue/drowsiness/impaired mental performance	72 hrs[a]
Cetirizine	NA	10 mg qd	AR, UR, ANA	Minimal sedation	7–10 days[a]
Fexofenadine	NA	60 mg bid 180 mg qd	AR, UR, ANA	None	5–7 days[a]
Loratadine	NA	10 mg qd	AR, UR, ANA	None	7–10 days[a]
Azelastine	IA	2 sprays bid	AR	Some sedation possible	7 days[a]
Budesonide	IS	200 µg/puff 2 puffs qd	AS	Steroid side effects and oral thrush	
	NS	32 µg/spray 2 sprays qd	AR	Steroid side effects	
Flunisolide	IS	250 µg/puff 2 puffs bid	AS	Steroid side effects and oral thrush	
	NS	25 µg/spray 2 sprays bid	AR	Steroid side effects	
Fluticasone	IS	44–220 µg/puff 2 puffs bid or qd	AS	Steroid side effects and oral thrush	
	NS	50 µg/spray 2 sprays qd	AR	Steroid side effects	
Mometasone	NS	50 µg/spray 2 sprays qd	AR	Steroid side effects	

(continued)

Table 12-1. (continued)

Medication	Class	Usual adult dosage	Indications	Major side effects	Other
Triamcinolone	IS	200 µg/puff[b] 4 puffs bid	AS	Steroid side effects and oral thrush	
	NS	55 µg/spray 1–2 sprays qd	AR	Steroid side effects	
Fluticasone/salmeterol mixture	IS/LBD	100, 250, 500 µg fluticasone/puff 50 µg salmeterol/puff 1 inhalation bid	AS	Steroid side effects, oral thrush, and must be used no more than 1 inhalation bid	
Salmeterol diskus	LBD	50 µg/inhalation 1 inhalation bid	AS	None Must not be used more than 1 inhalation bid	
Salmeterol inhaler	LBD	21 µg/puff 2 puffs bid	AS	None Must not be used more than 2 puffs bid	
Albuterol	SBD	90 µg/puff 2 puffs q6h prn	AS	May make patient shaky, nervous, and anxious	
Zafirlukast	LTA	20 mg bid (>12 y/o) For 7–11 y/o: 10 mg bid	AS, AR	None	

Montelukast	LTA	10 mg qhs	AS, AR	None
Zileuton	LTA	600 mg qid (>12 y/o)	AS, AR	May cause liver damage (need to monitor LFTs before initiation of and during therapy)
Ipratropium bromide	NAC	21 or 42 µg/spray 2 sprays q8h prn	NAR	Dry mouth, nasal mucosa, epistaxis
	IAC	18 µg/spray 2 puffs q8h prn	AS	Dry mouth, cough

ANA, anaphylaxis; AR, allergic rhinitis; AS, asthma; CA, classic antihistamine; IA, intranasal antihistamine; IAC, inhaled anticholinergic; IS, inhaled steroid; LBD, long-acting bronchodilator; LFTs, liver function tests; LTA, leukotriene antagonist; NA, newer antihistamine; NAC, intranasal anticholinergic; NAR, nonallergic rhinitis; NS, nasal steroid; SBD, short-acting bronchodilatory; UR, urticaria; y/o, years old.

[a]Time before skin testing that antihistamine should be discontinued.

[b]Out of the inhaler, but only 100 µg/spray is inhaled from the spacer-mouthpiece.

[c]Out of the inhaler, but only 108 mg/puff is inhaled from the mouthpiece.

   d. Patients with the hyper-IgE syndrome have a coarse facies and may
   have recurrent "cold" soft-tissue abscesses, which are abscesses that
   lack erythema.
2. Skin examination
   a. Urticaria, or hives, is a maculopapular erythematous, often pruritic,
   eruption in the cutaneous tissues.
   b. Angioedema is edema in the SC tissues and is often painful but not
   pruritic.
   c. Dermatographism (or dermographism) is the tendency to form
   wheal-and-flare responses (urticate) to firm pressure applied to the
   skin. These patients may have physical urticarias as the etiology of
   their recurrent skin rashes (see Urticaria/Angioedema, sec **II.A.2**).
3. Head, ears, eyes, nose, and throat. The anatomy of the nose must be
   clearly evaluated, looking for the presence of swollen and edematous
   turbinates, pale or blue-tinged nasal mucosa, polyps (whitish to clear
   sacs often hanging from the underside of the turbinates), and any septal
   deviation, ulceration, or perforation that may alter airflow.
4. Pulmonary. A thorough lung examination is required, including auscultation of the lung fields, listening for any evidence of wheezing or an
   increased expiratory phase. In some patients, the use of a forced expiratory maneuver helps to expose underlying wheezing that cannot be
   heard at rest.
III. Treatment
   A. Environmental control measures are the first and most important therapy
      for allergic disorders because these interventions limit or prevent exposure
      of patients to the allergens to which they are sensitive. Examples of appro-
      priate control measures include
      1. Pets (in particular, furred pets)
         a. Keep pet out of home or at least out of the bedroom.
         b. Remove carpeting.
         c. Wash the pet regularly.
      2. Dust mites
         a. Wash bedding in hot water ($\geq 130°F$) weekly.
         b. Use synthetic pillows, blankets, mattresses.
         c. Encase the pillows and mattress in dust mite–proof encasings.
         d. Maintain home humidity below 45%.
   B. Medications (Table 12-1).
   C. Corticosteroids represent potent medications for treating allergic disorders.
      1. Mechanisms of action of steroids include inhibiting the production of
         cytokines, which effectively prevents the late-phase response. Steroids
         do not block the immediate-phase response and are not a contraindica-
         tion to skin testing.
      2. Side effects. Long-term use of steroids is associated with side effects.
         The risk of side effects is much greater with systemic (oral) steroids
         than with topical (inhaled) steroids.
         a. Posterior capsular cataracts are associated with prolonged use, and
            annual ophthalmologic examinations are recommended for patients
            on any continual steroid dose (inhaled or oral).
         b. Adrenal suppression occurs with extended use of oral (any dose) or
            high-dose inhaled steroids (see Chap. 17). Short courses (less than a
            month) of oral steroids do not appear to have a significant effect on
            the HPA axis.
         c. Osteoporosis is a risk of corticosteroid use; patients should be
            encouraged to take supplemental calcium and may require bone den-
            sity scans to evaluate their risk.
         d. Newer studies suggest that **growth retardation** in the pediatric pop-
            ulation **does not** occur with moderate inhaled corticosteroid doses
            (*N Engl J Med* 2000;343:1054, 1064).

D. Immunotherapy

1. **Indications** are for **allergic rhinitis, asthma with or without an allergic rhinitic component,** and **venom hypersensitivity**. The mechanisms of action are still under investigation.

2. **Treatment** consists of initial SC injections that contain increasing doses of the allergen extracts to which the patient is sensitive. Once the "buildup" phase is completed (this period is variable), the patient is kept at a maintenance dose for several years. The required length of therapy is variable (usually at least 3–5 years). Immunotherapy should only be prescribed by an allergist after the patient's response to a battery of skin tests or, under special circumstances, based on the results of in vitro testing.

3. **Adverse reactions** are usually mild, with only localized pruritus, erythema, and edema. However, some reactions can be severe enough to include asthmatic flares, diffuse urticaria, and even anaphylactic shock. The highest risk of a reaction is during the initial buildup phase; however, a reaction may occur at any dose. A physician and staff who are experienced in treating anaphylactic shock and an emergency cart **must** be immediately available. The risk for a reaction from an injection is greatest in the 20–30 minutes following the shot, and patients should not be allowed to leave the office until this period has passed. Any time that a patient has had a significant reaction, immunotherapy should be held, pending discussion with an allergist. The only exception to this rule is venom immunotherapy, in which the risk of a reaction is greatest for up to 60 minutes after the shot, and therefore, patients need to wait for an hour before leaving the office.

Anaphylaxis

I. Introduction

A. **Definition.** Anaphylaxis (severe systemic allergic reaction) represents the rapid release of mast cell mediators, preformed as well as newly synthesized (see Allergy, sec. I). The symptoms of anaphylaxis may be related to one or, more commonly, multiple organ systems and are among the most rapid and profound of the allergic reactions; without rapid treatment, they may prove to be fatal. Although the office management is essentially identical, anaphylaxis can be divided into two broad categories: **true anaphylactic** reactions, which require the presence of IgE-type antibodies, and **anaphylactoid** reactions (often referred to as **pseudoallergic reactions**), which are the result of the release of mast cell mediators by any means other than IgE mediated.

B. **Epidemiology.** Anaphylactic reactions are not rare. Common causes of anaphylaxis and their incidence are shown in Table 12-2.

II. Pathophysiology.
The rapid release of vasoactive mediators rapidly results in a loss of vascular tone, resultant pooling in the splanchnic bed, and functional hypovolemia. Because of increased capillary permeability, fluid and colloid are lost into the extravascular space. The net result of these two alterations is a profound decrease in BP. Other manifestations of anaphylaxis include (1) the lower-respiratory tract: **bronchospasm** with wheezing and shortness of breath; (2) the upper-respiratory tract: **laryngeal edema** as well as profuse nasal discharge, watery itchy eyes, and marked postnasal drip; (3) GI tract: **nausea, vomiting, diarrhea, and abdominal cramping**; (4) genitourinary: **uterine cramping**; and (5) skin: **urticaria and angioedema**. Rarely, the patient experiences anaphylactic-induced pulmonary edema and acute CHF (cardiac anaphylaxis).

III. Classification and diagnosis of anaphylaxis.
Anaphylactic reactions can be classified according to the severity of the reaction. The most common classification is given in Table 12-3. Keeping this classification in mind helps the physi-

Table 12-2. Estimated incidence or prevalence of acute anaphylactic reactions

Cause	Incidence or prevalence
General cause	1/2700 hospitalized patients
Chymopapain	2% of females; 0.2% of males
Insect sting	0.4–0.8% of U.S. population
Radiographic contrast material	1/1000–14,000 procedures
Penicillin (fatal outcome)	1.0–7.5/million treatments
General anesthesia	1/300 treatments
Hemodialysis	1/1000–5000 treatments
Immunotherapy (severe reaction)	0.1/million injections

Modified from TC Sim. Anaphylaxis. How to manage and prevent this medical emergency. *Postgrad Med* 1992;92:277.

cian in the differential diagnosis of anaphylaxis. In addition, anaphylaxis may be monophasic, biphasic, or, in rare cases, prolonged. As noted previously, classic allergic reactions may have an early and a delayed or late phase. This is also true for anaphylactic reactions, and it is not uncommon to see a patient who was successfully treated for anaphylaxis have a **second**, often as profound, reaction 4–12 hours following the initial anaphylactic reaction. The **criteria** for the diagnosis include at least one of the following: laryngeal edema, bronchospasm or hypotension, and the presence of other distinctive signs of allergy, such as urticaria or angioedema, or both; sneezing or rhinorrhea (often profuse); nausea; vomiting or diarrhea; and uterine cramping. In addition, a history of recent exposure to the agent is associated with anaphylaxis. A few conditions that might **mimic** anaphylaxis include vasovagal syncope, hyperventilation syndrome, globus hystericus, hereditary angioedema, carcinoid syndrome, systemic mastocytosis, and fictitious anaphylaxis.

IV. **Treatment of anaphylaxis** includes prevention, recognition, prompt institution of therapy, and early transport to an emergency care facility.

Table 12-3. Classification of anaphylactic/anaphylactoid reactions according to severity

Grade	Skin	GI	Respiratory	Cardiovascular
I	Pruritus, urticaria, flush, etc.	None	None	None
II	Pruritus, urticaria, flush, etc.	Nausea	Dyspnea Hypotension	Tachycardia
III	Pruritus, urticaria, flush, etc.	Vomiting Defecation	Bronchospasm Cyanosis	Shock
IV	Pruritus	Vomiting	Respiratory	Cardiac

A. Prevention is one of the most important aspects of treatment for the practitioner. Emphasis should include instructing the patient that most severe reactions (including those to food, drugs, stinging insects, and radiocontrast media) rarely go away. If these reactions are identified, the patient should be advised to avoid that agent in the future. Individuals who are food sensitive should read all labels for prepared food and inquire for the presence of that food at restaurants. The "Food Allergy Network" (see Resources, sec. **II**) can help individuals by identifying food that contains potent allergens and in designing meals that avoid those allergens. In addition, every patient who has experienced anaphylaxis in the past should have an Epi-Pen prescribed and carry it with him or her at all times. A medical alert bracelet or necklace that identifies important allergens (especially drug allergy) is also an important preventive measure.

B. Recognition. Perhaps the most important aspect of the treatment of anaphylaxis is the early recognition that a reaction has occurred. Indeed, the physician should always err on the side of identifying a reaction when one may not have occurred rather than waiting to see if the reaction will become more profound. True anaphylaxis rarely goes away without treatment.

C. Prompt institution of therapy. The hallmark of the treatment of anaphylaxis is the rapid introduction of **epinephrine** and **fluids** with other therapeutic agents added later. Indeed, most studies of fatal anaphylaxis have demonstrated failure to introduce these measures as a major contributor to the adverse outcome.

D. Prompt transport to an emergency care facility. The outpatient treatment of anaphylaxis should be directed toward stabilizing the patient to assure a patent airway and maintain an adequate BP. Once this has been established, the patent should be rapidly transported to an emergency care facility. The outpatient setting is not equipped to treat the more serious and prolonged forms of anaphylaxis.

E. Drugs used in the treatment of anaphylaxis.

    1. Adrenergic or sympathomimetic agonists. The most important agent for the treatment of anaphylaxis is **epinephrine**, and this agent should be used as soon as the reaction is recognized. The usual doses for epinephrine are shown in Table 12-4. It is important to remember that in most cases SC or IM epinephrine is adequate, with recent data suggesting that IM administration is preferred. There is no need for IV therapy

Table 12-4. Doses for epinephrine in the treatment of anaphylaxis

Minor to moderate manifestations	Dose and route
Type I or II	0.3–0.5 mg (1:1000) SC or IM adults
	0.01 mg/kg (1:1000) SC or IM children
	Repeat every 12–20 min × 4
Severe reaction—type III	0.5–1.0 mg (1:1000) SC or IM adults
	0.01–0.02 mg/kg SC or IM children
	Repeat every 3 min × 4
Severe reaction—type IV	0.1–1.0 mg (1:10,000) IV adults
	0.01–0.02 mg (1:10,000) IV children
Continuous IV therapy—if intermittent therapy fails	0.1–1.0 µg/kg/min; titrate to maintain BP
Upper-respiratory compromise	1.0–4.0 mg (racemic) by inhalation (meter-dose inhaler or nebulizer)

unless a type IV reaction occurs. **IV epinephrine should always be given using 0.1 mg/ml or 1:10,000 aqueous** rather than the 1:1000 concentration. Intermittent epinephrine can be repeated at 15- to 20-minute intervals, and after four doses, if necessary, can be followed by continuous IV therapy until the BP is stabilized. Other sympathomimetic agents that may be useful include terbutaline (given SC or IM), dopamine, dobutamine, and norepinephrine. In general, these agents are used in profound and prolonged anaphylactic reactions and are beyond the scope of this chapter.

2. **Fluids.** Establishment of IV access and the institution of fluid replacement therapy should be accomplished as soon as epinephrine has been given. Two types of fluids are available for therapy: colloid [albumin, hydroxyethyl starch (Hetastarch), pentastarch, dextrans, and blood and blood products] and crystalloid (dextrose, saline, and Ringer's lactate). The choice between colloid and crystalloid has received significant attention. In general, colloid has the benefit of increasing oncotic pressure, which has been lost due to capillary leakage. Colloid solutions have been associated with increased oxygen saturation and less increase in lung water than crystalloid solutions. Some colloid solutions are associated with adverse side effects, such as anaphylactoid reactions (dextrans) and infectious diseases (blood and blood products). Of the colloid solutions, hydroxyethyl starch is the preferred solution. An initial infusion of 500 ml is followed by crystalloid therapy. The choice of crystalloid solution is arbitrary, and any of the solutions mentioned above is adequate. Sufficient solution should be given to maintain the BP.

3. **Antihistamines.** H_1-type antihistamines (Table 12-1) are a useful adjunct for the treatment of anaphylaxis, particularly for patients who experience urticaria or generalized skin pruritus. These can be given intravenously, intramuscularly, or orally. However, **antihistamines are not a substitute for epinephrine and fluids**. One should not give an antihistaminic and then wait to see if it is effective, even in mild anaphylaxis. The combination of IV H_1- and H_2-blocking agents has been reported to be effective in patients who are taking beta-blockers (including eyedrops) and who may not respond to the usual doses of epinephrine (see sec. **IV.E.5**), although H_2-blocking agents are usually more effective for prophylaxis against anaphylaxis.

4. **Corticosteroids have no place in the acute treatment of anaphylaxis**, because they have little or no effect on the acute phase of allergic reactions. Steroids may lessen the late-phase reaction, and these agents should be used as an adjunct once the patient has been stabilized. The use of IV methylprednisolone (Solumedrol), 1–2 mg/kg every 6 hours; IV hydrocortisone hemisuccinate (Solu-Cortef), 100 mg every 4 hours; or oral hydrocortisone, 4–6 mg/kg every 4–6 hours, has been shown to be helpful in patients with anaphylaxis.

5. **Other agents.** Several pharmacologic agents may be useful in the office treatment of anaphylaxis. Glucagon, 1 mg IV, may be effective in patients who take beta-blockers. Patients who experience significant bronchospasm, such as asthmatics, should receive a short-acting β agonist. Less effective are anticholinergic agents such as ipratropium bromide (Atrovent), and IV theophylline or aminophylline.

6. **Other therapeutic measures.** Patients with acute anaphylaxis are often hypoxic. Thus, the rapid establishment of an adequate airway is critical. Aerosolized racemic epinephrine can be tried in patients who have laryngeal edema; however, if this is not available or is not rapidly effective, use of an endotracheal tube, if available, and the physician is practiced in its use; a cricothyroid puncture; or tracheotomy may be necessary. The establishment of an airway should be accompanied by the use of oxygen therapy.

V. The office emergency kit. Any physician who may need to treat anaphylaxis should establish a basic emergency kit. This should include (1) epinephrine: 1:1000 aqueous for SC and IM use and 1:10,000 aqueous for IV use; racemic epinephrine: meter-dose inhaler or nebulizer use; (2) IV fluids: colloid and crystalloid; (3) large-bore IV catheter; (4) tourniquet; (5) oxygen with face mask or nasal prongs; (6) Ambu-bag; and (7) additional medications: H_1 antihistamines, H_2 antihistamines, corticosteroids.

VI. Summary of immediate treatment measures for anaphylaxis. The practitioner should have a high index of suspicion for an anaphylactic reaction. Once the diagnosis is suspected, a coordinated series of measures should be instituted. These include the following: (1) Establish an airway; (2) administer aqueous epinephrine; (3) establish IV access and administer fluids—most often colloid followed by crystalloid; (4) query patient regarding prior anaphylaxis; (5) query patient regarding concomitant medications (especially beta-blockers); (6) if indicated, administer H_1 and H_2 antihistaminics, glucocorticoids, or glucagon; and (7) arrange for rapid transport of the patient to an emergency care facility.

Venom Hypersensitivity

I. Introduction. Estimates suggest that 7% of the population in the United States have specific IgE against *Hymenoptera* venoms. Only insects with true stingers are included within the order *Hymenoptera*. Some examples are yellow and bald-faced hornet, yellow jacket, paper wasp, honeybee, and fire ants. A sting introduces roughly 20–50 μg venom protein. Included in this mix of proteins are many vasoactive amines, alkaloids, and species-specific proteins, such as hyaluronidase, acid phosphatase, and phospholipase A.

II. Diagnosis

  A. History

    1. Type of insect. It is important to try and identify the stinging insect, as this will guide skin testing and ultimate therapy. It is also helpful to determine if the patient was stung once or multiple times and by one or more insects.

    2. Site of sting. The location of the sting may be important in determining whether or not a systemic reaction occurred. It can also aid in identification of the insect involved. For example, honeybees usually sting when they are stepped on and are not normally known to attack people. Yellow jackets, however, attack people when their food source is threatened. This usually happens in the late fall, when they can be found scavenging for food in garbage containers.

    3. Types of reaction. Two types of reactions to stings occur.

      a. Large local reactions are characterized by induration, erythema, and pain at the sting site. The area involved can spread to regions of the body that are directly adjacent to the sting site, but, as long as these sites are contiguous, the reaction is still considered local. These reactions are often quite dramatic and may last for up to a week, but they rarely progress and need no further evaluation.

      b. Systemic reactions include any reactions that occur away from the initial sting site. For example, facial urticaria immediately following a sting on the left hand is considered a systemic reaction, whereas edema of the entire left arm is not considered as such. Systemic reactions can include urticaria, bronchospasm, laryngeal edema, hypotension, and other symptoms of anaphylaxis. Most patients who have a severe reaction have no history of venom-induced anaphylaxis. In patients with a history of a systemic reaction, 60% have a similar reaction with a re-sting, whereas only 11% have a worse reaction.

   B. Skin testing
   1. **Skin testing** with various concentrations of the venoms is used to deter-
      mine sensitivity to *Hymenoptera* venoms. False-positive skin test results
      are possible due to venom cross reactivity. **RAST inhibition** is a serum
      test that involves adding specific antigens to determine the level of cross
      reactivity. Usually, this test isolates the important insects.
III. Treatment
   A. Local reactions require supportive care of ice, compression, and elevation.
      In severe local reactions, corticosteroids (usually 0.5 mg/kg prednisone) are
      sometimes prescribed to help decrease the edema and irritation. In addition,
      antihistamines (see Table 12-1 for medications and doses) can help alleviate
      the pruritus that is often associated with a sting.
   B. Systemic reactions need to be aggressively treated, acutely and chronically.
      1. **Acute** treatment of a systemic reaction includes the liberal use IM
         (preferable) of SC epinephrine (Table 12-4) to treat anaphylaxis rapidly.
         β Agonists are useful if bronchospasm develops from the sting
         (Albuterol meter-dose inhaler or by nebulization). Antihistamines are
         also helpful in the acute treatment to block the effects of histamine
         release. Corticosteroids (0.5–1.0 mg/kg prednisone for 7–10 days) are
         helpful as well in the treatment of acute stings. These medications help
         abrogate the edema as well as help modify a late-phase response from
         occurring.
      2. **Chronic** therapy involves treating the patient with venom immunother-
         apy, which has been shown to reduce the patient's risk of a systemic
         reaction from a subsequent sting to that of the general population. In
         addition to immunotherapy, any patient who has had a systemic reac-
         tion to a sting should have self-injectable epinephrine (Epi-Pen) pre-
         scribed and be taught how to use it appropriately. Besides epinephrine,
         these patients should have antihistamines with them at all times. Also,
         it is a good idea to encourage patients to wear a medical alert bracelet
         that identifies them as venom allergic.
   C. Special issues regarding immunotherapy. Once patients begin venom
      immunotherapy, they are protected from subsequent stings—even if they
      are just in the buildup phase of the injections. The maintenance dose of
      the injections usually contains 100 μg venom proteins—roughly 1.5–2.0
      times the amount in a single sting. The question of **how long** a patient
      should continue to receive immunotherapy is still under investigation.
      Some physicians treat for 5 years and then discontinue the shots, whereas
      others continue immunotherapy until the patient's skin tests become neg-
      ative or at least a logfold less reactive. The patient, primary care physi-
      cian, and allergist should all be involved in the decision of when to
      discontinue immunotherapy.

Urticaria and Angioedema

I. Introduction. Urticaria is an erythematous maculopapular eruption in the
superficial layers of the dermis and is associated with pruritus. It can further
be divided into acute and chronic lesions based on the temporal nature of the
rash. **Acute** urticaria is any urticarial episode that lasts for less than 6 weeks;
chronic urticaria is an episode that has lasted for at least 6 weeks. An urticarial
episode consists of a period when hives are present daily or nearly daily. It
should be noted that a given crop of hives will likely be present only for a short
period, but the patient may have multiple crops of hives during the episode.
Angioedema, by contrast, consists of edema in the deep layers of the dermis
and is usually characterized by **pain** rather than pruritus. Urticaria and
angioedema often coexist in the same patient.

II. Diagnosis
A. Clinical findings
1. **History.** Determine whether the urticaria is **acute or chronic**. It is also important to determine whether the lesions are **pruritic or painful**. Because vasculitis may present with urticarial lesions, it is critical to determine if the individual crops of hives **last more than 24 hours** and if they **resolve with scarring**. Both of these conditions are associated with urticarial vasculitis, not urticaria.
2. **Physical examination.** Specifically, the physician should look for evidence of thyroid disease, collagen vascular disease, occult infection, or malignancy. Several types of urticaria can develop from physical causes. These **physical urticarias** can be diagnosed during the examination by using various maneuvers to reproduce each of them. For example, cold urticaria can be diagnosed by placing an ice cube on the forearm for 4 minutes. The cube is then removed and the arm observed for 10 minutes. A hive that develops at the same location where the ice cube was indicates a positive test.
B. Differential diagnosis. The differential diagnosis depends on whether the urticaria is acute or chronic.
1. **Acute.** Most of the inciting agents that lead to acute urticaria can be easily identified because of the close temporal relationship between exposure and hive development. Often the patient has already identified the responsible agent before seeking medical attention. Agents that often cause acute urticaria include **foods** (peanuts and shellfish, for example), **medications** (such as penicillin), **infections** (usually viral infections), and **physical** causes. The physical urticarias arise from various physical stresses and can be reproduced in the office by repeating the stress. Offending agents include **cold, heat, pressure, sun, water, vibration, cholinergic stimulation, and exercise**. In some patients, exercise is a trigger only when closely preceded by eating.
2. **Chronic.** The inciting agents that lead to chronic urticaria are much more difficult to identify because the temporal relationship is not as clear as in acute urticaria. These patients tend to be more emotionally and physically affected by their disease and its chronicity. Chronic urticaria has been attributed to **medications** (such as nonsteroidal anti-inflammatory drugs), **collagen vascular disease** (for example, systemic lupus erythematosus), **neoplasia, autoimmune diseases, and chronically eaten foods**. The autoimmune phenomenon that is most often associated with urticaria is **thyroid disease**. Patients may be hypo-, hyper-, or even clinically euthyroid but usually have **antithyroid peroxidase autoantibodies** (also known as **antimicrosomal antibodies**). In these patients (including the clinically euthyroid), treatment with physiologic doses of thyroid hormone often leads to resolution of the urticaria.
3. Current research suggests that 30–50% of patients with chronic urticaria have **autoantibodies** directed **against** either **IgE** or the **high-affinity IgE receptor (FcεRI)**. These patients do not respond well to antihistamines alone and often require corticosteroids for relief of their hives. Further treatment options for these patients are still being investigated. **Idiopathic urticaria**, the largest set of urticarias, is a catchall group that represents those cases in which no etiology for the urticaria can be discerned.
C. Workup
1. The **usual tests** that are performed to evaluate the differential for chronic urticaria are outlined below.
   a. CBC with differential
   b. Sedimentation rate
   c. Liver function tests (to evaluate for hepatitis)
   d. Antinuclear autoantibody screen
   e. Antithyroid peroxidase (or antimicrosomal) antibodies

       f. Urinalysis (to evaluate for urinary tract infection)

       g. In the future, it may become customary to evaluate for anti-IgE or anti-FcεRI autoantibodies, or both. Currently, it is not normally performed due to the lack of a commercially available test, and more recent data suggest that properly performed autologous skin testing is more useful than laboratory tests in diagnosing anti-FcεRI autoantibodies.

    2. Skin and RAST testing. Although the specific antigens that are responsible for urticaria are often hard to discern, it may be helpful in some patients to perform skin or RAST testing. These tests tend to be more useful in patients with acute urticaria in whom a specific food or medication is believed to be the offending agent. As mentioned previously, skin testing is the preferred modality to evaluate for allergy; however, some patients with urticaria have such severe skin disease that RAST testing may be more feasible.

    3. Food additives. In addition to specific food allergens, urticaria can develop from sensitivity to food additives. The only reliable test for sensitivity to food additives is a double-blind placebo-controlled challenge. These are usually performed in an allergist's office and take several hours to complete.

III. Treatment

  A. The most important therapeutic intervention is to **avoid the inciting agent(s)** and/or **treat the underlying condition**.

  B. Pharmacologic options include the use of **antihistamines**, often in escalating doses, to control the pruritus and urticarial flares. In addition to the traditional H_1-receptor antagonist antihistamines (see Table 12-1 for medications and doses), patients may benefit from the addition of an H_2-receptor antagonist (cimetidine, ranitidine, famotidine, etc.). **Tricyclic antidepressants**, such as doxepin (starting dose approximately 10–25 mg daily), are often used because of their strong antihistaminic activity. Because these medications are often sedating, they should be given shortly before or at bedtime. Finally, **corticosteroids** can be used (often prednisone, 0.5 mg/kg daily). Steroids alleviate urticarial flares; however, the numerous side effects that are associated with their chronic use limit the feasibility of corticosteroids in chronic urticaria.

  C. In patients with **chronic idiopathic urticaria**, it is helpful to control their urticaria with appropriate doses of medications and then to withdraw the medications after a specified duration of time (6 weeks to 6 months) to evaluate for the continued presence of urticarial lesions. If the hives recur, restart the medications for another period of time.

IV. Angioedema (without urticaria)

  A. Angioedema without urticaria usually presents as a **painful, nonpruritic swelling** of the deep dermis. The most often **affected areas** are the soles of the feet, palms of the hands (including the thenar eminence), buttocks, and face (including the larynx, lips, tongue, and periorbital regions). Attacks often occur after even minimal trauma and may progress around the body. The greatest danger with angioedema is that it may involve the larynx and can lead to complete obstruction of the airway.

  B. Diagnosis. In most cases angioedema is due to either a drug [usually an angiotensin-converting enzyme (ACE) inhibitor, an angiotensin II receptor (AII-R) inhibitor, aspirin, an antibiotic, or a nonsteroidal anti-inflammatory drug] or a deficiency in the complement component C1 esterase inhibitor (C1INH).

    1. Angioedema from an **ACE inhibitor or AII-R inhibitor** can occur at any point during a course of treatment and necessitates discontinuation of the drug, even if it is not the cause, because these drugs can enhance angioedema caused by other factors. Clearly, all drugs of the same class need to be avoided; however, it is less clear whether sensitivity to one class necessitates avoidance of the other. However, several case histories have been reported in which angioedema has developed in patients with ACE inhibitor–induced angioedema when treating with an AII-R therapy (*Ann Pharmacother* 1999;33:936). Therefore, if possible, it is probably best to avoid both classes of medications if a patient develops sensitivity to one of them.

2. A **deficiency in C1INH** can be either **acquired or hereditary** (known as **hereditary angioedema**). The acquired form of the disease is often associated with a hematologic malignancy and the subsequent production of an autoantibody that blocks the function of C1INH.

   a. To evaluate for a possible deficiency in C1INH, a **C4 level** can be obtained. This is low even between attacks in hereditary angioedema. Further evaluation includes a **quantitative C1INH level**. If this is not significantly decreased, a **functional C1INH level** should be obtained. This is reduced in either acquired or hereditary forms. Finally, **mixing studies** and an **anti-C1INH antibody enzyme-linked immunosorbent assay (ELISA)** can be obtained to evaluate for the presence of an inhibiting autoantibody (often associated with an underlying hematologic malignancy).

   b. Patients with known or suspected angioedema due to a complement deficiency should be evaluated by an allergist/immunologist.

V. **Treatment**

A. **Avoidance** of the causative agent is the primary treatment in drug-induced angioedema. As mentioned above, a reaction to an ACE inhibitor or AII-R inhibitor may be reason to avoid all drugs of both classes. In cases in which angioedema is secondary to a malignancy, **treatment of the underlying disease** leads to resolution of the angioedema.

B. **For chronic therapy** of hereditary angioedema, **androgens** (usually stanozolol) can be used. These increase the levels of C1INH and prevent attacks of angioedema. These patients should be referred to an allergist/immunologist for diagnosis and therapy. Because of their masculinizing effects, androgens should be particularly avoided in the treatment of females. Primary care physicians should not attempt to treat hereditary angioedema.

C. **For acute therapy** of angioedema, **epinephrine** can be used. This leads to vasoconstriction and acute reduction in the edema. Unfortunately, patients with hereditary angioedema usually respond poorly to epinephrine alone. In these cases, **fresh frozen plasma (FFP)** (which contains C1INH) can be given; however, in some patients this worsens the swelling. **Purified C1INH** is in clinical trials; when commercially available, it could be used to acutely treat patients with angioedema. As **preparation for surgery**, patients can be given FFP or C1INH before the operation to prevent peri- and postoperative angioedema.

D. **Supportive therapy** is always important. Laryngeal angioedema may develop, and therefore it is always important to safeguard the airway. Some patients may even require intubation or tracheostomy during their attacks.

Drug and Food Allergies

I. **Introduction.** Allergic reactions to drugs represent a major contributor to the spectrum of adverse drug reactions. To the practitioner, this is particularly important, as studies have suggested that as many as 40% of all hospitalizations in the United States are in one way or another related to an adverse drug reaction. This, coupled with the large number of therapeutic agents that a single patient may be taking, often provides a therapeutic dilemma for the practitioner.

A. **Classification** of adverse reactions include

1. **Reactions related to the pharmacologic properties of the drug** such as side effects, toxic reactions, and drug interactions. Because these

reactions are based on the chemical properties of the drug, they occur in all patients if a sufficient amount of drug is given. Therefore, in many cases the reaction may be lessened by alteration in the dose of the drug.

Reactions due to toxic metabolites may mimic immunologic reactions or side effects. In this case, the biotransformation product rather than the drug itself is the offending agent. The reaction to sulfa-containing drugs (mostly sulfamethoxazole in patients who are HIV positive) is an example of this reaction. These reactions are different from other side effects, and the method for abrogating the reaction differs from that of other types of adverse drug reactions.

2. **Idiosyncratic reactions** are adverse effects with an unknown mechanism. They are seen in susceptible individuals, but the basis for the susceptibility is not known. These reactions may occur at any point during therapy. The reactions may be mild, such as the facial dyskinesis that is seen with phenothiazines, or devastating, such as the aplastic anemia with chloramphenicol. What is clear is that idiosyncratic reactions almost invariably recur if the drug is reintroduced. The physician should always be aware of the potential for an idiosyncratic reaction; however, fear of such a reaction should not prevent the use of a therapeutic agent that is clearly necessary.

3. **Immunologically based reactions.** Adverse reactions may be the result of production of antibodies or cytotoxic T cells directed against the drug or a biotransformation of the drug. The types of reactions include contact sensitivity of fixed drug reactions (type IV or cell-mediated reaction); tissue-specific reactions due to T-cell immunity, such as drug-induced hepatitis; tissue-specific damage due to IgG antibodies (type II or III); and drug allergy due to IgE antibodies (type I). Other reactions are believed to have an immunologic basis, but the exact mechanism has not been elucidated. Examples include drug fever and erythema multiforme minor and major (Stevens-Johnson syndrome) and toxic epidermal necrolysis.

B. **Mechanism of drug allergy.** The majority of therapeutic agents are low-molecular-weight organic compounds and alone are not capable of inducing the production of either antidrug antibodies or T cell proliferation. It is only when the drug (or more likely one or more of its biotransformation products) reacts covalently with a tissue protein (or carbohydrate) that becomes a hapten that it is capable of inducing an immune response. The actual immunogen (allergen) may be the hapten itself, the hapten-protein conjugate, or a tissue protein that has been altered by interaction with the drug such that it is now recognized by the body as foreign. Because a chemical bond must occur between the drug and tissue protein, the propensity of that drug to bind to protein either in its native state or following metabolism determines the allergenic potential of that drug. Thus, beta-lactam antibiotics are very reactive with tissue protein and are major allergens, whereas cardiac glycosides are very unreactive, and true allergy to this class of drugs is rarely seen. The physician should keep in mind the potential for a specific drug class to react with protein, as this makes up one factor in the determination of which drug has caused a reaction among patients who are taking multiple therapeutic agents.

1. **Route of administration** is important in the induction phase of drug allergy. As is pointed out below (see sec. **III.D**), the parenteral administration of a drug has the highest potential for inducing an immunologic reaction. Oral administration is much less likely to result in an immunologic reaction to a drug. Application of a drug to the skin may result in a contact sensitivity (type IV) rather than the production of antidrug IgE.

2. It is important to remember that in all but the rarest cases, the **actual immunogen is not known.** This is important because the development of in vivo tests (skin tests) or in vitro tests (RAST or ELISA) is based on

a thorough knowledge of the chemical structure of the allergen. For the first-generation beta-lactam antibiotics (penicillins and first-generation cephalosporins), the immunogens are well described or are surmised from extensive skin testing. Thus, 75% of patients with a history of a penicillin reaction have a positive skin test to penicilloyl-polylysine (Pre-Pen), whereas 6% of patients react with penicillin G and 7% react with penicilloic acid. The latter two reagents are used to conjugate rapidly with tissue proteins and provide the appropriate antigen. With a knowledge of the allergens, this skin test has high sensitivity and specificity. Other drug classes have not been studied, and thus, the allergen(s) are not known. As noted in sec. **II.B**, it is possible to use the native drug as an allergen in the hopes that the drug or its metabolite will provide an appropriate allergenic structure; however, the predictive value of these tests is questionable.

II. Diagnosis. The diagnosis of drug allergy is based on a thorough history, physical examination, in vivo or in vitro testing, or both, and, when necessary, a provocative challenge.

A. History. The history should emphasize

1. **The drug or drugs that the patient had been taking at the time of the reaction.** If patients are experiencing the reaction at the time that they are seen, it is always a good idea to have them bring all of their drugs to the clinic. Patients often forget one or more of the drugs that they are taking, and the drugs that they are taking may not be the ones that have been prescribed. If the reaction occurred in the past, a chart review may be necessary.

2. **The type of reaction** and the potential for that reaction to be immunologic in nature. It is often helpful for the physician to make a list of the potential offending drugs and then to rank the drugs by allergenic potential. Although all drugs are potential allergens, as mentioned previously (see sec. **I.B**), some are much more allergenic than others.

3. **The severity of the reaction** is also very important, as it determines the steps that may have to be taken to abrogate a similar reaction. An anaphylactic reaction is much more significant than a minor skin rash.

4. **A history of reactions** to drugs is very helpful. Several groups have demonstrated that a patient who has had one reaction to a drug is more likely to have another than is a patient who has never reacted. For some patients, true reactions are seen to multiple drug classes and probably represent an increased ability to react to haptenated proteins. This has been referred to as the **multiple drug allergy syndrome**.

5. **A family history of drug allergy** is also a predictive factor. The relative risk of a drug reaction is multifold higher if the patient's mother or father has also had a drug reaction.

6. Finally, **the nature of concurrent illness** should be established to assure that the reaction is not the result of that illness and not the drug or drugs. For example, a facial rash in a patient with lupus erythematosus is most likely the result of the disease process and not a drug reaction.

B. In vivo or in vitro testing. Skin testing is the most important technique for the diagnosis of a true drug allergy. In the case of penicillin or the first-generation cephalosporins, skin testing is easily performed and highly predictive of an allergic reaction. Referral to an allergist/immunologist is necessary for skin testing to be performed. In vitro testing, such as RAST or ELISA tests, has the same drawback as skin testing, as it relies on knowledge of the actual allergen. These tests are further compromised by the amount of time that is necessary for the test to be performed (usually greater than 24 hours), and thus, they are not applicable to the acute situation. Evidence has demonstrated that skin testing may not be reliable within the first several weeks after a severe drug reaction, and this may be the one area in which in vitro testing is necessary.

C. **Provocative dose challenge.** A provocative dose challenge provides a method for determining a patient's sensitivity to a given drug or drug class and for initiating therapy to that drug. Indeed, in practice this is performed only when a decision to start the patient on the drug has been made. The challenge begins with a small (1 mg) dose of the drug and proceeds rapidly to higher doses. In practice, we generally base the dose for challenge on the dose of drug that is necessary for therapy. If the patient tolerates a 1-mg to 10-mg dose, then one-tenth the therapeutic dose followed by one-fourth the therapeutic dose and then one-half the therapeutic dose at 15- to 30-minute intervals are given. The provocative dose challenge should be performed in a medical setting where appropriate resuscitative measures are available.

III. **Therapy**

A. **The most effective therapy for drug allergy is the selection of an alternative drug class.** In the majority of cases, an effective therapeutic agent is available that does not cross react with the drug to which the patient is sensitive. In some cases, an alternative drug may be of the same drug class but lacks a reactive side chain. An example is the substitution of lisinopril or enalapril, which does not have a sulfonamide side chain, for captopril, which contains a sulfonamide. Similarly, ethacrynic acid may substitute for furosemide. The substitution of an alternative antibiotic, which may differ only in a reactive side chain, is often very effective and precludes the need for skin testing and desensitization. The selection of an alternative modality is also effective in anaphylactoid reactions. For example, the selection of a low-ionic-strength radiocontrast medium rather than the high-strength material decreases the potential for a reaction greatly. The selection of an alternative drug should always be the first consideration in approaching a drug-allergic patient.

B. **Provocative dose challenge.** As noted above (see sec. **II.C**), when skin testing or in vitro testing is not available, a provocative dose challenge is often effective. The physician should choose the drug class that is least likely to give a positive reaction. For example, patients who have a history of a reaction to a local anesthetic (which almost never causes a true allergic reaction) can receive a provocative challenge with the least reactive group of agents, those that do not contain a paraaminobenzoic acid ester group. Because preservatives such as parabens or additional agents such as β-adrenergic agonists can cause reactions, we recommend that the provocative challenge be carried out using **preservative-free solutions.** These are available as obstetric preparations of most local anesthetics. If a small (1-ml) dose of the local anesthetic does not provoke a reaction, this anesthetic can be used without hesitation.

C. **Pretreatment protocols.** For a number of drug classes that cause reaction by anaphylactic or anaphylactoid mechanisms, a pretreatment protocol is available to prevent or decrease any reaction that might occur. The protocol that is used in the reintroduction of radiocontrast media is presented in Table 12-5.

D. **Drug desensitization.** Drug desensitization provides a method to reintroduce a drug to which a patient is sensitive. This should only be performed under the supervision of an allergist/immunologist and only in a location that is capable of treating significant and potentially prolonged anaphylaxis. The desensitization procedure involves the introduction of minute amounts of the drug and then slowly increasing the dose (usually by doubling) every 15–20 minutes until a full therapeutic dose is achieved. As noted previously, the potential for a reaction is much less when oral medication is used. Therefore, when possible, the initiation of the desensitization procedure is by the oral route followed by parenteral medication if indicated. The mechanism by which the desensitization procedure works is not known, but evidence indicates that mast cells become resistant to the release of mediators by the drug but not by other allergens. The purpose of desensitization is to

Table 12-5. Protocol for pretreatment of patients with a history of radiocontrast media reactions

Time before the procedure	Drug and dose		
	Prednisone[a]	Cimetidine[b]	Diphenhydramine[c]
13 hrs	50 mg PO or IV	300 mg PO or IV	—
7 hrs	50 mg PO or IV	300 mg PO or IV	—
1 hrs[d]	50 mg PO or IV	300 mg PO or IV	50 mg PO or IV

[a]Other agents include methylprednisolone, 40 mg IV.
[b]Other agents include ranitidine, 150 mg.
[c]Other agents include chlorpheniramine, 10–12 mg.
[d]Can also add ephedrine, 25 mg PO, 1 hr before procedure.

prevent a potentially life-threatening reaction. The procedure does not prevent the appearance of mild skin reactions such as pruritus or urticaria. Importantly, the desensitized state lasts only as long as the drug is given. Once the drug has been stopped, the patient becomes sensitive again in 8–48 hours. It is not possible to predict when the patient will become sensitive; thus, **if the patient misses taking the drug for more than 12 hours, the procedure has to be repeated**. If the physician foresees a need to retreat with the same medication in a short period of time, the drug should be continued (usually orally) to avoid having to undergo another desensitization.

IV. **Summary.** Drug allergy represents a portion of the spectrum of adverse reactions to drugs. It is important always to question every patient concerning drug reaction. The diagnosis can be made using a quality history and physical examination, skin or in vitro testing when available, and provocative dose challenges if necessary. It is possible to reintroduce the drug if necessary using premedication protocols and drug desensitization. **Neither of these, however, is a substitute for a well-thought-out alternative drug.**

V. **Food allergies**

  A. **Introduction**

    1. Sensitivity to food is not uncommon, but **food allergy** is a term reserved for an immunologic-mediated (i.e., IgE-mediated) sensitivity to food. Food allergy is thought to occur in 2–4% of children and in fewer than 1–2% of adults.

    2. **Symptoms.** Patients may present with a number of varying symptoms. These can include urticaria/angioedema, asthmatic flares, abdominal cramping, diarrhea, rhinoconjunctivitis flares, and anaphylaxis.

    3. **Risks for death.** The risk of death from food allergies is increased (especially with children) when patients have asthma and are unaware that they have ingested a food to which they are sensitive, patients are away from home or a primary caregiver when the reaction occurs, and the time to epinephrine injection is greater than 30 minutes (*N Engl J Med* 1992;327:380).

  B. **Diagnosis**

    1. Determine what type of reaction occurred, and whether it was IgE mediated.

      a. **IgE-mediated food allergy.** Determine the **timing** of the reaction after ingestion of the suspected food. Most allergic reactions occur within 15–30 minutes of ingestion. Reactions that occur hours after eating are much less likely to represent an allergic response. Determine the **suspected foods** that are involved. In food allergy in adults, the most often offending agents are peanuts, tree nuts, and shellfish. In children, the common offending foods also include milk, wheat, soy, and egg.

    b. Non-IgE–mediated food sensitivities can also present as food intolerance. **Eosinophilic gastroenteritis** is a disorder that is characterized by eosinophilic infiltration of the bowel wall and peripheral eosinophilia. These patients often present with malabsorption and usually have allergic diseases as well. These patients should be evaluated and treated by a specialist. Several other **malabsorption syndromes** can masquerade as food allergies (see Chap. 14).

  2. Testing. As with any allergic disease evaluation, a positive test must correlate with the patient's history for that allergen to be associated with the patient's symptoms. These tests should be performed in an allergist/immunologist's office.

    a. Skin testing for the various food allergens is often performed. Because of the irritant nature of many food allergen preparations and the possibility of systemic reactions, only epicutaneous and not intradermal testing should be performed. In some cases, testing is done with fresh fruits or vegetables, which are pricked with the testing device. The device then is used to prick the patient.

    b. CAP-RAST testing allows for the determination of specific IgE against various food allergens. An area of current research is to identify what levels of specific IgE are associated with clinical disease.

    c. The gold standard for diagnosing food allergy is the **double-blind placebo-controlled food challenge**. These challenges can be dangerous and should be performed by allergists either in their clinic or in the hospital. If this food challenge does not show sensitivity to the suspected food, an open-label challenge with the food is usually performed.

    d. To evaluate for eosinophilic gastroenteritis or other malabsorption syndromes, **endoscopy** may be necessary (see Chap. 14).

C. Treatment

  1. Avoid the offending food.

  2. Educate the patient and family members/friends about how allergic reactions to foods occur, how to avoid these reactions, and how to treat when a reaction occurs. In children it is important that all potential caregivers (including, for example, the parents of the child's friend) understand the disease and how to avoid and treat reactions.

  3. To treat episodes, the patient (and caregivers) should always have immediately available **self-injectable epinephrine** (Ana-Kit or Epi-Pen). Any patients for whom self-injectable epinephrine is prescribed should have the proper use of the injector demonstrated to them in the physician's office. Before leaving the office, patients should prove to the physician that they understand the proper use of self-injectable epinephrine. They should also be aware that whenever they have used their epinephrine, they should seek immediate medical attention.

Rhinitis and Rhinoconjunctivitis

I. Introduction. Nearly one-fifth of the general population has a form of seasonal or perennial allergic rhinoconjunctivitis, or both, making it one of the most common chronic disorders. The disease tends to occur predominantly in childhood, and the onset is usually before puberty. Untreated, rhinoconjunctivitis can lead to several other diseases, including sinusitis, otitis media, and asthma.

II. **Differential diagnosis.** It should be noted that allergic rhinitis is just one component of the differential.
   A. **Inflammatory**
      1. **Allergic.** Rhinitis due to the presence of specific IgE against seasonal or perennial allergens, or both
      2. **Infectious.** Often associated with viral upper-respiratory infections
      3. **Nonallergic rhinitis with eosinophilia syndrome.** A not-well-characterized syndrome consisting of nasal eosinophilia in a patient with rhinitis and no evidence of allergic sensitization
      4. **Atrophic.** More common in elderly patients; occurs as a result of thinning of the nasal mucosa
   B. **Noninflammatory**
      1. **Vasomotor/gustatory.** This rhinitis tends to occur within minutes of exposure to cold or foods, or both (or even with the thought of eating).
      2. **Rhinitis medicamentosa.** This is a result of overuse of an intranasal decongestant (see sec. **IV.E.2**).
      3. **Hormonal etiology.** Pregnant patients and those with thyroid disease may have an associated nonallergic rhinitis. This rhinitis resolves with appropriate treatment of the thyroid disease or with the conclusion of the pregnancy.
   C. **Structural**
      1. **Foreign body.** Usually a unilateral rhinitis.
      2. **Tumor/granuloma/hypertrophic sinuses.** Often unilateral rhinitis (except with hypertrophic sinuses).
      3. **Cerebrospinal fluid leak.** This can be diagnosed because it is a unilateral rhinorrhea that contains glucose (nasal discharges have no glucose, but cerebrospinal fluid does).
      4. **Ciliary dysfunction.** Diagnosed by an abnormally increased sugar transit time ("saccharin test") from the anterior nares to the pharynx or by abnormal ciliary anatomy identified by electron microscopy of nasal mucosa biopsies.
III. **Diagnosis**
   A. **History.** Most important component for making the diagnosis:
      1. Determine the patients' **symptoms**. Are they having nasal discharge, nasal pruritus, sneezing, headaches, and/or bilateral or unilateral nares involvement? It is important to determine if other organ systems are involved (such as the lungs or eyes).
      2. Determine the **seasonality** of the patient's symptoms. Allergic sensitivity to tree, grass, and weed pollens tends to occur in the spring, summer, and fall, respectively, whereas allergies to dust mites, molds, and pets generally do not have a seasonal distribution.
      3. It is important to obtain a history of **aggravating and alleviating factors** of which the patient is aware. Often, patients know that their symptoms are worse when they visit a friend with a cat or, perhaps, when they dust or go outside. They might note that they are better in less humid environs, for example.
   B. **Physical examination** (see Allergy, sec. **II.C**).
   C. **Testing.** To identify the allergens to which a patient is sensitive, either **skin testing** (epicutaneous and intradermal) or **RAST testing** can be performed. However, it is important that any positive results be clinically correlated with the patient's symptoms.
IV. **Treatment**
   A. **Environmental control measures** are the most important therapeutic intervention that can be made. If patients are sensitive to dust mites, (ideally) they should remove all carpet in the home, use dust mite–proof encasings on their pillows and mattress, use synthetic pillows and comforters, wash all bedding in water with a temperature of 130°F or greater weekly, and keep home humidity less than 45%. Pet-sensitive patients should keep

their pets out of the house, if possible, or, if not, the animals should be excluded from the bedroom at all times. Cats and dogs that have access to the indoors should be washed on a regular basis.

B. Once environmental control measures have been undertaken, the next intervention is the use of a **nonsedating antihistamine** to block the symptoms associated with histamine release. The U.S. Food and Drug Administration considers loratadine and fexofenadine (both oral preparations) as the only nonsedating antihistamines, because their incidence of net sedation is less than 2%. Second-generation antihistamines with very low sedation are cetirizine (oral preparation; net sedation approximately 7%) and azelastine (nasal spray preparation only; net sedation approximately 6%). (Sedation information from 2001 *Physicians' Desk Reference*. See Table 12-1 for further details.)

C. To treat the underlying inflammation, intranasal anti-inflammatory medications can be used. **Intranasal nonsteroidal anti-inflammatory medications**, such as cromolyn sodium, are the safest agents to use and are now available over the counter. Unfortunately, for maximum effectiveness cromolyn sodium (2 squirts/nostril) needs to be used four times/day.

D. The most effective anti-inflammatory medications for rhinitis (not just allergic, but any inflammatory etiology) are **intranasal corticosteroids** (see Table 12-1 for doses). The same corticosteroids that are found in asthma inhalers are also available for intranasal inhalation. Improvement may occur within 24–48 hours of starting the medication but often takes up to a week before a full therapeutic effect is reached. The doses given are much lower than those used in asthma, and, therefore, risks of systemic side effects from intranasal steroids are much lower. The major side effect of these medications is epistaxis. If this occurs, the patient should stop using the nasal spray for several days until the bleeding stops (they can use intranasal saline during this period), and then they can restart the steroid spray. See Table 12-1 for further details.

E. Decongestants can also be used in rhinitis. Two forms exist.

    1. Oral decongestants (such as pseudoephedrine) are useful in treating nonallergic rhinitis, especially in patients whose major symptom is nasal congestion.

    2. Nasal decongestants (α-adrenergic medications), although available over the counter, should be avoided if possible. These medications provide immediate relief of nasal congestion; however, tachyphylaxis develops quickly. Because the withdrawal of the drug leads to a rebound hyperemia with worsening nasal congestion, patients' nostrils are often addicted to these medications by the time they see a physician (a condition known as **rhinitis medicamentosa**). If patients must use an intranasal decongestant, they should use it for **no more than 3 days at a time**. Addicted patients often require a short course of systemic corticosteroid therapy to get them off the decongestant. Once the systemic corticosteroids have been started, patients should stop using their nasal decongestant and start an intranasal corticosteroid regimen.

F. Immunotherapy is quite helpful in allergic rhinitis and can be thought of as a corticosteroid-sparing anti-inflammatory agent. See the therapeutic modality section (Allergy, sec. **III.D**) for details.

G. Intranasal anticholinergics are useful in patients with noninflammatory rhinitis. For example, an intranasal anticholinergic (ipratropium bromide 0.03%, 1–2 sprays/nostril) can be used 10–15 minutes before each meal to help alleviate gustatory rhinorrhea.

H. Antibiotics are not usually indicated in rhinitis unless there is reason to believe that the patient may have an underlying sinusitis. In these cases, an antibiotic that has good sinus penetration and is active against *Streptococcus pneumoniae*, *Haemophilus influenzae*, and *Moraxella catarrhalis* is indicated (mainly beta-lactam antibiotics—with or without a beta-lactamase

inhibitor—or a sulfa drug, quinolone, or macrolide antibiotic in beta-lactam–sensitive individuals).
   I. **Surgery** is reserved for those patients who have chronic sinusitis and in whom no other therapy is able to control their rhinitis. In many cases, the surgery provides only temporary relief and is not curative.

Asthma

The National Asthma Education and Prevention Program of the National Heart, Lung, and Blood Institutes of Health (NHLBI) released the Expert Panel Report 1, entitled *Guidelines for the Diagnosis and Management of Asthma*, in 1991. An updated report was released in 1997. A similar set of clinical practice guidelines, the Global Initiative for Asthma, was released in 1998. These guidelines resulted from a report based on the NHLBI/World Health Organization workshop on a global strategy for asthma management and prevention. These evidence-based guidelines for asthma prevention and management have defined a standard of care for patients with asthma. This chapter follows those guidelines. By definition, asthma is an inflammatory illness, and as such its prevention and treatment require that therapeutic interventions prioritize this established premise.

I. Diagnosis
   A. **Clinical presentation.** Asthma may have its onset in infancy through adulthood. Typically, the patient presents with a history of wheezing, cough, breathlessness, and chest tightness with breathing. These symptoms may be either intermittent or persistent, with severity that may be mild, moderate, or severe.
   B. **History.** The varied possible etiologies, "triggers" of either intermittent episodes or persistent asthma, and other factors that are responsible for continued symptoms of asthma require a careful and inquiring historic review as well as a complete general medical history. This historic review should include information relative to duration and circumstances of the onset of illness, family history, the home, work/school environment, the patient's perception of causative and contributory factors, and psychosocial issues. It is important to elicit and understand patients' perceptions and concerns regarding asthma.
   C. **Physical examination.** The physical examination of the upper airways highlights a search for evidence of sinusitis, nasal allergy, and nasal polyps. The chest examination may be normal, even during persistent asthma; however, often a forced expiratory maneuver uncovers wheezing. The most typical findings during severe asthma relate to the use of extrathoracic muscles, wheezing, or a prolonged expiratory phase of breathing.
   D. **Differential diagnosis.** Causes of airway obstruction other than asthma must be considered, particularly in patients in whom the history, physical examination, and pulmonary function studies do not confirm the diagnosis of asthma (Table 12-6).
   E. **Pulmonary function tests.** Objective measurement of pulmonary function is essential in the diagnosis and management of asthma. Although patients with asthma at times have normal pulmonary function, persistent asthma usually has a reduction in forced expiratory volume in 1 second (FEV_1). An inhaled bronchodilator may allow confirmation of the reversibility of the reduced FEV_1 by 12% or greater, a diagnostic characteristic of asthma. However, depending on its severity, persistent asthma may not be reversible until the medications have taken effect. The use of home monitoring with a peak expiratory flow rate (PEFR) meter can substantiate the diagnosis of asthma by demonstrating an intraday (a.m. to p.m.) variability in PEFR of 20% or greater. On occasion, when the diagno-

Table 12-6. Differential diagnosis of airway obstruction, excluding asthma

---

Localized obstruction
  Endobronchial tumor
  Endobronchial foreign body
  External bronchial compression
  Laryngeal obstruction
  Congenital anomaly
Generalized obstruction
  Chronic obstructive lung disease
  Cystic fibrosis
  Bronchiectasis
  CHF
  Churg-Strauss syndrome (angiitis and allergic granulomatosis)
  Carcinoid
  α_1-Antitrypsin deficiency
  Immotile cilia syndrome
  Pulmonary embolus

From PE Korenblat, HJ Wedner. *Allergy: Theory and Practice* (2nd ed). Philadelphia: WB Saunders, 1992, with permission.

sis is uncertain and the FEV_1 is normal or near normal and significant reversibility with a bronchodilator cannot be demonstrated, a bronchial inhalation challenge (methacholine challenge) can be useful in supporting or refuting the diagnosis of asthma.

F. Frequently, patients with varying degrees of asthma severity are seen as outpatients. Severity assessment can be based on FEV_1 or PEFR (<80% of personal best or predicted), symptoms of cough, breathlessness, wheeze, use of accessory muscles, and nighttime awakening. In severe asthma, oxygen saturation and blood gases are required.

II. Evaluation

A. Once one is secure in the diagnosis of asthma, it is important to use the history to help identify the causative and contributory factors. Asthma may result from an IgE or non-IgE–mediated process, or both (e.g., >80% of asthmatic children have an allergic component). Exposure to indoor allergens (e.g., animals, cockroaches, dust mites, mold spores) or outdoor allergens (e.g., pollen, mold spores), or both, is responsible for the majority of IgE-mediated asthma. The non-IgE etiologies and factors that are responsible for continued asthma encompass infection, medications (e.g., aspirin, nonsteroidal anti-inflammatory agents), or miscellaneous causes such as exercise-induced asthma, occupational exposures, pollution, irritant sensitivity, or tobacco use or exposure. The evaluation often requires allergy skin testing or, under certain circumstances, in vitro allergy testing (e.g., dermatologic difficulty that precludes applying tests to the skin or concerns of provoking a reaction because of an extreme sensitivity to the test antigen).

B. All too often, patients do not follow or fully understand instructions regarding medication use. It is important to review medication compliance and proper device utilization on **each** visit, particularly when asthma is not controlled.

C. During a new patient evaluation or during the evaluation of newly acquired asthma, under most circumstances, a recent chest x-ray should be obtained.

Table 12-7. Classify severity[a]: clinical features before treatment

	Symptoms	Nighttime symptoms	PEF
Step 4: Severe persistent	Continuous Limited physical activity	Frequent	≤60% predicted Variability >30%
Step 3: Moderate persistent	Daily Use β_2 agonist daily Attacks affect activity	>1 time/wk	60–80% predicted Variability >30%
Step 2: Mild persistent	≥1 time/wk but <1 time/day	>2 times/mo	≥80% predicted Variability 20–30%
Step 1: Intermittent	<1 time/wk Asymptomatic and normal PEF between attacks	≤2 times/mo	≥80% predicted Variability <20%

PEF, peak expiratory flow.
[a]The presence of one of the features of severity is sufficient to place a patient in that category.
Adapted from the National Asthma Education Prevention Program Expert Panel Report 2. *Guidelines for the Diagnosis and Management of Asthma*, National Institutes of Health, April 1997, and *Global Initiative for Asthma*, based on the Global Strategy for Asthma Management Prevention NHLBI/WHO Workshop Report, 1998.

The concurrent occurrence of chronic sinusitis with persistent and worsening asthma often requires radiographic evaluation. When evaluating for inflammatory sinus disease, particularly when surgical intervention is not anticipated to be required, a limited sinus CT is adequate and superior to sinus x-rays.

    D. Gastroesophageal reflux can precipitate cough and asthma. A history of symptoms that is compatible with gastroesophageal reflux is usually, but not invariably, present. Although pH monitoring and radiographic evaluation are most diagnostic, a clinical trial with a proton pump inhibitor (e.g., omeprazole, 20–40 mg qd, or lansoprazole, 15–30 mg qd) is often adequate to evaluate the role of gastroesophageal reflux in a particular patient.

III. Severity classification

    A. The **severity and chronicity of symptoms** guide the therapy of asthma (Table 12-7). The NHLBI guidelines sort asthma into the categories of intermittent and mild, moderate, and severe persistent asthma. The major goal of therapy is prevention of symptoms and of adverse long-term consequences of persistent asthma. Specifically, the guidelines state that the aim of treatment is to have minimal (ideally no) chronic symptoms (including nocturnal symptoms), minimal (infrequent) episodes with no emergency visits, minimal need for as-needed β_2 agonists, no limitations on activities—including exercise, a near-normal PEFR with variability of less than 20%, and minimal (or no) adverse effects from medicine. Periodic patient visits are necessary to assess and monitor the attainment of these goals and patient satisfaction with their asthma care and plan.

    B. Objective measurement of lung function. The care of the patient with asthma requires an interpretive understanding and availability of pulmonary function testing. Interventions based solely on history and physical examination, without objective measurement of lung function, often are misguided. Home peak flow monitoring accompanied by a written action plan allows informed physician-directed patient self-assessment of asthma.

IV. Therapy

A. The stepwise approach to managing asthma involves long-term control medications, quick-relief medications, and education (Table 12-8). A patient who is informed about the many aspects of asthma and provided with a simplified management program will have enhanced compliance. While following the stepwise approach to asthma management (Table 12-8), it is important to step therapy up during worsened asthma and to also step therapy down with improvement of symptoms and stability of lung function, as demonstrated by objective measures of lung function.

B. Relievers. Quick relievers (inhaled β_2 agonists) not only can be used for relief of symptoms, but their documented requirement (peak flow measurements or other pulmonary function studies) signals the possibility that the patient's long-term controllers may need to be altered.

C. Controllers. Persistent asthma requires the inclusion of a long-term controller medication. Long-acting bronchodilators may be required for control of asthma symptoms but should not be used as monotherapy in persistent asthma. The place of inhaled cromolyn sodium, nedocromil sodium, and inhaled and oral corticosteroids place in step therapy is well defined (Table 12-8). The leukotriene modifiers' (montelukast, zafirlukast, and zileuton) role in asthma management is less well defined in the NHLBI guidelines. The leukotriene modifiers have found consensus recommendation, based on scientific clinical trials, that they are appropriate medications for "add on" therapy (as have long-acting bronchodilators and theophylline). They can be used for incompletely controlled asthma in patients who use inhaled corticosteroids or in those who require high-dose inhaled corticosteroids, to lower the dose of inhaled corticosteroids while still maintaining asthma control. They have also been shown to diminish significantly the respiratory symptoms that occur from the ingestion of aspirin in sensitive patients and to lessen lower-airway responses to inhaled allergen, cold air, and exercise. Although controversial, there are limited data to support their use as monotherapy in mild persistent asthma. If a leukotriene antagonist fails to provide appropriate relief as monotherapy, an inhaled corticosteroid should be started. The combination of an inhaled long-acting bronchodilator and an inhaled corticosteroid, delivered simultaneously by the same device, provides a treatment option for all stages of persistent asthma.

D. Education. Patients require instruction in the proper technique of inhaler use and should be asked to demonstrate the technique on each subsequent office visit. They should also know how to avoid their asthma triggers and to understand the purpose of each of the medications prescribed for them.

E. Initial outpatient treatment of asthma exacerbation (Fig. 12-1). Inhaled β agonist, often by nebulization, should be administered at one dose every 20 minutes for 1 hour. Oxygen should be administered to achieve oxygen saturation of greater than 90%. Patients who require oral or inhaled corticosteroids for asthma control, who have had recent systemic corticosteroids, or who are severely ill at the time of presentation should be administered systemic corticosteroids.

F. Who should be hospitalized? Patients with a history of intubation for asthma must be considered candidates for hospital admission, and those who do not satisfactorily respond to initial therapy should be admitted to the hospital. The post–initial treatment presence of a pulsus paradox of greater than 12 mm Hg, PEFR or FEV_1 less than 50% predicted, oxygen saturation less than 90%, and carbon dioxide pressure greater than 42 mm Hg are indicators of an unsatisfactory response to therapy and thus the need for hospital admission.

G. Acute care discharge instructions. Patients should be provided with a PEFR meter and given written instructions in self-management based on

Table 12-6. Treatment of asthma in adults and children older than 5 years old

	Long-term preventive	Quick relief
Step 4: Severe persistent	Daily medications **Inhaled corticosteroid**, 800–2000 µg or more, and Long-acting bronchodilator: either **long-acting inhaled** β_2 **agonist** and/or sustained-release theophylline, or leukotriene modifier; may enhance control and allow control with lower doses of inhaled corticosteroids Corticosteroid tablets or syrup long term	Short-acting bronchodilator: **inhaled** β_2 **agonist** as needed for symptoms
Step 3: Moderate persistent	Daily medications **Inhaled corticosteroid**, ≥500 µg and, if needed, Long-acting bronchodilator: either **long-acting inhaled** β_2 **agonist**, sustained-release theophylline, or long-acting β_2 agonist tablets or syrup Consider adding antileukotriene, especially for aspirin-sensitive patients, and for preventing exercise-induced bronchospasm The addition of any one of these medications may provide more effective symptom control when added to low–medium dose steroid compared to increasing the steroid dose	Short-acting bronchodilator: **inhaled** β_2 **agonist** as needed for symptoms, not to exceed 3–4 times in 1 day
Step 2: Mild persistent	Daily medication Either **inhaled corticosteroid**, 200–500 µg, or cromoglycate or nedocromil or sustained-release theophylline; antileukotrienes can be considered, but their position in therapy at this step has not been fully established	Short-acting bronchodilator: **inhaled** β_2 **agonist** as needed for symptoms, not to exceed 3–4 times in 1 day
Step 1: Intermittent	None needed	Short-acting bronchodilator: **inhaled** β_2 **agonist** as needed for symptoms, but no more than 2 times/wk, exclusive of use for exercise-induced asthma; use of short-acting inhaled β_2 agonist more than 2 times/wk may indicate the need to initiate long-term controlled therapy

Adapted from the National Asthma Education Prevention Program Expert Panel Report 2. *Guidelines for the Diagnosis of Management of Asthma*, the National Institutes of Health, April 1997, and *Global Initiative for Asthma*, based on the Global Strategy for Asthma Management Prevention NHLBI/WHO Workshop Report, 1998.

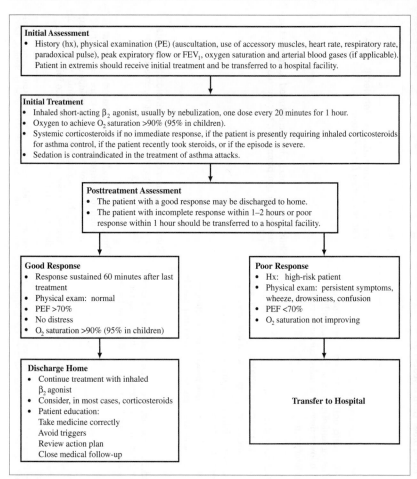

Fig. 12-1. Office management of asthma exacerbation. PEF, peak expiratory flow. (Adapted from *Global Initiatives for Asthma*, based on the Global Strategy for Asthma Management Prevention NHLBI/WHO Workshop Report, 1998.)

PEFR and symptoms. They should be cautioned to avoid their asthma triggers and to seek help with worsening symptoms or declining PEFR and be given an appointment for an outpatient follow-up visit within 7–10 days of discharge.

H. Specialty consultation. Consultation with an asthma specialist should be considered under a wide variety of circumstances: when the diagnosis is in doubt, when clinical conditions complicate asthma (e.g., sinusitis), when the patient does not respond optimally to therapy, in the presence of moderate or severe persistent asthma, when allergy evaluation is needed, and after either two emergency department visits or one hospital admission for asthma.

Resources

I. Physician
  A. National Institutes of Health
  1. National Institute of Allergy and Infectious Diseases
  NIAID Office of Communications and Public Liaison
  Building 31, Room 7A-50
  31 Center Dr. MSC 2520
  Bethesda, MD 20892-2520
  http://www.niaid.nih.gov
  2. National Heart, Lung, and Blood Institute
  NHLBI Information Center
  PO Box 30105
  Bethesda, MD 20824-0105
  301-592-8573; fax 301-592-8563
  http://www.nhlbi.nih.gov
  B. American Academy of Allergy, Asthma, and Immunology
  611 East Wells St.
  Milwaukee, WI 53202
  414-272-6071; fax 414-272-6070
  http://www.aaaai.org
  C. American College of Allergy, Asthma, and Immunology
  85 West Algonquin Rd., Suite 550
  Arlington Heights, IL 60005
  847-427-1200; fax 847-427-1294
  http://www.acaai.org

II. Patient
  A. Food Allergy Network
  10400 Eaton Pl., Suite 107
  Fairfax, VA 22030
  800-929-4040; fax 703-691-2713
  http://www.foodallergy.org
  B. Asthma and Allergy Foundation of America
  1125 15th St. NW, Suite 502
  Washington, DC 20005
  202-466-7643; fax 202-466-8940
  http://www.aafa.org
  C. American Lung Association
  1740 Broadway
  New York, NY 10019
  800-LUNG-USA
  http://www.lungusa.org
  D. Allergy and Asthma Network—Mothers of Asthmatics
  2751 Prosperity Ave., Suite 150
  Fairfax, VA 22031
  800-878-4403; fax 703-573-7794
  http://www.aanma.org

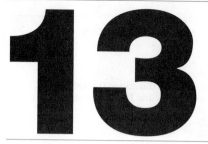

Gastrointestinal I: Common Complaints and Symptoms

Jayaprakash
Sreenarasimhaiah and
Joshua R. Korzenik

Approach to the Patient with Abdominal Pain

I. **Definition.** The varied presentation of **abdominal pain** in the ambulatory setting can often provide ample information to guide the identification of a specific etiology. Pain is a subjective sensation of discomfort, filtered through personality and psychological issues. Still, it usually has distinct characteristics that allow a careful history to reveal a cause. In assessing a patient with abdominal pain, categorization of pain is useful in terms of organ dysfunction (i.e., hepatobiliary, gastric, intestinal) as well as a mechanism (i.e., inflammation, obstruction, ischemia, neurogenic) to direct proper evaluation and therapy.

II. **History**

A. **Onset.** The initial evaluation should elicit the chronology of events and determine the duration of symptoms, whether acute or chronic (Table 13-1). An etiology can more often be identified for those with acute pain. In an outpatient assessment, the first consideration for a patient in acute pain is whether he or she can be adequately evaluated in that setting or whether an emergency room and possible hospitalization are more appropriate. The high frequency of functional bowel disease (irritable bowel syndrome) generates many office visits for chronic abdominal pain, but such a diagnosis should not be rapidly assumed without a thorough evaluation.

B. **Localization.** Some causes of abdominal pain can be well localized, particularly if they result from inflammation in the parietal peritoneum (Fig. 13-1).

1. **Esophageal disorders** can produce substernal pressure or pain. This can result in pain that radiates to the neck, jaw, arm, and back and may mimic cardiac angina.

2. Pain from the **GI tract** is more difficult to localize. The stomach, duodenum, and pancreas produce discomfort in the epigastrium; small-bowel obstruction or inflammation localizes to the periumbilical area; and colonic pain is less well localized to the lower abdomen.

3. **Stretching of the liver capsule or distention of the gallbladder** can generate right upper quadrant pain. Abdominal disease can produce referred pain, as shoulder pain can be caused by inflammation under the diaphragm.

4. **Non-GI abdominal pain.** Conversely, not all abdominal pain is due to GI disease. Radiation from the flanks or suprapubic pain can be clues to urinary tract disease. When upper abdominal pain is present, one must also consider pleural, pulmonary, or pericardial sources. In women, a gynecologic etiology may be found in lower abdominal symptoms (Table 13-2).

C. **Character of pain.** A nonspecific subjective description of the character of abdominal discomfort may not be helpful. Qualities such as sharpness, tearing, cutting, gnawing, burning, dullness, or boring can be found in various

Table 13-1. Causes of chronic abdominal pain

Pancreaticobiliary disease
  Cholelithiasis
  Choledocholithiasis
  Sphincter of Oddi dysfunction
  Chronic pancreatitis (particularly with chronic alcohol use)
Vascular disease
  Intestinal ischemia (postprandial)
Inflammatory disease
  Crohn's disease
  Ulcerative colitis
  Familial Mediterranean fever
Neurologic disease
  Abdominal migraines
  Abdominal epilepsy
  Nerve root radiculopathy (diabetes, spinal cord compression fractures)
Intermittent obstructive disease
  Internal or abdominal wall hernia
  Crohn's disease
  Adhesions
  Intussusception
Gynecologic disease
  Endometriosis
  Mittelschmerz (related to menstrual cycles)
Neoplastic
  Underlying neoplasm
Metabolic
  Heavy metal (lead) poisoning
  Acute intermittent porphyria (exacerbated by recent barbiturate use)
Functional bowel disease
  Irritable bowel disease

---

processes. **Colic** refers to the episodic buildup of pain that may be characterized by cramps.

  D. Relation to eating. Cholecystitis, pancreatitis, or gastric ulcers can produce postprandial pain. Peptic ulcers of the duodenum may improve with food ingestion. Intestinal angina may be associated with a fear of eating due to pain and can occur in older persons with mesenteric ischemia.

  E. Bowel habits. Patients should be questioned about any changes in bowel movements (new and long-standing) and changes in stool caliber and volume. Constipation can result in diffuse abdominal discomfort. Diarrhea can be accompanied by cramping. Patients with alternating complaints of diarrhea and constipation may have irritable bowel disease.

  F. Nausea and emesis. Nausea is a nonspecific symptom that signals an underlying etiology. Biliary processes, peptic ulcers at the gastric outlet, or bowel obstruction should be considered. Infectious sources with accompa-

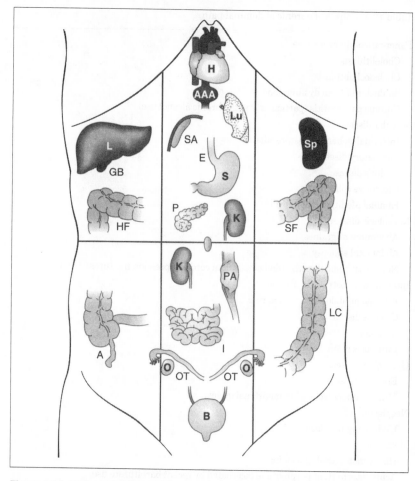

Figure 13-1. Differential diagnosis by abdominal quadrant (see Table 13-2 for localization of causes). Right upper quadrant: GB, gallbladder; HF, hepatic flexure (obstruction); L, liver. Right lower quadrant: A, appendix. Left upper quadrant: SF, splenic flexure; Sp, spleen. Left lower quadrant: LC, left colon. Epigastrium: AAA, abdominal aortic aneurysm; E, esophagus; H, heart; K, kidney; Lu, lung; P, pancreas; S, stomach and duodenum; SA, subphrenic abscess. Hypogastrium: B, bladder (cystitis, distended bladder); I, intestine; K, kidney; O, ovary; OT, ovarian tube; PA, psoas abscess.

nied diarrhea are sometimes discovered. However, this is a common physiologic response to a variety of systemic disorders and should not restrict the evaluation only to GI disease.

G. Hiccups can result from distention of the esophagus or stomach or irritation of the diaphragm.

H. Melena and hematochezia. Such history can give concern for ulcers, infections, or ischemia leading to intestinal bleeding. Melena (dark, tarry stools) usually signals an upper GI source, although it can occur during right-sided colonic bleeding. Hematochezia (bright red blood from the rectum) usually reflects a colonic source but sometimes presents during massive upper bleeding.

Table 13-2. Common causes of acute abdominal pain with localization

Right upper quadrant
Acute cholecystitis, cholangitis, choledocholithiasis
Biliary colic
Acute hepatic inflammation/distention, abscess

Right lower quadrant
Appendicitis
Infective terminal ileitis
Crohn's disease
Tubo-ovarian disorders
Ectopic pregnancy
Ruptured ovarian cyst
Salpingitis
Renal disorders
Right ureteric calculus
Pyelonephritis
Pyogenic sacroiliitis

Left upper quadrant
Splenic infarct/rupture/abscess
Splenic flexure ischemia

Left lower quadrant
Acute diverticulitis
Infectious or inflammatory colitis
Pyogenic sacroiliitis
Tubo-ovarian disorders

Central abdominal pain
Gastroenteritis, gastritis
Peptic ulcer disease/gastroesophageal reflux disease
Small intestinal colic
Acute pancreatitis
Myocardial infarction, pericarditis
Aortic dissection
Abdominal aortic aneurysm
Pneumonia

Diffuse abdominal pain
Acute infectious peritonitis
Appendicitis
Diabetic ketoacidosis
Diverticulitis
Inflammatory bowel disease and toxic megacolon
Perforated ulcer (gastric or duodenal)
Sickle cell crisis   (continued)

Table 13-2. (continued)

Spontaneous peritonitis in cirrhosis
Acute noninfectious peritonitis
Familial Mediterranean fever
Hemorrhagic pancreatitis
Postoperative states

Adapted from T Yamada, DH Alpers, L Laine, et al. (eds), *Textbook of Gastroenterology* (3rd ed). New York: Lippincott Williams & Wilkins, 1999:804.

- **I. Position.** Pain that is worse while supine can occur in pancreatic disease. Certain movements may result in abdominal pain due to musculoskeletal disorders or nerve root compression.
- **J. Urinary symptoms.** Dysuria, difficulty in passing urine, or hematuria may be present. Cystitis, pyelonephritis, obstructive uropathy, and nephrolithiasis can all result in significant abdominal discomfort.
- **K. Menstrual history.** Menstrual cycles, irregularity, or abnormalities in bleeding may generate abdominal pain or worsening of underlying GI disorders. Symptoms of inflammatory bowel disease or irritable bowel syndrome can clearly worsen during and around the time of menses. Pain that follows a close pattern of menstrual cycles may be due to underlying endometriosis (see Chap. 24).
- **L. Depression and anxiety.** When organic causes are eliminated, psychiatric causes should be considered. Irritable bowel syndrome may be present in some.
- **M. Red flags.** Pain that awakens the patient from sleep, fever, prolonged severe pain of more than several hours' duration, persistent emesis, changes in patterns or localization, and significant alterations in appetite or mental status should prompt a search for serious organic illness.
- **III. Physical examination**
  - **A. Inspection.** Assessment for signs of cachexia, pallor, position, and severity of distress provides clues for a systemic illness. Inspection of the abdomen may suggest the presence of ascites, masses, prior surgical procedures, or other abnormalities. Numerous cutaneous findings, known as **stigmata of liver disease** (described in Approach to Abnormal Liver Chemistries, sec. **II**), may reveal unrecognized underlying cirrhosis.
  - **B. Percussion.** Tympany can indicate gas-filled or dilated loops of bowel. Dullness can indicate a mass or, particularly in the flanks, is present in ascites. Detection of hepatomegaly or splenomegaly should be done on examination. Dullness above the left costal margin may indicate an enlarged spleen. Normal liver spans are usually 6–12 cm in the right midclavicular line and 4–8 cm in the midsternal line.
  - **C. Auscultation.** The quality and localization of bowel sounds are very nonspecific and usually unhelpful, but the presence or absence of sounds is important. High-pitched sounds may be present in bowel obstruction. Absent sounds may be a feature of ileus or a catastrophic abdominal event.
  - **D. Palpation.** Tenderness in particular locations can indicate visceral sources. For example, Murphy's sign is palpable tenderness in the right upper quadrant, which induces a midinspiratory catch in breathing. It is a sign of cholecystitis. The finding of tenderness during palpation that is absent to compression by the stethoscope during auscultation may indicate less severity of discomfort than the patient suggests or even a lack of real organic pain. Abdominal masses can also be detected on palpation. Mesenteric ischemia classically presents with pain that is out of proportion to findings on physical examination.
  - **E. Worrisome signs for surgical abdomen** include guarding and peritoneal signs (see Dyspepsia, sec. **III**), fever, Murphy's sign, iliopsoas sign, and absent or high-pitched bowel sounds.

IV. **Diagnostic testing**
A careful history and physical examination are essential since **laboratory testing rarely makes a diagnosis.**
   A. **Laboratory testing**
      1. **Leukocytosis** suggests an acute inflammatory response and is present in acute cholecystitis, intra-abdominal abscess, perforated viscus, intestinal infarction, pancreatitis, pelvic inflammatory disease, urinary tract infections, and pyelonephritis.
      2. **Anemia** must be correlated to history.
      3. **Hepatobiliary** diseases can be evaluated by bilirubin, amylase, lipase, alkaline phosphatase, and liver transaminases. These are described more extensively in Approach to Abnormal Liver Chemistries, sec. **III.**
      4. **Urinalysis** can be used to assess hydration, proteinuria, infection, and renal diseases.
   B. **Plain x-ray** (upright and lateral decubitus views) is essential if perforation or obstruction is suspected. In contrast to this typical obstructive series radiograph, a single view of the abdomen can overlook free air under the diaphragm, an important finding in an acute surgical abdomen.
   C. **Ultrasound** may show organomegaly or biliary duct disease.
   D. **CT scanning** is useful in some cases of mesenteric ischemia, but this diagnosis may require further evaluation with angiography.
V. **Management** for specific etiologies is discussed later. Nonspecific abdominal pain is usually self-limited. This requires reassurance and regular follow-up evaluations, particularly in irritable bowel syndrome. Further workup is usually not indicated. A patient in severe pain can be provided with some analgesics to alleviate distress while the etiology is being pursued, but close follow-up is essential.

Nausea and Vomiting

I. **Definitions.** Nausea and vomiting are nonspecific responses to a myriad of illnesses. An effortless return of gastric or esophageal contents without muscular or spasmodic contractions is known as **regurgitation**; a forceful contractile process is known as **emesis.**
II. **History**
   A. **Onset and duration.** The onset of nausea and emesis may coincide with other symptoms. Diarrhea that accompanies this can indicate an infectious gastroenteritis, although its presence is not necessary. Triggers that initiate symptoms can include smells, tastes, emotional or physical stress, headaches, or pain of any source.
   B. **Relationship to eating.** Vomiting that occurs soon after meals can be a result of gastric outlet obstruction. If delayed after meals, one should consider gastroparesis (particularly in diabetics) or proximal intestinal obstruction. Undigested food in emesis occurs in Zenker's diverticulum (pharyngoesophageal diverticulum) and achalasia (see Chap. 14). Emesis that consists of partially digested food or food consumed several hours earlier is more common in gastric outlet obstruction and gastroparesis.
   C. **Abdominal pain.** Generalized abdominal pain with or without complaints of abdominal distention should be evaluated for GI obstruction until proven otherwise. Nausea and vomiting accompanied by an initial periumbilical pain can be due to appendicitis. The pain can be temporarily relieved but recurs in the right lower quadrant. Right upper quadrant pain with nausea or even emesis can be due to biliary colic. Acute viral hepatitis A may have a similar presentation.
   D. **Medications.** Numerous medications report nausea and vomiting as an adverse effect. Predictably, nausea occurs with most chemotherapeutic

agents. Nausea is commonly seen with the use of nonsteroidal anti-inflammatory agents and many oral antibiotics, such as erythromycin, metronidazole, sulfa drugs, and tetracycline. Cardiovascular medicines that are commonly associated with nausea include digoxin (particularly when supratherapeutic), beta-blockers, and calcium channel antagonists. Drugs that act on the central nervous system include narcotic analgesics and therapies for Parkinson's disease.

E. **Labyrinthine disorders.** Symptoms of vestibular disturbances, such as vertigo, ear pain, visual disturbance, unsteady gait, or motion sickness, can initiate a mild or moderate sense of nausea.

F. **Neuropsychiatric**
1. **Central causes.** Patients or their family members sometimes describe disorientation, lethargy and headaches, or alterations in vision. All of these should make the clinician suspicious for an intracranial process, such as increased pressure, infection, or mass effect, resulting in a centrally mediated emesis.
2. **Headaches.** Nausea and emesis can frequently be either the prodrome or the initial manifestation of **migraine** headaches.
3. **Idiopathic.** Some patients give a history of a defined predictable symptom complex that includes severe nausea and emesis persisting for days followed by periods of normality for weeks to months. This entity is well known as **cyclical vomiting.** Nausea and emesis may be a response to emotional distress.

G. **Other causes.** Symptoms of CHF, particularly with passive hepatic congestion, can result in nausea. Nausea can be a systemic response to a focal infection elsewhere, such as appendicitis or pyelonephritis. Metabolic derangement such as diabetic ketoacidosis also commonly presents in this manner. Hyperemesis gravidarum is characterized by emesis during the first trimester of pregnancy [*Gastroenterology* 2001;120(1):263–286].

III. **Physical examination**
A. **Orthostatic hypotension** may be present in persistent emesis due to dehydration. Careful evaluation of heart rate and BP with positional changes must be monitored. Decreased skin turgor or dry mucous membranes are signs of significant fluid losses.
B. **Feculent odor of the breath** may be a finding in those with intestinal obstruction, gastrocolic fistula, and bacterial overgrowth. Zenker's diverticulum can result in halitosis. Oral examination might reveal poor dentition and enamel erosion in those with eating disorders such as bulimia.
C. **Auscultation of the abdomen** can be of limited value and has the primary aim of distinguishing the presence or absence of sounds. High-pitched noises may suggest a small-bowel obstruction. A succussion splash, the movement of gastric fluid within the stomach that is heard on auscultation, is sometimes noted in gastric outlet obstruction or gastroparesis.
D. **Palpation** may find areas of tenderness. Obstructive abdominal masses are sometimes noted. Murphy's sign may be useful for nausea of biliary origin.
E. **Blood** in the stool that is either occult or gross may be a clue to an ulcer located in the gastric outlet.

IV. **Diagnostic testing**
A. **Blood chemistry testing** can direct evaluation of a number of causes of nausea. Amylase and lipase (pancreatitis) and liver enzymes (hepatobiliary processes) can be helpful. Hyponatremia and uremia may contribute to these symptoms. Additionally, a pregnancy test should be obtained in women of childbearing age.
B. **Radiologic studies.** An obstructive series consisting of three views (upright, supine, and lateral decubitus) is important in searching for intestinal obstruction. Air fluid levels and a cutoff of bowel gas pattern may be seen. Free air that is seen particularly under the diaphragm is a sign of intestinal perforation. Upper GI series with or without a small-bowel follow-through can detect

mechanical sources of nausea and emesis. Pancreatitis may require confirmation by CT scan. On occasion, a radionuclide gastric emptying scan may be useful to diagnose motility defects. If an intracranial process is considered the culprit, CT scan or MRI examination of the brain may be pertinent.

   C. **Gastroenterologic studies.** After an initial search for and correction of common causes such as metabolic abnormalities or medications, one can consider more invasive studies for persistent symptoms. Structural anatomic lesions can be effectively diagnosed by esophagogastroduodenoscopy (EGD). Motility testing can demonstrate nausea or regurgitation due to esophageal functional disorders such as achalasia.

   D. **Psychiatric assessment** may become necessary for those in whom no organic causes have been described. Cyclical vomiting may require such evaluation.

V. **Management**

   A. Treating the **underlying process** is fundamental, but antiemetic agents may temporarily alleviate symptoms. Antiemetic agents such as **prochlorperazine** can be given starting at 5–10 mg PO tid/qid or 25-mg suppositories q12h. Prokinetic medication such as **metoclopramide** is usually started at 10 mg PO/IM/IV 1 hour before meals and at bedtime (qhs). A number of serotonin receptor inhibitors such as **ondansetron** are frequently used in emesis that results from chemotherapy. Anti–motion sickness agents such as **scopolamine** (0.5 mg/patch to be placed behind the ear once in 3 days) may benefit some. Prokinetic agents may also be useful for gastroparesis and intestinal dysmotility.

   B. **Indications for hospitalization.** Those who have clinical evidence of severe dehydration will likely benefit from intravenous rehydration. Concomitant emesis and diarrhea can result in severe fluid losses. Hypokalemia may need careful correction. Generally, very old and very young patients and those with diabetes or accompanying debilitating illness may require more than outpatient treatment.

Dysphagia and Odynophagia

I. **Definitions. Dysphagia** is a sense of difficulty with the passage of food from the pharynx to the stomach. This should be distinguished from globus, which is a subjective feeling of fullness in the throat that is not related to eating. **Odynophagia** is the presence of pain that may or may not accompany dysphagia. The **swallowing apparatus** consists of the pharynx, cricopharyngeus (upper esophageal sphincter), body of the esophagus, and lower esophageal sphincter. The upper one-third of the esophagus is composed of skeletal muscle, and the lower one-third consists of smooth muscle. An overlap of mixed muscle tissue exists in the middle.

II. **History**

   A. **Relation to food.** Some patients complain of dysphagia for particular foods only.

      1. If **solid foods** progressively become more difficult to swallow, whereas liquids pass with ease, one should consider a mechanical obstructive cause such as a malignancy or a benign stricture. In advanced obstruction, all substances may become difficult to swallow.

      2. If the onset of dysphagia involves **solids and liquids** together, esophageal motor defects such as achalasia or diffuse esophageal spasm must be considered. Those with achalasia may report regurgitation of undigested food several hours after a meal, particularly when lying down at night.

      3. **Intermittent dysphagia** for solids, usually meat or bread, can result from a mucosal abnormality of the lower esophagus known as **Schatzki's ring** [*J Clin Gastroenterol* 1998;7(4):285].

B. **Localization.** A subjective complaint of dysphagia sensed in the neck or at the sternal notch is unhelpful in localization. Such a sensation may be a referred symptom created by the obstruction of food anywhere in the swallowing apparatus.

C. **Pain**
   1. **Infections,** including monilial, herpetic, or other viral esophagitis, must be considered in patients who are debilitated or give a history of immunosuppression. The lack of orally visible *Candida* does not exclude the potential for esophageal infection. Herpetic esophagitis can be seen in immunocompetent persons as well.
   2. **Acute odynophagia** that accelerates over the course of a few days can be the result of pill-induced esophagitis or ulcers. Tetracycline, slow-release potassium tablets, alendronate, ferrous sulfate, quinidine, and nonsteroidal anti-inflammatory agents are well-known offenders.

D. **Other associated symptoms**
   1. **Weight loss** that is out of proportion to the quality and duration of dysphagia may suggest carcinoma. A history of heavy tobacco and alcohol use can be found in many patients with esophageal squamous cell carcinoma.
   2. **Tracheobronchial aspiration** may occur in those with brainstem neuromuscular diseases, achalasia, or severe gastroesophageal reflux. Tracheoesophageal fistula presents similarly.
   3. **Hoarseness** preceding dysphagia usually is of laryngeal origin. When it follows the onset of dysphagia, infiltration of the recurrent laryngeal nerve involvement by cancer or the effects of reflux should be considered.
   4. **Hiccups** can reflect a lesion in the distal esophagus, a process of diaphragmatic irritation, or gastric or esophageal distention.
   5. **Prolonged heartburn** that precedes the dysphagia is usually present in peptic strictures. These individuals may describe chronic antacid use. A spontaneous improvement of long-standing reflux symptoms can be worrisome for development of either a stricture or cancer (see Chap. 14, Esophageal Diseases, sec. I).
   6. **Chest pain** can occur in those with severe reflux, accounting for half of noncardiac chest pain (*Am J Med* 1991;90:576). It is also a manifestation of motor deficits such as diffuse esophageal spasm. The latter can be aggravated by either hot or cold liquids, cause frequent awakening at night, and has a potential to develop into achalasia. This symptom is often difficult to distinguish from cardiac disease, and a thorough history is necessary to elicit symptoms of angina as well as coronary risk factors.
   7. **Mucosal disease** may be present in those patients who provide a history of ingestion of caustic substances, previous radiation therapy, or occasionally prior tracheal intubation [*Med Clin North Am* 1999;3(1):97].

III. **Physical examination**
   Examination of the neck may reveal structural defects that result in dysphagia. Thyromegaly, spinal deformity, and neck masses may all be responsible. Skin examination is important for features of collagen vascular disease such as scleroderma or CREST (**c**alcinosis, **R**aynaud's phenomenon, **e**sophageal involvement, **s**clerodactyly, and **t**elangiectasias) syndrome, which is associated with dysphagia and impaired peristalsis (see Chap. 22). Oral lesions of pemphigus or epidermolysis bullosa may be found in some patients, causing dysphagia due to esophageal involvement.

IV. **Diagnostic testing**
   A. **Endoscopy.** When structural lesions are suspected, an endoscopy is useful as an initial test to visualize the mucosa directly. Biopsy of suspicious lesions can be performed, and therapy can be initiated.
   B. **Radiologic tests.** Barium swallow can be used in cases with high risks for sedation, patient anxiety, and anticoagulation concerns. This test can identify structural defects along the entire esophagus such as strictures, achalasia,

and sometimes rings. Video- and cinefluoroscopy can aid in the diagnosis of esophageal webs or motor disorders, such as cricopharyngeal spasm, pharyngeal paralysis, or achalasia. Modified barium swallow studies are used to evaluate real-time swallowing mechanisms at the oropharyngeal level. This may be needed to identify oropharyngeal dysmotility and aspiration.

C. **Ambulatory pH monitoring** has been used to determine if acid reflux is present. This is particularly useful if diagnosis by endoscopy or therapeutic medication trials is unclear. pH is recorded for 24 hours and is positive in those who have a pH of less than 4.5 for more than 6% of the time tested. Provocative testing such as the Bernstein acid perfusion test (using hydrochloric acid) is rarely used for reproduction of symptoms due to acid reflux, and its use is questionable.

D. **Esophageal manometry** may be useful in the workup of dysphagia, heartburn, or noncardiac chest pain to determine pressures of the upper and lower esophageal sphincters and functions of the smooth muscle. Achalasia, diffuse esophageal spasm, or scleroderma esophagus can all be diagnosed with this method. Nevertheless, manometry should not be a first-line test without prior structural evaluation, preferably by endoscopy or, alternatively, barium swallow radiography.

V. **Management**

A. Many patients with symptoms of **gastroesophageal reflux** are given acid suppression initially. Proton pump inhibitors are usually more efficacious than histamine-2 blocking agents. Omeprazole, 20 mg qd, or lansoprazole, 30 mg qd, are starting doses that can be doubled if no effect is seen in several weeks. New proton pump inhibitors with similar efficacy are now available, including rabeprazole, 20 mg qd, and pantoprazole, 40 mg qd. Additionally, esomeprazole (40 mg PO qd) and pantoprazole IV have recently become available. Some patients may achieve relief with one of the many inexpensive antacid preparations that are available over the counter (see Chap. 14).

B. **Achalasia** can be treated with agents, such as nitrates or calcium channel blockers, to reduce lower esophageal sphincter pressure. This is rarely effective. Pneumatic dilation under fluoroscopic visualization provides more sustained relief. Heller myotomy, a surgical procedure that dissects the smooth muscle of the hypertensive lower esophageal sphincter, provides excellent long-term improvement as well. Botulinum toxin injected during endoscopy into the sphincter may have acceptable results for those at high risk for other interventions.

C. **Strictures and rings of the esophagus** can be treated during endoscopy by bougienage, the passage of dilators with or without guidewire assistance.

D. **Symptomatic treatment** of odynophagia may include parenteral narcotic agents or topical viscous lidocaine. Hiccups usually are self-limited but in refractory cases may require phenothiazines such as **prochlorperazine** (5–10 mg PO/IV tid/qid prn) or **chlorpromazine** (Thorazine, 10–25 mg PO/IM q6h prn). **Baclofen** (5–60 mg PO daily) has also proved to be helpful.

Dyspepsia

I. **Definitions.** This nonspecific term, which is applied to many GI symptoms, includes a persistent or recurrent discomfort or pain located in the upper abdominal area. Symptoms described by the patient consist of bloating, heartburn, nausea, and food intolerance. Symptoms can be generalized broadly into two categories: peptic ulcer disease and nonulcer dyspepsia.

II. **History**

Nonspecific upper abdominal complaints suggest a broad range of processes, not necessarily implying any specific entities.

A. **Timing of pain** can sometimes suggest certain processes. Nocturnal pain that results in awakening several hours after ingestion of food is suspicious for peptic ulcer disease.
B. **Relation to food.** Pain in the preprandial state may be referred to by the patient as "hunger pain" and could signal peptic ulcer disease. Such pain may be relieved by food, particularly if a duodenal ulcer exists. Early satiety can result from ulcers at the gastric outlet, infiltrating tumors or any process, creating reduced gastric wall compliance. Intestinal angina, characterized by fear of eating because of subsequent abdominal pain, should always be considered in those with cardiovascular disease and the elderly.
C. **Previous peptic ulcer disease** may be reported by some patients with dyspepsia. Prior gastric surgery and a history of cigarette smoking or alcohol use may be risk factors.
D. **Nonulcer dyspepsia** is a diagnosis of exclusion. Patients may present with a symptom complex similar to that with peptic ulcer disease but more commonly have vague persistent discomfort with atypical features. Biochemical, clinical, and endoscopic abnormalities need to be excluded [*N Engl J Med* 1998;339(19):1376–1381].
E. **Radiation of pain** can be helpful in identifying an etiology. Pain boring directly through to the back and somewhat improved on leaning forward is characteristic of pancreatitis. Patients who appear ill with this type of pain may have a perforated peptic ulcer or a leaking abdominal aneurysm. Pain that is referred to the right shoulder blade may originate in the gallbladder or from any process that results in diaphragmatic irritation.
F. **Dysmotility** lacks pain as a significant feature. Rather, patients may complain of early satiety, recurrent retching or vomiting, or a bloated feeling in the upper abdomen that is not accompanied by visible distention. Gastroparesis and chronic idiopathic intestinal pseudo-obstruction are possible causes.
G. **Colonic symptoms**, such as constipation or diarrhea, tenesmus, or nonspecific lower abdominal discomfort, in association with upper abdominal complaints may be a clue to irritable bowel disease.
H. **Aerophagia** is a common occurrence that results in fullness, belching, or reflux-like symptoms. Unconsciously, an excess of air is swallowed during and between meals. Habitual gum chewing may be a contributing factor. Repetitive belching is frequently reported by the patient and usually alleviates much of the discomfort.
I. **Red flag symptoms** with dyspepsia include weight loss, GI tract bleeding, recurrent emesis, dysphagia, and use of nonsteroidal agents. Patients who are older than 45 years are more likely to have a structural cause. The presence of any of these features deserves further investigation.

III. **Physical examination**
Tenderness that is palpable can be noted in peptic ulcer disease and pancreaticobiliary disorders. Right upper quadrant tenderness that is increased with inspiration (Murphy's sign) indicates cholecystitis. Masses are occasionally detected. **Peritoneal signs** should be sought in any patient with acute complaints and an ill appearance. Rebound tenderness is discomfort induced by movement of an irritated peritoneum within the abdominal cavity during the release of pressure from palpation. This and guarding are classic peritoneal signs. Jaundice can suggest a hepatic or biliary process. Blood in the stool on examination, usually melena, may suggest a bleeding peptic ulcer. Occult fecal blood may also be present.

IV. **Diagnostic testing**
A. **Blood tests** can include a CBC if bleeding ulcers are suspected. Leukocytosis can be a clue for intra-abdominal infection. If suspected by history or physical examination, thyroid tests can be obtained to evaluate for hyper- or hypothyroid states. A fasting glucose can be obtained to screen for diabetes mellitus if gastroparesis is a suspected etiology.
B. **Endoscopy** of the upper GI tract is indicated for those with alarm symptoms and for whom trials with acid-suppressing medications are inadequate. If

mucosal abnormalities, such as peptic ulcers, erosive gastropathy, or duodenitis, are noted, testing for *Helicobacter pylori* is usually performed. Alternatively, testing of blood serology can be used to determine previous exposure (see Chap. 14).

   C. Radiography. Upper tract barium x-rays are not usually helpful unless ulcers are suspected. Gastroparesis can be demonstrated by gastric emptying scintigraphy but is usually suspected clinically. Ultrasound can be used for biliary tract examination. Otherwise, ultrasound and CT scan have low yield.

V. Management

   A. Various treatments are required based on the presentation. Symptoms that suggest **peptic ulcers** should be managed initially with acid suppression.

   B. Nonulcer dyspepsia often does not respond to specific treatment, although some may improve with acid suppression or tricyclic antidepressant use. In those without alarm symptoms (weight loss, dysphagia, bleeding, or recurrent emesis) and those younger than 45 years old, a 4-week empiric trial of histamine blocker or proton pump inhibitor should be prescribed. If the patient is older than 45 years and has new complaints or any alarm symptoms, an upper endoscopy should be performed initially. Eradication of *H. pylori* in this setting has been shown to have minimal benefit (*Am J Gastroenterol* 1996;91:1773).

   C. Dysmotility-like dyspepsia may benefit from prokinetic agents such as metoclopramide.

   D. Reflux should be treated symptomatically with a regularly scheduled course of antihistamine antacids or proton pump inhibitors for 4–6 weeks. Weight reduction, dietary changes, and elevation of the head of the bed can be useful [*Gut* 1999;45(Suppl I):132–135].

Constipation

I. Definition. Constipation is a subjective feeling of infrequency or difficulty in passing stools. An average Western diet results in bowel movements of at least three times/week. The frequency of bowel movements may decrease with age. The absolute inability to pass stools can be referred to as **obstipation**.

II. History

   A. Onset and duration. Recent significant alterations in bowel habits in an adult without previous problems should alert the clinician to search for organic causes. Intermittent constipation may be due to medications, dietary habits, or functional bowel disease. Those symptoms that do not relent should be carefully investigated for serious illnesses like an obstructive state secondary to a mass. Patients with a left-sided colonic mass may sometimes describe a gradual reduction of stool caliber.

   B. Pain or bleeding. When pain occurs with defecation, one should consider either inflammatory or obstructive causes such as diverticulitis, anal fissures, inflammatory colitis, thrombosed external hemorrhoids, and cancer. Bleeding can accompany all of these in variable degrees. Cramping abdominal pain with bloating relieved by defecation and sometimes accompanied by upper GI symptoms can be considered irritable bowel syndrome if organic pathology has been excluded. A sense of incomplete rectal evacuation is known as **tenesmus**. Some individuals may have a similar sensation resulting from proctitis or other inflammatory processes that affect the rectum.

   C. Genitourinary complaints. Some individuals, particularly postmenopausal women, describe constipation that accompanies urinary incontinence. Abnormal pelvic floor relaxation, rectocele, and cystoceles can all be present. Digital manipulation either through the vagina or the rectum may be described by the patient as a routine practice to stimulate bowel movements. A careful history regarding these issues should be acquired, as many patients may be embarrassed to reveal such details.

   D. Medications. New medications should be reviewed. Calcium channel blockers for hypertension remain a common culprit for constipation. The patient should be questioned about pain medications, particularly opiate products, nonprescription anticholinergic agents, and iron supplements. Laxative use and abuse should be ascertained, as some individuals may develop worsening constipation or a "cathartic colon."

   E. Diet. A 2-week diary of eating and bowel habits may be of assistance. Adequate intake of fiber and fluid (6–8 glasses daily) should be evaluated.

III. **Physical examination**

   Abdominal examination may reveal distention, tenderness, and masses. If tympanic distention is found, one must consider ileus or varying degrees of obstruction. **Perineal and rectal examination** is imperative. Visual inspection can identify external deformities, such as rectal prolapse and hemorrhoids. Perineal sensation and rectal sphincter tone and reflexes should be tested. Digital examination of the rectum can assess for fissures, distal fixed stenosis, masses, or fecal impaction. In those with concurrent genitourinary complaints, the examiner may be able to feel a rectocele, which can bulge anteriorly into the vagina, perineal descent, or rectal prolapse.

IV. **Diagnostic testing**

   A. Laboratory tests. Constipation can be exacerbated by disturbances in serum electrolytes. In particular, low potassium, magnesium, and abnormally low or high calcium may become clinically significant. If long-standing symptoms exist or history dictates, thyroid studies can be performed. Hyperglycemia may identify diabetics who may have a very slow transit time.

   B. Endoscopic studies. In new-onset or progressive constipation (especially in those patients older than 50 years), colonoscopy is essential to evaluate for colon cancer or strictures. Proctoscopy may be useful to identify rectal pathology such as hemorrhoids, fissures, and masses. Melanosis coli, a dark pigmentation that is most often seen in the distal colon, can be found in many patients who use an excess of anthroquinolone laxatives. Once mechanical sources are excluded, anorectal manometry can be used to determine functional disease.

   C. Radiologic studies. To exclude an obstructive colonic process, a barium enema may be helpful when combined with flexible sigmoidoscopy. In severe constipation, ingestion of radiopaque markers with serial radiographs can confirm colon transit time and sometimes differentiate colonic inertia from pelvic floor muscle disorders. Defecography can help visualize the voluntary and involuntary portions of defecation for many disturbances. Localization of dysmotility to areas such as the rectum or pelvic floor muscles may become evident (*Dis Colon Rectum* 1988;31:190). Radiologic findings that should prompt immediate attention include obstruction and megacolon (grossly dilated colon with significant abdominal distention).

V. **Management**

   A. Diet. Increased fiber intake is the most fundamental treatment of persistent idiopathic constipation. This increases stool bulk and stimulates intestinal motility. All ambulatory adults without signs of megacolon or mechanical obstruction should undergo a trial. Most individuals with constipation are able to achieve a positive response with 20–30 g of daily fiber supplementation (*Cleve Clin J Med* 1999;6691:41). Extensive patient education materials and counsel with a dietitian can be beneficial.

   B. Behavioral changes include the creation of a regular schedule for defecation.

   C. Pharmacologic agents

      1. **Enemas** can be safely used for acute constipation to achieve immediate relief. When constipation is severe, enemas are preferred to allow for more comfortable bowel movements. Saline enemas (120–240 ml) are nonirritating, whereas tap water enemas (500–1000 ml) can be irritating. Hard or impacted stool can be evacuated by oil retention enemas

such as cottonseed with dioctyl sodium sulfosuccinate (Colace, 120 ml). Manual disimpaction may also become necessary.

2. Bulk-forming laxatives should be first-line agents and include natural products such as **psyllium** (e.g., Metamucil, 1 tsp in liquid or 1 packet with liquid PO bid–qid). Synthetic products are **methylcellulose** (e.g., Citrucel, 1 tbsp in 8 oz water qd–tid) **or polysaccharide derivatives** (e.g., FiberCon, 1 g qid prn, 500-, 625-, 1000-mg tablets accompanied by 4–6 glasses of water).

3. Emollient laxatives such as **mineral oil** (15–45 ml PO q6–8h) should be used with caution due to the risk of aspiration and lipid pneumonia. Avoid use before bedtime. **Docusate salts** (50–200 g PO qd) should be given between meals to avoid malabsorption of fat-soluble vitamins.

4. Stimulant laxatives, such as **castor oil** (15–60 ml qd), **cascara** (1 tsp PO bid), and **senna** (2 tsp PO bid), and the diphenylmethylate substances, such as **bisacodyl** (10–15 mg PO qhs), can be tried for immediate results but should be avoided for chronic use.

5. Saline laxatives such as **magnesium citrate** (200 ml PO qid) and **Fleet Phospho-Soda** can be used in those with severe constipation if there are no contraindications.

6. For more refractory patients, hyperosmolar agents include **polyethylene glycol (GoLYTELY)**, which can be given as one glass daily, creates regular bowel movements. A similar product called **Miralax** (1 tsp in 8 oz water qd) is now available in a powder form. **Lactulose** (15–30 g PO q2–3h prn) can be used either acutely or long term. Nonabsorbable saccharides such as sorbitol can also be used for immediate results.

7. Stool softeners including **Colace** (100 mg PO bid) can be used along with bulk-forming therapy for maintenance [*J Clin Gastroenterol* 1999;28(1):11].

8. The routine long-term use of laxatives should be avoided except for fiber supplements, hyperosmolar agents, and stool softeners, which have an adequate safety profile.

9. **Surgical treatment** is reserved for rectal deformities, intestinal obstructions and masses, resuspension of rectal intussusception, or prolapse and pelvic floor disorders.

Diarrhea

I. **Definitions.** The normal Western diet results in stool output ranging from three times/week to three times/day. Not only is there a subjective increase in the frequency of stools but also the term refers to a more liquid consistency. Objectively, a stool quantity that exceeds 200 g/24 hours is defined as **diarrhea**. Traditionally, acute diarrhea has been designated as that which has been present for less than 2–3 weeks. The duration of chronic diarrhea is longer than this period.

II. **History**

A. **Timing.** The onset and duration should be determined. Relation to eating can be important in determining if the diarrhea is due to osmotic rather than secretory pathology (Table 13-3). The latter does not improve with fasting. Nighttime diarrhea can be a clue to organic causes, including infections, secretory diarrhea, and sometimes diabetic diarrhea. Functional diarrhea such as irritable bowel syndrome tends not to disturb the patient during sleep.

B. **Infectious contacts.** It should be ascertained from the patient if anyone else at work, home, or usual contact has similar symptoms. Restaurant outbreaks of bacterial gastroenteritis or hepatitis should be considered.

Table 13-3. Chronic diarrhea

	Osmotic diarrhea	Secretory diarrhea	Malabsorptive diarrhea
Causes	Ingestion of unabsorbed solutes	Hormonal	Intestinal mucosal disease
	Lactose intolerance	VIPoma	Celiac sprue
	Medications	Zollinger-Ellison	Whipple's disease
	Sorbitol	(gastrinoma)	Eosinophilic gastroenteritis
	Antacids	Carcinoid	Crohn's disease
	Magnesium laxatives	Bile salt malabsorption	Intestinal resection
	Maldigestion	Pancreatic cholera	Lymphatic obstruction
	Chronic intestinal ischemia	Collagen vascular disease	Small-bowel overgrowth
	Short-bowel syndrome	Intestinal lymphoma	Pancreatic insufficiency
	Gastrocolic fistula		
	Mucosal transport defects		
Symptoms and signs	Moderate volume of stool	Voluminous stool	Weight loss
	Improved with fasting	Little change with fasting	Signs of nutrient deficiency
		Nighttime symptoms	
Diagnosis	Increased osmolar gap [measured osmolality is 100 mOsm greater than twice the sum of stool cations (K and Na)]	Stool osmolality approximates serum osmolality	Fecal fat >7–10 g/ 24 hrs (in steatorrhea)
	Sometimes acidic stool pH	24-hr stool quantity >1 L	Anemia
		Usually neutral stool pH	Hypoalbuminemia

VIP, vasoactive intestinal polypeptide.

Those who travel may have had contact with unsanitary conditions and should be questioned carefully. A patient who reports **blood, mucus, or pus** in the diarrheal stool or fever, or both, may have an invasive bacterial pathogen.
- **C. Abdominal pain** can manifest as cramping during bowel movements. Localized pain to the lower quadrants or rectum, bleeding, tenesmus, and weight loss may be some of the features of inflammatory bowel disease. Pain is more commonly associated with Crohn's disease than ulcerative colitis. A nonspecific diffuse pain or discomfort may be reported in those with irritable bowel syndrome.
- **D. Malabsorption.** Patients with steatorrhea (fat malabsorption) often describe light-colored loose stools that are difficult to flush and stick to the toilet bowl. Fatty food intolerance may be seen in certain disorders of pancreatic exocrine insufficiency. Nighttime visual impairment and bone pain may be noted in fat-soluble vitamin malabsorption of vitamins A and D, respectively.
- **E. Volume of stool.** Frequent small volumes of stool output with urgency suggest a distal colorectal pathology. Larger volumes of stool with less frequency may be noted in small-bowel or proximal colonic disorders.

F. Medications. Antibiotic use within the preceding 6 weeks should be elicited as a predisposing factor for *Clostridium difficile* pseudomembranous colitis. The use of excessive alcohol, caffeine, or chocolates has been reported to be the cause of diarrhea in some. True food allergies are rare. Patients should be questioned about the use of sugar substitutes and sugar-free candy or chewing gum, as these may contain sorbitol. Fat substitutes such as olestra are also important sources.

III. Acute diarrhea
A. Infectious agents
1. **Viruses** such as Norwalk agent in adults and older children and rotavirus in young children can be implicated during certain seasons.
2. **Bacteria.** Enterotoxigenic bacteria include *Escherichia coli* (traveler's diarrhea), *Bacillus cereus*, *Clostridium perfringens*, and *Staphylococcus aureus*. Enteropathic agents can be quite invasive and include *Campylobacter*, *Salmonella*, *Shigella*, and certain species of *Yersinia*. A preformed toxin such as *S. aureus* can cause diarrhea, occurring within 12 hours of food ingestion. A lag time of up to 3 days may be noted in *Salmonella* [*Am J Gastroenterol* 1997;92(11):1962].
3. **Protozoa.** *Giardia* species can be acquired from spring water consumption during camping and travel to developing countries. Amebiasis is common in similar travelers and homosexual men.

B. Medications (see sec. II.F)

C. Bloody diarrhea. Invasive infections, particularly *Campylobacter* and *Shigella*, may be causative agents. Acute onset of watery diarrhea that becomes bloody within 24–48 hours and is accompanied by fever can suggest a hemorrhagic colitis caused by *E. coli* O157:H7. Inflammatory bowel disease or a drug-induced colitis are also possibilities. Older individuals with atherosclerosis may present in this manner with superior mesenteric artery or vein thrombosis. Ischemic colitis in those with previous hypotension should be considered.

D. Diverticular diarrhea can have features of left lower quadrant discomfort, rectal urgency, pain with defecation, tenesmus, and fever.

E. Fecal impaction may paradoxically cause diarrhea in the elderly or in those who consume narcotic pain medications. This is usually small liquid stool leakage around an impacted hard stool.

IV. Chronic diarrhea
A. Several categories of diarrhea exist, including **osmotic, secretory, malabsorptive, and inflammatory** (Table 13-3).

B. Those who describe **steatorrhea** may have short-bowel syndrome, malabsorption disorders, bacterial overgrowth, and fat-soluble vitamin deficiency (vitamins A, D, E, and K). Malabsorption may be due to pancreatic exocrine insufficiency, cirrhosis and bile duct obstruction, mucosal disease due to autoimmune enteropathies, celiac sprue, and Whipple's disease.

C. Secretory diarrhea includes vasoactive intestinal polypeptide (VIP)oma or the watery diarrhea-hypokalemia-achlorhydria (WDHA) syndrome, which can occur as non–beta cell pancreatic adenomas. Gastrinoma is the most common neuroendocrine tumor and produces large volumes of hydrochloric acid along with peptic ulcers and fat maldigestion.

D. Dumping syndrome is seen in postgastrectomy states. The initial phase of this syndrome is voluminous diarrhea shortly after eating. Within a few hours, some may experience the latent phase characterized by weakness, lightheadedness, flushing, and other features of hypoglycemia due to a reactive insulin release.

E. Irritable bowel syndrome can be characterized by alternating features of diarrhea and constipation, abdominal pain, and sometimes depression or anxiety (see Chap. 14).

F. Diabetic diarrhea can occur in those who have poorly controlled diabetes for longer than 5 years. Nighttime incontinence may be a feature. These patients usually have coexisting severe peripheral neuropathy and sometimes retinopathy and nephropathy.

G. Factitious diarrhea. Surreptitious use of laxatives can result in severe watery diarrhea, nausea, emesis, and weight loss. The majority of these individuals are women less than 30 years old who may have eating disorders such as anorexia nervosa or bulimia or middle-aged women with extensive medical histories who have secondary gains from chronically being in the sick role (*Clin Gastroenterol* 1986;15:723).

H. Previous GI surgery. Distal gastric resections can result in the dumping syndrome as previously described. Prior vagotomy can also result in diarrhea. Significant intestinal resection, particularly segments of the ileum that exceed 100 cm, can result in malabsorption and a bile acid–induced diarrhea [*Dig Dis* 1998;16(2):118].

V. Physical examination. Dehydration should be evaluated by searching for orthostatic hypotension, pulse changes, poor skin turgor, and dry mucous membranes. Cutaneous findings of systemic diseases may be present. Dermatitis herpetiformis, an intensely pruritic rash of grouped lesions found on the scalp, buttocks, and extensor surfaces, is associated with celiac sprue. Acrodermatitis enteropathica, characterized by a maculopapular erythema of the extremities and perineum along with alopecia, is sometimes seen in those with zinc and other mineral deficiencies.

VI. Diagnostic testing

A. A conservative workup should be used initially. The cost of testing all stool can become exorbitant in this usually self-limited illness. Testing should be used in those with severe unrelenting diarrhea, chronic diarrhea, immunocompromised states, or epidemiologic conditions such as community outbreaks.

B. Stool studies. Stool should be examined for ova and parasites and cultures. Prior antibiotic use, particularly within 6 weeks of onset of symptoms, should prompt the testing of stool for *Clostridium difficile* toxin. In those with persistent watery diarrhea, stool electrolytes and osmolality may be measured and correlated to an osmotic gap. Positive Sudan staining of the stool may indicate fat malabsorption and should be performed in the workup of chronic diarrhea or if history is suggestive. Fecal leukocytes are nonspecific and usually not helpful but may be a clue to an invasive infectious pathogen or a chronic inflammatory disease.

C. Blood tests. A CBC may help uncover anemia or infections. Electrolytes, BUN, and creatinine can assist in identifying the severity of dehydration or metabolic acidosis. A screening thyroid-stimulating hormone level can be measured in those with chronic diarrhea. Markers for inflammatory bowel disease, pANCA (**p**erinuclear **a**nti**n**eutrophilic **c**ytoplasmic **a**ntibody), and ASCA (**a**nti-**S**accharomyces **c**erevisiae mannan **a**ntibodies) are not yet supported with sufficient data to justify their routine use as a screening test [*Gut* 2000;46(1):58]. The presence of immunoglobulin A antiendomysial antibody is highly sensitive and specific for celiac sprue.

D. Sigmoidoscopy without enema preps can be a useful tool for those who have had diarrhea longer than 1 week and an initial negative workup. Abnormal mucosa can be noted, and random biopsies for infectious and inflammatory colitis can be done. If colitis is present, a full colonoscopy may become necessary to determine the extent of involvement. Upper endoscopy with small-bowel biopsies can be performed in chronic diarrhea to identify celiac sprue histologically.

VII. Management

A. Rehydration is the initial intervention for diarrhea. Oral rehydration is preferred with noncaffeinated and nonalcoholic products, but parenteral fluid administration may become necessary. A rehydrating solution can be created for use at home and includes 1 L water, 1 cup fruit juice, 4 tbsp sugar or honey, 1 tsp baking powder, and ¾ tsp salt. This may help resolve nausea, vomiting, and abdominal pain. Although not as effective for severe dehydration, commercial agents such as Gatorade and Pedialyte can be used in milder illnesses.

B. Symptomatic treatment

  1. **Kaolin and pectin-containing agents** (Kaopectate) may add bulk to stool.
  2. **Bismuth subsalicylate** has antisecretory, antimicrobial, and anti-inflammatory properties. When administered as two tablets (262 mg) every 30 minutes up to eight doses/day, it can help hasten the recovery of severe traveler's diarrhea.
  3. **Loperamide** is used as 4 mg initially followed by 2-mg capsules with a maximum of 8 mg/day. Lomotil (diphenoxylate plus atropine) can be given as 5 mg initially, then 2.5 mg after each loose stool to a maximum of 20 mg/day. Tincture of opium (0.6 ml q4h), belladonna/opium (1 suppository q12h prn), codeine (30–60 mg PO q4h prn), and paregoric can be used. All of these agents impair intestinal motility and should be avoided in bacterial infectious states, as they may delay clearance of the organism. They should also be avoided in advanced liver disease. Loperamide is the preferred opiate for treatment of diarrhea because it has the fewest side effects including CNS depression.
  4. **Anticholinergic agents** such as atropine hyoscyamine and products are useful to some, particularly with cramping that accompanies diarrhea.
  5. **Bulk-forming substances** such as psyllium and methylcellulose may ameliorate functional diarrhea.

C. Antibiotics are not required for most acute infectious diarrhea, which is usually self-limited. If the patient appears toxic or has a persistent diarrhea in which an organism is identified, however, antibiotics may be useful. In severe **traveler's diarrhea** that presents as dysentery with bloody stools and with or without fever, ciprofloxacin, 500 mg bid for 3–7 days, or trimethoprim-sulfamethoxazole, 1 tablet PO bid for 5 days, may hasten recovery. In simple watery traveler's diarrhea, antibiotics are not indicated.

D. Cholestyramine (4 g mixed in fluid every 12 hours with no other medications 1 hour before or 4 hours after dose) can improve refractory diarrhea of malabsorption or bile acid–induced diarrhea, which can occur as a result of distal small-bowel resections. Caution must be advised in drug interactions, as this agent can prevent the adequate absorption of many medications.

Lactose Intolerance

I. Definition. Many adults have malabsorption of lactose due to low levels of intestinal disaccharidases, which are essential for metabolism. This results in an osmotic diarrhea. The average adult on a Western diet ingests 300 g carbohydrate daily, 15 g of which is lactose. Lack of metabolic capacity is seen in a variety of groups, particularly those of Asian or African heritage. Northern Europeans and Native Americans are also commonly afflicted (see Chap. 3, sec. **XI.D**).

II. History. Symptoms of **abdominal pain** can be quite variable but are induced only by the ingestion of dietary lactose and disappear with avoidance. Many individuals experience cramping, distention, bloating, flatulence, diarrhea, nausea, or vomiting. For some, a threshold exists in which limited quantities of lactose are tolerable. Bowel movements are described as bulky, watery, and frothy in appearance. Secondary intolerance resulting from inflammatory mucosal injury may be reported in patients who have a history of radiation enteritis, tropical sprue, celiac disease, or *Giardia*. Worsening of symptoms of irritable bowel syndrome can sometimes be triggered by lactose ingestion in intolerant individuals.

III. Physical examination. Diffuse nonspecific tenderness may be present. Borborygmi or audible bowel sounds may be heard.

IV. Diagnostic testing

    A. History is the primary route to diagnosis. Lactose challenge and elimination diets can be added for confirmation [*J Clin Gastroenterol* 1999;28(3):208–216].

    B. Blood tests may indicate severity of dehydration or the presence of metabolic acidosis if diarrhea is severe.

    C. Lactose absorption testing has been replaced by **lactose breath hydrogen measurement**, which is occasionally useful when the diagnosis is unclear despite history and empiric therapy. Hydrogen is compared in the breath before ingestion of lactose and then at 30 minutes after intake (*Annu Rev Med* 1990;41:141).

V. Management

    A. Dietary changes. Reduction or restriction of lactose can be tried for a defined period to determine accuracy of the diagnosis. Substitution of alternative nutrients is needed. Acidophilus milk is not adequately lactose depleted, but lactose-free milk is available. Live culture yogurt containing beta-galactosidase is tolerated by many individuals.

    B. Enzyme supplementation can be accomplished by many nonprescription agents in the form of tablets or drops. These supplements have some therapeutic benefit but should not be used to determine a diagnosis. Calcium carbonate supplements should also be provided if the patient is lacking in other dietary sources of calcium.

Anorectal Complaints

I. Anorectal pain

    A. Hemorrhoids

        1. In the anus, the dentate line (mucocutaneous junction) divides the sensory and nonsensory regions. Internal hemorrhoids are found above this line, whereas external ones form below and can produce pain. Discomfort from hemorrhoids usually manifests as anal pruritus and sometimes pain. The most exquisite pain and bleeding occur with thrombosis of an external hemorrhoid. Internal hemorrhoids may produce mild discomfort, but significant pain is seen primarily in prolapse and strangulation. Bleeding is usually minimal, bright red, and found on the outside of stool or on toilet paper. Larger amounts of blood, uncommon in hemorrhoids, should suggest other etiologies.

        2. Treatment includes increased dietary fiber, which results in softer bulky stools and less straining. A stool softener may also be of benefit. Analgesic suppositories and witch hazel can help alleviate symptoms. Warm sitz baths given two to three times a day can reduce swelling. If thrombosis occurs, surgical incision and drainage provide prompt relief and can be easily performed in the clinic setting (*Dis Colon Rectum* 1995;38:687). Those with persistent symptomatic hemorrhoids despite medical therapy may benefit from referral to a gastroenterologist for endoscopic band ligation or to a surgeon for hemorrhoidectomy.

    B. Anal fissure. This painful linear ulcer, found in the anal canal, is a tear of the tissue or sphincter as a result of passage of hard stools. Although usually not seen well on colonoscopy, anoscopy identifies the posterior midline as the site of the tear in 90% of cases. Severe pain, however, often makes even this or a digital examination impossible. A simple visual inspection after spreading the buttocks can often identify a linear tear perpendicular to the dentate line. A lateral fissure found on examination may suggest

Crohn's disease, proctitis, leukemia, syphilis, tuberculosis, or carcinoma. Patients usually have underlying constipation. Complaints of frequent passage of bright red blood and pain with defecation are consistent with this diagnosis. A diet that is high in fiber, stool softeners, topical anesthetic ointments, and sitz baths are recommended. Chronic anal fissures can be quite disabling and may require a surgical anal sphincterotomy. Topical nitroglycerin or injection with botulinum toxin has achieved temporary relaxation of sphincter tone to permit healing.

C. **Perirectal fistula.** Patients present with a chronic purulent, foul-smelling discharge from the rectum or small openings in the perineum. Pain with defecation is reported along with intense pruritus. In the setting of diarrhea, abdominal pain, or rectal bleeding, the presence of a perirectal fistula should make one suspicious for Crohn's disease. Anoscopy or sigmoidoscopy can visualize the internal focus of a fistula, commonly, a red granular papule that is exuding pus. Antibiotics such as ciprofloxacin and metronidazole may aid in healing. Surgical excision and drainage often becomes necessary. If related to Crohn's disease, alternative medical therapy is available.

D. **Abscess.** If not treated early, this may develop into a serious infection. The presence of an abscess can raise suspicion for Crohn's disease or immune compromise with neutropenia. Patients particularly complain of acute pain in the rectum that is worse with sitting, defecation, or movement. On examination, fever may be present. A fluctuant tender area of mucosa is noted, with erythema, warmth, and often a foul-smelling discharge. **The need for surgical drainage is almost a certainty.**

E. **Rectal prolapse.** Patients frequently notice extrusion of the rectum during defecation and may report the need for manual reduction. Straining at the toilet is common. To the examiner, a prolapse is usually obvious during sitting or straining. On occasion, defecography can be used to confirm the diagnosis. Sigmoidoscopy or barium enema is recommended to exclude malignancy. Acutely, manual reduction must be attempted. Complete prolapse or frequent partial prolapse that concerns the patient must be repaired surgically (*Adv Surg* 1996;29:59).

F. **Rectosigmoid intussusception.** Hematochezia and pain may be the initial presentation. Endoscopic examination may discover a neoplasm or obstructing polyp at this site. Defecography is useful in diagnosing this process if structural lesions are not evident.

G. **Proctalgia fugax.** This is a condition found in young adults characterized by sudden brief episodes of severe rectal pain occurring along the midline. It can radiate upward into the abdomen. Occasionally, the pain is extreme, resulting in syncope. The underlying process is spasm of the levator ani musculature. Defecation or prolonged sitting can result in spasm. Treatment primarily involves reassurance to the patient that no serious organic illness is present. Local heat and massage may help.

II. **Fecal incontinence**

A. **History.** Many patients are embarrassed by incontinence and are therefore reticent to volunteer such symptoms. They may also accept this as a sign of aging. Some individuals may describe episodes of rectal urgency and fecal soiling of garments. This problem is inaccurately reported by some people as diarrhea. Poor flatus control is also frequently present. Those who experience urinary incontinence may have pelvic floor musculature relaxation or even neurologic disorders such as spinal neuropathies.

B. **Diagnosis.** Examination should include evaluation of the rectum for impacted stool, anal sphincter tone, and a neurologic examination. Endoscopic ultrasound can assess the sphincter for mechanical disruption. Perineal sensory disturbances, identifiable by nerve conduction studies, can be a sign of low back injury or degenerative disk disease with nerve damage.

C. Treatment. Fiber increases stool bulk and may be helpful in those with milder symptoms. If diarrhea is prominent and infectious sources are excluded, opiate antidiarrheals should be tried. Disimpaction in the appropriate setting may be of benefit. Some patients are taught techniques of pelvic floor muscle strengthening with biofeedback. In severe refractory illness, surgical repair may become the only option.

III. Pruritus ani. Recurrent itching sensation of the anus or perianal skin may be a manifestation of residual fecal material, hemorrhoids, rectal fistula, anal fissures, malignancy, psoriasis, or ingestion of certain foods such as tomatoes. Infections that cause these symptoms include pinworms, scabies, pubic lice, and certain sexually transmitted diseases. Treatment is aimed at the underlying pathology. Antimicrobial therapy is specific for the particular organism. Symptomatic therapy includes lanolin or witch hazel creams. Oral antihistamines such as diphenhydramine, 25 mg qhs, may help nocturnal symptoms. Short-term topical treatment with hydrocortisone cream 1% (not to exceed 2 weeks' duration) or zinc oxide ointment may also be useful.

IV. Palpable lump. Patients may notice unusual masses with defecation. External hemorrhoids or prolapsed internal ones may be culprit. Prominent anal papillae or external skin tags should also be considered. These may sometimes be a manifestation of Crohn's disease. On examination, both with digital palpation and anoscopy, one should look for evidence of an anal malignancy or anal polyps. These findings may require sigmoidoscopy or colonoscopy for full evaluation and biopsies. Rectal prolapse can be noted during sitting or straining. Hypertrophic anal papilla is one of the most common findings. In women, endometrioma may sometimes present in this manner.

V. Rectal bleeding. Bleeding amounts can be quite variable. Small amounts are commonly seen in hemorrhoids. Larger amounts deserve investigation for other causes, including lesions of the colon other than those of the rectum. Pain during bleeding can occur with prolapsed internal hemorrhoids, anal fissures, proctitis of various causes, and chronic radiation proctitis. Anoscopy or sigmoidoscopy, at a minimum, must be performed to exclude serious etiology. Significant amounts of bleeding, recurrent loss, or anemia should prompt a full colonoscopic evaluation. Severe hemorrhage, particularly in the elderly, those with co-morbidities, signs and symptoms of orthostatic hypotension, or an acute significant drop in blood count may need hospitalization for further management and treatment.

Colon Cancer Screening

I. Definition. Screening for cancer of the colon, an important task of preventive medicine, can reduce mortality. Although most individuals are asymptomatic, the clinician needs to stratify patients into groups of varying risk for cancer. Guidelines from the American Cancer Society and American College of Gastroenterology use these risks to determine the most optimal screening.

II. Screening for the average risk population

   A. Asymptomatic individuals older than 50 years should undergo annual fecal occult blood testing and a flexible sigmoidoscopy every 5 years (Table 13-4).

   B. Fecal occult blood test (see Chap. 14, Colonic Polyps and Neoplasia, sec. **II. A.1**).

   1. This is a simple examination of two samples from each of three consecutive stool tests for the presence of occult blood by the guaiac color change. Randomized trials have shown yearly testing to be superior to longer intervals in detecting significant colonic lesions. But these stud-

Table 13-4. Colon cancer screening recommendations

	FOBT	Flexible sigmoidoscopy	DCBE	Colonoscopy
Average risk	Annually after age 50 yrs	Every 5 yrs along with FOBT	No definite guidelines; some suggest annual FOBT + DCBE every 5 yrs	Once every 10 yrs
First-degree relative with (CRC)	Annually after age 40 yrs	Every 5 yrs at age 40 or 10 yrs before index relative	—	Age 40 yrs or 10 yrs before index relative; repeat in 10 yrs
History of adenomas	—	—	—	Repeat colonoscopy every 3–5 yrs
Single adenoma less than 1 cm	Annually after age 50 yrs	Every 5 yrs along with FOBT	—	Once every 10 yrs
History of nonadenoma polyps	Annually after age 50 yrs	Every 5 yrs along with FOBT	—	—
Familial adenomatous polyposis	—	Annually from puberty; colectomy for polyposis	—	Every 1–2 yrs in attenuated forms; fewer polyps and later cancer onset
Hereditary nonpolyposis coli	—	—	—	Every 1–2 yrs; annual examination if adenomas
Prior CRC that is completely resected	—	—	—	Once at 6–12 mos; then every 3–5 yrs

CRC, colorectal cancer; DCBE, double-contrast barium enema; FOBT, fecal occult blood test.

      ies have also shown poor reliability in detecting many polyps and as many as one-third of cancers. Positive predictive value of Hemoccult positivity in patients older than 50 years in several studies ranges from 20% to 30% in detecting cancer or polyps larger than 1 cm (*J Natl Cancer Inst* 1991;83:243).

2. Previously, an enthusiasm for hydration of stool samples had been present in the hopes of increasing sensitivity. Nonhydrated samples have a sensitivity of 50–80% and a specificity of up to 98% for colonic lesions. Current practice guidelines suggest that hydration results in an increase of sensitivity to 80–90% but decreases specificity and positive predictive value by greater than 10%. Therefore, hydration of stool has been shown to increase false positivity and is not recommended.

3. If the fecal occult blood test is **positive**, it is recommended that an examination of the entire colon be performed. Examination should preferably include **colonoscopy** or, alternatively, **double-contrast barium enema (DCBE) supplemented by flexible sigmoidoscopy.**

C. **Flexible sigmoidoscopy** (see Chap. 14, Colonic Polyps and Neoplasia, sec. **II.A.2**). Two-thirds of all colorectal neoplasms are within the reach of the sigmoidoscope, advanced to 60 cm. Polyps that are less than 1 cm in size can be biopsied. If adenomas are found that are either multiple or larger than 1 cm, the patient should undergo a full colonoscopic evaluation. Despite common clinical practice, a single small adenoma (less than 1 cm) does not require further colonic investigation. The presence of a large adenomatous polyp that exceeds 1 cm in the distal colon often heralds similar synchronous lesions more proximally (*N Engl J Med* 1992;326:653).

D. **DCBE.** DCBE, a radiographic method to detect polyps and lesions throughout the entire colon, serves only as a diagnostic entity without the ability to biopsy or remove suspicious lesions. Small polyps less than 1 cm and rectal lesions may be missed. Additionally, barium enema does **not** detect mucosal lesions such as angioectasia, which may be particularly important to recognize in those individuals who have iron deficiency without other identifiable sources. DCBE alone has not been evaluated in the reduction of mortality from discovering colorectal cancer. Increased sensitivity is achieved by combining this with flexible sigmoidoscopy. A thorough purging of the bowel is required. No sedation is used. Although it involves some discomfort and inconvenience to the patient, DCBE is likely a safer procedure than sigmoidoscopy or colonoscopy and does not require discontinuation of anticoagulants.

E. **Colonoscopy** (see Chap. 14, Colonic Polyps and Neoplasia, sec. **II.A.4**) can inspect the entire colon and reach the cecum in 95% of examinations. A bowel prep the evening before testing is needed. Aspirin and medications with antiplatelet effects should be discontinued 1 week before examination to avoid additional risks of bleeding from polypectomy. Oral iron supplements can interfere with visualization of the mucosa and should be stopped at least 3–4 days before the procedure. The clear advantage to this procedure is the ability to detect polyps of all sizes and either biopsy or remove them at the same setting. In fewer than 5% of examinations, adenomas larger than 1 cm can be overlooked. **Risks** include sedation, particularly cardiopulmonary compromise. Bleeding from polypectomy, biopsies, and other interventions are unusual but should be explained to patients. The risk of perforation is rare and approximates 1 in 1000 procedures. No studies in average-risk patients have been performed to determine reduction in mortality from colon cancer by colonoscopy alone. Nevertheless, colonoscopy alone in this group has been recommended every 10 years. Although insurance coverage is still uncertain, more evidence is mounting in favor of the superior efficacy of screening colonoscopy in contrast to flexible sigmoidoscopy in the asymptomatic adult (*N Engl J Med* 2000;343:162–168).

III. **Screening of high-risk populations**

A. **Prior adenomatous polyps**

1. **Multiple adenomatous polyps or those that exceed 1 cm** in size should prompt repeat colonoscopy **every 3 years** after initial examination.

2. **Large polyps**, those with **villoglandular features, or high-grade dysplasia** may necessitate a shorter interval based on physician judgment.

3. **Small single adenomas** less than 1 cm in size do not need colonoscopic follow-up.

B. **Prior colorectal cancer** (see Chap. 14, Colonic Polyps and Neoplasia, sec. **II.C**). If complete resection of a cancer is performed for cure, individuals should have repeat **colonoscopy every 3–5 years**. Carcinogenic embryonic antigen levels are annually tested by some practitioners for early detection of cancer recurrence. This should never be used as a primary screening measure. Testing should only be performed in this group if the patient is receptive to the consequent workup of an elevated result, which may include exploratory laparotomy (*Gastroenterology* 1997;112:594–642).

C. Family history

1. Individuals who have a first-degree relative, including a sibling, parent, or child, with colorectal cancer should be offered the same screening as those of average-risk groups but at an earlier age. Screening should begin either at age 40 years or 10 years before the youngest age of cancer appearance in the family. The history of a single relative with colon cancer who is older than 60 years of age does not increase the risk for a younger person.

2. **Familial adenomatous polyposis (APC)** (see Chap. 14, Colonic Polyps and Neoplasia, **sec. II.B.1**). This autosomal dominant disorder usually manifests with hundreds of colonic adenomas, although attenuated presentations may have only greater than 10 polyps.

3. **Inheritance of the mutated APC gene** can result in a 50% likelihood of developing adenomatous polyps by the age of 16. Polyposis has a 100% risk of transformation into colon cancer by age 40 years. **Genetic testing** is now commercially available, with counseling offered at specific referral centers, particularly for children of affected families. The false negativity of testing can be up to 20%, particularly if no other family member has been identified as a mutated gene carrier. Some families with an attenuated form of the disorder may benefit from testing to identify those individuals who may safely forego strict screening measures. Beginning at puberty, **annual flexible sigmoidoscopy** should be performed. If polyposis is discovered, the timing of colectomy should be discussed. This is usually not necessary before 20 years of age (*Gastroenterology* 1993;104:1535).

4. **Hereditary nonpolyposis colorectal cancer (Lynch syndrome).** The **Amsterdam** criteria must be met for the diagnosis of this syndrome (see Chap. 14, Colonic Polyps and Neoplasia, sec. **II.B.2**). Extracolonic malignancy usually involves the ovaries, endometrium, breast, renal pelvis, stomach, or small intestine. Genetic counseling and testing are available. Testing can be performed if the specific gene is known from evaluation of the parents but should not be offered at earlier than age 20 years. Complete examination by colonoscopy every 1–2 years should be performed between age 20–30 years or 5 years earlier than the youngest relative with cancer. If adenomatous polyps are discovered, annual examination is necessary. If cancer is found, a subtotal colectomy with annual examination is recommended [*Dis Colon Rectum* 1999;42(1):1].

Approach to the Patient with Jaundice

I. Definitions. Yellow pigmentation of the sclera and skin is noted by elevated levels of serum bilirubin (2.5 and 5 g/dl, respectively). **Carotenemia**, although rare, must be distinguished from jaundice. It has yellowing of the skin but not the eyes from ingestion of foods such as carrots, egg yolks, and sweet potatoes.

II. History

A. Onset. In ascribing an etiology to jaundice, an acute or chronic process should first be determined. Acute onset may indicate events such as hemolysis or biliary tract obstruction. Chronic or insidiously worsening jaundice may suggest intrahepatic or extrahepatic obstruction from malignant infiltration or metastatic disease. Primary biliary cirrhosis may also have gradual progression of jaundice.

B. **Pruritus.** Almost all patients complain of generalized itching with jaundice of at least 3–4 weeks duration.

C. **Abdominal pain. Charcot's triad** of fever, right upper quadrant pain, and jaundice can be the presentation of cholecystitis. The addition of mental status alteration and hypotension to this triad is known as **Reynold's pentad** and can indicate ascending cholangitis. A primary hepatic process is also possible. Pain in the midabdomen that radiates to the back may be present in pancreatitis.

D. **Painless jaundice** should raise suspicion for pancreaticobiliary disorders. Neoplasms of the pancreatic head may result in a partially obstructive biliary tree.

E. **Dark urine** is noted by many patients earlier than jaundice. It is an indication of increased urobilinogen.

F. **Weight loss** is an ominous presentation for pancreaticobiliary malignancy.

G. **Exposure to viruses** should be ascertained, particularly hepatitis. The patient should be asked about blood transfusion history, intravenous drug use, and sexual contacts. Travel history to areas that are endemic for hepatitis should be sought.

H. **History of prior cholelithiasis** should make the clinician consider possible choledocholithiasis. Even those with prior cholecystectomy have been reported to have common bile duct stones on occasion.

I. **CHF** and passive hepatic congestion can account for up to 10% of all jaundice in those older than 60 years of age [*Dig Dis* 1999;17(1):49].

III. **Physical examination**
Fever can be found in acute and chronic illness but may be suggestive of infection such as cholangitis. Stigmata of chronic liver disease should be sought on examination (see Approach to Abnormal Liver Chemistries, sec. **II**). Hepatomegaly greater than 15 cm in span can be found in passive congestion, malignant or fatty infiltration, or other infiltrative disorders. Splenomegaly is found in patients with portal hypertension and cirrhosis. It may also be found in those with hemolysis and a vast array of hematologic disorders and malignancies. Ascites may be present in cirrhosis of various causes and intra-abdominal malignancy from other viscera. CHF and pancreatitis may also be the source. A palpable distended gallbladder without tenderness (Courvoisier's sign) is commonly found in pancreaticobiliary malignancy with obstruction. Cutaneous findings include xanthomas, which may be seen in the chronic cholestasis of primary biliary cirrhosis. Gray-bronze discoloration of the skin may suggest hemochromatosis with hepatic involvement. Urticaria may be a sign of acute hepatitis B infection.

IV. **Diagnostic testing**

A. **Hemolysis** can be detected by CBC, peripheral smear examination, elevated reticulocyte count and lactate dehydrogenase, reduced haptoglobin, and predominantly indirect hyperbilirubinemia.

B. **Bilirubin** (see Chap. 14, Liver Diseases, sec. **I.C.2**) elevation can be prolonged despite convalescence of the acute illness because of its binding to albumin. Pure unconjugated hyperbilirubinemia that does not exceed 5 g/dl without hemolysis is seen in **Gilbert's syndrome**.

C. **Alkaline phosphatase** is more sensitive than bilirubin for extrahepatic obstruction. 5'-Nucleotidase and gamma glutamyl transpeptidase (GGT) levels can differentiate the source (see Chap. 14, Liver Diseases, sec. **I.B**).

D. **Liver disease markers** in the appropriate setting can be examined. These include antimitochondrial antibody (primary biliary cirrhosis), anti–smooth-muscle antibody and antinuclear antibody and immunoglobulins (autoimmune disorders), iron studies (hemochromatosis), viral hepatitis panel, and alpha-fetoprotein (hepatocellular malignancy) (*JAMA* 1989;262:3031).

E. **Paracentesis** should never be delayed in the patient with new-onset ascites. Using a syringe, peritoneal fluid for diagnostic testing can easily be acquired in the office setting. The initial studies should include a cell count to rule out infection. A serum-ascites albumin gradient can be derived from calculating the difference between relatively simultaneous serum and ascites measures. Values that exceed 1.1 indicate portal hypertension. Cytology can be sent on the remaining fluid.

F. **Ultrasound**, a readily available and noninvasive test, should be used initially for the rapid evaluation of the biliary system. It has 95% sensitivity for detection of cholelithiasis and acute cholecystitis, as well as 95% accuracy for identifying ductal dilation. The distinction between stones, tumors, and strictures is not as effective as that of a spiral **CT scan**. CT scan of this region is also excellent for liver parenchymal examination.

G. **Radionuclide imaging** is occasionally needed despite other noninvasive tests to recognize cystic or common duct obstruction in the setting of cholangitis.

H. **Endoscopic retrograde cholangiopancreatography**, an invasive procedure, is most useful in diagnosing and treating obstructive jaundice. Choledocholithiasis, cholangitis, intra- and extrahepatic strictures, and pancreatic ductal disease can all be managed.

I. **Liver biopsy** is helpful in diagnosing the etiology of liver disease in those with abnormal enzymes for greater than 6 months and if obstruction is excluded.

V. Management

A. **Treatment** is variable with the underlying illness.

B. **Pruritus** can be treated symptomatically by cholestyramine, 4–6 g; oral antihistamines (rarely effective); doxepin; or moisturizing topical agents. Ursodeoxycholic acid (13–15 mg/kg/day) can alleviate pruritus in those with primary biliary cirrhosis. Rifampin, 300 mg bid, benefits most individuals with chronic pruritus, and some may require phenobarbital, 120 mg/day.

C. **Hereditary disorders of unconjugated hyperbilirubinemia** such as Gilbert's syndrome need no treatment. Phenobarbital may be used to reduce bilirubin levels in those with Crigler-Najjar syndrome type II.

Approach to Abnormal Liver Chemistries

I. Laboratory evaluation, imperfect and incomplete by itself, must be integrated with the clinical history, physical examination, and setting. The sensitivity and specificity of each test must also be considered.

A. **History**

1. **Nonspecific symptoms** include nausea, vomiting, chills, fevers, anorexia, and weight loss. Fatigue alone is frequently reported as the primary presenting symptom by many individuals with liver disease. Spontaneous lack of desire for cigarettes in a previous smoker may indicate worsening liver disease.

2. **Medications.** A careful review of all medications (prescription and nonprescription agents) should be performed. **Acetaminophen, vitamin A, and herbal agents** may be hepatotoxic and should be reviewed. It should be noted that several nonprescription cold remedies contain acetaminophen. The use of as little as 4 g/day acetaminophen in an alcoholic individual has been shown to result in hepatocyte damage. Thought to be harmless for centuries, several Chinese herbal medicines that are used as health tonics, sedatives, analgesics, cathartics, and weight loss substances have now been proved to be hepatotoxins. An inquiry into the prescription medications should include duration, recent changes, and drug interactions. Nonsteroidal anti-inflammatory agents such as ibuprofen and diclofenac may

be overlooked as a common cause of increased transaminases (*Semin Liver Dis* 1990;10:322).

3. **Alcohol use.** Long-term use and binge drinking habits should be ascertained. In men, daily consumption that exceeds 80 g alcohol (72 oz beer, 9 oz liquor, or 30 oz wine) for 10–15 years can lead to cirrhosis. Lower levels, possibly 20–40 g/day, may have a similar effect in women.

4. **Hepatitis A** can be acute and subacute in presentation with a variable appearance. Transmission is fecal-oral, usually with a 2- to 4-week incubation period. Some individuals may never exhibit symptoms, whereas others present with nausea, vomiting, diarrhea, jaundice, and abdominal pain of various degrees. Many experience the prodrome of nonspecific GI complaints for up to 2 weeks before the onset of jaundice. During this prodrome, patients can transmit the illness. Homosexual men and day care workers are at increased risk for spreading this infection. Exposure from a particular restaurant should be ascertained and reported to the health department promptly. This form of hepatitis does not result in chronic disease.

5. **Hepatitis B and C.** Joint pains in the proximal interphalangeal joints, dysgeusia, and dysosmia may be the prodrome symptoms of hepatitis B in the patient with risk factors. Most infections of hepatitis C are asymptomatic in the acute phase. Risk factors are similar for both Hepatitides. Patients should be asked about blood transfusions, needle sticks particularly in health care providers, intravenous drug abuse, and tattoos. Sexual transmission is established in hepatitis B and less clear in hepatitis C. Patients with risk factors should be counseled regarding safer sex practices. Under current U.S. standards for careful testing of blood products, the risks of transfusion-related infection with hepatitis B are 1 in 63,000 and, with hepatitis C, 1 in 103,000 (*N Engl J Med* 1996;334:1685).

6. **Occupational risks.** Certain occupational exposures can result in hepatotoxicity. Chemicals such as arsenic are found in many industrial settings and in organic gardening. Agricultural workers may be at risk for insecticide poisoning.

7. **Jaundice and pruritus.** Patients notice jaundice themselves much later than those around them. Pruritus, which is usually generalized, is present in almost all cases of jaundice that exceed 3–4 weeks.

8. **Abdominal pain.** Abnormal liver tests combined with abdominal pain may reflect stretching of the liver capsule or an inflammatory/obstructing process in the biliary tree that produces right upper quadrant abdominal pain. Hepatitis or other illness that results in hepatomegaly can have similar discomfort. Right upper quadrant pain and fever with jaundice should raise the possibility of cholangitis. In general, a rapid intense right upper quadrant pain may imply choledocholithiasis but may also present as epigastric or upper back pain.

II. **Physical examination**
   Stigmata of liver disease. Physical findings in patients with chronic liver disease include parotid gland enlargement, spider angiomas (most commonly found on the trunk), palmar erythema, Dupuytren's contractures (fibrous contractures of the palmar fascia), gynecomastia, hepatomegaly or small liver size, splenomegaly, caput medusae, pulsatile liver edge, hepatic rub of malignancy, testicular atrophy, and generalized cachexia. **Murphy's sign** (right upper quadrant tenderness palpated during inspiration) may indicate cholecystitis. The findings are less dramatic in the setting of cholangitis because the area of pathology is protected by the ribcage from external palpation.

III. **Specific laboratory examinations**
   The frequently used connotation liver function tests is a misnomer. Not all the tests reflect true functions but may reflect hepatocyte death or other cellular injury.

A. Bilirubin (see Chap. 14, Liver Diseases, sec. **I.C.2**)

1. Virtually all bilirubin is unconjugated in a healthy state. Impaired excretion results in an increase in the conjugated form. The **total bilirubin usually exceeds 2.5 g/dl** if clinical icterus is apparent. An isolated indirect hyperbilirubinemia that does not exceed 5 g/dl with normal transaminases and no indications of hemolysis may be the result of a familial benign disorder known as Gilbert's syndrome (see Chap. 14, Liver Diseases, sec. **I.C.2**). This hyperbilirubinemia may occur during states of fasting and physiologic stress.

2. Bilirubin binds to albumin and can form a complex that remains intact for up to 3 weeks, the half-life of albumin. Patients who are in the convalescent phase of an acute hepatobiliary process may still remain jaundiced, with a persistently elevated bilirubin. Other laboratory indices may be improving, but reduction of bilirubin may lag behind.

B. Prothrombin time (see Chap. 14, Liver Diseases, sec. **I.C.3**). This index is a measure of the liver's synthetic function. Vitamin K–dependent factors of coagulation II, VII, IX, and X are reflected by this test. A normal value is dependent on intact synthesis and absorption of intestinal vitamin K. Cirrhosis, hepatitis, and cholestatic syndromes may have prolonged values. It is a useful prognosticator in patients with cirrhosis.

C. Albumin. This test is another index of hepatic synthesis. It has a half-life of 20 days, making it a better indicator of chronic rather than acute liver processes. Prealbumin has a half-life of 1.9 days but is not usually helpful clinically. Low levels may be present in some patients with poor nutrition. Levels do not often correlate accurately, however, and albumin should not be used as a primary assessment of a patient's nutritional state. Loss of this protein can occur through the GI tract or kidneys. A dilutional effect should also be considered in volume overload states. Albumin can be decreased during normal pregnancy and in acute and chronic inflammatory states.

D. Aminotransferases. AST, also known as SGOT, can be released into the blood from numerous tissues, including liver, cardiac and skeletal muscle, kidney, and brain. ALT, or SGPT, is more specific to liver, and serum levels rise with hepatocyte death. The highest elevations, in the thousands, are seen in viral hepatitis and toxin- or ischemia-induced hepatic injury. Elevation of AST and ALT in a 2:1 ratio or greater, high serum GGT, and an elevated mean corpuscular volume of red cells can be highly suspicious for alcoholic liver disease. Injury from alcohol almost never results in elevations that exceed 10-fold of the normal values.

E. Alkaline phosphatase. Elevated serum levels can arise from processes that affect the liver, skeletal system, intestines, placenta, kidneys, and leukocytes. The largest increases are seen in cholestatic syndromes. Intrahepatic and extrahepatic biliary ductal obstruction can result in a rise as well. Markedly increased levels without associated liver disease are sometimes seen in CHF, bone diseases, and Hodgkin's lymphoma. Rarely, low levels are found in patients who have hypothyroidism, zinc deficiency, Wilson's disease with acute hemolysis, and pernicious anemia.

F. Other chemistry tests include serum globulin, which should be correlated to the serum albumin. Hypergammaglobulinemia that exceeds 3.0 g/dl can be seen in autoimmune chronic hepatitis more frequently than in viral hepatitis. Serum immunoglobulin A levels can be elevated in alcoholic liver disease. Immunoglobulin M values can be predominant in primary biliary cirrhosis. Autoimmune hepatitis tends to have a larger immunoglobulin G fraction. Viral serology markers for hepatitis A, B, and C can be obtained if clinical suspicion is raised.

G. Summary of workup. One should begin by correlating the liver chemistry abnormalities to the clinical scenario. Acute liver injury should be differentiated from a more chronic state. Repeat testing for confirmation may be necessary, particularly when withholding aspirin, nonsteroidal anti-inflammatory agents, and alcohol for at least 72 hours. If alkaline phosphatase is increased and origin is uncertain, one should check serum GGT or 5'-nucleotidase, which are sensitive markers of hepatic injury, to confirm a hepatic source. Prolonged prothrombin time that is not correctable by vitamin K can reveal underlying liver disease. Hepatobiliary imaging such as an ultrasound or CT scan may become necessary in persistent abnormalities. If abnormalities persist for more than 6 months, chronic liver disease, including viral hepatitis, alcohol, autoimmune, and other causes, should be considered, with possible evaluation for a liver biopsy as well.

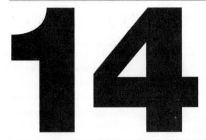

Gastrointestinal II: Diseases

Marc J. Bernstein
and Asif Hussain

Esophageal Diseases

I. **Gastroesophageal reflux disease (GERD)** is defined as any symptom or esophageal injury that results from the backwash of gastric contents into the esophagus. It is the most common esophageal disorder. More than 30% of Americans experience at least monthly episodes of heartburn. GERD is also the most common cause of noncardiac chest pain (*Am J Dig Dis* 1976;21:953, and *Gastroenterology* 1997;112:1448).

A. **Pathogenesis.** If the time that the esophageal mucosa is acidified, or the caustic potency of refluxed fluid, is increased, the risk of GERD increases. Three factors are widely known to increase acid reflux into the esophagus.

1. **Transient lower-esophageal sphincter relaxations.** These events are the physiologic response to gastric distension with air or food (commonly manifest as eructation for gas venting). They are responsible for the majority of the reflux events in normal individuals (*Gastroenterology* 1995;109:601).

2. **Hiatus hernias** are the most common anatomic disruption of the esophagogastric junction. A hiatus hernia exists when the proximal stomach has migrated cranially across the diaphragm and into the chest cavity. It is usually acquired in adulthood and is found in up to 15% of Americans (*Ann Intern Med* 1992;117:977).

3. **Hypotensive lower-esophageal sphincter.** This is not likely to be an isolated cause of GERD but probably contributes in a subset of patients. Lower-esophageal sphincter pressure is decreased by certain food ingredients (e.g., caffeine, chocolate, fatty foods, peppermint), some drugs (e.g., theophylline, narcotics, benzodiazepines, barbiturates), or personal habits (e.g., smoking, alcohol consumption) (*Gut* 1990;31:4).

B. **Presentation.** GERD symptoms are markedly variable. Still, the most frequently encountered symptoms are heartburn, acid regurgitation, and dysphagia (the combination of heartburn and acid reflux is more than 90% specific) (*Lancet* 1990;335:205). Common nonesophageal symptoms include pharyngitis/laryngitis, hoarseness, asthma, and chronic cough (*Am J Gastroenterol* 1999; 94:2812). Other GI disorders that may mimic GERD include esophageal motor disorders, peptic ulcer disease (PUD), infectious esophagitis (especially herpetic esophagitis), and pill esophagitis/ulceration (often from alendronate, aspirin, potassium chloride, quinidine, or tetracycline). When evaluating patients, it is important to realize the overlap of symptoms from GERD with symptoms from potentially dangerous cardiac and pulmonary disorders.

C. **Diagnosis.** Clinical history, 24-hour ambulatory pH monitoring studies, and upper-GI tract imaging studies are the basis for diagnosing GERD. When life-threatening pathologies are excluded, it is reasonable to presume GERD in a patient with characteristic symptoms that are relieved by antireflux therapy (*Gastroenterology* 1995;108:A137). Upper endoscopy has limited sensitivity but permits evaluation of gross mucosal injury and also allows for mucosal sam-

Table 14-1. Diagnostic tests for esophageal dysfunction

Test	Indications	Limitations
Barium esopha-gography	Initial evaluation of dysphagia without associated symptoms or overt esophageal obstruction Use of a 13-mm barium pill can provide important information	Limited assessment of mucosal detail No avenue for intervention Residual barium may inhibit follow-up endoscopic studies
Computed tomography	Assess for extrinsic lesions Staging of esophageal cancer	Limited sensitivity for the detection of lymphadenopathy
Endoscopy	Evaluation for mucosal disease of the esophagus Evaluation of odynophagia Screening/surveillance for Barrett's esophagus Mucosal biopsy Esophageal dilation Evaluation of suspected infectious esophagitis	Less sensitive than barium studies for assessment of mild to moderate luminal narrowing Relatively invasive
Endoscopic ultra-sonography	Assessment of submucosal lesions Staging of esophageal neoplasms	Inconvenient Limited clinical availability If dilation is required to use instrument, there is a high risk of perforation
Esophageal manometry	Evaluation of dysphagia not explained by results from other tests Assessment before fundoplication	Poor yield in evaluation of chest pain syndromes
Ambulatory pH monitoring	Assessing acid exposure/reflux as a cause of chest pain Monitor effectiveness of acid suppression in GERD Identification of GERD as a cause of extraesophageal symptoms such as asthma, cough, or hoarseness	Inconvenient Results may be variable 20% false-negative rate even in patients with esophagitis

GERD, gastrointestinal reflux disease.

pling to evaluate for histopathologic changes. Endoscopic techniques also provide a means for esophageal dilation if a stricture is encountered. Barium esophagography can show evidence of severe esophageal injury; however, this study is less useful in milder GERD. The use of barium liquid and pills may be more sensitive for the detection of esophageal narrowings than is endoscopy. Ambulatory pH monitoring (combined with a symptom diary) is particularly useful in the evaluation of patients who do not respond to typical therapies and who have minimal findings by other tests (*J Thorac Cardiovasc Surg*

Table 14-2. Dosing antacid therapy

Drug	Dose for GERD	Dose for active PUD	Maintenance therapy	Nonulcer dyspepsia
H$_2$RAs[a]				
Cimetidine	400 mg PO bid–qid[b]	800 mg PO qp.m.[c]	400 mg PO qa.m.	400 mg PO bid
Famotidine	20–40 mg PO bid[b]	40 mg PO qp.m.[c]	20 mg PO qa.m.	20 mg PO bid
Nizatidine	150 mg PO bid–qid[b]	300 mg PO qp.m.[c]	150 mg PO qa.m.	150 mg PO bid
Ranitidine	150 mg PO bid–qid[b]	300 mg PO qp.m.[c]	150 mg PO qa.m.	150 mg PO bid
Proton pump inhibitors				
Esomeprazole	40 mg PO qa.m.–bid[d]	40 mg PO qa.m.[e]	40 mg PO qa.m.	40 mg PO qa.m.
Lansoprazole	30 mg PO qa.m.–bid[d]	30 mg PO qa.m.[e]	15 mg PO qa.m.	30 mg PO bid
Omeprazole	20 mg PO qa.m.–bid[d]	20 mg PO qa.m.[e]	20 mg PO qa.m.	20 mg PO qa.m.
Pantoprazole	40 mg PO qa.m.–bid[d]	40 mg PO qa.m.[e]	40 mg PO qa.m.	40 mg PO qa.m.
Rabeprazole	20 mg PO qa.m.–bid[d]	20 mg PO qa.m.[e]	20 mg PO qa.m.	20 mg PO qa.m.

GERD, gastroesophageal reflux disease; PUD, peptic ulcer disease; H$_2$RAs, histamine-2 receptor antagonists.
[a]Doses should be modified in the setting of renal insufficiency.
[b]Lower doses are preferred for patients with nonerosive esophagitis; higher doses are preferred for patients with erosive esophagitis. Timing of dose might be between breakfast and lunch for the first dose and between dinner and bedtime for the second dose.
[c]Dose given between evening meal and bedtime. Therapy should be continued for 6–8 wks.
[d]Dose is titrated for individual patient needs. The first dose should be given before breakfast, and if needed the second dose should be given before the evening meal.
[e]Therapy should be continued for 4–6 wks.

1980;79:656, and *Gastroenterology* 1996;110:1982). Table 14-1 reviews tests that are commonly used to evaluate esophageal disease.
   D. **Treatment** should be organized in a stepwise approach, starting with conservative and then progressing to more aggressive treatments as needed.
      1. For some patients with mild or infrequent episodes of symptomatic GERD, **lifestyle modification** may be all that is required. Management recommendations along this line include (1) avoiding large meals, (2) avoiding eating 2–3 hours before lying down, (3) avoiding foods and beverages that can decrease the lower-esophageal sphincter pressure, (4) avoiding tight-fitting garments, (5) losing weight, and (6) elevating the head of one's bed (placement of 4- to 6-in. blocks underneath the legs of the bed is preferred over propping the head up with pillows).
      2. **Acid suppression.** Over-the-counter antacids (30 ml of a high-potency liquid antacid) may be sufficient for patients with very mild GERD. Histamine-2 receptor antagonists (H$_2$RAs) can be useful as well; large doses are often required. The proton pump inhibitors (PPIs) are clearly superior to the H$_2$RAs in providing rapid symptom relief and esophageal healing from GERD (*Gastroenterology* 1987;92:1306, and *Gastroenterol-*

ogy 1997;112:1798). Among patients for whom PPIs are required to provide relief, maintenance therapy with these drugs is commonly needed to achieve sustained freedom from symptoms (*N Engl J Med* 1995;333: 1106). Table 14-2 lists acid-suppressing agents and suggested doses. Adverse effects from acid-suppressing agents are discussed in Gastric and Duodenal Diseases, Peptic Ulcer Disease, secs. **F.2.a** and **F.2.b.**

3. **Promotility drugs** may be useful in the management of GERD. These medications enhance gastric emptying and increase lower-esophageal sphincter pressure. Metoclopramide (5–20 mg PO qac and qhs) can be helpful in the management of GERD. Downsides to therapy with metoclopramide include tachyphylaxis and CNS side effects (e.g., drowsiness, psychiatric symptoms, and extrapyramidal reactions). These side effects should sharply limit the use of metoclopramide for GERD. Cisapride has been largely removed from the American market because of concerns related to the potential induction of fatal cardiac dysrhythmias. Although intriguing drugs, prokinetic agents alone typically produce relief and sustain remission only in milder cases of GERD (*N Engl J Med* 1995;333:1106).

4. **Antireflux surgery** is an option that is appropriate in the management of patients with **well-established** GERD that is refractory to medical treatment or for patients who wish to avoid lifelong acid suppression (*N Engl J Med* 1992;326:786). Before one pursues this option, efforts to assess the clinical significance of reflux disease with endoscopy and 24-hour ambulatory pH monitoring must be performed. Esophageal manometry must also be done to assess for adequate esophageal motility; severe dysphagia can result if antireflux surgery is performed in a patient with poor esophageal peristalsis. Laparoscopic fundoplication has important safety and recovery time advantages over previously standard open surgical techniques.

E. **Complications of GERD.** The major complications of GERD are dysphagia (either with or without an esophageal stricture) and Barrett's metaplasia of the esophagus.

1. **Esophageal strictures** may result from chronic esophageal injury related to acid reflux. When dysphagia results, esophageal dilation is frequently needed. Some patients experience dysphagia from erosive or ulcerative esophagitis without an accompanying luminal narrowing; in this setting, a therapeutic trial of medical therapy without dilation is appropriate (*Gastroenterology* 1994;106:907). Dysphagia in a patient with GERD should also raise suspicion for other possible pathologies, including esophageal malignancy, Schatzki's ring (a mucosal ring of the distal esophagus that is invariably associated with a hiatus hernia), and esophageal webs (often associated with iron deficiency).

2. **Barrett's esophagus** is a metaplastic (not an inflammatory) condition of the esophagus. It is characterized by the transformation of squamous mucosa to columnar mucosa. Only Barrett's mucosa with specialized intestinal metaplasia (columnar mucosa with mucin-secreting goblet cells) is associated with a high (0.4–0.8%) annual incidence for the development of adenocarcinoma. Most authorities agree that patients with established Barrett's esophagus (who are candidates for esophagectomy) should have surveillance endoscopy with biopsies every 6–24 months to assess for dysplastic changes that are suggestive of degeneration toward malignancy. The frequency of the endoscopic evaluation might be based on the nature of the histologic changes. Additionally, some experts advocate a single upper endoscopy as surveillance for Barrett's metaplasia in patients who have experienced at least 10 years of GERD symptoms. Esophagectomy should be reserved for patients with established malignancy or for those who are confirmed to have high-grade dysplastic changes that persist after a trial of potent acid suppression (*Arch Intern Med* 1999;159:1411).

II. Motor disorders of the esophagus

A. Achalasia is the most common disorder of esophageal motility. Incomplete relaxation of the lower-esophageal sphincter with swallowing and the absence of esophageal peristalsis are the defining features. This disorder typically presents as chronically progressive dysphagia, first to solids and later to liquids. This is usually associated with weight loss.

1. The **diagnosis of achalasia** is suggested by barium esophagography that shows a dilated esophageal body with a "bird's beak" tapering at the lower-esophageal sphincter. Definitive establishment of achalasia is by esophageal manometry showing the defining features of the disorder. In evaluating patients with suspected idiopathic (probably autoimmune) achalasia, upper endoscopy is mandatory to exclude mass lesions of the gastric cardia that can produce a similar motility disorder of the esophagus, termed **pseudoachalasia**.

2. The **treatment of achalasia** is complex and requires a multidisciplinary approach with treatments tailored to individual patient needs. Therapeutic options include medical treatment with nifedipine or isosorbide dinitrate, endoscopic injection of the lower-esophageal sphincter with botulinum toxin, endoscopic pneumatic balloon dilation of the lower-esophageal sphincter, and surgical myotomy of the lower-esophageal sphincter that is usually accompanied by an antireflux operation. As a general rule, the more invasive options are associated with a higher risk of complications, but they offer a higher chance of providing immediate and sustained symptomatic improvement (*Am J Gastroenterol* 1999;94:3406).

B. Other primary motility disorders of the esophagus are much less defined than is achalasia. These disorders include **diffuse esophageal spasm** (potentially intense but nonperistaltic contractions) and **nutcracker esophagus** (a disorder characterized by high-amplitude but well-ordered esophageal peristalsis). These disorders may be the root of some chest pain syndromes, but they are difficult to diagnose. Manometry is diagnostically useful among fewer than 5% of patients (*Am J Gastroenterol* 1998;93:2359).

C. Systemic illnesses associated with esophageal dysmotility include systemic sclerosis, diabetes mellitus, intestinal pseudo-obstruction, and Chagas' disease. Preserved proximal esophageal motility (striated muscle), aperistalsis of the distal esophagus, and hypotension of the lower-esophageal sphincter (both of which are smooth-muscle functions under autonomic control) characterize esophageal involvement with systemic sclerosis. Because of this pattern of dysmotility, systemic sclerosis places patients at high risk of GERD and its complications. In these cases, aggressive medical therapy is preferred, but surgical therapy can be cautiously considered in extreme situations (*Surg Clin North Am* 1983;63:859).

III. Esophageal cancer

A. Incidence. The overall occurrence rate of esophageal malignancies has been static, although there has been a remarkable shift in the histopathology of these devastating tumors. Since the 1970s, the incidence of squamous cell esophageal tumors has diminished, but the risk of adenocarcinoma has increased (*JAMA* 1991;265:1287).

B. Diagnosis. Although barium esophagography can provide some information about esophageal pathology, endoscopy with biopsy is the primary method for the diagnosis of esophageal carcinoma. Esophageal tumors are usually discovered when endoscopy is performed to evaluate dysphagia or GI bleeding. Outside of surveillance for established cases of Barrett's esophagus, there are no validated screening guidelines for esophageal cancer (*Am J Gastroenterol* 1999;94:20).

C. Treatment. Staging plays a pivotal role in the management of esophageal cancers. Staging should follow TNM (tumor, nodes, metastases) guidelines. Endoscopic ultrasonography and CT scanning play pivotal roles in this evaluation. Patients with early disease (stages 0, I, and IIA) are usually cured with surgery alone. In advanced esophageal cancer (stages IIB and III), surgery with adjuvant and neoadjuvant radiation and chemotherapy (usually cisplatin and 5-fluorouracil) is associated with modest prolongation of survival but with high morbidity and low cure rates. For most patients with advanced regional or metastatic disease, palliative treatment with radiation, chemotherapy, and endoscopic techniques (laser ablation and stent placement) can improve dysphagia. Photodynamic therapy (the administration and local activation of laser-light–activated chemotherapy) is available, but its widespread application has yet to be standardized (*Am J Gastroenterol* 1999;94:20, and *Br J Surg* 1999;86:727).

Gastric and Duodenal Diseases

I. PUD

A. Ulcers are defects of the GI mucosa that extend through the muscularis mucosa into the submucosa or muscularis propria. Erosions are similar but more superficial defects. The unifying feature of peptic lesions is that their fundamental etiology is the interaction of gastric acid and pepsin. Peptic ulcers are common lesions with an annual incidence of approximately 1% in North America.

B. Etiology. Under normal conditions, mechanisms, including mucous/bicarbonate barrier, epithelial cell extrusion of acid with blood flow–mediated removal of absorbed acid, and the inherent barrier function of the epithelium, protect the lumen of the proximal GI tract from acid damage. When these mechanisms fail, epithelial cell injury can result. Even in the event of mucosal cell injury, ulcerogenesis is still inhibited by cellular restitution, cell replication, and wound healing. However, when the rate of cellular injury exceeds the protective and healing capacity of the mucosa, ulcer formation results. It is now understood that most ulcers develop in the setting of *Helicobacter pylori* infection or nonsteroidal anti-inflammatory drug (NSAID) use, or both. Less frequently, ulcers result from primary acid hypersecretory disorders or from other mucosal injury [*Aliment Pharmacol Ther* 1995;9(Suppl 2):59, *Ann Intern Med* 1994;120:977, *BMJ* 1997;315:1333, and *J Clin Gastroenterol* 1997;24:2].

  1. *H. pylori* are gram-negative, spiral-shaped, urease-producing bacteria that are trophic for the gastric epithelium. The organisms are resistant to acid lysis and, if untreated, cause a lifelong inflammatory response. *H. pylori* are adapted to an acid milieu and are much less able to survive in a neutral or basic environment. Through a complex mechanism of mucosal cell injury and induction of gastric acid secretion, these bacteria increase the risk of gastroduodenal ulcer, proximal GI tract lymphoma, and gastric adenocarcinoma [*Am J Gastroenterol* 1998;93:2330, and *Curr Opin Gastroenterol* 1998;14(Suppl 1):59].

  a. The **mode of transmission** of *H. pylori* infection remains uncertain. Available studies suggest person-to-person spread, with most infections acquired during childhood. Urban settings and poor sanitation are risk factors for infection. The rate of new infections in North America is dropping at present (*Am J Gastroenterol* 1998;93:2330).

  b. Many techniques are available to diagnose the presence of *H. pylori*. **Mucosal biopsy** with histopathologic examination is currently the most sensitive and specific test for the presence of *H. pylori* (approximately 95%). Such sampling requires the application of invasive testing to acquire tissue samples. Biopsy samples can also be placed in specialized agar gels to test for urease activity. These rapid urease tests are inexpensive, convenient, and relatively sensitive and specific (approximately 90%). Less invasive techniques may also have a role in the testing for *H. pylori*. **Urea breath tests** are extremely sensitive and specific tests for *H. pylori* that use ^{13}C or ^{14}C orally ingested urea; if urease activity is present in the stomach, the label can be detected in exhaled carbon dioxide. The urea breath techniques are the preferred test for noninvasively assessing for *H. pylori* eradication after treatment. With the agar urease and the urease breath tests, the risk of false-negative results among patients who take PPIs is high. By substantially increasing gastric pH, these drugs suppress *H. pylori* replication (and urease production) and thereby adversely affect the sensitivity of these tests. **Serologic testing** for immunoglobulin G (IgG; IgA and IgM measurements are less preferred) antibodies against *H. pylori* as an initial test is highly specific and sensitive for infection. Although antibody levels tend to fall after successful eradication, they can persist, so that the diagnostic value of a positive result after antibiotic therapy is reduced. A negative result confirms eradication (*Gastroenterology* 1995;109:136).

C. **Clinical presentation.** Symptoms of PUD are nonspecific and poorly sensitive markers. Patients can be entirely asymptomatic, with approximately 1–3% of adult patients having silent ulcers. The use of NSAIDs and the presence of diabetes can increase the risk for silent ulcers. Symptomatic patients may present with complaints, including abdominal pain, increased appetite, anorexia, weight loss, nausea/vomiting, heartburn, food intolerance, bloating, and belching. Complicated presentations that require emergency assessment include perforation, penetration, and brisk upper-GI hemorrhage. Up to 20% of patients who experience these serious complications may have been previously asymptomatic (*Gastroenterology* 1989;96:626).

D. **Diagnosis.** In young patients (<45 years) with symptoms suggestive of PUD who do not have alarm symptoms (such as weight loss, dysphagia, or early satiety), empiric serologic testing for *H. pylori* (with treatment if positive) and a therapeutic trial of acid suppression may be warranted (*Ann Intern Med* 1995;123:260). In older patients or those with concerning symptoms, imaging studies are standard. Imaging is also appropriately used for patients who have symptoms that are recalcitrant to a 6-week therapeutic trial with acid-suppressing drugs (*Gastroenterology* 1996;110:72). Imaging the gastric and duodenal mucosa can be done radiographically or endoscopically. Upper-GI barium radiography can have variable sensitivity and specificity that are greatly influenced by the experience of the radiologist and the technique used (air-contrast techniques are much more sensitive than single-contrast studies). Barium studies do not permit tissue sampling, and edematous mucosal folds may obscure dangerous pathology. On the whole, upper endoscopy is more sensitive and specific than are radiographic techniques, although with optimal radiographic techniques the sensitivities are comparable. After diagnosing PUD, it is imperative to segregate benign from malignant lesions. This is more important with gastric ulcers, as the incidence of gastric cancer substantially exceeds primary duodenal malignancies. For gastric ulcers, it is standard to exclude malignancy by extensive tissue sampling or follow-up endoscopy to ensure ulcer resolution (*Gastroenterology* 1993;105:1583).

E. **Zollinger-Ellison syndrome (ZES)** includes the triad of severe PUD, gastrin-secreting tumors, and gastric acid hypersecretion. The diagnosis should be considered among patients with ulcers that are distal to the duodenal bulb and multiple or medically refractory ulcers and patients with PUD accompanied by otherwise unexplained diarrhea. Approximately 90% of patients with gastrinomas have ulcers. The diagnosis of ZES is suggested by the clinical presentation along with serum tests that confirm the presence of a gastrinoma. Laboratory tests that are suggestive of ZES include a markedly elevated fasting serum gastrin (>1000 pg/ml), which, in the right clinical setting, establishes the diagnosis (*Annu Rev Med* 1995;46:395). Caution is necessary for interpreting serum gastrin levels as atrophic gastritis and the use of PPIs can both lead to profound hypergastrinemia (>1000 pg/ml). Provocative tests measure serum gastrin in response to intravenous secretin, intravenous calcium infusion, or ingestion of a test meal. The **secretin stimulation test** is the most widely standardized; therefore, it is the test of choice for evaluating patients with suspected gastrinomas but normal or minimally elevated serum gastrin levels (*Ann Intern Med* 1974;81:758). The **treatment of ZES** starts with aggressive acid-suppression therapy (lansoprazole, 60 mg PO qd to 90 mg PO bid, or omeprazole, 60 mg PO qd to 120 mg PO bid) (*Gastroenterology* 2000;118:S9). Exhaustive efforts should be pursued to locate the tumors when the diagnosis is established. The prognosis is guarded, as more than 50% of patients may die as a result of untreatable gastrinomas. Helpful imaging studies include OctreoScan (a nuclear medicine scan that uses a radiolabeled somatostatin analogue), CT scan, and mesenteric angiography. If ZES is diagnosed, even if a tumor is not located by imaging studies, surgical exploration should be pursued.

F. **Ulcer treatment.** When ulcers are diagnosed, *H. pylori* infection should be sought and, if present, should be treated. NSAIDs and aspirin should be discontinued if medically feasible. Therapy to eradicate *H. pylori* is all that is necessary for patients with low-risk PUD who become asymptomatic after treatment. This low-risk category includes nonsmoking patients who are able to avoid NSAIDs and who have had no complications of bleeding, penetration, or perforation (*Ann Intern Med* 1992;116:705). Acid-suppressing medication should be used as outlined in Table 14-2. Maintenance acid-suppression therapy should be used for patients with recurrent, refractory, giant, or complicated ulcers. Maintenance therapy is also advised for patients who smoke or continue to use NSAIDs, as well as for patients whose medical condition might be severely compromised by recurrent ulcers.

1. **Treatment/eradication of *H. pylori*.** The decision to test a patient for *H. pylori* must be accompanied by the intention to treat that infection if it is discovered (*Am J Gastroenterol* 1998;93:2330). Treatment of *H. pylori* requires the use of one or two nonantibiotic agents (usually colloidal bismuth and either a PPI or H₂RA). Many regimens have been tried and reported. Only those that have a better than 90% eradication rate should be standard. Two drug regimens have a lower success rate and should not be considered first line. Typically, metronidazole or clarithromycin is required, but resistant organisms have been detected. It is reasonable to start with either a metronidazole- or clarithromycin-containing regimen and, if infection is shown to persist, switch to a regimen based on the other drug (*N Engl J Med* 1995;333:984). Specific regimens to treat *H. pylori* are outlined in Table 14-3. Once *H. pylori* infection is treated, it is often appropriate to **retest** for successful eradication, especially for patients who have had a complicated ulcer and for those with persistent or recurrent symptoms (*Am J Gastroenterol* 1998;93:2330). The need for eradication testing is also important when maintenance therapy is to be avoided.

2. **Antiulcer pharmacology**

   a. **H₂RAs.** Cimetidine, ranitidine, famotidine, and nizatidine are drugs that suppress gastric acid secretion by blocking stimulating receptors on gastric parietal cells. These drugs are well absorbed after oral administration. They are cleared by hepatic and renal metabolism but poorly removed by dialysis. Although dose reduction is preferred when patients with renal disease are treated, dose reduction is probably not required in liver dysfunction (unless accompanied by renal failure). Cimetidine has rare side effects including gynecomastia. Cimetidine may also interfere with the metabolism of drugs that are processed through the cytochrome P-450 system (e.g., warfarin, theophylline, phenytoin, diazepam, and propranolol). Otherwise,

Table 14-3. Recommended protocols for eradication of *Helicobacter pylori*

Triple therapies (14-day therapy recommended)

Omeprazole, 20 mg PO bid; lansoprazole, 30 mg PO bid; rabeprazole, 20 mg PO bid; or ranitidine bismuth citrate, PO bid

and two of the following:

Amoxicillin, 1 g PO bid

Clarithromycin, 500 mg PO bid

Metronidazole, 500 mg PO bid

Quadruple therapy (7–14 day therapy recommended—longer duration of therapy may have slight cure rate advantage)

Omeprazole, 20 mg PO bid; lansoprazole, 30 mg PO bid; or rabeprazole, 30 mg PO bid

Tetracycline, 500 mg PO qid

Metronidazole, 500 mg PO tid

Bismuth subsalicylate, 2 tablets PO qid

Adapted from DY Graham. Therapy of *Helicobacter pylori*: current status and issues. *Gastroenterology* 2000;118:S2–S8.

these drugs are associated with only rare idiosyncratic reactions. Dosing recommendations are shown in Table 14-2.

  b. **PPIs.** Omeprazole, lansoprazole, rabeprazole, pantoprazole, and esomeprazole are powerful suppressors of gastric acid secretion. They work by reversibly inhibiting the parietal cell H^+K^+–adenosine triphosphatase. These drugs have an excellent therapeutic index. Only rarely do patients experience headache or idiosyncratic secretory diarrhea. Maximal acid suppression from PPIs usually occurs after 4 days of conventional administration. The PPIs are principally cleared by hepatic metabolism, and the safety profile of these drugs makes dose adjustment unnecessary. Dosing recommendations are shown in Table 14-2.

  c. **Sucralfate** is a topically active drug that in an acid environment forms a film to provide a protective barrier for the mucosa. The medication is usually administered at a dose of 1 g four times/day. Side effects are not severe but may include constipation.

G. **The role of NSAIDs.** The dose-related link between NSAIDs and GI injury, especially PUD, is well recognized. The two fundamental issues that arise are ulcer treatment and ulcer prevention.

  1. **Treatment of NSAID ulcers.** NSAID-induced ulcer disease can be treated with any approved therapy for ulcer disease. It is preferable to stop NSAID therapy when ulcer disease occurs. New selective cyclooxygenase-2 inhibitors may be preferred when NSAID therapy must be continued, although they do not eliminate the risk of ulcer, are costly, and may be associated with fluid retention. Maintenance doses of PPIs are the preferred antiulcer drugs when NSAIDs must be continued in the presence of ulcer disease (*N Engl J Med* 1998;338:727). Testing for and treatment against *H. pylori* is also recommended for NSAID users who have ulcers.

  2. **Prevention of NSAID ulcers.** A history of PUD, advanced age (>60 years), concurrent corticosteroid therapy, and anticoagulant therapy enhance the risk for NSAID-related GI complications (*Ann Intern Med* 1991;115:787, and *Am J Gastroenterol* 1998;93:2037). High-risk patients should be considered for ulcer prophylaxis if NSAIDs are

needed. **Misoprostol** is a synthetic prostaglandin that is effective in ulcer prophylaxis. Doses of 200 μg PO qid are most effective, but lower doses of 200 μg PO bid may also be beneficial. Although the higher doses are commonly associated with diarrhea and abdominal discomfort, the lower-dose regimens have an adverse effect profile that is only modestly worse than that of placebo. H_2RAs are probably effective at preventing NSAID-induced duodenal ulcers but do not seem to prevent gastric ulceration. On the other hand, PPIs are effective in preventing gastric and duodenal ulcers (*N Engl J Med* 1998;338:719).

Diseases of the Small Bowel and Colon

I. **Inflammatory bowel disease (IBD).** Ulcerative colitis (UC) and Crohn's disease (CD) are the most clinically important IBDs. They have similar epidemiologies in that both are most commonly diagnosed between ages 15 and 35 years, although onset can occur at any time in life and both genders are equally affected. UC is an idiopathic chronic disease that is defined by mucosal inflammation of the large bowel. The inflammatory changes always involve the distal rectum and extend proximally in a circumferential and uninterrupted distribution. The length of involved colon varies. In severe cases, the entire large bowel and distal portion of the terminal ileum may be involved. With long-standing disease, UC patients are at increased risk for the development of colorectal malignancy. This risk is especially high for patients with pancolonic inflammation and for those with an 8- to 10-year history of the disease. Even patients with limited disease may be at an increased cancer risk, but usually this higher risk begins 20 or 30 years into the disease history (*Gastroenterology* 1983;85:22). Patients who face this risk of malignancy should undergo annual colonoscopy, with surveillance biopsies performed to evaluate for dysplastic changes. CD is a distinct disease that is characterized by transmural intestinal inflammation. Unlike UC, CD can involve any part of the GI tract from the oropharynx to the anus, and the inflammatory process is usually asymmetric, with skip areas of normal tissue separating diseased intestinal segments. The transmural nature of CD presents a risk of internal or enterocutaneous fistula formation, abdominal abscess formation, and luminal stricture development from chronic scarring. Distinct pathologies distinguishing CD that involves only the colon from UC can be difficult.
   A. **Manifestations**
      1. Bloody diarrhea with associated rectal urgency and tenesmus is the hallmark presentation of active **UC**. Symptoms can be less marked or absent during relative remissions (*Medicine* 1966;45:391).
      2. The manifestations of **CD** vary sharply with the degree and segment of intestinal involvement. Characteristic symptoms include chronic or nocturnal diarrhea, abdominal pain, anorexia, weight loss, aphthous stomatitis, or potentially destructive perianal inflammation (*N Engl J Med* 1996;334:841).
      3. The systemic inflammation seen with IBD can be associated with **extraintestinal manifestations**. In some instances, the severity of these manifestations is directly related to disease (usually colonic) activity, and treatment of the IBD improves these extracolonic symptoms (*Dig Dis Sci* 1999;44:1). Malabsorption from IBD can also lead to systemic consequences.
         a. **Joint involvement.** Central arthropathies, including **ankylosing spondylitis** and **sacroiliitis**, are associated with CD more often than with UC. These diseases correlate poorly with the activity of the

underlying intestinal inflammation. On the other hand, IBD-associated peripheral arthropathies tend to flare with colonic inflammation. This acute inflammatory arthropathy occurs in approximately 10–15% of patients with an acute attack of colonic IBD. The joint involvement is usually asymmetric and affects larger joints (knees, hips, ankles, wrists, and elbows). Treatment of the underlying colitis usually improves this inflammatory arthritis (*Primary Care* 1984;11:271, and *N Engl J Med* 1959;261:259).

    b. Skin involvement. Several cutaneous manifestations are noted with IBD. **Erythema nodosum** (seen more often with CD than UC) is a painful, poorly demarcated nodular lesion that tends to be bilateral (but not symmetric). It is almost invariably related to the activity of colitis but may also be an adverse effect of sulfasalazine administration. **Pyoderma gangrenosum** (seen more often with UC than CD) is a debilitating skin disease characterized by irregular, blue-red ulcers with purulent necrotic bases. In declining order of frequency, these lesions are noted on the lower extremities, buttocks, abdomen, and face. Although treatment of the underlying colitis usually improves pyoderma, occasional patients have persistent problems even if the colitis is controlled (*Inflamm Bowel Dis* 1998;4:71).

    c. Ocular involvement. Episcleritis or anterior uveitis occurs in 5–8% of patients with active colitis. In addition to management of IBD, topical treatment with corticosteroid ocular preparations may also be beneficial.

B. The **diagnosis** of IBD is suspected on clinical grounds. Testing is necessary to segregate idiopathic IBD from other forms of mucosal inflammation and from noninflammatory disorders such as irritable bowel syndrome (IBS).

    1. In a patient with symptoms that are suggestive of **UC**, stool examination and sigmoidoscopy with biopsy should be performed. This confirms colonic inflammation, delineates the pattern of involvement, and aids in the exclusion of infectious causes. Rectal involvement with proximal symmetric extension strongly suggests UC. Colonoscopy and contrast enema may also be helpful, but the clinician should use caution with these tests in the setting of an active flare of IBD.

    2. The diagnosis of **CD** can be confirmed by endoscopic, radiographic, or pathologic studies that demonstrate the typical focal, asymmetric, transmural, and occasionally granulomatous features of CD. The mainstays of diagnosis include endoscopy (especially colonoscopy with attempted terminal ileoscopy) and contrast radiography (especially small-bowel follow-through or enteroclysis), which help to identify the pattern and character of mucosal disease. Findings of rectal-sparing, skip lesions, small-bowel (especially ileal) disease, luminal strictures, and deep linear mucosal ulcers suggest CD disease over UC (*Med Clin North Am* 1990;74:51).

C. Treatment. Medical therapies are the initial management of IBD. Surgical therapy is reserved to treat disease that is unresponsive to medical management and steroid-dependent disease (especially in the setting of steroid-induced complications). Colectomy is also indicated when dysplastic changes (unrelated to direct inflammation) are found in patients with colitis.

    1. Medical therapy. The general principles of medical management of CD and UC are the induction and maintenance of remission. The location of the intestinal disease activity and the nature of extraintestinal problems should be noted, and therapy should be appropriately targeted to maximize benefit while minimizing the chances of drug toxicity. The most often used medical therapies and dosages are outlined below and in Table 14-4 (*Am J Gastroenterol* 1997;92:204, and *Am J Gastroenterol* 1997;92:559).

Table 14-4. Oral and topical agents used in the management of inflammatory bowel disease

Drug	Indications	Dose	Adverse effects
Aminosalicylates			
Sulfasalazine	Ulcerative colitis: therapy of mild to moderate active disease and maintenance of remission Crohn's disease: therapy of mildly active disease limited to the colon; role in maintenance is debated	Active disease: 2–6 g PO qd, usually in 3–4 divided doses; start with low dose and titrate upward Maintenance: 2 g PO bid	Anorexia, dyspepsia, nausea, headache, hemolysis, reversible azoospermia, folate malabsorption, agranulocytosis, alopecia, hepatitis
Olsalazine	Same as sulfasalazine	500 mg PO bid	15% incidence of secretory diarrhea even with decreased colon inflammation in addition to side effects listed for Asacol
Asacol (enteric-coated mesalamine)	Same as sulfasalazine	Active disease: 1.6–6.4 g PO qd in 2–4 divided doses Maintenance: 800 mg PO bid	Rare side effects include headache, rash, drug fever, pneumonitis, pericarditis, cholestasis, and pancreatitis
Pentasa (controlled-release mesalamine)	Crohn's disease: mild to moderately active small-bowel disease with or without colonic involvement; role in maintenance is debated	1 g PO qid	Same as Asacol
Rowasa (mesalamine) suppository	Treatment and maintenance of ulcerative or Crohn's proctitis; may be used as adjunct to oral therapy	500 mg PR bid	—
Rowasa (mesalamine) enema	Treatment and maintenance of left-sided ulcerative colitis or distal colonic Crohn's disease; can be used as adjunct to oral therapy	60 ml (4 g) as overnight retention enema	—

Corticosteroids			
Prednisone	Treatment of mildly to severely active ulcerative colitis and Crohn's disease	40 mg PO qa.m. dose should be tapered	Sleep/mood disturbances, cutaneous changes, osteodystrophy, aseptic necrosis, hypertension, cataracts, glucose intolerance, immunosuppression
	Should not be used as maintenance		
Hydrocortisone suppository/foam	Mildly to moderately active ulcerative proctitis or Crohn's proctitis; can be used as adjunct to oral therapy	10–100 mg PR qd or bid	
Hydrocortisone suppository	Mildly to moderately active ulcerative proctitis or Crohn's proctitis; can be used as adjunct to oral therapy		
Immunomodulators			
6-mercaptopurine or azathioprine	Adjunctive therapy in the long-term treatment of active ulcerative colitis and Crohn's disease	6-mercaptopurine, 1.5 mg/kg qd	Nausea, drug fever, rash, arthralgia, bone marrow suppression, pancreatitis, hepatitis, immunosuppression
	Steroid-sparing therapy in patients with steroid-dependent Crohn's disease and select patients with ulcerative colitis	Azathioprine, 2.0–2.5 mg/kg qd	
Antibiotics			
Ciprofloxacin	Data supporting use of these drugs are limited	500 mg PO bid	Nausea, vomiting, headache, restlessness, rash, hepatitis
Metronidazole	Crohn's disease: induction of remission and maintenance of active disease, fistulous disease, and perianal disease	250 mg PO qid	Anorexia, nausea, vomiting, peripheral neuropathy, disulfiram-like response
	Ulcerative colitis: may be useful in maintenance		

Source: BE Sands. Therapy of inflammatory bowel disease. *Gastroenterology* 2000;118:S68–S82, with permission.

a. **Aminosalicylates.** 5'-ASA drugs are the initial selection to treat patients with IBD. They should be used with extreme caution when treating patients who have aspirin hypersensitivity. These drugs are indicated in the treatment of active CD and UC. In low doses, they are also particularly useful in decreasing the frequency of disease exacerbation in UC; the role of such maintenance therapy in CD is less established.

(1) **Sulfasalazine** reaches the colon intact, where it is metabolized by colonic bacteria to a sulfapyridine moiety (simply functions as a carrier for 5'-ASA but is responsible for toxicity) and 5'-ASA. This drug is useful only for the treatment of colonic disease. Most side effects of sulfasalazine are dose related but greatly limit its application. They include nausea/vomiting, headache, abdominal pain, azoospermia, and yellow discoloration of tears, sweat, and urine. Additionally, sulfasalazine interferes with normal folic acid absorption; therefore, patients who are treated chronically with this drug should be given a folate supplement. Sulfasalazine is relatively inexpensive, and therefore it is often the first-choice aminosalicylate to treat patients with IBD colitis.

(2) **Olsalazine** is a 5'-ASA dimer. Bacterial-mediated cleavage in the colon releases active drug. Although this might seem an ideal preparation, approximately 10–15% of patients who are given this drug have idiosyncratic secretory diarrhea that necessitates changing to a different aminosalicylate preparation.

(3) **Mesalamine** (5'-ASA) can be given orally only when protected by an enteric-coated or pH-mediated release capsule. Without such a capsule, the drug is promptly absorbed and degraded before it can exert its mucosal activity on the more distal intestine. Although access to oral mesalamine pills may be limited by expense, these controlled-release preparations are available and are useful in the treatment of small-bowel and colonic inflammation. With the absence of a sulfapyridine moiety, oral mesalamine preparations can be administered at high doses with few adverse effects. Because of their cost, these drugs are frequently reserved to treat patients with small-bowel inflammation or those who are intolerant to sulfasalazine. They are marketed under the trade names Asacol and Pentasa. Asacol is designed to release the mesalamine for topical activity in the colon. Pentasa is designed to release mesalamine into the small bowel. Therefore, Pentasa may be particularly useful in the management of patients with CD and jejunoileal involvement. Finally, mesalamine as a rectal suppository (to treat the distal 10–20 cm of the rectum) or an enema (to treat the distal 30–60 cm of the large intestine) is useful for the respective treatment of proctitis or left-sided colitis (*Drugs* 1999;57:383).

b. **Glucocorticoids** are commonly used in the management of IBD. They are most appropriately used concomitantly with other medical therapies. Topical and systemic preparations are used, but systemic therapy should be used sparingly and with extreme caution if infectious complications are not excluded. Steroids are not recommended for maintenance therapy because of the associated metabolic and osseous side effects. Typically, systemic steroids are reserved for patients with moderate to severe disease that is not controlled using 5'-ASA drugs. Common starting doses are prednisone, 20–40 mg/day, with higher doses offering little benefit but presenting markedly increased toxicity risks. If higher doses are pondered, hospitalization is likely needed. Once a therapeutic effect is seen, the clinician should pursue a taper over 2–3 months to attempt to eliminate the therapy (*Gastroenterology* 2000;118;S68). Topical steroids are available in suppository, foam, and enema forms. These are a useful primary therapy or adjunct in the management of patients with rectal or left colon disease.

c. **Immunosuppression. 6-Mercaptopurine (6-MP)** and its prodrug **azathioprine (AZA)** are becoming increasingly widely used in the management of IBD. These drugs are especially used to treat patients with CD who have recurrent disease flares or who are unable to be weaned from steroids without recurrent flares. These drugs are also useful for UC patients with similar difficulties. Once these drugs are selected, 3–6 months of administration may be required before the full therapeutic benefit is noted. An expected side effect of 6-MP and AZA includes occasional bone marrow suppression; therefore, the patient's CBC should be followed at least every 3 months. A common idiosyncratic effect of these drugs is pancreatitis. If pancreatitis develops, the drug should be immediately discontinued; repeat challenge with either 6-MP or AZA is contraindicated. On the other hand, if a patient is intolerant of 6-MP or AZA, for reasons other than pancreatitis, a trial with the other drug may be successful in up to 40%. Other immunosuppressing drugs, including methotrexate and cyclosporin, have been used successfully, but the availability of high-quality data is much less well established than with 6-MP or AZA (*Hepatogastroenterology* 1999;46:2265).

d. **Antibiotics.** Although data are limited, metronidazole has also been advocated in the armamentarium against colonic IBD. In some patients with perianal, fistulizing, or mildly active CD, monotherapy with this antibiotic may be partly helpful (*Am J Gastroenterol* 1984;79:533, and *Gut* 1991;32:1071). The long-term safety profile of chronic metronidazole therapy is poorly understood, however, and the clinician must be careful to monitor for neurologic toxicity. Ciprofloxacin has also been tested in IBD, and initial data suggest only a limited role (*Gastroenterology* 1998;115:1072).

e. **Infliximab.** This U.S. Food and Drug Administration–approved drug is a monoclonal antibody against tumor necrosis factor. It is administered as an intravenous infusion and clearly has some role in the management of patients with medically recalcitrant CD and fistulas from CD (*Inflamm Bowel Dis* 1999;5:119). However, the drug is very new, and preapproval studies are limited. Data related to using this drug to treat UC are emerging.

f. Although **antidiarrheal drugs** are safe in mild colitis, they should be avoided in the setting of a severe infectious or IBD-colitis, as they can increase the risk for the development of toxic megacolon.

2. **Surgical management.** The surgical management of UC and CD differs drastically. Surgical indications for UC are dangerous hemorrhage, toxic megacolon/perforation, severe uncontrollable colitis, or extraintestinal manifestations. Patients who are steroid dependent and experiencing intolerable side effects from medications should also be considered for colectomy, and surgery should be considered for UC patients with dysplastic mucosa noted on surveillance biopsies. Typically, surgery for UC is total colectomy. Unlike with UC, surgery for CD is limited resection of disease segments. CD typically recurs after surgical resection, and surgery should therefore be reserved for patients with medically unresponsive complications or refractory disease.

II. **Microscopic colitis.** Two disorders are commonly referred to as **microscopic colitis: collagenous colitis and lymphocytic colitis.** These most commonly affect middle-aged to elderly women and are manifest as episodic, profound watery diarrhea that may be accompanied by fecal incontinence. These disorders may be associated with diabetes mellitus, an elevated erythrocyte sedimentation rate

(ESR), or other autoimmune processes. The diagnosis can only be established when clinical suspicion leads to random biopsies of an otherwise normal-appearing colon; histologic changes confirm the diagnosis. Treatment is usually symptomatic with the use of antidiarrheal drugs (e.g., loperamide or diphenoxylate-atropine). In more refractory cases, colloidal bismuth, antibiotics, aminosalicylates, or even steroids are helpful (*Semin Gastrointest Dis* 1999;10:145).

III. Celiac disease (also termed **celiac sprue** or **gluten-sensitive enteropathy**) is a mucosal disease of the small intestine. Histologically, the disease is characterized by villous atrophy that is commonly associated with mild crypt hyperplasia and inflammatory infiltrate. Celiac disease is accompanied by an increased risk for the development of small-bowel lymphomas, especially with long-standing disease activity (*N Engl J Med* 1991;325:1709).

   A. Clinically, the disease varies with the extent of the histologic changes (usually the proximal intestine is affected first, with the abnormalities propagating down the small bowel). The **manifestations**, which are principally the result of malabsorption, include diarrhea, weight loss, lassitude, iron and other micronutrient deficiencies, and abdominal bloating/discomfort. Extraintestinal manifestations may include dermatitis herpetiformis, which is a chronic, usually symmetric eruption of vesicles, papules, and urticarial wheals.

   B. The **diagnosis of celiac disease** is most accurately established by tissue sampling, usually endoscopic biopsies of the proximal duodenum. Serologic tests also play a role. Serum IgA antiendomysial antibody assays have a 100% specificity and 85–90% sensitivity for the diagnosis of untreated celiac disease; the titers of these antibodies may fall dramatically with gluten avoidance (*Am J Gastroenterol* 1999;94:3079). Antigliadin antibody assays are also readily available but are less sensitive and specific for the diagnosis of sprue (*Gut* 1996;39:43).

   C. Treatment. Prompt symptomatic improvement is usually noted with dietary avoidance of gluten-containing cereal grains. The most common cause of poor response is inadvertent dietary noncompliance. Still, lymphoma and severe forms of the disease, termed **refractory sprue** and **ulcerative jejunoileitis** (both associated with a poor prognosis), must be considered in those with persisting symptoms in spite of gluten avoidance (*Dig Dis Sci* 1999;17:100).

IV. Infectious diarrheas are categorized based on whether they affect the small intestine or colon, species type (bacterial or viral), and invasiveness. The offending organisms are listed and characterized in Table 14-5.

   A. Noninvasive small-bowel bacterial pathogens include *Staphylococcus aureus*, *Bacillus cereus*, and *Clostridium botulinum*, which all rapidly cause disease because of a preformed enterotoxin. *S. aureus* and *B. cereus* are treated conservatively. The severe neurologic symptoms that can result from botulism can be treated with an antitoxin. *Clostridium perfringens* and *Vibrio cholerae* usually produce a diarrheal illness after a brief incubation period. These illnesses are treatable conservatively, but antibiotics may shorten the duration of illness, especially from cholera. Enterotoxigenic *Escherichia coli* is the most common cause of travelers' diarrhea, and treatment is conservative, although antibiotics can be used prophylactically (see Chap. 19).

   B. Invasive small-bowel bacterial pathogens include enteropathogenic *E. coli*, *Salmonella typhi*, *Yersinia enterocolitica*, and *Listeria*. Nontyphoidal *Salmonella* species account for up to one-half of the foodborne enteric illnesses in the United States. Symptoms include fever, nausea, vomiting, and diarrhea. The diagnosis is established by stool culture, and although most patients improve with conservative management, antibiotics (e.g., ampicillin, amoxicillin, trimethoprim-sulfamethoxazole, or quinolones) are used to treat elderly and severely ill patients.

   C. Viral illnesses that affect the small bowel include rotavirus and Norwalk virus. These cause a severe diarrheal illness in children and, less often, in adults. Treatment is conservative.

Table 14-5. Infectious enteritis and colitis

Organism	Incubation (hrs)	Predominant symptom	Pathogenicity	Implicated food	Treatment
Staphylococcus aureus	1–8	Vomiting	Preformed enterotoxin	Salad, pastry, meat	Conservative
Bacillus cereus emetic disease, diarrheal disease	1–6, 6–14	Vomiting, diarrhea	Preformed enterotoxin	Fried rice, meat, creamed foods, salad	Conservative
Clostridium botulinum	12–36	Neurologic symptoms	Preformed enterotoxin	Raw honey, improperly canned foods	Antitoxin
Clostridium perfringens	8–24	Diarrhea	Enterotoxin	Meat, pasta salads, dairy products	Conservative, antibiotics
Vibrio cholerae	12–72	Diarrhea	Enterotoxin	Seafood, water	Tetracycline
Enterotoxigenic *Escherichia coli*	24–72	Diarrhea	Enterotoxin	Salad, fruit, meat, pastry	Conservative
Salmonella (nontyphoid)	8–48	Diarrhea	Invasion	Eggs, poultry	Ampicillin, amoxicillin, ciprofloxacin
Salmonella (typhoid)	3–60 days	Fever	V_i antigen	Eggs, poultry	TMP/SMX, ciprofloxacin
Rotavirus	48–72	Diarrhea	Invasion	Seafood, fresh water	Conservative
Norwalk virus	24–48	Diarrhea	Invasion	Shellfish, drinking water	Conservative
Shigella	24–72	Diarrhea	Invasion, enterotoxin	Water, infected food	Ciprofloxacin, tetracycline

(continued)

Table 14-5. (continued)

Organism	Incubation (hrs)	Predominant symptom	Pathogenicity	Implicated food	Treatment
Campylobacter	24–144	Diarrhea, sometimes bleeding	Invasion, cytotoxin	Poultry, eggs, raw milk, water	Usually conservative; severe cases: erythromycin, fluoroquinolones
Enteroinvasive *E. coli*	?	Diarrhea, sometimes bleeding	Invasion, ?cytotoxin	Meat, fruit	Usually conservative
Enterohemorrhagic *E. coli* (*E. coli* O157:H7)	12–24	Diarrhea	Shiga-like toxin	Poorly cooked ground beef, unpasteurized dairy products	Conservative
Clostridium difficile	Usually associated with antibiotic administration	Diarrhea	Cytotoxin	None	Discontinuation of unnecessary antibiotics; administration of metronidazole or oral vancomycin

TMP/SMX, trimethoprim-sulfamethoxazole.

D. Among the most common **colonic bacterial infections** are invasive pathogens such as *Shigella* and *Campylobacter* species. Infection from these organisms can lead to diarrhea, fever, abdominal pain, and GI bleeding. The diagnosis is usually confirmed by stool cultures. Although conservative management is often successful, fluoroquinolones, tetracycline, and trimethoprim-sulfamethoxazole are useful in treating *Shigella*. The role of antibiotics to treat *Campylobacter* is less well established; because of resistance to other antibiotics, erythromycin is now the drug of choice. *E. coli* O157:H7 is another invasive pathogen that has been popularized by outbreaks related to contaminated ground beef. Infection with this organism can lead to abdominal pain, bloody diarrhea, and systemic complications that include the hemolytic-uremic syndrome; treatment is supportive. *Clostridium difficile* is a toxigenic bacterial pathogen that colonizes the colon when the usual colonic flora is altered by antibiotics or immunosuppressing medications. It causes severe diarrhea; bleeding rarely occurs. Treatment includes discontinuation of contributing antibiotics; 10-day treatment with metronidazole or oral vancomycin is commonly used as well. If relapse occurs after treatment of *C. difficile*, a prolonged course of antibiotics is likely to be successful [*Gastrointestinal and Liver Disease* (6th ed.) New York: Saunders, 1998:1594].

V. Colonic diverticular disease

A. Colonic diverticulosis is the presence of mucosal herniations through the colonic wall; therefore, these lesions are not true diverticula (true diverticula involve all cell layers) but rather pseudodiverticula. The etiology of diverticula is unclear but is probably multifactorial, related in part to age and low-fiber content of the diet.

1. **Incidence.** Diverticulosis is remarkably common among aging Western populations. Approximately 33% of Americans have diverticulosis by age 50 years, and in two-thirds diverticulosis develops by age 80 years.

2. **Manifestations.** The majority of patients with diverticulosis are asymptomatic. Some individuals note minor symptoms (such as abdominal bloating, irregular bowel habits, and mild abdominal discomfort) that are similar to symptoms from IBS. On the other hand, in 10–20% of patients, complications that include bleeding and diverticulitis may develop. Diverticulitis occurs with the self-contained perforation of a diverticular pouch, usually in the sigmoid colon (the location of 85% of these anomalies).

   a. Most cases of **diverticulitis** present as the abrupt onset of left-lower-quadrant abdominal pain. Patients may also have a low-grade fever and leukocytosis. In the event that the perforation is not contained, a localized abscess or frank peritonitis can develop.

   b. **Bleeding** occurs in up to 15–40% of patients with diverticulosis. Although it is usually minor, in 5% of patients massive bleeding that requires inpatient management may develop. Unlike with diverticulitis, most bleeding diverticula are in the right colon. The bleeding from these lesions may be clinically indistinguishable from bleeding caused by angiodysplasia, which also tends to be localized to the right colon.

3. **Diagnosis.** Most diverticula are diagnosed incidentally during colonoscopy or barium enema. When diverticulitis is suspected, the diagnosis should be presumed and treated based on clinical information. If further testing is needed, CT scan (or abdominal ultrasonography) helps to establish the diagnosis and to exclude the presence of an abscess. Water-soluble contrast enemas can also be performed during an episode of diverticulitis; however, this test has been largely supplanted by CT scanning because of its widespread availability. Barium enemas and endoscopy are relatively contraindicated during an episode of acute diverticulitis, but they can be safely performed as part of the evaluation of diverticular bleeding or approximately 6 weeks after the resolution of diverticulitis.

4. **Medical treatment.** The principal treatment for diverticulosis is dietary fiber supplementation. The ingestion of 20–30 g fiber/day may decrease the tendency for further diverticula to form. Most patients require a vegetable laxative supplement to ingest this amount of fiber (*Clin Gastroenterol* 1986;15:903). Most cases of mild diverticulitis can be successfully treated on an outpatient basis. Outpatient therapy includes a clear liquid diet for 48–72 hours and oral antibiotics (appropriate regimens combine a broad-spectrum antibiotic, such as sulfamethoxazole-trimethoprim, ciprofloxacin, or amoxicillin-clavulanic acid, with an antibiotic against anaerobic bacteria such as metronidazole) for 7–10 days (*Am J Gastroenterol* 1999;94:3110, and *N Engl J Med* 1998;339:1081). Patients with severe inflammatory manifestations require hospitalization.

5. **Surgical management.** Surgical resection of the affected colon is an option for patients with recurrent diverticular bleeding or recurrent diverticulitis or for patients who have had complications of diverticulitis (such as colonic stricturing or fistula formation). For the most part, surgery is not required after a first episode of diverticulitis, as patients have only a 20–30% chance of experiencing recurrent diverticulitis. This rule does not apply well to patients who experience the first episode of diverticulitis when they are younger than 40 years of age. These younger patients tend to follow a more aggressive course and have a 50–60% risk of recurrent diverticulitis; therefore, surgery may be an earlier consideration (*Am J Gastroenterol* 1999;94:3110).

VI. Irritable bowel syndrome is a functional GI disorder that is defined by abdominal pain, bloating, and variably disordered bowel habits. Complaints of abnormal stool form/consistency, mucus in the stool, fecal urgency, and incomplete evacuation of stool commonly accompany the IBS.

A. Formal criteria for the diagnosis of IBS, called the **Rome criteria**, have been established. By these criteria, symptoms must be present for 12 weeks, which need not be consecutive, in the preceding year of abdominal pain (*Am J Gastroenterol* 1996;91:2000). In addition to the symptoms listed above, the diagnosis of IBS relies on the reasonable exclusion of organic disease. Although psychological disturbance is not part of IBS, it greatly influences health care–seeking behavior. Among individuals with IBS, the coexistence of a psychological disorder (such as major depression) increases the tendency for an individual to seek medical attention.

B. **Prevalence.** IBS is the most common functional bowel disorder, affecting more than 24% of women and 19% of men. Functional GI disease is a major reason for primary care and gastroenterology office visits.

C. The **diagnosis** of IBS is based on clinical history. Testing for patients who are suspected of having IBS should follow standardized guidelines; appropriate testing includes CBC, ESR, stool samples for ova and parasites, fecal leukocytes, fecal-occult blood test, and sigmoidoscopy (colonoscopy for patients older than 45 years of age). Further evaluation may be desirable and should be based on specific symptoms that any patient experiences (*Gastroenterology* 1997;112:2120).

D. The **treatment** of IBS demands a physiologic and psychosocial approach. The trials that test different medical therapies are complicated, as patients with IBS have a 30–88% response rate to placebo treatments; nonetheless, some medical therapies have been widely applied.

1. The **therapeutic relationship** between patient and practitioner is critically important. Reassurance is an important tool, and this is most effective when the patient's fears are earnestly addressed in a nonjudgmental approach. A symptom diary may be invaluable in integrating patients into relationships in which they are collaborating in their own care.

a. **Dietary recommendations** often include avoidance of lactose and sorbitol (in some sugarless products); this is always a reasonable trial for patients with symptoms of bloating and diarrhea (*Gastroenterology* 1995;27:117). Calcium carbonate supplements (1000 mg/day) can be used for patients who are concerned about calcium intake on a lactose-restricted diet. Fiber supplementation is also routinely recommended for patients with mild diarrhea-predominant and mild constipation-predominant IBS. On the other hand, clinical trials of fiber supplementation have been flawed in design, have been complicated by a high dropout rate, and have shown little therapeutic difference between fiber supplementation and placebo. Although a therapeutic trial with fiber supplementation is safe and therefore a reasonable alternative for mild IBS, it is nevertheless unlikely to be useful for patients with severe symptoms.

   b. The **medical therapies** for IBS should largely be based on control of predominant symptoms. In the management of abdominal pain, narcotics should be avoided. Valid options include anticholinergic agents, such as hyoscyamine; tricyclic antidepressants, such as amitriptyline, imipramine, and desipramine (proven effective in some studies); and serotonin reuptake inhibitors, such as fluoxetine, sertraline, paroxetine, and fluvoxamine (not proven in studies but increasingly used in the setting of intolerance to tricyclic antidepressants) (*Aliment Pharmacol Ther* 1994;8:499). In the management of diarrhea, opioid derivatives such as loperamide and diphenoxylate are useful. Based on the clinical results of one study and because bile acid malabsorption was noted in up to 30% of patients, cholestyramine can be considered to be an effective treatment with diarrhea-predominant IBS [*Gastroenterology* 1998(Suppl);G0170]. In the management of constipation, periodic doses of stimulant laxative, such as cascara, bisacodyl, or senna, are safe; nevertheless, regular use is best avoided. When more routine laxative therapy is needed, osmotic laxatives, such as sorbitol, lactulose, or isotonic solutions that contain polyethylene glycol, are recommended. Dosages used may vary and can be adjusted as necessary to control symptoms.

Colonic Polyps and Neoplasia

I. A **colonic polyp** is any discrete tissue protrusion or growth from the mucosa into the lumen. Colonic polyps are classified as neoplastic (adenomas or adenocarcinomas) or benign (hyperplastic, hamartomatous, juvenile, and inflammatory). Approximately 75% of polyps are adenomas, which are defined as dysplastic lesions without frank malignancy. Although still benign, adenomas (if not removed) have an approximately 10% chance of degeneration to colon or rectal cancer over 5–10 years. This genetic and histologic transition is termed the **adenoma-to-carcinoma sequence**. The removal of adenomas prevents this malignant transition.

   A. The **incidence** of colonic polyps increases with age; approximately 40% of Westerners older than the age of 60 years have one or more polyps. Individuals with a personal or a family history (especially one or more first-degree relatives younger than 60 years of age) of colonic neoplasia face an especially high risk of polyp development. Although the prevalence of polyps may be higher in men than in women, this difference should not have a marked impact on clinical decisions.

   B. In American and European societies, **colorectal cancer** is the second leading cause of cancer mortality and the third most commonly diagnosed malignancy. If diagnosed before metastasis or local invasion, colon cancer can often be cured. Even in the setting of an isolated liver metastatic lesion, 25% of patients can achieve a 5-year survival with surgical resection and adjuvant chemotherapy. Even though colorectal cancers are often preventable and treatable, almost 130,000 cases are diagnosed in the United States each year, and mortality might exceed 55,000 of those cases (*Cancer* 1996;46:5).

II. In general, polyps and early cancers are **asymptomatic**. These early lesions are diagnosed by the application of **screening and surveillance methods**. On the other hand, large lesions can lead to obstruction, intussusception, modification of bowel habits, and diarrhea with resultant electrolyte abnormalities.

A. **Screening** for colonic neoplasia includes diagnostic evaluation for patients with symptoms of colorectal cancer or interval evaluation of patients without symptoms. The available screening techniques are listed below (*Ann Intern Med* 1993;119:836).

1. **Fecal occult blood testing (FOBT)** is a readily available test that detects the peroxidase activity of hemoglobin if sufficient quantities are present in the stool. Although FOBT has very limited sensitivity and specificity, it is partially effective, safe, and relatively inexpensive. Yearly FOBT (testing of two samples from three consecutive stools) is often recommended for all patients older than 40 years of age; still, it is not appropriately used in exclusion of other screening methods. Patients should be advised to avoid red meat (increases false-positives) and vitamin C preparations (increases false-negatives) around the time of FOBT. The significance of a positive FOBT on a stool or mucous sample obtained during digital rectal examination is entirely unproven. Follow-up evaluation of a positive FOBT should include colonoscopy; an alternative would be air-contrast barium enema (ACBE) combined with flexible sigmoidoscopy (*Gastroenterology* 1985;88:820).

2. **Flexible sigmoidoscopy** is an endoscopic assessment of the distal third of the large bowel. The utility of the test as a cancer screen is based on the imperfect assumptions that most colonic polyps are present in the lower colon and that if a significant lesion is located in the proximal colon (not examined by the sigmoidoscope) a herald lesion may be present in this lower part of the colon. Small hyperplastic polyps (diagnosed by biopsy) are not an indication for further evaluation; however, large polyps and those that are adenomatous should be further evaluated and removed by colonoscopy. Flexible sigmoidoscopy is routinely recommended every 5 years for patients 50 years of age and older, and this has been shown to decrease mortality from colorectal cancer (*N Engl J Med* 1992;326:653). Flexible sigmoidoscopy is also the recommended diagnostic test for young patients (<40 years) who have clinically insignificant bleeding that is most suggestive of a perianal or hemorrhoidal source. The risk of serious complication with sigmoidoscopy is 1:3000.

3. **ACBE or double-contrast barium enema** has 85–95% sensitivity for the diagnosis of neoplastic lesions. The utility of ACBE for the evaluation of patients with average risk for colorectal cancer is unproven, and recommendations for its application as a screening test are evolving. Still, an approach using ACBE every 5–10 years after age 50 years has gained limited support among screening experts (*Gastroenterology* 1997;112:594).

4. **Colonoscopy** provides a global endoscopic evaluation of the colon. It has a very high specificity and sensitivity for the detection of colonic neoplasia and allows for the endoscopic resection of most polyps. The majority of cancers cannot be removed endoscopically. Presently, the role of colonoscopy as a primary screening test is growing. The test is modestly invasive (approximately 1:1000 complication risk) and expensive. Until recently, colonoscopy had been reserved for patients who have a significant family history of colorectal cancer, positive FOBT, positive sigmoidoscopy, abnormal ACBE, overt lower-GI bleeding, or substantial change in abdominal or bowel symptoms (*N Engl J Med* 1993;329:1977).

B. Patients at increased risk for development of colorectal cancer include those with a first-degree relative who has sporadic colorectal cancer, a family history of familial adenomatous polyposis syndrome (APC), or a family history of hereditary nonpolyposis colon cancer (also termed **HNPCC or Lynch syndrome**).

    1. APC is an autosomal genetic disorder characterized by the formation of innumerable colonic polyps in the second or third decade of life and an inevitable tendency to development of colon cancer. Suspected individuals should undergo genetic testing, and if the gene is found or the test is inconclusive, flexible sigmoidoscopy should be performed annually until polyposis is confirmed. Once polyps develop, colectomy (rather than endoscopic resection of the polyps) is recommended to prevent colon cancer. Affected patients must also be screened for ampullary neoplasms.

    2. Lynch syndrome is an autosomal dominant trait manifest as the development of colorectal cancer without an antecedent history of colonic polyps. It is likely that polyps that lead to these tumors are flat and less well recognized and have more advanced histologic changes when detected and removed. The Amsterdam criteria include (1) the existence of three or more relatives with colorectal cancer (one of whom is a first-degree relative of the others), (2) colorectal cancer that spans at least two generations, and (3) one or more cancers diagnosed before age 50 years. For affected patients, colonoscopy is recommended every 1–2 years between the ages of 20 and 30 years and every year after age 40 years.

    3. Patients with long-standing IBD (especially UC) should undergo colonoscopy with surveillance biopsies to evaluate for dysplasia.

C. Surveillance is required for patients with a documented history of colonic polyps and colon cancer.

    1. Patients in whom adenomatous polyps are found and removed at colonoscopy should have a repeat colonoscopy at 3 years. If the first follow-up is normal or shows only a single, small (<1 cm) tubular adenoma, the next examination can be performed in 5 years. In select instances, shorter intervals may be appropriate based on physician judgment.

    2. Patients who have undergone resection of a colorectal cancer with curative intent (but who did not have a preoperative colonoscopy) should have a complete colonoscopy within 1 year of the resection. If the preoperative examination is normal, the colonoscopy should be offered at 3 years, and further follow-up should mirror the schedule outlined above.

III. The principal step in the **treatment of colorectal cancer** is surgical resection. Patients with rectal tumors frequently are treated with neoadjuvant radiation therapy that improves outcome and increases the chances that a primary anastomosis (without stoma) can be performed. Adjuvant chemotherapy clearly benefits a subset of patients with advanced tumors.

    A. Preoperative assessment should include imaging of the entire colon, preferably by colonoscopy or alternatively by contrast enema. CT scanning of the abdomen and plain chest radiography to evaluate for evidence of metastases are standard as well. The serum carcinoembryonic antigen should be checked preoperatively; although this blood test is not useful as a primary screening tool, serial measurements may detect early tumor recurrence.

    B. After resection, the stage of the tumor should be established. Postoperative chemotherapy with 5-fluorouracil and leucovorin (or levamisole) improves survival among patients with deeply invasive or metastatic tumors.

IV. Hemorrhoids are the dilation of a physiologic vascular cushion in the distal rectum. They are common abnormalities, affecting one-half of all Americans, and are more irritating than a life-threatening danger. Symptoms can include bleeding (occasionally severe), discomfort, pruritus ani, fecal soiling, and prolapse. Thrombosis of external hemorrhoids can cause bleeding and severe pain. Treatment (even with thrombosis) is usually conservative. Measures such as fiber supplementation, sitz baths, and local anesthetics are often used. Relatively rarely, surgical or local manipulations are required.

Liver Diseases

I. **Biochemical liver tests and biochemical assessment of liver function.** The evaluation of a patient for suspected liver disease involves two steps. These steps are (1) assessment of the type of liver injury and (2) assessment of the liver's degree of functional impairment. These steps involve both blood tests as well as clinical evaluation by history and examination. Once liver disease is suspected, it is often useful to segregate the disease into one of two categories: hepatocellular or cholestatic. **Hepatocellular injury** describes a primary hepatocyte injury. **Cholestatic disease** affects the production of bile and the delivery of bile to the duodenum. Early in the course of liver diseases, this differentiation is often diagnostically and therapeutically helpful. In more advanced liver diseases (regardless of etiology), distinctions become blurred and clinical consequences overlap. These tests and implications are listed in Table 14-6 (*Mayo Clin Proc* 1996;71:1089).

A. **Measurements of serum aminotransferases** are a critical tool in the screening and evaluation for liver disease. These tests include the aspartate aminotransferase (AST or SGOT) and alanine aminotransferase (ALT or SGPT). The ALT and AST can be elevated among patients with liver cell injury and perhaps less markedly so among patients with cholestatic liver diseases. Still, the AST is one of the earliest markers of acute biliary obstruction. Although the ALT is relatively specific for liver diseases, the AST can be elevated in a variety of liver and extrahepatic (muscle, blood cells, cardiac) injuries.

B. **Cholestatic markers.** Measurement of serum alkaline phosphatase is the most readily available marker that is somewhat specific for cholestatic liver injury. Unfortunately, the alkaline phosphatase is not perfectly specific for biliary processes—it can also be elevated in bone and less likely intestinal disease. Serum levels of 5'-nucleotidase and γ-glutamyltransferase (γ-GT) are supplemental tests that, if elevated, suggest a hepatic or biliary tree source of an elevated alkaline phosphatase. Heat fractionation can also segregate hepatobiliary from osseous forms of alkaline phosphatase. The γ-GT is frequently reported in many metabolic panels. Modest elevations of the γ-GT are nonspecific and, in the absence of other evidence of liver disease, might be disregarded.

C. The term **liver function test** is frequently used to refer to any serum measurement that relates to the liver. That is misleading, as liver function need not be compromised for some of these tests (e.g., aminotransferases) to be abnormal. Blood tests, including the serum albumin, bilirubin, and measurement of prothrombin time (PT), provide some assessment of the actual metabolic function of the liver. These blood tests are not sensitive detectors of liver failure; the liver has a large functional reserve, and routinely measured liver function may be within normal range until more than 80% of the inherent liver function is compromised.

1. **Albumin** is a serum glycoprotein that is synthesized by the liver. It serves as a carrier protein and as a means by which intravascular oncotic pressure is maintained. Although the serum albumin can be low in liver disease, it also can be low in protein-losing enteropathies, nephrotic syndrome, and almost any severe acute or chronic illness.

2. The serum **bilirubin** is frequently, but not invariably, elevated with bile duct obstruction or cholestatic liver injury. Care must be taken to assess that an elevated serum bilirubin represents a true hepatic or biliary abnormality. Most laboratory tests routinely report the serum bilirubin

Table 14-6. Characteristic patterns of liver test abnormalities[a]

Test	Hepatocellular injury	Cholestatic injury	Cirrhosis with hepatic insufficiency	Hemolysis or Gilbert's syndrome	Bone disease
Albumin	Normal, low	Normal, low	Low, very low	Normal	Normal
ALT and AST	Modest to marked elevation	Normal or mild to modest elevation	Normal, modest elevation	Normal	Normal
Bilirubin	Normal to high total and direct	High total and direct, may be normal	Normal, high total and direct	High total, normal direct	Normal
Alkaline phosphatase	Mild to modest elevation	Modest to marked elevation	Mild, modest elevation	Normal	Elevated
5'-Nucleotidase or γ-GT	Normal to modest elevation	Modest to marked elevation	Mild, modest elevation	Normal	Normal
Prothrombin time	Normal to marked prolongation	Normal to marked prolongation	Mild to marked prolongation	Normal	Normal
Platelet count	Normal	Normal	Low	Normal	Normal

γ-GT, γ-glutamyl transpeptidase.
[a]Although helpful, overlap of patterns prevents laboratory tests alone from being diagnostic.

as a total value that includes conjugated and unconjugated bilirubin. In typical bilirubin metabolism, serum bilirubin is conjugated by the liver and is thus rendered soluble and excretable by the kidney. This type of conjugated bilirubin is reported as direct bilirubin. Several disorders, such as hemolysis and inherited deficiencies of bilirubin glucuronosyl-transferase activity (e.g., Gilbert's syndrome), can produce elevation in total bilirubin, but with the unconjugated bilirubin accounting for the major portion of the elevation. In these situations, an extensive evaluation for liver or biliary disease may not be required. To evaluate patients with an elevated serum bilirubin but no other clinical, laboratory, or radiographic evidence of biliary obstruction (or liver disease), fractionation of direct and indirect bilirubin is the first step.

   3. The **PT** should be measured in all patients with suspected liver or biliary disease. Patients who have severe cholestasis may become deficient in fat-soluble vitamins; the deficiency of vitamin K can lead to prolongation of the PT. For these patients without other liver failure, the parenteral administration of vitamin K can produce overnight correction of coagulopathy. The PT can also be elevated because of primary hepatic insufficiency, disseminated intravascular coagulation, and pharmacologic anticoagulation.

D. A **CBC** may also provide information that is helpful in gaining insight regarding the chronicity and nature of any liver disease. Patients with advanced liver disease may have portal hypertension and associated hypersplenism. This can be manifest as leukopenia and thrombocytopenia. Although these abnormalities are not specific for liver disease, they can provide useful adjuncts in selected situations.

II. **Cirrhosis** is a histologic condition of the liver that is defined by extensive bridging fibrosis and the formation of regenerative nodules. Many patients with cirrhosis have clinically and, by routine laboratory assessment, normal liver function. On the other hand, portal hypertension and other forms of clinical decompensation from liver failure develop in some patients. The complications and management of common complications from cirrhosis are described below. Most patients who experience these complications should be managed in conjunction with an experienced hepatologist. Liver transplantation should be a consideration in many of these individuals as well.

A. **Gastroesophageal varices** are the result of portal hypertension. Shunting of blood results in dilated blood venous passages (characteristically in the distal esophagus and proximal stomach) that are exposed to high pressures. Approximately 20% of patients with cirrhosis and esophageal varices experience potentially life-threatening upper-GI hemorrhage from these abnormalities. If varices are present, lifelong therapy with nonselective beta-blockers, such as propranolol, nadolol, and timolol, decreases the risk of variceal bleeding (*N Engl J Med* 1991;324:1532, and *Am J Gastroenterol* 1998;93:2348). Unfortunately, there are few universally recognized parameters on which to base the dose of beta-blockade. Patients with an established history of variceal hemorrhage should be evaluated for long-term management that might include endoscopic obliteration of varices or vascular shunting procedures.

B. **Ascites** is the accumulation of fluid within the peritoneal cavity. Although it has many potential etiologies, it most commonly results from decompensated liver disease. The initial evaluation of ascites should include serologic tests of liver function and diagnostic paracentesis. Obtained ascites should be measured to calculate a **serum ascites albumin gradient (SAAG)**. The SAAG is calculated by subtracting the ascites albumin concentration (g/dl) from the serum albumin concentration (g/dl). A SAAG of greater than 1.1 g/dl suggests that portal hypertension from chronic liver disease (usually cirrhosis) is the cause of the ascites. Sodium restriction and diuretics, characteristically spironolactone (recommended starting dose 100 mg PO qd, with a maximal dose of 400 mg PO qd) and furosemide (recommended starting dose 40 mg PO qd, with a maximal dose of 160 mg PO qd), are used for the initial management of ascites. Care must be taken to avoid renal failure and electrolyte abnormalities (*Semin Liver Dis* 1997;17:249).

C. **Portosystemic (hepatic) encephalopathy (PSE)** is a central neurologic dysfunction that probably results from disordered clearance of neurotransmitters and gut-derived toxins. Initial manifestations can be subclinical and detected only by EEG or neuropsychiatric testing. More advanced manifestations can include sleep pattern disturbances and confusion. In severe cases, patients may become unresponsive. Seizures should not be considered a routine complication of hepatic encephalopathy. Physical examination findings commonly include asterixis, hyperreflexia, and an abnormal mental status examination. After shunting procedures for varices or ascites, patients face a 25% risk of new or worsening encephalopathy. The initial management of PSE is the elimination of medications (such as narcotics and sedatives) that may further contribute to an altered mental status. After this, lactulose can be administered and titrated to produce two to five soft bowel motions daily (usual starting dosage for lactulose, 30 ml PO bid); higher doses are not likely to be of benefit. Lactulose is a nonabsorbable disaccharide that alters the colonic flora and leads to the fecal excretion of amines and ammonia. Oral neomycin and metronidazole have also been used to alter bacterial flora and treat PSE (*N Engl J Med* 1997;337:473).

D. **Cholestasis** from liver failure may lead to fat-soluble vitamin deficiency, bone disease, jaundice, and pruritus. Therefore, cirrhotic patients should be monitored for fat-soluble vitamin deficiency, and, if present, appropriate water-soluble vitamin supplements should be provided. Pruritus from cholestasis can be quite disabling. Management options include the use of antihistamines, soothing lotions, and cool showers with pat drying of the skin to avoid excess drying. Further first-line medical options include the use of cholestyramine resin, 4 g PO bid–qid, or ursodeoxycholic acid, 13–15 mg/kg/day (*QJM* 1995;88:603).

E. **Hepatocellular carcinoma (HCCA)** is relatively uncommon in the general U.S. population but is seen more often among patients with end-stage liver disease. The biggest risk lies among patients with cirrhosis from hepatitis B, hepatitis C, hemochromatosis, and alcohol; other forms of liver failure have a lower risk. Symptoms are nonspecific and may simply be the worsening of other manifestations of cirrhosis. Therefore, screening should be performed at least annually for cirrhotic patients (especially those with hemochromatosis, viral hepatitis, or alcohol-induced liver disease) or patients with decompensation of previously stable liver disease. Screening techniques include quantitative measurements of serum alpha-fetoprotein (AFP) and imaging studies (ultrasound, contrast CT scan, and MRI scan). The AFP is normal in many patients with HCCA. Therefore, if a mass lesion is found by imaging studies, even with a normal or minimally elevated AFP, biopsy may be appropriate. The finding of a solid liver mass in a cirrhotic patient who has an AFP of greater than 1000 ng/ml is virtually diagnostic of HCCA. The treatment of HCCA is individualized. Some patients with small localized tumors can be considered for surgical resection (if compensated liver disease) or liver transplantation (if more advanced liver dysfunction). Directed therapies, including chemoembolization, alcohol injection of tumors, and ablation techniques, are rapidly evolving (*Lancet* 1999;353:1253, and *Digestion* 1998;59:556).

F. **Preoperative assessment.** Surgery, especially with general anesthesia, exposes cirrhotic patients to increased risk for mortality or hepatic decompensation (e.g., ascites, PSE, bleeding). If possible, for patients with acute hepatitis, surgery should be avoided. The extent of risk for patients with chronic liver disease is typically based on **Child-Pugh** grading of liver disease as outlined in Table 14-7. Additionally, intra-abdominal varices, coag-

Table 14-7. Child-Pugh classification

	Points		
	1	2	3
Encephalopathy	None	Asterixis/hyperreflexia or controlled with medical therapy	Obtundation or coma
Ascites	None	Medically controlled	Refractory to medical management
Bilirubin (mg/dl)	1–2	2.1–3.0	>3
Albumin (g/dl)	>3.4	2.8–3.4	<2.8
Protime (sec prolonged)	<4	4–6	>6

Grade A: 5–6 points.
Grade B: 7–9 points.
Grade C: 10 or more points.

Estimated surgical risk with general anesthesia

	Chance of decompensation	Liver-related mortality
Grade A	10–15%	0–10%
Grade B	20–50%	4–30%
Grade C	Almost 100%	20–75%

Source: CF Gholson, JM Provenza, BR Bacon. Hepatologic considerations in patients with a parenchymal liver disease undergoing surgery. *Am J Gastroenterol* 1990;85:487, with permission.

ulopathy, and thrombocytopenia may contribute to bleeding risks (*Am J Gastroenterol* 1990;85:487).

III. **Nonalcoholic steatohepatitis (NASH)** is a relatively newly identified pathology, but it may be responsible for abnormal aminotransferases in a substantial number of patients who are noted to have asymptomatic elevations of the ALT or AST. It is defined by steatosis (fatty infiltration of the liver) along with associated inflammation. The exact etiology and history of this disorder remain unexplained. Usually NASH produces no symptoms, but some patients may note mild right-upper-quadrant abdominal pain. Over many years, cirrhosis along with hepatic insufficiency develops in some NASH patients (*Gastroenterology* 1994;107:1103).

A. Before NASH is diagnosed, other forms of liver disease (especially hepatitis C and alcohol-induced liver disease) must be excluded. The **diagnosis** of NASH is suggested by the presence of risk factors, including obesity, hyperlipidemia, diabetes mellitus, and female gender. Still, these risk factors are not absolute and are not required for the diagnosis of NASH. Imaging studies, including ultrasound, CT, and MRI, may suggest steatosis but do not allow assessment for the presence of inflammation. To establish the presence of steatosis and inflammation definitively, liver biopsy is required.

B. No guidelines have been established for the **treatment** of NASH. Although weight loss and tight diabetic control are commonly recommended, any impact on NASH is likely to be small. Lipid-lowering agents have no established utility in treating NASH.

IV. **Alcohol-induced liver disease.** Alcohol is the leading cause of liver disease. Characteristically, alcoholic liver injury should only occur above threshold consumption (20 g ethanol/day in women and 80 g ethanol/day in men). Still, the sensitivity of liver to alcohol may be variable, and a history to attain the degree of alcohol consumption is notoriously inaccurate. Even among patients with chronic heavy alcohol consumption, the development of cirrhosis is not inevitable—only 10–20% of patients progress to cirrhosis (*Am J Gastroenterol* 1998;93:2022).

A. **Alcoholic hepatitis** is an acute or chronic illness characterized by necroinflammatory changes within the liver. Clinically, it may be asymptomatic and manifest only as elevated serum transaminases. Characteristically, the serum AST is elevated more substantially than the ALT; however, this pattern is not a foolproof means of establishing the diagnosis. More severe cases of alcoholic hepatitis may be associated with fever, abdominal pain, and complications of liver failure or portal hypertension.

B. **Alcoholic cirrhosis** is typically micronodular and results from chronic alcohol consumption. In the absence of telltale inflammation, it is histologically indistinguishable from any other forms of end-stage liver disease, and diagnosis is based principally on history.

C. The **treatment** of alcoholic liver diseases is simple. Alcohol abstinence and good nutrition are all that is available. Steroids have been advocated for select cases of extremely severe alcoholic hepatitis, but this remains hotly debated (*Gastroenterology* 1978;75:193, and *Gastroenterology* 1996;110:1847). Alcohol abstinence often requires aversion therapy with disulfiram as well as appropriate substance abuse supportive therapy.

1. In the setting of acute hepatitis complicated by liver dysfunction, often abstinence alone results in improvement.

2. Liver transplantation is the second-line option for those with persistent liver failure after alcohol consumption is discontinued. Typically, a 6- to 12-month abstinence period is required before transplantation. Although there is evidence that prolonged abstinence decreases alcohol recidivism after transplant, the application of this abstinence period does not affect long-term outcome after transplantation (*Transplantation* 1994;58:560).

V. **Hepatitis A** is caused by a picornavirus. The virus is spread from person to person via a fecal-oral route. In infected patients, an acute hepatitis develops that can vary from mild to very severe; there is no chronic hepatitis A. Although fulminant liver failure rarely results, it has been reported.

A. Characteristic **manifestations** of hepatitis A include elevated serum transaminases, fever, nausea/vomiting, abdominal pain, and cholestasis (manifest as jaundice and hyperbilirubinemia). The diagnosis is based on finding IgM antibodies to hepatitis A capsid protein; this test is typically ordered as HAVAB-IgM. Findings of a positive HAVAB-IgG or total, in the absence of an acute hepatitis, suggest immunity to hepatitis A rather than an acute infection. Table 14-8 delineates these tests.

B. The **treatment** of acute hepatitis A is supportive. Most patients can be treated on an outpatient basis, but hospitalization may be required for those who are unable to maintain hydration. Preparations for emergency liver transplantation should be considered for patients in whom coagulopathy and encephalopathy develop as a result of acute hepatitis A.

C. For nonimmune patients who are exposed to hepatitis A, highly effective **immunoprophylaxis** is available in the form of hepatitis A immune globulin. The immune globulin should be given to those who are exposed to the virus within a 2-week window; immunoprophylaxis after that is not appropriate. Hepatitis A immune globulin is derived from pooled human plasma and is given at a dose of 0.2 ml/kg. Although safe, immune globulin can cause pain at the injection site, arthralgias, and fever (*Vaccine* 1992; 10:S138). Effective vaccination is also available and is recommended for

Table 14-8. Blood testing for viral hepatitis

Serologic Testing for Hepatitis A

	Hep A-Ab IgM	Hep A-Ab total (IgM and IgG)	Serum transaminases/bilirubin
Acute hepatitis A	Positive	Positive	May be markedly abnormal
Immunity to hepatitis A (past infection or vaccination)	Negative (clears 3–4 mos after infection)	Positive	Normal

Serologic Testing for Hepatitis B

	HBsAg[a,b]	HBsAb	HBcAb-IgM	HBcAb-total (IgM + IgG)	HBeAg[c]	HBeAb	HBV-DNA (hybridization assay)	ALT/AST
Acute infection	Positive	Negative	Positive	Positive	Positive	Negative	Positive	Markedly elevated
Recovery from acute infection	Negative	Positive	Negative	Positive	Negative	Positive	Negative	Normal
Immunity from vaccination	Negative	Positive	Negative	Negative	Negative	Negative	Negative	Normal
Chronic infection	Positive	Negative	Negative	Positive	Positive	Negative	Positive	Modestly elevated or normal
Nonreplicative chronic carrier state	Positive	Negative/positive	Negative	Positive	Negative	Positive	Negative	Normal

Serologic Testing for Hepatitis C

	HCV-Ab RIA	HCV-RIBA	HCV-RNA by PCR	ALT/AST
Chronic infection	Positive	Positive	Positive	Modestly elevated, normal
False-positive Ab test	Positive	Negative	Negative	Normal
Resolved or subclinical infection	Positive	Positive	Negative	Normal

Ab, antibody; HBcAb, hepatitis B core antibody; HBeAg, hepatitis B envelope antigen; HBsAb, hepatitis B surface antibody; HBsAg, hepatitis B surface antigen; HBV, hepatitis B virus; HCV, hepatitis C virus; Hep A, hepatitis A; Ig, immunoglobulin; PCR, polymerase chain reaction; RIBA, recombinant immunoblot assay; RIA, radioimmunoassay.

[a]A small subset may have a mutant form of the virus that produces surface antigen that is not detected by routinely available assays.

[b]Positive patients should be screened for hepatitis D coinfection by hepatitis D virus antibody.

[c]A small subset may have a mutant form of the virus that does not express the envelope antigen.

high-risk populations (residents of high-risk population centers, men who have sex with men, residents and staff of institutions that serve the mentally handicapped, and restaurant workers). The hepatitis A vaccination typically is given as a series of two injections, and immunity is achieved in 95% with the first dose; this is increased to 99% after the second dose [*MMWR Morb Mortal Wkly Rep* 1996;45(RR-15):1].

VI. **Hepatitis B.** The causative virus of **hepatitis B** is a hepadnavirus. In the United States, the virus is now most commonly transmitted through intravenous drug use and by heterosexual exposures. In the Far East, vertical transmission continues to be a major health issue (*Semin Liver Dis* 1991;11:84).

A. **Pathogenesis.** Hepatitis B can cause an acute hepatitis, a chronic hepatitis, and a very low-grade chronic carrier state. The acute hepatitis can be quite severe. As a result, this is one of the most common causes of fulminant hepatic failure. Chronic viral activity can lead to cirrhosis and HCCA. The risk of chronic disease is less than 5% when the infection is developed in adulthood and greater than 90% when the infection is acquired during infancy or very early childhood. Although the clinical significance of the chronic carrier state is likely to be small, patients may still be at risk for reactivation of hepatitis B and the development of HCCA (*Hepatology* 1999;30:257).

B. The **diagnosis** of hepatitis B is necessarily complex and is based on a variety of serologic markers that assess disease activity and the immune response. These markers are listed in Table 14-8.

1. **Hepatitis B surface antigen** is the protein that forms the outer coat of the viral nucleocapsid (Dane particle). This antigen can be detected during the acute illness (1–2 weeks after infection), chronic hepatitis, and in the chronic carrier state. Although not invariably, the surface antigen usually disappears if the hepatitis is cleared. **Antibodies to the surface antigen (HBsAb)** may indicate prior exposure to or vaccination against hepatitis B. The presence of HBsAb does not perfectly correlate with viral clearance.

2. **Hepatitis B core antibody (HBcAb)** is present and measured in two forms, IgM and IgG. A positive **HBcAb-IgM** is the hallmark of acute hepatitis B infection. The presence of HBcAb-IgG is most consistent with a resolved past infection or a chronic carrier state.

3. **Hepatitis B envelope antigen (HBeAg)** is the hallmark of chronic active viral replication. Patients who are positive for HBeAg are believed to have active viral replication and are capable of transmitting the virus. Among patients with a resolved acute infection of a relatively inactive chronic carrier state, the HBeAg becomes negative and the **hepatitis B envelope antibody (HBeAb)** becomes positive. Occasional (1%) hepatitis B cases result from a precore mutant form of the virus. These patients do not have detectable HBeAg (but may have HBeAb), but they may have readily detectable viral replication by DNA assays.

4. The blood level of **hepatitis B DNA (HBV-DNA)** can be readily measured using a variety of methods. Of the available techniques, the hybridization technique and branched-chain DNA assays are the most clinically relevant. The sensitivity of this technique allows segregation of replicative from nonreplicative disease. Polymerase chain reaction assays of HBV-DNA may be too sensitive for clinical relevance.

C. **Treatment.** Supportive care is the principal treatment for acute hepatitis B. More specific therapies are indicated for patients with chronic disease. The goals of therapy are normalization of serum transaminases, clearance of HBeAg (for wild-type viral infection), clearance of HBV-DNA (for wild-type and precore mutant viral infection), and appearance of HBeAb.

1. **Interferon** is an immune modulator and antiviral drug that has potent activity against hepatitis B. It is only indicated for patients with active hepatitis and those who have an elevated serum ALT; it is ineffective in

the treatment of patients with normal serum transaminases. Side effects from interferon can be quite disabling. For patients who are able to complete therapy, approximately 30–40% have sustained treatment success (*N Engl J Med* 1997;336:347). Factors that suggest a good response to interferon therapy include active hepatitis (elevated ALT and necroinflammatory activity by liver biopsy), low levels of measurable viral DNA, non-Asian ethnicity, and infection that is acquired during adulthood (*Hepatology* 1999;29:971).

2. **Lamivudine (3-TC)** was initially developed as an antiretroviral drug. This nucleoside analogue is safe, and at a dose of 100 mg PO qd for 1 year it is remarkably effective at suppressing the viral replication in patients with chronic active hepatitis B. Unfortunately, viral infection usually recurs when lamivudine is discontinued, and sustained therapy is complicated by a high incidence for the development of drug-resistant mutant strains (*N Engl J Med* 1998;339:61). Still, some patients achieve sustained clearance of the virus (*N Engl J Med* 1999;341:1256).

3. **Hepatitis B immune globulin** is now recommended as postexposure prophylaxis for those who lack immunity to the virus. Additionally, highly effective recombinant vaccines are now readily available. The vaccine is administered as a three-dose series at months 0, 1, and 6. Successful vaccination is typically manifest as a positive HBsAb assay. Universal childhood vaccination against hepatitis B has become standard across the United States, and adult vaccination is recommended for high-risk populations.

VII. Hepatitis C is a relatively recently isolated RNA hepatatrophic virus. Chronic active hepatitis C is rapidly becoming a major health crisis in the United States and across the globe. Acute infection may produce a nonspecific viral illness. Although 15% of patients may clear the viral infection, in the majority a more sustained chronic hepatitis develops. The patients with chronic hepatitis are at risk for the slow development of cirrhosis, liver failure, and hepatocellular cancer. In approximately 20% of patients with chronic hepatitis C, cirrhosis develops over 2–3 decades.

A. **Prevalence.** Approximately 2% of Americans (about 4 million) have chronic hepatitis C. The large number of unrecognized cases and the limited use of available treatments magnify the scope of the problem. Liver failure from hepatitis C has become the leading indication for liver transplantation (*Semin Liver Dis* 1995;15:5).

B. Well-established modes of **transmission** of the virus include the transfusion of blood products before the early 1990s (when widespread testing for the virus became available), intravenous drug use, intranasal cocaine, and tattoos/body piercing. The risk of viral transmission in a monogamous sexual relationship is low (approximately 6% lifetime risk). The risk of vertical transmission from mother to child is also low (approximately 4%, but reports range from 0% to 25%) (*Hepatology* 1997;26:15S).

C. The **manifestations** of chronic hepatitis C are nonspecific. They include fatigue, myalgias, and arthralgias. Laboratory abnormalities include mildly elevated serum transaminases (usually less than two or three times upper limits of normal), but up to one-third of patients with chronic hepatitis C have normal ALT and AST. A small group of patients may have associated rheumatologic, renal, or dermatologic manifestations, such as cryoglobulinemia, glomerulonephritis, porphyria cutanea tarda, or lichen planus (*Semin Liver Dis* 1995;15:101).

D. The **diagnosis** of chronic hepatitis C requires a high index of suspicion. Patients with risk factors for hepatitis C should be tested by hepatitis C antibody test by radioimmunoassay, as should all patients with unexplained serum transaminase abnormalities or liver insufficiency. The hepatitis C virus (HCV)-Ab test can be falsely positive, and patients who test positive but have normal serum transaminases and no risk factors for hepatitis C should undergo confirmatory testing with either an HCV-recombinant immunoblot assay (HCV-RIBA) (a more specific antibody test) or detection of HCV-RNA by polymerase chain reaction. These tests are shown in Table 14-8.

E. Supplemental tests that are important in evaluating HCV infection include determination of HCV genotype, quantitative measurement of HCV-RNA, and liver biopsy. Information from these tests may be useful in predicting the course of HCV infection and the chances for successful therapy against HCV. Patients with genotypes other than 1 (70% of American HCV patients have genotype 1), low viral loads, and less advanced fibrosis by biopsy have the best chance for a good outcome with therapy (*Lancet* 1998;352:1456). It is important to note that although use of the HCV-RNA and genotype assays have become standard, some are not yet U.S. Food and Drug Administration approved, and the techniques/sensitivities are not standardized.

F. The **treatment** of HCV should be divided into conservative measures and then specific antiviral approaches.

1. **Conservative measures.** Patients should be urged and offered help in the discontinuation of alcohol consumption. Because hepatitis A can follow an especially virulent course among patients who are coinfected with chronic hepatitis C, it is worthwhile to ensure immunity to hepatitis A by checking the hepatitis A–Ab total; negative patients should be offered vaccination. Patients with cirrhosis from hepatitis C should be screened for HCCA, with annual determination of the serum AFP and imaging studies (either ultrasound or CT scan).

2. **Antiviral therapies.** Although several regimens are available, all present therapies against hepatitis C involve the subcutaneous administration of **interferon**. Interferons have immunomodulatory and antiviral effects. Interferon-based therapies are plagued by adverse side effects and poor response rates, and for those patients who do respond, there is a high risk for viral relapse when therapy is discontinued (*Hepatology* 1996;24:778). Side effects to interferon include pain at the injection site, fever, myalgias, worsening or unmasking of psychiatric disorders, thyroid abnormalities, bone marrow dysfunction, and worsening or unmasking of autoimmune processes. Contraindications include hepatic insufficiency, leukopenia, thrombocytopenia, established autoimmune disease, and uncontrolled psychiatric disease (including ongoing alcohol or substance abuse). **Ribavirin** is an antiviral agent that, when used in combination with interferon, can increase the chances of a sustained response; there is no role for ribavirin monotherapy to treat chronic hepatitis C (*N Engl J Med* 1998;339:1485). Side effects include hemolysis that can be potentially severe, dermatologic problems, and worsening of interferon complications. The techniques for administering interferon-based therapies are complex and beyond the scope of this chapter. Therapy should be pursued only by a primary physician particularly experienced in the treatment of hepatitis C who remains updated with rapidly evolving protocol changes or in conjunction with an experienced consultant.

VIII. Autoimmune hepatitis (AIH) is an idiopathic disorder characterized by immune-mediated necroinflammatory liver injury. The disease can lead to irreversible liver injury, and approximately 50% of patients are cirrhotic at the time of diagnosis. Immunosuppression therapies can be successful in preventing the progression to liver failure and improving liver function among patients who have active inflammation.

A. The **diagnosis** of the disorder is based on epidemiologic factors, laboratory findings, and liver biopsy. Other forms of liver disease (especially chronic viral infection) must be excluded. AIH displays a 4:1 female-male predominance and is often associated with extrahepatic autoimmune processes (e.g., arthritis, dermatitis, or thyroid disease). Important laboratory findings include elevated serum transaminases, hypergammaglobulinemia (IgG greater than 1.5 times the upper limit of normal), the presence of autoantibodies (antinuclear antibodies and anti–smooth-muscle antibodies are the most common among adult patients), and an elevated ESR. Although liver biopsy alone cannot establish the diagnosis, it can be helpful. Histologic findings that support the diagnosis include piecemeal necrosis and a dense plasma cell inflammatory infiltrate (*Hepatology* 1993;18:998).

B. Natural history. The mortality of untreated AIH probably exceeds 50% in 5 years. On the other hand, when remission is achieved and sustained with immunomodulatory therapy, survival is 90% at 10 years. Even responding patients who have cirrhosis at the time of diagnosis can expect this survival rate (*Gastroenterology* 1996;110:848). Patients who have evidence of liver failure (jaundice, ascites, portal hypertension) at the time of diagnosis often improve with treatment, and therefore these features should not discourage treatment if there is evidence of active necroinflammatory activity (as manifest by biopsy or blood tests).

C. The initial **treatment** of AIH is with corticosteroids. Usually, prednisone is started at a dose of 60 mg PO qa.m. AZA is generally administered as supplemental therapy, as it may speed remission and allows for steroid sparing when corticosteroids are tapered; blood tests are followed closely for evidence of relapse. Once remission is achieved, steroids can be slowly and carefully tapered. Except in the situation of treatment failure or the development of intolerable side effects, discontinuation of corticosteroids should not be considered in a period of less than 2 years, as there is a high risk of relapse. Many suggest continuing steroid-sparing therapies such as AZA indefinitely (*Hepatology* 1988;8:585, and *N Engl J Med* 1995;333:958).

IX. Cholestatic liver diseases are a heterogeneous group of disorders that are characterized pathogenically by dysfunction in the production of bile or the delivery of bile from the hepatocytes to the intestine. These disorders are diverse and result from immunologic, metabolic/drug, and infectious etiologies.

A. Primary biliary cirrhosis (PBC) is an idiopathic disorder characterized by intrahepatic bile duct inflammation. The disease is seen almost universally in women and is commonly associated with other autoimmune phenomena. In its earliest form, patients may be noted to have only isolated laboratory abnormalities (usually alkaline phosphatase). As the disease progresses, symptoms and laboratory findings of more marked cholestasis usually develop within 2–4 years; finally, cirrhosis and liver failure can occur. The diagnosis is suggested by the presence of **antimitochondrial antibodies**, which are present in 95% of patients with PBC, as well as elevated serum **IgM antibodies**. Characteristic liver biopsy findings in early disease include marked periductal inflammation ("florid bile duct lesion") and the presence of intrahepatic granulomas. As the disease progresses, marked bile duct proliferation can be seen; bile duct obliteration and finally biliary cirrhosis follow. Many therapies have been used to treat PBC, but so far **ursodeoxycholic acid** (15–20 mg/kg/day) has been the only drug that has been universally accepted as clinically worthwhile. It has been shown to improve liver function test abnormalities and liver biopsy appearance and, most important, to slow the progression of the disease (*N Engl J Med* 1996;335:1570).

B. Primary sclerosing cholangitis (PSC) is another idiopathic inflammatory disorder of the bile ducts. Unlike PBC, PSC is a macroscopic disorder that can affect the intra- and extrahepatic biliary system. The disease most often affects men (7:3 when compared with women) and is associated with superimposed IBD (usually UC) in 85% of patients with the disorder. The inflammation of PBC leads to bile duct stricturing. Over the course of an average of 9–17 years from diagnosis, patients are at risk for the development of secondary biliary cirrhosis. This time period may be punctuated by episodes of infectious cholangitis. The clinical progression of PSC is unpredictable. No specific drug treatments have been shown to slow or alter the progression of the disease. Treatment of IBD (even colectomy in UC patients) does not eliminate the risk for the development of PSC. Diagnosing PSC requires an appropriate index of suspicion. Although liver biopsy may suggest the **diagnosis** of PSC, cholangiography (usually endoscopic retrograde cholangiopancreatography) is the gold standard test. Management of patients with PSC includes conservative treatment of cholestasis, antibiotic therapy for episodes of cholangitis, and endoscopic (endoscopic retrograde cholangiopancreatography) dilation of strictures or placement of stents to treat mechanical obstruction. For appropriate patients with liver failure, with severe cholestasis that cannot be managed medically or endoscopically, or with recurrent episodes of bacterial cholangitis, liver transplantation is recommended (*N Engl J Med* 1995;332:924).

C. **Autoimmune cholangiopathy** is a disease that has overlapping features of AIH and PBC. For these patients, a trial of ursodeoxycholic acid might be warranted; alternatively, steroids can be considered in select patients.

D. Metabolic causes of isolated cholestatic liver injury include drug/hormonal effects and total parenteral nutrition **(TPN)–induced cholestasis**. In the case of drug-induced disease, discontinuation of therapy is necessary in some cases to avoid permanent liver injury (*Am J Gastroenterol* 1998;93:684). In the case of TPN-induced cholestasis, management options include (1) discontinuing TPN or decreasing TPN-supplied calories if feasible, (2) cycling TPN to hold infusion for 10 hours/day, (3) a therapeutic trial of metronidazole, or (4) a therapeutic trial of ursodeoxycholic acid.

E. **AIDS-related cholangiopathy** (most often caused by superimposed cryptosporidium infection) is a disorder that, like PSC, is characterized by biliary stricturing that is most readily diagnosed by cholangiography. The disorder is seen less commonly now that improved therapies have decreased the number of patients who have advanced AIDS.

X. **Metal overload disease**

A. **Hereditary hemochromatosis (HHC)** is a common genetic disorder that affects approximately 1% of individuals in populations of European ancestry. The underlying feature of the disorder is increased absorption of orally ingested iron from food. This excess iron is deposited in the liver, heart, and endocrine pancreas and can lead to injury and dysfunction. In the case of cirrhosis from hemochromatosis, patients are also at markedly increased risk for the development of HCCA.

1. **Symptoms.** Patients with early hemochromatosis are asymptomatic and may be detected only by routine blood test screening (usually a fasting transferrin saturation of >45% or, less often, ferritin >500). As the disease progresses, constitutive symptoms, including fatigue and more specific symptoms of arthritis, cardiac disease, diabetes, and liver failure, may develop. Cutaneous iron deposition can lead to bronzing of the skin, especially in sun-exposed regions (*N Engl J Med* 1993;328:1616).

2. Establishing the **diagnosis** of HHC is complex. Screening tests include the transferrin saturation and serum ferritin as outlined above (if these tests are abnormal, they should first be repeated in the fasted state). Patients with positive tests should undergo further testing that may include blood tests to assess for the C282Y gene mutation that is found in 85% of homozygous HHC patients. Liver biopsy may also suggest the diagnosis by measurement of the hepatic iron index and evaluation of the pattern of iron deposition in the liver (*N Engl J Med* 1999;341:1986, and *Ann Intern Med* 1999;130:953).

3. The **treatment** of HHC may seem archaic, but it is simple, and, if initiated before the development of cirrhosis, it is highly effective in preventing the progression of liver disease and minimizing the risk of malignancy. Initial treatment is weekly phlebotomy (500 ml blood) pro-

vided that the hemoglobin is above 10 g/dl (hemoglobin should be checked every week). If the hemoglobin falls to less than 10 g/dl, phlebotomy frequency should be decreased to every other week. The serum ferritin level is monitored every 1–3 months, and this frequent venesection is continued until the ferritin is less than 50 µg/L. Once the goal ferritin is achieved, phlebotomy is offered every 3–4 months.

B. **Wilson's disease** is a rare disease of copper overload in the liver. It affects approximately 1 in 30,000 individuals and can lead to acute and chronic liver failure as well as neurologic dysfunction. The diagnosis is suggested by a low serum ceruloplasmin (seen in 85% of patients) and elevated 24-hour urine copper level. If these tests are abnormal, a liver biopsy should be pursued, and, if appropriate, treatment with chelation therapy should be offered.

Outpatient Biliary and Pancreatic Disease

I. Cholesterol and pigment stones are the two principal chemical types of **gallstones**. Cholesterol stones account for 80% of the biliary stones in developed Western nations. Conditions that increase the risk of stones include female gender, obesity, Northern European or Native American ancestry, and a history of estrogen therapy. Factors that increase bile stasis, such as prolonged bowel rest, weight reduction, or some drugs (such as octreotide) also enhance the risk of cholesterol gallstone formation. Pigment stones, although less common than cholesterol stones, are frequently responsible for biliary pathology. These stones are seen with cirrhosis or hemolytic anemias. Most gallstone formation occurs in the gallbladder, which can provide a reservoir for bile stasis and for the precipitation of cholesterol or bilirubin calcium salts. Most gallstones are asymptomatic, but in 15–20% of patients complications from biliary obstruction caused by gallstones may develop. Uncomplicated biliary colic is the most common manifestation and is characterized by prolonged periods (hours) of right-upper-quadrant or epigastric pain that frequently radiates to the shoulder and may be associated with nausea/vomiting. More serious complications include frank biliary obstruction that can lead to cholangitis or pancreatitis. **Ultrasound** is the most sensitive test for the detection of gallstones. Cholecystectomy is the treatment of choice to prevent recurrent symptoms or complications. Dissolution therapy with ursodeoxycholic acid may be minimally effective (*N Engl J Med* 1993;328:412, and *Ann Intern Med* 1993;119:606).

II. **Pancreatic cancer.** Adenocarcinoma of the head or proximal portion of the pancreas is the most frequent cause of malignant biliary obstruction. The characteristic symptom is painless jaundice, and the diagnosis is usually established by contrast-enhanced CT scan. Ninety percent of patients with pancreatic cancer have local or distant tumor spread at the time of diagnosis. Also, most patients are elderly (the median age of diagnosis is in the eighth decade of life) and may have comorbid illnesses. These factors, when treating patients with pancreatic cancer, commonly place the emphasis on palliative therapies. Still, an experienced biliary surgeon should evaluate patients before abandoning curative efforts (*Gastrointest Endosc Clin N Am* 1995;5:217).

III. **Chronic pancreatitis** is permanent morphologic and functional damage to the pancreas. Alcohol consumption is the most common etiology in adults; cystic fibrosis (as a cause of pancreatic insufficiency) is gaining importance, as the survival associated with this disease is improving. Consequences occur if greater than 90% of pancreatic function is compromised and can include chronic abdominal pain, fat malabsorption from exocrine pancreatic insufficiency, and, in especially severe cases, glucose intolerance (*N Engl J Med* 1973;288:

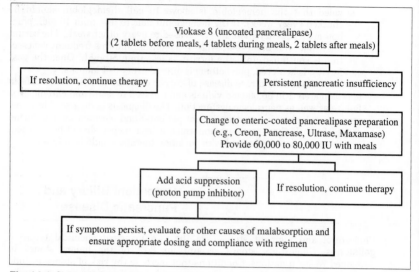

Fig. 14-1. Suggested algorithm for management of pancreatic insufficiency.

813). Diagnosis is based on clinical grounds, but some complicated testing is available. Enzyme supplementation is lifelong, complex, and expensive; the manufacture and formulation of specific enzyme supplements are poorly standardized, and therefore different preparations cannot be considered to be therapeutically equivalent. As lipase is highly sensitive to acid deactivation, acid suppression and enteric-coated enzyme formulations, although costly, are important in management. Fig. 14-1 lists a suggestive therapeutic algorithm for management.

15

Hematology

Lawrence T. Goodnough
and Morey A. Blinder

Approach to the Patient with Anemia

I. **Clinical presentation of anemia** can be accompanied by a variety of symptoms and signs, depending on the severity of anemia and the pace of its development. Pallor, tachycardia, dizziness, tinnitus, headaches, irritability, loss of concentration, fatigue, and weakness are common examples. Reduced exercise tolerance and even heart failure can be present with more severe anemia in some patients. Insidious onset of anemia over a prolonged interval may be accompanied by adaptive compensatory mechanisms that can lead to a virtually asymptomatic presentation.

II. **Initial evaluation**

   A. **History** is the most important part of the evaluation of anemia. Patient demographics (e.g., menstruating woman) provide important clues regarding potential sources of RBC loss. Dietary evaluation may unmask possible nutritional deficiencies. Pagophagia (obsessive consumption of ice) is a variant of pica that is specific to iron deficiency. The presence or absence of constitutional symptoms (fever, night sweats, weight loss, anorexia) is helpful in directing subsequent evaluation of possible underlying disease. A history of alcohol abuse, hematuria, hematochezia, melena, or hematemesis provides clues for blood loss. A careful drug history and family history are important as well.

   B. **Physical examination** can identify underlying accompanying pathology, such as **lymphadenopathy** or **hepatosplenomegaly**. Koilonychia (brittle, "spoon"-shaped fingernails) is pathognomonic for iron deficiency but occurs in only a fraction of patients. Other important findings are the presence of occult fecal blood, jaundice, bone tenderness, and neurologic symptoms.

III. **Laboratory evaluation** includes hemoglobin (Hb), hematocrit (Hct), mean corpuscular volume (MCV), reticulocyte (retic) count, and an examination of the peripheral blood smear.

   A. The **Hb and Hct** serve as an estimate of the RBC mass, but interpretation must take into consideration the volume status of the patient. Immediately after acute blood loss, the Hb is normal because compensatory mechanisms have not had time to restore normal plasma volume.

   B. The **MCV** determines the average RBC size and is useful for classifying anemia (microcytic, normocytic, and macrocytic for anemia with low, normal, and high MCV, respectively). Proper use of the MCV in establishing a diagnosis depends on examination of the peripheral smear for the following reasons: (1) Small and large cells may be present simultaneously, resulting in a normal MCV; (2) retics are larger than mature RBCs and will raise the MCV; and (3) abnormal cells may be present in numbers that are too small to affect the MCV.

   C. The **retic count.** The percentage of RBCs that are retics (normal 0.5–1.5%) is used to determine whether the anemia is due to underproduction or accelerated RBC destruction. This value is artifactually (i.e., not related to changes in marrow production) altered by the degree of anemia, so that calculating

$$\text{Corrected retic count} = \text{retic } (\%) \times \frac{\text{observed Hct}}{\text{expected Hct}}$$

A second artifact of the retic (%) is the early release of retics (which have a life span of 4 days) into the peripheral blood with increasing anemia. Thus,

$$\text{Retic index} = \frac{\text{corrected retic count}}{\text{no. days in peripheral blood}}$$

where retics exist in the peripheral blood for 1.0 day at normal Hcts and approximately 1.5, 2.0, and 3.0 days at Hct levels of 30%, 24%, and 18%, respectively. Retic responses require 3–7 days in new-onset anemias, with marrow responses defined as "appropriate" accompanied by a retic index that should be at least twofold greater than baseline in acute anemias and five- to eightfold greater in chronic compensated anemias. The retic count may also be reported as an absolute number, in which values greater than 100,000/μl are considered to represent an appropriate erythropoietic response.

D. **Examination of a well-prepared peripheral blood smear** is mandatory. Heterogeneity in RBC size (anisocytosis) and shape (poikilocytosis) may be seen. Specific morphologic abnormalities should be sought, as well as any abnormalities in the WBCs or platelets.

Anemias Associated with Decreased Red Blood Cell Production

I. **Iron deficiency** is the most common cause of anemia in the ambulatory setting. Menstrual loss or pregnancy is the most common etiology. In the absence of menstrual bleeding, GI blood loss is the presumed etiology in most patients, and the appropriate radiographic and endoscopic procedures should be pursued to identify a source and exclude occult malignancy.

A. **Clinical presentation.** Patients may present with fatigue, related to the universal importance of iron in cellular metabolism. A careful history to elicit blood loss (melena, hematochezia, hematemesis, menorrhagia) is essential.

B. **Laboratory evaluation** depends on patient demographics. Assuming opportunity for follow-up, a microcytic (MCV <80) anemia in the setting of a menstruating female needs only a baseline Hb/Hct that is repeated 2–4 months after initiation of oral iron therapy. Postmenopausal women and men require more detailed evaluation, including evaluation of potential RBC losses, commonly via the GI tract (peptic ulcer disease, colon carcinoma) or, rarely, the urinary tract (e.g., paroxysmal nocturnal hemoglobinuria). Because evaluating these patients may require considerable expense, laboratory studies are necessary to document iron deficiency before further evaluation.

1. **Iron, transferrin, and transferrin saturation** are traditionally used to diagnose iron deficiency anemia but are diagnostic only in marked, uncomplicated iron deficiency. In this setting, serum iron declines to below 50 μ/dl once iron stores are exhausted. Transferrin increases linearly to approximately 400 μ/dl once patients are in negative iron balance, so that transferrin saturation falls below 16% only when iron stores are exhausted.

2. **Ferritin** is the primary storage form for iron in the liver and bone marrow. It is in equilibrium with the iron pool in the plasma and is therefore

widely used as a surrogate marker of iron stores. A level of less than 10 ng/ml in women or 20 ng/ml in men is indicative of low iron stores. However, 25% of women with no stainable iron in the bone marrow have serum ferritin levels above this cutoff. Ferritin is an acute-phase reactant, so that normal levels may be seen in inflammatory states despite low iron stores. A serum ferritin of >200 ng/ml excludes iron deficiency, except in renal dialysis patients, in whom a cutoff of 400 ng/ml is used.

3. Flow cytometric analysis of retics allows precise measurements of **retic Hb content (Chr)**. In dialysis patients, Chr is 100% sensitive and 80% specific and is a more accurate predictor of response to iron therapy than serum ferritin or transferrin saturation. It is the strongest predictor of iron deficiency in children and should be considered an alternative to biochemical iron studies for diagnosis of iron deficiency in pediatric anemias.

4. A **bone marrow biopsy** that shows absent staining for iron is the definitive test for establishing iron deficiency and is helpful when the serum tests fail to confirm the diagnosis.

C. Treatment

1. **Oral iron therapy** in stable patients with mild symptoms consists of **ferrous sulfate**, 325 mg PO one to three times/day. Iron is best absorbed on an empty stomach, and between 3 mg and 10 mg elemental iron can be absorbed daily. Oral iron ingestion may induce a number of GI side effects, including epigastric distress, bloating, and constipation, so that noncompliance is a common problem. These side effects can be decreased by initially administering the drug with meals or once/day and increasing the dose as tolerated. Concomitant administration of vitamin C improves absorption by maintaining the iron in the reduced state.

2. **Parenteral iron therapy** may be useful in patients with (1) poor absorption (e.g., inflammatory bowel disease, malabsorption), (2) very high iron requirements that cannot be met with oral supplementation (e.g., ongoing bleeding), or (3) intolerance to oral preparations. The following formula can be used to approximate the amount of iron that is required to restore the Hb to normal levels and replenish the iron stores:

$$\text{Iron (mg)} = 0.3 \times \text{body weight (lb)} \times (100 - \text{Hb}[(g/dl)/14.8 \times 100])$$

Most patients require 1000–2000 mg iron to correct the deficit. Iron dextran and sodium ferric gluconate are the available parenteral agents. Iron dextran can be administered IM or IV. A single dose of IV iron dextran (diluted in 250–500 ml normal saline and infused at 6 mg/minute) has been used with few complications and is the generally preferred route (*J Lab Clin Med* 1988;111:566). IM and IV therapy of iron dextran may rarely be complicated by anaphylaxis; therefore, a 0.5-ml IM or IV test dose should be administered 1 hour before therapy is initiated. Delayed reactions to IV iron, such as arthralgia, myalgia, fever, pruritus, and lymphadenopathy may be seen within 3 days of therapy and usually resolve spontaneously or with nonsteroidal anti-inflammatory drugs (NSAIDs). A typical IM dosing schedule is 1 ml (50 mg) into each buttock per week until the total dose is administered. An alternative preparation, ferric gluconate, has been approved for intravenous administration. The side effect profile appears to be better than that of iron dextran, and ferric gluconate has not been reported to cause any deaths in more than 20 years of experience worldwide. The recommended dosage is 125 mg diluted in 100 ml normal saline infused IV over 1 hour. Ferric gluconate can also be administered undiluted by slow IV push over 10 minutes (12.5 mg/min). This can be repeated weekly until circulating iron (to a normal Hct) and storage iron (1–3 g) are replenished. Reticulocytosis should manifest within 3–7 days, with

RBC volume expansion equivalent to one blood unit (3 Hct percentage points) generated every 1–2 weeks.

II. **Megaloblastic anemia** is a term used to describe disorders of impaired DNA synthesis in hematopoietic cells but affects all proliferating cells. Almost all cases are due to folic acid or vitamin B_{12} deficiency.

A. **Folate deficiency** arises from a negative folate balance arising from decreased intake (alcoholism), malabsorption, or increased requirement (pregnancy, hemolytic anemia). Patients present with sleep deprivation, fatigue, and manifestations of depression, irritability, or forgetfulness. Patients on slimming diets, alcoholics, the elderly, and psychiatric patients are particularly at risk for nutritional folate deficiency. **Pregnancy and lactation** require higher (three- to fourfold) daily folate needs and are commonly associated with megaloblastic changes in maternal hematopoietic cells, leading to a dimorphic (combined folate and iron deficiency) anemia. Folate malabsorption can be seen in sprue. **Drugs** that can interfere with folate absorption include ethanol, trimethoprim, pyrimethamine, diphenylhydantoin, barbiturates, and sulfasalazine. Patients who are undergoing dialysis require enhanced folate intake because of folate losses. Patients with hemolytic anemia, particularly sickle cell anemia, require increased folate for accelerated erythropoiesis and can present with aplastic crisis (rapidly falling RBC counts) with folate deficiency.

B. **Vitamin B_{12} deficiency** occurs insidiously over 3 years or more, because daily vitamin B_{12} requirements are 1–3 µg, whereas total body stores are 1–3 mg. By the time that anemia due to vitamin B_{12} is clinically manifest, neurologic manifestations are commonly prevalent, with some element of incapacity. Because multivitamins now contain folic acid, the hematologic manifestations of vitamin B_{12} deficiency may be obscured, leading solely to neurologic presentations. Causes of vitamin B_{12} deficiency include total or partial (up to 20% of patients within 8 years of surgery) gastrectomy and pernicious anemia (PA). PA occurs in individuals who are older than 40 years (mean onset, age 60 years). Up to 30% of patients have a positive family history. PA is associated with other autoimmune disorders (Graves' disease 30%, Hashimoto's thyroiditis 11%, and Addison's disease 5–10%). Of patients with PA, 90% have antiparietal cell immunoglobulin G (IgG) antibodies, and 60% have anti-intrinsic factor antibodies.

C. **Physical examination** may indicate poor nutrition, pigmentation of skin creases and nail beds, or glossitis. Jaundice or splenomegaly may indicate ineffective and extramedullary hematopoiesis. Vitamin B_{12} deficiency may cause decreased vibratory and positional sense, ataxia, paresthesias, confusion, and dementia. Neurologic complications may occur even in the absence of anemia and may not resolve despite adequate treatment. Folic acid deficiency does not result in neurologic disease.

D. **Laboratory evaluation.** A macrocytic anemia is usually present, and leukopenia and thrombocytopenia may occur. The peripheral smear may show anisocytosis, poikilocytosis, and macro-ovalocytes; hypersegmented neutrophils (containing ≥5 nuclear lobes) are common. Lactic dehydrogenase (LDH) and indirect bilirubin are typically elevated, reflecting ineffective erythropoiesis and premature destruction of RBCs.

   1. **Serum vitamin B_{12} and RBC folate levels** should be measured. RBC folate is a more accurate indicator of body folate stores than serum folate, particularly if measured after folate therapy or improved nutrition has been initiated.

   2. **Serum methylmalonic acid and homocysteine (HC)** may be useful when the vitamin B_{12} or folate level is equivocal. Methylmalonic acid and HC are elevated in vitamin B_{12} deficiency; only HC is elevated in folate deficiency.

   3. A **Schilling test** may be useful in the diagnosis of PA due to vitamin B_{12} deficiency but rarely affects the therapeutic approach. Detecting antibodies to intrinsic factor is specific for the diagnosis of PA.

4. **Bone marrow biopsy** may be necessary to rule out myelodysplastic syndrome and hematologic malignancy. These disorders may present with findings similar to those of megaloblastic anemia on peripheral smear.
E. **Treatment** is directed toward replacing the deficient factor. Potassium supplementation may be necessary to avoid potentially fatal arrhythmias due to hypokalemia induced by enhanced hematopoiesis. Reticulocytosis should begin within 1 week of therapy, followed by a rising Hb over 6–8 weeks. Coexisting iron deficiency is present in one-third of patients and is a common cause for an incomplete response to therapy.
   1. **Folic acid,** 1 mg PO qd, is given until the deficiency is corrected. High doses of folic acid (5 mg PO qd) may be needed in patients with malabsorption syndromes.
   2. **Vitamin B_{12}** deficiency is corrected by administering cyanocobalamin. Unless the patient is severely ill (decompensated CHF due to anemia, advanced neurologic dysfunction), treatment with full doses of B_{12} (1 mg/ day IM) should await confirmation of diagnosis, because diagnosis mandates a commitment to lifelong therapy. After 1 week of daily therapy, 1 mg/week should be given for 4 weeks and then 1 mg/month for life. Patients who refuse or cannot take parenteral therapy can be prescribed oral tablets or syrup at 50 μg/day for life.
III. **Anemia of chronic renal insufficiency** is attributed primarily to decreased endogenous erythropoietin (Epo) production and may occur as the creatinine clearance declines below 50 ml/minute.
   A. **Laboratory evaluation** reveals a normal MCV in 85% of the cases. The Hct is usually 20–30%. If the patient's creatinine is greater than 1.8 mg/dl, the primary cause of the anemia can be assumed to be Epo deficiency, and an Epo level is unnecessary. Iron deficiency should also be evaluated in patients who are undergoing dialysis due to chronic blood loss.
   B. **Treatment** of anemia of chronic renal insufficiency has been revolutionized by recombinant human Epo. Therapy is initiated in predialysis patients who are symptomatic. Objective benefits of reversing the anemia include enhanced exercise capacity, improved cognitive function, elimination of RBC transfusions, and reduction of iron overload. Subjective benefits include increased energy, enhanced appetite, better sleep patterns, and improved sexual activity.
      1. **Administration of Epo** can be IV (hemodialysis patients) or SC (predialysis or peritoneal dialysis patients). A typical initial dose is 50–100 units/kg three times/week until the Hct reaches 32%; the average maintenance dose is 75 units/kg three times/week. Folate deficiency is universal in patients who are undergoing dialysis, and all such individuals should receive folate, 1 mg PO qd.
      2. **Adverse reactions** to Epo are uncommon. Hypertension may develop or worsen in patients while the Hct is increasing. Seizures may occur, although the etiology is not well characterized.
      3. **Suboptimal responses to Epo therapy** are a common phenomenon due to iron deficiency or aluminum toxicity, or both. Because anemia is a powerful determinant of life expectancy in patients on chronic dialysis, intravenous iron administration has become standard therapy in many individuals who receive Epo therapy and has also been shown to reduce the Epo dosage that is required to correct anemia. Aluminum intoxication blunts the response to Epo. Secondary hyperparathyroidism that causes bone marrow fibrosis and relative Epo resistance may also occur.
IV. **Anemia of chronic disease** often develops in patients with long-standing inflammatory diseases, malignancy, autoimmune disorders, and chronic infection. The etiology is multifactorial; defective iron mobilization during erythropoiesis, inflammatory cytokine-mediated suppression of erythropoiesis, and impaired Epo response to anemia all play a role. Anemia of chronic disease is also a common complication of therapy for the underlying disease (e.g., chemotherapy for malignancy, zidovudine for HIV infection).

    A. Laboratory evaluation. A normocytic, normochromic anemia is typical. Iron studies are difficult to interpret. Clinical responses to iron therapy can be seen in patients with ferritin levels of up to 100 ng/ml. A bone marrow evaluation for storage iron may be necessary to rule out an absolute iron deficiency accompanying an anemia of chronic disease. No laboratory test is diagnostic for the anemia of chronic disease.

    B. Treatment. Therapy for anemia associated with chronic disease is directed at the underlying disease and at eliminating exacerbating factors such as nutritional deficiencies and marrow-suppressive drugs. Epo therapy (150 units/kg SC three times/week) should be given when the Hct decreases below 30% or with symptoms of anemia. A single dose of 600 units/kg has been shown to be equivalent to 150 units/kg three times weekly in perisurgical patients, and once weekly dosing is commonly used in the oncology setting. Transfusion should be considered for patients with Hct levels of less than 24% or if symptomatic.

    C. Anemia in cancer patients who are receiving chemotherapy can be successfully prevented and treated with Epo at dosages of 100–150 units/kg three times/week. In anemic patients with myeloma or non–Hodgkin's lymphoma, a dosage of 200 units/kg/week is usually effective in those with residual marrow function (as indicated by a normal platelet count), whereas a dosage of 600 units/kg/week is recommended in those with a hypoproliferative anemia (*Blood* 1997;89:4248).

V. The **thalassemia syndromes** are inherited disorders characterized by reduced Hb synthesis associated with mutations in either the α- or β-chain of the Hb molecule. Affected individuals are of Mediterranean, Middle Eastern, Indian, African, or Asian descent.

    A. Beta thalassemia results in an imbalance between beta globulin (underproduced) and alpha globulin (excess), forming insoluble alpha tetramers and leading to ineffective erythropoiesis and hemolytic anemia. **Thalassemia minor (trait)** occurs with one gene abnormality with modest β-chain underproduction. Patients are asymptomatic and present with microcytic, hypochromic RBCs and Hb levels greater than 10 g/dl. **Thalassemia intermedia** occurs with abnormalities in both beta-globulin genes, so that the anemia is more clinically severe (Hb 7–10 g/dl). **Thalassemia major** (Cooley's anemia) is caused by severe abnormalities of both genes, so that anemia is fatal in infancy or requires lifelong transfusion support.

    B. Alpha thalassemia occurs with decreased function of one or more of the four alpha-globulin genes. Mild microcytosis and mild hypochromic anemia (Hb >10 g/dl) is seen with loss of one or two genes, whereas HbH disease (splenomegaly, hemolytic anemia, and beta-globulin tetramers) is seen with the loss of three genes. Treatment of HbH disease rarely requires transfusion or splenectomy, but oxidant drugs similar to those that exacerbate glucose-6-phosphate dehydrogenase deficiency should be avoided because increased hemolysis may occur (Table 15-1). Hydrops fetalis occurs with the loss of all four alpha-globulin genes.

    C. Clinical presentation. A family history of microcytic anemia or microcytosis is helpful. Splenomegaly may be the only physical manifestation.

    D. Laboratory. The MCV is low. Microcytic hypochromic RBCs are seen, along with poikilocytosis and nucleated RBCs. Hb electrophoresis is diagnostic.

    E. Therapy. Hb levels of 9–10 g/dl are required, and transfusions are necessary in the more severe forms of the disease to prevent the skeletal deformities that result from accelerated erythropoiesis. The resultant iron overload often requires chelation therapy (deferoxamine mesylate, 50–100 mg/kg/day) given by continuous SC infusion for 10–12 hours/day, along with vitamin C supplementation (100 mg PO) to enhance urinary iron excretion. Splenectomy should be considered in patients with accelerated (more than 2 units/month) transfusion requirements. Bone marrow transplant should be considered in young patients with thalassemia major who have human leukocyte antigen–identical related donors.

Table 15-1. Drugs that can induce RBC disorders

Sideroblastic anemia	Aplastic anemia[a]	Hemolytic episode in G6PD deficiency	Immune hemolytic anemia		
			Autoantibody	Hapten	Immune complex[b]
Chloramphenicol	Acetazolamide	Dapsone	α-Methyldopa	Akfluor 25%	Amphotericin B
Cycloserine	Antineoplastic agents	Furazolidone	Cephalosporins	Cephalosporins	Antazoline
Ethanol	Carbamazepine	Methylene blue	Diclofenac	Penicillins	Cephalosporins
Isoniazid	Chloramphenicol	Nalidixic acid	Ibuprofen	Tetracycline	Chlorpropamide
Pyrazinamide	Gold salts	Nitrofurantoin	Interferon-alpha	Tolbutamide	Diclofenac
	Hydantoins	Phenazopyridine	L-Dopa		Diethylstilbestrol
	Penicillamine	Primaquine	Mefenamic acid		Doxepin
	Phenylbutazone	Sulfacetamide	Procainamide		Hydrochlorothiazide
	Quinacrine	Sulfamethoxazole	Teniposide		Isoniazid
		Sulfanilamide	Thioridazine		p-Aminosalicylic acid
		Sulfapyridine	Tolmetin		Probenecid
					Quinidine
					Quinine
					Rifampin
					Sulfonamides
					Thiopental
					Tolmetin

Note: Data compiled from multiple sources. Agents listed are available in the United States.
G6PD, glucose-6-phosphate dehydrogenase.
[a]Drugs with more than 30 cases reported; many other drugs rarely are associated with aplastic anemia and are considered low risk.
[b]Some sources list mechanisms for many of these drugs as unknown.
Source: SN Ahya, K Flood, S Paranjothi (eds), *The Washington Manual of Medical Therapeutics* (30th ed). Philadelphia: Lippincott Williams & Wilkins, 2001, with permission.

Anemias Associated with Increased Red Blood Cell Loss or Destruction

I. **Clinical presentation.** Patients with abrupt onset of anemia, in contrast to chronic insidious anemia, tolerate diminished red cell mass poorly. The anemia may be relatively mild (i.e., Hct >30%), but the patient can present with symptoms of fatigue, malaise, dizziness, syncope, or angina. Acute blood loss most commonly occurs in the GI tract (gastritis due to alcohol or NSAIDs, diverticulosis, or peptic or gastric ulcer disease) and may be accompanied by epigastric symptoms, nausea and vomiting, and diarrhea or melena.

II. **Physical examination** may reveal vital sign changes indicative of hypovolemia (hypotension, tachycardia) due to blood loss or an increased cardiac output as a compensatory mechanism. Occult sites of blood loss are seen in patients with hip fracture or retroperitoneal bleeds.

III. **Laboratory evaluation.** If presentation is within 5 days of onset, the only abnormal laboratory value may be decreased Hct. Retic response requires 3–5 days, after which an elevated retic count indicates an appropriate erythropoietic response to RBC loss or destruction. LDH and bilirubin are increased with more prolonged clinical onset. Serum haptoglobin is decreased with hemolysis due to clearance of intravascular Hb. With severe hemolysis, free Hb can be measured in the plasma, and urine hemosiderin can be detected in the urine with more chronic hemolysis. Examination of the peripheral smear is an important clue to detect hemolysis. Intravascular hemolysis reveals red cell fragmentation (schistocytes, helmet cells), whereas spherocytes indicate extravascular, immune-mediated hemolysis. Polychromatophilia and nucleated RBCs can be seen with intense hemolysis and erythropoiesis. Evaluation for hemolysis includes the direct Coombs' test [direct antibody testing (DAT)] for the presence of antibody attached to red cells; the indirect Coombs' test indicates the presence of free antibody in the plasma.

IV. **The sickle cell diseases** are a group of hereditary Hb disorders in which the Hb undergoes sickle shape transformation under conditions of deoxygenation. The most common are homozygous sickle cell anemia (HbSS) or other heterozygous conditions (HbSC, HbS–beta thalassemia). A large number of individuals give a positive history for sickle cell trait because of newborn screening programs for hemoglobinopathies. **Sickle cell trait** is present in 2.5 million people in the United States, occurring in 8% of African-Americans. No hematologic findings are associated with sickle cell trait, which is a benign hereditary condition. Nevertheless, some risks of exposure to hypoxia have been reported in patients with sickle cell trait, including high altitude (splenic infarction, cerebrovascular complications) and basic training of military recruits (increased incidence of sudden death related to extreme exertion and dehydration). A monograph on sickle cell disease is available and provides useful guidelines (National Institutes of Health Publication No. 95-2117 at http://www.nhlbi.nih.gov/health/prof/blood/sickle).

    A. **Clinical manifestations** are variable but are all related to chronic hemolysis and vascular occlusion. Delayed growth and development occur in the pediatric years; other pediatric complications include cerebrovascular accidents and splenic autoinfarction, resulting in increased susceptibility to encapsulated bacterial infections. Renal medullary infarction results in chronic polyuria due to impaired urinary concentration, leading to a chronic risk of dehydration. Cholelithiasis is present in more than 50% of patients, primarily due to bilirubin stones. Osteonecrosis of the femoral heads occurs in 10% of patients. Chronic leg ulceration is also seen. In general, patients with HbSC disease have a less severe course, presenting with splenomegaly and higher levels of Hb.

B. Laboratory. Hb electrophoresis distinguishes HbSS from other abnormal Hb. The Hct ranges from 5 to 10 g/dl in HbSS disease. The MCV may be slightly elevated due to chronic reticulocytosis. Leukocytosis (10,000–20,000/µl) and thrombocytosis (>450,000/µl) are common, due to enhanced stimulation of the marrow compartment and to autosplenectomy. Peripheral smear shows sickle-shaped RBCs, target cells (particularly in HbSC and HbS–beta thalassemia), and Howell-Jolly bodies, indicative of functional asplenism. Microcytosis is seen in HbS–beta thalassemia. The degree of anemia and reticulocytosis is generally milder in HbSC disease.

C. Prevention and health maintenance

    1. Dehydration and hypoxia should be avoided because they may precipitate or exacerbate sickling. Intense exercise, traveling to high altitudes, and flying in unpressurized aircraft should be avoided.

    2. Folic acid, 1 mg PO qd, should be administered to all patients with sickle cell disease because of chronic hemolysis.

    3. Antimicrobial prophylaxis with penicillin VK, 125 mg PO bid up to age 3 years, then 250 mg PO bid until 5 years, is effective in reducing the risk of infection. Patients who are allergic to penicillin should receive erythromycin, 10 mg/kg PO bid. In most patients, antimicrobial prophylaxis should be discontinued after 5 years of age (*J Pediatr* 1995;127:685).

    4. Immunizations against the usual childhood illnesses should be given to children with sickle cell disease, including hepatitis B vaccine. After 2 years of age, a polyvalent pneumococcal vaccine should be administered. Yearly influenza vaccine is recommended.

    5. Ophthalmologic examinations are recommended yearly in adults because of the high incidence of proliferative retinopathy, which leads to vitreous hemorrhage and retinal detachment.

    6. Surgery and anesthesia. Local and regional anesthesia can be used without special precautions. With general anesthesia, measures to avoid volume depletion, hypoxia, and hypernatremia are crucial. For major surgery, RBC transfusions to increase the Hb concentration to 10 g/dl seem to be as effective as more aggressive regimens in most circumstances (*N Engl J Med* 1995;333:206).

D. Infections in adults typically occur in tissues that are susceptible to vaso-occlusive infarcts (bone, kidney, lung). Treatment of osteomyelitis and urinary tract infections should be based on results of culture data. *Staphylococcus, Salmonella,* and enteric organisms are the most common. Pneumonia is most likely to be caused by *Mycoplasma, Staphylococcus aureus,* or *Haemophilus influenzae* and must be distinguished from acute chest syndrome (see sec. **F.2**).

E. Complications of chronic hemolysis

    1. Aplastic crisis presents with a sudden decrease in Hb level. The retic index is inappropriately low (<3%), reflecting suppression of erythropoiesis. The most common etiology in pediatric patients is infection with parvovirus B19; viral syndromes (including Epstein-Barr virus and hepatitis) and bacterial infections can also suppress erythropoiesis and cause an aplastic crisis. **Folate deficiency** should also be suspected because of the chronic increased requirements for erythropoiesis. Patients with suspected aplastic crisis require hospitalization. Therapy includes folate, 5 mg/day, as well as RBC transfusions.

    2. Cholelithiasis, primarily with bilirubin stones, is present in more than 50% of adult patients. Acute cholecystitis should be treated medically, and cholecystectomy should be performed when the attack subsides. Elective cholecystectomy for asymptomatic gallstones is controversial.

F. Acute vaso-occlusive complications

    1. Vaso-occlusive pain crises are the most common manifestation of sickle cell disease. Pain is typically in the long bones, back, chest, and abdomen. These crises are precipitated by stress, including vasoreactivity of the microvascular system along with dehydration or infection, or both, and generally last for 2–6 days. Although a given individual tends to have a consistent pattern of presentation, wide variability is found among patients. Patient-specific factors related to the ability to cope with stress and chronic illness also contribute to the clinical variability. Generally, one-third have very mild disease with rare painful episodes, characterized by lower Hb values and higher fetal Hb levels. One-third of patients have intermediate severity, requiring a handful of hospitalizations yearly. Another one-third with severe disease have recurrent severe episodes that require frequent emergency room treatments and more than six hospitalizations a year. **Outpatient management** consists of rehydration (oral fluids, 3–4 L/day), evaluation for and management of infections, analgesia, and, if needed, antipyretic and antibiotic therapy. **Morphine** (0.3–0.6 mg/kg PO q4h) is the drug of choice for moderate to severe pain. Outpatient pain management is a complex problem that may require multidisciplinary approaches, including social services, psychiatric consultation, and anesthesia pain services, to minimize the use of narcotic medications. Transfusion therapy has no role in the treatment of uncomplicated vaso-occlusive crises. **Indications for hospitalization** include inability to ingest adequate oral fluids, requirement for parenteral opioids or antibiotics, a declining Hb level associated with inadequate erythropoiesis, or hypoxia.

2. **Acute chest syndrome** occurs when hypoxia (<90% oxygen saturation) leads to increased intravascular sickling and irreversible occlusion of the microvasculature (predominantly pulmonary) circulation. Patients with lung pathology, such as acute pneumonia, are particularly at risk. **Individuals with suspected acute chest syndrome require immediate hospitalization** and aggressive transfusion therapy, including red cell exchange.

3. **Hepatic/splenic sequestration** crises occur with acute splenic or hepatic enlargement due to blood congestion. Clinical presentation consists of sudden pain in the affected organ, a rapidly falling Hb level, and hypovolemia leading to shock or sudden death. Splenic sequestration usually occurs in individuals with an intact spleen, such as infants with HbSS or adults with HbSC or HbS–beta thalassemia. Hospitalization and aggressive transfusion therapy, including red cell exchange, are indicated.

4. **Priapism** refers to painful erection due to vaso-occlusion. Primary treatment is hydration and analgesia. Persistent erections for more than 24 hours may require transfusion therapy or surgical drainage.

G. **Chronic organ damage**
   1. **Osteonecrosis** of the femoral and humeral heads may cause considerable morbidity in approximately 10% of patients. Treatment consists of local heat, analgesics, and avoidance of weight bearing. Hip and shoulder arthroplasty may be effective in decreasing symptoms and improving function.
   2. **Stroke** occurs most commonly in children younger than 10 years and is usually caused by cerebral infarction. Long-term transfusions to maintain the HbS concentration at less than 50% for at least 5 years reduce the incidence of recurrence.
   3. **Leg ulcers** should be treated with rest, leg elevation, and intensive local care. Wet to dry dressings should be applied three to four times/day. A zinc oxide–impregnated bandage (Unna boot), changed weekly for 3–4 weeks, can be used for nonhealing or more extensive ulcers.
   4. **Renal tubular defects** caused by sickling in the anoxic hyperosmolar environment of the renal medulla may lead to isosthenuria (inability to concentrate urine) and hematuria in sickle cell trait and disease. These

conditions predispose patients to dehydration, which increases the risk of vaso-occlusive events.

H. Pregnancy is associated with increased spontaneous abortions or premature delivery, along with increased vaso-occlusive crises.

I. Hydroxyurea therapy (15–35 mg/kg PO daily) has been shown to increase levels of fetal Hb and decrease the frequency of vaso-occlusive crises by 50% in adults with sickle cell disease.

V. Red cell enzyme deficiencies. The most common hereditary enzyme deficiency is glucose-6-phosphate dehydrogenase deficiency, a sex-linked disorder that typically affects men. RBCs that are deficient in this enzyme are more susceptible to hemolysis via oxidant stress, triggered by infections or drug exposure (Table 15-1), leading to chronic or episodic hemolysis.

    A. Clinical presentation. A mild form of the disease is seen in approximately 10% of African-American men. A more severe form is the Mediterranean variant, in which hemolysis is precipitated when susceptible individuals ingest fava beans and present with fatigue, jaundice, and bilirubinuria.

    B. Laboratory. Peripheral smear shows "bite cells," and special stains can show precipitated Heinz bodies within RBCs. Diagnosis is made by demonstrating reduced levels of the enzyme. Because older senescent cells with lower enzyme levels hemolyze first during the acute hemolytic episode, a younger population of RBCs may result in a falsely elevated (normal) enzyme level. Diagnosis may have to await recovery from the hemolytic episode.

    C. Treatment. Acute hemolytic episodes are largely intravascular and self-limited. Therapy, including hydration and transfusion, is therefore supportive. Identification and removal of oxidant stresses such as drugs are paramount.

VI. Autoimmune hemolytic anemia (AIHA) is caused by antibodies to RBCs, which cause a shortened RBC life span. The diagnosis rests on the detection of RBC-bound antibody. "Warm" AIHA refers to IgG antibodies that react best at 37°C, whereas in "cold" AIHA, antibodies (usually IgM) are most reactive at lower temperatures.

    A. Warm-antibody AIHA may be idiopathic or associated with an underlying malignancy (lymphoma, chronic lymphocytic leukemia), collagen vascular disorder, or drugs (Table 15-1).

        1. Clinical presentation. Mild cases may present with stable Hb levels and profound reticulocytosis. In fulminant cases with an RBC life span of less than 5 days, the anemia can be severe and the compensatory erythropoiesis inadequate, with a presentation of a rapidly declining Hb, fever, chest pain, and dyspnea. Jaundice, icterus, and dark urine reflect elevated indirect bilirubin from Hb degradation.

        2. Laboratory evaluation shows a positive DAT for IgG, with 80% of patients having antibodies detectable in the serum (positive indirect Coombs' test). Plasma haptoglobin is decreased, LDH is increased, and the peripheral smear shows spherocytes.

        3. Therapy is directed at identifying and treating any underlying cause. Steroid therapy (prednisone, 1–2 mg/kg/day) and splenectomy for patients with refractory disease is used to decrease the immune clearance of RBC.

    B. Cold-antibody AIHA is associated with episodic cold-induced hemolysis, resulting in cyanosis of the ears, nose, fingers, and toes precipitated by the cold. Cold agglutinin disease is the most common syndrome. It may be chronic and associated with a B-cell neoplasm (lymphoma, chronic lymphocytic leukemia, Waldenström's macroglobulinemia) or acute and caused by an infection (*Mycoplasma*, mononucleosis). The cold agglutinin is a monoclonal IgM antibody. IgM and C3 are present on the RBC, but the DAT identifies only the presence of C3. IgG is negative on the DAT. The anemia is often mild and stable because serum complement inhibitors (C3 inactivator) limit complement activation on the RBC membrane. Exposure to cold, however, can precipitate acute hemolysis in some patients, and avoidance of exposure to cold is of the utmost importance. The disease is otherwise generally characterized by mild anemia with exacerbations, remissions, and prolonged survival. Additional evaluation to identify and treat any underlying malignancy is key.

VII. Drug-induced hemolytic anemia is caused by one of three different mechanisms. Treatment consists of discontinuing the offending agent. Medications that are known to cause these effects are listed in Table 15-1.

   A. Drug-induced autoantibodies present similarly to warm AIHA. The DAT is positive for IgG. α-Methyldopa is the best-known example.

   B. Haptens form when a drug (usually an antimicrobial) coats RBC membranes, forming a new antigenic determinant. If antibodies against the drug are present and the patient receives the drug (particularly at high doses), a DAT-positive hemolytic anemia may result.

   C. Immune complexes occur in most cases of drug-induced hemolysis. IgM (occasionally IgG) antibodies may develop against a drug and form a drug-antibody complex that adheres to the RBCs. Because the antibody is usually IgM, the DAT is positive only for C3.

VIII. Microangiopathic hemolytic anemia is a morphologic classification in which fragmented RBCs are seen on peripheral blood smear. Extrinsic processes that cause RBC fragmentation and hemolysis include fibrin strand deposition [disseminated intravascular coagulation (DIC)], damaged endothelium [thrombotic thrombocytopenic purpura (TTP)], hemolytic-uremic syndrome, and the preeclampsia/eclampsia syndromes; malfunctioning heat valves; and improper use of blood warmers. Therapy is directed at the underlying process that is causing hemolysis.

Other Red Blood Cell Disorders

I. Myelodysplastic syndrome is an acquired, malignant clonal disorder that precedes the onset of acute leukemia, sometimes for many years. The morphologic classifications are based on findings on the peripheral smear and bone marrow biopsy: (1) refractory anemia, (2) refractory anemia with ringed sideroblasts, (3) refractory anemia with excess blasts, (4) refractory anemia with excess blasts in transformation, and (5) chronic myelomonocytic leukemia. Myelodysplastic syndrome usually occurs in the elderly, and a history of environmental exposure to chemicals (benzene, gasoline), radiation, or alkylating chemotherapy agents is sometimes present. Presentations range from mild cytopenias without symptoms to severe pancytopenia. Progression to marrow failure or acute leukemia commonly occurs.

   A. Laboratory. Anemia is the predominant manifestation, but leukopenia and thrombocytopenia may also occur. The diagnosis is established by demonstrating abnormal hematopoietic cells in the bone marrow.

   B. Therapy is supportive. Long-term transfusion therapy may lead to iron overload. Deferoxamine chelation may be necessary after 50–100 units of RBC transfusions. Only 20% of patients respond to Epo, because endogenous levels of Epo are usually high (>200 μ/ml). Patients with refractory anemia with ringed sideroblasts may be responsive to pyridoxine (50–200 mg/day PO).

II. Aplastic anemia is an acquired disorder of hematopoietic stem cells, presenting in people of all ages not only as anemia but also as pancytopenia. Approximately one-third of patients have a history of drug exposure (Table 15-1) or viral infection (e.g., hepatitis, Epstein-Barr virus, cytomegalovirus). Therapy is supportive, with early referral for possible stem cell transplantation. Transfusions should be minimized and, when administered, should be leukodepleted and from nonfamily members.

III. Polycythemia vera is a hematologic malignancy with excess proliferation of all hematopoietic elements but presents primarily with increased RBC mass. The average age at presentation is 60 years. Patients have a variety of symptoms, including weight loss (secondary to hypermetabolism), weakness, gouty arthropathy, pruritus, and CNS symptoms (headaches, dizziness). Physical examination reveals hepatosplenomegaly as well as hypertension and ruddy cyanosis.

A. Laboratory. Elevated levels of Hb, WBCs (66%), and platelets (50%) are seen. RBC morphology often reflects iron deficiency due to chronic, occult GI hemorrhage, and megathrombocytes may be seen. Iron replacement sometimes is necessary before the elevated RBC mass becomes truly manifest. The leukocyte alkaline phosphatase is elevated in 70% of patients. A direct measurement of RBC mass (chromium 51 labeling) is necessary to document absolute polycythemia and rule out factitious or relative polycythemia. Clinical factors that could cause secondary polycythemia (hypoxemia, right-to-left shunts) need to be considered.

B. Therapy. With reduction of RBC mass via chronic phlebotomy to an Hct of less than 45%, prolonged survival is now the rule. Nevertheless, thrombotic events are characteristic and account for the most common cause of death in patients who are managed by phlebotomy alone. Elderly patients and those with a history of thrombosis are therefore candidates for myelosuppressive therapy, such as radioactive phosphorus (phosphorus 32) or chlorambucil therapy.

Platelet Disorders

I. Thrombocytopenia is defined as a platelet count of less than 150,000/μl. Quantitative thrombocytopenia should be confirmed by an examination of the peripheral smear to rule out pseudothrombocytopenia due to anticoagulant or temperature effect.

A. Clinical presentation. Patients with platelet counts greater than 50,000/μl rarely have symptoms or signs of bleeding, unless medications that inhibit platelet function (aspirin, NSAIDs) are ingested. Spontaneous bleeding occurs when platelet counts are less than 10,000–20,000/μl manifest first by petechiae in the gravity-dependent lower extremities. Mucosal or serosal bleeding, epistaxis, or GI bleeding may also occur. The history may be negative, but concurrent illnesses or constitutional symptoms that suggest an underlying disease are clues for further evaluation. A careful and detailed medication history is key.

B. Laboratory. The CBC indicates whether the thrombocytopenia is isolated or whether anemia, leukopenia, or pancytopenia is present. The mean platelet volume can be helpful: The presence of large (mean platelet volume >12 femtoliters), young platelets suggests increased destruction, whereas normal-sized or small platelets suggest underproduction. A useful diagnostic strategy is to categorize thrombocytopenia into disorders of increased consumption or decreased production. A bone marrow examination to evaluate the presence or absence of an adequate number of platelet precursors (megakaryocytes) is usually performed to help make this distinction.

C. Underproduction of platelets is indicated by a reduced number of megakaryocytes.

1. Viral suppression is probably the most common etiology of mild (between 100,000/μl and 150,000/μl) thrombocytopenia. The effect is transient, and recovery is prompt after clearance of the viral infection.

2. Drug-induced thrombocytopenia can be caused by many drugs, and is almost always due to an increase in platelet destruction (see sec. **D.3**).

Thrombocytopenia is a common side effect of chemotherapy and radiation therapy. Ethanol intake is another common cause of suppression of a megakaryopoiesis.

3. **Infiltration of the marrow** by neoplasia can cause thrombocytopenia and may be one of the initial manifestations of an underlying malignancy. Clues to such a myelophthisic process can be seen on peripheral smear. Abnormally shaped RBCs (including teardrop cells), early WBC precursors (myelocytes), nucleated RBCs, and megakaryocytic fragments are occasionally seen. A bone marrow examination is indicated for further evaluation.

D. **Increased destruction** of platelets may be due to consumption or immune clearance.

1. **Immune (idiopathic) thrombocytopenic purpura (ITP)** is a disorder caused by production of antiplatelet antibodies.

a. **Clinical presentation.** Occasionally, patients present unexpectedly when a routine CBC reveals an isolated thrombocytopenia, but most patients have a positive bleeding history, such as menorrhagia, epistaxis, or mucocutaneous manifestations.

b. **Laboratory.** The platelet count is usually less than 100,000/µl, and thrombocytopenia can be severe (<5000/µl). Bone marrow examination confirms the presence of adequate numbers of megakaryocytes, indicating a consumptive process. Platelet-associated IgG can be demonstrated in more than 80% of patients, but its nonspecificity makes this test unhelpful. In the absence of a diagnostic test, ITP is a diagnosis of exclusion. Other possible immunologic or nonimmunologic mechanisms should be considered. The possibility of drug-induced thrombocytopenia is particularly important (Table 15-2).

c. **Therapy** may not be necessary in patients whose platelet counts remain above 50,000/µl. If platelet counts are lower and if bleeding manifestations occur, glucocorticoid therapy (prednisone, 1 mg/kg/day) is initiated. Hospitalization is indicated for severe (<10,000/µl) thrombocytopenia or in patients with serious hemorrhage (e.g., funduscopic evidence of hemorrhage). Platelet therapy should also be considered in such individuals. Up to 80% of patients respond to corticosteroid therapy; once the response occurs the steroid can be tapered slowly over several months. Patients who maintain normal platelet counts or those who have mild (>30,000/µl) thrombocytopenia may not require any further therapy. Intravenous immune globulin (IVIG; 1 g/kg IV daily for 2 days) and splenectomy should be considered in patients without an initial response or in those who cannot be tapered off glucocorticoid therapy because of recurring significant thrombocytopenia. Pneumococcal, meningococcal, and *H. influenzae* type B vaccine should be administered at least 2 weeks before splenectomy. The 10–20% of patients who relapse after splenectomy can be successfully managed with further glucocorticoid therapy. The possibility of an accessory spleen should be investigated.

d. **ITP during pregnancy** may be difficult to distinguish from gestational thrombocytopenia. IVIG is the initial therapy with platelet counts of less than 10,000/µl during the first trimester or less than 30,000/µl during the second or third trimester. Glucocorticoid therapy can be complicated by gestational diabetes and hypertension. Even with successful management of the platelet count of the mother, passive transfer of antibodies against platelets to the fetus causes neonatal thrombocytopenia in up to 20% of neonates. The role for cesarean section versus vaginal delivery is controversial.

e. **HIV and AIDS** patients develop ITP up to 10% and 30% of the time, respectively, and are responsive to corticosteroid therapy. Splenectomy is useful for patients with refractory disease. Therapeutic plasma exchange with immunoabsorbent columns may be effective.

Table 15-2. Drugs implicated in immune thrombocytopenia

Antibiotics	**Antiarrhythmics**
Penicillins	Quinidine
Penicillin	Procainamide
Ampicillin	Lidocaine
Methicillin	Digoxin
Cephalosporins	Amiodarone
Cefotetan	**Antihypertensives**
Cephalothin	Furosemide
Gentamicin	Hydrochlorothiazide
Vancomycin	Spironolactone
Trimethoprim	Acetazolamide
Sulfonamides	Captopril
Anti-inflammatory drugs	α-Methyldopa
Acetaminophen	**Anticonvulsants**
Aspirin	Phenytoin
Ibuprofen	Carbamazepine
Indomethacin	Valproic acid
Diclofenac	**Anticoagulants**
Piroxicam	Heparin
Sulindac	Low-molecular-weight heparin
Iodinated contrast agents	**Other drugs**
Tolmetin	Tricyclic antidepressants
Antihistamines	Cocaine
Cimetidine	Heroin
Ranitidine	Quinine
Chlorpheniramine	Sulfonylureas

2. **Posttransfusion purpura** is a rare but life-threatening clinical syndrome. A profound thrombocytopenia and a clinical presentation that can otherwise be mistaken for ITP develop. The key history is a previous blood transfusion within 7–10 days of presentation. The vast majority of patients with posttransfusion purpura are women who, via previous pregnancies, were exposed to the PL^{A1} platelet antigen, which is present in 98% of the population (including father and child) but is absent in the patient. Acutely, the diagnosis is made similar to that for ITP, except for the positive history for recent transfusion. Therapy must not wait for the confirmatory test, which is a serum assay for antibody to PL^{A1}. After treatment returns the platelet count to normal levels, direct platelet testing confirms that they are PL^{A1} negative. In contrast to ITP, platelet transfusions should not be administered unless PL^{A1}-negative platelets can be procured. Treatment is with IVIG or plasmapheresis.

3. **Drug-induced thrombocytopenia** has been described with many commonly prescribed medications (Table 15-2). Only the most essential medications should be continued when patients present with a clinical

picture that is consistent with drug-induced thrombocytopenia. IVIG therapy can be given if the thrombocytopenia is severe. Heparin is the most common agent producing thrombocytopenia. Mild thrombocytopenia is common (up to 5% of patients) with heparin and is not always immune mediated. **Heparin-induced thrombocytopenia** is a more specific syndrome, suggested by platelet count declines of more than 50% or an absolute count of less than 100,000/μl, usually within 6–12 days of initiation of therapy. In a small subset of patients, severe thrombocytopenia develops, along with life-threatening arterial or venous thrombosis. Heparin should be discontinued immediately in this setting.

    4. TTP is a life-threatening, hematologic emergency characterized by aggregation and consumption of platelets in the microvasculature.

        a. Clinical presentation. Patients present with a variety of complaints related to the clinical pentad of fever, thrombocytopenia, CNS symptoms and signs (headache, impaired sensorium ranging from confusion to coma, or seizures), anemia, and renal dysfunction. A careful history may reveal a several-week course that may have been preceded only by a viral syndrome ("idiopathic" TTP). A variant of TTP is induced by *Escherichia coli* subtype 157, a bacterial contaminant of improperly prepared meat. This is more abrupt in presentation, including GI symptoms (bloody diarrhea), and may have a more predominant renal component (hemolytic-uremic syndrome). Other variants include pregnancy-associated TTP, TTP due to drugs such as cyclosporin A, and TTP associated with systemic lupus erythematosus.

        b. Laboratory. Microangiopathic hemolytic anemia is always present, with schistocytes seen on peripheral smears. A markedly elevated LDH is also common, indicative of accelerated cell turnover and tissue hypoxia. Serum creatinine may be elevated, and coagulation studies are normal.

        c. Treatment. Immediate transfer to a facility with plasma exchange capabilities is indicated. Plasma infusions (up to 12 units daily) are indicated during any delay in transfer. Platelet transfusions are considered contraindicated, but this is controversial.

II. Thrombocytosis is an absolute elevation of the platelet count (>500,000/μl).

    A. Reactive thrombocytosis is a raise in the platelet count in response to splenectomy, iron deficiency, GI bleeding, chronic infectious or inflammatory conditions, and malignancy. Platelet counts of up to 1,000,000/μl can be seen. Patients are not considered at risk for thrombosis or bleeding, and no specific therapy is required. Treatment of the underlying disorder can normalize the platelet count.

    B. Essential thrombocythemia is a clonal proliferative disorder (similar to polycythemia vera) of hematopoietic stem cells.

        1. Clinical presentation. Patients present with marked elevation (>600,000/μl) in platelet counts with no apparent evidence of an underlying condition for reactive thrombocytosis and absence of the Philadelphia chromosome on bone marrow cytogenetic analysis. They are usually asymptomatic but may present with (and are slightly predisposed to) thrombosis and mucosal bleeding.

        2. Treatment with aspirin (325 mg PO qd) is safe, but its additional benefit to cytoreduction is unclear. Cytoreduction to a target platelet count of 400,000/μl can be achieved with anagrelide or hydroxyurea. Interferon-alpha can be used in pregnancy. Patients older than 60 years, those with prior thrombosis, or those with cardiovascular risk factors require cytoreduction.

III. Disorders of platelet function are suggested by a prolonged bleeding time in the face of a normal platelet count.

A. Acquired disorders

1. **Drug induced.** A single low dose of aspirin (81 mg) irreversibly inhibits aggregation physiology of all circulating platelets. Other NSAIDs reversibly inhibit platelet function while the drug is in plasma phase. Bleeding manifestations generally are rare, but easy bruisability or occult GI bleeding can occur. Patients should discontinue aspirin 5–7 days before elective surgery. Other NSAIDs should be discontinued for 24–48 hours (representing 4–5 half-lives). **Ticlopidine** is an agent that is used for inhibiting platelet function but can cause neutropenia. **Clopidogrel** is an alternative, as it causes less neutropenia. Ticlopidine should be held for 10 days before elective surgery because of its long half-life. The bleeding time is not predictive of postoperative bleeding. Platelet transfusion compensates completely for aspirin-induced platelet dysfunction and should be reserved for patients with significant bleeding.

2. **Uremia** is associated with inhibition of platelet function in patients with renal failure. Any role of platelet dysfunction for risk of bleeding is probably additive to other confounding factors such as the presence of substantial (Hct <28%) anemia (which itself affects platelet-vascular endothelial cell interaction), heparin anticoagulation for dialysis, or anatomic reasons for hemorrhage. Treatment is more intensive dialysis. Platelet transfusion therapy does not treat the platelet dysfunction, because transfused platelets become dysfunctional in uremic plasma. **Desmopressin** (diamino-8-D-arginine vasopressin, DDAVP) given intravenously (0.3 µg/kg in 50 ml normal saline over 30 minutes) causes von Willebrand's factor (vWF) release from vascular endothelial cells, thereby facilitating platelet adhesion in the microcirculation. Cryoprecipitate (10–20 units) also improves platelet dysfunction. RBC transfusion to Hct levels of greater than 28% are also associated with improvement in platelet function.

B. Inherited disorders of platelet function are very rare, except for von Willebrand's disease (vWD; see Disorders of Hemostasis, sec. **III.C**).

Disorders of Hemostasis

I. Approach to the bleeding patient

A. Clinical presentation. Patients with bleeding disorders present with a variety of manifestations. Mild, previously unrecognized disorders can present unexpectedly after otherwise minor trauma, dental manipulations, routine surgery, miscarriage, or otherwise uncomplicated pregnancy and delivery. A previous personal or family history of abnormal bleeding may provide important clues regarding inherited disorders. A careful history of therapeutic medications is important to determine whether an acquired coagulation disorder is present, including hemorrhagic complications related to anticoagulation therapy.

B. Physical examination. In general, platelet-related disorders present with mucocutaneous manifestations such as epistaxis, gingival bleeding, skin (petechia, prolonged bleeding from cuts), and GI manifestations. Patients with coagulopathies can present similarly but may present with serosal bleeds, either spontaneous or secondary to trauma, particularly in joints but also in retroperitoneal, pleural, or oral cavities.

C. Laboratory evaluation includes a CBC and platelet count to establish the activity and severity of hemorrhage and the presence or absence of thrombocytopenia. **Prothrombin time (PT)** and **partial thromboplastin time (PTT)** are important screening assays. The PTT is used to determine whether a disorder of the intrinsic coagulation pathway, such as hemophilia A or B, vWD, or factor XI deficiency disease, is possible. The PT is used to determine whether a disorder of the extrinsic pathway such as factor VII deficiency or multiple coagulation factor abnormalities (anticoagulant therapy, liver disease) is present. The **international normalized ratio** has been developed to allow comparison (and standardization) of PT assays that may use different thromboplastin reagents. It is to be used only for monitoring patients who are receiving warfarin therapy. The thrombin time is used to evaluate the possible effect of heparin or circulating anticoagulants such as fibrin degradation products on the conversion of fibrinogen to fibrin, such as is seen in patients with DIC. If the initial PT or PTT, or both, are abnormal, further specialized assays should be performed, including (1) mixing studies (a 1:1 dilution of normal plasma with the patient's plasma) to detect the presence of circulating anticoagulants (or inhibitors) directed against certain coagulation factors and (2) assays for specific coagulation factor activity, such as antihemophiliac factor (factor VIII deficiency, or hemophilia A), Christmas factor (factor IX, or hemophilia B) deficiency, or vWF. A screen for DIC is performed in patients who are suspected of having generalized and systemic activation of the coagulation system. This is seen in obstetric complications (retained dead fetus syndrome, amniotic fluid embolus, abruptio placentae), trauma, hemolytic transfusion reactions, severe liver dysfunction, or sepsis syndromes. DIC screens include PT, PTT, thrombin time, assays for fibrin degradation products, fibrinogen level, and fibrinopeptide A levels.

 II. **Acquired disorders of coagulation**
  A. **General treatment considerations.** Patients who are bleeding significantly require urgent or emergent care, including hospitalization and consultation with specialists. Therapy can be targeted for patients with known disorders (Table 15-3) but may be presumptive until a specific diagnosis is established. Plasma therapy can be administered to patients who have abnormal PT or PTT assays and clinically significant hemorrhage. The most common

Table 15-3. Coagulation factor concentrates

Product	Low purity (<1 IU/ml)	Intermediate purity[a]	High purity[b]	Activated products
Factor VIII	Cryoprecipitate	Humate-P	Alphanate SD	—
		Koate-HP	Hemophil-M	
		Hyate-C (porcine)	Monoclate-P	
			Recombinate[c]	
			Bioclate[c]	
			Kogenate[c]	
			Helixate[c]	
			Monarc M	
Factor IX	—	Konyne	Mononine	Autoplex T
		Proplex T	Alphanine SD	FEIBA VH
			BeneFIX[c]	
Factor VII	—	—	—	VIIa concentrate

[a]Concentration for factor VIII products: 5–40 IU/ml; for factor IX products: 2–50 IU/ml.
[b]Concentration for factor VIII products: >1000 IU/ml; for factor IX products: >150 IU/ml.
[c]Recombinant product.

setting in adults is patients with **liver disease** (cirrhosis or acute fulminant hepatitis), who have multiple coagulation deficiencies, along with consumptive elements due to impaired reticuloendothelial system clearance of substances that activate the coagulation system. Another common presentation is in patients with **warfarin overdose.** Parenteral vitamin K (10 mg SC or IV daily) administration is the first treatment consideration in patients with liver disease and in individuals with warfarin (a vitamin K antagonist) overdose. For patients with life-threatening or otherwise substantial hemorrhage, plasma therapy is given at an initial dosage of 15 ml/kg, which provides approximately an additional 25–35% of each coagulation factor.

- **B. Vitamin K deficiency** can be caused by malabsorption states or poor dietary intake combined with antibiotic-associated loss of intestinal bacterial production (e.g., intubated or cachectic patients treated with prolonged and multiple antibiotic regimens). Warfarin induces an iatrogenic functional state of vitamin K deficiency by interfering with conversion to its active (reduced) state. Vitamin K is required by hepatocytes to complete synthesis of clotting factors II, VII, IX, X, and the natural anticoagulant proteins C and S. Manifestations of vitamin K deficiency are bleeding and prolongation of PT that are out of proportion to the PTT.
- **C. Liver disease** is indicated by evidence of liver dysfunction, such as elevated direct bilirubin or decreased levels of serum albumin; clinical evidence of impaired liver metabolism such as hepatic encephalopathy, jaundice, or icterus; acute liver inflammation (e.g., markedly elevated ALT and AST); or evidence of cirrhosis (portal hypertension with hepatosplenomegaly).
- **D. Acquired inhibitors of coagulation.** Antibody (inhibitors) directed against factor VIII can arise spontaneously (1) in women who are several weeks postpartum after a normal labor and delivery, (2) in patients with collagen vascular disease such as systemic lupus erythematosus, (3) in elderly patients, and (4) in patients with known inherited coagulation disorders, particularly factor VIII deficiency. Drug-induced inhibitors against a variety of other coagulation factors are much less common. Treatment is difficult and is indicated only when patients have hemorrhage or are scheduled for surgery. For low-titer inhibitors, high-dose porcine or recombinant factor VIII concentrate therapy to override the inhibitor can be successful in pediatric patients or adults with smaller blood volumes. Factor IX concentrate is given for minor bleeding. Activated factor concentrates (Table 15-3) coupled with therapeutic plasma exchange may be required in patients with serious hemorrhage. Factor VIIIa has been approved for use in hemophilia patients with inhibitors. The recommended dose is 90 μg/kg IV q2–3 hours.

III. Inherited disorders of coagulation

- **A. Antihemophiliac factor (factor VIII) deficiency (hemophilia A)** accounts for 85% of X-linked bleeding disorders, caused by a mutation at the factor VIII locus that leads to impaired synthesis of the procoagulant moiety of the factor VIII molecule. The clinical phenotype of the individual patient depends on the functional level of factor VIII activity: severe (<1%), moderate (1–5%), or mild (>5%) hemophilia. A positive family history (males with bleeding disorders on the maternal side of the family tree) can be elicited in up to 75% of male patients who present with abnormal PTT and hemorrhage. Twenty-five percent of factor VIII–deficient males result from mothers who became carriers as a result of spontaneous factor VIII mutations; these patients have a negative family history. Patients with mild or moderate hemophilia may present with hemorrhage only when challenged by trauma or invasive procedures (dental extractions, surgery). Severe hemophiliacs present with spontaneous serosal, particularly joint, hemorrhage.
    - **1. Laboratory.** PTT is prolonged, and PT is normal. Factor VIII levels are low. Patients who are known to have factor VIII deficiency should always be evaluated for a possible factor VIII inhibitor (using a mixing assay) before an elective surgery or invasive procedure is performed.

2. **Treatment** is designed to increase factor VIII to hemostatic levels. Some commercially available concentrates are summarized in Table 15-3. For life-threatening hemorrhage (CNS, perioperative, or trauma), initial doses are administered to achieve 200% factor VIII levels, so that nadir factor VIII levels (at 8–12 hours) remain at 80–100%. Severe bleeding (joint, muscles) or milder hemorrhage (lacerations, dental procedures) requires initial factor VIII dosage to achieve levels of 100% and 50%, respectively, to maintain nadir levels of 25–50%. Every unit/kg factor VIII administered increases the plasma factor VIII activity by 2%, so that 100 units/kg factor VIII is an appropriate initial dose for life-threatening hemorrhage, and 25–50 units/kg factor VIII therapy can be initiated for milder to moderate circumstances or hemorrhage. Subsequent factor VIII (at 50% initial dosage) is administered q6h for the initial 24 hours, and q8–12h thereafter, if necessary. The DDAVP (0.3 μg/kg IV q6h for a total of 6 doses) results in a two- to threefold increase in factor VIII levels and can be used in patients with mild hemophilia who have mild bleeding (e.g., dental extractions). ε-aminocaproic acid (Amicar, 5 g q6h PO) can also be used for dental procedures but is contraindicated if urologic bleeding is present.

B. **Christmas factor (factor IX) deficiency** or **hemophilia B** accounts for 15% of patients with an X-linked bleeding disorder. Clinical presentations are similar to those of factor VIII deficiency. DDAVP is not helpful for patients with factor IX deficiency. The initial dosage of factor IX is the same as for factor VIII; subsequent doses (at 50% initial levels) are administered q24h.

C. **vWD** is the most common inherited bleeding disorder, occurring in nearly 1% of the population. The spectrum of the disease is heterogeneous, due to different mutations of the large vWD gene. The vWF molecule affects platelet adhesion to vascular endothelium and the factor VIII levels in plasma, so that bleeding manifestations can occur even when vWF levels are "mildly" affected (5–15% levels). Mucocutaneous bleeding (epistaxis, oral cavity, GI, skin lacerations) and menorrhagia are most common, rather than the spontaneous joint hemorrhages that are seen in patients with hemophilia A or B. Many patients with mild vWD may not be recognized until they are challenged by trauma or surgical procedures later in life. The diagnosis should be suspected in any patient with unexpected or unusual bleeding after surgery or invasive procedures.

1. **Laboratory** classification of vWF is divided into three main types: Type 1 vWD accounts for up to 80% of patients who have a partial quantitative deficiency. The PTT and bleeding times are abnormal, reflecting diminished procoagulant factor VIII levels and platelet function (ristocetin cofactor) activity. Type 2 vWD patients tend to have normal procoagulant factor VIII activity but more severe qualitative platelet dysfunction. Type 3 vWD patients have more severe quantitative deficiencies of procoagulant factor VIII and platelet dysfunction.

2. **Treatment.** DDAVP can be useful in type 1 or type 2 patients with mild vWD and minor bleeding episodes. Tachyphylaxis to DDAVP develops after four doses (over 24 hours). Oral contraceptives are useful in women with menorrhagia. Patients with moderate to severe hemorrhage require plasma product therapy; Humate-P (Table 15-3) is richest in vWF. Initial doses are 100–200 units/kg for moderate to severe (including surgery) hemorrhage, followed by 50% initial dosage q12h.

Monoclonal Gammopathies

I. **Monoclonal gammopathy of unknown significance (MGUS)** refers to the presence of a monoclonal protein (M protein) in the absence of a known related disease, such as multiple myeloma or amyloidosis.

A. Clinical presentation. M protein is commonly found as a result of a serum protein electrophoresis assay. The incidence of MGUS increases with age; the median age is 64 years, and 3% of persons over 70 years of age have an M protein. Two-thirds of patients who present initially with an M protein are classified as having MGUS, whereas 14% and 8% are diagnosed as having multiple myeloma or amyloidosis, respectively. The remainder of cases are associated with Waldenström's macroglobulinemia, lymphoma, chronic lymphocytic leukemia, or "smoldering" multiple myeloma.

B. Laboratory. The M protein is detected by electrophoresis, with a median concentration of 1.7 g/dl (range, 0.3–3.2 g/dl). IgG (74%) is most common, followed by IgM (16%) and IgA (10%). A bone marrow examination may show a mild increase (3–10%) in plasma cells in patients with MGUS. A urine immunoelectrophoresis assay should be done to look for Bence Jones (light chain) proteinuria. Underlying plasma cell dyscrasias must be ruled out. The presence of abnormal plasma cell morphology, increased (>10%) plasma cells in the bone marrow, anemia, an elevated (>3 g/dl) M protein, lytic bone lesions, hypercalcemia, Bence Jones proteinuria, or renal impairment indicates the possibility of a malignant monoclonal gammopathy.

C. Prognosis. MGUS develops into malignancy in 16–33% of patients over a 10- to 20-year interval, respectively, and multiple myeloma develops in two-thirds of these individuals. Patients with MGUS should therefore be followed indefinitely. Initial follow-up depends on the level of M protein; if it is less than 2 g/dl, 6 months of follow-up and annually thereafter are appropriate. If it is greater than 2 g/dl, 3-month intervals for 1 year to determine a stable M protein is appropriate, followed by yearly thereafter. Increases of more than 0.5 g/dl or the presence of Bence Jones proteinuria requires closer follow-up or evaluation for an underlying plasma cell dyscrasia, or both.

II. Malignant plasma cell dyscrasias

A. Multiple myeloma is an IgG monoclonal disorder that can present with an unexpected skeletal fracture (long bone or vertebral body), newly diagnosed renal failure (due to Bence Jones proteinuria), hematologic abnormalities (anemia, neutropenia, thrombocytopenia), hypercalcemia, or a combination of these. Evaluation is as for MGUS.

B. Waldenström's macroglobulinemia is an IgM monoclonal disorder with a more lymphoproliferative presentation, characterized by mild hematologic abnormalities and accompanied by lymphadenopathy or splenomegaly, or both. The IgM gammopathy can lead to hyperviscosity (CNS, visual, cardiac) manifestations. Evaluation is as for MGUS.

C. Amyloidosis is an infiltrative disorder due to light-chain deposition into connective tissues. Weakness, fatigue, macroglossia, peripheral neuropathy, renal insufficiency, and CHF are common initial presentations. An M protein is found in 90% of patients. Patients may have a mildly prolonged PT or PTT due to an acquired factor X deficiency. Diagnosis is made by positive stains for amyloid protein in biopsy tissue.

16

**Oncology and
Palliative Care**

Michelle Z. Schultz

Approach to the
Cancer Patient

All patients who face a possible cancer diagnosis have four basic questions: (1) Is it really cancer? (2) How much cancer is there? (3) What can be done about it? (4) Can it be cured, or, if not, how much time do I have? Answering these questions forms the basis of cancer management.

I. **Diagnosis.** With very rare exceptions, the diagnosis of cancer requires evaluation of a tissue sample by a pathologist. Either cytology or histopathology is mandatory to prove that a cancer exists. This information is important for several reasons. Clearly, a diagnosis of cancer affects every aspect of a patient's life, ranging from ability to obtain insurance to far-reaching psychosocial issues. In addition, the treatment of cancer requires aggressive interventions that carry inherent risks of short- and long-term morbidity and even mortality. Therefore, a firm diagnosis must be established before administration of potentially lethal therapy. Finally, tissue diagnosis precisely defines the histopathologic subtype of malignancy [such as small-cell vs. non–small-cell lung cancer (NSCLC)] and thus dictates therapy. Prognostic information can also be obtained at the time of biopsy (e.g., the depth of invasion of a melanoma or the presence of estrogen receptors on a breast cancer).

II. **Extent of disease.** Determining the extent of a solid tumor or lymphoma is a process called **staging**. This process often requires extensive radiographic analysis for clinical staging or gross and microscopic examination of surgical specimens for pathologic staging. As discussed below for specific cancers, the staging guides treatment recommendations. The American Joint Committee on Cancer (AJCC) has adopted a detailed staging system based on local tumor characteristics (T), involvement of regional lymph nodes (N), and distant metastatic spread (M). TNM staging guidelines are published in the *AJCC Cancer Staging Manual* (5th ed. Philadelphia: Lippincott–Raven, 1997). Completion of staging often occurs after a definitive surgical procedure (e.g., colectomy or lymph node dissection). Thus, staging and treatment are interdependent.

III. **Treatment.** Many of the most prevalent solid tumors are best managed through a multidisciplinary approach involving surgeons, medical oncologists, radiation oncologists, and others. Different options are often available, and patients should be involved in the decision-making process. The goals of treatment, be they cure, prolongation of survival, or improvement in quality of life, should be agreed on in advance. In situations in which different approaches may yield similar results (e.g., prostatectomy vs. radiation), an informed decision is required from the patient. Treatment recommendations should be carefully tailored to individual patient needs, taking into account comorbidities and psychosocial issues.

A. **Surgery.** Resection of all apparent cancer remains the mainstay of treatment for most solid tumors. **Resectability** should be determined by clinical staging. In addition, **operability** is decided by the individual's fitness to undergo the necessary procedure. For example, a lung cancer patient's advanced chronic obstructive pulmonary disease may preclude pneumonectomy. Oncologic surgery may include sampling or formal dissection of regional lymph nodes for prognostic and therapeutic purposes. Finally, surgery may be indicated for palliation, such as diverting colostomy for a tumor that is obstructing the bowel.

B. Radiation therapy is used as definitive or curative therapy in a variety of circumstances, including early stages of cancers of the larynx or prostate or Hodgkin's disease. Additionally, it is indicated to reduce local recurrence and possibly prolong survival after surgery for some cancers, including those of the breast and rectum. Palliative radiation therapy is useful for symptom management, such as pain from bone metastases or neurologic deficits from CNS involvement.

C. Systemic therapy. In contrast to surgery and radiation therapy, which have local effects, **chemotherapy, hormonal therapy, and immunotherapy** are used with the intent of treating actual or potential tumors throughout the body.

  1. **Adjuvant therapy** refers to the use of systemic therapy in conjunction with seemingly curative therapy (usually surgery) to improve disease-free and overall survival by eliminating undetected local and micrometastatic tumor deposits. Because there is no way to measure response to this therapy, the duration of treatment is determined empirically by prior clinical trials. Furthermore, there is no way to confirm whether an individual patient absolutely benefits from systemic adjuvant therapy. In view of potential side effects from systemic adjuvant therapy, the patient must make an informed decision as to whether to undergo treatment. Cancers for which adjuvant systemic therapy has been confirmed to improve survival in conjunction with surgery include colorectal cancer, breast cancer, ovarian cancer, and osteosarcoma. The benefits in other primary sites are less well defined. Similarly, hormonal therapy is an effective adjuvant for breast cancer and may improve outcome for patients with locally advanced prostate cancer who are undergoing primary radiation therapy.

  2. **Neoadjuvant therapy** refers to systemic therapy and sometimes radiotherapy that is administered before definitive therapy (usually surgery). One advantage of neoadjuvant therapy is the ability to measure tumor sensitivity to given agents. In addition, the surgical procedure and its complications may be minimized and organ function may be preserved. The neoadjuvant approach is sometimes used for diseases such as esophageal, rectal, lung, and bladder carcinomas and osteosarcomas.

  3. **Combined-modality therapy** usually refers to combinations of chemotherapy and radiotherapy that are used to treat bulk disease. Surgery may be part of the initial plan or may be reserved to salvage nonresponding tumors that remain resectable. Combined-modality therapy with chemotherapy and radiation improves survival for some patients with locally advanced lung, esophageal, head and neck, pancreatic, and cervical cancers. Combinations of chemotherapy and radiation may be curative and simultaneously preserve organ function by avoiding surgery in cancers of the larynx and anus.

  4. **Primary or induction chemotherapy** is used as the main modality to bring about remission. Chemotherapy alone may be curative in germ cell tumors and certain lymphomas. After successful induction chemotherapy, acute leukemias require **consolidation** with more intensive chemotherapy. Very high doses of chemotherapy may ablate the bone marrow, requiring rescue with **allogeneic** or **autologous** bone marrow stem cells to repopulate the marrow. Allogeneic transplants have been curative in selected patients with chronic myelogenous leukemia (CML) and acute myeloblastic and lymphoblastic leukemias (AML and ALL). Autologous stem cell rescue has been most successful for aggressive lymphomas. Its use in other situations remains investigational.

5. **Immunotherapy** refers to pharmacotherapy with agents that are intrinsic to the immune system. High concentrations of these biological response modifiers stimulate the immune system to kill cancers. Examples include **interferon-alpha, interleukin-2,** or **monoclonal antibodies.** Toxicities range from fevers and flu-like symptoms to anaphylaxis and capillary leak syndromes. Tumor vaccines and gene therapies remain experimental.

D. **Palliative therapy** is administered with the primary goal of improving symptoms and quality of life. Prolongation of survival is a secondary goal, which may or may not be achieved, but cure is not the intent. Chemotherapy, hormonal therapy, radiotherapy, immunotherapy, and surgery are all useful for palliation. However, patient selection for such interventions is crucial. For patients with advanced cancer whose functional capacity [termed **performance status (PS)**] is considerably limited, aggressive treatment may be detrimental rather than beneficial.

E. **Supportive care** of cancer patients entails management of all of the symptoms related to the cancer itself and of toxicities of treatment, expected and unexpected. It also includes the multidisciplinary care of psychosocial issues. The goals of supportive care are to optimize quality of life and minimize the morbidity and mortality of cancer treatment. Specific symptoms and complications are discussed in Supportive Care of Cancer Patients.

F. **Clinical trials** are available for many disease sites and stages. Because cancer treatment modalities are far from ideal, clinical research is vital to test new strategies for improving survival and quality of life. Patients who participate in clinical trials receive treatments that are theorized to be at least as good as, if not better than the standard of care. Informed consent must always be obtained, and patients have the right to withdraw at any time.

IV. **Prognosis.** An individual's prognosis is based on staging, comorbidities, PS, and response to treatment. Although it is possible to predict curability or median survival, longitudinal follow-up is often required to get a more accurate sense of prognosis for a given patient. Even when the outlook is not good, a direct and compassionate discussion of prognosis is essential. This allows the patient and family to form realistic goals to guide health care decisions.

Therapy of Common Malignancies

Comprehensive discussions of treatment options for all cancers are beyond the scope of this book. The following is an overview of treatment considerations for the most common solid tumors. More detailed treatment explanations for these and other cancers can be obtained from the National Cancer Institute's CancerNet Web site at http://www.cancernet.nci.nih.gov (Table 16-1).

I. **Breast cancer** should be considered a systemic disease from the early stages in the majority of cases. The management of breast cancer is a multidisciplinary effort between surgeons, medical oncologists, and radiation oncologists.

A. **Early-stage breast cancer** defines small tumors in the breast with or without spread to axillary lymph nodes. Due to screening and high public awareness, the majority of new breast cancers in the United States now present at this stage. Prognostic factors that predict risk of recurrence and guide treatment decisions are the size of the primary tumor, number of lymph nodes involved, and presence of hormone receptors [estrogen (ER), and progesterone (PR)]. Although the majority of patients enjoy prolonged disease-free survival, it is difficult to use the word **cure,** as relapse may occur years or, rarely, decades later.

1. **Surgery.** Wide local excision (**lumpectomy**) is indicated in the majority of cases. In combination with **radiation therapy,** such **breast-conserving therapy** has demonstrated equivalence to **modified radical mastectomy** for local control and overall survival. Axillary lymph node dissection is

Table 16-1. Web sites for oncology and palliative care

Agency for Healthcare Research and Quality (AHRQ)	http://www.ahrq.gov/clinic
American Society of Clinical Oncology (ASCO)	http://www.asco.org
American Cancer Society (ACS)	http://www.cancer.org
American Gastroenterological Association	http://www.gastro.org
Centers for Disease Control and Prevention (CDC)	http://www.cdc.gov
National Cancer Institute (NCI)	http://www.cancernet.nci.nih.gov
National Hospice and Palliative Care Organization (NHPCO)	http://www.nhpco.org

indicated for prognostic purposes. **Sentinel node biopsy** may replace full node dissection. This procedure minimizes morbidity by using a dye or radioactive colloid injected at the primary site to identify the lymph node most likely to contain metastases. If negative, the remaining axillary nodes need not be dissected. Modified radical mastectomy should be performed for multifocal disease or per patient preference, with discussion of immediate or delayed reconstruction options. **Noninvasive breast cancer** (ductal carcinoma in situ) is more often detected mammographically. Lumpectomy with radiation is sufficient for most patients, but simple mastectomy is preferred if the cancer is multicentric.

2. **Radiation therapy** significantly reduces the risk of local recurrence and is essential for patients who are treated with lumpectomy. Postmastectomy adjuvant radiation can be considered for all premenopausal node-positive patients and for postmenopausal women with four or more positive nodes. A course of radiation takes approximately 6 weeks and may be complicated by radiation changes in the skin and lymphedema of the ipsilateral arm.

3. **Adjuvant systemic therapy.** Almost all women with **invasive breast cancer** are candidates for adjuvant therapy. Patients with node-negative, ER-positive tumors of 1 cm or less have an excellent prognosis and usually do not receive adjuvant chemotherapy but can be considered for adjuvant hormonal therapy. Individualized recommendations for treatment options should be discussed with patients based on risk of recurrence, age, and menopausal status.

   a. **Hormonal therapy.** For patients whose tumors express ER or PR, **tamoxifen** for 5 years decreases the risks of recurrence by up to 50%. Additionally, there is a reduction in the risk of second primary breast cancers. Tamoxifen can be used alone for patients with lower risks of relapse or for those who decline or cannot tolerate chemotherapy. It is often added after chemotherapy for higher-risk patients.

   b. **Chemotherapy** reduces the annual rate of recurrence of breast cancer by 25–28% and the annual rate of death by 16–25%. A wide variety of active regimens are available, often containing cyclophosphamide, anthracyclines, or taxanes. The optimum chemotherapy combinations and duration are still being investigated.

   c. **Follow-up** after completion of therapy is important for detection of recurrent disease and second primary breast cancers. Surveillance guidelines are published by the American Society of Clinical Oncology.

      (1) History and physical examination every 3–6 months for 3 years, then every 6–12 months for 2 years, then annually

      (2) Breast self-examination monthly

      (3) Mammography annually starting 6 months after radiation therapy

4. Routine laboratory studies, chest x-ray, bone scan, CT scan, liver ultrasound, or tumor markers are not recommended.

B. **Metastatic breast cancer** remains incurable. The median survival is 2–3 years, but this is a diverse disease that ranges from rapidly progressive to very indolent. More than 20% of patients survive for 5 years, and up to 10% live for 10 years or more. Palliative therapy is highly effective in alleviating symptoms and may have a modest survival benefit. For patients with ER-positive disease that involves bone, soft tissue, or lung, hormonal therapy is effective in two-thirds of cases, with a toxicity profile much less than that of chemotherapy. In addition to tamoxifen, hormonal manipulations include **aromatase inhibitors** such as **anastrozole** or **letrozole** for postmenopausal patients or **ovarian ablation** [oophorectomy, gonadotropin-releasing hormone (GnRH) analogues] for premenopausal patients. Chemotherapy is indicated for those with ER-negative disease or visceral involvement (e.g., liver, lymphangitic spread to the lungs, multiple sites, etc.) or after hormone failure. Numerous active agents are available that can be used alone or in combinations. Patients whose tumors overexpress the Her2/neu receptor may benefit from monoclonal antibody therapy with **trastuzumab (Herceptin)**. Monthly administration of **pamidronate** reduces skeletal-related events, such as pathologic fractures and spinal cord compression, and may reduce bone pain.

II. **Lung cancer** is the leading cause of cancer death in men and in women, and results of treatment remain inadequate for the majority of patients. Lung cancer is histologically divided into small-cell, which disseminates early on, and non–small-cell (NSCLC; squamous, large-cell, and adenocarcinomas), which may be cured by surgery when localized.

A. **Non–small-cell lung cancer.** Stage and PS have crucial importance in the selection of therapy for NSCLC. Patients with localized disease (stages I and II) are candidates for surgical resection. Those with comorbidities that preclude resection can be considered for definitive radiotherapy. Locally and regionally advanced (stage III) patients with good PS are most often treated with combined chemoradiotherapy, which prolongs survival over radiotherapy alone. This approach provides palliation in the majority of patients and long-term survival in a minority. Individuals with metastatic disease (stage IV) cannot be cured. Stage IV patients with good PS may benefit from chemotherapy, which has demonstrated modest survival benefits and improved quality of life over supportive care alone. Radiation therapy often palliates symptomatic local or distant disease.

B. **Small-cell lung cancer** is usually an aggressive disease, with median survivals of only 2–4 months without treatment. However, it is more sensitive to chemotherapy and radiation than is NSCLC. Chemotherapy prolongs survival significantly and is the mainstay of treatment. Staging is divided into only two groups. Those with **limited-stage** disease have tumor that is confined to one hemithorax, the mediastinum, and the supraclavicular nodes and is encompassable within a single radiotherapy port. With concurrent chemoradiotherapy the median survival improves to 16–24 months, with up to 20% of patients surviving long term. Patients with **extensive-stage** disease do not fit the criteria for limited disease. Thoracic radiotherapy does not improve outcome in these patients, and therefore treatment generally consists of chemotherapy alone. Despite complete remission rates of 20–30%, almost all patients relapse, and median survival is only 6–12 months. The CNS is frequently involved. To decrease the risk of CNS relapse, prophylactic cranial irradiation is sometimes offered to patients with limited-stage disease who achieve complete remission. Radiation therapy can palliate symptoms from brain metastases, superior vena cava obstruction, and so forth, for patients whose cancers are refractory to chemotherapy.

III. **Colorectal cancer** is the second leading cause of cancer death in the United States, with outcome dependent on stage. Staging is based on the degree of penetration of the tumor through the bowel wall and the involvement of regional lymph nodes. Stage I tumors do not extend through the bowel wall or involve lymph nodes and have a high cure rate with surgery alone. Stage II tumors penetrate through the bowel wall, whereas stage III denotes lymph node involvement. Patients with stage IV tumors have metastatic disease.

A. Surgery is the mainstay of treatment and provides detailed staging information that is necessary to predict prognosis and guide further therapy. The majority of patients with resectable disease are cured, although relapse rates may exceed 50% in node-positive cases.

B. Adjuvant therapy. Substantial evidence has shown that postoperative adjuvant **chemotherapy** with a 5-fluorouracil (5-FU)–based regimen benefits patients with stage III colon cancer, with up to a 33% reduction in mortality. The benefits for patients with stage II colon cancer remain uncertain. For those with rectal cancer, there is a considerable risk of local recurrence due to the inability to obtain wide radial margins in the bony pelvis. For this reason, **radiation therapy** is a standard component of treatment for stage II and III rectal cancer. 5-FU combined with radiation therapy reduces local failure rates and improves overall survival in these patients. **Neoadjuvant chemoradiation** may reduce surgical morbidity and allow for preservation of sphincter function.

C. Follow-up. After potentially curative treatment of colorectal cancer, surveillance may result in early detection of recurrent disease. Isolated local recurrences or solitary metastases in the liver or lungs may be resectable, resulting in long-term survival rates of approximately 20%. Surveillance guidelines are published by the American Society of Clinical Oncology.

    1. Carcinoembryonic antigen (CEA) should be measured every 2–3 months for 2 years or more in asymptomatic patients who are potential surgical candidates. Although not all tumors produce CEA, a normal preoperative CEA level does not preclude this surveillance.

    2. History and physical examination are recommended every 3–6 months for 3 years, then annually. Abnormalities should prompt further testing.

    3. Colonoscopy to rule out additional synchronous primary tumors is recommended within 1 year of diagnosis. Follow-up colonoscopy should be performed every 3–5 years.

    4. Laboratory and radiology. The guidelines recommend **against** routine surveillance of liver enzymes, CBC, fecal occult blood testing, chest x-ray, and CT scan.

D. Metastatic disease. Inoperable recurrent or metastatic disease is incurable. Palliative chemotherapy with 5-FU plus leucovorin or irinotecan, or both, may lead to improvements in survival and quality of life for patients with good PS.

IV. Prostate cancer is the most frequently diagnosed cancer in men but not the most lethal. It can be cured when localized and responds to hormonal therapy when widely metastatic. Management is complex because the natural history of prostate cancer is quite variable. Additionally, as the disease is frequently diagnosed in elderly men (median age, 72 years), many patients with prostate cancer ultimately die of other causes. Nonetheless, approximately 37,000 men in the United States die of prostate cancer annually. Prognosis depends on the extent of tumor and the degree of differentiation (Gleason grade). Tumors that spread beyond the capsule or that are poorly differentiated are more likely to metastasize. Although widely variable, the median survival of patients with metastatic disease is only approximately 3 years. Therefore, younger men with localized disease and without major comorbidities are candidates for definitive therapy. Older patients, those with low-grade tumors, and those with other life-threatening illnesses may warrant close observation alone. Such **watchful waiting** produces survival rates that are similar to those seen with surgery or radiation in selected patients.

A. Organ-confined disease. Definitive therapy options for organ-confined disease (stage I and II) include **prostatectomy**, external beam **radiotherapy**, or interstitial **brachytherapy**, with similar survival results in nonrandomized comparisons. Pelvic lymph node sampling before prostatectomy may spare unnecessary surgical morbidity for patients with nodal involvement, who are rarely cured.

1. **Surgery.** Radical prostatectomy with sparing of the neurovascular bundles is associated with cancer-specific survival that approaches 90% in appropriate patients with organ-confined disease, but this falls off rapidly with high-grade histology or extracapsular spread. Complications of surgery include impotence, urinary incontinence, urethral stricture, and, rarely, fecal incontinence. In a national survey of Medicare patients, more than 30% reported using pads or clamps for urinary incontinence and 63% reported problems with wetness. The incidence of impotency ranges from 35% to 75%, increasing with age and extracapsular spread. Accidents with fecal leakage may occur in 15–30% of patients.

2. **External beam radiation therapy** is associated with similar survival to surgery when patients are carefully matched for stage, age, and comorbidities. However, it has often been reserved for older, more infirm patients or those with more advanced disease. Complications include cystitis, proctitis, urinary and sexual dysfunction, and urethral stricture. The incidence of proctitis, including frequent bowel movements or bleeding, ranges from 10% to 30%. Cystitis, hematuria, and/or urethral stricture occur in fewer than 15% of patients. The rate of urinary incontinence that requires pads or clamps is less than 10%. Sexual function is preserved in approximately 80% of patients after the first year but diminishes with time to about 30–60% after 5 or more years.

B. **Locally advanced disease.** External beam radiation is recommended for locally advanced (stage III) prostate cancer. Adjuvant hormonal therapy should be considered, as it has been demonstrated to prolong survival in some series.

C. **Metastatic disease.** Hormonal therapy is beneficial for patients with advanced disease. Although not curative, it provides excellent palliation in the majority of individuals. Treatment is typically instituted at the time of diagnosis of advanced disease, as delaying until symptoms appear is associated with an increased risk of spinal cord compression, pathologic fractures, and obstructive uropathy. Hormonal therapy consists primarily of testicular androgen suppression via bilateral **orchiectomy** or **GnRH analogues** (leuprolide or goserelin). Estrogenic therapy is equally effective but associated with cardiovascular risks at high doses. **Antiandrogens** (flutamide, bicalutamide, and nilutamide) are useful to block the tumor flare that is associated with the initiation of GnRH analogues. The **combined androgen blockade** that is produced by the addition of these drugs remains of uncertain long-term benefit. Withdrawal of antiandrogens may lead to decline in prostate-specific antigen level in some patients. Palliative chemotherapy has been demonstrated to improve quality of life in symptomatic **hormone-refractory** patients with good PS.

Supportive Care
of Cancer Patients

Supportive care focuses on controlling the multitude of symptoms that are experienced by cancer patients, whether related to the cancer itself, adverse effects of cancer therapy, or intercurrent illnesses. Many cancer symptoms can be alleviated by treatment of the cancer with chemotherapy, radiation therapy, surgery, or other modalities. However, these treatments commonly lead to new problems or worsening of existing ones such as fatigue and anorexia. Occasionally, patients have few or no cancer symptoms but require treatments that induce significant toxicity (e.g., adjuvant therapy for breast cancer). In addition to physical symptoms, many experience psychological distress, including depression, anxiety, and fear. **Palliative care** is a subset of supportive care that is aimed at relieving symptoms and suffering without aiming to prolong life. The focus of palliative care is to improve quality of life for terminally ill patients. The following discussion includes guidelines for supportive and palliative care. *The Oxford Textbook of Palliative Medicine Second Edition* (New York: Oxford University Press, 1996) is an excellent resource for more extensive discussion of these topics.

I. **Treatment-related toxicities.** For most cancer treatments, the likelihood of side effects is high, and many are predictable. Supportive care in this setting must always include primary and secondary prevention of toxicities whenever possible. Examples include prophylactic antiemetics, empiric broad-spectrum antibiotics for neutropenic fever, or nutritional supplements for anorectic patients.

II. **Disease-related symptoms.** Although some cancers are asymptomatic at onset, in virtually all patients a wide variety of symptoms eventually develop. In the advanced stages of disease, the most common symptoms include pain, anorexia, fatigue, dyspnea, and depression. Mental status changes often occur in the terminal phase.

III. **Management.** The following reviews several of the most common and predictable symptoms for which supportive care is essential. All of these principles can be applied to noncancer patients as well.

A. **Nausea and vomiting (N/V)** are complex phenomena that are mediated by several neurotransmitters in the GI tract and the brain, including acetylcholine, dopamine, histamine, and serotonin. A wide variety of antiemetic agents are available that prevent and treat N/V by blocking these signals. The cortex also controls learned responses such as anticipatory N/V with chemotherapy or that related to anxiety.

1. **Chemotherapy-induced N/V.** Several classes of antiemetics are often combined for synergistic control of chemotherapy-induced N/V. For highly emetogenic chemotherapy agents such as **cisplatin**, patients are premedicated with **dexamethasone**, 10 mg, and a serotonin antagonist such as **ondansetron**, 8 mg, or **granisetron**, 1–2 mg. Because of the typical delayed emesis for up to 72 hours, **dexamethasone**, 4 mg, and dopamine antagonists such as **prochlorperazine**, 10 mg, are prescribed four times a day around the clock for 3 days. Benzodiazepines such as **lorazepam**, 1 mg every 6 hours as needed, can be added as well, especially if anticipatory N/V has occurred in the past. For less emetogenic regimens, **prochlorperazine**, 10 mg every 6 hours, can be taken orally as needed. **Prochlorperazine** can also be administered intravenously or intramuscularly, 10 mg every 6 hours, or per rectal suppository, 25 mg every 8 hours, as needed for vomiting that precludes oral administration. Oral **ondansetron**, 4–8 mg two to three times a day, or **granisetron**, 1 mg one to two times a day, can be quite effective but is expensive and thus is often reserved for refractory cases.

2. **Radiation** to the abdomen or pelvis may cause N/V via small-bowel irritation. A similar approach to that of chemotherapy-induced N/V should prove effective.

3. **Nonchemotherapy medications.** N/V is a common temporary side effect of **opioid analgesics**, generally lasting only approximately 72 hours with regular dosing. However, it may persist in some patients and may occasionally require a shift to another opioid. Toxic levels of other agents such as **digoxin** or **phenytoin** may produce N/V. **Prochlorperazine**, 10 mg every 6 hours as needed, is generally adequate. Nonsteroidal anti-inflammatory drugs (NSAIDs) may lead to esophagitis or gastritis, producing considerable N/V along with dyspepsia. Liquid antacids, 1–2 tablespoons every 2 hours as needed; histamine-2 receptor blockers such as **ranitidine**, 150 mg one to two times a day; or proton pump inhibitors such as **lansoprazole**, 15–30 mg/day, can be used.

4. **GI dysmotility** occurs in a variety of disorders, including opioid analgesic therapy, peritoneal carcinomatosis, autonomic neuropathy from diabetes mellitus, or spinal cord injury. The prokinetic agent **metoclopramide**,

10–20 mg every 6 hours, may improve symptoms. Severe constipation may result in N/V that resolves with successful catharsis (see below).

5. **Antihistamines** and **anticholinergics** may control opioid- or anesthesia-induced stimulation of the vestibular apparatus. Examples include **hydroxyzine**, 25–50 mg every 6 hours, or **scopolamine**, 0.1–0.4 mg IV every 4 hours or one to three transdermal patches every 72 hours, respectively.

6. **Other agents.** Although their antiemetic mechanisms of action are not well understood, these medications have been beneficial for many patients with refractory N/V. **Corticosteroids** such as dexamethasone, 10-mg IV bolus followed by 4 mg every 6 hours IV or PO, is typically used to treat nausea from increased intracranial pressure. Similar doses may also be useful for chemotherapy- or radiation-induced emesis or for other refractory cases. The synthetic cannabinoid **dronabinol**, 2.5–5.0 mg every 8 hours, is beneficial for some patients but may cause sedation, hallucinations, or other mental status changes. **Benzodiazepines** such as lorazepam, 0.5–2.0 mg every 4–6 hours, are often prescribed in addition to traditional antiemetics. Intestinal obstruction may require bowel rest with nasogastric suctioning or even palliative surgery.

B. **Myelosuppression** occurs predictably after most solid tumor chemotherapy regimens. Nadirs occur 10–14 days after dosing, and recovery is usually rapid. Subsequent cycles of chemotherapy are typically held until recovery of the neutrophil count to greater than 1500 and platelet count to greater than 100,000.

1. **Neutropenia.** No treatment is necessary for uncomplicated neutropenia. Immediate broad-spectrum antibiotic therapy must be instituted empirically for febrile episodes. Coverage for *Pseudomonas* is critical, requiring agents such as **cefepime**, 2 g IV every 12 hours, or **levofloxacin**, 500 mg/day. The latter can be given orally to carefully selected outpatients who appear to be very stable. WBC growth factors can be given on subsequent cycles to avoid dose reductions or treatment delays (e.g., **granulocyte colony-stimulating factor**, 300–480 μg/day for 10 days).

2. **Thrombocytopenia** is rarely clinically significant and is less common than neutropenia. Platelet transfusions are only required for patients who have platelet counts below 10,000 or who are actively bleeding.

3. **Anemia** is a common sequela of chemotherapy and may produce or exacerbate fatigue and dyspnea. Transfusions are reserved for symptomatic patients or those with hemoglobin below 8 g/dl. **Erythropoietin** starting at 40,000 units weekly during chemotherapy may obviate the need for transfusions and minimize fatigue (see Chap. 15).

C. **Stomatitis** is painful inflammation and ulceration of oral mucosa that may be superinfected with *Candida* and serves as a portal of entry for bacteria. Management consists of mouth rinses with salt or baking soda solutions. Popular concoctions, often termed **magic mouthwash**, combine equal portions of **viscous lidocaine, diphenhydramine,** and **magnesium–aluminum hydroxide antacids** with or without **nystatin** and are dosed at 30 ml swish and spit every 6 hours. For esophagitis the mixture should be swallowed. Severe cases may be palliated by **sucralfate** slurries, 1 g every 6 hours, and may even require **opioid analgesics**.

D. **Diarrhea,** defined as an increase in the number of bowel movements over baseline, can lead to life-threatening dehydration and electrolyte abnormalities. Etiologies include infections, malabsorption, medications (including chemotherapy), and abdominal or pelvic radiotherapy. The mainstays of pharmacotherapy for diarrhea that is related to chemotherapy or radiation are the synthetic opioids, **loperamide (Immodium)** and **diphenoxylate-atropine (Lomotil)**. The starting dose of these agents is two tablets, followed by one tablet after each diarrheal stool. For refractory cases, **octreotide**, a somatostatin analogue, can be started at 100 μg SC every 8 hours and titrated as needed. Finally, it should be noted that **overflow incontinence** from obstipation may occur, requiring disimpaction rather than antidiarrheal agents.

E. **Constipation.** The etiology of constipation is often multifactorial. Contributing factors include medications (opioids, anticholinergics, calcium channel blockers, iron, calcium), mechanical obstruction, hypercalcemia, spinal cord injury, autonomic dysfunction, dehydration, and physical inactivity. Constipation is common with all opioids, and pharmacologic tolerance rarely develops. Symptoms may be so severe that patients opt to discontinue pain medications. To avoid this, a stimulant laxative such as **senna** or **casanthranol**, two tablets two to three times/day, should be started prophylactically at the initiation of all opioid therapy. These agents are also available combined with the stool softener **docusate**. Refractory constipation may require the addition of osmotic cathartics such as **lactulose** or **sorbitol**, 30 ml four times/day prn, or **magnesium citrate**, one-half to one bottle as needed. The prokinetic agent **metoclopramide**, 10 mg four times/day, aids in the dysmotility that is associated with opioids or autonomic neuropathies. Lubricant stimulants, including **mineral oil** or **glycerin suppositories**, and large-volume **enemas** may be required as well. Dietary interventions and stool softeners alone are rarely sufficient. Bulk-forming agents such as psyllium should be avoided in debilitated anorectic patients.

F. **Anorexia and cachexia.** Loss of appetite, weight loss, and malnutrition are common to most chronic illnesses in the late stages and are extremely frustrating to patients and their caregivers. Nutritional supplements are widely used. Pharmacotherapy is limited to **megestrol acetate**, 800 mg/day; **dronabinol**, 2.5 mg q8–12h; or corticosteroids such as **prednisone**, 20 mg each morning. These drugs may achieve weight gain and improve the patient's sense of well-being temporarily but will eventually fail. In the terminal stages of an illness, it is essential to clarify for patients and caregivers that this is an expected part of their disease and that dying patients do not experience feelings of starvation. Artificial feeding of anorectic patients does not improve energy levels or prolong survival and may lead to N/V, bloating, or aspiration. Therefore, tube feedings and parenteral nutrition are rarely indicated in the care of dying patients.

G. **Fatigue, malaise, and generalized weakness** are extremely common symptoms of underlying disease and treatment. Management is difficult, centering around minimizing sedating medications and optimizing nutrition, fluids, and electrolytes. Pharmacotherapy is of limited benefit. Corticosteroids such as **prednisone**, 20 mg each morning, may enhance feelings of well-being and increase energy but may produce multiple side effects. Their efficacy may wane after 4–6 weeks, but, due to adrenal suppression, they should be continued until death. Psychostimulants such as **methylphenidate**, 5 mg at 9 a.m. and noon, may be useful for opioid-induced sedation.

H. **Insomnia** is frequently due to medications, depression, anxiety, or physical distress. Treatment of unrelieved pain or other symptoms may suffice. Avoidance of caffeine, excess alcohol, and prolonged bed rest is advisable. Pharmacotherapy includes **benzodiazepines** such as **lorazepam**, 0.5–2.0 mg at bedtime; **antihistamines** such as **diphenhydramine or hydroxyzine**, 25–50 mg at bedtime; or sedating antidepressants such as **trazadone**, 50 mg, or **amitriptyline**, 25–50 mg at bedtime.

I. **Depression** occurs in 25–75% of cancer patients. Although it is underdiagnosed, it is not inevitable. Risk factors for major depression include pain or other symptoms, progressive physical impairment, and medications such as steroids or benzodiazepines. The diagnosis should be suspected for patients with pain that does not respond as expected. Treatment consists of psychotherapy and pharmacotherapy. For rapid improvement, psychostimulants such as **methylphenidate**, 5 mg at 9 a.m. and noon, start working within hours to days. **Tricyclic antidepressants** and **selective serotonin reuptake inhibitors** are usually effective in 2–4 weeks. A wide variety of antidepressants are available (see Chap. 29).

J. Dyspnea is a subjective feeling of breathlessness or suffocation. Similar to pain, the only reliable measure of dyspnea is patient report. Respiratory rate and pulse oximetry do not correlate with subjective accounts. The prevalence of dyspnea in terminally ill patients is up to 74%, and the differential diagnosis is extensive. The underlying cause should be treated when possible. Otherwise, pharmacologic and nonpharmacologic interventions should be attempted.

1. **Opioids.** Low doses of opioids have central and peripheral action. Relief of dyspnea is not related to slowing of the respiratory rate, as low doses of opioids do not cause respiratory suppression. For opioid-naïve patients, relief of severe dyspnea can be achieved with **morphine**, 5–15 mg q4h orally, and the dose should be titrated as needed. Patients who are receiving chronic opioids require increases over baseline doses.

2. **Benzodiazepines** are valuable for acute or subacute dyspnea associated with anxiety. They can be combined safely with opioids if titrated gradually. For example, a starting dose of **lorazepam**, 0.5–2.0 mg q4–6h, may be helpful.

3. **Other.** Oxygen therapy, or more simply opening the window or turning on a fan, may be beneficial. Keeping the room cool and less crowded may help as well. Behavioral approaches include reassurance, relaxation techniques, distraction, or hypnosis.

Pain Management

Pain is a common symptom of cancer, affecting more than 50% of all cancer patients and more than 70% of patients with advanced cancer. Half of all cancer patients report moderate to severe pain, and 30% report excruciating pain. With vigilant attention to patients' needs, adequate control of pain can be achieved in the vast majority of cases. Guidelines for cancer pain management are available through the Agency for Health Care Policy and Research (Publication No. 94-0593) and the American Cancer Society (*CA Cancer J Clin* 1994;44:262). Many of the principles used for cancer pain management can be applied to chronic noncancer pain as well.

I. **Assessment.** Pain is best relieved if the underlying source can be treated. In cancer patients this might pertain to healing of stomatitis or palliative radiation to a painful bone metastasis. Even when the source of pain cannot be remedied, the treatment depends on specific characteristics and intensity of the pain. A thorough pain evaluation should include description of the location, sites of radiation, alleviating and exacerbating factors, quality (e.g., dull, stabbing, burning), and intensity of the pain. Physical examination should assess bony tenderness, range of motion, presence of masses, and neurologic function. Visual analogue scales are useful for grading pain intensity and measuring degree of relief. Pertinent radiographic studies should follow. Adequate analgesia, including opioids, should be prescribed during the workup and not reserved until after confirmation of incurable cancer.

II. **Step-wise therapy.** Following the protocol of the World Health Organization's **analgesic ladder** can relieve more than 90% of cancer pain. It should be noted that patients who present with severe pain may go right to Step 2 or even Step 3. Adjuvant agents (see below) can and should be added at any level, depending on the type of pain. NSAIDs are often continued along with opioids, especially for bone pain.

A. **Step 1.** For mild to moderate pain, nonopioid analgesics, such as **aspirin, acetaminophen**, or **NSAIDs**, should be used. The efficacy of these agents is limited by a ceiling dose above which toxic effects predominate.

B. **Step 2.** The "weak opioid analgesics" are typified by fixed combinations of acetaminophen or aspirin with **codeine, oxycodone**, or **hydrocodone** (Table 16-2). The maximal dose of these combinations is two tablets every 4

Table 16-2. Commonly used opioid analgesics for chronic pain

Generic name	Trade name(s) and formulations[a]	Recommended dosing interval
Morphine		
Sustained release	MS Contin, 15, 30, 60, 100, 200 mg	q12h
	Oramorph SR, 15, 30, 60, 100 mg	q12h
	Kadian, 20, 50, 100 mg	q12–24h
	MSIR tablets, 5, 15 mg	q3–4h
Short acting	Roxanol, 20 mg/ml elixir	q2–4h
	Various elixirs, 1, 2, 20 mg/ml	
Oxycodone		
Sustained release	Oxycontin, 10, 20, 40, 80 mg	q12h
Short acting	OxyIR or Roxicodone tablets, 5, 10 mg	q3–4h
	Roxicodone elixir, 5 mg/ml	
	Oxyfast elixir, 20 mg/ml	q2–4h
With APAP	Tablets, mg oxycodone/mg APAP	
	Percocet, 2.5/325	
	Percocet, 5/325	
	Percocet, 7.5/500	
	Percocet, 10/650	
	Roxicet, 5/325 or 5/500	
	Tylox, 5/325	
	Elixir, mg oxycodone/mg APAP	
	Roxicet, 5/325/5 ml	
Codeine	Various	q4–6h
	Tablets, 15, 30, 60 mg	
	Elixir, 15 mg/5 ml	
With APAP	Tablets, mg codeine/mg APAP	q4–6h
	Tylenol #2, 15/325	
	Tylenol #3, 30/325	
	Tylenol #4, 60/325	
Hydrocodone, with APAP	Vicodin, Lortab (5 mg hydrocodone/325 mg APAP)	q4–6h
Hydromorphone	Dilaudid	q3–4h
	Tablets, 1, 2, 3, 4, 8 mg	
	Elixir, 5 mg/ml	
	Suppository, 3 mg	
Meperidine	Demerol	Not recommended for chronic pain
Fentanyl		
Transdermal	Duragesic patch, 25, 50, 75, 100 µg/hr	q72h
Transmucosal	Actiq oralet (lollipop), 200, 300, 400 µg	q2h
Methadone	Various	q8h
	Tablets, 5, 10, 40 mg	
	Elixir, 5 mg/5 ml, 10 mg/5 ml, 5 mg/ml, 10 mg/ml	

APAP, acetaminophen.
[a]The most frequently prescribed brands and formulations are listed. This is not a comprehensive list.

Table 16-3. Equivalent opioid doses (mg)

Opioid	Oral	Parenteral
Morphine	60	20
Hydromorphone	15	3
Meperidine	600	150
Methadone	40	20
Codeine	360	N/A
Oxycodone	40	N/A
Fentanyl	25 μg/hr[a]	0.2

N/A, not applicable
[a]Only available as 72-hr transdermal patch. Dose is based on 24-hr oral opioid dose.

> hours because of the potential toxicity of the nonsteroidal or acetaminophen component. This step is used for patients with intermittent pain that requires intermittent dosing.
>
> **C. Step 3.** The "strong opioids" used at this level are often available on sustained-release formulations or have long half-lives. Pure opioids, such as **morphine, hydromorphone, methadone,** or **fentanyl,** have no maximum dose and should be titrated upward until pain is relieved or side effects become intolerable. Regular around-the-clock dosing is preferred at this step.

III. Guidelines for opioid use in chronic pain
  A. Start with the lowest effective dose.
  B. Use around-the-clock dosing to avoid peaks and valleys (periods of pain from low serum levels and periods of toxicity from excess serum levels).
  C. **Sustained-release** preparations are ideal for prolonged periods of pain relief and improved compliance.
  D. Titrate doses to adequate analgesia or intolerable side effects. For uncontrolled pain, increase the daily dose by up to **50%** every 24–48 hours for oral preparations.
  E. Always prescribe immediate-release formulations for **breakthrough pain.** Use one-fourth to one-third of the total daily dose every 2–4 hours.
  F. Keep regimens as simple as possible. Avoid multiple opioids.
  G. Side effects differ from patient to patient. When side effects are intolerable, opioid rotation should be attempted. **Equianalgesic doses** must be used to maintain pain relief (Table 16-3).
  H. Educate patients and families about dosing principles and side effects, and reassure them about addiction.

IV. Examples
  A. A patient whose chronic pain is controlled on ten daily Percocets (containing 5 mg oxycodone each) could be switched to sustained-release morphine, 30 mg q12h, or a fentanyl patch, 25 μg/hr q72h.
  B. A patient's pain is poorly controlled on sustained-release morphine, 30 mg bid, and two Percocets every 4 hours. The 24-hour morphine equivalent of the current regimen is at least 120 mg. Increase morphine to 180 mg/day or 90 mg bid. Add immediate-release morphine, 30 mg q3h prn for breakthrough pain.
  C. Pain is controlled on sustained-release morphine, 120 mg bid, but the patient has nausea and excess sedation. One should try sustained-release oxycodone, 80–100 mg bid, or a fentanyl patch, 100 μg/hr q72h.

V. Alternative routes of administration. Patients may be unable to swallow pills or even liquids for a variety of reasons. The **transdermal** fentanyl patch may provide sustained pain relief in such cases. In the final few days or hours of life, patients may obtain prolonged pain relief by administration of sustained-release morphine or oxycodone tablets **per rectum**. Concentrates of morphine or oxycodone, 20 mg/ml, can be administered in small enough volumes for **sublingual** absorption, even in obtunded patients. Very rapid onset of pain relief may be obtained by dissolving the fentanyl transmucosal oralet (sometimes referred to as a **lollipop**) through the buccal mucosa. However, the duration of action of this fentanyl preparation is brief and costs several dollars per dose. **Patient-controlled analgesia** pumps can include a basal infusion and bolus, allowing patients to self-administer IV or SC opioids at predetermined limits of time and dose. This is a good way to control refractory pain rapidly and to get an accurate assessment of a patient's 24-hour opioid requirements. However, it is very expensive and usually reserved for short inpatient admissions. When converting back to oral analgesics, one should be sure to correct for decreased bioavailability (Table 16-2).

VI. **Common side effects of opioids.** Constipation can be severe, and tolerance to this rarely develops. One should always prescribe prophylactic stimulant laxatives such as **senna**, two tablets bid. N/V may occur initially or with rapid titration. Antiemetics such as **prochlorperazine**, 10 mg q6h prn, are useful until tolerance develops, usually in a few days. Sedation, lightheadedness, confusion, or hallucinations may occur. Tolerance generally develops after a few days of steady-state levels, but symptoms may persist with intermittent dosing. Physical dependence occurs with chronic opioid use and is not equivalent to addiction. Withdrawal symptoms can be avoided by tapering off rather than abruptly discontinuing opioids.

VII. **Pharmacologic adjuncts to analgesics.** Anticonvulsants and tricyclic antidepressants may provide relief of **neuropathic pain**, which is due to direct nerve injury such as spinal cord compression or postherpetic neuralgia. Typically described as burning, stabbing, or shooting pain, neuropathic pain may be difficult to control with opioids or NSAIDs alone. A neuropathic component should be suspected for any pain that is poorly controlled despite high opioid doses.

A. **Anticonvulsants** appear to work by suppressing neuronal firing. **Gabapentin**, which has demonstrated efficacy for neuropathic pain due to malignancy, diabetic neuropathy, and multiple sclerosis, has a wide therapeutic window. Starting at 300 mg tid, the dose can be titrated as high as 1200 mg tid. **Carbamazepine**, 100–200 mg bid to tid, or **phenytoin**, 100 mg tid, may also be effective, although with a narrower therapeutic window.

B. **Tricyclic antidepressants** may be effective immediately at doses well below those for depression (e.g., **amitriptyline**, 25–50 mg bid). Because of their sedating effects, they have added benefit for patients with insomnia.

C. **Corticosteroids** can improve pain control from nerve compression, visceral distension, or severe bone pain. For malignant spinal cord compression, high-dose **dexamethasone** (20- to 100-mg IV bolus, then 4–10 mg IV 4 times daily) relieves pain and decreases the likelihood of permanent cord damage along with rapidly instituted radiation therapy.

VIII. **Nonpharmacologic modalities** in addition to analgesics may significantly improve control of chronic pain. Cutaneous stimulation (e.g., heat, cold, or massage) is a simple technique that family members can apply. Neurostimulatory techniques, including **transcutaneous electrical nerve stimulation (TENS)** or **acupuncture**, are effective in selected patients. **Physiatry consultation** may be useful to provide simple exercises, assistive devices, or immobilization with a sling or brace, depending on the source of pain. **Psychological therapies** involve relaxation techniques, biofeedback, behavior therapy, or support groups.

IX. **Invasive techniques** are usually reserved for truly refractory pain in patients with a life expectancy of at least several months. Neuroablative techniques (**nerve blocks, rhizotomy**, or **cordotomy**) may provide control of intractable pain. **Epidural or intrathecal** infusion of anesthetics or opioids may provide relief when the required doses of systemic opioids are unduly toxic. All of these maneuvers are expensive, carry innate risks, and require consultation with an experienced anesthesiologist or neurosurgeon.

Hospice Care

Hospice is a philosophy of care based on a coordinated program of support services for terminally ill patients and their families. Palliative care is provided with the aim of improved quality of life and a comfortable death. Any patient with a limited life expectancy (approximately 6 months or less) may be eligible for hospice care. Although the majority of hospice patients have cancer, those with other advanced illnesses, such as CHF, pulmonary diseases, or dementia, may benefit from this approach. The interdisciplinary hospice team consists of nurses who are trained in pain and symptom management, home health aides, social workers, chaplains, and volunteers. The referring physician may remain involved in medical decisions unless transfer to the hospice medical director is desired. Care is generally given in the home but can be imparted in nursing homes or hospitals if necessary. Medicare hospice benefits also include complete coverage for all medications that pertain to the hospice diagnosis, durable medical equipment, and oxygen. Most hospice agencies provide 24-hour on-call service, brief respite care, and bereavement counseling for 1 year after the patient dies. More information about hospice care and availability can be obtained from the **National Hospice and Palliative Care Organization** (http://www.nhpco.org).

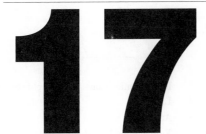

Endocrine Diseases

William E. Clutter

Evaluation of Thyroid Function

I. **Introduction.** The major hormone secreted by the thyroid is **thyroxine (T_4)**, which is converted in many tissues to the more potent **triiodothyronine (T_3)**. Both are bound reversibly to plasma proteins, primarily **T_4-binding globulin (TBG)**. Only the unbound (free) fraction enters cells and produces biological effects. T_4 secretion is stimulated by **thyroid-stimulating hormone (TSH)**. In turn, TSH secretion is inhibited by T_4, forming a **negative feedback** loop that keeps free T_4 levels within a narrow normal range. Diagnosis of thyroid disease is based on clinical findings, palpation of the thyroid, and measurement of plasma TSH and thyroid hormones (*Clin Chem* 1999;45:1377). **Thyroid palpation** determines not only the size and consistency of the thyroid but the presence of nodules, tenderness, or a thrill.

II. **Plasma TSH assay is the initial test of choice in most patients with suspected thyroid disease.** TSH levels are elevated in even mild primary hypothyroidism and are suppressed to less than 0.1 µU/ml in even subclinical hyperthyroidism (i.e., thyroid hormone excess that is too mild to cause symptoms). Thus, **a normal plasma TSH level excludes hyperthyroidism and primary hypothyroidism.** However, TSH levels usually are within the reference range in secondary hypothyroidism and are not useful for detection of this rare form of hypothyroidism. Because even slight changes in thyroid hormone levels affect TSH secretion, **abnormal TSH levels are not specific for clinically important thyroid disease**, which should usually be confirmed by plasma thyroid hormone measurement.
   A. **Plasma TSH is elevated mildly** (up to 20 µU/ml) in some euthyroid patients with nonthyroidal illnesses and in subclinical hypothyroidism.
   B. **TSH levels may be suppressed to less than 0.1 µU/ml** in nonthyroidal illness, in subclinical hyperthyroidism, in some euthyroid elderly patients, and during treatment with dopamine or high doses of glucocorticoids. Also, TSH levels remain lower than 0.1 µU/ml for some time after hyperthyroidism is corrected.

III. **An estimate of plasma free T_4** confirms the diagnosis of clinical hypothyroidism in patients with elevated plasma TSH and confirms the diagnosis and assesses the severity of hyperthyroidism when plasma TSH is less than 0.1 µU/ml. Plasma free T_4 concentrations can be measured by immunoassay or by calculation of the T_4 index. Measurement of total plasma T_4 alone is not adequate, because TBG levels are altered in many circumstances.

IV. **Effect of nonthyroidal illness on thyroid function tests.** Many illnesses alter thyroid tests without causing true thyroid dysfunction. These changes must be recognized to avoid mistaken diagnosis and therapy (*Thyroid* 1997;7:125).
   A. The **low T_3 syndrome** occurs in many illnesses, during starvation, and after trauma or surgery. Conversion of T_4 to T_3 is decreased, and plasma T_3 levels

Table 17-1. Effects of drugs on thyroid function tests

Effect	Drug
Decreased T$_4$	
True hypothyroidism (TSH elevated)	Iodine (amiodarone, radiographic contrast)
	Lithium
Decreased TBG (TSH normal)	Androgens
Inhibition of T$_4$ binding to TBG (TSH normal)	Furosemide (high doses)
	Salicylates
Inhibition of TSH secretion	Glucocorticoids
	Dopamine
Multiple mechanisms (TSH normal)	Phenytoin
Increased T$_4$	
True hyperthyroidism (TSH <0.1 μU/ml)	Iodine (amiodarone, radiographic contrast)
Increased TBG (TSH normal)	Estrogens, tamoxifen
Inhibited T$_4$ to T$_3$ conversion (TSH normal)	Amiodarone
	Propranolol (high doses)

T$_3$, triiodothyronine; T$_4$, thyroxine; TBG, T$_4$-binding globulin; TSH, thyroid-stimulating hormone.

are low. It may be an adaptive response to illness, and thyroid hormone therapy is not beneficial.
   B. The **low T$_4$ syndrome** occurs in severe illness. It may be due to decreased TBG levels, inhibition of T$_4$ binding to TBG, or suppressed TSH secretion. **TSH levels decrease early in severe illness,** sometimes to less than 0.1 μU/ml. During recovery they rise, sometimes to levels higher than the normal range (although rarely higher than 20 μU/ml).
V. **The effects of drugs on thyroid function tests** (Table 17-1). **Iodine-containing drugs (amiodarone and radiographic contrast media)** may cause hyperthyroidism or hypothyroidism in susceptible patients. Many drugs alter thyroid function tests, especially plasma T$_4$, without causing true thyroid dysfunction (*N Engl J Med* 1995;333:1688). In general, plasma TSH levels are a reliable guide to determining whether true hyperthyroidism or hypothyroidism is present.

Hypothyroidism

I. **Etiology. Primary hypothyroidism** (due to disease of the thyroid itself) accounts for more than 90% of cases (*Lancet* 1997;349:413). **Chronic lymphocytic thyroiditis (Hashimoto's disease;** *N Engl J Med* 1996;335:99) is the most common cause and may be associated with Addison's disease and other endocrine deficits. Its prevalence is greatest in women and increases with age. **Iatrogenic hypothyroidism** due to thyroidectomy or radioactive iodine (RAI) therapy also is common. Transient hypothyroidism occurs in postpartum thyroiditis and subacute thyroiditis, usually after a period of hyperthyroidism. Drugs that may cause hypothyroidism include iodine, lithium, alpha interferon, and interleukin-2. **Secondary hypothyroidism** due to TSH deficiency is uncommon but may occur in any disorder of the pituitary or hypothalamus. However, it rarely occurs without other evidence of pituitary disease.

II. **Clinical findings.** Most symptoms of hypothyroidism are nonspecific and develop gradually. They include **cold intolerance**, fatigue, somnolence, poor memory, constipation, menorrhagia, myalgias, and hoarseness. Signs include **slow tendon-reflex relaxation**, bradycardia, facial and periorbital edema, dry skin, and nonpitting edema (myxedema). Mild weight gain may occur, but hypothyroidism does not cause marked obesity. Rare manifestations include hypoventilation, pericardial or pleural effusions, deafness, and carpal tunnel syndrome. Laboratory findings may include hyponatremia and elevated plasma levels of cholesterol, triglycerides, and creatine kinase. The ECG may show low-voltage and T-wave abnormalities.

III. **Diagnosis.** Hypothyroidism is readily treatable and should be suspected in any patient with compatible symptoms, especially in the presence of a goiter or a history of RAI therapy or thyroid surgery.

A. **In suspected primary hypothyroidism, plasma TSH is the best initial diagnostic test.** A normal value excludes primary hypothyroidism, and a markedly elevated value (>20 μU/ml) confirms the diagnosis. If plasma TSH is elevated moderately (5–20 μU/ml), plasma free T_4 should be measured. A low free T_4 confirms clinical hypothyroidism. A clearly normal free T_4 with an elevated plasma TSH indicates subclinical hypothyroidism, in which thyroid function is impaired but increased secretion of TSH maintains plasma T_4 levels within the reference range. These patients may have nonspecific symptoms that are compatible with hypothyroidism and a mild increase in serum cholesterol and low-density lipoprotein cholesterol levels. They develop clinical hypothyroidism at a rate of 2.5%/year. **Thyroid imaging with ultrasound or radionuclide scan is not useful in diagnosis of hypothyroidism.**

B. **If secondary hypothyroidism is suspected** because of evidence of pituitary disease, plasma free T_4 should be measured. Plasma TSH levels are usually within the reference range in secondary hypothyroidism and cannot be used alone to make this diagnosis. Patients with secondary hypothyroidism should be evaluated for other pituitary hormone deficits and for a mass lesion of the pituitary or hypothalamus.

C. **In severe nonthyroidal illness,** the diagnosis of hypothyroidism may be difficult. Plasma total T_4 and T_4 index often are low. The validity of free T_4 immunoassays in such patients has not been clearly established (*Clin Chem* 1996;42:188). **Plasma TSH still is the best initial diagnostic test.** Marked elevation of plasma TSH (>20 μU/ml) establishes the diagnosis of primary hypothyroidism. A normal TSH value is strong evidence that the patient is euthyroid, except when there is evidence of pituitary or hypothalamic disease, in which case free T_4 should be measured. Moderate elevations of plasma TSH (<20 μU/ml) may occur in euthyroid patients with nonthyroidal illness and are not specific for hypothyroidism.

IV. **Therapy. T_4** is the drug of choice (*N Engl J Med* 1994;331:174). The usual replacement dose is 100–125 μg PO qd, and most patients require doses between 75 and 150 μg qd. In elderly patients, the average replacement dose is somewhat lower. The need for lifelong treatment should be emphasized.

A. **Initiation of therapy.** Young and middle-aged patients should be started on 100 μg qd. In otherwise healthy **elderly patients**, the initial dose should be 50 μg qd. Patients with **heart disease** should be started on 25 μg qd and monitored carefully for exacerbation of cardiac symptoms.

B. **Follow-up and dose adjustment**

1. **In primary hypothyroidism, the goal of therapy is to maintain plasma TSH within the normal range.** After 6–8 weeks, plasma TSH should be measured. The dose of T_4 then should be adjusted in 12- to 25-μg increments at intervals of 6–8 weeks until plasma TSH is normal. Thereafter, annual TSH measurement is adequate to monitor therapy. Overtreatment, indicated by a plasma TSH below the normal range,

should be avoided, as it increases the risk of osteoporosis (*J Clin Endocrinol Metab* 1996;81:4278) and atrial fibrillation (*Endocrinol Metab Clin North Am* 1998;27:51).

2. **In secondary hypothyroidism, plasma TSH cannot be used to adjust therapy.** The goal of therapy is to maintain the **plasma free T$_4$** near the middle of the reference range. The dose of T$_4$ should be adjusted at 6- to 8-week intervals until this goal is achieved. Thereafter, annual measurement of plasma free T$_4$ is adequate to monitor therapy.

3. **Coronary artery disease** may be exacerbated by treatment of hypothyroidism. The dose should be increased slowly, with careful attention to worsening angina, heart failure, or arrhythmias. If cardiac symptoms worsen despite medical therapy, coronary revascularization (which can be done safely in hypothyroid patients) should be considered.

C. **Difficulty in controlling hypothyroidism.** Most often, difficulty is due to **poor compliance** with therapy. Observed therapy may be necessary in some cases. Other causes of increasing T$_4$ requirements include (1) **malabsorption** due to intestinal disease or **drugs that interfere with T$_4$ absorption** (e.g., cholestyramine, sucralfate, aluminum hydroxide, ferrous sulfate); (2) **other drug interactions** that increase T$_4$ clearance (e.g., rifampin, carbamazepine, phenytoin) or block conversion of T$_4$ to T$_3$ (amiodarone); (3) **pregnancy**, in which T$_4$ requirement increases in the first trimester; and (4) gradual failure of remaining endogenous thyroid function after treatment of hyperthyroidism.

D. **Subclinical hypothyroidism** (see sec. **III.A**) should be treated with T$_4$ if any of the following are present (*Ann Intern Med* 1998;129:141): (1) symptoms compatible with hypothyroidism, (2) a goiter, (3) hypercholesterolemia that warrants treatment, or (4) plasma TSH of greater than 10 μU/ml. Untreated patients should be monitored annually, and T$_4$ should be started if symptoms develop or serum TSH increases to greater than 10 μU/ml.

E. **Surgery.** Although hypothyroidism increases the risk of minor perioperative complications, there is little increase in the risk of serious complications or mortality. Emergency surgery need not be delayed, but treatment of hypothyroidism should be started (see sec. **A**); the initial doses can be given IV. Elective surgery should be postponed until hypothyroidism has been treated for several weeks.

F. **Urgent therapy** is rarely necessary for hypothyroidism. Most patients with hypothyroidism and concomitant illness can be treated in the usual manner (see secs. **A** and **B**). However, hypothyroidism may impair survival in critical illness by contributing to hypoventilation, hypotension, hypothermia, bradycardia, or hyponatremia. Such patients should be admitted to the hospital for therapy of hypothyroidism and the concomitant illness.

1. **Confirmatory tests should be obtained before thyroid hormone therapy is started** in a severely ill patient, including serum TSH and free T$_4$.

2. **T$_4$,** 50–100 μg IV, can be given q6–8h for 24 hours, followed by 75–100 μg IV qd until oral intake is possible. **Such rapid correction is warranted only in extremely ill patients. Vital signs and cardiac rhythm should be monitored carefully** to detect early signs of exacerbation of heart disease.

3. Hydrocortisone, 50 mg IV q8h, usually is recommended during rapid treatment with thyroid hormone, on the grounds that such therapy may precipitate adrenal failure.

Hyperthyroidism

I. **Etiology** (*Lancet* 1997;349:339). **Graves' disease** (*N Engl J Med* 2000;343:1236) causes most cases of hyperthyroidism, especially in young patients. **Toxic multinodular goiter** (MNG) is a common cause in older patients. Unusual causes include **iodine-induced hyperthyroidism**, usually precipitated by drugs (e.g., amiodarone or radiographic contrast media), thyroid adenomas (which present as a single nodule), subacute thyroiditis (painful tender goiter with transient hyperthyroidism), postpartum thyroiditis (nontender goiter with transient hyperthyroidism), and surreptitious ingestion of thyroid hormone. TSH-induced hyperthyroidism is extremely rare.

II. **Clinical findings.** Symptoms include **heat intolerance**, weight loss, weakness, palpitations, oligomenorrhea, and anxiety. Signs include **brisk tendon reflexes**, fine tremor, proximal weakness, stare, and eyelid lag. Cardiac abnormalities may be prominent, including sinus tachycardia, atrial fibrillation, and exacerbation of coronary artery disease or heart failure. In the **elderly**, hyperthyroidism may present with only atrial fibrillation, heart failure, weakness, or weight loss, and a high index of suspicion is needed to make the diagnosis. Graves' disease may also cause two signs that are not found in other causes of hyperthyroidism: **proptosis** (exophthalmos) and **pretibial myxedema**.

III. **Diagnosis.** Hyperthyroidism should be suspected in any patient with compatible symptoms, as it is a readily treatable disorder that may become highly debilitating.

A. **Plasma TSH is the best initial diagnostic test, as a TSH level of higher than 0.1 µU/ml excludes clinical hyperthyroidism. If plasma TSH is lower than 0.1 µU/ml, plasma free T$_4$ should be measured** to determine the severity of hyperthyroidism and as a baseline for therapy. If plasma free T$_4$ is elevated, the diagnosis of clinical hyperthyroidism is established.

B. **If plasma TSH is lower than 0.1 µU/ml but free T$_4$ is normal**, the patient may have clinical hyperthyroidism due to **elevation of plasma T$_3$ alone**; therefore, plasma T$_3$ should be measured. Other explanations include suppression of TSH by **nonthyroidal illness**. A third-generation TSH assay with a detection limit of 0.01 µU/ml may be helpful in patients with suppressed TSH and nonthyroidal illness. Most patients with clinical hyperthyroidism have plasma TSH levels that are lower than 0.01 µU/ml in such assays, whereas nonthyroidal illness rarely suppresses TSH to this degree. Finally, **subclinical hyperthyroidism** may lower TSH to less than 0.1 µU/ml, and therefore suppression of TSH alone does not confirm that symptoms are due to hyperthyroidism.

C. **Differential diagnosis** (Table 17-2) affects the choice of therapy and is based on (1) the presence of **proptosis** or **pretibial myxedema**, which indicates Graves' disease (although many patients with Graves' disease lack these signs); (2) **palpation of the thyroid** to determine whether a diffuse or nodular goiter is present; most hyperthyroid patients with a diffuse nontender goiter have Graves' disease; (3) history of recent **pregnancy, neck pain**, or **iodine administration**, which suggests causes other than Graves' disease; or (4) in rare cases, **24-hour RAI uptake** (RAIU), which is needed to distinguish Graves' disease or toxic MNG (in which RAIU is elevated) from postpartum thyroiditis, iodine-induced hyperthyroidism, or factitious hyperthyroidism (in which RAIU is very low). **Thyroid imaging with ultrasound or radionuclide scan is not useful in diagnosis of hyperthyroidism.**

Table 17-2. Differential diagnosis of hyperthyroidism

Signs	Diagnosis
Diffuse, nontender goiter	Graves' disease (rarely postpartum silent thyroiditis)
Multiple thyroid nodules	Toxic multinodular goiter
Single thyroid nodule	Thyroid adenoma
Tender painful goiter	Subacute thyroiditis
Normal thyroid gland	Graves' disease (rarely postpartum thyroiditis or factitious hyperthyroidism)

IV. **Therapy** (*Ann Intern Med* 1994;122:281). Some forms of hyperthyroidism (subacute or postpartum thyroiditis) are transient and require only symptomatic therapy. Three methods are available for definitive therapy: RAI, thionamides, and subtotal thyroidectomy, none of which controls hyperthyroidism rapidly. **During treatment, patients are followed by clinical evaluation and measurement of plasma free T$_4$.** Plasma TSH is useless in assessing the initial response to therapy, as it remains suppressed until after the patient becomes euthyroid. Regardless of the therapy used, all patients with Graves' disease require lifelong follow-up for recurrent hyperthyroidism or development of hypothyroidism.

A. **Symptomatic therapy.** β-adrenergic antagonists are used to relieve such symptoms of hyperthyroidism as palpitations, tremor, and anxiety until hyperthyroidism is controlled by definitive therapy or until transient forms of hyperthyroidism subside. The initial dose of **atenolol**, 25–50 mg qd, or **propranolol**, 20–40 mg qid, is adjusted to alleviate symptoms and tachycardia. β-adrenergic antagonist therapy should be reduced gradually, then stopped as hyperthyroidism is controlled. Verapamil at an initial dose of 40–80 mg tid can be used to control tachycardia in patients with contraindications to β-adrenergic antagonists.

B. **Choice of definitive therapy**

1. **In Graves' disease, RAI therapy is the treatment of choice for almost all patients.** It is simple, highly effective, and causes no life-threatening complications. However, it **cannot be used in pregnancy. Propylthiouracil (PTU) should be used to treat hyperthyroidism in pregnancy**, but it provides long-term control of hyperthyroidism in fewer than one-half of patients and carries a small risk of life-threatening side effects (see sec. **D.3**). Thyroidectomy should be used only in patients who refuse RAI therapy and who relapse or develop side effects with thionamide therapy.

2. **Other causes of hyperthyroidism.** Toxic MNG and toxic adenoma should be treated with RAI (except in pregnancy). Transient forms of hyperthyroidism due to thyroiditis should be treated symptomatically with atenolol. Iodine-induced hyperthyroidism is treated with thionamides and atenolol until the patient is euthyroid.

C. **RAI therapy.** A single dose permanently controls hyperthyroidism in some 90% of patients, and further doses can be given if necessary. A **pregnancy test** is done immediately before therapy in potentially fertile women. Usually, 24-hour RAIU is measured and used to calculate the dose. Thionamides interfere with RAI therapy and should be stopped at least 3 days before treatment. If iodine treatment has been given, it should be stopped at least 2 weeks before RAI therapy. Most patients with Graves' disease are treated with 8–10 mCi, although treatment of toxic MNG requires higher doses.

1. **Follow-up.** Usually, several months are needed to restore euthyroidism. Patients are evaluated at 4- to 6-week intervals, with assessment of clinical findings and plasma free T$_4$. If thyroid function stabilizes within the normal range, the interval between follow-up visits is increased gradually to annual intervals.

   a. **If symptomatic hypothyroidism develops**, T$_4$ therapy is started (see Hypothyroidism, sec. **IV**). Mild hypothyroidism after RAI therapy may be transient, and asymptomatic patients can be observed for a further 4–6 weeks to determine whether hypothyroidism will resolve spontaneously.

   b. **If symptomatic hyperthyroidism persists** after 6 months, RAI treatment is repeated.

2. **Side effects. Hypothyroidism** occurs in 30% or more of patients within the first year and continues to develop at a rate of approximately 3%/year thereafter. A slight rise in plasma T$_4$ may occur in the first 2 weeks after therapy, owing to release of stored hormone. This development is

important only in patients with **severe cardiac disease**, which may worsen as a result. Such patients should be treated with thionamides to restore euthyroidism and to deplete stored hormone before treatment with RAI. No convincing evidence has been found that RAI has a clinically important effect on the course of Graves' eye disease. It does not increase the risk of malignancy. No increase in congenital abnormalities has been found in the offspring of women who conceive after RAI therapy, and the radiation exposure to the ovaries is low, comparable to that from common diagnostic radiographs. Concern for potential teratogenic effects should not influence physicians' advice to patients.

D. **Thionamides.** Methimazole and PTU inhibit thyroid hormone synthesis. PTU also inhibits extrathyroidal conversion of T_4 to T_3. Once thyroid hormone stores are depleted (after several weeks to months), T_4 levels decrease. These drugs have no permanent effect on thyroid function. **In the majority of patients with Graves' disease, hyperthyroidism recurs** within 6 months after therapy is stopped. Spontaneous remission of Graves' disease occurs in approximately one-third of patients during thionamide therapy, and, in this minority, no other treatment may be needed. Remission is more likely to occur in mild, recent-onset hyperthyroidism.

1. **Initiation of therapy.** Before starting therapy, patients must be warned of side effects and precautions. Usual starting doses are **PTU**, 100–200 mg PO tid, or **methimazole**, 10–40 mg PO qd; higher initial doses can be used in severe hyperthyroidism.

2. **Follow-up.** Restoration of euthyroidism takes up to several months. Patients are evaluated at 4-week intervals with assessment of clinical findings and plasma free T_4. If plasma free T_4 levels do not fall after 4–8 weeks, the dose should be increased. Doses as high as **PTU**, 300 mg PO qid, or **methimazole**, 60 mg PO qd, may be required. Once the plasma free T_4 level falls to normal, the dose is adjusted to maintain plasma free T_4 within the normal range. No consensus exists on the optimal duration of therapy, but periods of 6 months to 2 years are used most commonly. Regardless of the duration of therapy, patients must be monitored carefully for recurrence of hyperthyroidism after the drug is stopped.

3. **Side effects** are most likely to occur within the first few months of therapy. **Minor side effects** include rash, urticaria, fever, arthralgias, and transient leukopenia. **Agranulocytosis** occurs in 0.3% of patients who are treated with thionamides. Other life-threatening side effects include **hepatitis**, vasculitis, and drug-induced lupus erythematosus. These complications usually resolve if the drug is stopped promptly. **Patients must be warned to stop the drug immediately if jaundice or symptoms that are suggestive of agranulocytosis (e.g., fever, chills, sore throat) develop** and to contact their physician promptly for evaluation. Routine monitoring of WBC is not useful for detecting agranulocytosis, which develops suddenly.

E. **Subtotal thyroidectomy.** This procedure provides long-term control of hyperthyroidism in most patients. Surgery may trigger a perioperative exacerbation of hyperthyroidism, and patients should be prepared for surgery by one of two methods.

1. **A thionamide** is given until the patient is nearly euthyroid (see sec. **D**). Supersaturated potassium iodide (SSKI), 40–80 mg (1–2 gtt) PO bid, is then added, and surgery is scheduled 1–2 weeks later. Both drugs are stopped postoperatively.

2. **Atenolol, 50–100 mg qd**, and SSKI, 1–2 gtt PO bid, are started 1–2 weeks before surgery is scheduled. The dose of atenolol is increased, if necessary, to reduce the resting heart rate below 90 beats/minute. Atenolol, but not SSKI, is continued for 5–7 days after surgery.

3. **Follow-up** includes patient evaluation at 4–6 weeks after surgery, with assessment of clinical findings and plasma free T_4 and TSH. If thyroid

function is normal, the patient is seen at 3 and 6 months, then annually. If symptomatic hypothyroidism develops, T_4 therapy is started (see Hypothyroidism, sec. **IV**). Mild hypothyroidism after subtotal thyroidectomy may be transient, and asymptomatic patients can be observed for a further 4–6 weeks to determine whether hypothyroidism will resolve spontaneously. Hypothyroidism persists or recurs in 3–7% of patients.

4. **Complications** of thyroidectomy include **hypothyroidism** in 30–50% of patients and **hypoparathyroidism** in perhaps 3%. Rare complications include permanent vocal cord paralysis due to recurrent laryngeal nerve injury and perioperative death. The complication rate appears to depend on the experience of the surgeon.

F. **Subclinical hyperthyroidism** (*Endocrinol Metab Clin North Am* 1998;27:37) is present when the plasma TSH is suppressed to less than 0.1 µU/ml, but the patient has no symptoms that are definitely caused by hyperthyroidism and plasma levels of T_4 and T_3 are normal. Subclinical hyperthyroidism increases the risk of atrial fibrillation in the elderly and predisposes to osteoporosis in postmenopausal women and should be treated in these groups of patients (see sec. **C**). Whether other patients should be treated is unclear (*Ann Intern Med* 1998;129:144).

G. **Urgent therapy** is warranted when hyperthyroidism exacerbates heart failure or coronary artery disease and in rare patients with severe hyperthyroidism complicated by fever and delirium (*Endocrinol Metab Clin North Am* 1993;22:263). Such patients should be admitted to the hospital for therapy.

1. **PTU**, 300 mg PO q6h, should be started immediately.

2. **Iodide (SSKI**, 1–2 gtt PO q12h) should be started approximately 2 hours after the first dose of PTU to inhibit thyroid hormone secretion rapidly.

3. **Propranolol**, 40 mg PO q6h (or an equivalent dose IV), should be given to patients with **angina or myocardial infarction**, and the dose should be adjusted to prevent tachycardia. Propranolol may benefit some patients with heart failure and marked tachycardia but can further impair left ventricular function. In patients with clinical heart failure, it should be given only during invasive monitoring of left ventricular filling pressure.

4. **Plasma free T_4** is measured every 3–4 days, and treatment with iodine is discontinued when free T_4 approaches the normal range. RAI therapy should be scheduled 2 weeks after iodine is stopped (see sec. **C**).

H. **Hyperthyroidism in pregnancy.** If hyperthyroidism is suspected, plasma TSH should be measured. Plasma TSH declines in early pregnancy, but rarely to less than 0.1 µU/ml. If TSH is less than 0.1 µU/ml, the diagnosis should be confirmed by measurement of plasma free T_4. **RAI is contraindicated in pregnancy**, and therefore patients should be treated with **PTU** (see sec. **D**). The dose should be adjusted to maintain the plasma free T_4 near the upper limit of the normal range. The dose required often decreases in the later stages of pregnancy. Atenolol, 25–50 mg PO qd, can be used to relieve symptoms while awaiting the effects of PTU. The fetus and neonate should be monitored carefully for hyperthyroidism.

Euthyroid Goiter

I. **Introduction.** The diagnosis of euthyroid goiter is based on palpation of the thyroid and on evaluation of thyroid function. If the thyroid is enlarged, the examiner should determine whether the enlargement is diffuse or multinodular or whether a single nodule is present. All three forms of euthyroid goiter are common, especially in women. Imaging studies, such as thyroid scans or ultrasonography, provide no useful information in addition to palpation of the thyroid and should not be performed. Furthermore, 20–50% of people have nonpalpable thyroid nodules that are detectable by ultrasound. These nodules rarely have any clinical importance, but their incidental discovery may lead to unnecessary diagnostic testing and treatment (*Endocrinol Metab Clin North Am* 2000;29:187).

II. **Diffuse goiter.** Almost all euthyroid diffuse goiters in the United States are due to **chronic lymphocytic thyroiditis** (Hashimoto's thyroiditis; *N Engl J Med* 1996;335:99). As Hashimoto's disease also may cause hypothyroidism, plasma TSH should be measured even in patients who are clinically euthyroid. Small diffuse goiters usually are asymptomatic, and therapy seldom is required. Symptomatic diffuse goiters may shrink with suppression of plasma TSH to the lower limit of the normal range by T_4 therapy. If T_4 is not given, the patient should be monitored regularly for the development of hypothyroidism.

III. **MNG** is common in older patients, especially women. Most patients are asymptomatic and require no treatment. In a few patients, hyperthyroidism (toxic MNG) develops (see Hyperthyroidism, sec. I). In rare patients, the gland compresses the trachea or esophagus, causing dyspnea or dysphagia, and treatment is required (*N Engl J Med* 1998;338:1438). T_4 treatment has little, if any, effect on the size of MNGs and is rarely indicated. **RAI therapy** reduces gland size and relieves symptoms in most patients. Subtotal thyroidectomy can also be used to relieve compressive symptoms. The risk of malignancy in MNG is low, comparable to the frequency of incidental thyroid carcinoma in clinically normal glands. Evaluation for thyroid carcinoma with needle biopsy is warranted only if one nodule enlarges disproportionately.

IV. **Single thyroid nodules** are usually benign, but a small number are thyroid carcinomas (*N Engl J Med* 1998;338:297). Clinical findings that increase the likelihood of carcinoma include the presence of cervical lymphadenopathy, a history of radiation to the head or neck in childhood, and a family history of medullary thyroid carcinoma or multiple endocrine neoplasia syndromes type 2A or 2B. A hard fixed nodule, recent nodule growth, or hoarseness due to vocal cord paralysis also suggests malignancy. However, most patients with thyroid carcinomas have none of these risk factors, and **nearly all single thyroid nodules should be evaluated with needle aspiration biopsy**. Patients with thyroid carcinoma should be managed in consultation with an endocrinologist. Nodules with benign cytology should be re-evaluated periodically by palpation and biopsied again if they enlarge. T_4 therapy has little or no effect on the size of single thyroid nodules and is not indicated (*Ann Intern Med* 1998;128:386). **Imaging studies cannot distinguish benign from malignant nodules and should not be performed.**

Adrenal Failure

I. **Etiology.** Adrenal failure may be due to disease of the adrenal glands (**primary adrenal failure, Addison's disease**), with deficiency of cortisol and aldosterone and elevated plasma adrenocorticotropic hormone (ACTH), or to ACTH deficiency caused by disorders of the pituitary or hypothalamus (**secondary adrenal failure**), with deficiency of cortisol alone (*N Engl J Med* 1996;335:1206).

A. Primary adrenal failure most often is due to **autoimmune adrenalitis**, which may be associated with other endocrine deficits (e.g., hypothyroidism). Infections of the adrenal gland such as **tuberculosis** and **histoplasmosis** may cause adrenal failure. **Hemorrhagic adrenal infarction** may occur in the postoperative period, in coagulation disorders and hypercoagulable states and in sepsis. Adrenal hemorrhage often causes abdominal or flank pain and fever; CT scan of the abdomen reveals high-density bilateral adrenal masses. Adrenoleukodystrophy causes adrenal failure in young males. In patients with **AIDS**, adrenal failure may develop owing to disseminated cytomegalovirus, mycobacterial or fungal infection, adrenal lymphoma, or treatment with ketoconazole, which inhibits steroid hormone synthesis.

B. **Secondary adrenal failure** is due most often to **glucocorticoid therapy**; ACTH suppression may persist for a year after therapy is stopped. Any disorder of the pituitary or hypothalamus can cause ACTH deficiency, but usually other evidence of these disorders can be seen.

II. **Clinical findings.** Findings in adrenal failure are nonspecific and, without a high index of suspicion, the diagnosis of this potentially lethal but readily treatable disease is missed easily. Symptoms include **anorexia, nausea, vomiting, weight loss**, weakness, and fatigue. **Orthostatic hypotension** and **hyponatremia** are common. Usually, symptoms are chronic, but **shock** that is fatal unless treated promptly may suddenly develop. Often, this **adrenal crisis** is triggered by illness, injury, or surgery. All these symptoms are due to cortisol deficiency and occur in primary and in secondary adrenal failure. **Hyperpigmentation** (due to marked ACTH excess) and **hyperkalemia and volume depletion** (due to aldosterone deficiency) occur only in primary adrenal failure.

III. **Diagnosis.** Adrenal failure should be suspected in patients with hypotension (including orthostatic hypotension), persistent nausea, weight loss, hyponatremia, or hyperkalemia.

A. The **short cosyntropin (Cortrosyn) stimulation test** is used for diagnosis (*Clin Endocrinol* 1996;44:147). Cosyntropin, 250 µg, is given IV or IM, and **plasma cortisol is measured 30 minutes later**. The normal response is a stimulated plasma cortisol higher than 20 µg/dl. This test detects primary and secondary adrenal failure, except within a few weeks of onset of pituitary dysfunction (e.g., shortly after pituitary surgery).

B. The **distinction between primary and secondary adrenal failure** usually is clear. Hyperkalemia, hyperpigmentation, or other autoimmune endocrine deficits indicate primary adrenal failure, whereas deficits of other pituitary hormones, symptoms of a pituitary mass (e.g., headache, visual field loss), or known pituitary or hypothalamic disease indicate secondary adrenal failure. If the cause is unclear, the **plasma ACTH** level distinguishes primary adrenal failure (in which it is elevated markedly) from secondary adrenal failure. Most cases of primary adrenal failure are due to autoimmune adrenalitis, but other causes should be considered. Evidence of adrenal enlargement or calcification on abdominal CT indicates that the cause is infection or hemorrhage. Patients with secondary adrenal failure should be tested for other pituitary hormone deficiencies and should be evaluated for a pituitary or hypothalamic tumor.

IV. **Therapy**

A. Adrenal crisis with hypotension must be treated immediately. These patients should be admitted to the hospital for therapy and be evaluated for an underlying illness that precipitated the crisis.

   1. If the diagnosis of adrenal failure is known, hydrocortisone, 50 mg IV q8h, should be given, and 0.9% saline with 5% dextrose should be infused rapidly until hypotension is corrected. The dose of hydrocortisone is decreased gradually over several days as symptoms and any precipitating illness resolve, then is changed to oral maintenance therapy. Mineralocorticoid replacement is not needed until the dose of hydrocortisone is less than 100 mg/day.

   2. If the diagnosis of adrenal failure has not been established, a single dose of dexamethasone, 10 mg IV, should be given, and a rapid infusion of 0.9% saline with 5% dextrose should be started. A Cortrosyn stimulation test should be performed (see sec. III.A). Dexamethasone is used because it does not interfere with subsequent measurements of cortisol. After the 30-minute plasma cortisol measurement, hydrocortisone, 50 mg IV q8h, should be given until the test result is known.

B. **Outpatient maintenance therapy** in all patients with adrenal failure requires cortisol replacement with prednisone; most patients with primary adrenal failure also require replacement of aldosterone with fludrocortisone (Florinef).

1. **Prednisone**, 5 mg PO every morning and 2.5 mg PO every evening, should be started. Patients should initially be evaluated every 1–2 months. The dose of prednisone is adjusted to eliminate symptoms and signs of cortisol deficiency or excess, with most patients requiring between 5 mg every morning and 5 mg bid. Eventually, annual follow-up is adequate unless an acute illness develops. Concomitant therapy with rifampin, phenytoin, or phenobarbital accelerates glucocorticoid metabolism and increases the dose requirement.

2. **During illness, injury, or the perioperative period, the dose of prednisone must be increased.** For minor illnesses, the patient should double the dose for 3 days. If the illness resolves, the maintenance dose is resumed. Vomiting requires immediate medical attention, with IV glucocorticoid therapy and IV fluid. Patients can be given a prefilled syringe of dexamethasone, 4 mg, to be self-administered IM for vomiting or severe illness if medical care is not immediately available. **For severe illness or injury**, hydrocortisone, 50 mg IV q8h, should be given, with the dose tapered as severity of illness wanes (*N Engl J Med* 1997;337:1285). The same regimen is used in **patients who are undergoing surgery**, with the first dose of hydrocortisone given preoperatively. Usually, the dose can be reduced to maintenance therapy 3–4 days after uncomplicated surgery.

3. **In primary adrenal failure, fludrocortisone**, 0.1 mg PO qd, should be given, along with liberal salt intake. During follow-up visits, supine and standing BP and serum potassium should be monitored. The dose of fludrocortisone is adjusted to maintain BP (supine and standing) and serum potassium within the normal range; the usual dose is 0.05–0.30 mg PO qd.

4. **Patients should be educated** in management of their disease, including adjustment of prednisone dose during illness. They should wear a medical identification tag or bracelet.

Cushing's Syndrome

I. **Etiology.** Cushing's syndrome (the clinical effects of increased glucocorticoid hormone) most often is **iatrogenic**, due to therapy with glucocorticoid drugs. **ACTH-secreting pituitary microadenomas (Cushing's disease)** account for approximately 80% of cases of endogenous Cushing's syndrome. **Adrenal tumors** and **ectopic ACTH secretion** account for the remainder.

II. **Clinical findings** (*N Engl J Med* 1995;332:791) include truncal obesity, rounded face, fat deposits in the supraclavicular fossae and over the posterior neck, hypertension, hirsutism, amenorrhea, and depression. More specific findings include **thin skin, easy bruising, reddish striae, proximal muscle weakness, and osteoporosis**. Diabetes mellitus develops in some patients. Hyperpigmentation or hypokalemic alkalosis suggests Cushing's syndrome due to ectopic ACTH secretion.

III. **Diagnosis** is based on increased cortisol excretion and lack of normal feedback inhibition of ACTH and cortisol secretion (*Endocrinol Metab Clin North Am* 1999;28:191).

A. The **overnight dexamethasone suppression test** (1 mg dexamethasone given PO at 11:00 p.m.; plasma cortisol measured at 8:00 a.m. the next day; normal plasma cortisol level <2 µg/dl) or **24-hour urine cortisol** measurement can be done as a screening test. Both tests are very sensitive, and a normal value virtually excludes the diagnosis.

B. An abnormal screening test indicates the need to perform a **low-dose dexamethasone suppression test**. Dexamethasone, 0.5 mg PO q6h, is given for 48 hours, and urine cortisol is measured during the last 24 hours. Failure to suppress urine cortisol to less than the normal reference range is diagnostic of Cushing's syndrome. Testing should not be done during severe illness or depression, which may cause false-positive results. Phenytoin therapy also causes false-positive **dexamethasone** suppression test results by accelerating metabolism of dexamethasone. **Random plasma cortisol levels are not useful for diagnosis,** because the wide range of normal values overlaps that of Cushing's syndrome. After the diagnosis of Cushing's syndrome is made, tests to determine the cause should be done in consultation with an endocrinologist.

Incidental Adrenal Nodules

I. **Introduction.** Adrenal nodules are a common incidental finding on abdominal imaging studies. Most incidentally discovered nodules are benign adrenocortical tumors that do not secrete excess hormone, but the differential diagnosis includes adrenal adenomas that cause Cushing's syndrome or primary hyperaldosteronism, pheochromocytoma, adrenocortical carcinoma, and metastatic cancer.

II. **Clinical evaluation.** The patient should be evaluated for symptoms and signs of Cushing's syndrome (see Cushing's syndrome, sec. I). Hypertension suggests the possibility of primary hyperaldosteronism or pheochromocytoma. Episodes of headache, palpitations, and sweating suggest pheochromocytoma. Hirsutism suggests the possibility of an adrenocortical carcinoma.

III. **Radiologic and laboratory evaluation.** The imaging characteristics of the nodule may suggest a diagnosis (e.g., benign adrenocortical nodule) but are not specific enough to obviate further evaluation (*Endocrinol Metab Clin North Am* 2000;29:27).

 A. **Patients who have potentially resectable cancer elsewhere** and in whom an adrenal metastasis must be excluded may require needle biopsy of the nodule. Pheochromocytoma should be excluded with measurement of plasma metanephrines or 24-hour urine catecholamines before biopsy.

 B. In other patients, the diagnostic issue is **whether a syndrome of hormone excess or an adrenocortical carcinoma is present.** Plasma potassium and dehydroepiandrosterone sulfate and 24-hour urine catecholamines should be measured, and an overnight dexamethasone suppression test or 24-hour urine cortisol should be performed.

IV. **Management.** Patients with hypertension and hypokalemia should be evaluated for **primary hyperaldosteronism** by measuring the ratio of plasma aldosterone (in ng/dl) to plasma renin activity (in ng/ml/hr) in a single blood sample. This sample can be obtained in an ambulatory patient without special preparation. If the ratio is less than 20, the diagnosis of primary hyperaldosteronism is excluded, whereas a ratio greater than 50 makes the diagnosis very likely. Patients with an intermediate ratio should be further evaluated in consultation with an endocrinologist. Abnormalities of cortisol secretion should be evaluated further (see Cushing's Syndrome, sec. **III.B**). If there is clinical or biochemical evidence of a pheochromocytoma, the nodule should be resected after appropriate α-adrenergic blockade with phenoxybenzamine. Elevation of plasma dehydroepiandrosterone sulfate or a large nodule suggests adrenocortical carcinoma. A policy of resecting all nodules greater than 4 cm in diameter appropriately treats the great majority of adrenal carcinomas while minimizing the number of benign nodules removed unnecessarily (*Endocrinol Metab Clin North Am* 2000;29:159). Most incidental nodules are less than 4 cm in diameter, do not produce excess hormone, and do not require therapy. At least one repeat imaging procedure 3–6 months later is recommended to ensure that the nodule is not enlarging rapidly (which would suggest an adrenal carcinoma).

Hypercalcemia

I. Introduction. Approximately 50% of serum calcium is ionized (free), and the remainder is complexed, primarily to albumin. Changes in serum albumin alter total calcium concentration without affecting the clinically relevant ionized calcium level, and if serum albumin is abnormal, clinical decisions should be based on ionized calcium levels. Calcium metabolism is regulated by **parathyroid hormone (PTH)** and metabolites of **vitamin D**. **PTH increases serum calcium** by stimulating bone resorption, increasing renal calcium reabsorption, and promoting renal conversion of vitamin D to its active metabolite calcitriol (1,25-dihydroxyvitamin D [1,25(OH)$_2$D]). Serum calcium regulates PTH secretion by a negative feedback mechanism; hypercalcemia suppresses PTH release. **Vitamin D** is converted by the liver to 25-hydroxyvitamin D [25(OH)D], which in turn is converted by the kidney to 1,25(OH)$_2$D. The latter metabolite increases serum calcium by promoting intestinal calcium absorption and plays a role in bone formation and resorption. Other factors that raise serum calcium include PTH-related peptide (*N Engl J Med* 2000;342:177), which acts on PTH receptors, and some cytokines produced by plasma cells and lymphocytes.

II. Etiology (Table 17-3). More than 95% of cases are due to primary hyperparathyroidism or malignancy.

A. Primary hyperparathyroidism causes most cases of mild hypercalcemia in ambulatory patients (*N Engl J Med* 2000;343:1863). It is a common disorder, especially in elderly women. Approximately 85% of cases are due to an adenoma of a single gland, 15% to enlargement of all four glands, and 1% to parathyroid carcinoma. Familial syndromes that include primary hyperparathyroidism (e.g., the multiple endocrine neoplasia syndromes) cause enlargement of all four glands.

B. Malignancy causes most severe, symptomatic hypercalcemia. Common causes of malignant hypercalcemia (*Endocrinol Rev* 1998;19:18) include **breast carcinoma** (which is usually metastatic to bone when hypercalcemia occurs); **squamous carcinoma** of the lung, head and neck, or esophagus (which may produce humoral hypercalcemia without extensive bone metastases); and **multiple myeloma**. Renal, bladder, and ovarian carcinoma may also cause hypercalcemia. Most malignant hypercalcemia is due to secretion of PTH-related peptide by the tumor, except for myeloma, in which hypercalcemia is mediated by cytokines.

Table 17-3. Major causes of hypercalcemia

Common
    Primary hyperparathyroidism
    Malignancy
Uncommon
    Sarcoidosis, other granulomatous diseases
    Drugs
        Vitamin D toxicity
        Lithium
        Calcium carbonate (milk-alkali syndrome)
    Hyperthyroidism
    Familial benign hypercalcemia

C. **Other causes of hypercalcemia** are uncommon and are almost always suggested by the history or physical examination. Thiazide diuretics cause persistent hypercalcemia only in patients with increased bone turnover, for example, due to mild primary hyperparathyroidism. Sarcoidosis and other granulomatous disorders may cause hypercalcemia by excessive synthesis of 1,25-(OH_2)D. Familial benign hypercalcemia is a rare autosomal dominant disorder that causes asymptomatic hypercalcemia from birth. It is due to a genetic defect in the calcium-sensing receptor on parathyroid cells and should be suspected if there is a family history of asymptomatic hypercalcemia.

III. **Clinical findings**

A. Most **symptoms of hypercalcemia** are present only if serum calcium is above 12 mg/dl. Mild hypercalcemia causes polyuria, whereas chronic hypercalcemia may cause nephrolithiasis. Severe hypercalcemia may cause renal failure. **GI** symptoms include anorexia, nausea, vomiting, and constipation. **Neurologic** findings include weakness, fatigue, confusion, stupor, and coma. **ECG manifestations** include a shortened QT interval. Polyuria combined with nausea and vomiting may cause marked dehydration, which impairs calcium excretion and may cause rapidly worsening hypercalcemia.

B. **Presentations of primary hyperparathyroidism** include (1) in the majority of patients, mild, asymptomatic hypercalcemia found incidentally; (2) nephrolithiasis; (3) decreased bone density (and rarely a specific bone disorder, osteitis fibrosa); and (4) symptoms of hypercalcemia.

IV. **Diagnosis.** Mildly elevated serum calcium levels should be repeated and the **serum ionized calcium** should be measured to determine whether hypercalcemia is actually present.

A. **The history and physical examination** should focus on (1) the **duration of hypercalcemia** (if present for more than 6 months without obvious cause, primary hyperparathyroidism is almost certain); (2) history of **renal stones** (which are not seen in hypercalcemia of malignancy); (3) **symptoms and signs of malignancy,** for example, a breast mass or a history of breast cancer, cough or hemoptysis, or weight loss; (4) clinical evidence for any of the unusual causes of hypercalcemia such as use of calcium supplements, vitamin D, or lithium; and (5) family history of hypercalcemia or other components of multiple endocrine neoplasia syndromes.

B. **Laboratory evaluation.** The **serum intact PTH level** should be measured. If serum PTH is elevated in a patient with hypercalcemia, the diagnosis of primary hyperparathyroidism is confirmed. Intact PTH is suppressed to below the reference range or to the lower part of the reference range in all other causes of hypercalcemia except familial benign hypercalcemia. If the PTH level is suppressed, evaluation for other causes of hypercalcemia should be directed by clinical findings and may include a chest x-ray, bone scan, and serum and urine protein electrophoresis. **Severe symptomatic hypercalcemia is usually due to malignancy, and the cancer is almost always clinically apparent.** Vitamin D intoxication can be confirmed by measurement of elevated serum levels of 25(OH)D, and the diagnosis of sarcoidosis as the cause of hypercalcemia is supported by elevated serum levels of 1,25(OH_2)D. In rare cases in which the diagnosis remains unclear, measurement of serum levels of PTH-related peptide may help to confirm or exclude malignancy.

V. **Therapy.** Patients with symptoms of hypercalcemia or serum calcium levels greater than 13 mg/dl should be admitted to the hospital for evaluation and therapy. Treatment of severe hypercalcemia includes measures that increase calcium excretion and decrease resorption of calcium from bone. Their purpose is to relieve symptoms while the cause of hypercalcemia is found and either treated or corrected.

A. **Extracellular fluid volume restoration.** Severely hypercalcemic patients are almost always dehydrated, and the first step in therapy is extracellular fluid (ECF) volume repletion with 0.9% saline to restore the glomerular filtration rate and promote calcium excretion. At least 3–4 L should be given in the first 24 hours, and a positive fluid balance of at least 2 L should be achieved.

B. Saline diuresis. After ECF volume is restored, infusion of 0.9% saline (100–200 ml/hr) promotes calcium excretion. **Serum electrolytes,** calcium, and magnesium should be measured q6–12h. Furosemide adds little to the effect of saline diuresis and may prevent adequate restoration of ECF volume. It should not be given unless clinical evidence of heart failure develops.

C. Pamidronate is a bisphosphonate that inhibits bone resorption and should be used if symptoms or a serum calcium of greater than 12 mg/dl persist after initial volume repletion. A dose of 60–90 mg in 1 L 0.9% saline is infused over 4 hours. Serum calcium should be measured daily. Hypercalcemia abates gradually over several days and remains suppressed for 1–2 weeks. Treatment can be repeated when hypercalcemia recurs. Side effects include asymptomatic hypocalcemia, hypomagnesemia, and hypophosphatemia and transient low-grade fever.

D. Glucocorticoids are effective in hypercalcemia due to **myeloma, sarcoidosis,** and **vitamin D intoxication.** The initial dose is prednisone, 20–50 mg PO bid, or its equivalent. It may take 5–10 days for serum calcium to fall. After serum calcium stabilizes, the dose should be gradually reduced to the minimum needed to control symptoms of hypercalcemia.

VI. Management of primary hyperparathyroidism

A. The only effective therapy for primary hyperparathyroidism is parathyroidectomy. However, in the asymptomatic majority of patients, surgery may not be indicated. The natural history of asymptomatic hyperparathyroidism is not fully known, but in many patients the disorder has a benign course, with little change in clinical findings or serum calcium for years (*N Engl J Med* 1999;341:1249). The major concern in these patients is the possibility of progressive loss of bone mass and increased risk of fracture. Deterioration of renal function is also possible but unlikely in the absence of nephrolithiasis. Currently, it is impossible to predict the patients in whom problems will develop.

B. Indications for parathyroidectomy include (1) symptoms due to hypercalcemia, (2) nephrolithiasis, (3) hip or spine bone mass by dual-energy radiography more than 2 standard deviations below the gender-specific mean peak bone mass (a T score less than –2), (4) serum calcium of more than 12 mg/dl, (5) age younger than 50 years, and (6) infeasibility of long-term follow-up. Surgery is a reasonable choice in otherwise healthy patients even if they do not meet these criteria, because experienced surgeons have a success rate of 90–95% with low perioperative morbidity, and correction of hyperparathyroidism is followed by an increase in bone mass (*N Engl J Med* 1999;341:1249) and a decrease in the risk of fracture (*BMJ* 2000;321:598). Preoperative localization of an adenoma may permit a limited neck dissection, which further decreases the risk of complications.

C. Asymptomatic patients who do not meet criteria for parathyroidectomy or who refuse surgery can be followed by assessing clinical status, serum calcium and creatinine levels, and bone mass at 1- to 2-year intervals. Surgery should be recommended if any of the above criteria develop or if there is progressive decline in bone mass or renal function. In postmenopausal women, strong consideration should be given to estrogen replacement, which probably helps preserve bone mass in these patients.

Hyperprolactinemia

I. Etiology (Table 17-4). In women, the most common causes of pathologic hyperprolactinemia are prolactin-secreting pituitary **microadenoma** (i.e., an adenoma with a diameter of less than 1 cm) and **idiopathic hyperprolactinemia.**

Table 17-4. Major causes of hyperprolactinemia

Pregnancy and lactation
Prolactin-secreting pituitary adenoma (prolactinoma)
Idiopathic hyperprolactinemia
Drugs
    Dopamine antagonists (phenothiazines, metoclopramide, methyldopa)
    Others (verapamil, cimetidine, some antidepressants)
Interference with synthesis or transport of hypothalamic dopamine
    Hypothalamic lesions
    Pituitary macroadenomas
Primary hypothyroidism
Chronic renal failure

       In men, the most common cause is prolactin-secreting **macroadenoma**. Hypothalamic or pituitary lesions that cause deficiency of other pituitary hormones often cause hyperprolactinemia.

  II. Clinical findings. In women, hyperprolactinemia causes **amenorrhea** or irregular menses and **infertility**. Only approximately one-half these women have **galactorrhea**. Prolonged estrogen deficiency increases the risk of osteoporosis. In men, hyperprolactinemia causes **androgen deficiency** and infertility but not gynecomastia. **Mass effects** of a large pituitary tumor (e.g., headaches, visual field loss) and **hypopituitarism** are common in men with hyperprolactinemia.

 III. Diagnosis. Hyperprolactinemia is common in young women, and plasma prolactin should be measured in women with amenorrhea, whether or not galactorrhea is present. Mild elevations should be confirmed by repeat measurements. The history should include medications and symptoms of pituitary mass effects or hypothyroidism. Laboratory evaluation should include **plasma TSH** and a **pregnancy test**. Prolactin levels greater than 200 ng/ml occur only in prolactinomas, and levels between 100 and 200 ng/ml strongly suggest this diagnosis. Levels lower than 100 ng/ml may be due to any cause except prolactin-secreting macroadenoma, and such levels in a patient with a large pituitary mass indicate that it is not a prolactinoma. Testing for hypopituitarism is needed only in patients with a macroadenoma or hypothalamic lesion and should include measurement of plasma free T_4, a Cortrosyn stimulation test (see Adrenal Failure, sec. **III.A**), and measurement of plasma testosterone in men. **MRI** of the pituitary should be performed in most cases, as nonfunctional pituitary or hypothalamic tumors may present with hyperprolactinemia.

 IV. Therapy (*Endocrinol Metab Clin North Am* 1999;28:143)

    A. Microadenomas and idiopathic hyperprolactinemia. Most patients are treated because of **infertility** or to prevent **estrogen deficiency** and **osteoporosis**. Some women may be observed without therapy by periodic follow-up of prolactin levels and symptoms. In most patients, hyperprolactinemia does not worsen, and prolactin levels sometimes return to normal. Enlargement of microadenomas is rare.

       1. Dopamine agonists suppress plasma prolactin and restore normal menses and fertility in most women. Initial doses are **bromocriptine**, 1.25–2.5 mg PO qhs with a snack, or **cabergoline**, 0.25 mg twice/week. Doses are adjusted by measurement of plasma prolactin at 2- to 4-week intervals to the lowest dose that suppresses prolactin to the normal range. Maximally effective doses are 2.5 mg bromocriptine tid and 1.5

mg cabergoline twice/week. Initially, patients should use barrier contraception, as fertility may be restored quickly. **Side effects** include **nausea** and **orthostatic hypotension**, which can be minimized by increasing the dose gradually and usually resolve with continued therapy. Side effects are less severe with cabergoline.

2. **Women who want to become pregnant** should be managed in consultation with an endocrinologist.

3. **Women who do not want to become pregnant** should be followed with clinical evaluation and plasma prolactin every 6–12 months. Every 2 years, plasma prolactin should be measured after bromocriptine has been withdrawn for several weeks to determine whether the drug still is needed. Follow-up imaging studies are not warranted unless prolactin levels increase substantially.

4. **Transsphenoidal resection** of prolactin-secreting microadenomas is used only in the rare patients who do not respond to or cannot tolerate bromocriptine. Prolactin levels usually return to normal, but up to one-half of patients relapse.

B. **Prolactin-secreting macroadenomas.** Such lesions should be treated with a **dopamine agonist**, which usually suppresses prolactin levels to normal, **reduces tumor size**, and **improves or corrects abnormal visual fields** in some 90% of cases. The dose is adjusted as described in sec. **A.1**, except that if mass effects are present, the dose should be increased to maximally effective levels over a period of several weeks. Visual field tests, if initially abnormal, should be repeated 4–6 weeks after therapy is started. Pituitary imaging should be repeated 3–4 months after initiation of therapy. If tumor shrinkage and correction of visual abnormalities are satisfactory, therapy can be continued indefinitely, with periodic monitoring of plasma prolactin. The full effect on tumor size may take more than 6 months. Repeat imaging probably is not warranted unless prolactin levels rise despite therapy.

1. **Transsphenoidal surgery** is indicated to relieve mass effects and to prevent further tumor growth if the tumor does not shrink or if visual field abnormalities persist during dopamine agonist therapy. However, the likelihood of surgical cure of hyperprolactinemia due to a macroadenoma is low, and most patients require further therapy with a dopamine agonist.

2. **Women with prolactin-secreting macroadenomas should not become pregnant** unless the tumor has been resected surgically, as the risk of symptomatic enlargement during pregnancy is 15–35%. Barrier contraception is essential during dopamine agonist treatment.

Male Hypogonadism

I. **Introduction.** The testes have two distinct but related roles: (1) secretion of testosterone (the major androgen) by the Leydig cells, which produce and maintain sexual characteristics, and (2) production of spermatozoa by the seminiferous tubules, a process that requires high local concentrations of testosterone. The testes are regulated by the pituitary gland, which secretes the gonadotropins, luteinizing hormone (LH), and follicle-stimulating hormone. Gonadotropin secretion is regulated by the hypothalamus via secretion of LH-releasing hormone and by negative feedback by gonadal hormones. Hypogonadism due to disease of the testes results in diminished feedback on the pituitary and increased secretion of gonadotropins. If hypogonadism is due to disorders of the pituitary or hypothalamus, serum gonadotropin levels are within or below the reference range. Male hypogonadism may present with **androgen deficiency** or **infertility** due to oligospermia (low sperm count). Androgen deficiency is always associated with infertility, but oligospermia often occurs in men with normal testosterone levels.

Table 17-5. Major causes of androgen deficiency

Testicular disorders
    Klinefelter's syndrome
    Orchitis (mumps, other viruses)
    Trauma
    Drugs (including alcohol)
    Autoimmune testicular failure
Hypothalamic-pituitary dysfunction
    Congenital luteinizing hormone–releasing hormone deficiency (Kallman's syndrome)
    Hyperprolactinemia
    Cushing's syndrome
    Other pituitary or hypothalamic disorders
    Chronic illness
Combined defects
    Hepatic cirrhosis
    Chronic renal failure

    II. Etiology (Table 17-5). Male hypogonadism may be due to disorders of the testes or to dysfunction of the pituitary or hypothalamus. Cirrhosis and chronic renal failure impair gonadotropin secretion and testicular function.
        A. Testicular disorders. Klinefelter's syndrome (47,XXY karyotype) occurs in approximately 1 in 500 male births. Seminiferous tubules fail to develop normally, and because of this, the testes are small and firm with no spermatogenesis. The degree of androgen deficiency ranges from mild to severe. Klinefelter's syndrome usually presents as delayed puberty or persistent gynecomastia after puberty. **Viral orchitis** in adults, most often due to **mumps,** can cause testicular atrophy. It usually causes infertility alone, but androgen deficiency occurs in severe cases. **Alcohol** causes testicular dysfunction directly and by causing hepatic cirrhosis. Drugs that impair androgen synthesis or action include ketoconazole, cimetidine, and spironolactone. **Infertility without androgen deficiency** is usually idiopathic but may be due to milder forms of the disorders that cause androgen deficiency or to cryptorchidism that was not corrected early in childhood. **Azoospermia** (complete absence of sperm in the ejaculate) with normal testosterone levels may be due to obstruction or absence of the vas deferens.
        B. Hypothalamic-pituitary dysfunction. Any disorder of the hypothalamus or pituitary may cause androgen deficiency alone or combined with other pituitary hormone deficiencies. **Hyperprolactinemia** in men (see Hyperprolactinemia) is usually due to a prolactin-secreting pituitary macroadenoma. **Kallman's syndrome** (congenital deficiency of LH-releasing hormone) presents as failure of puberty. Other pituitary hormones are usually intact. Most patients have **anosmia** (lack of sense of smell).
    III. Clinical findings. Androgen deficiency in adult men most often presents as **decreased libido.** Growth of facial and body hair may be diminished. Impotence (erectile dysfunction) with a normal libido is usually due to neurologic or vascular disorders or to drugs rather than to androgen deficiency.
    IV. Evaluation
        A. The history should include the age at onset of puberty, libido, potency and frequency of intercourse, frequency of shaving, testicular injury or infection, past fertility, medications, and chronic illnesses. Physical signs may

include testicular atrophy (testes less than 15 ml in volume or less than 4 cm in greatest diameter), decreased facial and body hair, gynecomastia, and lack of sense of smell.

B. Laboratory studies. Androgen deficiency is confirmed by measurement of **serum testosterone**. If testosterone is low, **serum LH** should be measured. An **elevated serum LH** indicates a testicular cause of androgen deficiency. **If LH is not elevated**, hypothalamic or pituitary dysfunction is responsible, and serum **prolactin** should be measured, secretion of other pituitary hormones should be assessed, and the pituitary and hypothalamus should be imaged. Men with infertility but normal serum testosterone levels should be evaluated by **semen analysis**. The most important characteristic is sperm concentration, with the normal range considered to be greater than 20 million/ml. Interpretation is complicated by variability of the sperm count in normal men. Oligospermia should be confirmed by at least two semen analyses.

V. Treatment

A. Androgen deficiency is treated by **injections of testosterone ester** (testosterone enanthate or cypionate), 150–250 mg IM every 2 weeks. In most men, a dose of 200 mg is satisfactory. **Testosterone patches** (Androderm) can be used instead; the usual dose is one 5-mg patch/day. Skin irritation at the site of the patch may occur. **Androgel** (1% testosterone gel) can be applied topically. The starting dose is 5 g once daily, and the dose may be adjusted based on serum testosterone levels. Side effects of androgens include acne and gynecomastia. Men older than age 50 years should undergo regular screening for prostate cancer. Patients should be followed at 6- to 12-month intervals, with assessment of their clinical response. Measurement of serum testosterone is only necessary if there is an inadequate clinical response to therapy.

B. Infertility due to testicular disorders such as idiopathic oligospermia is not correctable. Patients with azoospermia and normal levels of testosterone and gonadotropins should be evaluated for obstruction of the vas deferens in consultation with a urologist. Patients with hypogonadism due to pituitary or hypothalamic disorders who desire fertility should be referred to an endocrinologist for treatment.

Hirsutism

I. Introduction. Hirsutism is the growth of dark terminal hair in a male pattern in a woman (*Lancet* 1997;349:191). It is a common complaint and may indicate androgen excess. However, there is a broad range of hair growth in normal women, and many patients with hirsutism have no evidence of androgen excess.

II. Etiology. Androgen excess can originate from the ovaries or adrenals. Exogenous androgens can also cause hirsutism. By far the most common cause is the **polycystic ovary syndrome**, which includes hirsutism, infertility, and amenorrhea or irregular menses that are not due to another identifiable disorder (*Endocrinol Metab Clin North Am* 1999;28:397). These patients do not ovulate, and the ovaries contain multiple cystic follicles. Hirsutism and menstrual irregularity usually begin at puberty. A wide range of abnormality is found in this syndrome, from mild hirsutism alone (sometimes called **idiopathic hirsutism**) to amenorrhea with enlarged ovaries. These women are resistant to insulin, and the resulting high insulin levels play a role in stimulating ovarian androgen production. Rare ovarian tumors may produce hirsutism. **Adrenal causes** of hirsutism include Cushing's disease, congenital adrenal hyperplasia, and, rarely, adrenal carcinoma.

III. Clinical findings. Even slight increases in androgen production can cause noticeable hair growth in women. More severe androgen excess causes **virilization**: frontal and temporal **balding**, laryngeal enlargement and **deepening of**

the voice, **increased muscle mass**, **clitoral enlargement**, and suppression of gonadotropins leading to **amenorrhea**. Virilization suggests a serious underlying cause.

IV. **Clinical evaluation.** The major issue in evaluating hirsutism is whether a woman is one of the small minority with a serious cause such as Cushing's syndrome or an ovarian or adrenal tumor. The history should include the age at onset of hirsutism, symptoms of virilization, any abnormality of menses, and fertility. The physical examination should include the extent of hair growth, signs of Cushing's syndrome or virilization, and palpation for ovarian enlargement. Serum **total and free testosterone** should be measured. Testing for Cushing's syndrome should be performed if there are any symptoms or signs to suggest this disorder (see Cushing's syndrome, sec. **II**). Multiple ovarian cysts are a common finding in women with normal menses and no hirsutism, and ultrasound of the ovaries should not be performed unless an ovarian tumor is suspected.

   A. Almost all patients with no evidence of virilization and mild elevation of free testosterone have a disorder that falls within the spectrum of polycystic ovary syndrome. They can be treated for this without further evaluation.

   B. Patients with evidence of virilization or with serum total testosterone levels greater than 200 ng/dl may have an ovarian or adrenal tumor and should be further evaluated in consultation with an endocrinologist.

V. **Therapy.** Patients with mild hirsutism may not require medical therapy if cosmetic measures such as plucking or shaving produce a satisfactory result. The response of hair growth to drug therapy is slow and often incomplete.

   A. **Oral contraceptives** suppress ovarian androgen production and may improve hirsutism.

   B. In women with the polycystic ovary syndrome, drugs that improve insulin resistance may reduce androgen production and improve menstrual abnormalities and fertility. **Metformin**, 500–1000 mg bid, can be used in patients with normal renal function (*J Clin Endocrinol Metab* 2000;85:139). It should be started at a dose of 500 mg qd and the dose gradually increased over a several-week period. Side effects include diarrhea, nausea, and abdominal cramps. Lactic acidosis is very rare in patients with serum creatinine of less than 1.5 mg/dl. Patients should be followed at 3- to 6-month intervals, with assessment of hair growth, menstrual regularity, and serum free testosterone.

   C. **Spironolactone**, 25–100 mg bid, is an androgen and aldosterone antagonist that can reduce excess hair growth (*J Clin Endocrinol Metab* 2000;85:89). Side effects include irregular menses, nausea, and breast tenderness. It should not be used in patients with renal dysfunction because it may cause hyperkalemia. Combination therapy with an oral contraceptive may be more effective and allows regular menses. Patients should be followed at 3- to 6-month intervals, with assessment of hair growth, menstrual regularity, and serum potassium.

18

Diabetes Mellitus

Samuel Dagogo-Jack

Diabetes Mellitus

Diabetes mellitus (DM) is a group of metabolic disorders that results in hyperglycemia. These disorders have different etiologies but a common manifestation, hyperglycemia, which is associated with acute and chronic complications regardless of underlying etiology. The occurrence of acute and long-term complications of DM can be prevented or markedly reduced by a treatment regimen that results in normalization or near-normalization of blood glucose levels.

I. **Classification of DM and related disorders** [*Diabetes Care* 2001;24(Suppl 1):S5].

   A. **DM** encompasses disorders with well-defined etiologies and others that are less well understood.

      1. **Type 1 diabetes** accounts for fewer than 10% of all cases of DM, tends to occur in younger subjects, and is caused by severe insulin deficiency, which in most cases is due to an immune-mediated destruction of the pancreatic islet β cells. The risk factors for autoimmune β-cell destruction include inheritance of disease susceptibility genes (human leukocyte antigen haplotypes) in the major histocompatibility locus and possible exposure to environmental triggers. Islet cell autoantibodies can be detected in most but not all patients, indicating that the etiology of β-cell failure is idiopathic in a small subset of patients. To control blood glucose and prevent diabetic ketoacidosis (DKA), and to preserve life, there is an obligate need for exogenous insulin. Transient episodes of insulin independence ("honeymoon phase") or reduced insulin requirement may occur early in the course of type 1 DM.

      2. **Type 2 diabetes** accounts for more than 90% of all cases of DM. It is usually a disease of older adults but is being diagnosed with increasing frequency in younger age groups including children, in whom (as in adults) obesity constitutes a major risk factor. Other hallmarks of type 2 DM in childhood include ethnicity (non-Caucasian ancestry), female preponderance, acanthosis nigricans, and absence of ketoacidosis. Insulin resistance and relative insulin deficiency are characteristic findings in persons with type 2 DM. Obesity, physical inactivity, and genetic predisposition increase the risk for insulin resistance; the etiology of the insulin secretory defect in type 2 DM is not well understood. Endogenous insulin production may be sufficient to prevent ketogenesis under basal conditions, but DKA can develop during stress.

      3. **Other specific types** of DM include maturity-onset diabetes of the young (MODY), which results from various genetic mutations that impair β-cell function; those caused by genetic defects in insulin action; and DM associated with endocrinopathies (e.g., Cushing's syndrome and acromegaly), pancreatic exocrine disease, drugs, and other syndromes. Some of these may be obvious (e.g., glucocorticoid-induced

DM), but the majority are so rare that a systematic search is unwarranted in routine clinical practice.

   4. **Gestational DM** (GDM) occurs in approximately 4% of pregnant women and usually resolves after delivery. Nonetheless, women with a history of GDM remain at increased risk for development of type 2 DM later in life (see Diabetes in Pregnancy).

B. **Diagnosis of DM.** The diagnosis of DM can be established using fasting or postprandial plasma glucose levels.

   1. **Plasma glucose of 126 mg/dl or greater after an overnight fast** (no food for at least 8 hours preceding the test) is consistent with a diagnosis of diabetes. This should be confirmed with repeat testing on a different day.

   2. **Symptomatic persons with plasma glucose of 200 mg/dl or greater.** The presence of symptoms of marked hyperglycemia (polyuria, polydipsia, unexplained weight loss, sometimes with polyphagia, blurred vision, certain infections) together with a finding of a random plasma glucose of 200 mg/dl or greater establishes a diagnosis of DM.

   3. **Plasma glucose of 200 mg/dl or greater at 2 hours after ingestion of oral glucose (75 g).** The oral glucose tolerance test (OGTT) can be confounded by variables such as physical activity, illness, stress, carbohydrate intake, and the length of the antecedent fast. To be reliable, the OGTT should be performed under unstressed conditions in persons with unrestricted physical activity and a daily carbohydrate intake of more than 150 g who have been fasting for no less than 8 hours and no longer than 14 hours before the test. Plasma glucose is measured at baseline and again at 2 hours after glucose ingestion. A normal response is a 2-hour plasma glucose of less than 140 mg/dl. For practical purposes, the OGTT should be reserved for asymptomatic persons with equivocal fasting plasma glucose results.

C. **Impaired glucose tolerance (IGT) and impaired fasting glucose (IFG)** refer to intermediate metabolic states between normal glucose tolerance and DM. IGT is defined by a 2-hour OGTT plasma glucose that is greater than 140 mg/dl but less than 200 mg/dl, and IFG is defined by a fasting plasma glucose of 110 mg/dl or greater but less than 126 mg/dl. IFG and IGT appear to be risk factors for type 2 diabetes through their association with the insulin resistance syndrome (syndrome X), the components of which include abdominal obesity, dyslipidemia, and hypertension. The case for specific therapeutic intervention in persons with IGT or IFG has not been established, but studies that evaluate the roles of diet, exercise, and medication to improve insulin sensitivity are in progress. Nonetheless, exercise and dietary modification are appropriate recommendations for physically inactive or overweight persons.

D. **Screening for DM** is recommended for all persons at age 45 years or older [*Diabetes Care* 2000;23(Suppl 1):S20].

   1. **Screening for type 1 DM** using autoantibodies or other markers of β-cell dysfunction is currently not appropriate because of the low incidence of type 1 DM and the lack of effective therapy for euglycemic persons with positive islet autoantibodies.

   2. **Screening for type 2 DM**, using plasma glucose measurement, is appropriate because of the high prevalence of undiagnosed type 2 DM and associated complications. Screening is recommended for all persons at age 45 years or older; normal tests should be repeated at 3-year intervals.

   3. **Screening should be considered at a younger age** or be performed more frequently in persons with risk factors such as obesity, family history of DM, history of GDM, or delivery of a baby who weighs greater than 9 lb.

   4. **Enhanced screening** also is appropriate for individuals from high-risk ethnic populations (Native American, Asian-American/Pacific Islander, Hispanic-American, African-American), and those with a history of hypertension, dyslipidemia, or previous IGT or IFG.

5. **The OGTT and fasting plasma glucose** are both suitable screening tests, but the fasting plasma glucose is preferred because it is more efficient, more convenient, and less expensive.

II. **Principles of management of DM.** The therapeutic goals are alleviation of symptoms, achievement of metabolic control, and prevention of acute and long-term complications of diabetes. An individualized, multimodality regimen that leads to normalization (or near-normalization) of fasting and postprandial plasma glucose levels offers the best chance of accomplishing these goals. The mnemonic **MEDEM** (**m**onitoring, **e**ducation, **d**iet, **e**xercise, **m**edications) should be used to recall the modalities of diabetes care.

A. **Monitoring** indices of diabetes control provides valuable feedback, facilitates optimization of care, and promotes an essential alliance between patients and the diabetes care team.

1. **Hemoglobin A_{1c} (HbA_{1c})**, the best-characterized glycohemoglobin, is formed by an irreversible combination of glucose with the NH_2 terminus of the β chain of HbA in erythrocytes. Thus, HbA_{1c} provides a reliable, integrated measure of blood glucose profile over the preceding 2–3 months. Because the concentration of HbA_{1c} in healthy people is approximately 4–6%, current recommendations stipulate a goal of less than 7% for patients with diabetes.

2. **Self-monitored blood glucose (SMBG)** is an important (but underused) tool of diabetes management and education. SMBG (up to four times or more daily) is recommended for patients with type 1 DM. The optimal frequency has not been established for patients with type 2 DM, but regular SMBG is recommended. The minimum frequency and timing of SMBG can be negotiated with patients who have limited resources. The results of SMBG should be reviewed, with appropriate feedback, during office visits.

3. **Urine glucose** correlates poorly with blood glucose, is dependent on renal glucose threshold (150–300 mg/dl), and should only be used for monitoring diabetes therapy if SMBG is impractical.

4. **Ketone bodies** can be detected in blood or urine during states of excessive production (e.g., DKA, starvation, alcohol intoxication). **Blood ketones** are used to confirm DKA. **Ketonuria** tends to reflect ketonemia, and therefore monitoring for urine ketones using Ketostix or Acetest tablets is recommended for all diabetic patients during febrile illness or persistent hyperglycemia or if signs of impending DKA (e.g., nausea, vomiting, abdominal pain) develop.

B. **Education** is integral to successful management of diabetes. Effective diabetes education entails conceptual and practical elements. Conceptually, the nature of diabetes and the overall treatment objectives should be communicated to and comprehended by the patient. Practical elements of diabetes education include diet planning; routine self-management skills; techniques for monitoring of glucose and ketones; prevention, recognition, and correction of hypoglycemia; and management of diabetes during travel, emergencies, and intercurrent illness. Diabetes education should be reinforced at regular intervals and extended to live-in partners and close family members.

C. **Dietary modification** through medical nutrition therapy is essential to total diabetes care. Broadly, nutritional principles are similar to those advocated for health promotion in the general populace. However, persons with diabetes require an individualized dietary intervention, guided by state of glycemic control, body weight, lipid profile, BP, and other metabolic end points.

1. **Total calories** should be adequate to maintain reasonable weight; caloric restriction is appropriate in overweight persons. The composition and especially timing of meals should not vary markedly from day to day.

2. **Protein** intake should constitute 10–20% of total calories in patients with diabetes, as in healthy subjects. Patients with diabetic nephropa-

thy usually are allowed a protein intake of 0.8 g/kg/day (approximately 10% of total calories), equivalent to the adult recommended dietary allowance. With deterioration in renal function, further restriction in protein intake (0.6 g/kg) may be beneficial in some patients.

3. **Total fat** intake should be less than 30% of total calories, with saturated fat restricted to less than 10% of total calories. Cholesterol intake should be less than 300 mg/day. Further reduction in the intake of saturated fat and cholesterol should be advised in patients with hypercholesterolemia.

4. **Carbohydrate** allowance varies depending on glucose, lipid, and weight considerations and should be individualized.

5. **Dietary fiber** improves bowel emptying and may offer protection against colon cancer and other GI disorders; an intake of 20–35 g/day is recommended (see Chap. 13, Constipation, sec. **V.A**).

6. **Sodium** intake of 3 g/day or less is advisable; restriction to 2.4 g/day or less is recommended for persons with hypertension. Excessive amounts of sodium (>400 mg/single serving or >800 mg/meal) should be avoided.

7. **Alcohol intake** should be limited to two drinks per day for men and one drink per day for women, as recommended in the Dietary Guidelines for Americans [*Diabetes Care* 2000;23(Suppl 1):S43]. One alcoholic beverage is counted as two fat exchanges in the meal plan. Alcohol inhibits gluconeogenesis, which increases the risk for hypoglycemia.

8. **Vitamins, minerals, and micronutrient supplements** are not necessary if the diet is adequate and balanced (see Chap. 3). No specific micronutrients, herbal extracts, enzyme preparations, intermediary metabolites, or proprietary food supplements have been proved to alter the pathophysiology or outcome of DM. Therefore, care must be taken to ensure that unproven remedies, promoted in the popular press and available over the counter, do not distract the patient with diabetes from embracing established therapies.

9. **Nonnutritive sweeteners**, such as saccharin, aspartame, acesulfame K, and sucralose, do not add calories; they can be used to flavor beverages in place of sucrose, fructose, or other sugars.

10. **Tobacco** use should be discouraged because of the additive risk for macrovascular disease in diabetes; smoking cessation interventions (see Chap. 1) should be offered to persons who are unable to quit on their own.

D. **Regular exercise** increases insulin sensitivity, reduces fasting and postprandial blood glucose, lowers HbA_{1c}, improves lipid profile, and offers numerous metabolic, cardiovascular, and psychological benefits in diabetes patients. Risks include fluctuations in blood glucose, exacerbation of preexisting heart disease, worsening of proliferative retinopathy and proteinuria, and foot trauma in patients with peripheral neuropathy. With careful screening and attention to meal planning, drug dosing, and glucose monitoring, exercise should be safe for most patients with diabetes.

1. **Screening with exercise-stress ECG** is recommended for all patients aged 35 years or older. Dilated funduscopy to identify proliferative retinopathy and testing for microalbuminuria and peripheral or autonomic neuropathy should be performed. Positive results should lead to appropriate modification of exercise regimen. High-impact routines increase the risk of foot trauma and are best avoided in patients with peripheral neuropathy.

2. **Exercise prescription** should be tailored to the individual patient's physical condition and personal preference and should always include 5- to 10-minute warm-up and cool-down periods. Aerobic exercise (e.g., walking, cycling, swimming) of moderate intensity (50–75% of maximal effort) for 20–45 minutes, three or more times per week, is recommended. Use of proper footwear should be emphasized.

3. **Pre- and postexercise monitoring** of blood glucose with appropriate adjustments to drug dosage and caloric intake can help prevent wide

swings in blood glucose. Insulin injection sites should be selected carefully to avoid too-rapid absorption from exercising body parts.
E. **Medications** that are used for treating diabetes include insulin and oral agents. Patients with type 1 DM require lifelong insulin therapy, whereas type 2 DM patients respond initially to oral antidiabetic agents but may require insulin as the disease progresses. The oral agents include insulin secretagogues (sulfonylureas and repaglinide); metformin, which is a biguanide; α-glucosidase inhibitors; and insulin sensitizers or thiazolidinediones. Medications for diabetes are most effective if prescribed as part of a comprehensive management plan that includes dietary and exercise counseling.

Drugs Used for Treatment of Diabetes Mellitus

I. **Insulin** (Table 18-1). Exogenous insulin is required lifelong by patients with type 1 DM insulin therapy and is also indicated during pregnancy and in selected type 2 DM patients. Insulin formulations differ according to pharmacokinetic properties, structure (animal or human), and concentration. Following subcutaneous injection, there is individual variability in the duration and peak activity of insulin preparations and day-to-day variability in the same subject. In general, rapid-acting insulins have a peak activity at 2–4 hours and an effective duration of action of 6–8 hours, intermediate-acting insulins have a peak activity at 6–12 hours, and long-acting insulins have a 14- to 24-hour span of maximal activity.
A. **Rapid-acting insulins** include regular insulin, semilente, and lispro. Regular insulin can be administered IV, IM, or by the more familiar subcutaneous route. Absorption of IM injection is variable and undependable, especially in hypovolemic patients. IV regular insulin should be given by continuous infusion for the treatment of hyperglycemic crises; an IV bolus of regular

Table 18-1. Approximate kinetics of human insulin preparations after subcutaneous injection

Insulin type	Onset of action (hrs)	Peak effect (hrs)	Duration of activity (hrs)
Rapid acting			
Lispro	0.25–0.50	0.50–1.50	3–5
Regular	0.50–1.00	2–4	6–8
Intermediate acting			
NPH	1–2	6–12	14–18
Lente	1–3	6–12	16–20
Long acting			
Ultralente	4–6	10–16	18–24
Glargine	4–6	6–24[a]	24

NPH, neutral protamine Hagedorn.
Note: Insulin dosage and individual variability in absorption and clearance rates affect pharmacokinetic data. Human insulins may peak earlier and be dissipated faster than porcine or bovine insulins. Duration of insulin activity is prolonged in renal failure.
[a]After a lag time of approximately 5 hrs, glargine has a flat peakless effect over a 24-hr period.

insulin exerts only a transient effect that lasts at most 30 minutes. Subcutaneous injection of regular insulin or semilente has an onset of action within 1 hour. **Insulin lispro** is a human insulin analogue that is absorbed very rapidly (within 15 minutes) from subcutaneous sites, reaches peak plasma levels within 1 hour, and has a shorter duration of action than regular insulin (approximately 3–4 hours).

B. **Intermediate-acting insulins** include neutral protamine Hagedorn (NPH; isophane) and lente (zinc). These insulins are released slowly from subcutaneous sites and reach peak activity after 6–12 hours, followed by gradual decline.

C. **Long-acting insulins.** Ultralente insulin and protamine zinc insulin (PZI) are absorbed more slowly than the intermediate-acting preparations. **Glargine** is a bioengineered human insulin analogue with absorption kinetics that results in an extended duration of action. Administered at bedtime, glargine provides a steady basal supply of circulating insulin over approximately 24 hours.

D. **Species.** Pork and beef pancreata were the major sources of insulin until it became possible to produce insulin of the same amino acid sequence as native human insulin by recombinant DNA technology or by chemical synthesis. Human insulin preparations are less immunogenic than animal preparations.

E. **Concentration.** Most insulins now contain 100 units/ml (U-100). A U-500 preparation is available for the rare patient with severe insulin resistance.

F. **Mixed insulin therapy.** Rapid-acting insulins (regular and lispro) can be mixed with intermediate-acting (NPH and lente) or long-acting (ultralente) insulins in the same syringe for convenience. The rapid-acting insulin should be drawn first, cross contamination should be avoided, and the mixed insulin should be injected immediately. PZI and glargine should not be mixed with other types of insulin. Commercial premixed preparations of rapid- and intermediate-acting insulins are available and can be used for patients who are unable or unwilling to do the mixing themselves.

G. **Subcutaneous insulin delivery** is accomplished using disposable syringes with fine hypodermic needles; less widely used devices include insulin pens and pumps. Alternative routes for insulin delivery (e.g., oral, nasal) are under development.

   1. **Sites of injection.** The anterior abdominal wall, thighs, buttocks, and arms are the preferred sites for subcutaneous insulin injection. Absorption is fastest from the abdomen, followed by the arm, buttocks, and thigh, probably as a result of differences in blood flow. Injection sites should be rotated within the regions rather than randomly across separate regions, to minimize erratic absorption. Clean techniques should be adopted, and areas of scarring, ulceration, or infection should be avoided. Exercise or massage over the injection site may accelerate insulin absorption.

   2. **Insulin pens** use cartridges (or "fountains") that contain 150 or 300 units of either regular insulin, lispro, NPH, or mixed insulin. The desired dose is selected by turning a dial on top of the pen and injected via a disposable needle by pushing a button at the lower end of the pen. Prefilled disposable insulin pens are also available.

   3. **Portable insulin infusion pumps** deliver continuous insulin via an indwelling subcutaneous needle or cannula in the abdominal wall. These programmable pumps contain a reservoir of rapid-acting insulin and provide predetermined basal and premeal boluses of insulin throughout the day.

H. **Complications of insulin therapy** include hypoglycemia, weight gain, and allergic reactions.

   1. **Iatrogenic hypoglycemia** is a limiting factor to aggressive efforts to achieve optimal glycemic control, especially in patients with type 1 DM. All patients with diabetes should be familiar with the warning symptoms of hypoglycemia and be taught to respond appropriately to such episodes (see Office Management of Diabetes Mellitus, sec. **VI**).

   2. **Weight gain.** Factors that contribute to weight gain include improvement in glycemic control, limitation of glycosuria, reversal of catabolic state, fluid retention, and anabolic effects of insulin. Caloric restriction and increased physical activity are advisable.

3. **Insulin allergy** may be triggered by constituents of animal insulins or additives to NPH and PZI formulations (e.g., protamine). Intermittent use of insulin is a known risk factor. Manifestations include local erythema, induration, or pruritus. Urticaria and anaphylaxis may also occur. Skin tests are helpful in diagnosis, and desensitization protocols are available for patients who must be treated with insulin (*Med Clin North Am* 1978;62:663).

4. **Insulin antibodies** occur in persons who have been exposed to exogenous (especially nonhuman) insulin. Rarely, these antibodies can be associated with insulin resistance. If this occurs in a patient treated with animal insulin, a change to human insulin may be beneficial.

5. **Lipodystrophy** at insulin injection sites is an occasional finding. **Lipoatrophy** that leads to indentations at injection sites might be due to impurities in insulin preparations and is reversible by injecting small doses of purified insulin around the lesions. **Lipohypertrophy** results from too-frequent use of the same site for insulin injection; this complication can be avoided by site rotation.

II. **Oral antidiabetic agents** (Table 18-2). Several classes of oral agents are now available for therapy of type 2 DM. The ideal treatment for type 2 diabetes should improve insulin secretion and action and prevent, delay, or reverse long-term complications. Because none of the available agents fulfills these requirements, antidiabetic medications often need to be used in combination for optimal results. **None of the oral antidiabetic agents is approved for use in pregnancy.**

A. **Insulin secretagogues** include sulfonylurea, meglitinide, and amino acid derivatives.

1. **Sulfonylureas** lower blood glucose by augmenting insulin secretion. Treatment with equivalent doses of different sulfonylurea drugs (Table 18-2) gives similar results, the mean decrease in fasting blood glucose being approximately 60 mg/dl. Sulfonylureas should be taken 30–60 minutes before food and should never be administered to patients who observe a voluntary or imposed fast. Therapy should be initiated with the lowest effective dose and increased gradually over several days or weeks to the optimal dose. Dose titration should be guided by results of SMBG initially and later by HbA_{1c} measurement. Some type 2 DM patients do not respond to sulfonylurea therapy (primary failure), whereas others, because of progressive β-cell dysfunction, fail to do so after having responded for several years (secondary failure). Hypoglycemia and weight gain are notable side effects of sulfonylureas. Hypoglycemia carries a worse prognosis when induced by sulfonylureas with a long duration of action (e.g., chlorpropamide), especially in the elderly. Sulfonylureas are contraindicated in patients with type 1 DM, in persons with renal insufficiency, and in those with a history of allergy to sulfonamides.

2. **Repaglinide**, a meglitinide analogue, augments the physiologic secretion of insulin in response to a meal. This drug can be used as a single agent or in combination with metformin in patients with type 2 DM. The initial dose is 0.5 mg PO with two to four meals daily. The drug should be taken within 30 minutes before meals and skipped if no meal is eaten. Each extra meal should be preceded by an additional dose of repaglinide. A higher initial dose, 1–2 mg PO with two to four meals daily, should be used for patients with poorly controlled diabetes (HbA_{1c} >8%) and a history of medication with other antidiabetic agents. The initial dose can be doubled at weekly intervals up to a maximum of 16 mg/day in divided doses. Repaglinide is eliminated mostly by the liver, and serum drug levels accumulate in patients with hepatic dysfunction. The main adverse effects are hypoglycemia and weight gain. As with

Table 18-2. Characteristics of oral antidiabetic agents

Drug	Daily dose range	Dose(s)/ day	Duration of action (hrs)	Main adverse effects
Sulfonylureas				Hypoglycemia, weight gain
First generation				
Tolbutamide	0.5–2.0 g	2–3	12	
Acetohexamide	0.25–1.5 g	1–2	12–24	
Tolazamide	0.1–1.0 g	1–2	12–24	
Chlorpropamide	0.1–0.5 g	1	36–72	
Second generation				
Glyburide	1.25–20.0 mg	1–2	16–24	
Glipizide	5–40 mg	1–2	12	
Glimepiride	1–8 mg	1	24	
Meglitinide				Hypoglycemia, weight gain
Repaglinide	1–16 mg	2–4	1–2	
Amino acid derivative				Hypoglycemia, weight gain
Nateglinide	180–360 mg	3	~1.5	
Biguanide				GI intolerance, lactic acidosis
Metformin	1.0–2.5 g	2–3	6–12	
α-Glucosidase inhibitors				GI intolerance
Acarbose	75–300 mg	3	N/A	
Miglitol	75–300 mg	3	N/A	
Thiazolidinediones				Fluid retention, hepatotoxicity
Rosiglitazone	2–8 mg	1–2	12–24	
Pioglitazone	15–45 mg	1	24	

N/A, not applicable because agents do not act systemically.

sulfonylureas, primary and secondary drug failure related to progressive β-cell dysfunction limit the efficacy of repaglinide. Glycemic response should therefore be monitored closely.

3. **Nateglinide** (*Diabetes Care* 2000;23:202), a derivative of the amino acid D-phenylalanine, is chemically distinct from the other insulin secretagogues. A dose of 120 mg PO tid taken within 1–30 minutes before breakfast, lunch, and dinner rapidly augments endogenous insulin secretion, resulting in a limitation of postprandial hyperglycemia. A lower dose, 60 mg PO tid, may be considered in elderly or frail patients with diminished food intake. Nateglinide is indicated as initial therapy or in combination with metformin in patients with type 2 DM. The insulin secretory response to nateglinide is most pronounced after a meal and is minimal in the fasting state. Nateglinide should be skipped if no meal is planned; however, additional doses are **not recommended** to cover snacks or extra meals. Nateglinide is rapidly eliminated ($T_{1/2}$ = 90 minutes) by hepatic and renal mechanisms, but its pharmacokinetics are unchanged in patients with

renal dysfunction and mild hepatic impairment. Therefore, no dosage adjustment is necessary in such patients. The drug is well tolerated and appears to pose minimal risk for hypoglycemia or weight gain.

B. Metformin, the only biguanide in current clinical use, inhibits hepatic glucose output and stimulates glucose uptake by peripheral tissues. Glycemic control on chronic metformin monotherapy is comparable to that achieved using sulfonylurea, but metformin therapy is associated with a modest weight loss and low risk of hypoglycemia. Metformin may also have beneficial effects on lipid and lipoprotein metabolism as well as fibrinolysis.

1. **Metformin therapy is initiated** with a single 500-mg or 850-mg tablet, taken with food; the dose is then advanced slowly every 1–2 weeks until optimal glycemic effect is achieved or the maximal dose (2000–2550 mg/day) is reached.

2. **Insulin is required for the glucose-lowering effect of metformin.** Thus, some patients who had responded initially to metformin may fail to do so with continued therapy, probably as a result of progressive β-cell failure.

3. **Adverse effects of metformin** include GI symptoms, which usually abate with time, and lactic acidosis, which can be fatal. Risk factors for lactic acidosis include renal dysfunction, hypovolemia, tissue hypoxia, infection, alcoholism, hepatic dysfunction, and cardiorespiratory disease. Metformin is not toxic to the liver or kidney, but its metabolism and elimination require normal hepatic and renal function. Thus, to prevent drug accumulation (and the attendant risk of lactic acidosis), metformin should be avoided in patients with hepatic or renal dysfunction and persons with pre-existing risk factors for lactic acidosis. A serum creatinine of 1.5 mg/dl in men (1.4 mg/dl in women) or higher precludes the use of metformin. Elderly patients should have a glomerular filtration rate (estimated from a 24-hour urine creatinine clearance) of 70 ml/min or higher to be eligible for metformin therapy. Metformin-treated persons with normal baseline hepatic and renal function do not require frequent monitoring of liver enzymes or serum creatinine, because no direct toxicity is expected. Annual or semiannual confirmation of normal hepatic and renal status should suffice in the absence of intercurrent illness or risk factors for hepatic or renal dysfunction. Metformin appears in breast milk and is best avoided in nursing mothers.

C. α-Glucosidase inhibitors reversibly block the intestinal enzymes that break down starches into monosaccharides and thereby delay the digestion and absorption of carbohydrates.

1. **Acarbose** and **miglitol** decrease postprandial hyperglycemia when administered with food in patients with diabetes. Both drugs exert maximal effects at a dosage of approximately 150 mg/day, but each drug should be initiated at low doses **(25 mg PO qd–tid)** and increased slowly in weekly steps of 25 mg to minimize GI intolerance. Patients should be instructed to take the medication at the first bite of food. Monotherapy with α-glucosidase inhibitors has a low risk of inducing hypoglycemia but seldom results in optimal glycemic control.

2. **Dose-related adverse effects** of α-glucosidase inhibitors include bloating, flatulence, loose stools, and other symptoms of carbohydrate malabsorption. Acarbose therapy has been associated with significant elevation in the levels of circulating liver enzymes, especially at the 300-mg/day dose range. The elevated enzymes usually return to baseline after withdrawal of drug. Periodic monitoring of transaminases, therefore, is recommended during therapy with α-glucosidase inhibitors. **Hypoglycemia** in patients who receive combination regimens that include α-glucosidase inhibitors should be treated preferentially with **glucose (dextrose)** rather than sucrose or other carbohydrates that cannot be digested in the presence of these drugs.

D. Thiazolidinediones increase tissue sensitivity to insulin, thereby improving glycemic control. Endogenous (or exogenous) insulin is required for expression of their antidiabetic effect. The risk of hypoglycemia is low during monotherapy but can be increased when thiazolidinediones are used in combination with exogenous insulin or sulfonylurea. Hepatotoxicity has been observed with members of the thiazolidinedione family, and therefore routine monitoring of liver function is mandatory. Thiazolidinediones are contraindicated in patients with active liver disease. Edema and decreases in hematologic indices observed during thiazolidinedione therapy probably result from increased plasma volume. Correction of ovulatory defects after thiazolidinedione therapy in premenopausal women with polycystic ovary disease and insulin resistance can lead to unexpected pregnancies. Therefore, effective contraceptive practice is recommended.

   1. Rosiglitazone is used alone as an adjunct to diet and exercise or in combination with metformin for treatment of type 2 diabetes. The usual starting dose is 4 mg PO qd (or 2 mg PO bid) taken with or without food. This can be advanced to 8 mg PO qd (or 4 mg PO bid) after 12 weeks if glycemic response is inadequate. Increased plasma volume, decreases in hematologic indices during the first 4–8 weeks, and edema are notable adverse effects. Use of rosiglitazone is not recommended in patients with significant heart disease (New York Heart Association class III and IV cardiac status). Although data from preapproval clinical trials suggest a low propensity for hepatotoxicity, regular monitoring of hepatic transaminases is required in patients who are treated with rosiglitazone.

   2. Pioglitazone is used as a single agent (together with diet and exercise), or in combination with sulfonylurea, metformin, or insulin, in patients with type 2 diabetes. The initial dose is 15 mg or 30 mg PO qd, taken with or without food; this can be increased after several weeks to 45 mg PO qd for optimal effect. Adverse effects include decreases in hematologic indices during the initial 4–12 weeks, increased plasma volume, and edema. Use of pioglitazone is not recommended in patients with significant heart disease (New York Heart Association class 3 and 4 cardiac status). Although data from preapproval clinical trials suggest a low risk for hepatotoxicity, regular monitoring of hepatic transaminases is required during pioglitazone therapy.

III. Drug combinations. Concurrent use of two or more medications from different oral antidiabetic drug classes often is necessary to achieve optimal glycemic control, especially in persons with type 2 diabetes.

   A. Widely used regimens include sulfonylurea plus metformin and thiazolidinedione plus sulfonylurea or insulin. The combination of a sulfonylurea and metformin (Glucovance) is now available in varying dosages. Addition of an α-glucosidase inhibitor to sulfonylurea, metformin, or insulin can also be considered. Nateglinide can be added to metformin to optimize glycemic control. Three-drug regimens (e.g., sulfonylurea, metformin, and thiazolidinedione) may be necessary in some patients with refractory hyperglycemia.

   B. Regimens that combine bedtime NPH insulin with daytime sulfonylurea or metformin have been effective in some patients. The primary objective is to improve glycemic control by exploiting the additive or synergistic effects of individual agents when used in combination. Properties such as effect on insulin resistance, hepatic glucose production, insulin secretion, body weight, serum lipid levels, and so forth can be used to select drug combinations.

   C. Combination therapy is most effective if initiated as part of a comprehensive diabetes care plan that includes emphasis on diet and exercise. The efficacy, safety, and tolerability of any chosen combination regimen should be evaluated at frequent intervals.

   D. A parsimonious approach to the length of the combination chain is recommended. Regimens that have three or more drugs for control of diabetes might be too cumbersome for the average patient, who likely is also taking other medications for concomitant ailments.

Office Management
of Diabetes Mellitus

I. Initial office evaluation of persons with DM [*Diabetes Care* 2000;24(Suppl 1):S35]. The tasks to be accomplished during the initial office visit include (1) elicitation of a detailed history that is pertinent to DM, (2) a diabetes-focused comprehensive physical examination, (3) establishment of relevant baseline laboratory values, and (4) formulation of a management plan.

    A. History (Table 18-3). The presence and severity of symptoms of hyperglycemia and symptoms that are suggestive of acute or chronic complications of diabetes should be documented. In addition, details of previous regimens for diabetes, use of medications that alter glucose metabolism, and cardiovascular risk factors should be obtained. The patient's understanding of diabetes and current self-care practices (dietary modification, exercise, glucose monitoring) also should be assessed.

    B. Physical examination (Table 18-3). The height, weight, and body mass index (BMI, weight in kg divided by square of height in meters) should be recorded. [The upper limit of normal BMI is 25 kg/m^2; persons with BMI higher than 25 kg/m^2 but less than 27 kg/m^2 are overweight, and those with BMI higher than 27 kg/m^2 are obese (for management of obesity see Chap. 3).] The state of hydration, nutrition, and overall health should be noted, and the BP should be recorded. The systemic examination should be comprehensive but focused on diabetes and its complications; it is helpful to proceed methodically from head to toe. Examination of the feet should include inspection of dorsum, sole, and interdigital spaces for evidence of deformity, trauma, ulceration, or infection; palpation for calluses, arterial pulsations, and local skin temperature; and testing for sensation with a monofilament.

    C. Laboratory evaluation (Table 18-3) during the initial office visit should include measurement of fasting plasma glucose (or random plasma glucose in symptomatic patients) if the diagnosis of diabetes is not secure. For established diabetic patients, glycohemoglobin should be obtained, together with urinalysis, fasting serum lipid profile, and serum creatinine. Microalbuminuria should be assessed using either a timed urine specimen or the microalbumin-creatinine ratio in a spot urine sample: A normal ratio is less than 30 mg microalbumin per gram creatinine.

    D. The initial management plan (Table 18-3) sets short- and long-term goals. Self-management education (including home blood glucose monitoring and testing for urine ketones), dietary intervention, and lifestyle modification (exercise, smoking cessation, etc.) should be initiated. Other key components of the initial plan include selection of medications for control of diabetes and associated conditions, screening for complications, appropriate referrals, and follow-up arrangement. It is advisable to involve family members and enlist their cooperation in the implementation of the various management tasks.

II. Type 1 diabetes. The treatment goal is normalization (or near-normalization) of blood glucose, as indicated by average preprandial blood glucose values of 80–120 mg/dl, bedtime blood glucose of 100–140 mg/dl, and HbA$_{1c}$ value of 7% or lower [*Diabetes Care* 2001;24(Suppl 1):S34]. This degree of glycemic control is associated with the lowest risk for diabetic retinopathy, nephropathy, and neuropathy (*N Engl J Med* 1993;329:978). Insulin therapy is required lifelong and can be initiated on an outpatient basis in otherwise competent patients who are not acutely ill and have no evidence of DKA. This therapy should be introduced as part of an individualized comprehensive strategy, using the mnemonic **MEDEM** to recall key components of care (see Diabetes Mellitus, sec. II). A team approach (with inputs from diabetes educators, dietitians, nurse practitioners) usually is necessary to impart the required education, dietary counseling, and self-care skills effectively.

Table 18-3. Evaluation during initial office visit for diabetes mellitus (DM)

History

Symptoms of DM

Medications for DM and other conditions

Self-management and monitoring skills

Acute and chronic complications

Family history

Lifestyle and coronary risk factors

Relevant laboratory data

Physical examination

Height, weight, vital signs

Eyes (preferably with dilation)

Oropharynx, gums, and teeth

Neck (including thyroid gland)

Heart, lungs, abdomen

Neurologic examination

Skin and extremities (especially feet)

Laboratory evaluation

Fasting plasma glucose

Glycohemoglobin

Fasting lipid profile

Serum creatinine

Urinalysis

Electrocardiogram

Other (e.g., thyroid-stimulating hormone, if indicated)

Management plan

Short- and long-term goals

Medications

Medical nutrition therapy

Lifestyle changes

Self-management education

Monitoring instructions

Continuing support and follow-up

Modified from American Diabetes Association. Clinical practice recommendations. *Diabetes Care* 2001;24(Suppl 1):S1.

Close contact between physician and patient is critical for successful outpatient management, particularly in newly diagnosed patients.

  A. **Initial insulin dosage** for optimal glycemic control is approximately 0.5–1.0 units/kg/day for the average nonobese patient. Usually, a conservative initial total daily dose is calculated and administered, using one of several options, to provide insulin supply throughout the day. The initial dose is then adjusted, based on SMBG values. Insulin requirement decreases during the transient β-cell recovery (honeymoon phase) that occurs after initiation of insulin therapy in some patients.

1. **Conventional insulin regimen** uses a mixture of rapid- and intermediate-acting insulins (so-called split-mixed) administered before breakfast and before the evening meal. Empirically, two-thirds of the total daily dose is injected in the morning and one-third in the evening, and approximately two-thirds of each injection comprises intermediate-acting insulin and one-third is rapid-acting insulin ("rule of thirds"). This regimen should be modified for patients with unusual work schedules or eating patterns. Adjustments to individual components of each injection are then made using data from self-monitored preprandial and bedtime blood glucose values.

2. **Multiple daily insulin injections** provide approximately 40–50% of the total daily insulin dose as basal supply, administered as one or two injections of long-acting or intermediate-acting insulin. The remainder is given as three doses of rapid-acting insulin taken before the main meals, roughly in proportion to the carbohydrate content. An allowance of 1.0 unit/10 g carbohydrate consumed is typical. The multiple daily insulin injection regimen is an effective option for intensifying diabetes control when the conventional regimen proves ineffective. It also allows greater flexibility with the timing and portions of meals.

3. **Continuous subcutaneous insulin infusion (CSII)** is a tool for intensive diabetes control in selected patients. It provides 50% of total daily insulin as basal insulin and the remainder as multiple preprandial boluses of insulin, using a programmable insulin pump. As with basal-bolus regimen, the premeal insulin doses are estimated from the carbohydrate content of the meals.

   a. **Initiation of CSII** is most appropriate in highly motivated and capable persons with considerable experience in diabetes self-care. **Self-monitoring of blood glucose** at least four times/day (before each meal and at bedtime) is a prerequisite for CSII.

   b. **Outpatient training and conditioning** are required to determine suitability for and proficiency in the CSII regimen.

   c. **Complications of CSII** include skin infection at infusion sites (30%), ketoacidosis from interrupted insulin delivery (15%), and hypoglycemia.

B. **Monitoring.** Patients with type 1 diabetes should perform self-monitoring of blood glucose three to four times a day. HbA_{1c} should be obtained approximately every 3 months.

III. **Type 2 diabetes.** Glycemic control is set at the same goal for type 1 and type 2 diabetes: average preprandial blood glucose values of 80–120 mg/dl, bedtime blood glucose of 100–140 mg/dl, and HbA_{1c} of 7% or lower [*Diabetes Care* 2001;24(Suppl 1):S34]. This degree of glycemic control protects against long-term complications in patients with type 2 diabetes (*Lancet* 1998;352:837). Obesity is prevalent, contributes to insulin resistance, and may require specific therapy in persons with type 2 diabetes. A comprehensive approach, tailored to individual needs, using the expertise of diabetes educators, dietitians, and other members of the diabetes care team, is strongly recommended. The mnemonic **MEDEM** can be used to recall key components of diabetes care (see Diabetes Mellitus, sec. **II**). Genuine commitment to the patient's overall well-being promotes adherence to the multiple behavioral and self-care tasks that are expected of the diabetic patient. Excellence in diabetes care requires frequent patient contacts between office visits, which can be accomplished by means of telephone, fax, or the Internet. Such contacts enable the diabetes care team to respond promptly to laboratory test results, review SMBG data, adjust medications, and assess compliance with lifestyle and pharmacologic interventions. These interactions also have a heuristic impact on patients, build trust between the patient and caregivers, and may help modify behavior.

A. **Nonpharmacologic measures** including dietary and exercise interventions are key components of type 2 diabetes management. Medications are added as needed but must not supplant lifestyle modification.

   1. **Dietary intervention** (see Diabetes Mellitus, sec. **II.C**). Restriction of total and saturated fat intake, with augmentation of complex carbohydrates and dietary fiber, has been demonstrated to enhance insulin action. Similarly, weight reduction improves insulin sensitivity. Specific dietary goals should take into account an individual's current weight, desirable weight, comorbid conditions, and lifestyle factors.

   2. **Exercise** (see Diabetes Mellitus, sec. **II.D**). Type 2 diabetes is more prevalent among sedentary persons compared with physically active persons. Physical activity enhances insulin sensitivity, and inactivity induces relative insulin resistance. The insulin-sensitizing effect of exercise can be demonstrated acutely and thus may be independent of weight loss.

B. **Pharmacologic therapy** (see Drugs Used for Treatment of Diabetes Mellitus, sec. **II**, and Table 18-2). Dietary modification, physical activity, and weight reduction (in the obese) constitute the foundation of type 2 diabetes therapy; all medications are adjuncts to these lifestyle measures. Glycemic control is set at the same goal (HbA$_{1c}$ $\leq 7\%$) for type 1 and type 2 diabetes, and antidiabetic medications, in conjunction with lifestyle modification, increase the likelihood of attaining this goal for the long term.

   1. **Newly diagnosed** type 2 diabetes patients should initially be offered diet and exercise therapy and be monitored closely for evidence of response or decompensation. Approximately 25% of such patients respond with improvement in glycemic control for variable periods; these patients may not require medication(s) for as long as their HbA$_{1c}$ remains at 7% or lower. Patients who present initially with marked hyperglycemia or complications require concurrent introduction of lifestyle and pharmacologic therapies.

   2. **Initial choice of medication** (see Drugs Used for Treatment of Diabetes Mellitus, sec. **II**) for control of uncomplicated hyperglycemia in patients with type 2 diabetes is a matter of clinical judgment. Maximal doses of sulfonylureas, metformin, and thiazolidinediones give comparable glucose-lowering effects when used as initial monotherapy. Insulin secretagogues such as sulfonylureas and repaglinide exert their glucose-lowering effects acutely, but approximately 20% of patients do not respond to these agents ("primary failure"). On the other hand, the maximum effects of metformin or thiazolidinediones may not be observed until several weeks after initiation of therapy. Because residual insulin secretory capacity is a prerequisite for the glucose-lowering effects of metformin and thiazolidinediones, many patients with advanced type 2 DM do not respond satisfactorily to these agents. Also, patients with abnormal renal or hepatic function at baseline are not candidates for metformin or thiazolidinedione therapy. α-Glucosidase inhibitors can be considered as initial therapy in patients with mild, predominantly postprandial hyperglycemia or persons in whom intolerance to the other agents develops. Insulin can be used as the initial drug in patients with severe hyperglycemia and is the drug of choice in pregnancy and for patients who present with acute diabetic crises.

   3. **Long-term oral therapy** for type 2 diabetes requires the use of multiple agents in combination (see Drugs Used for Treatment of Diabetes Mellitus, sec. **III**) because of progressive insulin resistance and β-cell failure (*JAMA* 1999;281:2005). Approximately 60% of patients who respond initially to treatment with sulfonylurea or metformin require a second agent within 3 years to maintain HbA$_{1c}$ at 7% or lower. Medications for combination therapy should be selected from drug classes that lower blood glucose by different mechanisms to ensure additive or synergistic effects.

4. **Bedtime NPH insulin with daytime sulfonylurea or metformin** has been advocated for patients whose diabetes is poorly controlled despite maximal doses of sulfonylurea or metformin. Although the merit and cost effectiveness (compared with switching to full doses of insulin) are debatable, this approach can be considered in patients who are not in acute metabolic crisis. It is a practical option for the patient with type 2 diabetes who is unwilling to accept standard insulin regimens. A low initial dose (approximately 12 units) of NPH insulin is given at bedtime (approximately 2100 hours) and increased by two to four units every few days, while continuing maximal doses of the oral agent, until a desirable fasting blood glucose level is achieved.

5. **Insulin treatment of type 2 diabetes is indicated** for severe hyperglycemia, DKA and nonketotic hyperosmolar crisis, and persistent hyperglycemia despite maximal doses of oral agents. Insulin is the drug of choice during pregnancy and is also commonly prescribed for renally impaired patients in whom sulfonylureas and metformin are contraindicated. Effective insulin regimens for patients with type 2 diabetes include single or multiple daily injections of various proportions of short- and intermediate- or long-acting insulins. Large doses (>100 units/day) usually are required to achieve optimal glycemic control in type 2 DM. The risk of insulin-induced hypoglycemia is low in this population, but weight gain can be considerable. No evidence has been found that exogenous insulin therapy increases cardiovascular risk in the type 1 (*N Engl J Med* 1993;329:978) or type 2 (*Lancet* 1998;352:837) DM population.

6. **Monitoring.** Patients with type 2 diabetes should perform SMBG regularly. Those who are treated with insulin or sulfonylurea should perform SMBG one or more times/day because of the associated risk of hypoglycemia. Patients whose diabetes is controlled with diet or other oral agents, or both, should perform SMBG daily to several times a week. The optimal frequency of self-testing depends on stability of glycemic control and can be negotiated with the patient. HbA_{1c} should be obtained approximately every 3 months.

IV. **Follow-up care for DM.** The recommended frequency of office visits for DM patients is at least quarterly, except for patients in excellent glycemic control, who can be seen every 6 months. More frequent visits and contacts often are necessary to stabilize patients with newly diagnosed diabetes or those who experience metabolic decompensation. The following tasks should be accomplished during follow-up visits.

A. **Interval medical history**, including hospital admissions and symptoms of hyperglycemia, hypoglycemia, diabetes complications, and cardiovascular disease, should be obtained. Compliance with and tolerability of current antidiabetic medication(s) should be documented. Recent infections or medications for intercurrent ailments should be recorded. In addition, the diet and exercise plans that are established during the initial visit should be reviewed for compliance and efficacy.

B. **SMBG records** should be reviewed with noticeable interest, and appropriate feedback should be provided for the patient's edification. Patients who neglect to bring in SMBG records should be encouraged to transmit the results by telephone or fax to enable appropriate adjustments to diabetes therapy. Those who habitually forget to bring in SMBG records or do not self-monitor at all should be courteously reprimanded and encouraged to change their ways. Socioeconomic barriers to implementation of diabetes self-care recommendations should be identified and addressed whenever possible. Correspondence with third parties may often be necessary to ensure coverage for the cost of diabetes self-care supplies; the physician should be a zealous advocate for patients in such situations.

C. **Physical examination**, focusing on pertinent organ systems, should be performed. A deliberate search for diabetes-related clinical findings (e.g., dehy-

Table 18-4. Routine follow-up and surveillance for chronic complications of diabetes

Complications	Method	Frequency	Goal
Hyperglycemia	Hemoglobin A_{1c}	Every 3 mos	<7%
Retinopathy	Dilated funduscopy	Yearly	Normal retina
Nephropathy	Microalbuminuria[a]	Yearly	<300 mg/day or <30 mg/g creatinine
Neuropathy	Light touch sensation (monofilament)	Every visit	Intact sensation
Hypertension	Sphygmomanometry	Every visit	<130/85 mm Hg
Dyslipidemia	Fasting lipid profile	Yearly	LDL <100 TG <200
Heart disease	Electrocardiogram[b]	Yearly	No ischemic changes
Diabetic foot	Clinical examination	Every visit	No ulceration

LDL, low-density lipoprotein cholesterol; TG, triglycerides.
[a]Timed overnight urine or spot urine (microalbumin-creatinine ratio).
[b]More aggressive cardiac testing is warranted in diabetes patients with symptoms of or additional risk factors for coronary artery disease.

dration, hypertension, skin lesions, eye changes, impaired sensation, foot ulceration, etc.) should be undertaken.

   D. Surveillance for specific chronic complications of diabetes (Table 18-4) should be implemented, in accordance with the Standards of Care recommendations for people with diabetes [*Diabetes Care* 2001;24(Suppl 1):S33].

   E. HbA$_{1c}$ level should be documented, and the result (together with SMBG records) should be used to modify the management plan established during the initial office visit. Referrals to other caregivers (e.g., podiatry, ophthalmology, nephrology, cardiology, etc.) should be initiated, as appropriate.

V. Perioperative considerations. Patients with DM undergo surgical procedures at a higher rate than do nondiabetic persons (*Arch Intern Med* 1999;159:2405). Although the stress of surgery frequently leads to deterioration of glycemic control, major surgical procedures often require a period of fasting during which oral antidiabetic medications cannot be used. Careful attention must therefore be paid to the DM patient who is undergoing a surgical procedure. Elective surgery preferably should be scheduled after acceptable glycemic control has been achieved. Whenever possible, surgery should be scheduled for early morning to minimize prolonged fasting.

   A. Patients who are managed with diet alone may require no special intervention if diabetes is well controlled. Fasting and intraoperative blood glucose should be monitored. If fasting plasma glucose is 200 mg/dl or greater, small doses of SC short-acting insulin (regular or lispro) or IV infusion of insulin and 5% dextrose in water (D5W) should be considered, depending on the duration and extent of surgery.

   B. Patients treated with oral antidiabetic agent. Sulfonylureas should be discontinued 1 day before surgery; other oral agents should be withheld on the operative day. Blood glucose should be monitored before and after surgery and during surgery for extensive procedures. Perioperative hyperglycemia (>200 mg/dl) can be managed with small SC doses of short-acting insulin (regular or lispro). Care must be taken to avoid hypoglycemia. For minor procedures, diabetes medications can be restarted once the patient starts eating. In patients who are exposed to iodinated radiocontrast dyes, metformin therapy is withheld for 72 hours postoperatively and restarted after documentation of normal serum creatinine and absence of contrast-induced nephropathy. For extensive or stressful major procedures, hyperglycemia can be managed using IV insulin infusion (see sec. **D**).

C. **Insulin-treated patients** can skip the morning dose of SC insulin on the day of surgery, depending on the nature of the operation. Patients who are treated with long-acting insulin can be switched to intermediate-acting forms 1–2 days before elective surgery. Close perioperative blood glucose monitoring is crucial to avoid extremes of glycemia.

1. **Patients who are undergoing minor surgery** of short duration require no special intervention if fasting plasma glucose is 100–200 mg/dl. Glucose levels should be monitored every hour intraoperatively and immediately after surgery. Perioperative hyperglycemia can be managed with small SC doses of short-acting insulin (regular or lispro). The usual insulin regimen can be resumed once oral intake is established.

2. **Patients who are undergoing major surgery** should have preoperative measurement of blood glucose, serum electrolytes, and urine ketones. Ideally, metabolic and electrolyte abnormalities (e.g., hyponatremia, dyskalemia, acidosis) should be corrected before surgery. For patients who are treated with conventional insulin regimens, one-third to one-half of the total daily dose of insulin can be administered SC before surgery, depending on ambient glucose levels. Patients who are treated with multiple doses of short-acting insulin can have one-third of their usual prandial dose of insulin, whereas patients who are using an insulin pump can continue their usual basal rate of infusion.

D. **IV insulin infusion** is an alternative to SC insulin for the management of diabetes in patients who are undergoing major procedures.

1. **Initial insulin infusion rate** can be estimated as one-half of the patient's total daily insulin dose expressed as units/hour. Regular insulin, 0.5–1.0 unit/hour, is an appropriate starting dose for most patients with type 1 diabetes; D5W (or D10W), 100 ml/hour, should also be started. An initial infusion rate of 1–2 units/hour can be used in patients treated with oral antidiabetic agents who require perioperative insulin infusion.

2. **Maintenance infusion rates** for insulin and dextrose are determined using hourly blood glucose measurements; the goal is to maintain intraoperative plasma glucose in the 100- to 200-mg/dl range.

3. **Potassium chloride**, 10 mEq, is added to each 500 ml dextrose to maintain normokalemia in patients with normal renal function.

4. **The duration of insulin and dextrose infusions** depends on the clinical status of the patient. The infusions should be continued postoperatively until oral intake is secure, after which the usual diabetes treatment can be resumed. It is prudent to give the first dose of SC insulin 30 minutes before the IV route is disconnected.

VI. Hypoglycemia. Mild episodes of iatrogenic hypoglycemia are frequent during therapy of DM using insulin or insulin secretagogues. The risk for development of severe hypoglycemia that requires external assistance is increased threefold during intensive insulin therapy in patients with type 1 DM who typically have defective counterregulatory responses. In contrast, severe hypoglycemia occurs in only approximately 2% of patients with type 2 DM during intensive therapy with insulin or oral agents.

A. **Risk factors** for iatrogenic hypoglycemia include skipped meals, physical exertion, misguided therapy, alcohol ingestion, and drug overdose. Recurrent episodes of hypoglycemia impair recognition of hypoglycemic symptoms, thereby increasing the risk for severe hypoglycemia.

B. **Diagnosis.** Mild hypoglycemia usually is perceived and handled competently by an experienced patient, whereas severe hypoglycemia often requires external intervention (e.g., glucagon injection, IV dextrose) or results in altered mentation, seizure, or coma. In the hierarchy of symptoms, autonomic symptoms of hypoglycemia (e.g., tremulousness, sweating, palpitations, hunger) precede neuroglycopenic symptoms (e.g., impaired concentration, irritability, blurred vision, lethargy) and development of seizure or coma. Secretion of counterregulatory hormones accounts for the early autonomic warning symptoms, which may be blunted in patients with defective counterregulation. Plasma or capillary blood glucose should be obtained, whenever feasible, to confirm hypoglycemia.

C. **Treatment.** Isolated episodes of mild hypoglycemia may not require specific intervention. Recurrent episodes require a review of lifestyle factors: Adjustments may be indicated in the content, timing, and distribution of meals; timing and intensity of exercise; and medication dosage and timing. Severe hypoglycemia is an indication for supervised treatment in a hospital environment; the duration of inpatient care usually is guided by the patient's mental status and need for parenteral glucose.

1. **Readily absorbable carbohydrates** (e.g., glucose and sugar-containing beverages) can be administered orally to conscious patients for rapid effect. Alternatively, milk, candy bars, fruits, cheese, and crackers may be adequate in some patients with mild hypoglycemia. Hypoglycemia associated with acarbose or miglitol therapy should be treated with glucose because these agents block the digestion of sucrose and other carbohydrates. Glucose tablets and other readily absorbable foods and beverages should be readily available to patients with DM at all times.

2. **Intravenous dextrose** is indicated for severe hypoglycemia, patients with altered consciousness, and during restriction of oral intake. An initial bolus, 20–50 ml, of 50% dextrose should be given immediately, followed by infusion of D5W (or D10W) to maintain blood glucose above 100 mg/dl. Aggressive and prolonged IV dextrose infusion, together with close inpatient observation, is warranted in sulfonylurea overdose in the elderly and in patients with defective counterregulation.

3. **Glucagon**, 1 mg IM (or SC), is an effective initial therapy for severe hypoglycemia in patients who are unable to maintain oral intake or in whom an IV access cannot be secured immediately. Vomiting is a frequent side effect, and therefore care should be taken to prevent the risk of aspiration of gastric contents. A glucagon kit should be available to patients with a history of severe hypoglycemia; family members and roommates should be instructed in its proper use.

4. **Education** regarding etiologies of hypoglycemia, preventive measures, and appropriate adjustments to medication, diet, and exercise regimens are essential tasks to be addressed during hospitalization for severe hypoglycemia.

5. **Hypoglycemia unawareness** and the related syndrome of defective glucose counterregulation result from recurrent episodes of iatrogenic hypoglycemia. Patients who are undergoing intensive diabetes therapy are particularly at risk. Inability to sense the autonomic warning symptoms of hypoglycemia predisposes to the development of neuroglycopenia, lethargy, stupor, seizures, and coma. Patients with hypoglycemia unawareness should be encouraged to monitor their blood glucose frequently and take timely measures to correct low values (<60 mg/dl). In patients with very tightly controlled diabetes, slight relaxation in glycemic control and scrupulous avoidance of hypoglycemia can restore the lost warning symptoms. β-Adrenergic blockers can mask hypoglycemic symptoms, but these agents are not contraindicated in diabetic patients who have a genuine need for them.

6. **Medical identification**, worn on a conspicuous anatomic region (e.g., wrist, neck), facilitates delivery of appropriate care in patients with altered consciousness.

VII. Indications for hospital admission include newly diagnosed type 1 diabetes, newly recognized diabetes in pregnancy, complications of diabetes, and other acute medical conditions. Inpatient care is particularly appropriate in the following situations:

A. DKA, as indicated by a plasma glucose of 250 mg/dl or greater in association with an arterial pH of less than 7.30, a serum bicarbonate level less than 18 mEq/L, and ketonuria or ketonemia.

B. Hyperosmolar nonketotic state, usually suggested by marked hyperglycemia ($\geq$400 mg/dl) and elevated serum osmolality (>315 mOsm/kg), often accompanied by impaired mental status.

C. Hypoglycemia (<50 mg/dl), especially if induced by a sulfonylurea drug or resulting in coma, seizures, or altered mentation.

Diabetes Mellitus in Pregnancy

Approximately 4% of pregnancies are complicated by diabetes. Increased maternal sensitivity to the anabolic effects of insulin occurs during the first half of pregnancy; insulin sensitivity declines in the second half. The midgestational insulin resistance predisposes to GDM and increased insulin requirement in women with prepregnancy diabetes. GDM and diabetes in pregnancy are associated with adverse obstetric, perinatal, neonatal, and long-term outcomes if they are not treated adequately. Ideally, every pregnancy in a known diabetic woman should be planned so that meticulous control can be instituted well in advance of conception. Collaboration with an obstetrician who is skilled in the management of pregnancy and delivery in pregnant diabetic women is invaluable.

I. Diagnosis of GDM [*Diabetes Care* 2001;24(Suppl 1):S77] is suggested by the presence of symptoms, discovery of glycosuria, or the results of routine screening for diabetes.

A. Initial screening and risk assessment should be undertaken at the first prenatal visit. Women with risk factors for GDM (e.g., obesity, history of GDM, family history of DM, high-risk ethnic group) should undergo glucose testing at the earliest opportunity. Those who test negative at initial screening should be retested at 24–28 weeks of gestation.

B. Glucose testing at 24–28 weeks of gestation is recommended for most women, except those who are at low risk for diabetes. A plasma glucose level greater than 140 mg/dl at 1 hour after a 50-g oral glucose load constitutes a positive screening test. A fasting plasma glucose of greater than 105 mg/dl (normal range during pregnancy, 60–80 mg/dl) also suggests GDM, which should be confirmed with a repeat test.

C. Confirmatory testing for patients with a positive screening test and those with equivocal fasting plasma glucose levels consists of a standard OGTT. Diagnostic values for the 3-hour, 100-g OGTT are 95 mg/dl (fasting), 180 mg/dl (1 hour), 155 mg/dl (2 hours), and 140 mg/dl (3 hours).

D. A single-step approach consisting of an OGTT without prior glucose screening may be more efficient and cost effective in certain high-risk populations (e.g., Native Americans).

II. Management of GDM consists initially of dietary and lifestyle modification. All patients are taught self-monitoring skills and encouraged to maintain regular physical activity. If the patient maintains fasting (<90 mg/dl) and postprandial (<120 mg/dl) blood glucose levels that are normally observed in nondiabetic pregnancies and is free from ketonuria, dietary measures are continued. Patients who are unable to maintain normal blood glucose levels around the clock or have persistent ketonuria require intensive insulin therapy.

A. **Dietary modification** should be individualized. An additional caloric allowance of 300–400 kcal/day above basal requirements is appropriate during pregnancy. Weight-loss diets are not generally prescribed during pregnancy, but obese women (BMI >30 kg/m^2) might benefit from moderate caloric restriction (approximately 1800 kcal/day).

B. **Exercise** of moderate intensity improves diabetes control and should be encouraged in women with an active lifestyle who are carrying an uncomplicated pregnancy. Heart disease, hypertension, microvascular disease (especially proliferative retinopathy, nephropathy, and autonomic neuropathy), and hypoglycemia unawareness are relative contraindications to exercise.

C. **Women with type 2 diabetes who become pregnant** may have been treated with oral agents or insulin, or both, before pregnancy. Ideally, diabetes control should be excellent (HbA_{1c} <7%) several months before conception. None of the oral antidiabetic agents is approved for use in pregnancy; thus, insulin therapy remains the only option.

D. **Insulin therapy** is indicated for patients with prepregnancy diabetes and diet-treated women with GDM who are unable to maintain normoglycemia. The goal is achievement of excellent metabolic control, as indicated by normal blood glucose levels around the clock and absence of starvation ketosis. (Ketoacidosis and ketonuria have been associated with increased adverse fetal outcomes.) Sufficient insulin, usually in multiple doses of rapid- and intermediate-acting insulin (see Office Management of Diabetes Mellitus, sec. **II.A**) and regular meals are required to achieve this goal. Hypoglycemia and ketosis should be avoided: Omission of a single meal in a pregnant woman can result in significant lipolysis and ketogenesis.

E. **Self-monitoring of blood glucose** should be performed four to six times/day (fasting, 2 hours after each meal, at bedtime) to guide insulin therapy. Less frequent SMBG can be considered in women with diet-controlled GDM.

F. **Obstetric management.** Determination of timing and mode of delivery is made by the attending obstetrician, based on overall maternal health and results of fetal monitoring.

Chronic Complications of Diabetes Mellitus

Chronic complications of DM include those due to hyperglycemia-mediated small-vessel disease (microvascular) and syndromes that result from multifactorial large-vessel disease (macrovascular). Diabetic patients with evidence of chronic complications are best managed in consultation with appropriate specialists.

I. **Microvascular disease.** The diabetes-specific microvascular disorders include retinopathy, nephropathy, and neuropathy; their development can be prevented or delayed by meticulous control of hyperglycemia. Owing to the long period (approximately 7 years) of asymptomatic or undiagnosed type 2 DM, one or more microvascular disorders already have developed in up to 25% of type 2 DM patients by the time of diagnosis.

A. **Diabetic retinopathy** includes background retinopathy (microaneurysms, retinal infarcts) and proliferative retinopathy. Background retinopathy usually is not associated with loss of vision, but the development of macular edema or proliferative retinopathy (particularly new vessels near the optic disc) requires elective laser therapy to preserve vision. Annual examination by an ophthalmologist is recommended from the outset for all type 2 DM patients and beginning at puberty or after 5 years of diagnosis for patients with type 1 DM.

B. **Diabetic nephropathy** is preceded by microalbuminuria (30–300 mg albumin/24 hrs), a potentially reversible state. Microalbuminuria precedes overt proteinuria (>300 mg albumin/day) by several years in type 1 and in type 2 diabetes. The mean duration from diagnosis of type 1 diabetes to development of overt proteinuria is 17 years, and the time from the occurrence of proteinuria to end-stage renal failure averages 5 years. Annual screening for microalbuminuria should be performed from the outset in type 2 DM patients and beginning at puberty or after 5 years of diagnosis in patients with type 1 DM. Measurement of microalbumin-creatinine ratio (normal <30 mg albumin/g creatinine) in a random urine sample is acceptable for screening. Intensive control of diabetes and hypertension and administration of angiotensin-converting enzyme (ACE) inhibitors are effective interventions for delaying the progression of incipient or established diabetic nephropathy.

   C. **Diabetic neuropathy** encompasses a wide variety of focal and diffuse neurologic syndromes.

   1. **Peripheral neuropathy**, the best-recognized example of diabetic neuropathy, presents with paresthesias, numbness, tingling, pain, and burning sensation in a glove-and-stocking distribution. Predominantly motor deficits, such as muscle weakness and atrophy, may also occur. Diabetic peripheral neuropathy is a major risk factor for foot trauma, ulceration, Charcot's arthropathy, and limb amputation. Sensation in the lower extremities should be documented at least annually, using either a light-touch monofilament or a tuning fork. Diabetic neuropathic pain may respond to (1) improvement in glycemic control and (2) tricyclic antidepressant (e.g., imipramine or amitriptyline, 10–25 mg PO qhs initially, increased gradually to 75–150 mg PO qhs), (3) anticonvulsants (e.g., carbamazepine, 100–400 mg PO bid), or topical capsaicin (0.075%) cream. Night cramps can be treated with quinine sulfate, 200–300 mg PO qhs.

   2. **Autonomic neuropathy** may manifest as orthostatic hypotension, cystopathy, or gastroenteropathy.

      a. **Orthostatic hypotension** is treated symptomatically, using supportive measures, semirecumbent sleeping posture, and volume expansion with sodium chloride, 1–4 g PO qid, and fludrocortisone, 0.1–0.3 mg PO qd.

      b. **Diabetic cystopathy** (neurogenic bladder) presents with symptoms of urinary urgency, incontinence, and retention. Recurrent urinary tract infections are common, and chronic antibiotic therapy may be required. Urologic evaluation to exclude other causes of bladder dysfunction is appropriate. Patients with urinary urgency sometimes find relief from antispasmodic therapy with oxybutynin, 5 mg PO tid. Intermittent self-catheterization may be necessary in patients with significant retention.

      c. **Diabetic gastroenteropathy** may present with gastroparesis or diarrhea. Diarrhea should be evaluated thoroughly before being attributed to diabetes. Empiric trial of broad-spectrum antibiotic (e.g., tetracycline, 250 mg PO qid, or azithromycin, 250 mg PO qd) is appropriate after exclusion of other causes of diarrhea. **Diabetic gastroparesis** leads to early satiety, nausea, and vomiting. Patients with severe nausea and intractable vomiting should be admitted for inpatient management. Less severe gastroparesis may respond to outpatient therapy with antiemetic (prochlorperazine, 5–10 mg IM or PO qid or 25 mg PR bid) or prokinetic (metoclopramide, 10–20 mg PO 30–60 minutes before meals and at bedtime) agents. Erythromycin, 125–500 mg PO qid, can also be tried, and amitriptyline, 25 mg PO qhs, has been helpful in some patients with cyclical vomiting.

II. Macrovascular complications of DM include coronary artery disease, stroke, and peripheral vascular disease. Coronary artery disease occurs at a younger age and may have atypical clinical presentations in patients with diabetes. DM is considered an independent risk factor for coronary artery disease. Moreover, myocardial infarction carries a worse prognosis and angioplasty gives less satisfactory results in diabetic patients compared to nondiabetic individuals. For these reasons, an **ECG** should be obtained yearly, and there should be a low threshold for ordering periodic stress tests in diabetic patients aged 35 years or older. **Risk factors for macrovascular disease** include insulin resistance, hyperglycemia, hypertension, dyslipidemia, dysfibrinolysis, cigarette smoking, and obesity.

A. **Insulin resistance** is associated with a twofold increase in the risk for macrovascular disease in persons with IGT and a three- to fourfold increase in patients with type 2 diabetes. Physical activity, dietary modification, and therapy with certain medications (e.g., thiazolidinediones and metformin) improve insulin sensitivity, which may have a beneficial effect on the risk for macrovascular complications. Therefore, maintenance of regular physical activity and optimal dietary modification (see Diabetes Mellitus, sec. **II.C** and **II.D**) are appropriate recommendations for reduction of macrovascular risk in DM patients.

B. **Hyperglycemia.** Glycemic control should be optimized using a comprehensive approach. The goal is maintenance of HbA_{1c} levels of less than 7%. The mnemonic **MEDEM** can be used to recall key components of diabetes control.

C. **Hypertension.** Adequate control of BP results in significant reduction of microvascular and macrovascular complications of diabetes. The BP goal in patients with DM is 130/85 mm Hg or lower. This goal should be pursued vigorously, using drugs from the available antihypertensive classes, none of which is contraindicated in persons with diabetes. Patients with evidence of microalbuminuria should be treated preferentially with drugs that inhibit ACE to preserve renal function.

D. **Dyslipidemia** associated with DM (*Diabetes Care* 1998;21:160) typically is characterized by hypertriglyceridemia, decreased high-density lipoprotein cholesterol (HDL-C) levels, and a preponderance of small, dense low-density lipoprotein cholesterol (LDL-C) particles. Total LDL-C levels in DM patients usually are not significantly different from those of nondiabetic persons. However, the predominant small, dense LDL particles in DM patients probably are associated with increased atherogenicity compared with the large, buoyant LDL particles seen in healthy persons. DM is considered an independent risk factor in the evaluation of dyslipidemia (*JAMA* 2001;285:2486–2497).

1. **Management of dyslipidemia** in DM patients consists initially of optimization of glycemic control, physical activity, and dietary modification.

2. **Lipid-lowering drugs** (see Chap. 5) should be added if nonpharmacologic measures fail to control lipid profile to the desired target. The lipid goals for patients with DM are LDL-C levels of 100 mg/dl or lower, HDL-C levels of 45 mg/dl or higher, and triglyceride levels of less than 200 mg/dl in fasting plasma specimens.

E. **Cigarette smoking** should be actively discouraged (see Chap. 1).

F. **Obesity** should be treated initially with nonpharmacologic interventions. Patients whose BMI is 27 kg/m^2 or higher are candidates for adjunctive pharmacotherapy (see Chap. 3).

G. **Impaired fibrinolysis and hypercoagulation** associated with diabetes increase the risk for thromboembolic disease. **Aspirin, 81–325 mg/day**, is of proven benefit in secondary prevention of myocardial infarction and ischemic stroke in DM patients.

H. **Treatment of peripheral vascular disease** consists of lower-extremity exercise, palliative medications, and vascular surgery.

1. **Graded walking exercises**, up to the point of claudication, promote the development of collateral circulation in the lower extremities.

2. **Low-dose aspirin**, 81–325 mg PO qd, is routinely prescribed.

3. **Palliative therapy with hemorheologic agents** can be considered in appropriate instances.
    a. **Pentoxifylline, 400 mg PO tid**, may provide relief for some patients with intermittent claudication. Pentoxifylline is contraindicated in patients with cerebral or retinal hemorrhage; it may also potentiate the actions of antihypertensives and anticoagulants and should be used with extreme caution in patients who are taking such medications.
    b. **Cilostazol, 100 mg PO bid**, also relieves claudicant pain. This drug, an antiplatelet and a phosphodiesterase III inhibitor, is contraindicated in patients with CHF of any severity; it should be used with caution in individuals with hepatic dysfunction and those who are receiving anticoagulants. A lower dose, 50 mg PO bid, should be used in patients receiving concurrent medications that inhibit CYP3A4 and CYP2C19 (e.g., ketoconazole, diltiazem, erythromycin, omeprazole). Grapefruit juice also inhibits the hepatic enzymes (CYP3A4 and CYP2C19) that are responsible for cilostazol metabolism and is best avoided during medication with cilostazol.
4. **Referral for surgical evaluation** is indicated in patients with intractable claudication, rest pain, or pregangrenous and gangrenous lesions of the lower extremity.

III. **Miscellaneous complications**
   A. **Erectile dysfunction** may result from a combination of diabetic neuropathy, vascular insufficiency, and endocrinologic or psychological factors. Glycemic control should be intensified, and specialist referral should be considered if the problem persists. If endocrinolgic evaluation proves negative and other treatable causes have been excluded, a trial of the phosphodiesterase V inhibitor, sildenafil, 50–100 mg PO precoitally, may be appropriate. **Sildenafil should not be used concurrently with nitrates** to prevent severe and potentially fatal hypotensive reactions (see also Chap. 25).
   B. **The diabetic foot** results from chronic neuropathy, vascular insufficiency, and infection. Poorly managed foot ulcers may result in gangrene formation and limb loss through amputation. Patient education should emphasize prevention: daily foot examination, use of proper footwear, and caution with self-pedicure. The exposed feet should be inspected and palpated during every office visit; significant findings, such as calluses, hammer toes, other deformities, and soft-tissue lesions, should trigger referral for specialized foot care. Patients with active foot ulcers should be treated aggressively; hospitalization for parenteral antibiotic therapy and local wound care often is necessary for optimal results.

Metabolic Effects
of Medications for
Comorbid Conditions

Approximately 40% of patients with diabetes have hypertension. Other comorbidities that are frequently seen in patients with diabetes include hyperlipidemia, heart disease, degenerative joint disease, chronic obstructive pulmonary disease (COPD), sleep apnea, depression, and peptic ulcer disease. These conditions often require chronic treatment, and some of the drugs used could affect insulin sensitivity, β-cell function, lipoprotein metabolism, and hepatic glucose production. It is advisable to select therapeutic agents for concurrent ailments that have neutral or beneficial effects on carbohydrate and lipid metabolism, whenever possible. Protease inhibitors used in the treatment of patients infected with HIV have been associated with the development of new-onset diabetes. The HIV-protease inhibitors appear to induce insulin resistance, and the clinical presentation is consistent with that of type 2 diabetes.

I. **Antihypertensive drugs** are generally well tolerated, and no particular class of agents is contraindicated in patients with diabetes. Diuretics and beta-blockers decrease cardiovascular morbidity and mortality in hypertensive subjects. Moreover, beta-blockers prevent reinfarction and sudden death in patients with a previous history of myocardial infarction, and ACE inhibitors confer a survival advantage in patients with heart failure. For these reasons, therapy with beta-blockers and ACE inhibitors should be offered to diabetes patients with the appropriate cardiovascular indications. The ACE inhibitors are specifically indicated for the preservation of renal function in patients with microalbuminuria and diabetic nephropathy. Although no antihypertensive drugs are specifically contraindicated in diabetes, virtually every class of agents has some notable effect(s) in patients with diabetes.

A. **Thiazide diuretics** are associated with exacerbation of insulin resistance, probably from hypokalemia, in patients with diabetes. Thiazides and furosemide also are associated with variable elevations in serum triglycerides, LDL and very LDL-C levels, and reduction in HDL-C levels. These lipid changes usually return to normal with continued diuretic therapy, except in patients with underlying lipoprotein disorders. As these effects may be dose related, the use of smaller doses (e.g., 6.25–25.0 mg thiazide) is advisable. Rarely, a switch from thiazide to nonthiazide diuretic may be necessary to optimize glycemic control.

B. **Beta-blockers** can mask hypoglycemic symptoms and prolong recovery from insulin-induced hypoglycemia. Also, increases in serum triglycerides and decreases in serum HDL-C levels occur during therapy with beta-blockers. Measures of tissue sensitivity to insulin indicate a decrease of approximately 25% following treatment with beta-blockers. Induction of insulin resistance and dyslipidemia is observed with nonselective as well as with β_1-selective agents. Thus, dose adjustment in diabetes medications may be warranted for optimal glycemic control in patients who receive concurrent treatment with a beta-blocker.

C. **ACE inhibitors** may precipitate acute renal failure in patients with bilateral atherosclerotic renovascular disease or exacerbate hyperkalemia in patients with diabetes-associated type IV renal tubular acidosis. Also, ACE inhibitors (such as calcium channel blockers, α_1-blockers, and vasodilators) can worsen orthostatic symptoms in patients with diabetic autonomic neuropathy. Glucose tolerance is not adversely affected during therapy with ACE inhibitors; in fact, improvement in insulin sensitivity may occur. Also, ACE inhibitors do not have adverse effects on lipid metabolism. The **angiotensin II receptor blockers** appear to have a comparable profile on carbohydrate and lipid metabolism, as do the ACE inhibitors.

D. **Calcium channel blockers** and other agents that cause a relaxation of arteriolar smooth muscle can worsen orthostatic hypotension in patients with diabetic autonomic neuropathy. Calcium channel blockers have a neutral or favorable effect on serum lipids. Rarely, use of calcium channel blockers has been associated with hyperglycemia, but, in general, the calcium channel antagonists have no adverse effects on glucose tolerance or insulin sensitivity.

E. **Other antihypertensive agents.** α_1-Blockers, such as prazosin and terazosin, have been reported consistently to decrease insulin resistance and improve glucose tolerance. Hydralazine, alpha-blockers, and labetalol (a combined alpha- and beta-blocker) have either neutral or favorable effects on plasma lipoprotein profiles. Centrally acting antihypertensive agents, such as guanabenz, guanfacine, and clonidine, are not associated with adverse effects on carbohydrate or lipid metabolism. The potent arteriolar vasodilator diazoxide causes hyperglycemia by inhibiting insulin secretion but does not affect tissue responses to exogenous insulin.

II. **Lipid-lowering drugs.** 3-Hydroxy-3-methylglutaryl coenzyme A (HMG CoA) reductase inhibitors and fibrates (e.g., gemfibrozil, fenofibrate) are well tolerated and do not adversely affect glycemic control. Patients who are treated with oral antidiabetic agents and bile acid resins (e.g., cholestyramine, colestipol) should be instructed to take their diabetes medications 1–2 hours before or 4–6 hours after ingestion of resin to prevent potential drug interactions. Nicotinic acid impairs glucose tolerance and worsens hyperglycemia in patients with diabetes. Therefore, antidiabetic drug doses should be adjusted to restore glycemic control in patients who require concurrent treatment with nicotinic acid.

III. **Bronchodilators** that are used for treatment of asthma and COPD, and over-the-counter cold remedies and nasal decongestants, can have appreciable effects on carbohydrate metabolism.

A. β_2**-Adrenergic agonists.** Catecholamines stimulate glycogenolysis and lipolysis, transiently increase insulin and glucagon secretion, inhibit peripheral glucose utilization, and predispose to hyperglycemia. Epinephrine, isoproterenol, terbutaline, and over-the-counter decongestants (containing sympathomimetic drugs) are capable of elevating blood glucose. The clinical impact of these effects is unclear, but a thorough medication history should be obtained in diabetic patients with persistent hyperglycemia. Inhaled agents are far less likely to affect metabolic control than is oral or parenteral medication.

B. **Theophylline**, in conventional doses, can augment circulating catecholamine levels, thereby predisposing to hyperglycemia. The clinical translation of this might be an increased need for antidiabetic medication in a patient who receives theophylline therapy for COPD. On the other hand, overdosage with theophylline can stimulate insulin secretion and predispose to hypoglycemia. The latter effect is probably mediated by an indirect β-adrenergic mechanism and does not occur during therapy with conventional doses of theophylline.

IV. **Anti-inflammatory agents.** Systemic glucocorticoid therapy impairs diabetes control by multiple mechanisms. Glucocorticoids inhibit peripheral glucose utilization, stimulate lipolysis, and increase hepatic glucose production. Compared with systemic therapy, inhaled corticosteroids are far less likely to cause adverse metabolic effects in patients with diabetes. When systemic therapy is unavoidable, as in patients with acute severe asthma or transplant recipients, close monitoring of blood glucose with adjustments in antidiabetic therapy is appropriate. Hyperglycemia sometimes is noted in patients who receive nonsteroidal anti-inflammatory drugs; the mechanism for this finding is obscure.

V. **Oral contraceptive drugs** that contain estrogen and progesterone combinations have been reported to induce insulin resistance. The contraceptive-induced insulin resistance usually is mild and reversible and can be minimized by selecting preparations with low estrogen and progesterone content. Usually, no adjustment of diabetes therapy is necessary in women who take oral contraceptives. **Estrogen replacement therapy** in menopausal women is not associated with significant alteration of glycemic control in women with diabetes.

Web Sites

---

http://www.diabetes.org
http://www.niddk.nih.gov
http://www.diabetes.com
http://www.idf.org
http://www.mdcc.com
http://www.shapeup.org

19

Infectious Diseases

Thomas C. Bailey and
J. Russell Little

General Principles of Therapy

I. **Determining whether antibiotic treatment is indicated is the first principle in outpatient treatment of infectious diseases.** In direct response to high rates of use of antibiotics, the rate of drug resistance in bacteria is increasing. Overuse and misuse of antibiotics are commonplace and result from a variety of cultural and economic factors (*Ann Intern Med* 2000;133:128). Antibiotics are most often prescribed inappropriately for upper respiratory tract symptoms, which are often viral or noninfectious in origin. In such cases, the role of the physician is to educate the patient regarding the nature of the illness and steps that can be taken to relieve symptoms. A directed history and physical examination are necessary before an antibiotic is prescribed. Antibiotics should not be prescribed for expediency or placebo effect.

II. **Criteria for antibiotic selection.** When an antibiotic is chosen, selection should take into consideration the prevalence of particular pathogens in a given host and region, local susceptibility patterns of those organisms, drug-drug interactions, tolerability, pharmacokinetics, pharmacodynamics, and cost.

III. **Assessment of therapy.** Some infections respond slowly, even when optimal therapy is used. When the expected response to treatment does not occur, however, therapy must be re-evaluated. The following questions should be asked: (1) Is the suspected or isolated organism really the etiologic agent? (2) Is adequate antimicrobial therapy being given (i.e., the appropriate drug, dosage, and route)? (3) Is the antimicrobial penetrating to the site of infection (e.g., is drainage, removal of a foreign body, or relief of obstruction necessary)? (4) Have resistant or superinfecting pathogens emerged? (5) Is a persistent fever due to an underlying disease, a complication (e.g., phlebitis), a drug reaction, or another process?

Specific Infectious Diseases

I. **Respiratory tract infections**
   A. **Upper respiratory tract infections**
      1. **Sinusitis** is a recurrent symptom complex that is usually triggered by episodic viral upper respiratory infections (URIs). Acute sinusitis is determined by symptoms ≤8 weeks and contrasts with chronic sinusitis (symptoms for ≥8 weeks). Blockage of the sinus ostia is usually caused by excessive secretions or mucosal edema that prevent drainage and ventilation of the individual sinus cavities. Common predisposing factors include URI, allergic rhinitis, dental disease, pressure changes

(e.g., air flight), swimming, and certain systemic illnesses (e.g., AIDS, immune globulin deficiency states, cystic fibrosis), or nasal polyps, nasal tumors, foreign bodies, deviated nasal septum, and so forth. Acute purulent sinusitis is usually caused by pneumococci, nontypeable *Haemophilus influenzae*, or *Moraxella catarrhalis* (less commonly *Staphylococcus aureus*). Patients with chronic sinusitis are more likely to have polymicrobial infections with aerobes as well as strictly anaerobic bacteria.

2. **Acute sinusitis** follows the seasonality of colds, and the causative viral agents are usually not identified.

   a. **History.** Risk factors for the development of sinusitis include osteomeatal occlusion of the normal drainage from the sinus due to nasal septal deviation, tumors, and most importantly, allergic or viral inflammatory reactions within the sinus cavity. The most common clinical manifestations of acute sinusitis are persistent coryza and postnasal drip that worsens progressively after several days, with the onset of headache, fever, and local pain and tenderness over the affected sinus. Patients with sphenoid sinusitis can present with severe frontal, temporal, or retro-orbital headache that radiates to the occiput.

   b. **Diagnosis.** The frontal and maxillary sinuses can be palpated directly. Ethmoid tenderness can be evaluated by pinching the bridge of the nose. The sphenoid is the hardest sinus to evaluate on examination because of its inaccessible posterior location. Examination of the inside of the nose may show pus or possibly drainage emerging from one of the turbinates. Findings that have been found predictive of sinusitis are maxillary toothache, colored or purulent nasal discharge, face pain or tenderness, poor response to decongestants, and inability to transilluminate the sinus. When chronic or recurrent sinusitis is present, especially if it is refractory to medical therapy, a sinus CT scan is the most efficient radiographic test to confirm the diagnosis of sinusitis and to evaluate its extent and severity. Sinus tap is rarely necessary for diagnosis, but it may be indicated for patients with persistent refractory infection or severe underlying disease such as AIDS.

   c. **Complications.** The most feared complications of sinusitis are extension of infection into bone, the orbit, and/or the CNS. Frontal headache and swelling over the frontal sinus ("Pott's puffy tumor") indicate probable osteomyelitis and mandate the use of prolonged antibiotics and débridement of necrotic bone. Extension into the orbit or the cavernous sinus is a rare but serious complication. Orbital cellulitis, sinusitis, and acidosis in diabetic patients suggest the possibility of invasive fungal infection caused by one of the *Zygomycetes* (mucormycosis). Consideration of cavernous sinus involvement or mucormycosis should dictate hospital admission, prompt radiographic evaluation of the extent of invasive disease, and ear-nose-throat surgical consultation.

   d. **Treatment of acute sinusitis**

      (1) **Decongestants.** Most cases of uncomplicated infection and mild symptoms can be managed with a 10-day course of decongestants alone (phenylephrine or oxymetazoline nasal spray). Comparative studies have shown no significant differences in cure rates at 14 days in patients treated with decongestants with or without amoxicillin. This inconsistent response to antimicrobial therapy may be related to a viral etiology of the infection.

      (2) **Antibiotics.** A bacterial etiology is suggested by significant fever with purulent nasal discharge, face pain, tenderness, or periorbital swelling. These patients should be treated promptly with antibiotics (see sec. **I.A.2.d.4**). Failure to respond to an adequate course of first-line oral antibiotics [e.g., amoxicillin or trimethoprim-sulfamethoxazole (TMP/SMZ)] may dictate a need for a broadened antimicrobial spectrum. Anaerobic bacteria are part of the

mouth and upper-airway normal flora (*Prevotella, Porphyromonas, Bacteroides, Peptococcus, Fusobacterium*), but sinus infection may also reflect extension of infection from the maxillary molar teeth. This mixed flora usually responds to one of the combination antimicrobials that contains a beta-lactam and a beta-lactamase inhibitor [e.g., amoxicillin-clavulanate (Augmentin), 875 mg PO bid, for 10 days].

(3) Surgery. Surgical drainage or intravenous antibiotics, or both, are a final therapeutic option for sinusitis. If surgical drainage is performed, the surgeon should be alerted to the need to obtain fungal as well as aerobic and anaerobic bacterial cultures at the time of operation, because organisms such as *Aspergillus fumigatus* or other fungi may be causative agents.

(4) Antibiotics for the treatment of sinusitis

Antibiotic	Recommended adult dosage (normal renal function)
Ampicillin	250–500 mg PO q6h
Amoxicillin	250–500 mg PO q8h
Amoxicillin-clavulanate	875 mg PO q12h
Clarithromycin	250–500 mg PO q12h
Loracarbef	200–400 mg PO q12h

Other agents that can be used successfully for the treatment of acute sinusitis include TMP/SMZ, 1 tablet DS PO q12h; azithromycin, 500-mg PO load and 250 mg PO qd thereafter; levofloxacin, 250–500 mg PO qd; or gatifloxacin, 400 mg PO qd. **The customary duration of antimicrobial therapy for acute sinusitis is 10 days.**

3. **Chronic sinusitis** (symptoms lasting more than 8 weeks) is mainly the result of refractory sinus obstruction that prevents the resolution of bacterial infection despite appropriate antibiotic therapy. Consequently, the management of chronic sinusitis must focus on correction of the obstruction, which may require operative intervention. Chronic bacterial sinusitis is typically polymicrobial, often including anaerobic and enteric gram-negative organisms. This mandates a longer course of therapy (oral antibiotics for a minimum of 1 month) and the choice of antibiotics that will be effective against common anaerobes (often beta-lactamase producers) as well as the usual gram-positive airway flora. Oral amoxicillin-clavulanate is reasonable therapy, but only if accompanied by spontaneous or induced sinus drainage.

4. **Allergic fungal sinusitis.** Most patients with allergic fungal sinusitis have a history of atopy or asthma. Optimal therapy usually requires surgical drainage or débridement, or both, and the choice of appropriate antibiotic therapy (if needed) may require the aid of an infectious disease specialist.

5. **Pharyngitis, URI.** Among adults with a chief complaint of sore throat, frequently implicated agents include beta-hemolytic streptococci (groups A, C, and G), viruses, *Mycoplasma*, and *Chlamydia* species. *Mycoplasma* and *Chlamydia* each comprise about 10% of cases. A large fraction do not reveal any pathogen.

a. **The beta-hemolytic streptococci**

(1) **Risk factors and transmission.** Acute pharyngitis caused by **group A streptococci (GAS)** is transmitted from person to person. The nasopharynx is the major natural reservoir for GAS, and infection arises from close contact with a GAS carrier.

School-aged children have the highest carriage rates, and household spread is common.

(2) Typical GAS pharyngitis is a sore throat that occurs during midwinter or early spring, associated with fever, tonsillopharyngeal erythema and exudate, swollen tender anterior cervical lymphadenopathy, an elevated WBC count, and the absence of cough, rhinitis, or laryngitis. Even with this constellation of findings, the diagnostic accuracy of GAS pharyngitis is not more than 20–30% in adults, although it is higher in children.

(3) Diagnosis. Throat culture can improve the accuracy of diagnosis. The optimal site for throat culture is the surface of the posterior pharynx, not the tongue, hard palate, or buccal mucosa. Even one or two doses of antibiotic therapy may account for some false-negative cultures. The GAS rapid antigen detection tests can be performed in minutes, and they have a sensitivity and specificity approaching that of the throat culture. When the rapid GAS antigen test is positive, the symptomatic patient can be treated appropriately. When the rapid antigen test is negative, the use of a second swab for confirmatory culture is recommended to avoid missing a GAS infection. This is particularly important if there are many GAS infections in the community or if rheumatogenic or nephritogenic strains are known to circulate. Since antibodies to GAS do not peak until 4–5 weeks after the symptomatic illness, this serologic test has no role in the diagnosis of acute pharyngitis.

(4) Screening. Household contacts of a symptomatic patient with GAS pharyngitis need not be screened for GAS carriage unless they are also symptomatic or if the index case has acute rheumatic fever.

(5) Approach to therapy of the patient with acute pharyngitis. Because pharyngitis with GAS is usually a self-limited condition that lasts 3–5 days in untreated individuals, it is reasonable to consider the benefits of treating this infection. Potential benefits include (1) slight reduction in the duration or severity of symptoms, or both; (2) prevention of local suppurative complications such as peritonsillar abscess; (3) prevention of spread of GAS to family members or other contacts; and (4) prevention of acute rheumatic fever or glomerulonephritis. Individualized clinical judgment should play a role in the decisions of which patients to culture or antigen test, or both, and which patients to treat. Antigen testing plus culture (the latter only for those with a negative antigen test) has been found to be cost effective (in children) and should be coupled with the strategy to administer antibiotic only if the laboratory test is positive. Practice guidelines from the Infectious Diseases Society of America (IDSA) for the diagnosis and management of GAS pharyngitis are available at the IDSA Web site (http://www.idsociety.org, and *Clin Infect Dis* 1997;25:574).

(6) Treatment of acute streptococcal pharyngitis. Beta-lactam–resistant GAS has not occurred, and penicillin remains the drug of choice for acute pharyngitis. Treatment for adolescents and adults should be penicillin V (250–500 mg PO qid or tid for 10 days) or, for penicillin-allergic patients, erythromycin estolate (250–500 mg PO bid or tid, maximum daily dose 1 g) for 10 days.

B. Bronchitis. Of all cases of chronic obstructive pulmonary disease (COPD), 90% fall into the category of chronic bronchitis. Bronchitis is characterized by productive cough and evidence of airway infection. The absence of abnormalities on chest radiography can usually distinguish bronchitis from pneumonia. Bacterial and viral pathogens are common etiologic agents in acute bronchitis and acute exacerbations of chronic bronchitis.

1. **Acute bronchitis, viral causes.** Clinical features of acute bronchitis include cough, purulent sputum, fever, and prominent constitutional complaints. This constellation of findings leading to a diagnosis of bronchitis often results in the administration of antibiotics even though it is generally caused by viral infection. Bronchitis is therefore one of the most common causes of antibiotic abuse (*Lancet* 1995;345:665). Bronchitis, however, can often precipitate acute respiratory decompensation in patients with advanced COPD, and under these circumstances empiric antibiotic therapy and even hospitalization can be justified. Among the viral agents that cause acute bronchitis, influenza deserves special consideration. Although viral culture of the nasopharynx remains the gold standard for confirming influenza viral infection, several rapid diagnostic tests are commercially available. Such tests have high sensitivities and specificities, respectively, and include tests that detect only influenza type A or tests that detect influenza A as well as B viruses.

2. **Treatment of viral bronchitis.** Four prescription antiviral agents are approved for treating uncomplicated influenza. Amantadine (200 mg PO qd for 10 days) and rimantadine (100 mg PO q12h for 10 days) are approved for prophylaxis and treatment of influenza A, and the neuraminidase inhibitor drugs, zanamivir and oseltamivir, are approved to treat influenza A and B but are not approved for prophylaxis. However, zanamivir (*N Engl J Med* 2000;343:1282) and oseltamivir (*JAMA* 2001;285:748) have demonstrated significant efficacy in prevention of household spread of symptomatic influenza in controlled clinical trials. Zanamivir is not generally recommended for patients with underlying airways disease (asthma or COPD) because it is self-administered as an inhaled particulate and there is a risk of serious adverse respiratory events. The recommended dosage for oseltamivir is 75 mg PO every 12 hours for 5 days. Zanamivir is self-administered, inhaled by mouth with a delivery device provided by the manufacturer, and the recommended dose is 10 mg (2 blister contents, q12h for 5 days).

3. **Influenza vaccination.** Despite the use of rapid diagnostic tests and available prophylactic medications, **influenza vaccination remains the most important measure to protect patients against influenza**. Persons at particularly high risk for complications of influenza are those ≥65 years of age, adults, and children with chronic disorders of the pulmonary or cardiovascular system and chronic metabolic diseases. Women in their second or third trimesters of pregnancy should be immunized.

4. **Other treatable pathogens that cause acute bronchitis** less commonly than viruses include *Mycoplasma pneumoniae*, *Chlamydia pneumoniae*, and *Bordetella pertussis*. *Mycoplasma* and *Chlamydia* infection are relatively common in young adults. Patient complaints usually include sore throat, constitutional symptoms, and cough that may persist for up to 6 weeks. Patients with *Chlamydia* infection complain of sore throat, hoarseness, and persistent cough (very similar to *Mycoplasma* infection). Microscopic examination of the sputum yields mononuclear cells and scant bacteria. *Mycoplasma* immunoglobulin M titers are usually elevated after 7 days, and there may be a cold agglutinin titer greater than 1:64. *B. pertussis* and *B. parapertussis* are the etiologic agents of whooping cough, but adult patients who have been immunized in childhood retain partial immunity, resulting in atypical features of infection that resemble acute bronchitis. Some patients notice a barking cough, sometimes associated with posttussive vomiting. Any patient with severe paroxysmal cough should be evaluated for pertussis with a sputum culture.

5. **Chronic bronchitis.** The definition of chronic bronchitis is "a productive cough with sputum production for 3 months/year for at least 2 con-

secutive years without an underlying etiology such as tuberculosis (TB) or bronchiectasis." The differential diagnosis of chronic productive cough includes several noninfectious entities (see Chap. 11). Etiologic agents are the same as for acute bronchitis, but the bacterial etiologies are relatively more frequent.

6. **Acute exacerbations of chronic bronchitis.** In patients who experience this clinical phenomenon, bacterial infections are commonly suspected but difficult to prove. Viral infections are definitely a common cause of exacerbations of chronic bronchitis. The sputum from patients with chronic bronchitis shows large numbers of neutrophils at all stages of the illness, and it has not been shown to change during exacerbations despite the patients' common perception that their sputum volume and purulent character are increased. Cultures of sputum from patients with chronic bronchitis may yield common respiratory pathogens, but evidence is lacking that this yield is different in patients with or without symptomatic exacerbations of their chronic bronchitis. Because the pathogenic role of these organisms remains in doubt, most experts recommend antibiotic therapy only for those patients with severe symptoms and those with fever.

7. **Management of bronchitis.** Most patients with acute bronchitis can be reassured and provided with symptomatic therapy, such as nonnarcotic cough suppressants [e.g., guaifenesin (Robitussin), 5 ml PO q4h prn for 5–7 days] or decongestants (e.g., chlorpheniramine/phenylephrine, 1–2 tablets PO q12h for 5–7 days), or both. Occasional patients with prolonged cough and typical upper-airway symptoms may prompt a clinical diagnosis of either *Chlamydia* or *Mycoplasma*, and both of these organisms are susceptible to macrolides (clarithromycin, 250–500 mg PO bid for 7–10 days, or azithromycin as a "Z-pack," 500 mg for the first day and 250 mg PO qd for four days); doxycycline, 100 mg PO every 12 hours for 7–10 days; or a fluoroquinolone (e.g., levofloxacin, 500 mg PO qd for 7–10 days). There are no clinical studies, however, that support the use of these agents in the absence of an etiologic diagnosis. Pertussis can be treated with erythromycin base (250–500 mg PO tid for 7–10 days), but when given late in the course of symptoms there is minimal benefit. The antibiotics that are favored for acute exacerbations of chronic bronchitis are amoxicillin (500 mg PO q8h), doxycycline (100 mg PO bid), or TMP/SMZ (1 tablet DS PO bid). The usual course of therapy is 5–7 days.

C. **Community-acquired pneumonia**

1. **Epidemiology of community-acquired pneumonia (CAP) and of pneumococcal disease.** Pneumonia is the sixth leading cause of death in the United States and the most common infectious cause. *Streptococcus pneumoniae* is the most common cause of CAP, and it is responsible for two-thirds of all cases of bacteremic pneumonia. Prospective studies evaluating the causes of CAP in adults, however, have failed to identify the cause of 40–60% of cases. Among immunocompetent adults, cigarette smoking was the strongest independent risk factor for invasive pneumococcal disease in a large multicenter North American study (*N Engl J Med* 2000;342:681). The high prevalence of smoking and a quadrupling of the risk of invasive pneumococcal infection in smokers should increase the motivation for smoking cessation programs and for pneumococcal immunization despite the absence of specific recommendations for this risk group (*N Engl J Med* 2000;342:732).

2. **Causes of CAP.** The most common causes of CAP have been traditionally divided into two categories, the "typical" and "atypical" agents. Typical etiologic agents include *S. pneumoniae, H. influenzae, S. aureus, Klebsiella pneumoniae,* and other gram-negative bacilli and anaerobic bacteria. Atypical agents are *Legionella* species, *M. pneumoniae,* and *C. pneumoniae.* **Pneumococcal pneumonia** is the most common cause of

CAP, and it is generally believed that many cases of culture-negative CAP are caused by the pneumococcus. The rate of false-positive cultures is also high, however, due to nasopharyngeal colonization with pneumococci. Despite the disappointing inadequacy of the diagnostic microbiology, it is reassuring that the majority of CAP cases of unknown etiology respond to a 10-day treatment course with clarithromycin, 500 mg PO every 12 hours; doxycycline, 100 mg PO every 12 hours; or levofloxacin, 500 mg PO qd. All patients with pneumonia should undergo chest radiography, and a follow-up chest radiogram should be considered after 2–3 days of therapy, especially if clinical improvement has not occurred. One must be wary that radiographic findings usually clear more slowly than clinical findings. **Practice guidelines** for the management of CAP in adults are available at the IDSA Web site (http://www.idsociety.org) or in print form (*Clin Infect Dis* 1998;26:811). These include recommendations for routine Gram stain and culture of expectorated sputum, which are at variance with the American Thoracic Society guidelines (*Am Rev Respir Dis* 1993;148:1418). ***H. influenzae*** (usually not type B), ***S. aureus***, and gram-negative bacilli each account for 3–10% of CAP cases. Interpretation of the diagnostic microbiology is complicated for these organisms due to common upper respiratory tract colonization.

3. **Diagnosis of CAP.** The diagnostic approach to the immunocompetent adult patient with CAP begins with a clinical evaluation followed by radiography and microbiologic testing. Pneumonia caused by the pneumococcus is most often associated with cough, sputum production, and fever. A parapneumonic effusion is present in the majority of patients, but empyema is an uncommon complication. No combination of physical examination findings can reliably define the presence of pneumonia. However, the absence of abnormal vital signs or lack of abnormalities on chest auscultation substantially reduces the likelihood of pneumonia.

   a. **The diagnosis of CAP without chest radiographic confirmation** should be considered only if there are significant clinical manifestations such as a new cough with abnormal vital signs and localized auscultatory findings. Given this risk and the cost of inappropriate therapy, the IDSA guidelines recommend that a chest roentgenogram be obtained for the routine evaluation of CAP. Establishing an etiologic diagnosis (by Gram stain and culture of expectorated sputum) is important. This is more strongly recommended for patients who require hospitalization.

   b. **Management of CAP.** A key decision facing the clinician is whether to hospitalize the patient with CAP. The general consensus is that approximately 75% of patients with pneumonia can be treated appropriately in the outpatient setting. Widely endorsed **prediction rules** (*N Engl J Med* 1997;336:243) suggest that if the patient is older than 50 years of age and has comorbid illness (especially neoplastic or liver disease), altered mental status, respiratory rate greater than 30, systolic BP less than 90 mm Hg, and/or arterial pH less than 7.35, elevated BUN, or depressed serum sodium, he or she should probably be treated and monitored in the hospital. Pulse oximetry and arterial blood gas determinations are also helpful in determining the severity of infection.

   c. **Serologic studies are usually not helpful** in the initial diagnostic evaluation of patients with CAP. Urine antigen tests have been shown to be sensitive and specific for detecting *Legionella pneumophila* serogroup 1, which accounts for approximately 70% of cases of Legionnaires' disease in the United States. A positive culture or urine antigen test is virtually diagnostic.

4. **Treatment for CAP.** Empiric therapy for outpatients is based primarily on clinical evaluation. The selection of antibiotics in the absence of an

etiologic diagnosis depends on multiple variables. For the treatment of outpatients, the generally preferred agents can be given orally and include a macrolide, for example, clarithromycin (500 mg PO q12h) or azithromycin (500 mg loading and 250 mg qd thereafter), or erythromycin base (250–500 mg PO q6h). Doxycycline (100 mg PO q12h) is also an option, but not for children younger than 8 years of age, or an oral beta-lactam such as cefuroxime (250–500 mg PO q12h), amoxicillin (250–500 mg PO q8h), or a combination of amoxicillin and potassium clavulanate (875 mg PO q12h). The new fluoroquinolones, for example, gatifloxacin (400 mg PO qd), should be limited to adults (1) for whom one of the above regimens has already failed, (2) who are allergic to alternative agents, or (3) who have documented infection with multidrug-resistant pneumococci. If aspiration pneumonia is suspected, IV ampicillin-sulbactam (Unasyn) is preferred, but cefuroxime (500 mg PO q12h), cefpodoxime (200–400 mg PO q12h), or cefprozil (250–500 mg PO q12h) are alternative options. If a penicillin-susceptible pneumococcus is the cause of CAP, penicillin V (500 mg PO q8h) or amoxicillin (500 mg PO q8h) is the preferred antimicrobial. For intermediate penicillin resistance, parenteral agents suggested by in vitro susceptibility test results are preferred. If the pneumococcal isolate is highly resistant to penicillin, agents based on aggregate susceptibility test results in the community should be chosen for parenteral therapy.

a. **The question of duration of antimicrobial treatment for CAP** remains open. This decision is usually based on the pathogen, response to treatment, comorbid illness, and complications. The IDSA guidelines recommend treatment of bacterial infections, such as those caused by *S. pneumoniae*, until the patient has been afebrile for 72 hours. Pneumonia caused by *Chlamydia* or *Mycoplasma* species should probably be treated for at least 2 weeks, and the same is true for Legionnaires' disease in immunocompetent patients. **Recommendations for changing to oral from intravenous antibiotics include the following:** The patient's condition should be improving clinically, and he or she should be hemodynamically stable, able to ingest drugs, and have a functional GI tract.

b. **Preventive therapy.** The currently available pneumococcal polysaccharide vaccines have shown an aggregate efficacy of ≥60% in preventing bacteremic pneumococcal infection in immunocompetent adults (*Arch Intern Med* 1994;154:2666). Their efficacy tends to decline with age. Despite controversies over vaccine efficacy, the death rate associated with bacteremic pneumococcal infections in persons older than 64 years of age remains high. The IDSA guidelines recommend vaccination for patients with risk factors for pneumococcal disease. Revaccination with pneumococcal polysaccharide vaccine has been recommended for immunocompromised persons older than 10 years of age and if more than 5 years have elapsed since the first vaccination. Revaccination for immunocompetent persons is recommenced for those ≥65 years of age, if the person received his or her first vaccination before age 65, and if more than 5 years have elapsed since the first dose [*MMWR Morbid Mortal Wkly Rep* 1997;46(RR-8, ACIP):1]. Even if these guidelines are followed, there is a significant risk of pain, tenderness, and erythema at the revaccination site. Pneumococcal and influenza vaccine (the latter just before or during the winter flu season) should be administered during hospitalization whenever possible. Immediately after an episode of pneumonia, there is no contraindication for the use of either vaccine. The protein conjugate pneumococcal vaccine (Prevnar) is clearly protective in neonates (<2 years of age), but efficacy in older children or adults remains unclear.

II. Mononucleosis typically occurs in older children and adolescents and is usually caused by the Epstein-Barr virus (EBV). It presents with fever, malaise, pharyngitis, cervical lymphadenopathy, and splenomegaly. The differential CBC shows atypical lymphocytes. Liver tests may be abnormal with a cholestatic pattern. Tests for heterophil antibody (e.g., Monospot) are usually positive but can be negative early in the course of disease. Cytomegalovirus (CMV) is a cause of heterophil-negative mononucleosis, as is primary HIV infection. Complications of EBV or CMV mononucleosis include hemolytic anemia, immune-mediated thrombocytopenia, encephalopathy, and Guillain-Barré syndrome. Airway obstruction and splenic rupture can occur with EBV mononucleosis. Treatment for typical EBV mononucleosis is symptomatic (acetaminophen or nonsteroidal anti-inflammatory agents for fever or pain). Prolonged convalescence is unnecessary, although contact sports should be avoided until splenomegaly resolves. Steroids (40–60 mg prednisone daily for 7–14 days) may be indicated to alleviate airway obstruction and immune-mediated complications. Antiviral therapy is not indicated except for acute HIV.

III. Varicella-zoster virus is a herpes group virus that causes varicella (chickenpox) and zoster (shingles).

    A. Diagnosis. Chickenpox in adults occurs in nonimmune individuals, usually following exposure to an infected child. Crops of vesicular lesions on an erythematous base ("dewdrops on a rose petal") occur at various stages of evolution, from vesicles to crusted pustules. Fever is usually present. Zoster (shingles) presents as a painful vesicular eruption in a dermatomal distribution. Trigeminal zoster, particularly involving the ophthalmic branch, may result in eye involvement and warrants formal ophthalmologic consultation to exclude this. Dissemination to skin and viscera may occur in immunocompromised individuals. These infections do not usually present a diagnostic dilemma. If the diagnosis is in doubt, a scraping from the base of a vesicle can be submitted on a glass slide for a direct fluorescent antibody test.

    B. Treatment. Because even immunocompetent adult patients can become quite ill and are at risk for varicella pneumonia, such individuals should be treated with acyclovir, 800 mg qid, or famciclovir, 500 mg tid for 5 days. Pulmonary involvement may be suggested by cough or dyspnea and should prompt a chest radiograph. Immunocompromised hosts with varicella and immunocompetent hosts with pneumonia should be treated with acyclovir, 10 mg/kg intravenously every 8 hours for 8–10 days. Treatment of disseminated zoster in immunocompromised individuals is the same as with varicella, using parenteral acyclovir. Ocular zoster in immunocompetent individuals also warrants parenteral therapy. In normal hosts, localized zoster can be treated with a 7-day course of valacyclovir, 1 g tid; famciclovir, 500 mg tid; or acyclovir, 800 mg five times/day. Oral agents are most effective in decreasing symptoms when treatment is initiated with 48 hours of lesion onset. Use of prednisone as adjunctive therapy is controversial. Postherpetic neuralgia can be severe and require narcotics for relief. Neuralgia may respond to tricyclic antidepressants (amitriptyline 12.5–25.0 mg qhs, titrate as required), gabapentin (100–400 mg tid), or topical capsaicin (0.025% cream to affected areas three to five times/day). For persistent neuralgia, topical lidocaine patches, neural blockade, nonpharmacologic approaches, and referral to pain clinic are other options to consider.

IV. Bites

    A. Dog and cat bites are a common occurrence and account for a large number of emergency room and office visits [*Arch Intern Med* 1997;157(17):1933]. The majority of these bites are caused by a known animal and occur most commonly on the extremities. A large proportion of bites become infected. Infection is predicted by presentation more than 8 hours after the bite, older age, and puncture wounds. Puncture wounds may be associated with septic arthritis, tenosynovitis, or abscess. Infected bites may have localized cellulitis with purulent discharge. A minority of patients have fever, adenopathy, or lymphangitis. Usual pathogens include *S. aureus*, streptococci, *Pas-*

teurella multocida, *Eikenella corrodens*, various aerobic gram-negative rods, and anaerobes. Initial treatment consists of irrigation and débridement. Most wounds should not be closed. Edematous wounds should be elevated, and hand wounds can be splinted. Antibiotic treatment consists of **amoxicillin-clavulanate**, 500 mg PO tid, or **ampicillin-sulbactam**, 1.5–3.0 g IV every 6 hours. An alternative regimen for beta-lactam–allergic patients includes a **quinolone** (e.g., ciprofloxacin, 500 mg bid, plus **clindamycin**, 450 mg qid). **Tetanus immunization should be up to date.** For bat or wild carnivore bites, or unprovoked dog or cat bites, rabies immunization (rabies immune globulin plus human diploid cell vaccine series) should be considered after consultation with the local health department.

- **B. Spider bites** may cause discomfort and a local reaction. In the United States, bites from the black widow (*Lactrodectus mactans* and *hesperus*) and the brown recluse spider (*Loxosceles reclusa*) may become clinically significant. More than half of black widow spider bites occur in California, while the brown recluse spider populates areas in the south central and southeastern United States. Identification of spider type is helpful in determining treatment. Tetanus prophylaxis should be administered for all spider bites.

    - **1. Black widow.** The female black widow characteristically has bright red or orange markings on the ventral abdomen contrasted against a glossy black body. Bites may be unprovoked, cause local pain or numbness, and cause systemic symptoms within minutes or hours due to a neurotoxin in the venom. With severe envenomations, seizures, respiratory distress, diffuse muscle spasms, and shock can occur. Abdominal rigidity can be striking although no abdominal tenderness on palpation may be present. Symptoms generally peak and resolve within several days. Treatment is largely symptomatic and supportive, focusing on wound care, pain relief, and muscle relaxation. In selected patients (small children, elderly, debilitated, or patients with a chronic illness) cautious administration of an equine serum antivenom may be appropriate in severe or life-threatening envenomations.

    - **2. Brown recluse.** The brown recluse spider can be identified by a dark violin pointing backward on the dorsal thorax against a tan or brown body. Bites can be variably painful. Shortly thereafter, the site may become erythematous with a central clearing and subsequent bleb or vesicle formation may ensue. With severe envenomations, fever, nausea, vomiting, hemolysis, thrombocytopenia, and shock can be present. Treatment is directed at local wound care with the use of antihistamines and analgesics as needed. Early local excision, oral dapsone, and steroids have been helpful in some circumstances, but are not standard treatment strategies. With systemic symptoms or severe necrosis, appropriate referral may be necessary.

- **C. Insect bites** (see Chap. 26).

- **D. Human bites** are managed in much the same manner as animal bites. Clenched-fist injuries often result in septic arthritis, tenosynovitis, or fasciitis. Assessment of HIV risk and need for HIV prophylaxis should be considered.

- **V. Travel medicine**

    - **A. General measures.** Food and waterborne diseases are the number one cause of illness in travelers. Viruses, bacteria, or parasites can cause travelers' diarrhea. Travelers should be instructed on common-sense measures to prevent illness, including washing hands often with soap and water; drinking only bottled or boiled water or carbonated drinks in cans or bottles; and avoiding tap water, fountain drinks, ice cubes, unpasteurized dairy products, and food purchased from street vendors: "Boil it, peel it, or forget it." If drinking unbottled water is necessary, it may be made safer by filtering through an "absolute 1-μ or less" filter and adding iodine tablets to the filtered water. If diarrhea occurs, in most cases it resolves spontaneously. Over-the-counter antidiarrheal agents can be taken in the absence of fever.

If fever or bloody diarrhea occurs, a quinolone antibiotic such as ciprofloxacin, 500 mg bid for 5 days, may be beneficial.

B. Protection from insect-borne diseases can be achieved by remaining in well-screened areas, using repellents and permethrin-impregnated mosquito nets, wearing long-sleeved shirts and long pants from dusk through dawn, and using insect repellent that contains DEET (diethylmethyltoluamide) in 30–35% strength for adults and 6–10% for children. In areas with schistosomiasis, travelers should not swim in fresh water [Centers for Disease Control and Prevention (CDC). *Health information for international travel 1999–2000.* Atlanta, GA: DHHS; **http://www.cdc.gov/travel/index.htm**; CDC voice information service 888-232-3228, fax information service 888-232-3299, or 1-877-FYI-TRIP (394-8747)].

C. **Malaria** is caused by protozoa of the genus *Plasmodium.* It is endemic to most of the tropical and subtropical world.

   1. **Malaria prophylaxis** is important to consider if traveling to Mexico, Central and South America, Dominican Republic, Haiti, Africa, parts of the Middle East, Asia, and a few countries within Eastern Europe. For travel to areas of risk where chloroquine-resistant *Plasmodium falciparum* has **not** been reported, once-a-week use of **chloroquine** (500 mg salt) is recommended. Chloroquine prophylaxis should begin 1–2 weeks before travel to malarious areas. It should be continued weekly during travel in malarious areas and for 4 weeks after a person leaves such areas.

   2. For travel to areas of risk where chloroquine-resistant *P. falciparum* exists, weekly use of **mefloquine** (250 mg salt) is recommended. Mefloquine prophylaxis should begin 1–2 weeks before travel to malarious areas. It should be continued weekly during travel in malarious areas and for 4 weeks after a person leaves such areas. Persons who travel to areas where drug-resistant *P. falciparum* is endemic and for whom mefloquine is not recommended may elect to use doxycycline. **Doxycycline** (100 mg PO daily) and atovaquone/proguanil (**Malarone**) are the only available effective prophylactic drugs for travelers to malaria-endemic areas of Thailand that border Myanmar and Cambodia. Travelers who use doxycycline should be cautioned about the risk of photosensitivity. Doxycycline prophylaxis should begin 1–2 days before travel to malarious areas. It should be continued daily during travel in malarious areas and for 4 weeks after the traveler leaves such areas. *Plasmodium vivax* and *Plasmodium ovale* parasites can persist in the liver and cause relapses for as long as 4 years after routine chemoprophylaxis is discontinued. **Atovaquone,** 250 mg, plus **proguanil,** 100 mg, can also be taken beginning 1–2 days before entering a malarious area and continued for 7 days following return. Primaquine decreases the risk of relapse of these forms of malaria. **Primaquine,** 1 tablet daily, is administered after the traveler has left a malaria-endemic area, usually during or following the last 2 weeks of prophylaxis. Because the risk of relapse to the usual traveler is small, prophylaxis with primaquine is generally indicated only for persons who have had prolonged exposure in malaria-endemic areas (e.g., missionaries and Peace Corps volunteers).

   3. **Malaria** begins as a nonspecific illness characterized by fever and chills, headache, myalgias, arthralgia, nausea, vomiting, or diarrhea. Left untreated, the illness may proceed to severe anemia, thrombocytopenia, pulmonary edema, hypoglycemia, encephalopathy, and death. Malaria should be suspected when illness occurs in a patient who has recently visited an endemic area. **Diagnosis** is made by identification of the parasites in a blood smear stained with Giemsa stain. Current information on the incidence of resistance in various regions of the world, prophylaxis, and treatment issues can also be obtained from the CDC, 1-877-FYI-TRIP (394-8747).

4. **P. falciparum malaria**, the most severe form of the disease, is a medical emergency. Chloroquine resistance is widespread. To date, the only areas of the world where there has been no documented resistance are Central America, Haiti, the Dominican Republic, and Egypt. Sulfadoxine-pyrimethamine (Fansidar) resistance occurs in Southeast Asia and the Amazon. Because of the widespread distribution of chloroquine resistance in *P. falciparum*, chloroquine resistance should be presumed in patients in whom *P. falciparum* malaria develops unless a careful history reveals travel only to areas where resistance does not occur. Chloroquine resistance should also be presumed in patients with severe infections (parasitemia >5% or mental status changes) and in those in whom malaria develops despite chloroquine prophylaxis.

   a. **Treatment.** Presumed **chloroquine-resistant** *P. falciparum* malaria should be treated with two drugs: quinine sulfate, 650 mg PO tid, and doxycycline, 100 mg PO bid, for 3 days. Sulfadoxine-pyrimethamine, three tablets PO as a single dose, can be substituted for tetracycline unless the patient acquired the disease in an area of Fansidar resistance. Patients who acquire *P. falciparum* in Thailand or surrounding countries should receive a 7-day course of quinine and tetracycline. Proguanil, four tablets PO once a day for 3 days, is also an option. Severe *P. falciparum* infection (see above), requires parenteral therapy with tetracycline, 250 mg IV qid, and quinidine gluconate, 10 mg/kg IV over 1–2 hours, followed by 0.02 mg/kg/minute as a continuous infusion (*N Engl J Med* 1989;321:65). Patients who require quinidine IV should be monitored for hypotension and arrhythmias in an intensive care setting. When the level of parasitemia falls to less than 1% and the patient is able to take oral medication, quinine sulfate and tetracycline can be given orally to complete a 3-day course of therapy. For parasitemias greater than 10%, exchange transfusion should be considered.

   b. *P. falciparum* malaria that is acquired in areas where chloroquine resistance does not occur can be treated with **chloroquine base**, 600 mg (1000 mg chloroquine phosphate) PO, followed in 6 hours by 300 mg PO and an additional 300 mg PO qd for 2 days. **Non-*Falciparum* malaria** is less severe and usually responds to oral chloroquine. Patients with *P. vivax* or *P. ovale* infection may relapse several months after their initial illness because of the persistence of dormant forms (hypnozoites) in the liver. After screening for glucose-6-phosphate dehydrogenase deficiency, these should be eradicated with primaquine, 15 mg base PO qd for 14 days. Relapses should be treated with chloroquine and primaquine.

D. **Vaccines** (see also Chap. 1). The following vaccines should be considered for the traveler. Specific recommendations regarding vaccines can be obtained from local health departments or the CDC (http://www.cdc.gov/travel/vaccinat.htm).

   1. **Diphtheria-tetanus.** After completion of a primary series, a booster should be administered once every 10 years for life.

   2. **Hepatitis A.** Consider for all travelers except those who are traveling to developed countries in Europe, Japan, Australia, New Zealand, or Canada.

   3. **Hepatitis B virus (HBV).** Consider for long-term travelers (staying >6 months) who are going to intermediate- or high-prevalence areas and any short-term travelers who may have contact with blood or body fluids (e.g., health care workers) if they have not had the vaccine previously.

   4. **Polio.** After completion of a primary series, CDC recommends an additional dose once in adult life if traveling to a country where the disease occurs (no Western Hemisphere countries).

   5. **Measles.** The CDC recommends a dose of measles vaccine for persons born in or after 1957 who have not had two doses on or after the first birthday. Exceptions include pregnant women and other persons for

whom it is contraindicated (e.g., those who are severely immunocompromised), who should not get measles vaccine. Vaccination is not necessary for persons with documentation of physician-diagnosed measles or serologic evidence of measles immunity.

6. **Meningococcus.** Consider if traveling during December–June to the savanna areas of sub-Saharan Africa ("meningitis belt"). It should also be considered for travelers to Saudi Arabia during the Hajj and Umra.

7. **Typhoid.** Consider for travelers to developing countries and those who are staying in areas of questionable sanitation.

8. **Yellow fever.** Yellow fever is endemic in sub-Saharan Africa and portions of South America. Some countries require a certificate of vaccination if traveling directly from the United States, and some require a certificate only if a traveler arrives from an infected area. Check with the CDC to determine if any country on the traveler's itinerary is currently infected with yellow fever.

9. **Japanese encephalitis.** This vaccine should generally be considered for travelers who visit Asia, the Indian subcontinent, and the Western Pacific for 30 days or longer.

10. **Rabies.** Consider for travelers who might be exposed to wild or domestic animals through work or recreation, except in countries listed as "rabies free."

Gastrointestinal Infections

Epidemiology of diarrheal illness. Foodborne diseases cause approximately 0.75 episodes of acute diarrheal illness/person/year in the United States. Unfortunately, known pathogens account for fewer than 20% of foodborne illnesses. The IDSA has published guidelines for the diagnosis and management of infectious diarrhea (*Clin Infect Dis* 2001;32:331), and these guidelines are also available on the Web (http://www.idsociety.org). A U.S. governmental Web site monitors the epidemiology and severity of GI infections (http://www.cdc.gov/ncidod/dbmd/foodnet). Adequate evaluation of a patient who presents with a diarrheal illness requires questioning about the severity and type of illness (febrile, hemorrhagic, nosocomial, persistent, inflammatory), exposures (travel; ingestion of raw or undercooked meat, seafood, or milk products; contacts who are ill; day care or institutional exposure; recent antibiotic use), and whether the patient is immunocompromised.

I. **Definitions. Diarrhea** is defined as an increase in the water content, volume, or frequency of stools. **Community-acquired or travelers' diarrhea** should prompt consideration of (culture or test for) *Shigella, Campylobacter, Escherichia coli* O157:H7, and *Clostridium difficile* toxins, or, for patients with seafood or seacoast exposure, *Vibrio* species. **Nosocomial diarrhea** is dominated by *C. difficile* as the causative agent. **Persistent diarrhea** is one that occurs for more than 7 days and is usually caused by intestinal parasites, including *Giardia, Cryptosporidium, Cyclospora,* or *Isospora belli* (also *Microsporidium* and *Mycobacterium avium* complex if the patient is immunocompromised). CMV can produce acute or subacute, sometimes bloody, diarrhea that is most often acquired as a result of blood transfusion or unprotected sex.

II. **Clinical approach to the patient with diarrhea.** The primary focus should be on the patient rather than on any particular etiology. Generally, patients with bloody diarrhea, peritoneal signs, or high fever associated with symptoms of gastroenteritis should be considered candidates for hospitalization. Patients with tachycardia, postural hypotension, weakness, confusion, and poor skin turgor should be referred for emergency care and parenteral rehydration. For the great majority of patients who do not require hospital care, the first concern should be their ability to cooperate with oral correction of dehydration, acidosis, and hypokalemia. Oral rehydration is underused in the United States, where IV hydration has become a reflex response. The composition of oral rehydration solution (ORS), recommended by the World Health Organization (WHO), consists of 1 L water containing 3.5 g sodium chloride, 2.9 g trisodium citrate or 2.5 g sodium bicarbonate, 1.5 g potassium chloride, and 20 g glucose or 40 g sucrose. WHO-ORS is a product of Jianas Bros. (St. Louis, MO), and other formulations, Rehydrolyte, Pedialyte, and Oral Electrolyte Solution (Ross Laboratories, Columbus, OH) or generic solutions are available over the counter.

III. **Major subgroups and etiologies of diarrheal diseases in the United States**
   A. **Toxigenic diarrheas** are caused by bacterial strains that elaborate enterotoxins that cause dehydrating diarrhea with little or no fever. Non–cholera vibrios contaminate shellfish (oysters, clams, mussels, and crabs) harvested from coastal waters. The most recent data indicate oyster contamination rates of 10–30%. *Vibrio vulnificus* produces the most severe illness, especially in patients with liver disease. Infection with this or other vibrios can also be acquired by contamination of pre-existing body surface wounds through direct contact with organisms in seawater. **Recommended empiric therapy** includes ciprofloxacin (750 mg PO, single dose), doxycycline (300 mg PO, single dose), or TMP/SMZ (1 tablet DS PO bid for 3 days). These diarrheas are often associated with midabdominal pain. They may be associated with soft-tissue infection with or without bacteremia or sepsis.
   B. *E. coli* is part of the normal GI flora, but it may cause diarrheal disease. The hemorrhagic colitis–producing *E. coli* (O157:H7 and others) are cytotoxin-producing strains that also cause the hemolytic-uremic syndrome. Prepared meat products and hamburger are the principal sources. Transmission of these *E. coli* strains from person to person is uncommon but has been documented in day care centers and nursing homes. Antimicrobial treatment is generally **withheld** from these patients, because there are studies that indicate more serious clinical features in recipients of antibiotic therapy with only slightly shorter duration of diarrhea. It should be kept in mind that the inflammatory bowel diseases such as ulcerative colitis or Crohn's disease can sometimes present acutely with symptoms that mimic infectious diarrhea, except that the course is likely to be prolonged rather than self-limited. The same is true for patients with lactase deficiency or with a first episode of irritable bowel syndrome. Ischemic bowel disease can also produce a noninfectious diarrheal syndrome, generally in elderly patients with symptoms of bloody diarrhea and abdominal pain.
   C. **Invasive diarrhea** is caused by *Shigella* species, *Salmonella* species, *Listeria monocytogenes*, and enterohemorrhagic *E. coli* strains.
      1. **Shigellosis** is transmitted from person to person. It is often clinically indistinguishable from salmonellosis. Household pets (turtles and lizards) may play a role in transmission. Poultry, meats, eggs, and dairy products have been implicated in focal outbreaks or epidemics. The stools are often bloody with abundant WBC. Tenesmus (rectal pain) and lower-abdominal pain are typical with these organisms. The diarrhea is initially watery, followed after a few days by multiple small-volume bloody mucoid stools. **Treatment** of *Shigella* enteritis is TMP/SMZ (1 tablet DS PO bid for 3 days) or ciprofloxacin (500 mg PO bid for 3 days).
      2. *Salmonella* infections are also associated with foodborne outbreaks. Eggs and chickens are common food sources. **Treatment** of *Salmonella* and *Shigella* infection is generally supportive because the process is usually self-limited; however, antibiotics may be indicated in severe cases, especially in children (not quinolones in children), immunocompromised patients, and the elderly. Ciprofloxacin (500 mg PO bid), ofloxacin (400 mg PO bid), or TMP/SMZ (1 tablet DS PO bid) is recommended for 3–7 days. Ampicillin-resistant strains of *Salmonella* and *Shigella* are common.

D. Typhoid fever is a disease of humans only. Infection is generally via contaminated water and, less commonly, food. Four *Salmonella typhi* syndromes are recognized: gastroenteritis, enteric fever, bacteremia, and enteric carriage. Long-term human carriers are the source of *S. typhi* infections. The reservoir site is usually the biliary tree, and carriage is more common in patients with gallbladder calculi. A third-generation cephalosporin (e.g., ceftriaxone, 2 g IV qd) should be elected, although resistant strains have been reported. Asymptomatic *S. typhi* carriers (>1 year by definition) should receive treatment in an effort to minimize the risk of spread to other individuals. No antibiotic has been shown to be consistently successful, but treatment of enteric carriage should be attempted with either ciprofloxacin (500–750 mg PO bid) or amoxicillin (6 g PO qd) plus probenecid (2 g PO qd), for 6 weeks. **Antimotility drugs** can also be used for the symptomatic treatment of patients with acute diarrhea in whom fever is absent or low grade and stools are not bloody. The dose of loperamide (Imodium) is two tablets (4 mg) PO initially, then one tablet after each unformed stool, not to exceed 16 mg/day, or give diphenoxylate (Lomotil), two tablets qid for ≤2 days. Both drugs may facilitate the development of hemolytic-uremic syndrome in patients who are infected with enterohemorrhagic *E. coli*. Fluids should be used aggressively with antimotility agents.

E. Listeriosis is a serious bacterial infection caused by eating food contaminated with *L. monocytogenes*. Foodborne outbreaks have been recognized in the United States with increasing frequency and have been traced by the CDC to uncooked vegetables, milk and milk products (even after pasteurization), fish, and fresh or processed chicken or beef. Long incubation periods (mean, 31 days) are typical, but one report documents an outbreak of a febrile gastroenteritis syndrome due to ingestion of *Listeria*-contaminated chocolate milk, and the median incubation time was only 20 hours (*N Engl J Med* 1997;336:100). Rates of serious *Listeria* infection are highest among infants and adults older than 60 years of age. In pregnant women, fetal infection with abortion may result. More severe infections, including bacteremia or meningitis, or both, occur in immunocompromised patients. The CDC has noted a high case fatality rate (23%) from foodborne listeriosis. If foodborne *Listeria* infection is suspected, hospitalization and parenteral therapy with ampicillin and an aminoglycoside or TMP/SMZ should be considered.

F. *Campylobacter* and *Yersinia*. Animal reservoirs include dogs, birds, cattle, sheep, and swine, but chickens account for 50–70% of human infections with *Campylobacter jejuni*. Infection can usually be related to undercooked contaminated food. *Yersinia enterocolitica* epidemics have been traced to contaminated milk and ice cream, as well as lake water and streams. Animal sources include puppies, cats, chickens, horses, and cows. *Yersinia* enteritis often clears without specific therapy. *Campylobacter* and *Yersinia* gastroenteritis can be treated with ciprofloxacin (500 mg PO bid for 3–5 days) or TMP/SMZ (1 tablet DS PO bid for 3–5 days), erythromycin (250–500 mg PO qid for 5 days), or doxycycline (100 mg PO bid for 7 days).

G. Other bacterial causes of diarrhea are *Aeromonas* species and *Plesiomonas shigelloides*. *Aeromonas* are ubiquitous environmental organisms that are found mainly in fresh and brackish water during summer months. Well water and spring water for drinking are also potential sources. *P. shigelloides* infection is associated with consumption of raw oysters or with travel to Mexico or the Orient. In most cases of diarrhea that are associated with these agents, no antibiotic therapy is indicated, but severe cases can be treated successfully with TMP/SMZ (1 tablet DS PO bid for 3 days) or with ciprofloxacin (500 mg PO bid for 3 days).

H. Viral diarrhea is caused by the caliciviruses such as the Norwalk agent, now recognized as the most common cause of outbreaks of acute nonbacterial gastroenteritis throughout the world [*J Infect Dis* 2000;181(Suppl 2):S254]. In the United States, these outbreaks occur commonly among children in day care centers. Except for the Norwalk agent, the etiology is generally not identified. The Norwalk virus causes approximately 40% of the nonbacterial epidemics of gastroenteritis in the United States. It does not produce a specific pattern of illness but has a short incubation period of 24–48 hours. Clusters occur in nursing homes, hospitals, and cruise ships as well as other institutional living arrangements. Transmission is by person to person spread, but infants are generally spared. Raw shellfish and contaminated drinking water are potential sources. **Rotavirus** is responsible for 35% of diarrhea cases in hospitalized children. It is spread by the fecal-oral route and is more common during the winter months in the United States. Older children and adults may be asymptomatic carriers. Antigen detection kits are available for identification of rotavirus, but this organism is rarely found in adults. Only supportive or symptomatic therapy is available for the viral diarrheas.

I. Parasitic etiologies of diarrhea seen in the United States

   1. ***Giardia lamblia*** is a ubiquitous protozoan that contaminates water or food and spreads from person to person by the fecal-oral route. Outbreaks tend to occur among travelers to wilderness areas or to developing countries. They are also more likely to occur among children in day care centers, in male homosexuals, and in institutionalized populations. Reservoirs include dogs, cats, sheep, and beavers. Treatment is metronidazole (250–500 mg PO tid for 5–10 days) or quinacrine (100 mg PO tid for 7–10 days).

   2. ***Entamoeba histolytica*** enteric infections result in an estimated 50 million cases worldwide annually. Like *Giardia*, it is most often spread from contaminated water sources or by person to person by fecal-oral transmission. It tends to occur in travelers, institutionalized persons, male homosexuals, and immigrants. Malnutrition, young age, pregnancy, malignancy, and glucocorticoid use are risk factors for more severe disease. Treatment for tissue phase infection is with metronidazole (500–750 mg PO or IV tid for 5–10 days) followed by a luminal agent such as iodoquinol (650 mg PO tid for 21 days) or paromomycin (25–30 mg/kg/day for 7 days).

   3. ***Cryptosporidium parvum*** is mainly an infection of patients with AIDS and other immunocompromised patients, but it is distributed worldwide, with a higher prevalence in underdeveloped countries. Waterborne infection and person-to-person or animal-to-person transmission are important epidemiologic factors. Outbreaks occur in families, day care centers, or health care facilities. Treatment for cryptosporidiosis in immunocompetent patients is generally unnecessary.

   4. ***Cyclospora cayetanensis*** was recognized in the United States after an outbreak that was caused by the importation of contaminated raspberries. Food and waterborne outbreaks have been reported previously. Established cases of *Cyclospora* infection should be reported to the CDC. Treatment with TMP/SMZ (1 tablet DS PO bid for 3 days) is generally effective in HIV-positive as well as normal hosts. Ciprofloxacin treatment is only slightly less effective.

   5. **Other causes** include *I. belli* and *Balantidium coli*, which are rare in the United States. These intestinal parasites are more likely to produce subacute or chronic symptoms. Treatment is with TMP/SMZ (1 tablet DS PO bid), but optimal duration has not been established. Ciprofloxacin is also effective.

J. Nosocomial diarrhea. *C. difficile* strains that secrete enterotoxins are the major cause of nosocomial diarrhea in the United States. Elderly debilitated patients or those in intensive care units are most frequently affected. Prior use of antibiotics, especially cephalosporins, other beta-lactams, or clindamycin, is a major risk factor, but nosocomial diarrhea may follow the use of any antibiotic and has also been noted after administration of cancer chemotherapeutic agents. Environmental contamination with bacterial spores promotes horizontal spread on the hands of medical personnel. Treatment is preferably with oral metronidazole (250–500 mg PO tid for 10–14 days) and should include discontinuation of all other antibiotics, if possible.

K. Food poisoning and travelers' diarrhea. The greatest risk is associated with travel to Latin America, Asia, and Africa. Intermediate risk is associated with travel to Southern European countries, Israel, and some Caribbean islands. Low-risk areas include Canada, the United States, Northern Europe, Australia, New Zealand, Japan, and most Caribbean islands. Travelers' diarrhea is a consequence of ingesting a fecally contaminated food or beverage. Particularly risky foods are raw vegetables, undercooked meat or fish, tap water, ice, unpasteurized milk or other dairy products, and peeled fruit. A good rule to follow when traveling in high-risk countries is never to eat any food unless you can peel it or have it thoroughly cooked. Short-term self-limited diarrhea is the rule even without treatment, but most prefer to take 3–5 days of TMP/SMZ (1 tablet DS PO bid) or ciprofloxacin (500 mg PO bid), and this usually shortens the symptomatic period.

    1. *Bacillus cereus* food poisoning usually occurs with foods that were contaminated before cooking and their subsequent maintenance at warm but not high temperature, which permits growth of the vegetative bacterial forms in the food before ingestion. When vomiting also occurs (usually within a few hours), it is almost always the result of ingestion of contaminated fried rice. Treatment with antibiotics is of no value.

    2. Mushroom poisoning. This form of food poisoning is caused by *Amanita* species of mushrooms, but it has similarities to *B. cereus* enteritis in time of onset and symptoms (vomiting and diarrhea). *Amanita* toxin, which is tasteless and not destroyed by cooking, results in hepatic and renal failure. Treatment is gastric lavage, activated charcoal, and fluid and electrolyte replacement (*Can Med Assoc J* 1997;157:431).

    3. Botulism is the result of *Clostridium botulinum* wound infection or ingestion of preformed *C. botulinum* exotoxin in contaminated, usually home-canned food. The incubation period is 12–36 hours after ingestion, and the usual clinical presentation is the acute onset of bilateral cranial nerve palsies followed by symmetric descending muscle weakness. Older patients have a higher fatality rate. Treatment is equine antitoxin, available from the CDC, which should be notified of all cases (telephone: 404-639-3670).

    4. *Clostridium perfringens* is responsible for another form of food poisoning. Outbreaks tend to involve large gatherings such as neighborhood or institutional picnics where meat or poultry has been precooked and then reheated only to a serving temperature, not cooking temperature. This results in germination of clostridial spores followed by growth and the secretion of potent exotoxins, which cause diarrhea and abdominal cramps. The syndrome is self-limited, and mortality is extremely rare. Antimicrobial therapy is not indicated.

    5. Other causes of food poisoning include biological chemical toxins (e.g., shellfish), heavy metals such as cadmium or arsenic, or the common seasoning agent, monosodium L-glutamate. These can be suspected from the clinical history, but only the heavy metals can be detected by assay. Treatment is determined by etiology.

IV. Diarrheas in the immunocompromised host

    A. Fecal-oral protozoal agents, such as those that cause cryptosporidiosis and microsporidiosis, have become less common in HIV-infected patients because of the availability of potent antiretroviral therapy. Microsporidia such as *Enterocytozoon bieneusi* and *Encephalitozoon intestinalis* are causes of chronic diarrhea. The mode of transmission is unknown, although homosexuals and foreign travelers are at greatest risk. Recommended therapy for microsporidiosis is albendazole (400 mg PO bid). *C. parvum* continues to be a common cause of diarrhea in those with advanced HIV infection, who are noncompliant or who refuse antiretroviral therapy. Specific treatment for *C. parvum* diarrhea is often unsuccessful, although improvement generally occurs with the immunologic reconstitution that accompanies successful highly active antiretroviral therapy (HAART). Some anecdotal reports suggest improvement with administration of the nonabsorbable aminoglycoside, paromomycin (2–4 g/day PO in divided doses). Another common cause of chronic recurring diarrhea in AIDS patients is enteric infection with MAC. GI involvement with *M. avium* complex (MAC) is a manifestation of disseminated MAC infection, and successful control (treatment with clarithromycin and ethambutol) is usually dependent on coadministration of HAART with resultant immune reconstitution.

  B. HIV enteropathy is a poorly characterized process that is attributed to HIV infection of small-intestinal mucosal cells seen mainly in patients with advanced or untreated HIV infection. Institution of HAART or symptomatic antimotility therapy is the major therapeutic option.

Fungal Infections

I. *Candida* species. *Candida albicans* is part of the normal GI flora, but it can be recovered in the absence of infection from the skin, sputum, female genital tract, and urine of patients with indwelling bladder catheters. Practice guidelines for the treatment of candidiasis are available at the IDSA Web site (http://www.idsociety.org) or in print format (*Clin Infect Dis* 2000;30:662).

  A. Thrush. This is a specific form of oral mucosal candidiasis. It occurs commonly in patients with relatively advanced AIDS, other immunodeficiencies, and children (e.g., asthma treated with inhaled steroids). It appears as white curd-like patches on the tongue and buccal mucous membranes. When patches are scraped off with a tongue blade, they leave a raw, bleeding painful surface. The diagnosis can be made visually and confirmed by microscopic examination of the lesion scraping, which reveals masses of hyphae and yeast. Culture is not recommended routinely because *Candida* grow in samples obtained from the mouth or throat in the presence or absence of thrush. Treatment is with oral nystatin (500,000 units "swish and swallow" 3–5 times/day), clotrimazole troches dissolved in the mouth five times/day, or oral fluconazole (100–400 mg PO qd). Itraconazole (PO or IV) or even IV amphotericin B (AMB) may rarely be required, especially in patients with chronic or extensive refractory candidiasis.

  B. Esophageal candidiasis. This infection may occur independently of oral candidiasis in AIDS or other immunocompromised states. A definitive diagnosis can be established by endoscopy. It sometimes coinfects the esophagus along with herpes simplex virus (HSV) or, less commonly, CMV. Treatment is usually successful with fluconazole (200–400 mg PO or IV qd for 10–14 days).

  C. *Candida* vaginitis occurs in women without any known predisposition, although it is most common in patients who are pregnant, have received antibiotics, or have diabetes mellitus. Vaginal carriage of *Candida* is higher among women who use oral contraceptives, and this seems to be directly related to the estrogen dosage, although the mechanism is unclear. Recurrent symptomatic infection is a significant problem that is generally unrelated to the development of resistance to antifungals. Some patients can only be cured after discontinuation of oral contraceptives. Either thick or thin vaginal discharge may be noted. Erythema of the vagina and labia is usually present. Dysuria generally denotes urethral involvement. Many intravaginal products provide adequate therapy for the nonimmunocompromised patient. These include clotrimazole vaginal cream or tablet; miconazole cream, suppository, or tablet; butoconazole cream; and terconazole suppository. They should be applied at bedtime. Courses of topical therapy are usually 3 days. Seven-day courses are only marginally better. A single oral dose of 150 mg fluconazole is more expensive but preferred by many patients.

D. Cutaneous candidiasis. Intertrigo is a common skin infection that affects moist skin surfaces such as the groin and axilla and under pendulous breasts, skin folds, or any areas of skin redundancy and maceration due to collected moisture, often seen in obese persons. Treatment is recommended with nystatin powder applied bid with or without the addition of an oral azole such as fluconazole (100–400 mg PO qd).

E. Candida paronychia and onychomycosis. *Candida* is a common cause of focal purulent infection at the lateral or proximal margins of fingernails or less commonly of toenails. Frequent immersion of the hands in water is a risk factor, and **paronychia** occur predominantly in laundry and kitchen workers. Artificial acrylic fingernails of health care workers have been shown to be more likely to harbor *Candida* (and other pathogens) than native nails. A possible role of artificial nails in the transmission of nosocomial pathogens has been suggested, but no predisposition to development of paronychia has been reported. Treatment of paronychia should include avoidance of all wet work and treatment with oral azole therapy such as itraconazole (200 mg PO qd for 1–4 weeks). Chronic paronychia can be treated with thymol 2–4% in absolute alcohol bid–tid. Surgical marsupialization is recommended for refractory cases. **Onychomycosis** is a result of chronic nailbed fungal infection. Untreated, it leads to thickening and discoloration of the nail. Treatment of onychomycosis is with itraconazole (200 mg PO qd) for 4–6 months (fingernails) or 10–18 months (toenails).

F. Disseminated candidiasis. Risk factors for invasion of the vascular system by *Candida* species include injection drug use, central venous catheters (especially when total parenteral nutrition is administered), and pressure monitoring devices. Treatment with antibacterial agents may also enhance the growth of fungal organisms including *Candida* species. Disseminated *Candida* infection almost always prompts hospitalization, and if an intravenous catheter is present, removal of the catheter is of primary importance. IV antifungal therapy is recommended, and this may require AMB (0.5–0.7 mg/kg IV qd) rather than fluconazole or itraconazole, especially if *Candida krusei, Candida glabrata*, or other relatively azole-resistant organisms are isolated.

II. Tinea infections are commonly known as **ringworm**. They are infections of the keratinized tissues, including the skin (any body site), hair, and nails. The etiologic agents are referred to as **dermatophytes**. Inflammation of the infected area is often greatest at the advancing margin, leaving some central clearing, with an irregular raised border of the skin lesion. Most ringworm infections cause little disability, and it is not uncommon for patients to report that lesions have been present for decades. The most common tinea infection in adults is athlete's foot (**tinea pedis**). This usually starts in the interdigital spaces, but it may spread to the undersurface and lateral aspects of the toes. The skin usually cracks and may become macerated with resultant itching. Other common sites of ringworm infections are the bearded area of men (**tinea barbae** or "barber's itch") or the face (**tinea faciei**), the body (**tinea corporis**), the groin (**tinea cruris**), the scalp (**tinea capitis**), or the nails (**tinea unguium**). Tinea infections are more common in prepubescent children and are highly contagious within this age group.

A. The **diagnosis** is made most rapidly by microscopic examination of hair, nail, or skin scrapings, but culture should also be done. In tinea capitis, ultraviolet light, which causes infected sites to fluoresce, is helpful in selecting infected hairs for examination and culture.

B. Another common dermatophyte infection of adults is **onychomycosis**, fungal infection of the nails. The most common pattern is distal and subungual. Associated thickening and discoloration (white, yellow, brown) of the nail are usually present. This infection has to be distinguished from onychomycosis caused by *Candida* species. *Candida* usually produces little nail plate thickening, and toenail infection is rare. Dermatophyte infection of the nails can be distinguished from psoriasis by its sparing of one or more nails. Psoriasis typically affects all nails on an affected extremity.

III. **Treatment of tinea infections** (also see Chap. 26)

A. **The treatment of tinea capitis** requires a systemic antifungal such as griseofulvin or an azole to penetrate the hair follicle. The usual dose of griseofulvin is 1 g PO qd of the microcrystalline preparation or 0.5 g PO qd of the ultramicrosized drug. Daily dosage should be ingested with a fatty meal or milk to enhance absorption. It may be necessary to increase the dose to a maximum of 24 mg/kg/day in some individuals whose initial response is unsatisfactory. The treatment should be continued until 2–3 weeks after clinical cure, usually 6–8 weeks. Alternatives to griseofulvin that are effective include ketoconazole, itraconazole, fluconazole, and terbinafine. Reported cure rates for tinea capitis are 88–94% in patients who are treated with itraconazole (100 mg PO qd). Doses of 400 mg qd itraconazole have been used to treat dermatophyte infections in adults, but one must be wary with all azole use of potential hepatotoxicity and drug interactions (e.g., increased effects of warfarin anticoagulation).

B. **For tinea pedis**, cure rates are high with terbinafine (not U.S. Food and Drug Administration approved for pediatric use). Terbinafine is available for topical use and as an oral preparation (250 mg PO qd). It is also important to control the hyperhidrosis of tinea pedis by the use of talcum or antifungal powders (undecylenic acid or tolnaftate powders), thick absorbent socks, and nonocclusive shoes. In severe or refractory cases, or both, a secondary bacterial infection must be ruled out. *S. aureus* and *Pseudomonas aeruginosa* are common in this area, and they can be controlled by antibacterial soaks (0.25% acetic acid) or topical phenolated resorcinol (Castellani's paint).

C. **Fungal infections of the nails (onychomycosis)** require systemic therapy, and the azole drugs have superseded griseofulvin as the agents of choice. Itraconazole has broad-spectrum activity, is incorporated into the nail, and persists there for 6 months after discontinuation of therapy (*Dermatol Clin* 1997;15:121). Mycologic cure rates vary between 40% and 80% for fingernails and between 3% and 38% for toenails (*Arch Dermatol* 1992;128:243). A treatment course of 4–6 months for fingernails and 10–18 months for toenails is required [*Fitzpatrick's Dermatology in General Medicine* (5th ed, vol II). New York: McGraw-Hill, 1999:2337–2357].

IV. **Systemic fungal infections.** The four major systemic infections in the United States are blastomycosis, histoplasmosis, coccidioidomycosis, and cryptococcosis. Blastomycosis and histoplasmosis are seen in the Mississippi and Ohio River Valleys and along the St. Lawrence River in the United States and Canada. Coccidioidomycosis occurs in the semiarid areas of the southwestern United States, including Arizona, New Mexico, and parts of California, Utah, and Nevada. Cryptococcosis and sporotrichosis have worldwide geographic distribution. Practice guidelines for the use of antifungal drugs and the management of patients with systemic fungal infections are available at the IDSA Web site (http://www.idsociety.org) or in print form (*Clin Infect Dis* 2000;30:653).

A. **Blastomycosis** is caused by the dimorphic fungus, *Blastomyces dermatitidis*. Organisms are inhaled to produce a primary pulmonary infection, which then disseminates to the skin, to the skeletal system, and less commonly to the

CNS and genitourinary systems. Symptoms of pulmonary blastomycosis include fever, night sweats, weight loss, productive cough, hemoptysis, and pleurisy. Radiography may reveal primarily upper-lobe disease with a fibronodular appearance or smooth-walled cavities. A mass lesion resembling lung carcinoma is not unusual. The first and sometimes only clinically evident site of systemic infection may be the skin. The characteristic cutaneous lesion is raised, verrucous, crusted, and usually located on the face or upper extremities. Biopsy of the advancing edge of a skin lesion often provides diagnostic histopathology and a positive fungal culture. **Treatment** options (IDSA guidelines: *Clin Infect Dis* 2000;30:679, or http://www.idsociety.org) include either itraconazole (400 mg PO qd or IV) or an initial treatment period with AMB (2.5–3.0 g IV over 2–3 months) for severely ill patients. With satisfactory clinical improvement, the patient who is initially treated with AMB can be switched to itraconazole to complete at least 6 months of total antifungal therapy. When prescribing oral itraconazole tablets, it is important to instruct the patient to arrange his or her dosage after meals or after an acidic beverage such as cola. Itraconazole liquid, however, is well absorbed independent of an acid environment. Serum itraconazole blood level measurement is available (Mayo Clinic) to confirm adequate absorption at the outset of therapy.

B. **Histoplasmosis** is caused by another dimorphic fungus, *Histoplasma capsulatum*, which is found worldwide (sparing Europe), with a high prevalence in the midwestern United States. This organism has been isolated from soil samples near starling roosts or accumulated bat droppings. Skin testing for delayed-type hypersensitivity to *H. capsulatum* has provided evidence that untreated primary infection with this fungus is very prevalent in the midwestern United States. Some individuals show residua of healed primary infection, represented by multiple calcified nodules in the lungs or spleen, or both. Symptomatic histoplasmosis is observed in children, farmers, construction workers, and others who are involved in outdoor activities. Some patients have an unusual form of mostly mediastinal involvement, with granulomatous, fibrocaseous lymph nodes that adhere to and compress mediastinal structures, creating a syndrome termed **mediastinal fibrosis**. **Disseminated histoplasmosis** is an important opportunistic infection in AIDS patients. It can be rapidly progressive and difficult to diagnose. Bone marrow aspiration or liver biopsy that shows the organisms and a positive fungal culture can lead to a prompt diagnosis. The urine *Histoplasma* antigen assay has also proved to be valuable in AIDS patients as an aid to diagnosis, but it is generally not helpful in normal hosts with histoplasmosis. Therapy in seriously ill patients with disseminated disease should be with IV AMB. (IDSA guidelines: *Clin Infect Dis* 2000;30:688, or http://www.idsociety.org.) Fluconazole (400 mg IV or PO bid) or itraconazole (400 mg IV or PO qd) has been shown to be an effective alternative to AMB in patients who do not have life-threatening disease and as a maintenance preventive therapy (200 mg PO qd of either azole) to avoid relapse in AIDS patients.

C. **Coccidioidomycosis** is the major endemic mycotic infection in the southwestern United States and northern Mexico. The causative micro-organism is *Coccidioides immitis*, and most infections are asymptomatic or self-limited, resolving over a period of weeks to months without specific treatment. It may progress, however, to chronic pulmonary disease or disseminate to bones, skin, and the CNS. Primary infection is probably very prevalent in the endemic area and results in either a mild self-limited URI or moderate to severe illness with fever, cough, malaise, anorexia, pleuritic pain, and skin eruption that are typical for erythema nodosum or erythema multiforme. For patients outside the endemic regions, diagnosis depends on obtaining an accurate travel history. Chest radiographs typically show single or multiple infiltrates, with hilar adenopathy and pleural effusions in a minority of cases. In 5–10% of patients, however, immune defenses fail to eradicate the infection, which progresses to chronic pulmonary disease with possible dissemination to other sites. This chronic form of infection is more frequent in diabetic or African-American men, pregnant women, or immuno-compromised patients. The lungs typically have one or more thin-walled cavities or nodules that are suggestive of malignancy. A definitive diagnosis requires microbiological evidence that *C. immitis* is present in the tissues (seeing spherules or obtaining a positive culture). Spherules do not take up Gram stain but are readily visualized with KOH, calcofluor, or Papanicolaou stain. Typical cultures can be positively identified promptly with DNA probes (*J Clin Microbiol* 1995;33:2913). Serologic testing is sensitive and specific. Repeated serologic testing during or after the first 2 months of illness increases the possibility of establishing a diagnosis. **Treatment** of early coccidioidomycosis may be unnecessary, but itraconazole (400 mg PO qd) or fluconazole (400–600 mg PO qd) for 3–6 months may be effective in shortening the symptomatic interval. (IDSA guidelines: *Clin Infect Dis* 2000;30:658, or http://www.idsociety.org.) Comparative trials have not been done. For progressive or disseminated infection, AMB (0.5–0.7 mg/kg/day IV) is the drug of choice. Treatment induction with amphotericin can often be followed with oral azole therapy when the patient has clearly improved and outpatient therapy is permissible.

D. **Cryptococcosis** is caused by a yeast (*Cryptococcus neoformans*) that is distributed worldwide in soil and pigeon droppings. Soluble capsular material that is shed in blood or spinal fluid may be detected by the cryptococcal latex agglutination test. Although infection begins with inhalation, *C. neoformans* has a propensity to spread to the CNS, producing symptoms and signs that are typical of meningitis. However, pulmonary cryptococcosis may cause a cough, fever, dyspnea, and multiple nodular lung densities. All patients with pulmonary cryptococcosis should have a lumbar puncture to establish whether the organism has spread to the meninges. Skin lesions that mimic molluscum contagiosum or acne may develop in patients with disseminated infection. Immunosuppressed patients (lymphoma, AIDS, organ transplant recipients, and those receiving corticosteroids or chemotherapy) are at greatest risk for cryptococcosis. The role of fluconazole has been firmly established for primary and maintenance therapy in AIDS patients, but its role in other patients has not been studied systematically. An **initial course** of AMB (0.7 mg/kg/day IV) with or without flucytosine (50–100 mg/kg/day PO in four divided doses) is generally indicated (IDSA guidelines: *Clin Infect Dis* 2000;30:710, or http://www.idsociety.org). When the patient is clinically stable and follow-up cultures are negative, antifungal therapy can be switched to fluconazole (400 mg PO qd). A 10-week course of intensive therapy is standard, and for AIDS patients lifelong maintenance therapy with fluconazole (200 mg PO qd) is indicated.

E. **Sporotrichosis** occurs as a nodular, pustular skin lesion, but it may disseminate. The causative organism is *Sporothrix schenckii*. In nature, the organism is a saprophyte of decaying wood and vegetable matter, and cutaneous infection is often linked to gardening and skin punctures or abrasions from cats, thorns, splinters, or tools. Most patients with sporotrichosis present with a cutaneous ulcer that is only minimally painful. The lymphatics are typically involved, and there may be red streaking of the skin or regional lymph node swelling, or both. Formation of secondary nodules (evolving to ulcers) occurs along the lymphatic channels. Pulmonary sporotrichosis usually produces cough and pulmonary infiltrates on chest radiographs. Fever and weight loss are relatively uncommon. Septic arthritis may occur as a manifestation of disseminated infection, and it usually follows an indolent course. Affected skin or lymph node biopsy can provide material for histopathology and culture. Growth on *S. schenckii* on Sabouraud's glucose agar generally occurs in 3–5 days, and the microscopic morphology of the yeast cells (oval or cigar shaped) is very distinctive. **Treatment** of lymphocutaneous sporotrichosis with a saturated solution of potassium iodide is generally successful and is considered the treatment of choice (5 drops PO tid for the first week, escalating the dose gradually, weekly to the maximum dose of 40–50 drops PO tid for 3–6 months). (IDSA guidelines: *Clin Infect Dis* 2000;30:684, or http://www.idsociety.org.) The mechanism of its efficacy is unknown. Itraconazole (100–200 mg/day PO for 3–6 months), however, has become a favored treatment for lymphocutaneous infection, and it has also been used successfully for the treatment of septic arthritis due to *S. schenckii*. Even disseminated sporotrichosis is rarely life threatening in nonimmunocompromised hosts. However, pulmonary sporotrichosis is typically chronic and progressive and probably should be treated with IV AMB or high-dose itraconazole.

Sexually Transmitted Diseases

History taking from male and female patients should attempt to determine the presence or absence of genital drainage or discharge; dysuria; sores or other lesions on or near the genitalia; the presence of warts, growths, or bumps on or near the genitalia; any rash; testicular pain or discomfort; abdominal, rectal, or pelvic pain; and the presence of any oral or pharyngeal symptoms. All patients should be queried about sex with men or women, or both; number of partners in the past year; sites of exposure (vaginal, penile, oral, rectal); condom use; known contact with sexually transmitted diseases (STDs); any drug allergies; and, for women, menstrual history. Barrier methods should be encouraged.

I. **Urethritis and cervicitis syndromes**
   A. **Gonorrhea** typically causes urethritis in men and cervicitis in women. Symptoms in men generally include purulent urethral discharge and dysuria, although some patients may be asymptomatic. Vaginal discharge occurs, but many women are asymptomatic.
      1. **Diagnosis.** Genital infection can be documented by gram-negative diplococci within WBC in urethral or endocervical smear, positive culture for *Neisseria gonorrhoeae* from urethral or endocervical swab, positive urethral or endocervical DNA probe test, or positive DNA amplification test for *N. gonorrhoeae* by ligase chain reaction or polymerase chain reaction test performed on an endocervical, urethral, or urinary specimen. Anorectal gonorrhea can be documented by an anoscopic sample showing gram-negative intracellular diplococci or a positive rectal culture for *N. gonorrhoeae*. Pharyngeal gonorrhea can only be documented by a positive pharyngeal culture for *N. gonorrhoeae*.
      2. **Treatment.** Recommended antigonococcal agents are single doses of ceftriaxone (125 mg IM) or cefixime (400 mg PO, not recommended for pharyngeal infection), ciprofloxacin (500 mg PO), or ofloxacin (400 mg PO). Quinolones are contraindicated in patients younger than 18 years old. Spectinomycin, 2 g IM, is an alternative therapy (not recommended for pharyngeal infection). Recommended concomitant therapy for *Chlamydia trachomatis* is single-dose azithromycin (1 g PO) or doxycycline (100 mg PO bid for 7 days). Where the results of diagnostic probe tests are not promptly available, empiric therapy for *N. gonorrhea* and *C. trachomatis* is encouraged.
      3. **Disseminated infection.** Patients with disseminated gonococcal infection should be referred for hospital admission for IV antibiotics. The diagnostic evaluation often includes cultures of blood, mucosal sites, skin lesions, and joint aspirates. The patient's sex partners should be evaluated.
   B. **Chlamydial infection.** *C. trachomatis* is a major cause of urethritis in men and cervicitis in women.
      1. **Diagnosis** should include a urethral or endocervical genetic probe test (Pace2 or Gen-Probe) or direct fluorescent antibody test that is positive

for *C. trachomatis* (Micro Trak), urethral or endocervical culture positive for *C. trachomatis* (not generally available), or a DNA amplification test such as polymerase chain reaction or ligase chain reaction performed on urine or an endocervical or urethral specimen.

2. **Treatment** is single-dose azithromycin (1 g PO) or doxycycline (100 mg PO bid for 7 days).

C. **Nongonococcal urethritis and mucopurulent cervicitis.** These syndromes mimic infection with *N. gonorrhoeae*, and most cases are negative on testing for *C. trachomatis*. Other agents that have been implicated include *Mycoplasma hominis, Ureaplasma urealyticum, Trichomonas vaginalis*, and occasionally HSV. The recommended therapeutic approach is to provide adequate coverage for possible *C. trachomatis* infection and then treatment for *T. vaginalis* in patients who do not respond. Treatment for *C. trachomatis* is either single-dose azithromycin (1 g PO) or doxycycline (100 mg PO bid for 7 days). Treatment of *T. vaginalis* is single-dose metronidazole (2 g PO). Simultaneous treatment of sex partner(s) is desirable.

D. **Bacterial vaginosis** (see Chap. 24)

E. **Trichomoniasis** (see Chap. 24)

F. **Vulvovaginal candidiasis.** This "yeast infection" is suggested by the presence of vulvovaginal soreness, dyspareunia, vulvar pruritus, external dysuria, and thick or "cheesy" vaginal secretions. Speculum examination may reveal candidal plaques that are adherent to the vaginal mucosa, with erythema or edema of the introitus. In contrast to bacterial vaginosis and trichomoniasis, the vaginal pH in vulvovaginal candidiasis is usually less than 4.5.

1. **The diagnosis** can be made by inspection of the typical vaginal lesions or by observation of fungal elements (budding yeast and pseudohyphae) in a KOH preparation.

2. **Treatment** is usually indicated if clinical features are present, even if yeast is not seen on microscopic examination. A positive culture may be misleading because 10–20% of women normally have yeast in the vagina. Treatment is with single-dose fluconazole (150 mg PO) or intravaginal azole cream or suppository such as clotrimazole or miconazole.

II. **Genital ulcer syndromes**

A. **Syphilis** is characterized by one or more painless, superficial ulcerations, that is, "chancres." These lesions are seen in the genital, anorectal, or pharyngeal sites. A chancre typically has raised, sharply demarcated borders; a red, smooth, nontender base; and scanty serous secretions. Regional lymphadenopathy may be present. The average time between exposure and chancre development is 3 weeks. Spontaneous resolution of lesions generally occurs in 3–6 weeks, even without treatment. The rash of **secondary syphilis** is macular, maculopapular, or papular, typically involving the palms, soles, and flexor areas of the extremities. The trunk, back, shoulders, abdomen, and face are commonly involved, and mucous patches may develop. The average time from exposure to onset of secondary symptoms is 6 weeks. **Latent syphilis** is diagnosed serologically in the absence of primary or secondary symptoms. Early disease (<1 year) is differentiated from late disease (>1 year) for treatment purposes. If a negative serology within the past year cannot be documented, the patient should be treated for late latent disease. **Tertiary syphilis** is rare but may be manifest as mucocutaneous/osseous lesions (gummas), cardiovascular lesions (aortitis), or neurologic involvement (neurosyphilis). Whereas neurosyphilis is generally a late complication, syphilitic meningitis may occur within the first few weeks of infection or at any time thereafter.

1. **Diagnosis.** The classic diagnosis of syphilis is dark-field microscopy of lesion exudate, but this is seldom available and is quite insensitive. Rapid plasma reagin (RPR) or the VDRL blood tests are often reactive within 1–2 weeks of onset of the chancre, but up to 30% may have negative RPR at the time of initial examination (chancre present). Also,

false-positive tests occur in a variety of conditions (e.g., systemic lupus erythematosus, pregnancy).

2. **Treatment** of adults with syphilis has become highly standardized. For primary, secondary, and early latent infection (<1 year duration), single-dose benzathine penicillin G (2.4 million units IM) is recommended. Alternatives include doxycycline (100 mg PO bid for 14 days), tetracycline (500 mg PO qid for 14 days), erythromycin (500 mg PO for 14 days, less effective), or ceftriaxone (250 mg IM qd for 8–10 days, less effective). For the treatment of adults with late syphilis (>1 year duration—except neurosyphilis), benzathine penicillin G (2.4 million units IM weekly for 3 weeks) is recommended. Alternatives are tetracycline (500 mg PO qid for 28 days) or doxycycline (100 mg PO bid for 28 days).

   For neurosyphilis, aqueous penicillin G (18–24 million units daily IV, 3–4 million units q4h for 14 days) is followed by a single dose of benzathine penicillin G (2.4 million units IM at the completion of IV therapy). A recommended alternative regimen is procaine penicillin (2.4 million units IM daily) plus probenecid (500 mg PO qid for 10–14 days) followed by a single dose of benzathine penicillin G (2.4 million units IM) at the completion of IV therapy. No data support the use of ceftriaxone, 1–2 g IV daily.

3. **For all stages of syphilis, penicillin is the treatment of choice.** For pregnant patients with a history of penicillin allergy, penicillin skin testing and desensitization are recommended, because alternative medications do not treat the fetus. Follow-up after treatment should be as outlined below.

   a. For **early syphilis**, there should be a clinical examination and repeat serology at 6 and 12 months. The RPR should show a fourfold decrease in titer within 6 months of treatment. One must consider treatment failure or reinfection if symptoms persist or recur or if nontreponemal titer increases fourfold.

   b. For **late syphilis**, there should be repeat serologies at 6, 12, and 24 months, and one should evaluate for neurosyphilis if the nontreponemal titer increases fourfold, if initially high titer ≥1:32 fails to fall fourfold in 12–24 months, or if signs or symptoms of neurosyphilis develop.

   c. For **neurosyphilis**, there should be repeat serologies at 3, 6, 12, and 24 months and follow-up lumbar puncture at 6-month intervals until the cell count is normal. Retreatment should be considered if cell count has not decreased at 6 months or cerebrospinal fluid (CSF) is not entirely normal at 2 years.

   d. For syphilis at any stage in **HIV-positive patients**, follow-up with clinical examination should be performed in 1 week and repeat serology in 3, 6, 9, 12, and 24 months, and then yearly, even if RPR becomes negative.

B. **Genital herpes.** HSV types 1 and 2 typically produce painful grouped vesicles on or near the genitalia. Over several days the lesions evolve into shallow ulcers, which generally heal within 1–2 weeks. HSV-1 and HSV-2 can be sexually transmitted, but most genital infections are caused by HSV-2. The clinical courses of acute first-episode genital herpes among patients with HSV-1 and HSV-2 infections are similar. The first episode of genital herpes in patients who have had prior HSV-1 infection is associated with less severe systemic symptoms and faster healing than primary genital herpes. Virtually any genital ulcer may be herpetic regardless of clinical characteristics. Virologic typing can be important because HSV-1 recurs less frequently than HSV-2. Extragenital lesions of HSV commonly develop during the course of primary genital herpes. They are most frequently located in the buttock, groin, or thigh areas. CNS involvement may be manifested as aseptic meningitis, transverse myelitis, or sacral radiculopathy. This can result in episodes of spinal or meningeal symptoms that recur over many years. These complications occur more commonly in women than in men. Reactivation of HSV-2 infection shows a steady but gradual decrease in recurrence rates over time. One study reported that reactivation of genital herpes decreased from an average of five to eight a year to two a year over a 5- to 8-year period.

1. **Diagnosis** relies on detection of grouped, tender vesicular or pustular lesions on an erythematous base. Lymphadenopathy, fever, headache, myalgias, urethritis, or cervicitis are variably present. Recurrences usually cause fewer lesions and less frequent occurrence of systemic symptoms. Most patients with genital HSV are asymptomatic or have mild or nonspecific symptoms. Laboratory diagnosis should rely mainly on HSV culture, which should be included in the diagnostic workup of all genital ulcers. The sensitivity of the culture depends greatly on how the specimen is obtained and handled. Vesicular fluid is rich in virus and should be submitted whenever possible. Unopened vesicles can be aspirated with a tuberculin syringe. Alternatively, the lesion can be unroofed with a scalpel blade and the vesicular fluid soaked up with a cotton, rayon, or Dacron swab. Calcium alginate swabs should not be used because this is inhibitory to HSV.

2. **Treatment** for genital HSV can be with several effective agents: acyclovir (400 mg PO tid for 7–10 days), famciclovir (250 mg PO tid for 7–10 days), or valacyclovir (1 g PO bid for 7–10 days). Early treatment usually reduces the symptomatic interval and may result in accelerated healing. **Suppressive therapy** may be recommended for patients with recurrent symptomatic infection, that is, acyclovir (400 mg PO bid), famciclovir (250 mg PO bid), valacyclovir (250–500 mg PO bid), or valacyclovir (1 g PO qd). Suppressive therapy with antiviral agents may not show benefit until 4–6 months of treatment. In many patients it may only shorten the symptomatic periods by 1–2 days. Treatment is recommended for 1 year, after which the need for continued suppressive therapy should be reassessed. Patients should be counseled that mild episodes may continue to occur and that they will remain infectious even though they are receiving therapy. Routine STD evaluation is recommended for all sex partners.

C. **Chancroid** is caused by infection with *Haemophilus ducreyi*. The typical lesions are painful, nonindurated, excavated genital ulcers with undermined borders. Tender, enlarged inguinal lymph nodes are often present. These may suppurate, or pus containing the organism may be aspirated from the resultant buboes, but techniques for culture are only 50–75% sensitive. Fever and other systemic symptoms are generally absent. Chancroid is worldwide in distribution but rare in the United States outside the endemic areas in New York City and the Gulf Coast states, where 90% of cases are in non-Caucasian uncircumcised men. Extragenital chancroid is rare. Prostitute contact is common. The incubation period may vary, but the median range is 5–7 days. It is essential to exclude syphilis in all cases of suspected chancroid.

1. **Laboratory diagnosis** relies on culture or Gram stain from a lymph node aspirate. A positive culture provides a definite diagnosis, whereas a smear of aspirated pus showing typical, small gram-negative bacilli provides only a presumptive diagnosis. Gram stain of ulcer exudate may be misleading and is not recommended. Simultaneous workup for syphilis, HSV, and HIV is recommended.

2. **Treatment** is single-dose azithromycin (1 g PO), single-dose ceftriaxone (250 mg IM), ciprofloxacin (500 mg PO bid for 3 days, contraindicated if the patient <18 years old), or erythromycin base (500 mg PO qid for 7 days). The patient should be re-examined in 2–3 days and then weekly until healed.

D. **Lymphogranuloma venereum** is caused by *C. trachomatis* serovars L1, L2, or L3. It is usually characterized by unilateral tender inguinal lymphadenopathy, sometimes with urethritis or transient genital ulceration, or both.

1. **Laboratory diagnosis** relies on isolation of an appropriate lymphogranuloma venereum strain that most laboratories are not equipped to perform

or type-specific chlamydial serology that may be diagnostic on a single serum specimen, although acute and convalescent sera are preferred.

   2. Recommended treatment is doxycycline (100 mg PO bid for 3 weeks) or erythromycin base (500 mg PO qid for 3 weeks). Azithromycin in multiple doses over 2–3 weeks may be effective, but clinical data are lacking. Sex partners during the 30 days before onset of symptoms should undergo routine STD examination, including *Chlamydia* cultures and serology.

E. Granuloma inguinale (donovanosis) is a progressive ulcerative condition caused by the intracellular gram-negative bacterium *Calymmatobacterium granulomatis*. It is endemic to India, Papua New Guinea, southern Africa, and central Australia. Painless, beefy-red ulcers are typical, without lymphadenopathy.

   1. Laboratory diagnosis relies on a tissue crush preparation or biopsy showing classic bipolar-staining Donovan bodies. The organism cannot be grown in standard culture media.

   2. Treatment is TMP/SMZ (1 tablet DS PO bid for 3 weeks), ciprofloxacin (750 mg PO bid for 3 weeks), or erythromycin base (500 mg PO qid for 3 weeks). In general, therapy should be continued until all lesions have completely healed. An aminoglycoside (e.g., gentamicin, 5 mg/kg IM or IV qd) should be added if lesions do not respond after the first few days of oral therapy.

III. Exophytic processes

A. Anogenital warts. Warts are caused by human papillomavirus, and some have been linked epidemiologically to cervical cancer. The diagnosis is usually made by inspection, which reveals typical "cauliflower" masses, usually involving the external genitalia, perineum, or perianal area. The differential diagnosis includes molluscum contagiosum or condyloma lata (secondary syphilis). A dermatologic consultation may be desirable for evaluation and biopsy of a lesion. A weak acetic acid solution (3–5%) can be used to highlight exophytic warts on the skin surface. The lesions turn white as the solution dries (do not apply to mucous membranes). Routine STD evaluation for all sex partners is recommended, including cervical cytology for female partners of infected men. The **treatment** of warts is typically with application of liquid nitrogen, podophyllin (10–25% in tincture of benzoin), or trichloroacetic acid. Liquid nitrogen is applied by a 10- to 15-second spray followed by a thaw and a single repeat application. Podophyllin is applied once or twice a week and washed off 1–4 hours after each application. Surgical removal of warts may be necessary for extensive disease.

B. Molluscum contagiosum is a benign papular lesion caused by the molluscum contagiosum virus. It can be transmitted sexually or nonsexually through close physical contact. Typical lesions are firm, small (1- to 5-mm diameter), fleshy papules that are often umbilicated. A firm white "pearl" is sometimes expressed on compression, followed by bleeding from the lesion. Very similar skin lesions may occur with disseminated *C. neoformans* or less commonly by *H. capsulatum*. In healthy patients, this is a self-limited infection and lesions usually resolve spontaneously. **Successful treatment** of lesions may be with liquid nitrogen or trichloroacetic acid in the same fashion as described for warts. For those with concomitant HIV infection, more aggressive treatment and referral to a dermatologist may be appropriate.

IV. Systemic STD syndromes

A. Pelvic inflammatory disease. This syndrome occurs in women and is caused by upper genital tract infection. It is characterized by pelvic pain, cervical motion tenderness, and systemic signs and symptoms of infection. The patient's complaints may also include dyspareunia, vaginal discharge, and menorrhagia or metrorrhagia. *N. gonorrhoeae* and *Chlamydia* are the most common causes, although polymicrobial pelvic abscess disease is also common. Severe cases may present as tubo-ovarian abscess or perihepatitis. The differential diagnosis includes acute appendicitis, ectopic pregnancy, septic abortion, and ovarian torsion. Some patients with pelvic inflammatory disease require hospitalization for IV antibiotics and possible surgical intervention. Treatment regimens use coverage for *N. gonorrhoeae* and *C. trachomatis*, but many of these infections are polymicrobial, containing anaerobes such as *Bacteroides* species.

   1. CDC guidelines for **hospital admission** should be reviewed prior to consideration of outpatient treatment. They are as follows: (1) Surgical emergencies cannot be excluded; (2) the patient is pregnant; (3) outpatient therapy has failed; (4) the patient is unable to follow or tolerate outpatient treatment; (5) the illness is severe, with nausea, vomiting, and high fever; (6) tubo-ovarian abscess is strongly suspected; or (7) the patient is immunodeficient. Hospitalized patients should be treated for at least 2 weeks with IV or PO antibiotics, or both.

   2. **Outpatient treatment** should be one of the following: (1) ofloxacin (400 mg PO bid) plus metronidazole (500 mg PO tid for 14 days) or (2) single-dose ceftriaxone (250 mg IM) plus doxycycline (100 mg PO bid for 14 days). The patient should be advised to remove an intrauterine device if present, abstain from sexual intercourse for 2 weeks, and comply with bed rest for 1–3 days or until pain is significantly improved. A follow-up examination within 72 hours is essential to assure that an adequate response to therapy has occurred. All sex partners within the past 3 months should be examined.

B. HBV (see Chap. 14). Patients with this sexually transmitted infection complain of malaise, fever, loss of appetite, abdominal pain, nausea, vomiting, jaundice, dark urine, arthralgias, or polyarthritis, but up to 50% may be asymptomatic. The physical examination may detect right upper quadrant abdominal tenderness, hepatic enlargement, or scleral or cutaneous jaundice.

   1. **Laboratory diagnostic studies** should include serologic testing for HBV, including hepatitis B surface antigen. Other useful diagnostic tests include hepatitis A immunoglobulin M, hepatitis C virus (HCV)–enzyme-linked immunosorbent assay test, CBC, and liver function tests. HBV is the only STD for which a 90% effective vaccine is available. Epidemiologic studies suggest that in the United States, 40–60% of cases of HBV infection are sexually transmitted.

   2. **Treatment** for acute HBV is supportive. Adequate fluid intake should be encouraged, as well as bed rest and abstinence from sexual contact until symptoms subside. A routine STD evaluation including HBV serology is recommended for all sex partners.

C. HIV infection (see Human Immunodeficiency Virus Infection and Acquired Immune Deficiency Syndrome).

Cellulitis

Cellulitis is an inflammatory condition of the skin and subcutaneous tissues. The organisms that are most often involved are GAS (*Streptococcus pyogenes*). Less often, streptococci that belong to other groups (group B in neonates as well as adults and groups C and G in adults) or *S. aureus* are the etiologic agents. **Erysipelas** is also caused by the pyogenic streptococci but can be distinguished clinically from cellulitis by its sharply demarcated raised border. It most often occurs on the face.

I. Cellulitis is a clinical diagnosis. Typical local features include (1) confluent erythema of the skin; (2) swelling of the involved area and warmth to the touch; (3) a usually tender affected area, possibly also with tender regional lymphadenopathy; and (4) lymphangitis, which is relatively uncommon. Vesicles, bullae, petechiae, and ecchymoses may also be seen in the affected area. The most common site for cellulitis is the skin over the tibial surface of the lower leg; however, any area of skin may be involved. The advancing edge of cellulitis (unlike erysipelas) is not elevated or well demarcated. Systemic findings, such as fever, rigors, and generalized myalgias, are common. Cellulitis may begin without any obvious portal of bacterial entry, or it may be induced by local trauma or radiation therapy or through sites involved with athlete's foot (tinea pedis). Cellulitis caused by GAS may occur as an immediate or delayed postoperative wound infection. Initial bouts of lower-extremity cellulitis predispose to recurrent bouts in roughly the same distribution. This is also notable in patients whose saphenous veins have been removed for coronary artery bypass surgery. Episodes of recurrent cellulitis in the same distribution also tend to occur in patients with congenital or hereditary lymphedema. Pain in the affected area is typical and may be severe and discordant with the physical findings. Such patients deserve consideration of short-course narcotic analgesia (e.g., acetaminophen/oxycodone).

II. **Treatment of cellulitis.** Immobilization and elevation of the affected area are important parts of the treatment. Mild and early cellulitis can be treated with oral therapy with cephalexin (0.5–1.0 g qid) or dicloxacillin (0.5 g qid) for 10–14 days or until objective and subjective improvement occur. For many patients who are suspected of having streptococcal cellulitis, penicillin VK (0.5 g PO qid) provides reasonable coverage. If staphylococcal infection is suspected or when there are no clues to etiology, dicloxacillin (0.5 g PO qid) is preferred. In patients who are allergic to penicillin, clindamycin (300 mg PO qid) or erythromycin (0.5 g PO qid) is an alternative. Patients who fail to respond may require hospital admission and parenteral antibiotics. Necrotizing fasciitis is a serious infection of subcutaneous tissues, not primarily the skin. It is commonly caused by GAS, but a second variety is polymicrobial and involves the genitalia (Fournier's gangrene), head, or neck. Necrotizing fasciitis requires hospitalization, parenteral antibiotics, and early surgical débridement.

III. **Exotic causes of cellulitis.** Erysipeloid is an uncommon form of cellulitis caused by *Erysipelothrix rhusiopathiae*. This infection generally occurs in persons who handle saltwater fish, shellfish, poultry, meat products, or hides. The organism is usually introduced through an abrasion on the hands and produces a violaceous painful area beginning 1 week after the injury. It does not ulcerate but has raised borders and may show central clearing. Occasionally, an adjacent joint is involved. Culture of a skin biopsy from the advancing margin of the lesion permits identification of the organism that is penicillin susceptible. Rare cases of cellulitis secondary to *S. pneumoniae* bacteremia have been reported. The **Enterobacteriaceae** and some fungi may produce cellulitis in immunocompromised or neutropenic patients. Clinically similar infections are caused by *Vibrio* species or *Aeromonas* species, which may progress rapidly to extensive cutaneous necrosis that requires prompt and extensive débridement. Bacteremia is common, and *V. vulnificus* may enter the circulation through the GI tract (e.g., after eating fresh oysters) rather than through a skin laceration or abrasion.

Tuberculosis

TB is a systemic disease caused by *Mycobacterium tuberculosis*. Pulmonary disease is the most frequent clinical presentation. Lymphatic involvement, genitourinary disease, osteomyelitis, and miliary dissemination may occur, as well as meningitis, peritonitis, and pericarditis. TB is more common among debilitated and otherwise immunocompromised patients (e.g., alcoholics and patients with AIDS). The prevalence of TB is highest among immigrants from Asia, Africa, the Pacific Islands, and Latin America.

I. **Diagnosis of TB** is established by culturing the organism from sputum, sterile fluids, urine, or tissue or, in culture-negative cases, by an appropriate response to antituberculous therapy. Sputum samples should be obtained on 3 separate days and submitted for acid-fast stain and mycobacterial culture. Positive fluorochrome or acid-fast smears are presumptive evidence of active TB, although nontuberculous mycobacteria and some *Nocardia* species may give positive results with these techniques.

II. **Treatment of TB** should be undertaken with the guidance of an expert and may include hospitalization to initiate therapy, patient education, and respiratory isolation for patients with pulmonary disease. The local health department should be notified of all cases of TB so that contacts can be identified and arrangements for directly observed therapy (DOT) can be made.

   A. **Chemotherapy.** Antituberculous therapy is based on two principles: (1) Multidrug therapy must be prescribed because of the emergence of drug resistance when a single drug is used, and (2) extended therapy is necessary because of the prolonged generation time of mycobacteria (>20 hours). Treatment recommendations follow those of the American Thoracic Society and the U.S. Public Health Service (*Am J Respir Crit Care Med* 1994;149:1359).

   1. **Pulmonary disease** can be treated with the following regimen (adult doses).

   a. **Initial therapy** includes **isoniazid (INH)**, 5 mg/kg/day (maximum 300 mg qd), and **rifampin**, 10 mg/kg/day (maximum 600 mg qd), for 6 months plus **pyrazinamide (PZA)**, 15–20 mg/kg/day (maximum 2 g qd), for the first 2 months with fully susceptible isolates. **Ethambutol**, 15–20 mg/kg/day, is also given initially until susceptibility results are known. Ethambutol should not be omitted from the initial regimen unless the community rate of INH resistance where the patient acquired the disease is known to be less than 4% and the patient has not received prior treatment and has had no known exposure to drug-resistant disease. In most cases, four-drug initial therapy is required. **Streptomycin**, 15 mg/kg/day IM (maximum 1 g), is an alternative to ethambutol. After 2–8 weeks of daily therapy and clinical response, medication can also be given twice a week under **DOT**: INH, 15 mg/kg (maximum 900 mg); rifampin, 10 mg/kg (maximum 600 mg); PZA, 50 mg/kg (maximum 4 g); and ethambutol, 50 mg/kg each visit. When daily therapy is given for the first 8 weeks, ethambutol can be discontinued once sensitivity results demonstrate susceptibility to all major drugs. If twice-weekly therapy is chosen after 2 weeks of daily therapy, ethambutol is retained in the regimen for a total of 2 months. **DOT is strongly encouraged for all patients, and intermittent therapy should only be given by DOT.**

   b. **Response to therapy** is monitored clinically, with serial sputum smear and culture examinations and chest radiographs. **Sputa** should be obtained every 2 weeks until smear negative and thereafter monthly until culture negative. A minority of patients is culture negative at 1 month, but 95% of patients should be culture negative after 3 months of therapy. **Chest radiographs** are obtained at diagnosis, after 2–3 months of therapy, and at completion of therapy.

   2. **Drug resistance.** All initial isolates should be submitted for susceptibility testing. Patients with persistently positive cultures after 3 months of therapy should have repeat susceptibility testing. Initial isolates with documented isolated resistance to INH should be treated with rifampin, ethambutol, and PZA for 6 months. Isolates that are resistant to INH and rifampin [multidrug-resistant (MDR)-TB] should be treated with at least three agents to which the isolate

is known to be susceptible for a minimum of 12 months beyond the last positive culture. An injectable agent is usually included in the regimen for the first 4–6 months of therapy. Treatment of MDR-TB requires the management of a TB expert.

3. **Extrapulmonary disease** can be treated in generally the same manner as pulmonary disease. However, miliary, bone and joint, and meningeal disease in children should be treated for 1 year.

4. **Immunosuppressed patients** should be treated with INH and rifampin for at least 6 months, supplemented initially by PZA and ethambutol. PZA is continued for 2 months. Ethambutol can then be discontinued if the isolate is known to be fully susceptible. Patients who are slow to respond should be treated for 9 months or longer. Because of complex interactions of rifampin with antiretroviral agents, an expert with experience in treating HIV and TB should treat patients with TB and HIV coinfection.

5. **Pregnant patients** should be treated in the standard fashion, except that PZA and streptomycin should not be used.

B. **Corticosteroid administration** in TB is controversial. Prednisone, 1 mg/kg PO qd initially, has been used in combination with primary antituberculous drugs for life-threatening complications such as meningitis and pericarditis.

III. **Screening and treatment for latent TB infection.** A positive tuberculin skin test in the absence of TB disease indicates latent TB infection (**LTBI**). In up to 5% of individuals whose intermediate-strength purified protein derivative (PPD) skin tests convert from negative to positive, active disease develops within 2 years of conversion if left untreated. The lifetime risk of disease is approximately 10%. Treatment of LTBI reduces this risk, but the potential for hepatotoxicity must be considered in these individuals, particularly among patients who are older than 35 years of age. The current approach to screening emphasizes targeted tuberculin testing among persons at highest risk for recent LTBI or with clinical conditions that increase the risk for TB. These groups are most likely to benefit from treatment regardless of age. Testing is discouraged among persons at lower risk for TB (*Am J Respir Crit Care Med* 2000;161:S221).

A. **Criteria for a positive PPD** are (1) a 5-mm induration for patients with HIV infection or other defect in cell-mediated immunity, contacts of a known case, patients with chest radiographs that are typical for tuberculosis, and patients who chronically receive 15 mg or more prednisone daily for 1 month or more; (2) a 10-mm induration for recent (within 5 years) immigrants from endemic areas, prisoners, the homeless, parenteral drug abusers, nursing home residents, and patients with chronic medical illnesses; and (3) a 15-mm induration for individuals who are not in a high-prevalence group (and therefore who should not have been tested).

B. **Treatment of LTBI. INH**, 5 mg/kg (maximum 300 mg) PO qd (adult dosage) with **pyridoxine** (B$_6$), 50 mg qd, for 6–9 months should be considered for all persons **regardless of age** who (1) develop a tuberculin skin test conversion (10-mm increase) within 2 years of a previously negative PPD; (2) have a positive PPD and are at high risk of developing active disease, including recent immigrants (within 5 years) from high-prevalence countries; intravenous drug users; patients with silicosis, diabetes mellitus, HIV/AIDS, or end-stage renal disease; individuals with hematologic, lymphoreticular, or head and neck or lung malignancy or conditions associated with rapid weight loss or chronic malnutrition; and patients who are receiving chronic immunosuppressive therapy equal to 15 mg prednisone equivalent; and (3) have a positive PPD (5 mm) and are household members or close contacts of patients with active disease. Patients with **HIV disease or fibrotic lesions on chest x-ray** should receive 9 months of INH. **Contacts** with a negative PPD who are at high risk for tuberculosis, particularly children, should also be treated, but treatment can be stopped if a repeat PPD at 3 months is negative. Untreated contacts with a nonreactive PPD should have a repeat PPD after 3 months.

C. Monitoring of INH. All patients should be informed that they should discontinue INH and seek medical care if anorexia or nausea develops. Monthly clinical monitoring for signs and symptoms of disease is indicated for all persons who are prescribed INH. For persons with risk factors for hepatotoxicity (e.g., underlying liver disease, daily alcohol use, HIV, pregnancy or postpartum, or use of other potentially hepatotoxic drugs), monthly monitoring of the ALT and AST is indicated, with discontinuation of INH for elevations greater than three times the upper limit of normal if associated with symptoms and five times the upper limit of normal if asymptomatic.

D. Alternatives to daily INH. INH can be prescribed twice weekly (15 mg/kg, maximum 900 mg) if given by DOT. If INH cannot be given, **PZA**, 20 mg/kg/day (maximum 2 g), plus **rifampin**, 10 mg/kg/day (maximum 600 mg), can be given for 2 months as an alternative. Attention must be paid to drug-drug interactions with this regimen. For example, rifampin renders birth control pills and many other drugs less active. Further, due to reports of serious hepatotoxicity, this regimen is not recommended for patients with underlying liver disease or those who have had INH-associated injury. No more than a 2-week supply should be dispensed at one time, and ALT, AST, and bilirubin should be monitored at 2, 4, and 6 weeks of treatment (*MMWR Morb Mortal Wkly Rep* 2001;50:722–725). For patients who are intolerant of INH or are contacts to patients with isolated INH resistance, rifampin, 600 mg qd, can be given for 4 months, again with attention paid to drug-drug interactions.

E. Treatment of LTBI after MDR-TB exposure. This is a complex issue and should be undertaken with the guidance of a TB expert. Options range from using two drugs to which the organism is known to be susceptible, for example, a quinolone or PZA plus ethambutol for 6–12 months, to simple observation in low-risk patients.

Human Immunodeficiency Virus Infection and Acquired Immune Deficiency Syndrome

I. HIV infection and AIDS. Human immunodeficiency virus type 1 is a human retrovirus that infects lymphocytes and other cells that bear the CD4 surface marker. Infection leads to lymphopenia, CD4 lymphocyte deficiency and dysfunction, impaired cell-mediated immune response, and polyclonal B-cell activation with impaired B-cell responses to new antigens. This immune derangement gives rise to AIDS, which is characterized by opportunistic infections and unusual malignancies. Transmission is primarily by sexual and parenteral routes. **Major risk groups** therefore include sexual contacts of infected persons, IV drug users, and children born to HIV-infected mothers.

II. Treatment of AIDS includes specific antiretroviral therapy, prevention and treatment of opportunistic infections, and neoplastic complications. Because treatment of HIV disease is complex and rapidly evolving, it is best managed by an expert with experience in treating such patients. The information presented here is not intended as a substitute for expert care. Excellent sources of information for physicians who wish to familiarize themselves with HIV care include http://www.hivinsite.org and http://www.hivatis.org.

A. **Management of the HIV-positive patient.** Patients with HIV infection may present acutely near the time of seroconversion or at a late stage with an AIDS-defining complication. Initial assessment of patients should be targeted to the determination of the degree of immunodeficiency with particular attention to the need for initiation of antiretroviral therapy and of prophylactic therapy against ***Pneumocystis carinii* pneumonia** (PCP).

B. **Primary HIV infection.** Initial infection with HIV type 1 may be associated with a mononucleosis-like syndrome, aseptic meningitis, spinal vacuolar myelopathy, peripheral neuropathy, and subacute encephalitis. As many as 90% of patients who are acutely infected with HIV experience at least some symptoms of the acute retroviral syndrome and can thus be identified as candidates for early therapy. Acute HIV infection is often not recognized in the primary care setting, however, because of the nonspecific nature of the symptoms. Maintaining a high index of suspicion is required.

C. **Initial assessment.** Most patients are asymptomatic initially. In some, recurrent oral candidiasis, lymphadenopathy, weight loss, fevers, night sweats, and chronic diarrhea may develop. History and physical examination should focus on such complications. Abnormal laboratory findings may include anemia, thrombocytopenia, and leukopenia. The most important initial laboratory tests are measurement of the CD4 (T4) lymphocyte count (normal range for adults is 600–1500 cells/mm^3) and HIV RNA viral load. CD4 counts of less than 500 cells/mm^3 usually indicate HIV-associated immune deficiency.

D. **Antiretroviral therapy.** Symptomatic HIV infection that is exhibited by an AIDS-defining illness or thrush is an indication for antiretroviral treatment regardless of CD4 count or HIV RNA load. Asymptomatic individuals with CD4 counts of less than 500 or HIV RNA greater than 20,000 by polymerase chain reaction should be offered therapy. Asymptomatic patients with CD4 counts of greater than 500 and HIV RNA less than 20,000 can be followed closely off antiretroviral therapy.

E. Typical **HAART** regimens for initial therapy consist of a triple or quadruple drug regimen, including one of the following nonnucleoside reverse transcriptase inhibitors (NNRTI) or protease inhibitors (PI): efavirenz (NNRTI), indinavir (PI), nelfinavir (PI), or ritonavir (PI) **plus** saquinavir (PI), **in conjunction with** one of the following pairs of nucleoside reverse transcriptase inhibitors (NRTI) stavudine + lamivudine, stavudine + didanosine, zidovudine + lamivudine, or zidovudine + didanosine. Choice and use of these agents are beyond the scope of this manual. However, the primary care physician who is treating patients with HIV disease in conjunction with an HIV expert should familiarize him- or herself with the toxicities of these agents and drug-drug interactions to avoid.

F. **Prophylactic measures. Because TB is an important complication of HIV infection, screening is warranted at the time of initial assessment.** Patients often become anergic as the degree of immune deficiency progresses. In such patients, chest radiography should be performed. Immunizations such as annual influenza vaccine, pneumococcal vaccine, and, for HBV-seronegative patients, HBV vaccine can also be offered. Prophylaxis against PCP (TMP/SMZ DS or dapsone, 100 mg qd) is indicated when the CD4 count is less than 200 cells/mm^3, when the percent of CD4 lymphocytes is less than 20% of the total lymphocyte count, or if the patient has thrush regardless of CD4 count.

G. For patients with CD4 counts of less than 50 cells/mm^3, weekly azithromycin (1200 mg) should be given as prophylaxis against infection with MAC. If immune reconstitution with HAART occurs with sustained CD4 counts of greater than 200 cells/mm^3, PCP and MAC prophylaxis can be discontinued.

H. Complications of HIV infection
1. Viral infections
  a. CMV infection is common in patients with AIDS. Manifestations include viremia with fever and constitutional symptoms, chorioretinitis, esophagitis, gastritis, enterocolitis, pancreatitis, acalculous cholecystitis, bone marrow suppression, necrotizing adrenalitis, and upper and lower respiratory tract infections. Therapy with **ganciclovir, 5 mg/kg IV every 12 hours**, is effective for chorioretinitis and GI disease but is associated with significant hematologic toxicity. Relapse after discontinuation of the drug is common, usually necessitating maintenance therapy until sustained immune reconstitution occurs with CD4 counts of greater than 200 cells/mm^3. It is usually necessary to discontinue zidovudine when systemic ganciclovir is given. Concomitant granulocyte colony-stimulating factor can be used as a possible means of ameliorating ganciclovir myelotoxicity. Patients with retinitis who are intolerant of systemic ganciclovir may benefit from intravitreal administration of the drug by an experienced ophthalmologist. Foscarnet is indicated for patients who have a documented ganciclovir-resistant CMV strain or who are failing ganciclovir therapy.
  b. Other herpetoviridae. HSV infection has been associated with esophagitis, proctitis, pulmonary disease, and large, atypical, persistent cutaneous ulcerations. IV acyclovir is usually effective for these problems, but relapses are frequent. **Varicella-zoster virus** may cause typical dermatomal lesions or may disseminate. Recurrent disease, meningoencephalitis, and cranial neuritis have been reported. Acyclovir, 800 mg 5 times/day, or famciclovir, 500 mg tid, are the treatments of choice. Evidence of EBV infection is common in patients with AIDS, particularly hairy leukoplakia. Oral acyclovir may be effective but should be reserved for symptomatic cases.
  c. JC virus is a papovavirus that is associated with **progressive multifocal leukoencephalopathy**. It is characterized by altered mental status, visual loss, weakness, and abnormalities of gait. Nonenhancing hypodense lesions are seen on CT of the head, but MRI is more sensitive. Polymerase chain reaction testing of CSF is often positive for JC virus. No effective therapy has been identified, but the course may be significantly altered by HAART.
2. Bacterial infections are common in patients with AIDS and often recur or follow an atypical or aggressive course despite adequate therapy. Therapy must be individualized, but in general, intense initial therapy followed by prolonged suppression is often necessary.
  a. Nontyphoidal salmonellae (especially *Salmonella typhimurium*) are associated with invasive disease that often recurs or persists despite appropriate antibiotics (*Ann Intern Med* 1985;102:186). Initial IV therapy with ampicillin, ceftriaxone, TMP/SMZ, or another agent should be followed by long-term oral suppressive therapy based on susceptibility testing (e.g., amoxicillin, 500 mg PO tid); even then, relapse may occur as soon as therapy is discontinued.
  b. Syphilis. The natural history of syphilis may be altered by HIV infection. Reactivation of previously treated disease, active disease with negative serology, asymptomatic neurosyphilis, and relapse after standard therapy have all been reported. The optimal management of syphilis in this setting remains unclear. Lumbar puncture of seropositive patients, IV penicillin G for any suspected infections, and long-term maintenance therapy are all potentially necessary measures.
  c. Bacterial pneumonias occur with increased frequency and are usually due to *S. pneumoniae*, *H. influenzae*, or group B streptococcus.

Pneumonia due to gram-negative enteric organisms occurs in advanced HIV disease. Chest radiographs may reveal typical lobar pneumonia, but diffuse interstitial infiltrates similar to PCP have been reported. These infections usually respond to specific antibiotic therapy, but relapses are not uncommon.

3. **Mycobacterial infections**

   a. *Mycobacterium tuberculosis.* TB occurs with increased frequency in patients with AIDS, particularly among substance abusers, immigrants from high-prevalence countries, and the urban poor. Atypical radiographic patterns and extrapulmonary disease are quite common; apical cavitary disease is uncommon in advanced HIV disease (see Tuberculosis for TB disease treatment recommendations). INH for 9 months should be considered in any HIV-positive patient with a reactive (5-mm in duration) PPD skin test. PZA plus rifampin for 2 months is an alternative if the patient is not taking a PI or NNRTI (please see Tuberculosis, sec. **III.D**).

   b. **MAC** is one of the most frequently occurring opportunistic pathogens in patients with AIDS. Generalized infection and GI disease are the most common manifestations. The organism can be cultured from blood, bone marrow, and tissue from the GI tract. Treatment with clarithromycin, ethambutol, and rifabutin is often effective. For patients with CD4 counts less than $50/mm^3$, MAC can be prevented by giving azithromycin, 1200 mg, once a week.

4. **Fungal infections**

   a. **Candidiasis.** Persistent oral, esophageal, and vaginal infections are common, but dissemination is rare in the absence of other risk factors such as IV catheters. The severity and frequency of mucocutaneous candidiasis increase with declining immune function. Topical therapy with clotrimazole troches PO five times/day for 14 days is effective for oral thrush. Esophagitis should be treated with fluconazole (200 mg one time followed by 100 mg PO qd for 14 days; higher doses up to 400 mg qd may be required in some patients). Vaginal candidiasis can be treated with fluconazole, 150 mg PO one time. Frequently recurring thrush can be prevented with fluconazole, 100 mg PO qd.

   b. *C. neoformans* is the most common cause of fungal CNS disease in patients with AIDS. Symptoms may be mild, and therefore the threshold for performing a lumbar puncture should be low. Initial treatment is with AMB and flucytosine for 2–3 weeks, followed by fluconazole, 400 mg qd for 8–10 weeks. Following acute treatment, lifelong maintenance therapy is required with fluconazole, 200 mg qd. Response is usually monitored clinically and is generally slow. Repeat lumbar puncture is indicated for clinical deterioration. In addition to routine CSF chemistries, cell count, cryptococcal antigen, and culture, the CSF opening pressure should be measured to assess the possibility of intracranial hypertension as a complication.

   c. *H. capsulatum* is an important pathogen in patients with AIDS from endemic areas and may cause disseminated disease and septicemia. Pancytopenia may result from bone marrow involvement. A cumulative dose of AMB, 1.5–2.0 g, is given initially for severely ill patients. For patients who are intolerant of AMB, liposomal AMB (Ambisome) can be considered. Itraconazole is effective for secondary prophylaxis.

   d. *C. immitis* also occurs in patients with AIDS from endemic areas. Extensive pulmonary disease with extrapulmonary spread is common. Fluconazole, 400 mg qd, is appropriate for the treatment of coccidioidal meningitis. Lifelong maintenance is required.

5. **PCP** remains the most common opportunistic infection in patients with AIDS and a leading cause of morbidity and mortality. Extrapulmonary

disease has been described, particularly in patients who receive aerosolized pentamidine for prophylaxis.

a. The **treatment of choice for PCP is TMP/SMZ**, 5 mg/25 mg/kg PO or IV every 6–8 hours for 21 days. Rashes commonly occur in patients with AIDS who are treated with TMP/SMZ but may not require a change in therapy (*Ann Intern Med* 1988;109:280). Pentamidine, 4 mg/kg infused over 2 hours IV qd for 21 days, is also effective and is used in patients who cannot tolerate TMP/SMZ or fail to respond during the first 5–7 days of TMP/SMZ therapy. Dapsone-trimethoprim and clindamycin-primaquine can also be used for moderate disease.

b. **Prophylactic therapy** [TMP/SMZ, 160 mg/800 mg (1 double strength tablet) PO qd, or dapsone, 100 mg PO daily, or pentamidine, 300 mg each month by aerosol] is indicated for patients who recover from PCP and for HIV-infected patients with CD4 lymphocyte counts of less than 200 cells/mm^3.

c. In patients with well-documented PCP and **moderate to severe disease** (arterial oxygen pressure <75 torr on room air), prevention of respiratory failure and survival benefit have been demonstrated with adjunctive use of **steroids** (*N Engl J Med* 1990;323:1451). Prednisone (or equivalent parenteral methylprednisolone if the patient is unable to take oral medication), 40 mg PO bid for 5 days, followed by 40 mg PO qd for 5 days, followed by 20 mg PO qd for the duration of anti-*Pneumocystis* therapy is recommended.

6. **Protozoal infections**

a. *Toxoplasma gondii* typically causes multiple CNS lesions with encephalopathy and focal neurologic findings. Treatment with sulfadiazine, 25 mg/kg PO every 6 hours (or TMP/SMZ, 5 mg/25 mg/kg PO or IV q6–8h), plus pyrimethamine, 100–150 mg PO on day 1, then 50–75 mg PO qd, often results in improvement, but indefinite therapy is needed to prevent relapse. Folinic acid, 5–10 mg PO qd, can be added to minimize hematologic toxicity. For patients who are intolerant of sulfonamides, clindamycin, 600 mg PO qid, can be substituted.

b. *Cryptosporidium* and *I. belli* may cause protozoal enteric infections in patients with AIDS. *I. belli* infection can be treated with TMP/SMZ, 160 mg/800 mg PO qid for 10 days and then bid for 3 weeks (*N Engl J Med* 1986;315:87). Relapses are not uncommon. Shorter courses of TMP/SMZ therapy followed by prophylaxis with pyrimethamine-sulfadoxine may also be effective (*J Infect Dis* 1988;157:225). No therapy has proved to be effective for cryptosporidiosis.

7. **Neoplasms** associated with AIDS include non-Hodgkin's lymphomas and Kaposi's sarcoma. Primary CNS lymphomas are common and may be multicentric. The treatment of these conditions is beyond the scope of this manual.

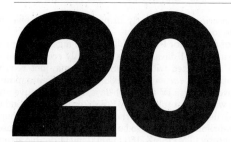

Kidney and Urinary Tract Disorders

Tom Tanphaichitr,
Gopa Green,
and Marvin Grieff

Laboratory Assessment

I. **Assessment of renal function.** Creatinine is a metabolite of skeletal muscle that is freely filtered at the glomerulus and undergoes no significant tubular resorption. It is secreted to a small degree by the renal tubules into the urine. Its production is relative to an individual's muscle mass. Serum creatinine (Scr) varies inversely with glomerular filtration rate (GFR). Any elevation of Scr above the normal range (0.6–1.2 mg/dl) should alert the physician to the presence of reduced GFR and renal insufficiency.

A. **Estimation of GFR.** Because Scr is a function of muscle mass and is dependent on age, gender, and size, it can often be difficult to assess the degree of renal impairment from Scr alone. Renal function, or GFR, can be clinically assessed more accurately by calculating or measuring the creatinine clearance (CrCl). This estimation of GFR is only accurate if the Scr is stable and in steady state. As renal disease progresses toward end stage, these methods become less accurate as creatinine is increasingly secreted by the diseased proximal tubules, causing overestimation of true GFR.

1. **The Cockcroft-Gault CrCl formula** takes age, weight, and gender into account to estimate GFR from a measurement of Scr:

$$\text{CrCl} = \frac{(140 - \text{age}) \times \text{lean body weight (kg)} \ (\times 0.85 \ \text{for females})}{72 \times \text{Scr(mg/dl)}}$$

This formula estimates CrCl in ml/min (normal: 100–125 ml/min for males and 85–100 ml/min for females). This rapid estimation of GFR is useful in adjustment of drug dosages for decreased renal function based on Scr.

2. **24-hour urine collection for CrCl** is the most accurate estimate of GFR in clinical practice. Patients should be instructed to discard their first morning urine and then begin the 24-hour urine collection, ending the collection with inclusion of the following morning's first void.

$$\text{CrCl} = \frac{\text{urine creatinine(mg/dl)} \times \text{urine volume(ml)}}{\text{Scr(mg/dl)} \times \text{time}(1440 \ \text{min for a 24-hr collection})}$$

The amount of total creatinine in the collection can be used to assess the adequacy of the collection; an adequate 24-hour urine collection contains 15–20 mg/kg creatinine for females and 20–25 mg/kg for males.

B. **Determination of chronicity.** The diagnosis of chronic renal failure (CRF) is suggested by a stable elevated Scr for greater than a few months. Acute renal failure (ARF) should be assessed urgently because it can often be reversed. The diagnosis of ARF is suggested by a history of sudden onset (days to weeks before presentation) of hypertension, edema, hematuria, or proteinuria. Further investigation in the determination of ARF versus CRF includes urinalysis and renal ultrasound. The finding of symmetrically small kidneys (<10 cm) on ultrasound images favors CRF, with the notable exceptions of diabetic nephropathy, polycystic kidney disease, amyloidosis, and HIV nephropathy, in which the kidneys may be enlarged. In patients with clearly established CRF, an acute deterioration of renal function must prompt an evaluation for causes of superimposed ARF, which are usually reversible.

II. **Urinalysis** begins with the interpretation of colorimetric reactions on a reagent strip that has been dipped into fresh urine. A microscopic examination of the urine sediment should be performed if there is abnormal renal function, a positive dipstick for hematuria or proteinuria, or evidence for a urinary tract infection (UTI). Ten to 12 ml of a freshly voided specimen should be centrifuged at 1500–3000 rpm for 3–5 minutes, then inverted and the supernatant drained. The pellet can be gently resuspended in the remaining few drops and one drop transferred to a microscope slide, covered with a coverslip, and viewed at 100×–400× to examine the formed elements in the urine.

A. **Hematuria.** The dipstick can detect as few as four RBCs/high-power microscopic field. Free hemoglobin or myoglobin in urine, as can be seen with hemolysis or rhabdomyolysis, catalyze the same dipstick reaction. These conditions should be suspected when the urine dipstick is positive for occult blood in the absence of RBCs on microscopic examination of the urine sediment. False-negative tests result from the presence of substances such as ascorbic acid (ingestion of >200 mg/day vitamin C) that diminish the oxidizing potential of the reagent strip. Detection of hematuria by dipstick should always be confirmed by microscopic examination of the urine. The presence of dysmorphic RBCs or RBC casts (an "active" urine sediment) or the coexistence of proteinuria suggests that the hematuria is of glomerular origin.

B. **Proteinuria.** Persistent proteinuria on more than one occasion should be investigated further. Because the dipstick only detects albumin, in cases of strong suspicion for light-chain excretion (e.g., elderly patients with anemia and high globulin fractions) a sulfosalicylic acid test should be performed to detect non-albumin proteins in the urine. A false-positive dipstick test may result from highly alkaline urine or high urinary concentration of penicillin, cephalosporins, or iodinated radiocontrast agents.

C. **Leukocyte esterase and pyuria.** The presence of positive leukocyte esterase (sensitivity, 75–96%) on dipstick or significant pyuria (≥ 8 leukocytes/mm^3) on a centrifuged specimen suggests a UTI. The presence of pyuria with a negative urine culture could suggest urethritis if the patient complains of dysuria or urgency. Pyuria in the presence of increasing Scr (ARF) suggests the diagnosis of acute interstitial nephritis. Leukocyte casts in the setting of a UTI indicate pyelonephritis.

D. **Bacteriuria and urine nitrite.** The detection of urine nitrite by dipstick suggests a UTI, although this technique may not detect gram-positive organisms or yeast. False positives can occur by contamination of the urine sample by vaginal flora. Bacteriuria (≥ 1 bacteria/mm^3) by microscopy of a fresh uncentrifuged specimen suggests a UTI.

Hematuria

Hematuria is defined by the presence of more than four RBCs/high-power microscopic field. Blood in the urine that is visible as red, pink, or cola-colored urine is referred to as **macroscopic or gross hematuria.** Hematuria should be divided etiologically into two categories: **glomerular** versus **nonglomerular.** Initial investigation of hematuria begins with a complete history and physical examination, which may serve to guide further laboratory testing. All patients with hematuria should have a urinalysis, including both a reagent dipstick and microscopic analysis.

I. History

A. Nonglomerular hematuria. Common causes of nonglomerular hematuria include benign prostatic hypertrophy, kidney stones, urinary tract tumors, and infection, but the differential diagnosis is broad (*JAMA* 1986;256:224). Patients may be entirely asymptomatic except for hematuria or they may have associated symptoms, which aid in diagnosis. Colicky pain at the costovertebral angle or flank with radiation to the groin usually indicates a ureteral stone. A history of dysuria or urinary frequency suggests a UTI, which is usually accompanied by leukocytes or bacteria in the urinalysis. Urinary hesitancy, dribbling, or weak urinary stream accompanies bladder outlet obstruction from a stone, enlarged prostate, or tumor. A family history of nephrolithiasis and a history of inflammatory bowel disease or bowel resection (hyperoxaluria) should also be sought in such cases. A history of heavy physical activity may explain transient (<48 hours) microscopic hematuria. Patients with polycystic kidney disease usually also have a family history of this disease. A history of sickle cell disease or sickle cell trait should be obtained in African-American patients, as vascular sickling, particularly in the renal medulla, can cause RBC extravasation.

B. Glomerular hematuria. The presence of hematuria along with a history that may suggest glomerular disease should prompt referral to a nephrologist. A history of hematuria 1–2 weeks after pharyngitis or skin infection suggests poststreptococcal glomerulonephritis. Bacterial infectious endocarditis, sepsis, abscesses, or infection of an indwelling foreign body such as a ventriculoatrial shunt can be associated with a proliferative glomerulonephritis. Other infectious diseases such as viral hepatitis (hepatitis B and C) and syphilis can also cause a variety of glomerulopathies. Immunoglobulin A nephropathy can present with episodic gross hematuria in the setting of upper respiratory infections. Immune complex–mediated glomerular diseases such as systemic lupus erythematosus or systemic vasculitis can present with arthritis, arthralgias, fever, or rashes. A family history of deafness and renal failure is a feature of hereditary nephritis or Alport's syndrome. As many of these glomerular diseases are associated with ARF and require specific treatment, a nephrologist should be involved early in the care of patients presenting with glomerular hematuria.

C. Medications. Patients taking systemic anticoagulant medications only present with hematuria if there is an underlying nonglomerular lesion that necessitates further evaluation, such as a stone, tumor, or infection. Exposure to cyclophosphamide may lead to hemorrhagic cystitis and, less commonly, bladder cancer, even after cessation of the medication.

II. Physical examination should start with measurement of BP. The presence of edema and hypertension strongly favors glomerular causes of hematuria. Rashes, arthritis, or heart murmurs can often be found with systemic vasculitis, autoimmune glomerulonephritis, and infectious endocarditis-related glomerulonephritis. Digital rectal examination may reveal an enlarged prostate, carcinoma, or prostatitis.

III. Urinalysis is used to determine if the hematuria is glomerular or nonglomerular. The presence of dysmorphic RBCs or RBC casts (an "active" urine sediment) or the coexistence of proteinuria suggests that the blood is coming from the glomerulus of the kidney. Other findings on the urinalysis may indicate UTI.

IV. Laboratory evaluation should include an assessment of renal function with Scr. An elevated Scr in the presence of hematuria requires urgent investigation. If the sediment is "active," a nephrologist should be consulted. If the sediment is not "active," a renal ultrasound should be performed to exclude urinary tract obstruction, which may be due to either stones, tumor, or prostatic disease. Hemoglobin electrophoresis should be obtained in African-American patients with hematuria without prior diagnosis of sickle cell disease or sickle cell trait.

V. Radiologic evaluation. Patients whose urinalysis does not reveal proteinuria or RBC casts should have a renal ultrasound. Patients younger than 40 years of age with a normal ultrasound should be referred to a nephrologist for further investigation. Because of an increased risk of urologic malignancy, patients older than 40 years of age with a normal ultrasound should undergo intravenous pyelogram, urine cytology, and further evaluation by a urologist (often including cystoscopy). In cases in which cystoscopy reveals bleeding from only one ureteral orifice, hematuria may be explained by unilateral vascular lesions such as arteriovenous fistula, hemangioma, or varices of the kidney or ureter. Renal angiogram may be performed to document these lesions, if indicated.

Proteinuria

I. Proteinuria is defined as urinary protein excretion greater than 150 mg/day. It is usually initially detected by reagent dipstick, which indicates the presence of albumin in the urine. Proteinuria is a marker of a wide variety of renal diseases. Any proteinuria that is detected by dipstick should be further evaluated. To aid in the determination of the etiology of proteinuria, an accurate quantitation of urinary protein excretion should be performed.

    A. A 24-hour urine collection for protein can accurately quantify the amount of daily protein excretion in the urine. Concurrent collection of urine creatinine should also be done to ensure the completeness of the collection. The amount of creatinine excreted stays relatively constant at 15–20 mg/kg for females and 20–25 mg/kg for males with stable weight and diet.

    B. Spot urine protein-creatinine ratio can be used to rapidly estimate the amount of protein excretion in 24 hours. This test uses a random spot urine sample for protein (mg/dl) and creatinine (mg/dl) concentrations to calculate urine protein-creatinine ratio. The resulting unitless ratio closely approximates the amount of daily protein excretion in $g/1.73\ m^2$ body surface area. A normal ratio is less than 0.15 (<150 mg/day). Although this test is less cumbersome to perform than the 24-hour urine collection, the results can be unreliable in patients at either extremes of muscle mass. Also, this test is not as accurate for predicting conditions that cause variable amounts of proteinuria/day (e.g., postural proteinuria or diabetic nephropathy).

II. Diagnostic approach. A positive dipstick test should be repeated at least once at a 1-week interval. Conditions that are associated with functional proteinuria, such as fever, emotional stress, heavy physical exercise, or acute medical illness, should be excluded before the test is repeated. Functional proteinuria is usually transient and is most likely related to changes in renal hemodynamics. If the proteinuria is transient, no further investigation is required.

    A. History and physical examination in patients with persistent proteinuria should focus on signs and symptoms of conditions associated with proteinuria, such as hypertension, diabetes mellitus (DM), or connective tissue diseases. Medications should be reviewed. Nonsteroidal anti-inflammatory drugs (NSAIDs) are associated with a variety of renal diseases and should be discontinued in the presence of proteinuria pending further evaluation.

    B. Microscopic examination of the urine sediment should be done once proteinuria is considered persistent (positive dipstick on more than one occasion). Urine sediment should be carefully examined for other signs of glomerular disease such as hematuria or RBC casts.

    C. Laboratory testing should include Scr and a 24-hour urine collection for protein. Abnormal values of renal function tests or proteinuria >150 mg/24 hours suggest intrinsic renal disease. Patients older than 30 years of age should also have a serum and urine protein electrophoresis to exclude paraproteinemia, which may be caused by multiple myeloma. Proteinuria of 3.5 g or greater in 24 hours is referred to as **nephrotic-range proteinuria**. When accompanied by hyperlipidemia, hypoalbuminemia, and edema, this condition is called **nephrotic syndrome**. Proteinuria of this magnitude is almost always of glomerular origin. In adults, accurate diagnosis often requires a renal biopsy. **Orthostatic proteinuria** is defined as proteinuria with less than 75 mg of urinary protein excretion while recumbent. Total urinary protein does not usually exceed 1.5 g/day. This condition has a good prognosis, is uncommon in patients older than 30 years of age, and can be diagnosed with a split urine collection for protein.

III. **Nephrology referral.** Persistent proteinuria that is associated with abnormal renal function tests, active urine sediment (hematuria, RBC casts), or nephrotic-range proteinuria (>3.5 g/day) strongly suggests progressive renal involvement. The differential diagnosis is vast, and therapeutic options depend on an accurate diagnosis of the etiology often requiring renal biopsy. Persistent proteinuria with normal renal function and non–nephrotic-range proteinuria follows a more indolent course. Nevertheless, approximately 40% of these patients experience progression of disease with long-term follow-up. Therefore, all cases of persistent proteinuria should be referred to and comanaged with a nephrologist.

Urinary Tract Infections

I. **Acute uncomplicated cystitis in women.** Patients with uncomplicated UTI have no evidence of upper tract infection (e.g., absence of fever or flank pain) and low risk of primary therapeutic failure. Affected patients present with dysuria, urgency, frequency, suprapubic pain, and/or hematuria. Fever ($\geq 37.8°C$), typically absent in uncomplicated cystitis, makes either complicated cystitis or pyelonephritis more likely.

A. **Laboratory evaluation** includes reagent dipstick and a microscopic examination of the urine, with culture if indicated (see Laboratory Assessment, sec. II). Patients with urethritis or vaginitis also may complain of dysuria, but only those with cystitis or urethritis have pyuria. A positive urine dipstick for leukocyte esterase detects pyuria, whereas a positive nitrite test suggests the presence of at least 10^5 bacteria/ml in the urine. A negative urine dipstick in the presence of UTI symptoms should trigger a microscopic examination of the urine for leukocytes and bacteria. Urine cultures are generally not necessary in women with uncomplicated cystitis, as the causative organisms are predictable and culture results only become available after the patient's symptoms have greatly improved or resolved. Urine cultures are required if there is any concern for a complicated UTI. Quantitative culture often yields more than 10^5 bacteria/ml, but colony counts as low as 10^2–10^4 bacteria/ml may indicate infection in women with acute dysuria (*Ann Intern Med* 1993;119:454). Uncomplicated UTIs in women are caused by *Escherichia coli* in 80% of cases and by *Staphylococcus saprophyticus* in 5–15% of cases.

B. **Treatment.** Trimethoprim-sulfamethoxazole (TMP/SMX) DS (160 mg/400 mg) PO bid, a first-generation cephalosporin (e.g., cephalexin), or a fluoroquinolone for 3 days is effective for uncomplicated UTIs in women. It is unclear whether increased hydration or cranberry juice have any role in the treatment of UTI. Patients with severe dysuria may benefit from urinary analgesia with phenazopyridine, 200 mg PO tid for 1–2 days. If symptoms do not resolve soon after therapy, a urine culture should be performed, and the diagnosis should be reassessed.

II. **Acute complicated cystitis.** Any patient with a risk factor for upper UTI or for whom an empiric 3-day course of antibiotics may not suffice should be assumed to have complicated cystitis. Risk factors include (1) prior urinary tract instrumentation, or urinary tract abnormality; (2) hospital-acquired infection; (3) DM; (4) immunosuppression; (5) multiple drug-resistant urinary pathogens; (6) symptoms for more than 7 days; and (7) age ≥ 65 years. Presenting symptoms of fever, flank pain, nausea, and vomiting suggest extension of the infection beyond the bladder to the upper tract, or pyelonephritis (see sec. **VIII** below).

A. **Laboratory evaluation** should include Scr, urinalysis using a reagent dipstick and microscopy, and a urine culture, including antibiotic sensitivity testing. Pyuria is present in almost all patients with complicated cystitis. Blood cultures should be obtained if the patient is febrile to rule out the presence of urosepsis.

B. **Treatment** should be begun empirically after the urine culture is obtained to cover a broad spectrum of gram-negative organisms using a fluoroquinolone such as ciprofloxacin, 500 mg PO bid, or levofloxacin, 500 mg PO qd. Parenteral therapy (e.g., ciprofloxacin, 400 mg IV bid) is indicated in patients who cannot take oral medications and in the case of multiply resistant uropathogens. When quinolones are contraindicated (e.g., pregnancy, allergy to quinolones), ceftriaxone, 1–2 g IV qd, may be used. Admission to the hospital is recommended in the presence of significant disability, inability to take oral medications, or noncompliance. Once drug sensitivities are known, it may be possible to switch to a less broad-spectrum antibiotic. The recommended duration of therapy for complicated cystitis is 7–14 days.

C. **Radiologic evaluation** should be considered if there are no signs of improvement within 48 hours of initiation of antibiotic therapy. Renal ultrasound or CT may detect anatomic urinary tract abnormalities or other pathology.

III. **Recurrent cystitis in women.** Young women who present with an initial episode of cystitis may experience recurrent infections in up to 20% of cases. Exogenous reinfections account for more than 90% of recurrences. Relapses with the original infecting organism that occur within 2 weeks of cessation of therapy should be cultured and re-treated for 10–14 days with an antibiotic based on bacterial sensitivity. In patients with three or more episodes/year, TMP/SMX SS qd or every other day is usually sufficient to decrease recurrences if there are no known urologic abnormalities or other predisposing factors.

A. **Honeymoon cystitis** should be considered in women with relapses that correlate with sexual intercourse. TMP/SMX SS (80 mg/200 mg) or cephalexin (250 mg) after coitus may provide adequate prophylaxis. An alternative method of contraception might decrease the frequency of reinfection in women who use a diaphragm and spermicide (*N Engl J Med* 1996;335:468).

B. **Postmenopausal women** may be predisposed to frequent UTIs due to postvoid residual urine, which is often associated with bladder or uterine prolapse. Lack of estrogen may also cause changes in the vaginal mucosa that promote colonization by *E. coli*. Antimicrobial prophylaxis, topical vaginal estrogen cream, or both decrease the frequency of recurrent infections in postmenopausal women with three or more UTIs/year (*N Engl J Med* 1993;325:753).

IV. **UTIs in men.** Men who present with acute uncomplicated UTIs may not necessarily have an underlying urologic abnormality. Patients present with dysuria, urgency, frequency, suprapubic pain, and/or hematuria. In men, risk factors for UTI in the absence of urologic abnormality include homosexuality, intercourse with an infected female partner, and lack of circumcision. The diagnosis may be made on the basis of symptoms along with a urinalysis, including microscopic examination of the urine. A pretreatment urine culture should be obtained. Urethritis should also be considered in sexually active men, especially in the presence of a negative urine culture. Treatment is similar to that of acute uncomplicated cystitis in women except that a 7-day course of treatment is warranted. If there is a prompt response to therapy, urologic evaluation is unlikely to be useful. Urologic studies are appropriate when treatment fails, in the event of recurrent UTI, or when pyelonephritis occurs. Prostatitis should also be considered in the event of recurrent UTIs.

V. **Asymptomatic bacteriuria** is defined as a positive mid-stream urine culture with greater than or equal to 10^5 colony-forming units/ml in patients without UTI symptoms. Treatment is justified in the following situations: before urologic surgery, after removal of a bladder catheter, in young children with vesicoureteral reflux, and in pregnant women. Anatomic changes of the urinary tract in pregnant women increase the risk of pyelonephritis with asymptomatic bacteriuria to 20–40%. Asymptomatic bacteriuria of pregnancy should be treated with 3 days of antibiotics. Penicillins and cephalosporins are safe in pregnancy, as are sulfonamides (except late in the third trimester when they may increase the risk of neonatal jaundice). Fluoroquinolones and tetracyclines are contraindicated during pregnancy. No evidence supports the routine screening of urine or treatment of asymptomatic bacteriuria in other settings, including in diabetic or elderly patients.

VI. **Acute prostatitis** (see Chap. 25) may occur spontaneously in young men or may be associated with an indwelling urethral catheter. It usually presents with fever, chills, dysuria, and a tense or boggy tender prostate. Vigorous prostatic massage should not be performed because it may induce bacteremia. Urine culture often reveals the causative pathogen. The most common pathogens in acute bacterial prostatitis include *Enterococcus*, *S. aureus*, *S. epidermidis*, or gram-negative organisms, including *E. coli*, *Klebsiella*, and *Enterobacteriaceae*. In patients who are younger than 35 years old, the sexually transmitted pathogens *Neisseria gonorrhoeae* or *Chlamydia trachomatis* account for a large proportion of cases. Empiric treatment with fluoroquinolones provides excellent penetration into prostatic tissues and should usually continue for 14 days. Chlamydia may cause a chronic prostatitis that may require prolonged treatment for 4 weeks or longer.

VII. **Epididymitis** symptoms include unilateral testicular tenderness and swelling. It is usually caused by *N. gonorrhoeae* or *C. trachomatis* in sexually active young men and by gram-negative enteric organisms in older men. Therapy should be directed accordingly, with ceftriaxone and doxycycline in young men and TMP/SMX or ciprofloxacin in men older than 40 years. The duration of therapy is usually 10–14 days. Bed rest, scrotal elevation, and analgesics are useful therapeutic adjuncts.

VIII. **Pyelonephritis** may occur as a result of ascending bacterial infection from the bladder in an otherwise healthy individual. Anatomic genitourinary abnormalities predispose patients to development of pyelonephritis. Although the presence of genitourinary abnormalities is often not known when the diagnosis of pyelonephritis is made, the treatment plans must be altered accordingly if they are discovered.

A. **Acute pyelonephritis**
  1. **Diagnosis.** Patients present with a variety of symptoms, often including fever, nausea/vomiting, and flank pain or costovertebral angle tenderness. Symptoms of cystitis may or may not be present. Urine specimens characteristically demonstrate significant bacteriuria, pyuria, and occasional leukocyte casts. Urine cultures should be obtained in all patients, but 20% of affected patients have fewer than 10^5 colony-forming units/ml. Blood cultures should be obtained in patients who require hospitalization, as bacteremia may be detected in 15–20% of these patients. The causative agent is usually *E. coli*. In patients who are very ill or who do not respond clinically within 48 hours, ultrasonography, CT scan, or intravenous pyelography should be considered to rule out an anatomic abnormality, intrarenal abscess, emphysematous pyelonephritis, or a renal calculus.
  2. **Treatment.** Patients with mild to moderate illness who are able to take oral medications can be safely treated as outpatients with TMP/SMX or fluoroquinolones for 14 days. Patients with more severe illness,

those who are nauseated and vomiting, and pregnant patients should be treated initially with parenteral therapy. Appropriate empiric parenteral regimens include initial therapy with a fluoroquinolone or a third-generation cephalosporin (e.g., ceftriaxone). If enterococcal infection is suspected on the basis of a urine Gram stain, ampicillin, 1 g IV every 6 hours, with or without gentamicin, 1 mg/kg IV every 8 hours, is appropriate.

B. Patients with **pyelonephritis with anatomic abnormalities** that were either previously established or discovered by radiologic assessment during the treatment of the acute episode, as well as pregnant women, should be hospitalized for parenteral treatment. Intrarenal abscesses may require drainage or prolonged antimicrobial therapy. Emphysematous pyelonephritis requires immediate nephrectomy. Urinary tract obstruction (e.g., stones or tumor) manifests as hydronephrosis and should be relieved with percutaneous nephrostomy or other urologic maneuver as soon as possible to allow drainage of the collecting system.

Nephrolithiasis

I. Presentation. Kidney stones cause symptoms when they become lodged at some point in the urinary tract. They may present as hematuria, flank or groin pain, and predisposition to UTI. Flank pain may be accompanied by nausea, vomiting, and ileus. Patients often have a family history of kidney stones, a history of prior kidney stones, gout, inflammatory bowel disease, or recurrent UTIs. The differential diagnosis of acute flank pain includes appendicitis, cholecystitis, ectopic pregnancy, and dissecting aneurysm. Stationary stones may be entirely asymptomatic and may be detected as an incidental finding on radiographic studies. Oliguria and ARF may occur either when both kidneys are obstructed or when the patient has an obstructed single kidney.

II. Evaluation of an acute stone episode should include a urinalysis, an assessment of renal function with Scr and serum electrolytes, including serum calcium, and a radiologic assessment of the urinary tract. Hematuria is present in the majority of patients with kidney stones, but its absence does not exclude a symptomatic kidney stone. A plain abdominal radiograph is likely to detect a stone, as calcium stones (which represent 70–90% of all stones) and cystine stones are both radiopaque. Plain abdominal radiography may miss stones of intermediate opacity, such as uric acid stones. Spiral CT scanning without intravenous contrast has high sensitivity (up to 98%) for both radiopaque and radiolucent stones and has become the gold standard for diagnosis of stone disease. Other diagnostic tests that are commonly used include intravenous pyelogram or renal ultrasound, which should be used in the evaluation of the pregnant patient with suspected nephrolithiasis.

III. Treatment of the acute stone episode is based on the size of the stone that is causing symptoms. Although they cause pain, stones of 5 mm or less usually pass on their own, and the patient may only require oral analgesia and hydration. Intravenous ketorolac has been shown to be effective in relieving renal colic (*Ann Emerg Med* 1996;28:151). One approach is to prescribe standard doses of an oral narcotic (acetaminophen with codeine) and an NSAID. Patients who are unable to take oral analgesia or fluids should be admitted to the hospital. Stones of less than 5 mm that do not pass within 7 days, stones of more than 6 mm, those that cause obstruction, those in a patient with a single kidney, and the finding of stones in the presence of renal failure require urologic intervention. In all cases, patients should be instructed to strain their urine and save any stones that are passed for analysis. NSAIDs should be discontinued at least 3 days before anticipated lithotripsy to minimize risk of bleeding.

IV. **Metabolic evaluation of nephrolithiasis.** All patients with kidney stones should have a determination of serum calcium, assessment of stone composition, and dietary counseling. Patients with an elevated serum calcium should be evaluated for primary hyperparathyroidism or other causes of hypercalcemia, including malignancy and sarcoidosis. The extent of the metabolic evaluation that should be undertaken for the patient with a single calcium stone has not been established, but recurrent calcium nephrolithiasis warrants complete investigation. Patients with noncalcium stones should undergo evaluation after the first episode. Additional studies include at least two 24-hour urine studies for measurement of urine volume, pH, calcium, urate, oxalate, citrate, creatinine, and sodium. Urine studies should not be performed within 3–4 weeks of an acute stone episode or in the presence of UTI. A quantitative 24-hour urine for cystine should be collected if the composition of the stone is unknown. Yearly follow-up examination of the patient with nephrolithiasis includes abdominal radiographs to check for new stone formation or growth of existing stones and repeat metabolic studies to assess the effects of specific therapies. General information for patients and treating physicians on kidney stones can be found at the following Web site: http://www.niddk.nih.gov/health/kidney/pubs/whastone/whastone.htm.

V. **Dietary modification in stone prevention.** Dietary counseling should be provided to all patients with kidney stones to prevent further stone formation. Fluid intake should be increased to achieve daily urine volumes of greater than 2000 ml to increase the urine flow rate and lower the urine solute concentration. This often requires a fluid intake of at least 2400 ml/day (80 oz/day), as insensible losses can amount to another 1000 ml/day (or more in a hot climate). A simple rule to share with patients is that their urine should always be clear rather than yellow. Dietary calcium restriction may result in impaired bone mineralization and may actually increase the risk for nephrolithiasis by increasing the absorption and urinary excretion of oxalate (*N Engl J Med* 1993;328:833). Calcium supplementation should be avoided as well, as it may also increase the risk for recurrent stones (*Ann Intern Med* 1997;126:497). To decrease urinary calcium, which is a frequent constituent of stones, a low-sodium diet (100 mEq or 2300 mg/day) should be followed. A low-oxalate diet may decrease urinary oxalate. Oxalate is present in beets, rhubarb, spinach, chard, greens, endive, okra, tea, chocolate, cocoa, and nuts. A low-protein/low-purine diet decreases urinary uric acid excretion and may also decrease urinary calcium excretion.

VI. **Calcium stones** account for approximately 80% of all stones and are composed of calcium oxalate or calcium phosphate. Calcium stones are usually idiopathic but can occur with primary hyperparathyroidism, medullary sponge kidney, or distal renal tubular acidosis (in which there is metabolic acidosis, urine pH persistently >5.5, nephrocalcinosis, and a tendency to form calcium phosphate stones). The urinary findings in patients with idiopathic calcium stones include hypercalciuria, hyperuricosuria, hyperoxaluria (may also be seen in patients with inflammatory bowel disorders), and hypocitraturia. Hypercalciuria is present in approximately 50% of patients with calcium stones. Calcium stones also may precipitate around a uric acid nidus in patients with hyperuricosuria, even in the absence of hypercalciuria. Each urinary abnormality can be identified based on the results of the 24-hour urine studies and treated as follows.

A. **Hypercalciuria** (calcium excretion >4 mg/kg/day) is most often due to increased GI absorption of calcium but may also be caused by impaired renal tubular calcium reabsorption or excessive skeletal resorption as in primary hyperparathyroidism. Primary hyperparathyroidism that results in renal stone formation is an indication for parathyroidectomy. Except for primary hyperparathyroidism and distal renal tubular acidosis, all other causes of hypercalciuria are treated similarly. Patients should maintain a normal calcium intake (800–1000 mg/day). They should ensure adequate fluid intake and restrict sodium intake to 2300 mg/day. Patients may require addition of a thiazide diuretic (e.g., hydrochlorothiazide, 25–50 mg PO qd) to increase renal calcium reabsorption. A low-sodium diet tends to improve the efficacy of the thiazide. Careful follow-up is important in these patients to ensure that therapy has decreased calcium excretion and has not caused adverse alterations in serum electrolytes such as hypokalemia.

B. Hyperuricosuria (>0.75 g/24 hr in men; >0.7 g/24 hr in women) may also result in calcium stone formation as uric acid crystals may serve as a nidus for calcium oxalate or calcium phosphate precipitation. Allopurinol, 300 mg PO qd, has been shown to decrease calcium stone formation in the setting of hyperuricosuria (*N Engl J Med* 1986;315:1386).

C. Hyperoxaluria (urinary oxalate excretion >40 mg/day) often responds to dietary restriction. Patients with small bowel malabsorption due to intrinsic disease (e.g., inflammatory bowel disease), postresection, or jejunoileal bypass may absorb excessive oxalate, resulting in enteric hyperoxaluria. Dietary restriction of oxalate and oxalate binders such as oral calcium citrate or cholestyramine with meals may be useful. A 24-hour urine collection should be obtained within 2–4 weeks of initiating supplemental dietary calcium therapy to monitor for hypercalciuria. Primary hyperoxaluria is due to a genetic enzymatic defect in amino acid metabolism in which excess oxalate is produced. These patients have nonenteric hyperoxaluria that does not respond to dietary manipulation. They should be referred to a nephrologist for further management of renal stone disease.

D. Hypocitraturia (<250 mg/24 hr in men; <300 mg/24 hr in women) refers to an abnormally low level of urinary citrate excretion. Citrate is a potent inhibitor of calcium oxalate precipitation. Citrate excretion can be enhanced by therapy with potassium citrate, 20 mEq PO tid. Lemon juice is an inexpensive and well tolerated source of dietary citrate and has been shown to increase urinary citrate excretion. Four ounces of lemon juice in 2 L of water/day may be useful in patients with borderline low urinary citrates (*J Urol* 1996;156:907).

VII. Uric acid stone formation is favored by conditions of uric acid overproduction, low urinary volumes, and persistently acid urine pH. Conservative therapy involves maintenance of urine volumes of greater than 2 L/day through oral hydration, dietary purine restriction (i.e., meat, fish, and poultry), and alkalinization of urine to pH 6.5–7.0 with an oral alkali preparation, such as potassium citrate, 20 mEq PO tid. Allopurinol, 300 mg PO qd, can be used if these measures fail. The potential adverse effects of allopurinol include allergic reaction, interstitial nephritis, and, rarely, hepatitis. Probenecid and other uricosuric drugs should be avoided, as they may increase the risk of uric acid or calcium stones.

VIII. Cystine stones arise from an autosomal recessive inherited disorder of dibasic amino acid renal transport, resulting in an excess cystine in the urine. Cystine is formed from the disulfide linkage of two cysteine molecules. It is relatively insoluble in urine and often crystallizes to form radiopaque stones. These stones are resistant to lithotripsy and often require surgical stone extraction. Hexagonal cystine crystals may be detected on microscopic examination of the urine. Cystinuria is often discovered after analysis of a stone or quantitative urine testing for cystine. In general, patients with cystine stones should be followed by a nephrologist. The goal of treatment is to reduce the urinary cystine concentration below its solubility limit (250 mg/L). Urine volume should be greater than 3 L/day, and urine should be alkalinized to a pH of greater than 7.0 with potassium citrate. Tiopronin, penicillin, or captopril form disulfide bonds with cysteine and decrease the availability of free cysteine to form the insoluble cystine dimer. These medications may be useful in decreasing urinary cystine excretion.

IX. Infection stones (struvite) occur under conditions of high urinary pH and increased ammonia production, reflecting infection with urea-splitting organisms (e.g., *Proteus mirabilis*, *Klebsiella*). *E. coli* does not produce urease. These stones are usually composed of magnesium ammonium phosphate (struvite) or carbonate apatite and are often in the shape of a "staghorn," as they grow rapidly and typically extend to involve more than one renal calyx. These stones often occur in paraplegic or quadriplegic patients because of increased predisposition to UTIs. For antimicrobial treatment to be effective, the infected stone must be removed surgically, percutaneously, or by shock-wave lithotripsy.

Chronic Renal Failure

The U.S. Renal Data System reports that in 1997 more than 350,000 people in the United States were enrolled in the End-Stage Renal Disease (ESRD) program, with more than 75,000 new cases in that year alone. ESRD patients experience greater morbidity and decreased quality of life than the general population. For example, the life expectancy of a patient who is beginning dialysis after age 59 years is a mere 4.3 years, which is only slightly better than that of patients with lung cancer. Optimal pre-ESRD care involves early recognition of CRF, medical treatments directed toward slowing the progression of CRF to ESRD, prevention of factors that accelerate the progression of CRF, and timely referral of patients to nephrologists.

I. **Causes of CRF.** Because patients with renal insufficiency often lack symptoms until late in the course of their disease, recognition of its common causes is essential.

A. **DM** is the most common cause of ESRD in the United States, accounting for up to 36% of new ESRD patients. Typically, patients with diabetic nephropathy have a long-standing history of DM, often with manifestations of other vascular complications such as retinopathy and peripheral vascular disease. The earliest manifestation of diabetic nephropathy is **microalbuminuria** (urinary albumin excretion of >30 mg/24 hrs), a strong predictor for progression of renal disease as well as for increased risk of cardiovascular disease. Interventions that are initiated before the onset of overt proteinuria (>300 mg/day) are most effective in preventing complications of diabetic nephropathy. A spot urine for albumin-to-creatinine ratio is a rapid screen for microalbuminuria (>30 mg albumin/g creatinine) and should be performed annually in patients with DM.

B. **Hypertensive nephrosclerosis** occurs in patients with long-standing, uncontrolled hypertension. Unlike diabetic nephropathy, proteinuria rarely reaches the nephrotic range (>3.5 g/day) in this disorder.

C. **Tubulointerstitial nephritis** results from many different etiologies. Among the more common causes are medications (analgesics, NSAIDs, antibiotics, lithium), urinary reflux, and chronic UTI. Urine findings are commonly unremarkable, with mild or no proteinuria.

D. **Glomerulonephritis**, as a group, is a common cause of CRF. Patients may initially present with ARF, sudden onset of hypertension, edema, or active urine sediment (RBCs and casts). Early recognition of these signs should prompt referral to a nephrologist to prevent progression to CRF.

E. **Polycystic kidney disease** is characterized by markedly enlarged kidneys that contain multiple cysts of varying sizes. Family history is often informative as it is inherited in an autosomal dominant pattern, although new mutations may account for sporadic cases.

II. **Treatment.** CRF invariably progresses toward ESRD. Treatment is therefore aimed at deterring this progression and addressing the attendant complications of the disease.

A. **Delaying the progression of CRF**

1. **Hypertension** leads to accelerated progression of renal insufficiency from all causes by exacerbating increased intraglomerular pressure. Many patients with CRF are volume overloaded due to the diseased kid-

neys' impairment in excreting an ingested salt load as well as altered renal hemodynamics. Diuretics, therefore, are effective in treating hypertension as well as volume overload in patients with CRF. Patients with GFR of less than 30 ml/min usually require loop diuretics for effective diuresis. All classes of antihypertensives are effective in delaying renal disease progression when BP is persistently elevated. Angiotensin-converting enzyme (ACE) inhibitors and angiotensin II receptor blockers may also have a renal-protective property independent of their effect on systemic BP, especially in diabetic patients with proteinuria (*N Engl J Med* 1993;329:1456, and *N Engl J Med* 1996;334:939). A mean arterial BP goal of 100 mm Hg (approximately 130/85) is recommended, but patients with more than 1 g/day of proteinuria may benefit from a mean arterial pressure as low as 92 mm Hg (approximately 125/75) (*Ann Intern Med* 1995;123:754). Patients should be encouraged to follow daily weights and BPs with a home monitoring device in consultation with their physicians.

2. **Dietary protein modification.** In general, reduction of dietary protein intake (0.7–0.8 g/kg/day) has been thought to retard the progression of renal insufficiency, especially in the presence of clinical proteinuria. Recently, however, it has been documented that patients actually spontaneously restrict protein intake as GFR declines (*J Am Soc Nephrol* 1995;6:1386). Hypoalbuminemia, a marker of increased mortality in dialysis patients, can occur in some cases. Therefore, protein restriction should be undertaken only on a case-by-case basis in consultation with a renal dietitian.

3. **Glycemic control** (hemoglobin A_{1c} <7%) in diabetic patients has been shown to slow the progression of chronic renal disease, perhaps by reducing intraglomerular pressure (*N Engl J Med* 1999;341:1127).

4. **Avoidance of nephrotoxins.** Diseased kidneys are particularly vulnerable to further insult. NSAIDs and the newer cyclooxygenase-2 inhibitors deplete prostaglandins, which are important for renal hemodynamic compensation. They should not be used in patients with a GFR less than 60 ml/min (Scr ≥ 1.5 mg/dl), especially those who are receiving an ACE inhibitor or diuretics. Questions regarding over-the-counter use of NSAIDs are important at every follow-up visit. Aminoglycoside antibiotics, IV contrast studies, and other agents associated with nephrotoxicity should be avoided in patients with CRF. If a contrast study is absolutely necessary, patients should be well hydrated with IV fluids (0.45% saline at a rate of 1 ml/kg/hr) for at least 12 hours before and after the procedure. Nonionic, low osmolarity contrast agents should be used if available, with the amount of contrast administered limited as much as possible. **Acetylcysteine** (600 mg PO bid the day before and the day of the procedure) may be of benefit in preventing contrast nephropathy in patients with a Scr ≥ 2.5 mg/dl (*N Engl J Med* 2000;343:180).

B. **Management of complications of CRF**
   1. **Sodium and water.** A moderate sodium-restricted diet (3000 mg or 130 mEq sodium/day) is usually adequate to avoid salt and volume overload. Patients with CRF are less able to deal with acute changes in sodium load. They may become volume depleted as a result of continued renal sodium wasting when abruptly placed on a sodium-restricted diet (e.g., with hospital admission). Free water excretion is well maintained in CRF until near end stage. Fluid restriction is therefore appropriate only when hyponatremia develops. Urinary concentration is more often impaired. Patients may become hypernatremic if access to free water is restricted.
   2. **Metabolic acidosis** occurs as less of the acid load from dietary protein metabolism can be excreted due to progression of the renal disease. Sodium bicarbonate, 650 mg PO tid, should be started when serum bicarbonate falls below 20 mEq/L to prevent bone demineralization,

insulin resistance, increased protein catabolism, growth retardation, and exacerbation of secondary hyperparathyroidism. Sodium or potassium citrate preparations (e.g., Bicitra) should be avoided in CRF patients, because citrate enhances aluminum absorption. Aluminum accumulates in renal disease leading to neurotoxicity.

3. **Anemia** of CRF is associated with erythropoietin deficiency that develops as the GFR falls below 30 ml/min. Treatment with erythropoietin is usually initiated when the hemoglobin is less than 10 g/dl and other etiologies for anemia (i.e., iron deficiency, GI blood loss, myelodysplasia) have been ruled out. The initial dose of erythropoietin is 80–120 units/kg/wk SC, in divided doses two to three times/week, with the goal to maintain a hemoglobin of 11–12 g/dl. The rate of increase in hemoglobin is dose dependent but does not usually exceed 1 g/dl/wk. A perceptible increase in hemoglobin may take 2–3 weeks of treatment. Effective erythropoiesis also requires adequate iron stores. CRF patients receiving erythropoietin should have transferrin saturation and ferritin monitored monthly and receive either oral (200 mg elemental iron qd) or IV iron supplementation to keep transferrin saturation >20% and ferritin >100 ng/ml. CBCs should be followed at least monthly in patients receiving erythropoietin. When the hemoglobin is greater than 13 g/dl, the dose of erythropoietin should be reduced or held. In that case, hemoglobin levels should be followed weekly, because erythropoiesis decreases once erythropoietin is held and anemia may redevelop. A novel erythropoiesis-stimulating protein, darbepoietin alpha, can be administered weekly or every other week. It may prove to be more convenient and as effective as erythropoietin for the treatment of anemia of CRF.

4. **Secondary hyperparathyroidism** occurs as an adaptation to phosphorus retention in CRF and progresses as hypocalcemia develops from decreased availability of calcitriol. Elevation in parathyroid hormone (PTH) results in increased bone turnover and renal osteodystrophy. Oral calcitriol therapy (0.5–1.0 µg/day) can be started to control secondary hyperparathyroidism. Serum calcium should be monitored weekly and maintained at the upper limit of normal. Calcitriol should be held if the serum calcium is greater than 11 mg/dl or if the serum phosphorus is greater than 6.5 mg/dl. **Parathyroidectomy** is required when the parathyroid gland becomes autonomous and fails to respond to reduction in phosphorus levels or to calcitriol supplementation. Other indications for parathyroidectomy include an elevated serum calcium in the presence of hyperparathyroidism and a markedly elevated intact PTH level (>800–1000 µg/L).

5. **Hyperphosphatemia** occurs as GFR falls below 25–30 ml/min and the kidneys are unable to excrete excess phosphorus despite the development of secondary hyperparathyroidism. Precipitation of calcium phosphate in the kidneys and other tissues can lead to disease progression with attendant high morbidity. Hyperphosphatemia should be controlled by limiting phosphorus intake to approximately 800 mg/day. Because further reduction of intake becomes impractical, phosphorus binders should be started when the GFR is less than 30 ml/min. Calcium carbonate, 500 mg with each meal, can be initiated and titrated to keep the phosphorus level between 4.5 and 5.0 mg/dl. The calcium phosphate product (serum calcium in mg/dl × serum phosphorus in mg/dl) should be monitored monthly. A product of greater than 60 suggests a high risk of calcium-phosphorus coprecipitation and should initiate a prompt reevaluation of the patient's diet and medications.

III. **Referral.** Management of patients with CRF should be done in consultation with a nephrologist. A National Institutes of Health consensus statement on morbidity and mortality of dialysis suggests that referral to a nephrologist should be made when Scr reaches 1.5 mg/dl in women and 2.0 mg/dl in men. The renal team, consisting of nephrologists, renal nurse specialists, social workers, and renal dietitians, is equipped to assist the primary care physician with issues such as anemia management, calcium/phosphorus control, and dietary modification. More important, early referral allows more time for patients to make informed choices regarding forms of renal replacement therapy, including referral to a renal transplant center, if appropriate, and placement of vascular or peritoneal access for dialysis if indicated.

Urinary Incontinence

I. **Urinary incontinence (UI)** affects approximately 50% of the institutionalized elderly and 30% of those who live at home. It can lead to perineal rashes, decubitus ulcers, UTI, and sepsis. Psychosocially, it can lead to loss of self-esteem, restriction of activities, depression, and institutionalization.

II. **Pathophysiology**

   A. **Stress incontinence** is a common cause of UI in elderly women. It is caused by an incompetent sphincter mechanism. Urine leaks occur when the intraabdominal pressure increases with straining, coughing, laughing, or sneezing. A common cause of impaired sphincter mechanism is abnormal positioning of the urethra secondary to pelvic prolapse. Congenital, traumatic (spinal cord injury), iatrogenic (radiation), or medical (alpha-blocker) denervation of the sphincter muscles can also lead to stress incontinence.

   B. **Urge incontinence** occurs when detrusor overactivity overcomes normal central inhibition of bladder contraction. It can occur as a result of central nervous system dysfunction such as stroke or Parkinson's disease. Hyperexcitability of the afferent sensory pathway due to cystitis, atrophic vaginitis-urethritis-trigonitis, or bladder wall hypertrophy (chronic low-volume voiding) may also cause urge incontinence. Symptoms include urinary frequency, urgency, and nocturia.

   C. **Functional incontinence** occurs in patients with a normal detrusor and sphincter mechanism. Most often, this condition is due to lack of access to the toilet as a result of immobility, inability to articulate the need for urination (dementia or delirium), or the use of fast-acting, potent diuretics.

   D. **Overflow incontinence** is more common in men than in women as a result of bladder outlet obstruction caused by prostatic hypertrophy, fecal impaction, or urethral stricture. Alternatively, overflow incontinence can occur as a result of an atonic bladder that can no longer contract forcefully enough to empty itself. This is a result of damage to bladder nerves (e.g., diabetic neuropathy, radiation, or tumor) or medications that impair detrusor contraction (e.g., anticholinergics, calcium channel blockers). Patients usually complain of dribbling or incomplete emptying of the bladder.

III. **Diagnosis of UI**

   A. **History and physical examination** may identify readily reversible and transient causes of UI (Table 20-1). Often, a careful history can uncover causes of functional UI, such as lack of access or confusion. Symptoms of UTI can often be elicited from the history and treated empirically in females. Physical examination may reveal atrophic vaginitis or fecal impaction. Finally, a careful review of the patient's medications frequently reveals the offending agents (Table 20-2).

   B. **Further investigation** is needed if transient or functional causes have been excluded or if patients continue to experience UI. Symptoms of urge incontinence include urinary urgency, frequency, and incomplete emptying of the bladder. The amount of urine loss is small to moderate, and nocturia is also common. Stress incontinence is usually characterized by a momentary leakage of urine associated with maneuvers that increase intraabdominal pressure (e.g., laughing, coughing, Valsalva). Continued urine leakage after the intraabdominal pressure has returned to normal suggests urge incontinence.

Table 20-1. Causes of transient urinary incontinence (DIAPPERS)

Cause	Comments
Delirium/confusional state	Exclude underlying acute illness, infections, and medications
Infection (UTI)	Asymptomatic bacteriuria does not cause UI
Atrophic urethritis/ vaginitis	Vaginal erosion, telangiectasia, petechiae, and friability; may contribute to other causes of UI
Pharmaceutical	See Table 20-2
Psychological	Rare; causes UI only if severe (e.g., severe depression)
Excessive urine output	Large fluid intake, diuretic agents (including theophylline, caffeinated beverages, and alcohol), and metabolic disorder (e.g., hyperglycemia, hypercalcemia); nocturnal UI may be secondary to mobilization of peripheral edema when patient is supine
Restricted mobility	Often due to correctable conditions such as arthritis, pain, or fear of falling
Stool impaction	May cause fecal and urinary incontinence

UI, urinary incontinence; UTI, urinary tract infection.

1. **Urinalysis** should be obtained to exclude treatable conditions such as UTI or glycosuria that may exacerbate UI.
2. **Postvoid residual (PVR)** should be measured to detect bladder retention that can lead to overflow incontinence. Moreover, PVR can also serve to document the effectiveness of the treatment of transient causes of UI (e.g., withdrawal of anticholinergics or fecal disimpaction). PVR is usually measured by straight catheterization of the bladder after the patient has urinated. Postvoid volume is normally less than 50 ml. A volume of greater than 100 ml is abnormal.
3. **Referral to a urologist** should be made if the diagnosis of UI remains equivocal. A recent onset of irritative bladder symptoms that causes urgency, particularly if associated with hematuria, may suggest bladder malignancy and the need for urologic evaluation. Furthermore, incontinence that is associated with recurrent UTI, prostate irregularities or enlargement, pelvic prolapse, or a prior history of pelvic surgery most likely requires referral to either urology or gynecology.

IV. **Treatment.** The first step in treating UI is to identify transient or functional causes as described above. Many patients respond to simple measures such as providing easy access to the toilet, treatment of UTI, or discontinuation of offending medications. Once transient or functional causes have been excluded, treatment that is aimed at specific types of UI can be explored.

A. **Urge incontinence** is treated initially with behavioral therapies that are aimed at decreasing uninhibited bladder contraction and improving bladder capacity. A bladder training program may be designed to set a regular voiding interval; the patient is encouraged to suppress urgency between the set intervals. Once the patient maintains control of this schedule, the interval can be extended until the desired voiding schedule is achieved. Demented or cognitively impaired patients may be prompted to void at a standard interval. Second-line therapy involves medication with anticholinergic and antispasmodic properties, such as oxybutynin (2.5–5.0 mg qd–qid), imipramine (10–25 mg qd–tid), or dicyclomine hydrochloride (10–20 mg qd–qid). Medications can augment but not replace behavioral therapy. Their use is frequently limited by side effects, including dry mouth, confusion, orthostatic

Table 20-2. Medications that cause/exacerbate urinary incontinence

Medication (examples)	Potential effects on UI
Potent diuretics (furosemide, bumetanide)	Polyuria, frequency, urgency
Anticholinergics (dicyclomine, disopyramide, antihistamine)	Urinary retention, overflow incontinence, delirium, fecal impaction
Antipsychotics (thioridazine, haloperidol)	Anticholinergic actions, sedation, rigidity, immobility
Antidepressants (amitriptyline, desipramine)	Anticholinergic actions, sedation
Antiparkinsonian (trihexyphenidyl, benztropine)	Anticholinergic actions, sedation
Sedative-hypnotics (diazepam, flurazepam)	Sedation, delirium, immobility
Narcotics (opiates)	Urinary retention, fecal impaction, sedation, delirium
α-Adrenergic antagonists (prazosin, terazosin)	Urethral relaxation may precipitate stress incontinence in women
α-Adrenergic agonists (nasal decongestants)	Urinary retention in men
Calcium channel blockers	Urinary retention
Angiotensin-converting enzyme inhibitors	Associated cough may precipitate stress incontinence in women and in some men with prior prostatectomy
Alcohol	Polyuria, frequency, urgency, sedation, delirium, immobility
Vincristine	Urinary retention

UI, urinary incontinence.

hypotension, and urinary retention. Low doses of two medications can be combined to limit side effects.
B. **Stress incontinence** should also be initially treated with conservative measures. Fluid limitation and frequent voiding may keep bladder volume below the threshold at which UI occurs with increased intraabdominal pressure. Pelvic muscle exercises such as Kegel's exercises are effective in motivated patients. However, patients need to continue these exercises indefinitely. Topical estrogen (1–2 g topical qd) or oral estrogen replacement (0.625–1.25 mg qd) may increase the thickness of the urethral mucosa in postmenopausal women. α-Adrenergic agonists such as phenylpropanolamine (25–75 mg PO bid) can increase sphincter tone. Imipramine (10–25 mg PO qd–tid) has α-adrenergic and anticholinergic properties and can be used in patients with symptoms of stress and urge incontinence. Refractory cases should be referred to urology for formal urodynamic evaluation and surgical options.
C. **Overflow incontinence** due to bladder outlet obstruction should be referred to urology for surgical correction. α-Adrenergic antagonists such as prazosin (1–2 mg PO bid–tid), terazosin (2–12 mg PO qhs), doxazosin (1–8 mg PO qhs), or tamsulosin (0.4 mg PO qd) or the antiandrogen finasteride (5 mg PO qd), can be used to delay or avoid surgery in patients with urinary outlet obstruction from benign prostatic hypertrophy. UI due to atonic bladder must be decompressed with intermittent catheterization for 10–14 days

followed by voiding trials augmented by application of suprapubic pressure (Credé maneuver), Valsalva, or double voiding. Pharmacologic agents such as bethanechol (cholinergic agent) are rarely helpful. If these measures fail or if PVR remains large, intermittent catheterization must be continued. An indwelling bladder catheter is less desirable and is necessary in fewer than 2% of patients in extended-care facilities.

D. Treatment failure may occur despite a thorough investigation and exhaustive trials of treatment options. Unfortunately, these patients are left with palliative measures such as absorbent pads or undergarments. Condom catheters can be tried in men but can cause skin breakdown. Indwelling Foley catheters should only be used if necessary, for example to allow healing of decubitus ulcers.

Approach to an Abnormal Serum Potassium

I. Physiology. The serum potassium concentration reflects only extracellular potassium (65–70 mEq), which represents a small fraction of the larger intracellular potassium pool (3600 mEq). The typical dietary intake of potassium is 40–120 mEq/day. Regulation of the serum potassium concentration requires transcellular distribution and renal potassium excretion to balance dietary intake. Under certain circumstances such as diarrhea or sweating, extrarenal losses of potassium can be substantial. Abnormalities in serum potassium derive from a relative shift in the balance between intake, transcellular distribution, and excretion.

II. Hypokalemia (*N Engl J Med* 1998;339:451)

A. Manifestations. Symptoms of hypokalemia usually occur at potassium concentrations of less than 2.5 mEq/L, although EKG changes and arrhythmias, particularly with digitalis therapy, can be seen at more mildly decreased levels. Noncardiovascular manifestations of severe hypokalemia include malaise, fatigue, weakness, constipation, muscle cramps, ileus, and hyporeflexia. Other complications of hypokalemia include rhabdomyolysis and worsening of hepatic encephalopathy. Secondary metabolic effects can also include metabolic alkalosis, decreased urinary concentrating ability (polyuria, nocturia, and increased thirst), and glucose intolerance.

B. Causes of hypokalemia reflect a combination of inadequate intake of potassium in the setting of potassium losses in the urine, stool, or both. **Inadequate intake** of potassium (<10–20 mEq/day) over a prolonged period may produce a significant deficit and is usually seen with other nutritional deficiencies. **Extrarenal losses** may be of GI origin (fistulas, diarrhea, laxative abuse) or in sweat. **Renal losses** are usually due to diuretic use, hyperglycemia with secondary glycosuria and kaliuresis, or vomiting. Hypokalemia can develop in up to 50% of patients who receive loop or thiazide diuretics, although potassium levels of less than 3.0 mEq/L are not usually seen. The determination of potassium excretion in the urine is important if the etiology of hypokalemia is unclear. Hypokalemia with a urine potassium of less than 25 mEq/24 hours suggests decreased potassium intake or extrarenal losses. Hypokalemia with a urine potassium of greater than 25 mEq/24 hours is usually due to diuretics or vomiting, which leads to increased renal potassium wasting stimulated by metabolic alkalosis. If the patient has no history of diuretic use, vomiting, or other clear etiology of the hypokalemia and the urine potassium is greater than 25 mEq/24 hours, potassium repletion and referral to a nephrologist for further investigation are warranted. The differential diagnosis of hypokalemia includes hypomagnesemia, renal artery stenosis, mineralocorticoid excess, glucocorticoid excess, and Bartter's syndrome.

C. **Management of hypokalemia**
1. **Potassium replacement.** Severe hypokalemia (<2.5 mEq/L) requires immediate referral to a medical facility for treatment. Mild to moderate hypokalemia (2.5–3.5 mEq/L) necessitates potassium replacement. Patients receiving digoxin or who have preexisting cardiac ischemia, heart failure, or left ventricular hypertrophy are at risk of cardiac arrhythmia with mild to moderate hypokalemia and should be monitored closely. Three potassium salts are usually given for replacement: (1) potassium chloride (10–40 mEq PO or IV, with IV potassium repletion rate no greater than 10 mEq/hr), (2) potassium phosphate (given for phosphate replacement), and (3) potassium citrate (given for replacement of bicarbonate or citrate). Serum potassium levels should be serially monitored during potassium repletion, especially in patients with DM, renal insufficiency, or administration of NSAIDs, ACE inhibitors, or angiotensin II receptor antagonists.
2. **Patients on diuretics** usually require 20–60 mEq of supplemental potassium/day to maintain serum potassium concentrations within the normal range. Furthermore, hypokalemia persists despite aggressive potassium supplementation in approximately 10% of these patients. The safest and cheapest approach to preventing hypokalemia is to ensure adequate dietary intake. Table 20-3 lists foods with high potassium content. Another way to correct or prevent hypokalemia in a patient receiving diuretics is to use combination diuretic therapy with a potassium-sparing diuretic such as amiloride, triamterene, or spironolactone. It is important to monitor serum potassium levels when using these drugs, especially when giving potassium supplements in the presence of DM, or with renal insufficiency, as well as in patients who are receiving digoxin or nonsteroidal anti-inflammatory agents. It is prudent to avoid potassium-sparing diuretics in the presence of advanced renal insufficiency, ACE inhibitors, or angiotensin II receptor antagonists.

III. **Hyperkalemia**
A. **Manifestations.** Cardiac arrhythmias are the most serious manifestation of hyperkalemia, and the risk of a cardiac arrhythmia only partially correlates with the level of serum potassium. However, it is rare to see ECG evidence of hyperkalemia if the potassium is less than 5.5 mEq/L.
B. **Causes.** Hyperkalemia in the outpatient setting is usually due to a combination of excess potassium intake and decreased renal excretion. Transcellular shifts may rarely account for hyperkalemia in the setting of hyperglycemia with insulin deficiency or transient exercise-induced hyperkalemia. Acute and chronic renal insufficiency account for most cases of hyperkalemia due to impaired renal potassium excretion. In the majority of patients with mild to moderate chronic renal insufficiency, hyperkalemia only develops in the presence of excess potassium intake or the use of medications that further impair the kidney's ability to excrete potassium, such as potassium-sparing diuretics, NSAIDs, ACE inhibitors, angiotensin II receptor antagonists, and trimethoprim.
C. **Evaluation and management of hyperkalemia**
1. **Exclude pseudohyperkalemia,** which is a common cause of a spuriously high potassium level in a patient with no predisposing factors. Pseudohyperkalemia represents an artifactually elevated plasma potassium due to potassium movement out of cells before or after venipuncture. This may be seen when venipuncture is performed after repeated fist clenching or when the tourniquet is placed around the arm for a prolonged period. Hemolysis of the blood sample by the needle or in the tube may also cause pseudohyperkalemia.
2. **Management of hyperkalemia.** Because of the potential for a fatal arrhythmia, patients with a potassium level of greater than 5.5 mEq/L need immediate evaluation. Any patient who has new-onset or worsen-

Table 20-3. Foods with high potassium content

Highest content (>25 mEq/100 g)		Dried figs
		Molasses
		Seaweed
Very high content (>12.5 mEq/100 g)		Dried fruits (dates, prunes)
		Nuts
		Avocados
		Bran cereals
		Wheat germ
		Lima beans
High content (>6.2 mEq/100 g)	Vegetables	Spinach
		Tomatoes
		Broccoli
		Winter squash
		Beets
		Carrots
		Cauliflower
		Potatoes
	Fruits	Bananas
		Cantaloupe
		Kiwis
		Oranges
		Mangoes
	Meats	Ground beef
		Steak
		Pork
		Veal, lamb

Reprinted from F Gennari. Hypokalemia. *N Engl J Med* 1998;339(7):451–458, with permission.

ing renal insufficiency with an elevated serum potassium also needs immediate evaluation. Drugs that can elevate the potassium level should be stopped, including potassium supplements, ACE inhibitors, angiotensin II receptor blockers, potassium-sparing diuretics, and NSAIDs. Dietary counseling should also be given to reduce the intake of potassium-containing foods.

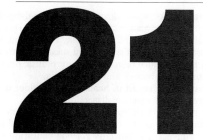

Musculoskeletal Complaints

Thomas M. DeFer

Neck Pain

I. **General considerations.** Neck pain is an extremely common symptom, but most episodes are short lived and seldom require medical care. Those patients who come to medical attention generally need only conservative treatment. With conservative therapy, more than half of the patients have improvement in neck pain within 2–4 weeks, and the majority are asymptomatic by 2–3 months.

II. **Etiology and pathogenesis.** By far, most neck pain is not serious and is musculoskeletal-biomechanical in origin, caused by minor trauma or age-related changes in the cervical spine. A much smaller number of patients have serious systemic diseases that affect the neck or referred pain.

  A. **Strain/sprain/spasm** of the paracervical musculature is an especially common cause of acute nonspecific neck pain, particularly in younger patients. It may develop after a prolonged period in an awkward position, sudden jarring neck movement related to minor trauma, or activities that require new, unusual, or repetitive neck movements.

  B. **Acute flexion-hyperextension neck injury (whiplash)** occurs most commonly after a rear-end car collision. For unclear reasons, whiplash tends to respond less well to therapy than do typical cervical sprains. After 12 months, 15–20% of patients remain symptomatic, with 5% severely affected (*Arch Neurol* 2000;57:590). Zygapophyseal joint pain has been suggested to be the most common cause for chronic neck pain after whiplash. Imaging tests are unrevealing. Fluoroscopically guided, controlled diagnostic blocks of the painful joint may establish the diagnosis.

  C. **Osteoarthritis/spondylosis.** Degenerative cervical spine changes generally begin in the fourth decade of life. Disk degeneration can result in posterior and lateral bulging. Osteoarthritis develops in the apophysial synovial joints. Osteophyte formation may occur, originating from the vertebral body, facet joints, and neural foramina margins. Occasionally, there is segmental instability or subluxation. This entire process is referred to as **cervical spondylosis**, and it is a common cause of **chronic mechanical neck pain** in older individuals. Encroachment on the neural foramina and spinal canal may result in **radiculopathy or cervical myelopathy**.

  D. **Degenerative cervical disk disease** increases with age and may result in neck pain with or without radiculopathy. Acute cervical disk herniations may also cause neck pain or radiculopathy, or both.

  E. **Cervical radiculopathy** may be caused by multiple processes, most commonly acute disk herniation, chronic disk degeneration, and cervical spondylosis. Radiculopathy is occasionally caused by a more serious condition such as malignancy or infection. Thoracic outlet syndrome, brachial plexus disorders, and upper-extremity peripheral nerve compression syndromes may mimic radicular symptoms.

  F. **Serious or systemic causes** of neck pain or radiculopathy, or both, are much less common and include vertebral osteomyelitis, epidural abscess, diskitis, meningitis, rheumatoid arthritis (RA), spondyloarthropathies, polymyalgia rheumatica, fibromyalgia, and primary or metastatic tumors. Cervical fractures are generally the result of significant trauma and may or may not present with neurologic symptoms. Osteoporotic fractures of the cervical spine are unusual.

G. **Other structures in the neck** may produce pain such as thyroiditis, pharyngitis, retropharyngeal or peritonsillar abscess, and carotodynia.

H. **Referred pain** to the neck may be the result of headaches, shoulder disorders, angina, esophageal disorders, and vascular dissection.

III. **Diagnostic evaluation.** In most patients, a thorough but focused history and physical examination are the primary diagnostic tools. An important goal is to detect symptoms and signs that suggest a potentially serious condition or a neurologic urgency. In the absence of such findings, special diagnostic tests are generally not indicated.

A. **The history** should focus on the mode of onset, nature, and location of the pain.

1. A history of **trauma** is important. Patients should also be asked about activities that may have preceded the pain (e.g., prolonged neck extension or flexion, twisting, new physical activity, sport, or job). Neck pain often does not develop until 12–24 hours after such activity. **Acute** neck pain that is unrelated to trauma suggests cervical strain or disk herniation (that may or may not be associated with radicular symptoms). **Chronic** neck pain with intermittent acute exacerbations (sometimes with radiculopathy) is often due to cervical spondylosis. Mechanical neck pain is typically exacerbated by movement and relieved by rest. Morning stiffness may be present in patients with an inflammatory arthropathy.

2. **Neurologic symptoms** are a vital component of the history.

   a. **Radiculopathy** may involve single, multiple, or bilateral roots. Sensory changes are usually more pronounced than motor symptoms. Patients may also complain of paresthesias that radiate from the neck into the arm. Weakness is the primary symptom of motor involvement. Extensive paralysis only occurs with multiple root involvement.

   b. Symptoms of **cervical myelopathy** (due to severe cervical spondylosis) generally develop slowly and intermittently. Patients complain of upper- and lower-extremity weakness and sensory changes. Spastic paraparesis of the legs and loss of sphincter control may eventually develop. In patients with RA, neck pain may indicate impending neurologic compromise. Forward subluxation of C1 can compress the spinal cord, resulting in sudden motor and sensory deficits at multiple levels.

   c. **Symptoms or history suggestive of a serious etiology**, such as malignancy or infection, should be carefully sought (e.g., fever, weight loss, very severe pain, pain unrelieved by rest, a history of cancer, long-term corticosteroid use, intravenous drug use).

B. **The physical examination** should include the entire cervical spine and surrounding areas (e.g., shoulders and head) and an appropriate neurologic examination. The range of motion (ROM) of the neck normally decreases with age. Lateral flexion of the neck may worsen radiculopathy symptoms, as may vertical pressure on the head (**Spurling's maneuver**). **Lhermitte's sign**, electric shock sensation down the spine into the arms and legs with spine extension, may be seen in cervical myelopathy/cord compression. Localized tenderness of the cervical spine and spasm of the paraspinal musculature may be present. The sensitivity and specificity of severe bony tenderness for fracture are unknown. When the patient has neurologic complaints, a thorough neurologic examination is necessary. Not all patients with radiculopathy have demonstrable findings on examination. **Cervical radiculopathy** has characteristic sensory changes and motor weakness (Table 21-1). Motor weakness in the upper and lower extremities, spasticity, hyperreflexia, clonus, Babinski's sign, and reduced sphincter tone are consistent with **cervical myelopathy**.

C. **Plain radiography** of the cervical spine should be used judiciously in patients with nonspecific mechanical neck pain. Use of plain radiographs in evaluating

Table 21-1. Features of cervical radiculopathy

Nerve root	Area of sensory change	Motor weakness	Reflex
C5	Upper lateral arm	Shoulder abduction	Biceps and brachioradialis
C6	Lower lateral forearm into thumb and index finger	Forearm supinators and pronators	Biceps and brachioradialis
C7	Dorsal and palmar surface of forearm into middle finger	Triceps and wrist extension flexion	Triceps
C8	Medial forearm into ring and little fingers	Intrinsic hand muscles	—

neck pain has two important limitations. First, cervical spondylosis is extremely common in asymptomatic individuals and increases with age. Second, plain radiographs are of very limited value in assessing nerve root or spinal cord compression. Nonetheless, plain films should generally be done in patients with radiculopathy to evaluate for serious bony abnormalities. Plain cervical spine films are warranted when a serious disorder is suspected or in cases that are related to significant trauma. If plain films are unrevealing but strong suspicion still exists, other imaging studies should be done.

  D. **CT or MRI** is recommended when tumor, infection, fracture, or other space-occupying lesion is strongly suggested by the clinical findings or in the setting of serious neurologic signs and symptoms. In the absence of severe or progressive neurologic symptoms, it is generally not necessary to do a CT or MRI for patients with typical radiculopathy. Many patients with cervical radiculopathy have substantial improvement in a few weeks. If symptoms have not improved with several months of conservative management and the patient is an appropriate potential candidate for surgery, CT or MRI may be useful.

  E. **Electrophysiologic tests** are usually not indicated in individuals with obvious radiculopathy. They are probably most useful when the cause of upper-extremity pain is unclear or surgery is being considered.

IV. **Treatment**

  A. Simple conservative therapy is appropriate for the majority of patients with **nonspecific mechanical neck pain**. In most cases, the pain improves in several weeks. A notable lack of quality data has been found to support the use of most conservative treatments, and many therapies are prescribed out of convention (*BMJ* 1996;313:1291).

    1. **Modest activity restriction** is generally believed to be appropriate. Patients should avoid activities that worsen their neck pain. Bed rest is not indicated, and patients should be encouraged to continue most daily activities. **Soft cervical collars** are also frequently recommended and may reduce symptoms in some patients. These collars are not particularly effective at reducing neck motion but may serve as a reminder to the patient to limit movements that can increase pain. Rigid cervical collars should not be prescribed by the untrained.

    2. **Manual therapies** (e.g., massage, manipulation, neck mobilization) may be effective for some patients, but the available literature regarding these treatments is extremely limited.

    3. **Physical medicine modalities** [e.g., electromagnetic therapy, infrared light, acupuncture, cervical traction, transcutaneous electrical nerve stimulation (TENS), laser treatments, spray and stretch vapocoolant] have not been studied in enough detail to assess adequately either effi-

Table 21-2. Nonsteroidal anti-inflammatory drugs

Chemical name	Trade name	Dosage	Frequency	Maximum dosage/day
Acetylsalicylic acid	—	325–500 mg	qid	None[a]
Celecoxib	Celebrex	100–200 mg	qd–bid	400 mg
Choline magnesium trisalicylate	Trilisate	1500 mg	bid	3000 mg[a]
Diclofenac[b]	Cataflam	50 mg	bid–tid	150 mg
	Voltaren	50–75 mg	bid–tid	150 mg
	Voltaren-XR	100 mg	qd	200 mg
	Arthrotec[c]	50–75 mg	bid–tid	150 mg
Diflunisal[b]	Dolobid	250–500 mg	bid–tid	1500 mg
Etodolac[b]	Lodine	300–500 mg	bid–tid	1200 mg
	Lodine XL	400–600 mg	qd	1200 mg
Flurbiprofen[b]	Ansaid	50–100 mg	bid–tid	300 mg
Ibuprofen[b]	Motrin	100–800 mg	tid–qid	3200 mg
Indomethacin[b]	Indocin	25–50 mg	bid–qid	200 mg
	Indocin SR	75 mg	qd–bid	150 mg
Ketoprofen[b]	Orudis	50–75 mg	tid	300 mg
Ketoprofen SR[b]	Oruvail	100–200 mg	qd	300 mg
Ketorolac[b]	Toradol	10 mg (PO)	q6h	40 mg[d]
		15–60 mg (IV/IM)	q6h	120 mg[d]
Meloxicam	Mobic	7.5–15.0 mg	qd	15 mg
Nambumetone	Relafen	500–750 mg	qd–bid	2000 mg
Naproxen[b]	Naprosyn	250–500 mg	bid	1000 mg
	Anaprox	275–550 mg	qd–bid	1100 mg
	Naprelan	375–500 mg	qd	1000 mg
Oxaprozin	Daypro	1200 mg	qd	1800 mg
Piroxicam[b]	Feldene	20 mg	qd	20 mg
Rofecoxib	Vioxx	12.5–25.0 mg	qd	25–50 mg[e]
Salsalate	Disalcid	500–1000 mg	bid–qid	3000 mg[a]
	Salflex	500–1000 mg	bid–qid	3000 mg[a]
Sulindac[b]	Clinoril	150–200 mg	bid	400 mg
Tolmetin[b]	Tolectin	200–600 mg	tid	1800 mg

[a]Dose can be adjusted to achieve salicylate level of 20–30 mg/dl.
[b]Available as generic.
[c]Combined with misoprostol, 200 µg/tablet.
[d]Combined duration of PO/IM/IV not to exceed 5 days.
[e]Rofecoxib, 50 mg PO qd, not to exceed 5 days.

cacy or effectiveness (*Cochrane Database Syst Rev* 2000;3:CD000961). Application of **local heat or ice** is an option for symptomatic relief.
4. **Pharmacotherapy** with **acetaminophen, nonsteroidal anti-inflammatory drugs (NSAIDs)** (Table 21-2), or **selective cyclooxygenase-2 (COX-2) inhibitors** may provide relief for nonspecific mechanical neck pain.

Narcotic analgesics may be an effective time-limited option for patients with acute severe neck pain. Some patients may find **muscle relaxants** effective, but sedation is a common side effect.

   5. **Surgery** has no role in the relief of neck pain secondary to cervical spondylosis in the absence of significant persistent neurologic involvement.

B. **Whiplash** does not respond as well to conservative treatments, but they are frequently used. For patients with chronic cervical zygapophyseal joint pain after whiplash confirmed with double-blind placebo-controlled local anesthesia, percutaneous radiofrequency neurotomy may provide lasting relief (*N Engl J Med* 1996;335:1721). A small study suggests that the acute treatment with high-dose methylprednisolone may be beneficial in preventing extensive sick leave after whiplash (*Spine* 1998;23:984).

C. **Neck pain with radiculopathy** is generally treated in a manner similar to that of nonspecific mechanical neck pain. Patients with prolonged severe radicular symptoms may benefit from surgical decompression. Those who are agreeable to surgery and are medically appropriate surgical candidates can be referred to a neurosurgeon. Patients with persistent radicular pain secondary to cervical spondylosis may respond to fluoroscopically guided therapeutic selective nerve root block (*Arch Phys Med Rehabil* 2000;81:741).

D. **Myelopathy** often requires surgical treatment and is best managed in conjunction with a neurosurgeon, neurologist, or both.

Low Back Pain

I. **General considerations.** Low back pain is one of the most common reasons for patients to seek medical attention. The lifetime incidence is estimated to be greater than 70%, with the highest prevalence in people 45–64 years of age. The medical and social costs of low back pain are enormous.

II. **Etiology and pathogenesis.** The vast majority of acute low back pain is believed to be mechanical in origin: myofascial or soft-tissue injury/strain, degenerative changes of the vertebrae and disks (spondylosis), spondylolisthesis, disk herniation with or without sciatica, spinal stenosis, and vertebral fracture. A very small number of patients have serious systemic diseases that affect the spine or have referred pain.

A. **Nonspecific mechanical low back pain.** In up to 85% of patients with low back pain, a specific diagnosis cannot be made. In most cases, it is attributed to some form of muscular strain or stress.

B. **Lumbar disk herniation** is common and increases with age. Of disk herniations, 95% occur at the L4–5 or L5–S1 levels. Disk herniation may result in low back pain, sciatica, or both. However, disk herniations may also be totally asymptomatic. Large midline disk herniations occasionally cause the cauda equina syndrome.

C. **Spinal stenosis** is usually caused by hypertrophy of the ligamentum flavum and facet joints, resulting in narrowing of the spinal canal, often at multiple levels. This narrowing may result in entrapment of nerve roots, with resultant symptoms in the legs. **Pseudoclaudication** or neurogenic claudication is characterized by back pain and pain and numbness of the lower extremities that worsen with walking and extension of the spine. Flexion of the spine may improve the symptoms. The discomfort typically lasts longer after walking than it does in true vascular claudication.

D. **Spondylosis** is generalized degenerative change of the spine, including disk degeneration, with disk space narrowing and osteoarthritic changes of the facet joints. Spondylosis is just as common in asymptomatic as in symptomatic individuals. In general, low back pain patients with spondylosis have the same prognosis as those without spondylosis. **Spondylolisthesis** is the forward movement of the body of one of the lower lumbar vertebrae on the vertebra below it or on the sacrum. Minor degrees of spondylolisthesis are fairly common and usually asymptomatic. Individuals with low back pain that is presumed to be secondary to spondylolisthesis usually follow a similar course as those with nonspecific low back pain. When the slippage is severe, it may cause back pain and radiculopathy.

E. Systemic causes. Low back pain has many potentially serious causes, but overall they are uncommon. The most common are malignancy and infection.

   1. Malignancy. Metastases from the breast, lung, or prostate are the most common causes. Multiple myeloma, lymphoma, and leukemia may also involve the spine, as can primary spinal cord tumors and extradural spinal tumors.

   2. Infectious causes include epidural abscesses, vertebral osteomyelitis, and diskitis. Endocarditis should be considered in patients with these infections. Although uncommon, *Mycobacterium tuberculosis* infection of the vertebral bodies (Pott's disease) is still occasionally seen.

   3. Metabolic bone disease, most notably **osteoporosis** (see Chap. 24), may cause compression fractures and should always be considered in older patients with low back pain.

   4. The **spondyloarthropathies** (ankylosing spondylitis, psoriatic arthritis, Reiter's syndrome, and reactive inflammatory arthropathy) may affect the spine. However, such individuals usually have other signs and symptoms that are attributable to these diseases.

   5. Abdominal aortic aneurysms may also result in low back pain and should be considered in older patients with a history of or risk factors for coronary artery disease.

F. Referred pain from other organ systems may present as back pain, including GI disorders (e.g., ulcer disease, pancreatitis, pancreatic cancer), genitourinary disorders (e.g., nephrolithiasis, pyelonephritis, prostatitis), gynecologic disorders (e.g., pelvic inflammatory disease, ectopic pregnancy, menstrual discomfort), and hip problems.

III. Diagnostic evaluation. In the vast majority of patients, the primary diagnostic tool is a careful but focused history and physical examination searching for **"red flags"** that suggest a potentially serious underlying condition or a neurologic urgency (Table 21-3). In the absence of red flags, special diagnostic tests are rarely indicated during the first month of pain (AHCPR publication 95-0643, 1994).

A. History

   1. Historic red flags are presented in Table 21-3.

   2. The sensitivity of the symptom of **sciatica**, defined as pain radiating into the buttocks and down the leg below the knee, is sufficiently high (0.95) that its absence makes a clinically significant lumbar nerve root compression unlikely (*JAMA* 1992;268:760). Disk herniation can cause isolated back pain.

   3. Although not very specific, a clear history of **pseudoclaudication** and age greater than 50 years points to **spinal stenosis**.

B. Key components of the **physical examination** for low back pain are temperature; inspection; palpation; ROM of the spine; limited sensory, motor, and reflex examinations; and straight leg-raising tests. Other portions of the examination are directed by the history obtained.

   1. Sensory involvement caused by a herniated disk should be dermatomal in nature. **Pinprick** is more accurate than light touch or temperature sensitivity. Sensory changes in L4, L5, and S1 dermatomes can be effectively detected on the medial, dorsal, and lateral aspects of the foot, respectively (Table 21-4).

   2. Ankle and great toe dorsiflexion should be tested. Weakness of these movements usually occurs together and typically suggests disk herniation at the L4–5 level. **Ankle plantar flexion** is an S1 function; however, only severe impairments are readily detectable.

Table 21-3. Red flags of low back pain

Age >50 years

History of cancer

Unexplained weight loss

Chronic steroid use

Pain duration >1 mo

Pain unresponsive to treatment for 1 mo

Pain unrelieved or worsened by rest

Intravenous drug use

Urinary tract or other infection

Fever

Bladder dysfunction

Saddle anesthesia

Unilateral or bilateral major motor weakness

Significant trauma relative to age

Rapidly progressive severe radiculopathy

Adapted from S Bigos, O Bowyer, G Braen, et al. Acute low back problems in adults. Clinical practice guideline no. 14. AHCPR publication 95-0642. Rockville, MD: Agency for Health Care Policy and Research, December 1994.

3. A diminished **knee reflex** may be seen with an upper-lumbar herniated disk. A reduced **ankle reflex** indicates involvement of the S1 nerve root.
4. A typical positive **straight leg–raising sign** reproduces or worsens the patient's sciatica symptoms between 30 and 60 degrees of leg elevation. Ipsilateral straight leg raising is only moderately sensitive (0.80) and nonspecific (0.40). **Crossed straight leg raising** is less sensitive (0.25) but highly specific (0.90). Straight leg raising and crossed straight leg raising can be done with the patient lying supine or sitting.
5. When neurologic symptoms other than sciatica are present, a complete neurologic examination is warranted. Patients with the **cauda equina syndrome** typically have saddle anesthesia, bilateral radicular findings, and decreased anal sphincter tone.

Table 21-4. Features of lumbosacral radiculopathy

Nerve root	Area of sensory change	Motor weakness	Reflex
L2	Upper anterior thigh	Hip flexion	—
L3	Anterior thigh	Knee extension and thigh adduction	—
L4	Lateral thigh, medial leg, and medial foot	Knee extension, thigh adduction, and dorsiflexion of foot	Knee
L5	Posterolateral thigh, lateral leg, dorsal foot	Dorsiflexion of great toe and foot	—
S1	Posterior thigh and leg, lateral and plantar foot	Plantar flexion of great toe and foot	Ankle

C. **Plain radiographs** of the lumbar spine are usually nondiagnostic and not necessary during the first month of acute low back pain when no red flags are found on the history and physical examination. Many asymptomatic patients have degenerative changes, whereas individuals with back pain may have completely normal films. Therefore, when degenerative changes are seen, it is very difficult to determine their significance. Plain films cannot detect nerve root impingement or spinal stenosis. When plain radiographs of the lumbar spine are nondiagnostic in patients with red flags, additional imaging studies such as CT or MRI should be strongly considered. Plain radiographs are probably advisable in all individuals with chronic low pain who have not had them done previously. They are also potentially indicated in any patient with chronic low back pain in whom clinical findings develop that are suggestive of tumor, infection, or fracture. Significant changes in symptoms or physical findings (particularly severe or progressive neurologic symptoms or signs) may also indicate the need for plain radiography.

D. **CT or MRI** should be done when tumor, infection, fracture, or other space-occupying lesion is strongly suggested by the clinical findings. In the absence of severe or progressive neurologic symptoms, it is generally not necessary to perform a CT or MRI for patients with sciatica, as many of these individuals have substantial improvement in 4–6 weeks. If symptoms have not improved in 1 month and the patient is an appropriate potential candidate for surgery, CT or MRI may be useful. Degenerative, bulging, and perhaps even herniated disks are believed to be indicative of the aging process of the spine. Given that many asymptomatic individuals have such findings, it can be difficult to determine their significance in symptomatic patients.

E. **Myelography and CT-myelography** are generally only indicated in special situations for preoperative planning in consultation with a surgeon.

F. **Bone scintigraphy** is rarely needed in the diagnostic evaluation of patients with low back pain. Bone scans may have a high yield for spinal metastases in patients with a known history of cancer. However, when they are positive, other diagnostic tests are usually required (i.e., CT or MRI).

G. **Electrophysiologic tests** are usually not indicated in individuals with obvious radiculopathy or in those with only low back pain. These tests appear to be most useful in the diagnostic evaluation of patients with leg pain when the diagnosis is unclear.

IV. **Treatment.** In the absence of red flags, treatment for most patients with acute nonspecific low back pain can be simple and conservative. Most patients improve in approximately 1 month with or without treatment. Pain that has persisted without improvement for over a month should be re-evaluated. The goals of treatment are to reduce pain, increase mobility, return to functioning at home, return to work, and prevent the development of chronic pain and disability.

A. **Education.** The overall good prognosis of acute low back pain should be stressed but not oversold. Although acute low back pain may rapidly and completely resolve, it certainly does not always do so, and recurrences are common. Patients should be encouraged to notify the physician if symptoms change significantly.

B. Some evidence has been found that **back schools** are better than placebo (but not more effective than other conservative treatments) for short-term relief of acute low back pain. Moderate evidence has been found that back schools have better short-term outcomes than do other conservative treatments for chronic low back pain (*Cochrane Database Syst Rev* 2000;2:CD000261).

C. Mounting evidence has demonstrated that **bed rest** may actually delay recovery and potentially contribute to the development of chronic back pain. Patients with acute nonspecific low back pain should be advised to continue ordinary activities as much as possible (*Br J Gen Pract* 1997;47:647). Patients with sciatica also should be encouraged to go about daily activities as much as tolerated (*N Engl J Med* 1999;340:418).

D. Activity restriction. It is reasonable to advise the patient to limit temporarily activities that are known to increase mechanical stress on the spine, including prolonged unsupported standing, heavy lifting, and bending or twisting the back while lifting.

E. Therapeutic exercise. Low-stress aerobic activities (e.g., walking, biking, or swimming) and trunk-conditioning exercises can safely be done during the first month of symptoms and may decrease pain, reduce recurrences, and improve functional outcomes. Exercise therapy for chronic low back pain is effective, but it is unclear exactly which specific conditioning exercises for the trunk muscles should be recommended (*Cochrane Database Syst Rev* 2000;2:CD000335).

F. Pharmacotherapy

    1. Acetaminophen is a reasonable first-line choice for the treatment of acute and chronic low back pain.

    2. There is strong evidence that **NSAIDs** are more effective than placebo in patients with acute nonspecific low back pain. There is moderate evidence that NSAIDs are effective for chronic low back pain (*Cochrane Database Syst Rev* 2000;2:CD000396).

    3. Selective COX-2 inhibitors have been shown to be as effective as traditional NSAIDs for other types of pain and are a reasonable but costly alternative for acute or chronic low back pain, with a lower incidence of serious GI toxicity (*JAMA* 2000;284:1247).

    4. Muscle relaxants are more effective than placebo in reducing the symptoms of acute nonspecific low back pain. Different types of muscle relaxants are probably equally effective (*Spine* 1997;22:2128).

    5. Tramadol (50–100 mg qid) is an alternative for patients who fail to respond to or who cannot take nonselective or selective NSAIDs, but side effects are common (e.g., nausea, constipation, drowsiness).

    6. Narcotic analgesics may be an effective time-limited option for patients with acute severe low back pain or sciatica that is not relieved by other medications. No convincing evidence has been found that narcotics are more effective than NSAIDs in promoting return to full activity (*Spine* 1996;21:2840). Many patients who take narcotic pain relievers have significant side effects, and the potential for dependence must be considered. The long-term use of narcotic analgesics in chronic nonspecific back pain is controversial.

    7. Tricyclic antidepressants are frequently prescribed for nondepressed individuals with chronic pain of many types, particularly of neurogenic origin. However, no study has clearly shown a tricyclic antidepressant to be superior to placebo. Some individuals have serious side effects from tricyclics, and this must also be considered.

G. Injection therapies have been tried in multiple different areas of the spine, including the facet joints, the epidural space, and soft tissue (trigger points, acupuncture points, or ligaments). Corticosteroids, local anesthetics, and saline have all been used.

    1. Trigger point injections. The theory of trigger points as a cause or perpetuator of low back pain is controversial at best. Evidence is insufficient to recommend for or against their use in either acute or chronic low back pain (*Cochrane Database Syst Rev* 2000;2:CD001824).

    2. Facet joint injections have been advocated for the treatment of the "facet joint syndrome." The syndrome is diagnosed clinically in patients with lumbar pain that improves with the injection of corticosteroid or local anesthetic into or near the facet joints. The efficacy of such treatment is unclear but can be considered in selected patients with chronic low back pain in whom more conservative treatment has failed.

    3. Epidural steroid injections have been recommended for subacute or chronic low back pain with and without sciatica. Results from multiple studies have been conflicting (*Anesth Intensive Care* 1995;23:564, and

Pain 1995;63:279). Epidural steroids can be considered for patients in whom conservative therapy has failed.

H. Other modalities

1. **Heat and ice.** As an option for symptomatic relief, patients can apply ice or heat locally for short periods several times a day.

2. A small amount of contradictory evidence is available regarding the use of **TENS and acupuncture-like TENS (ALTENS)** in acute low back pain. Therefore, these devices are not recommended for acute low back pain. Evidence is available to support the use of TENS and ALTENS for pain relief in the treatment of chronic low back pain, at least in the short term. ALTENS also appears to improve ROM in such patients (*Cochrane Database Syst Rev* 2000;2:CD000210).

3. From the limited data that are available, it appears that **traction** is ineffective for acute and chronic low back pain (*Spine* 1997;22:2756).

4. The use of **lumbar corsets and back belts** for the treatment of low back pain is controversial. At present, there is insufficient evidence to recommend for or against their use in either acute or chronic low back pain.

I. Surgical treatment

1. **Surgery for lumbar disk herniation.** There is good evidence that **surgical diskectomy** provides effective relief of sciatica for properly selected patients. Whether there is a significant difference in long-term outcomes is less clear. The primary benefit of diskectomy appears to be the more rapid relief of symptoms in those individuals in whom conservative therapy has failed (*Cochrane Database Syst Rev* 2000;2:CD001350).

2. **Surgical treatment for degenerative lumbar spondylosis** is especially controversial. Surgical treatments may include decompression, spinal fusion, or both. The data available are limited, sometimes of poor quality, and conflicting and often focus on technical rather than patient-centered outcomes. Unless there is evidence of cauda equina syndrome, severe nerve root compression, or significant spinal instability, this type of surgery should not be considered for acute low back pain. In patients with chronic low back pain that is thought to be due to lumbar spondylosis or low back and leg pain that are thought to be due to spinal stenosis unresponsive to conservative treatment, the possibility of surgery should be considered with extreme care (*Cochrane Database Syst Rev* 2000;2:CD001352).

Shoulder Pain

I. General considerations

A. Anatomy. The shoulder consists of three joints and two gliding planes. The joints are the **acromioclavicular, sternoclavicular, and glenohumeral**. The scapulothoracic surface and the subacromial space make up the gliding planes. The glenohumeral joint is very shallow and is the most commonly dislocated joint. The **rotator cuff** supports the glenohumeral joint and consists of four muscles: supraspinatus, infraspinatus, teres minor, and subscapularis. The tendons of these muscles blend with the shoulder joint capsule and insert on the greater and lesser tuberosities of the humeral head. The rotator cuff muscles assist in internal and external rotation and depress the humeral head during shoulder elevation. This action holds the humeral head down, minimizing impingement on the acromion process and the intervening tissues. The **subacromial bursa** lies deep to the deltoid muscle and superficial to the insertion point of the supraspinatus tendon. The long head of the biceps originates from the glenoid labrum. The **biceps tendon** passes out of the glenohumeral joint through the bicipital groove (between the tuberosities). The main function of the biceps is elbow flexion and forearm supination.

B. History and physical examination

  1. History. Intrinsic shoulder pain is typically worse at night and aggravated by lying on the affected shoulder. Motion of the shoulder generally increases the discomfort, particularly full forward flexed elevation and abduction to 90 degrees. A history of recent trauma, new physical activity (e.g., repetitive overhead arm motion), and prior dislocation are important. Patients with shoulder instability may complain that the shoulder has a disconcerting "going out" sensation.

  2. Physical examination of the shoulder should include observation, palpation of the bony and soft tissues, assessment of passive and active ROM, strength testing, and certain provocative tests. Normal **abduction** of the internally rotated (palm-down) shoulder is approximately 120 degrees and externally rotated (palm-up) 180 degrees. Normal **elevation** (forward flexion) of the shoulder is 180 degrees, **extension** 40 degrees, and **internal and external rotation** 90 degrees. If active ROM is limited, passive ROM should be carefully tested. **Cross-chest abduction** (touch the opposite shoulder) tests internal rotation and adduction. The **Apley scratch test** evaluates external rotation and abduction from above (scratch between the scapulae from above) or internal rotation and adduction from below.

C. Radiographs of the shoulder are frequently done, but they are often nondiagnostic. Anteroposterior (AP) views of the glenohumeral joint in internal and external rotation and an axillary view are typically done. Arthritis of the glenohumeral and acromioclavicular joints and calcification of the rotator cuff tendons can be visualized. Detection of shoulder dislocation may require special views.

II. Impingement syndrome

A. General considerations. The impingement syndrome causes the majority of painful nontraumatic shoulder problems. It is due to mechanical impingement of the rotator cuff structures by the humeral head against the subacromial structures. This is related to a continuum of inflammation, degeneration, and attrition of the rotator cuff structures, especially the supraspinatus tendon. As a result, the rotator cuff fails to prevent upward migration of the humeral head during shoulder elevation. Several interrelated conditions are involved in the impingement syndrome.

  1. Rotator cuff tendinitis refers to a spectrum of changes that affect the tendons of the rotator cuff, particularly the supraspinatus. Acute inflammation with hemorrhage and edema can occur secondary to trauma or overuse, particularly in younger patients. Acute rotator cuff tendinitis is sometimes associated with calcification of the supraspinatus and biceps tendons (**calcific tendinitis**). The pain of calcific tendinitis can be severe and may lead to a "frozen shoulder." With aging, the tendons undergo degenerative changes and attenuation related to chronic inflammation and repeated mechanical insults.

  2. Rotator cuff tears can occur suddenly secondary to falling on an outstretched arm or with lifting a heavy object. Tears can also occur more indolently in older patients with attrition of the rotator cuff or with a chronic inflammatory condition such as RA or the "Milwaukee shoulder" (progressive, destructive, shoulder arthropathy associated with bloody shoulder effusions and the deposition of basic calcium phosphate crystals).

  3. Subacromial bursitis and bicipital tendinitis may accompany rotator cuff tendinitis. In fact, it is often difficult to distinguish these entities, as they frequently occur simultaneously. Occasionally, the proximal biceps tendon **ruptures**.

B. History. Patients may have a history of repetitive overhead arm motion. Pain tends to be focal and anterior, occurring at night or when the patient is

lying on the shoulder. Activities such as throwing, working with arms overhead, and swimming aggravate the pain.

C. **Physical examination**

1. The **impingement sign** is elicited by passive forward flexion of the arm
   by the physician. Passive abduction to 90 degrees with internal rotation
   also causes pain.

2. The **apprehension sign** is elicited by having the patient point straight
   ahead with the shoulder in flexion; when the examiner exerts downward pressure on the upper arm, the patient's apprehension is evident
   due to impingement of the supraspinatus tendon.

3. The **drop arm sign** to demonstrate a rotator cuff tear is performed by
   assisting the patient in abducting and elevating the shoulder. When the
   examiner withdraws support of the upper arm, the patient is unable to
   hold the arm up if there is a complete tear of the rotator cuff.

4. The **supraspinatus liftoff test** demonstrates evidence of less advanced
   rotator cuff disease. The patient places the hand of the affected side on the
   small of the back, with the palm oriented posteriorly, and pushes against
   resistance. Normally, the patient should be able to push the examiner's
   hand away from the back. Weakness indicates rotator cuff disease.

5. **Yergason's sign** produces pain and tenderness over the bicipital groove
   with resisted supination of the forearm while the elbow is flexed and
   held at the side. Passive extension of the shoulder may also reproduce
   the pain of bicipital tendinitis.

6. **Speed's test** also identifies tendinitis or weakness of the long head of the
   biceps. The patient flexes the shoulder against resistance with the elbow
   extended and the forearm supinated. Pain is noted in the bicipital groove.

7. Rupture of the biceps tendon is evident as the "**Popeye sign,**" a mass of
   contracted muscle midway between the shoulder and the elbow.

D. **Imaging studies**

1. **Plain radiographs** are not necessary or appropriate in the initial evaluation of every patient with shoulder pain, especially if the history and
   physical examination suggest impingement. However, a radiograph
   should be obtained in patients who do not appear to be responding to
   conservative treatment. The primary value of a radiograph in this situation is to assess the degree of impingement, based on the vertical distance between the inferior aspect of the acromion and the superior
   aspect of the humeral head. Normally, the width of a ballpoint pen
   should "fit" in between the acromion and the humeral head. Narrowing
   of this space suggests that the patient has chronic rotator cuff disease,
   in which case response to conservative treatment may be inadequate.

2. **MRI**, or, in some centers, a diagnostic **ultrasound**, can assess the degree
   of supraspinatus tendon pathology. If the tendon is significantly narrowed or partially or completely torn, the patient should be referred to
   an orthopedist who is experienced in shoulder surgery.

E. **Treatment** goals are to reduce pain and improve shoulder function and ROM.
   The optimal management of impingement syndrome is unclear. Methodologi-
   cally strong trials are limited, and, therefore, it is difficult to provide evidence-
   based recommendations (*Cochrane Database Syst Rev* 2000;3:CD001156). The
   individual entities can be difficult to distinguish clinically, often coexist, and
   can overlap with other shoulder disorders. They are usually self-limited, and
   conservative treatments are generally sufficient. Some cases, however, are
   resistant to treatment, and recurrences can occur.

1. **Resting the shoulder** is reasonable. Patients should avoid activities and
   movements that aggravate the pain.

2. **Gentle ROM exercises** are usually recommended to maintain ROM and
   avoid adhesive capsulitis. Pendulum exercises are easy for patients to do
   at home and consist of flexing at the waist 90 degrees, supporting the
   upper body on a low table, and loosely swinging the arm like a pendu-

lum against gravity. The arc of movement is slowly increased over time. Referral to a physical therapist for careful strengthening of the shoulder muscles may be beneficial.

3. Evidence is insufficient to clearly support the use of **physiotherapy modalities** (e.g., ultrasound, laser, heat, cold, manipulation, and electrotherapy) (*BMJ* 1997;315:25). Application of **heat or ice** may be comforting.

4. **NSAIDs** are probably effective for the pain of impingement syndrome (*J Clin Epidemiol* 1995;48:691). No conclusive evidence has been produced in favor of a particular NSAID. **Selective COX-2 inhibitors** may also be effective and seem to be safer than typical NSAIDs, with a reduced risk of GI ulceration.

5. **Local corticosteroid injections** (subacromial bursa and rotator cuff region) are also frequently used and potentially effective (*Clin Exp Rheumatol* 1996;14:561). Methylprednisolone acetate, 40 mg, is a typical dose. Repeated injections should be avoided. Potential complications of steroid injections include infections, skin atrophy, and tendon weakening and rupture. Steroid injections may be inadvisable for patients with more than small rotator cuff tears.

6. **Referral to an orthopedist** who is experienced in shoulder surgery is appropriate for patients who are potentially accepting of surgery and who have prolonged pain and limitation of function. Early referral should be considered for all patients with moderate to large rotator cuff tears.

III. **Adhesive capsulitis (frozen shoulder)** may complicate any painful shoulder condition and has been associated with myocardial infarction, diabetes mellitus, apical lung cancer, cervical disk disease, metastatic lesions, and thyroid disease. However, such clinical associations are often lacking. The precise pathophysiology of adhesive capsulitis is not entirely clear but appears to involve initial hypervascular synovitis and subsequent fibrosis. What triggers this process is unknown (*Clin Orthop* 2000;372:95). It is not unusual for frozen shoulder to develop subsequently in the contralateral shoulder.

A. **History.** Adhesive capsulitis is most common in women in the fifth and sixth decades of life. The key historical feature is a painful and significant reduction in ROM. The onset can be fairly acute or chronic. As the condition progresses, pain subsides, but the limitation of ROM may become quite severe. After months of symptoms, some patients have a slow progressive improvement in ROM.

B. **Physical examination** is most notable for a marked loss of active and passive ROM.

C. **Radiographs** are typically normal but may show diffuse osteopenia.

D. **Treatment** with a long-term **physical therapy** program may be helpful, depending on patient motivation. **Corticosteroid injection** into the glenohumeral joint may be of some benefit, particularly early in the course. **NSAIDs** are a reasonable recommendation for patients with pain. Arthroscopic capsular release is sometimes recommended for recalcitrant cases but is of unproven value. Manipulation under anesthesia to improve ROM is seldom used.

IV. **Osteoarthritis** does not commonly occur as a primary process in the glenohumeral joint, with two exceptions: (1) rapidly progressive osteoarthritis of the shoulder in elderly women and (2) the Milwaukee shoulder (progressive, destructive shoulder arthropathy associated with bloody shoulder effusions and the deposition of basic calcium phosphate crystals). Secondary osteoarthritis may occur as a result of RA, trauma, repetitive manual labor, calcium pyrophosphate deposition disease, and long-standing rotator cuff tears (cuff-tear arthropathy).

A. The **history** is significant for a chronically painful shoulder with reduced ROM. Activity aggravates the pain. Patients may report previous trauma.

B. **Physical examination** reveals painfully reduced ROM and crepitus.

C. **Radiographs** may demonstrate joint space narrowing and, in more advanced cases, flattening of the humeral head, subchondral cysts, and marginal osteophytes.

    D. Treatment is generally conservative, including **NSAIDs** and **physical therapy**. Patients with advanced cases may require a total shoulder arthroplasty for pain relief.

V. Shoulder instability and dislocation. The shoulder joint is inherently unstable and the most commonly dislocated joint. Acute glenohumeral dislocation occurs most frequently in young active adults after a fall on an outstretched arm and results in anterior displacement of the humeral head. Recurrent dislocation is not unusual, with subsequent episodes requiring less force. Some patients have a chronic syndrome of glenohumeral instability with subluxation. This is often seen in athletes such as baseball pitchers.

    A. History of significant trauma (usually related to sports) and pain is elicited from patients with acute shoulder dislocation. Individuals with glenohumeral instability complain of a chronic feeling of the shoulder "going out" with certain activities and sometimes pain.

    B. Physical examination

        1. Patients with acute anterior dislocation have a loss of the shoulder's normally rounded appearance. The acromion process becomes the most lateral structure. A prominence of the humeral head is present anterior and inferior to the glenoid. ROM is painfully restricted. Patients with acute dislocation should have a detailed neurovascular examination, specifically the motor and sensory innervation of the axillary nerve.

        2. Glenohumeral instability is more difficult to demonstrate. Specific provocative maneuvers should be done.

            a. Anterior instability is most common and is suggested by a positive **anterior apprehension test**. With the shoulder initially at 90 degrees of abduction and neutral rotation, the arm is externally rotated (as in a throwing position), and the examiner applies slight anteriorly directed pressure from behind. The patient's discomfort is apparent through verbal and nonverbal cues. If the apprehension is significantly decreased by the application of posteriorly directed force during external rotation, this is a positive **relocation test**. Impingement produces a positive apprehension test, but it is not significantly altered by relocation.

            b. The **posterior apprehension test** is performed by having the patient flex the elbow and elevate the internally rotated shoulder to 90 degrees (hand on opposite shoulder). Posterior force is then applied to the elbow, and apprehension is apparent.

    C. Radiographs for acute dislocation should include AP and axillary views. With glenohumeral instability these are usually normal but may show subluxation with the patient holding weight. Other views may be needed (e.g., the West Point and Stryker notch views). CT or MRI may also be necessary.

    D. Treatment of acute shoulder dislocations is best handled by immediate **orthopedic consultation**. Patients with chronic glenohumeral instability are treated conservatively with a program of physical therapy and avoiding activities that provoke subluxation. Surgery may be indicated for some young patients and for those with continued intolerable symptoms.

Elbow, Wrist, and Hand Pain

I. Elbow pain

    A. General considerations. Elbow pain is a fairly common complaint in the ambulatory setting. Generally, only one of a few conditions is causative.

        1. History. Patients usually complain of pain but may also report stiffness or swelling, or both. A history of acute trauma is important and may suggest fracture, dislocation, or tendon rupture. Repetitive overuse is a major cause of elbow pain, and patients should be asked about recreational and occupational activities. The specific location of the pain may be the key to proper diagnosis. A history of weakness and sensory changes should also be sought.

2. **Physical examination** of the elbow should include inspection, palpation, ROM, and neurologic assessment. The point of maximal tenderness should be determined if possible. The normal range of extension and flexion is 0–140 degrees. Normal supination and pronation are 80 degrees each way. The neck, shoulder, and wrist should be examined to evaluate for referred pain.

3. **Radiographs** of the elbow typically include the AP and lateral views. In many cases plain films are nondiagnostic. They should probably be done in all patients with significant acute trauma to evaluate for dislocation and fracture. Special views are sometimes taken to evaluate the olecranon fossa and radial head. CT and MRI are occasionally indicated for better delineation of the bony and soft tissues.

B. **Lateral epicondylitis or tendinosis ("tennis elbow")** is the most common cause of elbow pain. The condition is caused by chronic overuse of the wrist extensors and supinators that originate from the lateral epicondyle. This results in repetitive microtears and angiofibroblastic degeneration or tendinosis of the origins of these muscles. No significant degree of inflammatory reaction appears to occur (*J Bone Joint Surg* 1999;81:259).

1. **History.** Patients complain of lateral elbow pain that worsens with certain activities. It is usually related to sports (e.g., racquet sports) or other repetitive uses that involve wrist extension and power gripping (e.g., carpentry or lifting with the palm facing down). It may develop acutely or more slowly. A direct blow to the outside of the elbow can also trigger lateral epicondylitis. Tenderness over the lateral elbow may be reported.

2. **Physical examination** of the elbow reveals maximal tenderness over the lateral epicondyle. Resisted wrist extension with the elbow extended often reproduces the pain.

3. **Radiographs** are usually nondiagnostic and unnecessary.

4. **Treatment** is almost always conservative. **Relative rest** (i.e., initially avoiding the activities that cause pain), **NSAIDs**, and a **compressive strap** worn just below the elbow ("tennis elbow splint") are often effective. Some patients find local application of ice comforting. Proper racquet size and backhand technique may also be of value. **Local corticosteroid injection** (e.g., 40 mg methylprednisolone) is an often-recommended alternative for patients who fail to respond to simple measures. It is generally believed to be effective, at least in the short term (*J Bone Joint Surg* 1997;79:1648). Surgery is rarely necessary.

C. **Medial epicondylitis or tendinosis ("golfer's elbow")** is very similar to but less common than lateral epicondylitis. It involves overuse and degenerative changes of the tendinous origins of the wrist flexor/pronator muscles at the medial epicondyle.

1. **History.** Patients complain of pain and tenderness over the medial epicondyle that is worsened by certain activities. It is also often related to sports (golf and throwing activities) and work.

2. **Examination** finds tenderness over the medial epicondyle. The pain may be reproduced by resisted wrist flexion.

3. **Radiographs** are unnecessary.

4. **Treatment** is similar to that for lateral epicondylitis. Local corticosteroid injection may be effective in the short term for those who do not respond to more conservative therapy (*J Bone Joint Surg* 1997;79:1648).

D. **Ulnar nerve entrapment (cubital tunnel syndrome)** results from compression of the ulnar nerve as it passes behind the medial epicondyle through the cubital tunnel, where it is very superficial. Direct pressure, repetitive elbow bending, prolonged elbow flexion, elbow arthritis, diabetes, and certain occupations and activities have all been associated with the condition. A firm direct blow to this area produces the familiar "funny bone" sensation.

1. **History.** Patients complain of medial elbow pain and sensory changes (numbness and paresthesias) in the ulnar nerve distribution, particularly the fourth and fifth digits. The symptoms may be worse at night. Weakness is sometimes reported.

2. **Physical examination** findings include sensory changes and weakness in the ulnar nerve distribution. Light touch and pinprick sensation are decreased in the ring and little fingers. Tapping the ulnar nerve where it passes behind the medical epicondyle causes pain along the inner elbow and paresthesias in the fourth and fifth digits (**Tinel's sign**). Full elbow flexion can produce a similar result (**elbow flexion test**). Reduced grip strength and intrinsic hand muscle weakness may be present. With prolonged nerve compression, atrophy of the intrinsic muscles may be seen.

3. **Radiographs** are generally unnecessary unless a bony abnormality causing nerve compression is suspected. **Nerve conduction studies and electromyography** may be useful when the diagnosis is uncertain or surgery is being considered.

4. **Treatment** is usually conservative. The elbow should be **kept straight** as much as possible. A **splint** can be worn at night to prevent flexion of the elbow during sleep. A cushioning **elbow pad** can be worn to protect the nerve during work. If possible, the patient's work environment should be altered to prevent further compression. A trial of **NSAIDs** is reasonable for pain. Surgery may be necessary for patients with recalcitrant symptoms.

E. **Olecranon bursitis** ("student's elbow") is a common condition that results from acute inflammation of the olecranon bursa. This bursa does not connect with the synovial cavity of the elbow. The cause may be infectious or noninfectious. The most common infectious agent is *Staphylococcus aureus*. Common noninfectious causes include repetitive trauma, gout, pseudogout, and RA. It can be difficult to differentiate an infectious from a noninfectious inflammatory bursitis.

1. **History.** Patients report a tender painful swelling of the posterior elbow that may develop acutely or more slowly. A history of trauma should be sought.

2. **Physical examination** is most notable for an obvious swelling ("goose egg") of the olecranon bursa, which may be quite large. Infectious and noninfectious causes may be indistinguishable on examination. Both can present with erythema, tenderness, and warmth. Marked findings are more likely to be traumatic or infectious in origin. Chronic or recurrent bursitis may be nontender.

3. **Radiographs** are usually not needed unless there has been significant trauma and fracture or dislocation is possible. **Aspiration of the bursal fluid** should be done to evaluate for infection. The fluid should be sent for Gram stain, culture, cell count, and crystal examination. Synovial fluid cell counts in infectious bursitis are generally lower (several thousand cells/ml) than in septic arthritis. The bursal fluid may be obviously bloody in cases of trauma.

4. **Treatment. Aspiration** of the olecranon bursa is not only diagnostic but also therapeutic. Fluid reaccumulation is not unusual in noninfectious cases, and repeat aspiration may be necessary. A **compression dressing** can be applied to help prevent recurrence, and an elbow pad can be used to prevent trauma. **NSAIDs** are frequently given. **Injection of 20 mg methylprednisolone** into the bursa may also reduce recurrence in patients with nonseptic olecranon bursitis (*Arch Intern Med* 1989;149:2527). Corticosteroid injection is contraindicated in infectious bursitis. Empiric **antibiotic treatment** (e.g., dicloxacillin or a cephalosporin) should be

given when infection is suspected pending culture results. Daily aspiration is usually necessary for septic bursitis.

II. Wrist and hand pain

A. General considerations. Wrist and hand complaints are common in primary care. Because of their obvious functional importance, careful diagnosis and treatment are particularly important.

1. **History.** Patients typically complain of pain, stiffness, swelling, weakness, numbness, and/or mass. The onset, progression, and location of the discomfort should be carefully detailed. A history of trauma may be important. The patient's hand dominance, occupation, activities, and hobbies may provide significant clues. The past medical history may suggest a systemic cause (e.g., a rheumatologic disease).

2. **Physical examination** of the hand and wrist should include inspection, palpation, ROM, and a neurologic assessment. The small joints of the hand should be examined individually. Careful inspection of the skin and nails may yield important hints to the diagnosis.

3. **Radiographs** of the hands and wrists may provide diagnostic information, particularly if arthritis is suspected. However, definitive changes may not be apparent until the disease has been present for an extended period of time. In cases of significant trauma, plain films are usually mandatory.

B. Stenosing tenosynovitis is an inflammation and thickening of tendons, sheaths, and synovium in the hand, sometimes with nodular enlargement of the tendon. It is frequently related to repetitive overuse, particularly those activities that involve gripping.

1. **Trigger finger or thumb** is caused by stenosing tenosynovitis of the flexor tendons of the fingers and thumb.

   a. **History.** Finger or thumb extension is limited when the affected tendon catches on the pulley at the base of the digit. This results in pain with use, and the affected digit can become painfully stuck in flexion. The finger may need to be forcibly extended with the other hand, often with a painful and audible pop.

   b. **Physical examination.** Palpation at the distal palmar crease may reveal a thickened tendon sheath or a tender nodule, or both, usually overlying the metacarpophalangeal (MCP) joint of the affected finger.

   c. **Radiographs** are unnecessary unless the patient has a history of injury or inflammatory arthritis.

   d. **Treatment** initially consists of **splitting** the MCP joint in extension and a short course of **NSAIDs. Corticosteroid injection** (methylprednisolone, 15–20 mg) with lidocaine into the flexor digital tendon sheath can also be effective (*J Hand Surg* 1995;20:628). Recurrence is common, and **surgical release** may be required.

2. **de Quervain's tenosynovitis** is a very similar condition that affects the tendons and sheaths of the abductor pollicis longus and the extensor pollicis brevis.

   a. **History.** Patients complain of pain, tenderness, and swelling on the radial side of the wrist in the region of the anatomic snuffbox. Ulnar deviation of the wrist and movement of the thumb exacerbate the pain, and a "squeaking" or "creaking" sensation may be described.

   b. **Physical examination. Finkelstein's sign** is diagnostic. The patient makes a fist enclosing the thumb; if this does not produce pain, the examiner forces the wrist into ulnar deviation as an additional stress. Focal tenderness is usually present over the radial styloid.

   c. **Radiographs** are usually unnecessary.

   d. **Treatment.** A short opponens **splint** is therapeutic, supplemented by **NSAIDs.** Refractory cases often respond well to **corticosteroid injection** (methylprednisolone, 20–30 mg) with lidocaine (*J Hand Surg* 1994;19:595). **Surgical release** is sometimes required.

C. **Dupuytren's contracture** is a fibroproliferative disorder that results in painless thickening and nodularity of the palmar aponeurosis. The flexor tendons of the hand are not primarily involved. The fibrosis of the palmar fascia draws the fingers (most commonly the ring and little finger) into flexion at the MCP joint. The condition generally affects men older than 40 years and appears to have a strong genetic component. It is also associated with diabetes, alcoholism, repetitive trauma, and seizure disorders.
   1. **History.** Affected patients complain of painless nodules in the palm, an inability to extend the fingers fully, and difficulty in picking up large objects.
   2. **Physical examination** reveals painless thickening and nodularity of the palmar fascia with flexion deformity of one or more fingers.
   3. **Radiographs** are unnecessary.
   4. **Treatment**. Apart from gently stretching the fingers, there is no known effective conservative treatment. Surgical treatment can be considered for the severely affected, but recurrences are common.
D. **Carpal tunnel syndrome** (CTS) is the most frequently occurring entrapment neuropathy. It results from compression of the median nerve as it passes through the carpal tunnel. It is most common in middle-aged women and usually affects the dominant hand. CTS is known to occur with increased frequency in patients with diabetes, amyloidosis, renal failure on hemodialysis, RA and other arthropathies of the wrist, pregnancy, hypothyroidism, and previous wrist trauma. It is often related to repetitive overuse of the hands and wrists.
   1. **History.** Patients usually complain of an aching pain in the wrist and hand, which may radiate up the forearm. Intermittent paresthesias and numbness in the median nerve distribution (palmar surface of the thumb, index, long, and radial side of the ring fingers) are typical. However, less-than-classic descriptions of the location of discomfort are not unusual. Symptoms are frequently worse at night and with overuse of the hands. The patient may describe "shaking out" the hand to improve the symptoms (the "flick sign"). Weakness, clumsiness, and a tendency to drop objects may also be reported. Patients should be questioned about trauma, work-related duties, hobbies, and activities.
   2. **Physical examination** classically reveals **decreased sensation** (hypalgesia) in the median nerve distribution, **weakness** of thumb abduction, and **Tinel's and Phalen's signs**. In Phalen's maneuver the wrists are held in unforced flexion for 30–60 seconds. Reproduction or worsening of the symptoms constitutes a positive test. Tinel's sign is the development of paresthesias in the median nerve distribution when the median nerve is tapped at the distal wrist crease. When compared to electrodiagnostic testing, however, Tinel's and Phalen's signs may have little diagnostic value (*JAMA* 2000;283:3110). Thenar atrophy can occur with long-standing CTS.
   3. **Radiographs** of the wrist are usually unnecessary unless trauma or arthritis is believed to be causative. **Electrodiagnostic testing** (median nerve conduction) is generally thought to be the gold standard for CTS, but false positives and false negatives do occur. Such testing should be considered when the diagnosis is uncertain or surgical treatment is being considered or in cases of work-related compensation.
   4. **Treatment** for most patients is initially conservative. Symptoms often improve with a simple **cock-up wrist splint** (worn primarily at night) and a course of **NSAIDs**. Work-related **ergonomic modifications** should be undertaken if necessary. If these simple measures fail, the patient can be referred for a single **corticosteroid injection** (40 mg methylprednisolone) with lidocaine (10 mg) into the area close to the carpal tunnel, which may be effective (*BMJ* 1999;319:884). Definitive treatment entails **surgical release**, a simple outpatient procedure in which the

flexor retinaculum is incised, relieving the pressure on the median nerve. Surgery is very effective in treating CTS, provided that the diagnosis has been confirmed electrodiagnostically.

E. **Ulnar nerve entrapment** can occasionally occur at the wrist as the nerve passes through the canal of Guyon. It may be caused by repetitive trauma (e.g., operating a jackhammer, using the hand as a hammer, resting the ulnar side of the wrist and hand on the edge of a desk or keyboard) or a space-occupying lesion (e.g., ganglion or lipoma). Patients may have sensory and motor changes in the ulnar distribution. When the ulnar nerve is tapped in the hypothenar area, there may be a Tinel's sign. In advanced cases there may be intrinsic hand muscle atrophy. Nerve conduction studies may help differentiate wrist entrapment from the more common elbow entrapment of the ulnar nerve. Treatment consists of **avoidance of repetitive trauma** or **surgical excision** of the offending mass.

F. **Arthritic conditions** of the wrist and hand are common. **RA** characteristically involves the wrist, MCP, and proximal interphalangeal joints. The erosive synovitis causes pain, stiffness, deformity, and loss of functionality. **Osteoarthritis** typically involves the distal interphalangeal and carpometacarpal joints (especially of the thumb). See Chap. 22 for a full discussion of the management of these conditions.

G. **Other causes**
   1. **Fingertip infections**
      a. **Paronychia** is the most common type of hand infection and is usually caused by *S. aureus*. It typically follows self-performed hangnail removal or an overly aggressive manicure. It is characterized by pain, tenderness, erythema, and swelling about the fingernail. Pus is sometimes present. Initial treatment consists of frequent **warm soaks** and oral antibiotic such as **cephalexin or dicloxacillin**. If improvement does not occur promptly or there is a visible pus collection, **surgical drainage** is warranted.
      b. **Felons** are a more serious infection of the entire distal pulp of the fingertip. Again, the most common organism is *S. aureus*. They are generally caused by a puncture wound to the thumb or index finger. Patients present with severe pain and tenderness, erythema, and tense swelling of the distal fingertip. Most felons require **surgical drainage**.
   2. **Subungual hematomas** result from trauma to the distal finger (e.g., from hammer or car door) and are generally quite painful. Radiographs to evaluate for distal phalangeal fractures can be obtained. Small subungual hematomas can be managed conservatively with elevation and ice. Patients with larger subungual hematomas or severe pain, or both, benefit from **nail trephination with electrocautery**. This method rapidly improves pain, is associated with very few complications, and provides a good cosmetic result (*J Accid Emerg Med* 1998;15:269).

Hip Pain

I. **General considerations.** Hip pain has many potential causes, but only a few are common. Pain may emanate from the hip joint, periarticular soft tissues, pelvic bones, and sacroiliac joint or be referred from another location (usually the lumbosacral spine).

A. **History.** Patients typically complain of painful limited ROM and difficulty in ambulating. The location of the pain can be the key to proper diagnosis. True hip joint pain usually affects the groin and radiates to the buttock. Bearing weight worsens the pain. Buttock pain alone without groin pain is likely to originate in the low back, sacroiliac joint, or ischial tuberosity. Lateral proximal thigh pain suggests trochanteric bursitis. Anterior thigh pain suggests lateral femoral cutaneous nerve entrapment. Pain that radiates down the posterior thigh is frequently due to lumbosacral radiculopathy. Patients with chronic progressive disease have increasing difficulty in ambulating and performing the activities of daily living.

B. **Physical examination.** The patient should be observed **standing and walking.** A limp or expression of pain may be demonstrative of the patient's complaint. The **abductor lurch (Trendelenburg's gait)** suggests intra-articular hip pathology. The patient shifts weight over the affected leg to unload weakened abductors. The **Trendelenburg's test** should be done. Ask the standing patient to raise the knee on the unaffected side so that weight is borne on the affected side. Normally, the pelvis elevates on the raised-knee side. A drop in the pelvis on the raised-knee side suggests weakness of the hip abductors on the straight-knee (affected) side. **Patrick's test, or the FABERE sign** (flexion-abduction-external rotation-extension), is performed by placing the supine patient's heel on the contralateral knee. The examiner then pushes the knee and thigh downward to put the hip into external rotation, producing pain in intrinsic hip disease. **Palpation** of the hip joint and surrounding area is done to elicit tenderness. **ROM** should be tested. Normal hip flexion is approximately 120 degrees; normal internal rotation is 30 degrees and external rotation 60 degrees. Hip joint pathology tends to affect internal rotation most. **Strength** of the adductors, abductors, and flexors should be tested. The lumbar spine and the sacroiliac joints should be examined. The groin is examined, looking for evidence of an inguinal or femoral hernia.

C. **Radiographs,** when indicated, should include AP and lateral views of the hip and an AP view of the pelvis. CT or MRI is occasionally needed to evaluate the hip further (e.g., occult hip fractures and osteonecrosis).

II. **Osteoarthritis of the hip joint** is very common and increases with age. It is characterized by loss of the articular cartilage of the joint. Predisposing factors include childhood hip disorders, leg-length anomalies, and work that involves heavy lifting and carrying.

A. **History.** Osteoarthritis of the true hip joint causes pain in the anterior groin, radiating down the anteromedial thigh, and is worse with weight-bearing. Pain may also occur in the lateral thigh or the buttock. The typical history is pain with activity that is relieved with rest. Patients may report pain that has been very slowly progressive over years. Difficulty in walking and performing activities of daily living may develop.

B. **Physical examination** is notable for painfully reduced ROM. Internal rotation is affected first. In time, extension, flexion, and abduction are also reduced. Joint contractures may eventually develop. An abductor lurch may be observed as a compensation for pain and secondary hip abductor weakness. Trendelenburg's and Patrick's tests may be positive.

C. **Radiographs** of the hip characteristically show joint space narrowing, osteophytes, cyst formation, and subchondral sclerosis.

D. **Treatment** depends on the severity of symptoms. See Chap. 22 for a more complete discussion of the treatment of osteoarthritis.

1. **Nonpharmacologic measures,** such as patient education and self-help programs, weight loss, use of a cane, physical therapy and exercise, and occupational therapy, should always be considered before medications are prescribed. Drug therapy is most effective when combined with nonpharmacologic strategies (*Arthritis Rheum* 2000; 43:1905).

2. **Acetaminophen** (1000 mg qid) is a reasonable choice for patients with mild to moderate pain and is probably comparable to the results obtained with NSAIDs.

3. **NSAIDs** at low analgesic doses can be tried in those patients who do not obtain adequate symptomatic relief with acetaminophen. If the lower dose is not effective, it can be increased to a full anti-inflammatory dose. No NSAID is clearly more effective than any other, although individual responses may vary (*Cochrane Database Syst Rev* 2000;2:CD000517). For those at increased risk of GI toxicity, an NSAID can be given in combination with **misoprostol** (200 µg tid–qid) or **omeprazole** (20 mg qd) (*N Engl J Med* 1999;340:1888). Many patients have side effects that are attributable to misoprostol (e.g., diarrhea and abdominal pain).

4. **Selective COX-2 inhibitors** are as effective as traditional NSAIDs and are a reasonable but more costly alternative with a lower incidence of serious GI toxicity (*JAMA* 2000;284:1247).

5. **Tramadol** (50–100 mg qid) is an alternative for patients who fail to respond to or who cannot take nonselective or selective NSAIDs, but side effects are common (e.g., nausea, constipation, drowsiness).

6. Surgical treatment with **total hip replacement** is often very effective and should be considered for patients with moderate to severe pain or disability, or both, who do not respond to medical treatment.

III. **Trochanteric bursitis** is another common cause of hip pain. It can occur in association with iliotibial band syndrome, hip joint pathology, previous hip surgery, leg-length discrepancy, and mechanical back pain.

A. **History.** Patients complain of lateral hip pain that may radiate down the leg. The pain is worse with exercise and at night, especially when the patient lies on the affected side. Some patients complain of a limp.

B. **Physical examination.** Local tenderness over the trochanteric prominence can be demonstrated, and hip ROM should be unrestricted.

C. **Radiographs** are usually unnecessary, as the diagnosis is made clinically.

D. **Treatment.** Trochanteric bursitis is slow to respond to therapy but almost never becomes chronic. **NSAIDs** often provide symptomatic relief, and **physical therapy** for modalities and iliotibial band stretching can be helpful. Patients should be encouraged to continue with stretching exercises at home. A **corticosteroid injection** (30–40 mg methylprednisolone) with local anesthetic (3 ml 1% lidocaine) into the greater trochanteric bursa usually brings at least temporary relief (*J Rheumatol* 1996;23:2104). Care should be taken to avoid a fluorinated corticosteroid preparation such as triamcinolone acetonide or hexacetonide, because these can result in atrophy of the skin and subcutaneous fat.

IV. **Avascular necrosis (osteonecrosis)** is the death of a variable amount of trabecular bone in the femoral head. The precise pathophysiology is not known, but it is unusual in the absence of known **risk factors**, which include corticosteroid treatment (especially in those with lupus), alcoholism, trauma or prior fracture, RA, sickle cell disease, myeloproliferative disorders, and radiation. A high index of suspicion should be maintained in patients with these risk factors. The condition may be bilateral. Severe avascular necrosis can cause collapse to the femoral head.

A. **History.** Pain tends to come on suddenly and can be severe, but the onset can be more gradual. A few patients may be asymptomatic. The pain is typically in the groin radiating to the buttocks and is increased with weightbearing.

B. **Physical examination.** Internal and external rotation of the hip are painful and sometimes reduced. The patient often has a limp.

C. **Radiographs** may show sclerosis of the femoral head. Collapse of the femoral head is seen in advanced cases. If initial radiographs are normal, an **MRI** should be considered because of its high sensitivity for this diagnosis.

D. **Treatment. Limited weightbearing** with a cane or walker may be sufficient for some patients, but **orthopedic consultation** should always be obtained to evaluate the need for surgical core decompression or total hip arthroplasty. If corticosteroid therapy remains necessary, efforts should be made to reduce the dose as much as possible.

V. Meralgia paresthetica is an entrapment neuropathy caused by compression of the **lateral femoral cutaneous nerve**. It may be related to one or more factors, including obesity, pregnancy, diabetes, wearing tight garments around the waist (e.g., pantyhose, tool belts), local surgery, trauma, repetitive hip extension (joggers, cheerleaders who do splits frequently), and, rarely, intrapelvic masses.

   A. History is remarkable for pain, burning, and dysesthesia in the groin and anterolateral thigh. The discomfort may extend to the lateral knee. No motor symptoms occur.

   B. Physical examination usually reveals hypoesthesia or dysesthesia, or both, in the lateral femoral cutaneous nerve distribution. Examination of the hip is normal unless coexistent hip pathology is present.

   C. Radiographs are generally not necessary.

   D. Treatment consists of eliminating the source of nerve compression or repetitive trauma. Weight loss in obese patients can be effective.

VI. Hip fractures are particularly common in elderly women and usually occur at the femoral neck or the intertrochanteric area. They are associated with a high morbidity and mortality. Age, Caucasian race, female sex, osteoporosis, and falls are common predisposing factors.

   A. History. Most patients report a fall and subsequent inability to walk. They have pain in the groin that radiates to the buttocks. A few patients may be able to walk with assistance, but pain increases with weightbearing.

   B. Physical examination classically reveals an externally rotated, abducted, and foreshortened leg. Ecchymosis or hematoma formation may be present at the hip.

   C. Radiographs. AP and lateral views of the hip and an AP view of the pelvis should be obtained. A view that is limited to the hip joint may miss pelvic fractures. Hip fractures are usually obvious, but plain films are occasionally negative. A bone scan, CT, or MRI may be necessary for diagnosis.

   D. Treatment is almost always **surgical**, and an **orthopedic consultation** is mandatory. A patient with an osteoporotic fracture should have bone density measured by dual x-ray absorptiometry as a baseline and should be started on medications to increase bone density and decrease the risk of subsequent fracture (see Chap. 24).

Knee Pain

I. General considerations. With normal use, the knee is subject to considerable wear and tear and is vulnerable to injury (often sports related). As such, knee pain is a common complaint. Degenerative disease, trauma, and inflammatory processes are the most frequent causes.

   A. History. Knee disorders usually present with one or more of the following: pain, stiffness, swelling, redness, warmth, tenderness, giving way, locking, and cracking. Acute knee pain is often traumatic, and the mechanism of injury should be detailed. An audible pop is sometimes heard. Subacute and chronic knee discomfort is also common. Patients should be carefully asked about exacerbating activities, sports, and prior episodes of trauma. The location of pain can be helpful. A history of pain in the contralateral knee or other joints, or both, can be important. Inflammatory conditions characteristically present with a large effusion and morning stiffness that improves with activity. With mechanical causes, pain is typically worsened with activity and improved with rest.

   B. Physical examination of the knee includes inspection, palpation, ROM, strength, and gait. Acute knee inflammation may make adequate examination difficult or impossible. Normal flexion of the knee is 135 degrees and extension 0 degrees.

1. The **bulge sign** can be used to detect **small knee effusions**. The patient's knee is extended flat on the examination table. Joint fluid is milked up into the suprapatellar pouch by moving the hand proximally along the medial side of the patella. The fluid is then milked down into the medial knee by moving the hand from above the lateral side of the patella along the lateral knee and down to the tibia. Excessive fluid creates a bulge medial to the patella.

2. The **anterior drawer test** and **Lachman's test** are used to test for **cruciate ligament instability**. Both knees should be tested for comparison. The anterior drawer test is performed with the patient supine and the knee flexed 90 degrees. The tibia is grasped with both hands and pulled anteriorly. Lachman's test is performed with the supine patient's knee in 20 degrees of flexion. The distal femur is stabilized with one hand while the other hand pulls the tibia forward. Excessive anterior displacement of the tibia and a less than sharp end point suggest anterior cruciate ligament (ACL) damage. Lachman's test is generally believed to be the more sensitive test.

3. **Stability of the collateral ligaments** should be tested in 20–30 degrees of flexion and full extension. One hand stabilizes the lateral side of the knee while the other hand applies abduction force to the distal leg or one hand stabilizes the medial side of the knee while the other hand applies adduction force to the distal leg. Excessive motion, usually with pain, signifies medial or collateral ligament damage.

4. **McMurray's test** can be used to detect meniscal tears. With the supine patient's knee in full flexion, the knee is slowly extended as the tibia is rotated internally and externally. A palpable or audible pop, often with pain, suggests a meniscal tear. This test is insensitive but fairly specific (*J Orthop Sports Phys Ther* 1995;22:116).

C. **Radiographs** of the knee are frequently done as a part of the evaluation of knee pain, but they are not always necessary. If the history and examination suggest a periarticular problem, plain films are unlikely to be diagnostic and are generally unnecessary. When a significant mechanical articular problem is suggested by the history and physical examination, plain films may be helpful. Standard films include AP and lateral views, and standing films should be obtained if possible. Detection of some fractures by plain radiography may require special views. Ligamentous and meniscal damage cannot be diagnosed with plain films. **MRI** may be useful in this situation if surgery is being considered in conjunction with an orthopedic consultant. The **Ottawa knee rules** or the **Pittsburgh decision rules** can be used to determine which patients with acute knee injuries require knee films (Table 21-5). A multicenter comparison found the sensitivity and specificity of the Ottawa rules to be 97% and 27%, respectively, and for the Pittsburgh rules 99% and 60%, respectively (*Ann Emerg Med* 1998;32:8).

II. **Osteoarthritis of the knee** is an extremely common condition and an important source of disability. Important associations include age, wear and tear, obesity, genetic factors, prior trauma (e.g., fractures, ligamentous injuries that cause instability, meniscal damage), and prior knee surgery. Osteoarthritis may affect any or all of the three compartments of the knee (medial and lateral tibiofemoral, patellofemoral). The medial compartment is the most commonly involved.

A. **History** is characterized by gradually developing knee pain that is worse with activity and improved with rest. Brief (less than 30 minutes) morning stiffness may occur, and patients may note trouble in walking, kneeling, climbing stairs, and getting into and out of chairs. Some may report a limp or a sensation of knee buckling. Symptoms may begin in one knee but often become bilateral. In some patients severe pain and disability eventually develop.

Table 21-5. Variables indicating the need for radiography after knee trauma

Ottawa knee rule

If any of the following factors are present:

    Age >55 yrs

    Tenderness at head of fibula

    Isolated tenderness of patella

    Inability to flex knee to 90 degrees

    Inability to walk four weightbearing steps immediately and in the emergency department

Pittsburgh knee rule

Fall or blunt trauma mechanism of injury plus either:

    Age >50 yrs, or

    Inability to walk four weightbearing steps in the emergency department

Adapted from IG Stiell, GA Wells, RH Hoag, et al. Implementation of the Ottawa knee rule for the use of radiography in acute knee injuries. *JAMA* 1997;278:2075–2079, and DC Seaberg, R Jackson. Clinical decision rule for knee radiographs. *Am J Emerg Med* 1994;12:541–543.

   B. Physical examination often reveals **tenderness** along the joint line, a **small effusion, crepitus** during knee motion, and sometimes palpable **osteophytes**. Patients with significant medial compartment disease often have a **varus** (bowleg) deformity when standing. Less commonly, a **valgus** (knock-knee) deformity may occur with lateral compartment disease.
   C. Radiographs should be obtained with the patient standing. Characteristic changes include asymmetric joint space narrowing, sclerosis, osteophytes, subchondral cyst formation, and varus or valgus deformity. Osteochondral loose bodies are sometimes seen.
   D. Treatment of knee osteoarthritis is very similar to that for the hip (see Hip Pain, sec. **II**). This includes **nonpharmacologic measures, acetaminophen, NSAIDs,** and **selective COX-2 inhibitors**. (Also refer to Chap. 22 for a more complete discussion of the treatment of osteoarthritis.)
     1. Weight loss is an important component of therapy.
     2. Exercise (aerobic walking or resistance exercise training) may modestly improve disability, physical performance, and pain in patients with knee osteoarthritis (*JAMA* 1997;27:25). Quadriceps strengthening is believed to be particularly important (*Arthritis Rheum* 2000;43:1905).
     3. Capsaicin cream (0.025% applied qid) may be an effective adjuvant treatment in some patients (*Clin Ther* 1991;13:383). Burning at the application site is common.
     4. Intra-articular corticosteroids (e.g., 40–60 mg methylprednisolone or up to 40 mg triamcinolone) may be of short-term benefit for some patients with acute flares of knee pain related to osteoarthritis (*Ann Rheum Dis* 1997;56:634). If there is any concern for infection, corticosteroid injection should be postponed until negative synovial fluid cultures are obtained. No single joint should be injected more than three or four times a year.
     5. Intra-articular hyaluronic acid derivative injections may be effective for the pain of knee osteoarthritis that has not responded to more conservative therapy (*Arthritis Rheum* 2000;43:1192). Two derivatives of hyaluronic acid have been approved by the U.S. Food and Drug Administration for the treatment of osteoarthritis of the knee: **hyaluronan (Hyalgan)** and **hylan GF-20 (Synvisc)**. These agents are given weekly

for three (hylan GF-20) or five (hyaluronan) injections. Some studies have shown efficacy comparable to that of NSAIDs for each medication. The effect takes longer to develop than with intra-articular steroids but may last considerably longer. These injections are often technically challenging, because patients with osteoarthritis of the knee typically have minimal effusion, making it difficult to be certain that the needle is within the knee joint.

6. **Chronic use of narcotics** may be appropriate in rare cases, especially for those who are not candidates for total joint arthroplasty.

7. **Orthopedic consultation for possible surgery** should be considered for patients with significant pain or disability, or both, that has been unresponsive to more conservative treatment.

III. **Acute monoarticular arthritis of the knee** is a fairly common presentation that requires a prompt and careful evaluation. The following discussion is generally applicable to acute monoarticular arthritis in other joints as well. The causes may be broadly classified as **noninflammatory or inflammatory**. Inflammatory conditions generally produce larger effusions and more heat and redness. Although septic arthritis typically presents with the most marked signs of inflammation, the differentiation can sometimes be quite difficult.

A. Important **noninflammatory causes** include trauma (e.g., fracture, meniscal tear, and ACL tear), hemarthrosis, sickle cell disease, and acute flares of osteoarthritis.

B. The **inflammatory conditions** can be divided into **noninfectious and infectious causes**. Noninfectious causes include RA, lupus, psoriatic arthritis, Reiter's syndrome, gout, and pseudogout. The most common infectious causes are gonococcal arthritis (especially in sexually active young adults) and *S. aureus*. Extra-articular infections, previous damage to the joint, prosthetic joints, serious underlying chronic illness, immunosuppression, corticosteroid therapy, and intravenous drug use are **predisposing factors** for septic arthritis.

C. **Evaluation** initially focuses on differentiating trauma, crystalline arthropathy, and, most importantly, infection. **Plain radiographs** are indicated for all patients with a history of trauma. **Aspiration** of the knee joint is mandatory unless the diagnosis is known with certainty. Synovial fluid should be sent for Gram stain, culture (including *Neisseria gonorrhoeae*), cell count and differential, and crystal analysis. An inflammatory fluid without crystals should raise a strong suspicion for infection, especially in a sexually active young adult (Table 21-6).

D. **Treatment.** Septic arthritis demands swift and aggressive treatment to minimize joint destruction. Unless there is an established diagnosis of noninfectious inflammatory arthritis (e.g., RA), strong consideration should be given to admission for empiric antibiotics until the synovial fluid cultures are negative. Definitive treatment of septic arthritis includes intravenous antibiotics (agent and duration determined by culture results), serial joint aspiration, and occasionally surgical drainage. Orthopedic consultation is

Table 21-6. Synovial fluid analysis

Classification	Color and clarity	Viscosity	WBC/ml
Normal	Clear, colorless	Viscous	<200
Noninflammatory	Clear, yellow	Viscous	200–2000
Inflammatory	Cloudy, yellow	Hypoviscous	2000–100,000
Septic	Purulent	Hypoviscous	>80,000

warranted for most large traumatic knee effusions. The treatment of other inflammatory arthropathies is discussed in Chap. 22.

IV. Patellofemoral pain syndrome (PFPS) is characterized by retropatellar or peripatellar pain and crepitation with certain activities. The condition is ill defined and poorly understood, but nonetheless **anterior knee pain** of this type is very common and may become chronic and limit activity. Multiple associations and predisposing factors have been proposed, including overuse/overloading, maltracking of the patella, patellar subluxation, obesity, malalignment of the knee-extensor mechanism, quadriceps weakness, and trauma. Many patients, however, have no such associations. The relationship of PFPS to chondromalacia of the patella is controversial. PFPS can occur without chondromalacia, and patients with chondromalacia may have no symptoms (*J Bone Joint Surg* 1999;81:355).

A. History. Patients complain of anterior knee pain with activities such as going down steps or hills, squatting, running, jumping, and prolonged sitting (the "theater sign").

B. Physical examination may reveal crepitus and malalignment of the patella with flexion and extension (patella tracks too far laterally). The patellar compression test supports the diagnosis. The examiner immobilizes the patella while the patient contracts the quadriceps muscle, pulling the patella proximally against the femoral condyles, reproducing the pain. Some quadriceps atrophy may also be present. A knee effusion is infrequently seen.

C. Radiographs of the patella (Merchant view) may show malalignment of the patella but are usually normal.

D. Treatment. Evidence-based treatment recommendations are difficult to make for PFPS. **Relative rest, acetaminophen, NSAIDs,** and **ice** are reasonable treatment options for most patients. Quadriceps training is generally believed to be of potential value. Knee taping and knee braces are advocated by some. Surgery may be appropriate for a few patients (e.g., those with serious chondromalacia or marked patellar maltracking or subluxation).

V. Ligamentous injuries are generally seen after trauma in athletic young adults. These injuries comprise a spectrum from torn and stretched ligamentous fibers to complete tear or rupture. Collateral and cruciate ligament injuries can occur alone or together, with or without meniscal damage.

A. History

1. **ACL tears** are usually caused by a significant **twisting injury**. A popping sensation may be described. Pain is immediate, quickly followed by the development of a large effusion, giving way, and great difficulty in walking.

2. **Collateral ligament tears** usually follow an **abduction or adduction force** (medial or lateral collateral ligaments, respectively). These patients complain of pain, stiffness, and localized swelling. Most are able to ambulate after the injury.

B. Physical examination of patients with acute ligamentous tears (especially ACL) can be quite difficult because of pain and swelling.

1. A sizable effusion and positive **anterior drawer** and **Lachman's tests** are usually present in ACL tears (see sec. **I.B.2**).

2. Application of **varus and valgus stress** in 20–30 degrees of flexion and with the knee in extension tests for collateral ligament damage (see sec. **I.B.3**).

C. Radiographs are usually normal but should be done to evaluate for avulsion fractures. **Arthrocentesis** in patients with ACL tears often produces bloody or serosanguineous fluid.

D. Treatment. If ligamentous injury is suspected, referral to an orthopedist or sports medicine specialist should be obtained. Initial conservative treatment includes **rest, ice, compression, elevation, NSAIDs, crutches,** and a **knee brace**. More specific treatment and possible surgical intervention should be directed by the orthopedic consultant.

VI. Meniscal tears typically occur after a **twisting injury**, and the medial meniscus is much more commonly affected. This type of injury can occur in isolation or with a medial collateral or ACL tear, or both. Older individuals may experience a degenerative meniscal tear after minimal trauma.

A. History. Patients usually report pain, swelling, and stiffness after a significant twisting injury. Pain may be referred to the popliteal area. Clicking, locking, or giving way may also be described. Most patients are able to walk after the injury.

B. Physical examination usually reveals an effusion. Tenderness may be present along the joint line near the tear. McMurray's test may be positive (see sec. **I.B.4**).

C. Radiographs are usually normal except for an effusion. An **MRI** is a more definitive test to prove the presence of a torn meniscus; however, false-positive results do occur.

D. Treatment. Orthopedic consultation is reasonable for most patients with a meniscal tear. Many patients heal with conservative treatment, which includes **rest, ice, compression, elevation, NSAIDs, and gradual return to activity**. Surgery should be reserved for patients who continue to have pain or locking, or both. In the presence of osteoarthritis of the knee, surgical treatment for a torn meniscus may actually lead to an intensification of knee pain, necessitating a total knee arthroplasty.

VII. Bursitis can occur at several locations in the knee. Bursae are synovially lined and produce a small amount of fluid that decreases friction between adjacent structures. Chronic overuse, trauma, and friction can result in inflammation. The pain of bursitis is typically worse with activity and improved with rest.

A. The **prepatellar bursa** lies between the skin and the patella. Prepatellar bursitis is usually caused by repeated trauma involving a lot of kneeling (e.g., "housemaid's knee" and "clergyman's knee"). It produces swelling directly above the patella. It should be evaluated with aspiration, as indolent **septic bursitis** can be present and may be complicated by surrounding cellulitis. Unlike septic arthritis, the synovial fluid in infectious bursitis often has a cell count of only a few thousand WBC, and therefore a high index of suspicion is needed to make the diagnosis. Patients without infection can be managed conservatively with avoidance of the inciting trauma, ice, and NSAIDs. When infection is likely or confirmed, antibiotic administration should be combined with daily aspiration of the bursa to be sure that the cell count falls and the Gram stain and culture become negative with treatment. Patients who are systemically ill should be admitted to the hospital for IV antibiotics. Surgical incision and drainage are rarely necessary.

B. The **pes anserine bursa** lies under the insertion of the hamstrings on the proximal medial tibia. It can become inflamed with overuse (e.g., walking or running) and in those with osteoarthritis of the knee. Pain occurs on the anteromedial aspect of the knee, and the area is exquisitely tender. Conservative treatment with relative rest, ice, and NSAIDs is frequently helpful. Local corticosteroid injection may also be effective.

VIII. Baker's cyst (popliteal cyst or semimembranosus-gastrocnemius bursitis) is a fluid-filled sac located in the popliteal fossa, usually on the medial side. It frequently connects with the joint cavity. It is often associated with knee effusions, posterior meniscal tears, and degenerative arthropathy (*Radiology* 1996;201:247). It is also very common in RA (*Clin Exp Rheumatol* 1995;13:633).

A. History. Many Baker's cysts are asymptomatic, but swelling, tenderness, and fullness behind the knee may be reported. Very large cysts can cause significant pain and even neurovascular compromise because of the pressure on surrounding structures. Some cysts become symptomatic only when they rupture, producing redness, swelling, warmth, pain, and tenderness of the calf.

B. Physical examination may reveal a prominence in the medial aspect of the popliteal fossa. In the situation of a ruptured cyst, inflammation of the calf occurs, potentially simulating thrombophlebitis.

C. Radiographs of the knee may show changes that are consistent with intra-articular pathology. Ultrasound can be used to visualize the cyst and evaluate for thrombophlebitis of the leg. MRI can also be used to visualize a Baker's cyst.

D. Treatment. Evidence-based treatment recommendations are very difficult to provide, as extremely few data are available. Mild to moderately symptomatic unruptured cysts can be treated with as-needed acetaminophen or NSAIDs. Some advocate knee joint aspiration (sometimes with corticosteroid injection) as effective treatment for more symptomatic individuals. Surgical treatment may be useful for a small number of patients. Ruptured cysts can be treated with relative rest, elevation, heat, and NSAIDs.

IX. Other causes

A. Iliotibial band friction syndrome is a common overuse injury in runners and cyclists. Repetitive movement of a tight iliotibial over the lateral femoral condyle causes friction and pain, particularly with climbing stairs and running down hills.

B. Tibial tubercle apophysitis (Osgood-Schlatter disease) generally presents in adolescents, with pain localized to the insertion of the patellar tendon at the tibial tubercle. It is often related to an ossicle of bone within the tibial tendon anterior to the tubercle. Pain usually resolves with time when the ossicle fuses with the underlying bone. Until that time, pain should limit athletic activity.

Ankle and Foot Disorders

I. General considerations. Ankle and foot problems are frequently encountered in the ambulatory setting. They are often related to mechanical abnormalities or inappropriate footwear.

A. History. The most common complaint is pain. Precise localization of the pain can be very important diagnostically. Medical history (e.g., diabetes mellitus, gout, RA, vascular disease, neuropathy, etc.), exacerbating and alleviating factors, chronicity, association with trauma, athletic and work activities, and footwear may provide valuable clues.

B. Physical examination. If possible, patients should be observed standing and walking with and without shoes. The shoes should be observed for type (e.g., severely pointed high heels) and unusual wear. ROM and inflammation of the joints should be assessed. Normal ankle dorsiflexion is 15 degrees and plantar flexion 55 degrees. Normal heel inversion is 35 degrees and eversion 20 degrees. One should take note of corns, calluses, ulcerations, and the appearance of the nails. Circulation and sensation should be evaluated.

C. Radiographs of the ankle and foot are sometimes useful but not always necessary. Standard films of the ankle include AP, mortise (30 degrees internal rotation), and lateral views. Standard foot films consist of AP and lateral views. Both should be obtained during weightbearing if possible.

II. Ankle pain

A. Ankle sprains are one of the most common injuries encountered. They are typically caused by inversion injuries and, therefore, usually involve the lateral ligaments. The severity of sprains can range from minimal to quite severe. Chronic ankle instability and recurrent injury after an ankle sprain is not uncommon.

1. **History.** Patients usually report a trip or fall that results in forced inversion of the ankle. Eversion injuries do occur but are much less common. Swelling, tenderness, and painful ambulation are common. Some patients have severe pain, an inability to walk, and/or ecchymosis.

2. **Physical examination** is notable for swelling, tenderness, and sometimes ecchymosis over the lateral collateral ligaments (deltoid ligament

Table 21-7. Variables indicating the need for ankle radiography

Any pain in the malleolar zone and any of the following:

  Bony tenderness at the posterior edge or tip of the lateral malleolus

  Bony tenderness at the posterior edge or tip of the medial malleolus

  Inability to bear weight immediately and in the emergency department

Adapted from IG Stiell, RD McKnight, GH Greenberg, et al. Implementation of the Ottawa ankle rules. *JAMA* 1994;271:827–832.

      for an eversion injury). Swelling may extend to involve the entire ankle. The medial and lateral malleoli should be palpated for tenderness. Discomfort with attempted manual inversion is obvious. Weightbearing may or may not be possible.

    3. **Radiographs** of the ankle are not always necessary and are often overused. The **Ottawa ankle rules** (Table 21-7) can be successfully used to determine when ankle films to evaluate for fracture are necessary, with a sensitivity of 100% and a specificity of 50%.

    4. **Treatment** for most ankle sprains is conservative, consisting of **rest, ice, compression, elevation,** and **NSAIDs.** An **air stirrup–type ankle brace** can be used for added support. As tolerated, weightbearing is permissible, but some patients require crutches. When the patient can bear weight without pain, increased activity can begin. Continued use of an air stirrup brace should be encouraged. Organized physical therapy for ankle strengthening after a sprain may be beneficial. Severe sprains require more intensive treatment, and an **orthopedic consultation** should be obtained for these patients. Use of an ankle support (semirigid orthosis or air stirrup) during sporting activities can reduce the risk of a recurrent sprain (*Cochrane Database Syst Rev* 2000;3:CD:000018).

  B. **Primary osteoarthritis** of the **tibiotalar (ankle) joint** is rare, but **secondary osteoarthritis** may develop after trauma or an inflammatory arthropathy such as RA. An effusion here suggests inflammatory arthritis, gout, or infection and should be aspirated to establish a diagnosis. In the case of osteoarthritis, a rigid brace to prevent movement of the ankle (e.g., Arizona brace) helps to reduce pain with walking. In the case of severe osteoarthritis, **orthopedic referral** for consideration of an arthrodesis should be obtained. Osteoarthritis of the **subtalar joint** can present with heel pain. An orthotic device is the preferred treatment.

III. **Heel pain**

  A. **Plantar fasciitis** is the most common cause of plantar heel pain. It is a painful inflammation of the insertion of the plantar fascia into the calcaneus. Plantar fasciitis is more common with a pronated foot and a flattened longitudinal arch, obesity, and excessive walking. Although it is usually an isolated problem, its presence may be a clue to a spondyloarthropathy such as Reiter's syndrome.

    1. **History.** Patients complain of pain under the heel, particularly when first rising in the morning or after a period of non-weightbearing.

    2. **Physical examination** discloses point tenderness over the plantar fascia insertion and for a short distance along the fascia.

    3. **Radiographs** are not necessary as a part of the initial evaluation. So-called heel spurs seen radiographically have no clinical significance.

    4. **Treatment** is almost always conservative and consists of a cushioning **heel insert** (can be purchased over the counter), **NSAIDs, ice,** and Achilles and plantar **stretching exercises.** Conservative treatment may require several weeks to months to be significantly effective. Local corticosteroid injections are sometimes used; however, there is only very lim-

ited quality evidence to support the use of this therapy (*Cochrane Database Syst Rev* 2000;4:CD:000416). A very few patients require more aggressive treatment and can be referred to a **podiatrist** or **orthopedic surgeon** if symptoms persist after prolonged conservative management.

B. Achilles tendinitis is a painful inflammatory condition of the Achilles tendon at or just proximal to its insertion onto the calcaneus. It usually affects young athletic individuals (e.g., runners and dancers). In older patients, degenerative changes in the tendon may be causative. Inflammation in this enthesis may also indicate a spondyloarthropathy, such as ankylosing spondylitis or Reiter's syndrome. Complete Achilles tendon rupture occasionally occurs.

1. **History** is notable for the insidious onset of pain in the Achilles tendon that is typically worsened by activity. Patients sometimes report a "squeaking" or "creaking" during plantar flexion.

2. **Physical examination** may reveal thickening and tenderness of the Achilles tendon. A protuberant posterolateral bony process of the calcaneus may also be present. "Pump bumps" (localized soft-tissue swelling) may occur where the shoe contacts the posterior heel.

3. **Radiographs** are not particularly helpful but may show calcification or periostitis where the Achilles tendon inserts onto the calcaneus.

4. **Treatment** is usually conservative and often includes **relative rest, heel lifts** (starting with $1/4$ in.), **ice, stretching exercises,** and **NSAIDs**. Corticosteroid injections are contraindicated because of the increased risk of tendon rupture. Patients who are unresponsive to conservative management may benefit from an **orthopedic or sports medicine consultation**.

C. Plantar fat pad atrophy causes diffuse heel pain with aging as reduced tissue elasticity and thickness of adipose tissue provide less "padding" for the inferior calcaneus. Shoes with **soft crepe soles** and **accommodative insoles** may be helpful.

D. Tarsal tunnel syndrome is characterized by paresthesias and dysesthesias on the bottom of the foot. It is caused by entrapment of the posterior tibial nerve in the area of the tarsal tunnel behind the medial malleolus. Symptoms may be worse with weightbearing and certain activities. Percussion over the posterior tibial nerve may reproduce the symptoms. Diminished sensation is sometimes demonstrable on the plantar surface of the foot. Radiographs are usually normal. **Referral to a podiatrist** for an **orthotic insert** may be helpful. **NSAIDs** may reduce local pain and inflammation.

IV. Mid- and forefoot pain

A. Hallux valgus is the most common great-toe malady and is characterized by the lateral movement of the first metatarsophalangeal (MTP) joint. The medial head of the first metatarsal enlarges with bony hypertrophy, and the bursa over it becomes inflamed as a "**bunion**." A marked female predominance is seen, probably because of constricting footwear; there may also be a hereditary predisposition. A similar condition may affect the lateral foot and fifth MTP joint and lead to "bunionette" formation.

1. **History.** Patients complain of pain, swelling, and deformity that are aggravated by shoe wearing. Numbness over the medial aspect of the great toe may also be reported.

2. **Physical examination** reveals medial deviation of the first metatarsal head and lateral deviation of the great toe phalanges. Impingement of the other toes is often present, and the second toe may override the great toe. Bunion formation is frequent, and there may be ulceration of the overlying skin.

3. **Radiographs**, although not entirely necessary, reveal the characteristic bony displacements.

4. **Treatment.** A **shoe with a wide toe box** is critical for symptom relief, sometimes supplemented by an insole. **Surgical treatment** may be appropriate in patients who are unresponsive to conservative measures.

B. **Hallux rigidus** entails pain and stiffness of the osteoarthritic first MTP, which must extend with each step. It usually affects older individuals. Restricted dorsiflexion of the first MTP is characteristic on examination. Radiographs typically show joint space narrowing and osteophyte formation. A **sole stiffener**, such as a steel shank, reduces motion at this joint and therefore reduces pain. A rocker-bottom sole can be used; however, it produces a gait that is difficult to get used to. **Surgical arthrodesis**, without a prosthetic implant, may be effective if conservative measures fail.

C. **Metatarsalgia** is a general term for pain under one or more of the metatarsal heads. It typically occurs when the pronated forefoot spreads out, and the second, third, and fourth metatarsal heads begin to bear weight with resultant **callus formation**. It may also be secondary to claw toe deformities (with distal migration of the plantar fat pad and subsequent exposure of the metatarsal heads) and cavus foot. Pain is often concentrated at the second metatarsal head. Relief can often be provided with a **metatarsal pad**, inserted into the shoe such that weightbearing occurs proximal to the metatarsal heads. In the presence of coexisting foot problems, such as pronation or osteoarthritis, it may be better to order a full-contact, custom-molded insole into which a metatarsal pad can be incorporated.

D. **Morton's neuroma** is characterized by pain in the web space between the third and fourth toes and is caused by compression on the interdigital nerve at this location. Plantar pain and dysesthesia of the affected toes are common. Walking and high-heeled, constrictive shoes worsen the symptoms. Squeezing the metatarsal heads may reproduce the discomfort. Characteristic changes of metatarsalgia may also be seen on examination. **Properly fitting footwear** with low heels can reduce pain. A **metatarsal pad** may also be effective. Some authorities advocate **local corticosteroid injection**. **Surgery** may be effective for patients who are unresponsive to conservative treatment.

E. **Gout**, and less commonly, **pseudogout**, can present as acute inflammation of the first MTP joint (**podagra**). Other commonly affected joints include the dorsum of the foot, the ankle, and the knee. Inflammation may be so intense as to resemble cellulitis, and localized exfoliation may occur as the attack resolves. The pain is typically quite severe. Fever and chills sometimes occur. Most patients are men. **Aspiration of the joint** for polarized microscopy crystal analysis is the definitive diagnostic test and helps to differentiate gout from septic arthritis. A common error is to misdiagnose painful noninflammatory first MTP osteoarthritis as gout, based solely on an elevated serum uric acid. Treatment typically entails **NSAIDs** in most cases. Refer to Chap. 22 for a more detailed discussion of the treatment of gout.

F. **Stress fractures** (fatigue fractures) of the metatarsals occur as a result of repetitive overuse. They are common in runners and dancers, and a recent increase in the level of activity is common. The second and third metatarsals are most commonly affected. Sudden or gradual onset of pain occurs in the forefoot near the metatarsals, which can be tender. Plain radiographs are negative the first 2 weeks, but after that callus may be seen. A bone scan is positive within the first week. MRI can detect very early stress fractures but is not usually required. Conservative treatment is generally effective: **rest, ice**, and **NSAIDs**. **Stiff-soled shoes** should be worn. Patients who do not respond may need immobilization.

G. **Pes planus (flat feet)** per se are not always symptomatic, but chronically pronated feet often lead to pain and further deformity. Flat feet may be related to multiple different foot problems, particularly posterior tibial tendon dysfunction, which is a common, but underdiagnosed, cause of ankle pain and foot deformity. It is characterized by sudden or progressive loss of strength of the posterior tibialis tendon with secondary progressive **flatfoot deformity**. The deformity is initially reversible but can become permanent. Multiple etiologies are possible, including **avulsion/rupture** of the tendon (usually traumatic), **partial tendon tear** and elongation, and **tendinitis**.

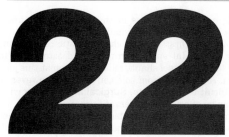

Rheumatologic Diseases

Richard D. Brasington

Approach to the Patient with Joint Pain

I. **History.** As with much of medicine, the history supplies the main clues to most rheumatologic diagnoses.
   A. **Nature of musculoskeletal pain.** An important issue to address early in the history is whether a given joint complaint is inflammatory or mechanical in nature. Characteristic inflammatory symptoms include swelling, heat, redness, morning stiffness, stiffness after inactivity, and sometimes fever. Mechanical symptoms include pain with activity that is relieved with rest, minimal morning stiffness, and lack of swelling or heat.
   B. **Location.** Next, distinguishing the specifics of which joints are involved helps narrow the differential diagnosis of arthritic complaints. Causes of monoarticular joint problems include infection, trauma, intra-articular hemorrhage, crystalline disease, overuse syndromes, and often osteoarthritis (OA). When joint symptoms are polyarticular, systemic inflammatory or autoimmune disease should be considered. Symmetric polyarticular symptoms suggest rheumatoid arthritis (RA), especially when the hands are involved. By contrast, asymmetric joint complaints are common for many of the seronegative spondyloarthropathies, such as Reiter's syndrome and psoriatic arthritis.

II. **Physical examination**
   A. **Gait.** Examine the patient walking away, turning, and walking back.
   B. **Hand.** Have the patient make a fist to see if the fingertips touch the palm. Inspect the dorsum of the hands, observe supination, and inspect the palmar side of the hands. Check power grip and pinch grip. Palpate the metacarpophalangeal joints.
   C. **Elbow.** See if the elbow can be completely extended and whether the patient can fully supinate and pronate the hands.
   D. **Shoulder.** Ask the patient to put both hands together above the head (without elevating the scapula), put both hands behind the head, and put both hands behind the back (normally the thumb tip can reach the tip of the scapula).
   E. **Cervical spine.** Have the patient touch the tip of the chin to the chest, look up, and look over each shoulder.
   F. **Lower spine.** Ask the patient to bend forward to touch the toes without bending the knees (see Seronegative Spondyloarthropathies, sec. **II.A**).
   G. **Hip.** The FABERE maneuver (flexion–abduction–external rotation) is performed by having the patient put the heel on the contralateral knee, with the examiner then pressing down on the medial knee, putting the hip into external rotation.
   H. **Knee.** The patient should be able to straighten the knee fully (extension) as well as to flex it so that the heel almost touches the buttocks.

   I. Ankle. One should look for limitations in flexion and extension as well as inversion and eversion.

III. Laboratory tests

   A. Basic principles. Very few rheumatologic laboratory tests are designed to serve as independent diagnostic tools. Rather, these tests should be used to test a hypothesis or ask a question to help support or dissuade a diagnosis. As such, test results must always be interpreted in a clinical context.

   B. The **erythrocyte sedimentation rate (ESR)** is a very nonspecific indicator of inflammation and is often elevated in inflammatory musculoskeletal conditions. Additionally, anemia can cause an increased ESR. As people age, their "normal" sedimentation rate increases.

   C. The **rheumatoid factor (RF)** is abnormal in 80% of cases of RA. However, this test can also be positive in Sjögren's syndrome, sarcoid, tuberculosis, bacterial endocarditis, chronic hepatitis, and other conditions in which immune complexes are formed. The RF is an immune complex of immunoglobulin (Ig) M that binds to the Fc portion of IgG.

   D. Antinuclear antibody (ANA) is a very sensitive test for patients with systemic lupus erythematosus (SLE) and may be abnormal in many other autoimmune diseases, such as scleroderma, Sjögren's syndrome, and polymyositis. Yet, because the specificity of the ANA is low, a positive ANA alone is not sufficient to make the diagnosis of SLE or a related disease.

   E. Antineutrophil cytoplasmic antibody (ANCA) is reported either as c-ANCA or p-ANCA. A positive ANCA should be further evaluated by an enzyme-linked immunosorbent assay (ELISA) to detect antibody to proteinase-3 (associated with c-ANCA) or myeloperoxidase (associated with p-ANCA). Antibody to proteinase-3 in significant titer is quite specific for Wegener's granulomatosis. However, antibody to myeloperoxidase is less specific and may be positive in conditions such as microscopic polyarteritis, polyarteritis nodosa, and pauci-immune glomerulonephritis.

   F. C-reactive protein (CRP) rises rapidly with inflammation and infection and falls quickly as inflammation resolves. Unlike the ESR, the CRP is not influenced by anemia and abnormal erythrocytes.

Osteoarthritis

OA is a common disease that affects approximately 20 million people in the United States. The usual joints that are involved in primary OA are the lower cervical spine, the lower lumbar spine, the first carpometacarpal joint of the thumb, the proximal interphalangeal (PIP) joints (Bouchard's nodes), and the distal interphalangeal (DIP) joints (Heberden's nodes) of the fingers, the hip, the knee, and the first metatarsophalangeal joint. Primary OA is rarely seen in the shoulders, elbows, wrists, metacarpophalangeal joints, and ankles. OA in these joints suggests a secondary cause (Table 22-1).

   I. Diagnosis. The typical history is one of mechanical pain, that is, pain with activity that is relieved with rest (pain at rest or at night is a sign of advanced disease). Morning stiffness may be present but usually lasts for less than 1 hour. Examination shows reduced range of motion. Mild swelling due to bony hypertrophy (especially at DIPs, PIPs, and knees) is common. Small to moderate-sized synovial effusions may be present in the knee. Routine laboratory tests are noncontributory, and synovial fluid tends to show a noninflammatory fluid, with a cell count of several thousand WBC/ml of mostly mononuclear cells. The classic finding on radiographic examination is joint space narrowing with subchondral sclerosis and hypertrophic bone formation at the joint margins (osteophytes/bone spurs). Periarticular osteopenia, erosions, and periosteal reaction are not seen.

Table 22-1. Causes of secondary osteoarthritis

Hemochromatosis (especially metacarpophalangeal joints)
Primary inflammatory arthropathy (e.g., rheumatoid arthritis)
Previous trauma to that joint
Calcium pyrophosphate deposition disease
History of manual labor

II. **Treatment.** The American College of Rheumatology has developed guidelines for the treatment of OA [*Arthritis Rheum* 2000;43(9):1905–1915].
  A. **Nonpharmacologic** measures include weight loss, use of a cane or walker, and exercises for range of motion and muscle strengthening. Quadriceps strengthening has been shown to reduce symptoms and retard progression of OA of the knee. A formal evaluation by a physical therapist should be considered, with the goal of muscle strengthening focused on muscle groups that are responsible for supporting the affected joints.
  B. **Pharmacologic therapy**
    1. **Simple analgesics** such as **acetaminophen**, 1000 mg qid, are often helpful and may be as beneficial as nonsteroidal anti-inflammatory drugs (NSAIDs) for some patients.
    2. **Selective cyclooxygenase (COX)-2 inhibitors**, such as **celecoxib**, 200 mg/day, or **rofecoxib**, 12.5–25.0 mg/day, can provide symptomatic pain relief with decreased GI toxicity. The Celecoxib Long-Term Arthritis Safety Study (CLASS) has shown that ulcer complications, such as GI bleeding and perforation, are significantly reduced in patients with OA and RA who are treated with celecoxib compared to traditional nonselective NSAIDs (ibuprofen and diclofenac). However, this benefit was lost for patients who took low-dose aspirin, an important consideration for those taking aspirin as primary and secondary coronary disease and stroke prevention (*JAMA* 2000;284:1247–1255). The VIGOR (Vioxx Gastrointestinal Outcomes Research) trial demonstrated a higher risk of myocardial infarction in patients who took rofecoxib than in those given naproxen, possibly attributable to the fact that at-risk patients in the study were not allowed to take daily low-dose aspirin. The VIGOR trial also showed that ulcers and ulcer complications were less frequent in RA patients taking rofecoxib compared to naproxen (*N Engl J Med* 2000;343:1520–1528).
    3. **NSAIDs** (Table 21-2) are commonly prescribed and have been specifically demonstrated to relieve the signs and symptoms of OA. However, risk factors for NSAID GI toxicity are important to consider (Table 22-2). Serious GI events, such as bleeding, perforation, and gastric outlet obstruction, usually occur without warning signs of dyspepsia. When necessary, NSAIDs should be initiated at lower doses (ibuprofen, 400–

Table 22-2. Risk factors for nonsteroidal anti-inflammatory drug–induced GI toxicity

Age
Duration and dose of nonsteroidal anti-inflammatory drug therapy
Concomitant treatment with warfarin (Coumadin) or corticosteroids
Poor general health
History of ulcer

600 mg tid–qid; naproxen, 375 mg bid; diclofenac, 50 mg bid), because these doses are associated with less GI toxicity. For patients at high risk for GI toxicity, prophylactic treatment with misoprostol, 200 µg bid–tid, or omeprazole, 20 mg/day, can be used.

4. **Glucosamine** is an important constituent of aggrecan and hyaluronan, the basic building blocks of articular cartilage. A study of glucosamine sulfate, 1500 mg PO qd, demonstrated that over a 3-year period, patients with OA of the knee obtained relief of symptoms that was superior to that of placebo (*Lancet* 2001;357:251–256). The results of this study cannot be generalized to glucosamine preparations other than glucosamine sulfate (such as glucosamine hydrochloride).

5. **Topical capsaicin** can be applied directly to painful osteoarthritic joints, especially the knees and the small joints of the hands. Therapy should be initiated with 0.025% cream applied three to four times a day and can be advanced to 0.075% if no relief is obtained from the lower strength. A burning sensation is common, and patients should be advised to wash the hands thoroughly after application and avoid touching the eyes, mouth, or genitals.

6. **More potent analgesics**, such as tramadol, propoxyphene, and narcotics, are sometimes indicated.

C. **Joint injection.** Another treatment is injection of medications directly into the affected joints. **Corticosteroids** may provide several weeks or months of relief, especially for OA of the knee. The first carpometacarpal joint may also respond but is relatively difficult to inject. Corticosteroid injections are often mixed 1:1 with a 1% lidocaine solution to provide immediate pain relief. The benefit of steroids usually occurs several hours to days later. By convention, injection of corticosteroids should be performed no more than three to four times a year/joint. Other agents, such as hyaluronate preparations (Hyalgan and Synvisc), may provide benefit that is comparable to that of NSAIDs for OA of the knee. At least three consecutive weekly injections should be given.

D. **Surgery.** Surgical consultation should be obtained for evaluation of joint replacements in patients who are suitable surgical candidates. Timing of surgery is based on symptoms.

Rheumatoid Arthritis

RA, the prototypical inflammatory arthritis, affects approximately 1% of the population and accounts for a significant degree of morbidity in affected patients. Although the fundamental etiology of RA is still unknown, much has been elucidated in the understanding of how the inflammatory process leads to joint damage. As a consequence, new therapies have been developed to reduce symptoms and the progression of disease.

I. **Diagnosis.** RA is a chronic, polyarticular inflammatory arthritis with a symmetric distribution that affects the hands and feet. The American College of Rheumatology has specified seven criteria associated with RA, of which at least four are necessary for diagnosis (Table 22-3). Factors that are associated with a poor prognosis include positive RF, multiple joints involved at presentation, radiographic changes at presentation, and extra-articular features such as vasculitis (leading to mononeuropathy), Felty's syndrome (granulocytopenia and splenomegaly, often with leg ulcers and recurrent infection), interstitial lung disease, ocular involvement, and pericarditis.

II. **Treatment.** Several important considerations in the treatment of a patient with RA should be addressed. Relief of symptoms of joint pain and swelling is important for the patient's quality of life. Additionally, treatment focused at retarding the development of joint damage is critical. Although pharmacologic treatment is the cornerstone for RA, nonpharmacologic treatment, such as physical therapy and occupational therapy, can also have a beneficial impact.

Table 22-3. Criteria for the diagnosis of rheumatoid arthritis[a]

Morning stiffness lasting longer than 1 hr

Swelling of three or more joints (observed by a physician)

Symmetric distribution

Involvement of the hand joints, especially the wrist, metacarpophalangeals, and proximal interphalangeals, sparing distal interphalangeals

Positive rheumatoid factor

Rheumatoid nodules on the extensor tendon surfaces, especially the olecranon

Radiographic changes, including periarticular osteopenia and erosions

[a]Four of seven criteria necessary for diagnosis.

A. **NSAIDs.** Most patients with RA benefit symptomatically from NSAIDs, generally in high doses. However, they do not prevent progression of bone and cartilage damage. Hence, the use of drugs that affect the progression of joint damage has become the standard in the treatment of RA.

B. **Disease-modifying antirheumatic drugs (DMARDs)** have the potential to retard the progression of disease. DMARDs should be instituted early (within the first few months of diagnosis), as evidence indicates that outcomes are improved for patients who are treated with DMARDs in the first 6–12 months of disease. Hence, initiation of therapy with NSAIDS (titrating to high doses) and DMARDs simultaneously can have a positive impact on the course of disease. Due to the complexities of these drugs and their side effects, consultation with a rheumatologist to plan, initiate, and monitor therapy may be helpful. Furthermore, many of these drugs may take several months to attain optimal clinical benefit.

1. **Methotrexate** is generally considered to be the DMARD of choice for most patients. From a starting dose of 7.5 mg PO once/week, the dose can be increased to 20–25 mg/week over a period of 8–12 weeks. If methotrexate is at least partially effective, it should be continued as other agents are added. Common side effects include stomatitis, nausea, and diarrhea. Supplementation with folic acid, 1–2 mg PO qd, can reduce side effects, although it may attenuate efficacy somewhat. Bone marrow suppression is uncommon but may occur at low doses in elderly patients. The risk of liver toxicity is increased by alcohol consumption, pre-existing liver disease, and possibly by diabetes and obesity. **Contraindications to methotrexate therapy include liver disease, abnormal liver function tests (LFTs), and regular alcohol consumption.** LFTs and CBCs should be checked every month until the dose is stable and every 2–3 months thereafter. Patients with baseline normal LFTs who abstain from alcohol are very unlikely to have methotrexate-induced hepatotoxicity. A biopsy should be performed in patients with persistent elevation of LFTs or a decrease in serum albumin to rule out methotrexate-induced hepatotoxicity.

2. **Hydroxychloroquine (Plaquenil)** is effective at doses of 400 mg PO qd. It is contraindicated in patients with renal or hepatic insufficiency. The risk of macular toxicity is extremely unusual provided that the dose does not exceed 6–7 mg/kg/day and rarely occurs before 5 years of treatment. Nonetheless, an ophthalmologist should perform a baseline examination and monitor the patient every 6–12 months. Nausea and skin discoloration occasionally occur. No evidence has shown that hydroxychloroquine prevents radiographic progression of disease.

3. **Sulfasalazine** should be initiated at 500 mg PO bid and gradually increased to 1000–1500 mg PO bid. An enteric-coated preparation improves GI tolerability. Monitoring for neutropenia and transaminase elevation

should be performed every 1–3 months. GI intolerance due to nausea or abdominal pain may occur. Sulfasalazine is contraindicated in patients with true sulfa allergy or glucose-6-phosphate dehydrogenase deficiency.

4. **Leflunomide (Arava)** is a pyrimidine synthesis inhibitor that has been shown to have efficacy comparable to that of methotrexate in the treatment of RA. A loading dose of 100 mg PO qd for 3 days is followed by maintenance therapy of 20 mg PO qd. Leflunomide is **teratogenic** and has a long half-life. Women who plan to become pregnant must discontinue the drug and complete a course of elimination therapy consisting of cholestyramine, 8 g tid for 11 days. Drug levels should be less than 0.02 mg/L on two separate occasions at least 14 days apart before pregnancy is considered. Diarrhea, nausea, and hair loss are also common side effects. Transaminases should be monitored monthly for liver toxicity. The daily dose can be reduced to 10 mg/day if the medication is not tolerated or if transaminase levels become elevated.

5. **Cyclosporine** is an inhibitor of T-cell activation with known clinical efficacy in the treatment of RA. However, its cost and potential for severe renal toxicity even in low doses have limited its use to severe refractory RA. A dose of 2–4 mg/kg/day, combined with methotrexate, may be effective in some patients.

6. **Tumor necrosis factor (TNF) blockers** are emerging as potent medications for the treatment of RA. They are generally well tolerated, and patients usually respond rapidly. TNF blockers are typically administered in conjunction with methotrexate therapy. Serious infections have occurred rarely; therefore, TNF blockers should not be given to patients with indolent chronic infections, such as osteomyelitis or tuberculosis, or to anyone with significant and active common infections. TNF blockers should be used in consultation with a rheumatologist.
   a. **Etanercept (Enbrel)** is a genetically engineered human fusion protein that consists of two molecules of the p75 TNF receptor. This drug is given by SC injection at a dosage of 25 mg twice/week.
   b. **Infliximab (Remicade)** is a chimeric antibody specific for human TNF that is administered intravenously at 3 mg/kg, given at initiation, 2 and 6 weeks, and every 8 weeks thereafter. Methotrexate should also be given; otherwise, efficacy declines with repeated dosing. An effect on radiographic progression of disease has been demonstrated.

7. Although **minocycline**, a tetracycline antibiotic, has demonstrated moderate efficacy for the treatment of RA in several clinical trials, its utility is controversial. Evidence has yet to support convincingly that RA is due to an infectious agent; therefore, it does not appear that minocycline's mechanism of action in RA is antimicrobial. Rather, its anti-inflammatory effect may be due to inhibition of matrix metalloproteinases. From a starting dose of 50 mg PO bid, the dosage can be increased to 100 mg PO bid. Dizziness is a fairly common side effect.

8. **Other DMARDs** that are less commonly used to treat RA include **gold salts, azathioprine, penicillamine,** and **cyclophosphamide.**

9. **Combination regimens** of multiple DMARDs or DMARDs plus biological agents are increasingly popular. Consensus among rheumatologists suggests that methotrexate should be part of every combination, if tolerated. Evidence indicates increased efficacy in the treatment of RA for the following combination regimens:
   a. Hydroxychloroquine, sulfasalazine, and methotrexate
   b. Cyclosporine and methotrexate
   c. Leflunomide and methotrexate
   d. Etanercept and methotrexate
   e. Infliximab and methotrexate

C. **Corticosteroids** (especially prednisone) in low doses are extremely effective for promptly reducing the symptoms of RA and can be considered to help patients recover their previous functional status. Unfortunately, short courses of oral corticosteroids produce only interim benefit, and chronic therapy is often necessary to maintain symptom management. Corticosteroids are appropriate in patients with significant limitations in their activities of daily living, particularly early in the course of disease while awaiting the efficacy of slow-acting DMARDs. Every effort should be made to taper to the lowest possible dose and to eliminate steroid therapy when feasible.

1. **Toxicities** of corticosteroids include weight gain, cushingoid features, osteoporosis (with fracture), avascular necrosis, infection, diabetes, hypertension, and increases in serum cholesterol levels. Keeping the daily dose of prednisone at 5 mg or less can often reduce toxicities.

2. **Bone loss** occurs rapidly in the first 6 months of corticosteroid treatment. Bisphosphonates, such as **alendronate** and **risedronate**, at 5 mg/day, have been shown to prevent corticosteroid-induced bone loss (*N Engl J Med* 1998;339:292–299, and *Arthritis Rheum* 1999;42:2309–2318). Alternatively, **etidronate**, 400 mg PO daily for 2 weeks every 3 months, or **pamidronate**, 30–60 mg IV every month, may be beneficial for steroid-induced bone loss in patients who cannot tolerate bisphosphonates (*N Engl J Med* 1997;337:382–387, and *Calcif Tissue Int* 1997;61:266–271). Supplementation with vitamin D (1–2 multivitamin tablets daily) and calcium (1200–1500 mg/day elemental calcium) is also important for osteoporosis prevention.

3. **Adrenal insufficiency** can be avoided by tapering corticosteroid doses slowly over several months.

D. **Immunoadsorption apheresis** with the Prosorba column has been shown to be effective in some patients with severe chronic RA and is an option to consider for those patients who fail to respond to more conventional treatment. The mechanism of action for this treatment is unclear. Consultation with a rheumatologist is advised.

E. **Ancillary medical services** can augment treatment strategies for patients with RA at any stage of disease.

1. **Occupational therapy** usually focuses on the hand and wrist and can help patients with splinting, work simplification, activities of daily living, and assistive devices.

2. **Physical therapy** assists in stretching and strengthening exercises for large joints such as the shoulder and knee, gait evaluation, and fitting with crutches and canes. Moderate exercise is appropriate for all patients and can help to reduce stiffness and maintain joint range of motion. In general, an exercise program should not produce pain for more than 2 hours after its completion.

3. **Orthopedic surgery** to correct hand deformities and replace large joints such as the hip, knee, and shoulder may benefit patients with advanced disease. The primary indication for reconstructive hand surgery is refractory functional impairment that limits activities of daily living. Total joint arthroplasty to replace the knee or hip should also be considered when pain cannot be controlled adequately with medications. The decision to pursue joint replacement in younger patients may be complicated by the likelihood that individuals may outlive their prosthetic joints, necessitating future surgery.

Infectious Arthritis and Bursitis

Infectious arthritis is generally categorized into gonococcal and nongonococcal disease. The usual presentation is with fever and an acute monoarticular arthritis, although multiple joints may be affected by hematogenous spread of pathogens. **Nongonococcal infectious arthritis** in adults tends to occur in patients with previous joint damage or compromised host defenses. In contrast, **gonococcal arthritis** causes one-half of all septic arthritis in otherwise healthy, sexually active young adults.

I. **General principles of treatment**

A. **Joint fluid examination**, including Gram stain of a centrifuged pellet, and culture are mandatory to make a diagnosis and to guide management. A joint fluid leukocyte count is useful diagnostically and as a baseline for serial studies to evaluate response to treatment (Table 21-6). Cultures of blood and other possible extra-articular sites of infection also should be obtained.

B. **Hospitalization** is indicated to ensure drug compliance and careful monitoring of the clinical response.

C. **IV antimicrobials** provide good serum and synovial fluid drug concentrations. Oral antimicrobials are not appropriate as initial therapy, and there is no role for intra-articular antibiotic therapy.

D. **Repeated arthrocenteses** should be performed daily or as often as necessary to prevent reaccumulation of fluid. Arthrocentesis is indicated to (1) remove destructive inflammatory mediators, (2) reduce intra-articular pressure and promote antimicrobial penetration into the joint, and (3) monitor response to therapy by documenting sterility of synovial fluid cultures and steadily decreasing leukocyte counts.

E. **Surgical drainage** or arthroscopic lavage and drainage are indicated for (1) septic hip; (2) joints in which either the anatomy, large amounts of tissue debris, or loculation of pus prevent adequate needle drainage (most commonly the shoulder); (3) septic arthritis with coexistent osteomyelitis; (4) joints that do not respond in 4–6 days to appropriate therapy and repeated arthrocenteses; and (5) prosthetic joint infection.

F. **General supportive** measures include splinting of the joint, which may help to relieve pain. However, prolonged immobilization can result in joint stiffness. An NSAID or selective COX-2 inhibitor is often useful to reduce pain and to increase joint mobility but should not be used until response to antimicrobial therapy has been demonstrated by symptomatic and laboratory improvement.

II. **Nongonococcal septic arthritis** is caused most often by *Staphylococcus aureus* (60%) and *Streptococcus* species. Gram-negative organisms are less common, except with IV drug abuse, neutropenia, concomitant urinary tract infection, and postoperatively. Initial therapy is based on the clinical situation and a carefully performed Gram stain, which reveals the organism in approximately 50% of patients (*N Engl J Med* 1994;330:769). With a positive Gram stain, antibiotic coverage can be focused accordingly. With a nondiagnostic Gram stain, antibiotics should be chosen to cover *S. aureus* and *Streptococcus* species and *Neisseria gonorrhoeae* in otherwise healthy patients, whereas broad-spectrum antibiotics are appropriate in immunosuppressed patients. IV antimicrobials usually are given for at least 2 weeks, followed by 1–2 weeks of oral antimicrobials, with the course of therapy tailored to the patient's response.

III. **Gonococcal arthritis** is more common than nongonococcal septic arthritis. The clinical spectrum of disease often includes migratory or additive polyarthralgias, followed by tenosynovitis or arthritis of the wrist, ankle, or knee and asymptomatic dermatitis on the extremities or trunk. In contrast to nongonococcal septic arthritis, Gram staining of synovial fluid and cultures of blood or synovial fluid often are negative. Bacteriologic assessment of the throat, cervix, urethra, and rectum may aid in establishing the diagnosis. Treatment is begun with an intravenous antibiotic for the first 1–3 days, generally ceftriaxone, 1 g qd, or ceftizoxime, 1 g q8h. Response to IV antibiotics is usually noted within the first 24–36 hours of treatment. After initial clinical improvement, therapy is continued with an oral antibiotic to complete 7–10 days of treatment. Ciprofloxacin, 500 mg bid, or amoxicillin clavulanate, 500–875 mg bid, can be used. Treatment of coexisting *Chlamydia* infection should also be considered.

IV. **Nonbacterial infectious arthritis** is common with many viral infections, especially hepatitis B, rubella, mumps, infectious mononucleosis, parvovirus, enterovirus, and adenovirus. It is generally self-limited, lasting for less than 6 weeks, and responds well to a conservative regimen of rest and NSAIDs. Arthralgias (often severe) or a reactive arthritis can be a manifestation of HIV infection. A variety of fungi and mycobacteria can cause septic arthritis and should be considered in patients with chronic monoarticular arthritis.

V. **Septic bursitis**, usually involving the olecranon or prepatellar bursa, can be differentiated from septic arthritis by localized, fluctuant superficial swelling and by relatively painless joint motion (particularly extension). Most patients have a history of previous trauma to the area or an occupational predisposition (e.g., "housemaid's knee," "writer's elbow"). *S. aureus* is the most common pathogen. Septic bursitis should be treated with aspiration, which can be repeated if fluid reaccumulates. Oral antibiotics and outpatient management are usually appropriate, and surgical drainage is rarely indicated. Preventive measures (e.g., knee pads) should be used in patients with occupational predispositions.

VI. **Lyme disease** is caused by the tick-borne spirochete *Borrelia burgdorferi*. Typical manifestations begin with an erythematous annular rash (erythema migrans) and flu-like symptoms. Arthralgias, myalgias, meningitis, neuropathy, and cardiac conduction defects may follow in weeks to a few months. Months later, an intermittent or chronic arthritis in one or a few joints, characteristically including the knee, may develop in untreated patients. The diagnosis is based on the clinical picture, exposure in an endemic area, and serologic studies. Unfortunately, serologic studies often give false-negative or false-positive results (*JAMA* 1992;268:891), and patients may remain seropositive for years after treatment. Antibiotic therapy is required. NSAIDs are a useful adjunct for arthritis. Vaccination should be considered for people living in high-risk areas who have frequent tick exposures.

Crystalline Arthritis

Deposition of microcrystals in joints and periarticular tissues results in **gout**, **pseudogout**, and **apatite disease**. A definitive diagnosis of gout or pseudogout is made by finding intracellular crystals in joint fluid examined with a compensated polarized light microscope. Urate crystals, which are diagnostic of gout, are needle shaped and strongly negatively birefringent. Calcium pyrophosphate dihydrate crystals seen in pseudogout are pleomorphic and weakly positively birefringent. Hydroxyapatite complexes, diagnostic of apatite disease, and basic calcium phosphate complexes can be identified only by electron microscopy and mass spectroscopy. In most cases, the arthritides associated with these compounds are suspected clinically but never confirmed.

I. **Gout** is caused by the accumulation of excess amounts of uric acid in the body, leading to deposition of monosodium urate crystals. This can produce four distinct clinical syndromes: (1) acute gouty arthritis, (2) chronic tophaceous gout, (3) urate nephropathy, and (4) urate renal lithiasis. All complications of gout result from hyperuricemia. In 90% of cases, this occurs as a result of underexcretion of urate, with overproduction accounting for the remainder. The renal handling of urate is complicated and involves glomerular filtration followed by reabsorption and secretion within the tubules. Alcohol and salicylates can promote hyperuricemia by impairing urate secretion, whereas dehydration and diuretics cause enhanced urate reabsorption. Gout occurs more commonly in men and is associated with hypertension, obesity, renal dysfunction, hyperlipidemia, and alcohol consumption. It occurs infrequently in premenopausal women and rarely in patients with RA. Organ transplant patients who take cyclosporine may have severe problems with gout.

A. **History.** Acute gouty arthritis presents with acute pain and swelling, usually of a single joint. Commonly affected joints include the great toe metatarsophalangeal joint (podagra), ankle, knee, or wrist. Episodes often occur at night and frequently accompany acute medical illnesses, postsurgical periods, dehydration, fasting, or heavy alcohol consumption. Pain may be severe, and immediate medical attention to provide pain relief is essential. Periarticular involvement is rare at presentation but may occur in longstanding cases. Intense periarticular inflammation with desquamation of skin may give the appearance of cellulitis.

B. **Diagnosis.** Gout is diagnosed by polarized microscopy of synovial fluid demonstrating bright, negatively birefringent, needle-shaped crystals (often found within a phagocytic polymorphonuclear leukocyte). Cell counts of synovial aspirates are usually consistent with an inflammatory arthritis (WBC = 2000–75,000, mostly polymorphonuclear leukocytes, see Table 21-6). Aspiration of superficial tophi with a 25-gauge needle can also provide diagnostic material.

C. **Treatment** is aimed at acute symptomatic relief and prophylaxis for recurrent disease. Drugs that are effective for the management of acute flares include the following.

   1. **NSAIDs** (Table 21-2) are particularly effective and are the treatment of choice for acute gout. They should be started in maximal doses and tapered over several days once the gouty flare has subsided. A common high-dose NSAID regimen is **indomethacin**, 50 mg PO qid given for several days until relief is obtained, followed by 50 mg tid for 2–3 days, 50 mg bid for 2–3 days, 50 mg/day for a few days, and then discontinuation. **Naproxen, ibuprofen, sulindac**, and other NSAIDs are also effective and are generally better tolerated than high-dose indomethacin.

   2. **Selective inhibitors of COX-2**, such as **celecoxib** and **rofecoxib**, have no effect on platelet function and therefore offer an advantage for patients who are receiving anticoagulants. However, these medications appear to have no advantage over traditional NSAIDs with respect to causing renal dysfunction in susceptible individuals. Therefore, COX-2 inhibitors should be used with great caution in patients with renal insufficiency, volume depletion, heart failure, or cirrhosis. Although there have been no trials of these agents for treatment of acute gout, rofecoxib, 50 mg PO once daily for a maximum of 5 days, or celecoxib, 200–400 mg PO bid, are appropriate doses. Ulcer complications are significantly less common with the COX-2 inhibitors than with traditional NSAIDs and should be considered in patients who are at high risk for NSAID-induced GI toxicity (Table 22-2).

   3. **Colchicine**, 0.6 mg PO every 1–2 hours until a maximum dose of 6 mg in 24 hours is reached, can be effective. Treatment with 1.2 mg/day can follow the loading dose. Oral colchicine is poorly tolerated because of diarrhea and abdominal cramping, and the dose should be reduced in patients with renal and hepatic impairment. Intravenous colchicine avoids GI toxicity but may cause severe myelosuppression. It should be avoided in patients with renal or hepatic insufficiency. The maximum recommended intravenous dose of colchicine is 2 mg in a single dose. Additional oral and intravenous colchicine should be avoided for at least 1 week after administration.

   4. **Adrenocorticotropic hormone gel**, 40–80 IU IM or SC, or **triamcinolone acetonide**, 40–100 mg IM, has been shown to be as effective as NSAIDs, and is an option for patients who cannot tolerate oral medications. The subcutaneous route is an advantage for anticoagulated patients, causing less hematoma formation than the intramuscular route.

   5. **Oral steroids** can be used when other therapies are contraindicated. Prednisone initiated at 60 mg/day and tapered rapidly can provide adequate symptomatic relief while avoiding toxicities of long-term steroid use.

6. **Intra-articular corticosteroids** are appropriate for large joints such as knees and ankles and an excellent choice for patients who are not good candidates for NSAIDs. Because the knee joint often has a tense effusion, aspiration of as much fluid as possible can bring immediate relief, followed by injection of 1–2 ml corticosteroid with an equal volume of 1% lidocaine. A volume of 1 ml is appropriate for the ankle.

D. **Prophylactic treatment** is advisable when patients have recurrent attacks. The patient should consider whether it is worth daily medication to prevent intermittent attacks. Colchicine, 0.6 mg once or twice daily, may be effective, as may low-dose NSAIDs such as indomethacin, 25 mg bid, or naproxen, 250 mg bid. In patients with multiple recurrent attacks, uric acid–lowering therapy may be beneficial. Allopurinol, a xanthine oxidase inhibitor, slows production of uric acid, and uricosuric agents such as probenecid increase renal excretion of uric acid. Traditionally, management should be dictated by the results of a 24-hour urine uric acid excretion, indicating probenecid for 600 mg/day or less and allopurinol for levels higher than 600 mg/day. However, as a practical point, allopurinol is much easier to administer than probenecid and is the treatment of choice for most patients.

1. **Allopurinol** is indicated for recurrent attacks that are not controlled with colchicine or NSAIDs. Other indications for allopurinol include the presence of tophi, renal stones, and severe hyperuricemia (>13 mg/dl). Asymptomatic hyperuricemia should not be treated with allopurinol. A starting dose of 100–150 mg/day can be increased after 2–4 weeks to 300 mg/day. Sometimes higher doses (400–600 mg/day) are required to bring the serum uric acid down to a target level of approximately 5 mg/dl or less. Allopurinol should not be started during an acute attack. Administration of prophylactic colchicine or low-dose NSAIDs before initiation of uric acid–lowering therapy may prevent the gouty attacks that sometimes accompany the initiation of allopurinol treatment. Although allopurinol should not be begun during an acute attack, it is not necessary to discontinue its use if a gout attack occurs after it is started. This medication is usually well tolerated, although elevated LFTs and a severe hypersensitivity syndrome can occur. The latter is more common with renal insufficiency and diuretic use. Patients must be educated that treatment with allopurinol is a lifetime commitment; it is quite common for patients in remission to conclude that their gout is resolved, only to experience recurrence once allopurinol has been discontinued. Allopurinol should never be given with azathioprine (Imuran), because allopurinol inhibits the metabolism of azathioprine and potentiates its effect. Tophaceous gout requires lifetime treatment with allopurinol. After months to years of treatment, tophi shrink, and osteolytic lesions in bone may heal.

2. **Probenecid** prevents tubular reabsorption of uric acid and can be used to enhance urinary excretion of uric acid provided that the baseline 24-hour urinary uric acid is 600 mg or less. Otherwise, increasing the urinary excretion of uric acid may precipitate uric acid kidney stones. Probenecid can be initiated at 500 mg PO daily and increased as needed, not exceeding 3000 mg in three divided doses. Normal renal function is necessary for probenecid to be effective. Salicylates antagonize the effect of probenecid, and even low-dose aspirin can negate its effect. Patients should maintain a high urine volume, and in some cases alkalinizing the urine may prevent stone formation.

II. **Pseudogout** is caused by deposition of calcium pyrophosphate crystals and tends to occur more often in elderly individuals. It may be precipitated by surgery and has been associated with hypothyroidism, hyperparathyroidism, diabetes, and hemochromatosis. Like gout, pseudogout tends to cause monoarticular attacks, especially in the knee. Symmetric involvement of the hands may mimic RA and is referred to as **pseudo-RA**. Periarticular inflammation can be severe, mimicking cellulitis. Polarized microscopy of synovial fluid reveals rhomboid-shaped crystals that are positively birefringent. Radiographic studies may demonstrate chondrocalcinosis (especially knee, wrist, and symphysis pubis) but alone are not diagnostic of pseudogout. Treatment is the same as for gout, except that there is no role for allopurinol or probenecid. Joint aspiration, alone or with steroid injection, often provides immediate relief of pain.

III. **Apatite disease** may present with periarthritis or tendonitis, particularly in patients with chronic renal failure. An episodic oligoarthritis also may occur, and apatite disease should be suspected when no crystals are present in the synovial fluid. Erosive arthritis may be seen, particularly in the shoulder (Milwaukee shoulder). The treatment of apatite disease is similar to that for pseudogout.

Systemic Lupus Erythematosus

SLE is a multisystem autoimmune disease of unknown etiology that commonly occurs in women of childbearing age. Manifestations of SLE are protean, and organ systems involved may include skin, heart, lungs, CNS, kidneys, hematopoietic system, and joints.

I. **Diagnosis.** The American College of Rheumatology has proposed 11 criteria for the diagnosis of SLE (Table 22-4). Accordingly, a diagnosis requires that at least four of them be present at some point through the course of the disease. Although these criteria were developed to define the diagnosis of SLE for clinical research purposes, they are sometimes useful in clinical practice to guide history and physical examinations of putative SLE patients. Laboratory tests may be useful to aid in the diagnosis and management of SLE when used appropriately.

A. The **ANA** is positive in virtually all patients with SLE (highly sensitive). Therefore, a negative ANA is useful to exclude SLE. However, a positive ANA test alone is of little significance. Regardless of how high the titer, an isolated positive ANA test is not diagnostic of SLE or any related disease.

B. **Antibodies to double-stranded DNA** are very specific for SLE, especially when present at high titers. Several techniques are available for measuring these antibodies. Two of the more common are the *Crithidia lucilia* fluorescent slide test and the ELISA test. High levels of anti-DNA antibody can correlate with disease activity, especially with lupus nephritis. Therefore, quantitative anti-DNA titers are sometimes useful in monitoring disease flares and response to treatment.

C. **Anti-Sm** is part of a panel of antibodies to **extractable nuclear antigens**. Although very specific for SLE, it is positive in a minority of patients.

D. **Serum complement measures, C3 and C4**, are sometimes abnormal in active SLE, especially in the setting of nephritis, and may rise and fall with disease activity. Like levels of anti-DNA antibodies, complement levels may be useful in following disease activity, especially in the setting of nephritis.

E. **Antiphospholipid antibodies** are important in diagnosing the **antiphospholipid syndrome**, characterized by fetal loss, venous and arterial thromboses, CNS events, and thrombocytopenia. Diagnosis of the phospholipid syndrome is relevant, as the treatment may necessitate lifelong anticoagulation.

1. **Anticardiolipin antibody** is measured by ELISA. IgG antibodies in significant titer are more predictive of clinical events than is IgM or IgA.

2. **False-positive VDRL (test for syphilis) or rapid plasma reagin** is a laboratory artifact due to antiphospholipid antibody binding to the phospholipid in the test reagent. The fluorescent treponemal antibody

Table 22-4. American College of Rheumatology criteria for the diagnosis of systemic lupus erythematosus[a]

Malar rash: fixed erythema sparing the nasolabial folds

Discoid rash: erythematous raised annular patches with scarring

Photosensitivity

Oral or nasal ulcers: observed by a physician

Nonerosive arthritis with inflammation

Pleuritis or pericarditis

Renal disorder

    Proteinuria greater than 500 mg/day

    Cellular casts

Neurologic disorders: especially seizures or psychosis

Hematologic disorder

    Hemolytic anemia with reticulocytosis

    Leukopenia (WBC <4000) on two occasions

    Lymphopenia (<1500) on two occasions

    Thrombocytopenia (<100,000) on two occasions

Immunologic disorder

    Anti-DNA antibody

    Anti-Sm antibody

    Antiphospholipid antibody

        Anticardiolipin antibody (immunoglobulin G or M)

        Lupus anticoagulant

        False-positive test for syphilis

Positive antinuclear antibody

[a]Four of eleven criteria must be present at some point through the course of disease.

absorption test should be negative, although a low-titer "beaded" pattern is sometimes observed.

3. The **lupus anticoagulant (LAC)** is a misnomer in two respects: It is not specific for lupus and promotes, not inhibits, coagulation. The activated thromboplastin time (PTT) assay is prolonged because antiphospholipid antibody binds and makes unavailable phospholipid that is needed for in vitro initiation of the coagulation cascade. A positive LAC is a more predictive test for clinical events due to antiphospholipid antibody than anticardiolipin antibody or VDRL. Two critical components define the LAC.
   a. Adding normal plasma does not correct the prolonged PTT.
   b. Adding platelet-rich plasma as a source of phospholipid adsorbs the antiphospholipid antibody and thereby normalizes the prolonged PTT.

4. The **dilute Russel viper venom time** is another method for detecting a LAC-like antiphospholipid antibody and is more sensitive than the LAC. Dilute Russel viper venom (rather than thromboplastin) is used to activate the intrinsic coagulation pathway. The assay performed in this manner becomes abnormal, with very small amounts of antiphospholipid antibody. Therefore, the dilute Russel viper venom time sometimes detects an antiphospholipid antibody that is missed by the LAC assay.

5. **Antibodies to** β_2**-glycoprotein 1** appear to be particularly predictive of events due to antiphospholipid syndrome. This test is available through reference laboratories.

II. **Treatment** for SLE is dependent on the clinical scenario. It is important to exclude alternative diagnoses such as infection and thrombosis in patients with lupus before aggressively treating a lupus flare. Initiation of conservative therapy is appropriate for mild symptoms. This includes sunscreen and sun avoidance for patients with photosensitivity, topical steroids for isolated skin lesions, and maintenance of adequate hydration. More severe cases of SLE may require prednisone in moderate (15–30 mg/day) or higher (40–60 mg) doses. Azathioprine and to a lesser extent methotrexate are used as steroid-sparing agents when unacceptably high doses of prednisone are required to control disease activity. Investigational new therapies for severe, treatment-unresponsive SLE include mycophenolate or immunoablation with or without stem cell transplantation. Symptom-specific treatments include the following.

A. **Arthritis** often responds to NSAIDs, although they must be used with caution in patients with decreased renal function. The addition of prednisone in low doses (5–10 mg/day) may be necessary. Long-term treatment with hydroxychloroquine often helps control arthritis (see Rheumatoid Arthritis).

B. **Rashes** may respond to topical corticosteroids (fluorinated topical steroids on the face should be avoided because of the risk of subcutaneous atrophy). If topical agents are not effective, systemic corticosteroids may be needed. Hydroxychloroquine is often beneficial in the long-term management of rash and may help to reduce the need for corticosteroids.

C. **Oral ulcers** can be treated with dental paste that contains benzocaine (Orabase B) or triamcinolone (Kenalog in Orabase) or an over-the-counter anesthetic oral rinse (e.g., Ulcer Ease).

D. Mild cases of **pleuritis** and **pericarditis** sometimes respond to NSAIDs, whereas more severe cases require corticosteroids.

E. The treatment of **renal disease** is complicated and is often assisted by a nephrologist. Either declining creatinine clearance or nephrotic range proteinuria is generally considered an indication for renal biopsy. Pathologic examination can confirm lupus nephritis, provide a World Health Organization class of nephritis, and determine the extent of activity and chronicity, all of which have an impact on prognosis. Furthermore, biopsy can help determine whether other factors, such as hypertension or diabetes, might be contributing to decreased renal function. For most serious renal lesions, periodic monthly cyclophosphamide is administered. High doses of corticosteroids, administered either orally or intravenously, are also commonly used.

F. For **hematologic** problems, such as hemolytic anemia, severe leukopenia, or thrombocytopenia, corticosteroids in moderate to high doses are required. Cyclophosphamide, danazol, dapsone, and splenectomy are sometimes needed. Thrombotic thrombocytopenic purpura may coexist with SLE, and therefore careful attention to the presence of schistocytes on peripheral blood smear is essential.

G. **Neuropsychiatric** disease is difficult to assess because there is no laboratory test or physical finding that can unequivocally support the diagnosis of CNS lupus. The diagnosis of neuropsychiatric lupus is based on clinical factors and is a diagnosis of exclusion. Most important, infection must be excluded. MRI may demonstrate a variety of abnormalities, but findings are not specific for SLE. It has been recognized that the antiphospholipid syndrome is the cause of many of the neurologic events in patients with lupus. Aggressive treatment with high-dose steroids may be necessary to help control symptoms of CNS lupus.

Seronegative Spondyloarthropathies

Spondyloarthropathies are a group of articular disorders characterized by involvement of the axial skeleton and negative test results for RF.

I. **The characteristic history** is that of inflammatory back pain. Five distinguishing symptoms include gradual onset, onset before the age of 40 years, morning stiffness, improvement with mild exercise, and duration of more than 3 months. When peripheral joint involvement is present, it is typically asymmetric and oligoarticular, generally in the lower extremities. Inflammation generally occurs where tendons insert on bone **(enthesopathy)** and produces "sausage digits" of individual fingers and toes (dactylitis), plantar fasciitis, and Achilles tendinitis. Nonarticular symptoms may include aphthous stomatitis, ocular inflammation such as conjunctivitis and iritis, and aortic dilatation.

A. **Ankylosing spondylitis**, the prototype of the spondyloarthropathies, is diagnosed in men much more commonly than in women, partly because the spine symptoms in women tend to be more subtle. Acute iritis produces severe eye pain and blurred vision and requires urgent referral to an ophthalmologist.

B. **Reiter's syndrome** entails a classic triad of arthritis, urethritis, and conjunctivitis, although "incomplete" Reiter's syndrome may occur. Onset classically follows nongonococcal urethritis or infectious diarrhea.

C. **Reactive arthritis** after infectious diarrhea with *Shigella*, *Salmonella*, or *Yersinia enterocolitica* may involve the spine and peripheral joints. The course may be extremely severe but tends to be self-limited and remits after a number of months.

D. **Psoriatic arthritis** has five basic presentations: spinal predominance, polyarticular small joint involvement (negative for RF), oligoarticular asymmetric large joint involvement, DIP joint predominance, and the rare arthritis mutilans with telescoping digits. In general, the severity of joint disease does not parallel that of the skin disease, except for the DIP pattern, which correlates with nail abnormalities. Significant arthritis may occur in the presence of trivial skin disease and perhaps in the absence of skin disease (psoriatic arthritis sine psoriasis).

E. **Ulcerative colitis and Crohn's disease** may be accompanied by inflammatory arthritis of two types. The peripheral joint variety tends to parallel the activity of the bowel disease, whereas the spondylitic pattern typically has an independent course of the bowel disease.

II. **Physical examination**

A. **Spine motion** may be simply assessed by having the patient bend forward with the knees extended and measuring the distance between the fingertips and floor (recognizing that hamstring tightness reduces the range of motion). To perform the modified Schober's test, one should make marks 10 cm above and 5 cm below the level of the sacral dimples. When the patient bends forward to touch the floor, the distance between these two marks should increase from 15 cm to at least 20 cm if normal spinal motion is present. The occiput-to-wall distance is assessed by having the patient stand with his or her back to the wall, attempting to touch the occiput to the wall, as a measure of neck extension. Chin-to-chest distance measures neck flexion.

B. **Peripheral joints** should be checked for diffuse fusiform swelling of fingers and toes (sausage digits or dactylitis) and asymmetric swelling of large joints, especially the knees and ankles.

C. **Ocular findings** in ankylosing spondylitis and Reiter's syndrome include redness and a pupil that reacts asymmetrically (synechia), indicating previous episodes of ocular inflammation.

   D. Skin findings in psoriasis are usually obvious, but the following areas should be specifically examined to look for subtle changes: the scalp, external auditory canal, umbilicus, and intergluteal cleft. Nail pitting and onycholysis may be seen. In Reiter's syndrome, circinate balanitis presents as an erythematous eruption on the glans penis (where psoriasis can also occur). It may be difficult to distinguish the skin findings of Reiter's syndrome from those of psoriasis. A characteristic hyperkeratotic eruption on the feet, keratoderma blenorrhagicum, is rarely seen in Reiter's syndrome.

 III. **Laboratory studies** are nonspecific. The RF is by definition negative, and the ESR is inconsistently elevated. Although the human leukocyte antigen B27 is present in more than 90% of Caucasians with ankylosing spondylitis, its frequency is much lower in the other spondyloarthropathies. Therefore, testing for B27 antigen is not appropriate in most cases, especially because it is present in approximately 8–10% of normal Caucasians. Radiographs to look for sacroiliitis (the sine qua non for the diagnosis of ankylosing spondylitis) include an anteroposterior view of the pelvis, sometimes supplemented by modified Ferguson views of the sacroiliac joints, taken with a 30-degree cephalad angle. Radiographs of peripheral joints show periostitis.

 IV. **Treatment**

   A. Physical therapy to improve and maintain spinal motion is extremely important. Because no treatment has been shown to prevent ankylosis of the spine, minimizing flexion deformity allows the spine to fuse in an erect posture.

   B. NSAIDs are the mainstay of symptomatic treatment. High doses are generally required (e.g., indomethacin, 50 mg qid; naproxen, 500 mg tid). NSAIDs should be used with caution in patients with inflammatory bowel disease, however.

   C. Sulfasalazine is efficacious in some patients for whom NSAIDs do not provide adequate relief (see Rheumatoid Arthritis).

   D. Methotrexate has a well-established role in treating psoriatic arthritis and is sometimes effective in the other spondylotic disorders. However, it must be recognized that methotrexate cannot be assumed to be as safe in the spondyloarthropathies as it is in RA. In fact, patients with psoriasis have an increased risk of fibrosis and cirrhosis from methotrexate and should undergo liver biopsy at cumulative dose intervals of 2.5–3.0 g.

   E. The **TNF blockers** etanercept and infliximab have been shown to be effective in providing symptomatic relief of disease in ankylosing spondylitis and psoriatic arthritis.

Scleroderma

The etiology of scleroderma is a poorly understood process that leads to pathologic changes of small-vessel vasculopathy (distinct from vasculitis) and fibrosis. The two major forms of this disease are diffuse scleroderma and limited scleroderma (known as the **CREST syndrome: c**alcinosis, **R**aynaud's phenomenon, **e**sophageal dysmotility, **s**clerodactyly, and **t**elangiectasias). The disease is characterized by fibrosis of skin and internal organs, especially the lungs, heart, kidneys, and GI tract.

 I. **Skin findings on physical examination** are key to the diagnosis. Patients with diffuse as well as limited disease may have sclerodactyly. In diffuse disease, skin in the upper arms may also be involved, as well as loss of facial wrinkles and perioral fibrosis. Raynaud's phenomenon is present in almost all patients with scleroderma but may be associated with other connective tissue diseases as well.

   A. Raynaud's phenomenon. The classic history is one of triphasic skin color change: pallor (vasospasm) followed by cyanosis (desaturation of tissue hemoglobin) followed by rubor (reactive hyperemia). Many patients note only two of these changes. Cold temperatures, tobacco smoke, stress, and certain medications may provoke symptoms. The nail fold capillaries can be visualized by coating the cuticle with a thin layer of clear surgical lubricant and looking through an ophthalmoscope set at +40. Dilatation or dropout of nail fold capillaries increases the likelihood that Raynaud's phenomenon will evolve into a systemic rheumatic disease (*Arch Intern Med* 1998;158:595–600).

B. The most important aspect of **treatment of Raynaud's phenomenon** is protecting the hands from cold temperatures. Glove liners of polypropylene or Thermax worn indoors or under gloves or mittens outdoors are helpful. Covering the head during cold weather is essential, because much of core body heat can be lost through the head, leading to lower body temperature in the extremities. A variety of vasodilating calcium channel blockers (especially dihydropyridines such as nifedipine or amlodipine) helps reduce recurrence and severity of Raynaud's symptoms. A regimen of desensitization to the cold has also been described (*J Rheumatol* 1985;12:953–956).

II. **Laboratory** findings include a positive ANA in most patients. Anticentromere antibody is a special subset of ANA, with a finely speckled pattern, and is seen in the majority of patients with limited disease. Anti-Scl 70 is an antibody to topoisomerase that is quite specific for diffuse disease but is found in a minority of patients.

III. **Treatment** is largely supportive and organ system specific, because there is no treatment that clearly alters the long-term course of this disease. Physical therapy is important to prevent or limit joint contractures. One study demonstrated that very low-dose penicillamine was no more effective than a therapeutic dose (*Arthritis Rheum* 1999;42:1194–1203).

A. **Skin.** Raynaud's phenomenon is treated symptomatically (see above). Some patients with scleroderma have extremely severe Raynaud's phenomenon, and more aggressive measures are undertaken, such as pharmacologic or surgical sympathetic blockade.

B. **Renal.** Azotemia, proteinuria, and a microangiopathic hemolytic anemia can develop in patients with scleroderma **renal crisis**. Hypertension must be managed aggressively, and the angiotensin-converting enzyme inhibitors are the drugs of choice primarily for their renoprotective properties. Corticosteroid treatment appears to be associated with the development of renal crisis.

C. **GI. Gastroesophageal reflux** can be treated with proton pump inhibitors or high-dose histamine-2 receptor blockers. Surgery to correct reflux should be avoided in these patients because of coexisting motility disorders. Mechanical dilatation is sometimes required for strictures. **Malabsorption** due to bacterial overgrowth can be treated with broad-spectrum antibiotics. Nutritional support is critical for patients with severe abnormalities of intestinal motility and malabsorption. Liquid supplements and total parenteral nutrition may be required.

D. **Pulmonary.** Scleroderma may manifest with interstitial lung disease, leading to hypoxemia and pulmonary hypertension. Data indicate that daily cyclophosphamide therapy for active alveolitis can reduce the progression of interstitial lung disease, although reduction in mortality has not been demonstrated (*Ann Intern Med* 2000;132:947–954). The intravenously administered prostacyclin analogue, epoprostenol (Flolan), which has been U.S. Food and Drug Administration approved for the treatment of primary pulmonary hypertension, may have some efficacy for the secondary pulmonary hypertension from the interstitial lung disease of scleroderma (*Ann Intern Med* 2000;132:425–434).

E. **Cardiac.** Myocardial fibrosis can result in congestive heart failure or arrhythmias if the conduction system is affected. Coronary artery vasospasm can cause angina that may be responsive to calcium channel blockers.

Sjögren's Syndrome

Sjögren's syndrome is a multisystem autoimmune disease characterized by dysfunction of exocrine glands. It may occur as a primary disorder or secondary to other rheumatic diseases such as RA, SLE, scleroderma, or inflammatory myopathy.

I. **History** is notable for the sicca symptoms of dry eyes and dry mouth. Parotid gland swelling may occur, and occasionally patients have symptoms of pancreatic insufficiency with diarrhea and malabsorption.

II. **Physical examination** shows a diminished corneal light reflex and reduced tear meniscus. Oral examination reveals a diminished or absent sublingual salivary pool, and the tongue and buccal mucosa may appear dry. The major salivary glands commonly are enlarged. Inflammatory arthritis and cutaneous vasculitis may also be associated with Sjögren's syndrome. Additionally, patients with Sjögren's syndrome often have symptoms of Raynaud's phenomenon (see Scleroderma, sec. **I.A**). Enlargement of lymph nodes, liver, or spleen raises the suspicion of lymphoma or other causes of secondary Sjögren's syndrome.

III. **Laboratory tests** associated with Sjögren's syndrome include serum tests of systemic autoimmunity, including +ANA, +RF, or the presence of SSA (anti-Ro) or SSB (anti-La) antibodies. Lymphocytic infiltration on biopsy of minor salivary glands from the inner surface of the lower lip helps support the diagnosis of Sjögren's syndrome.

IV. **Treatment.** Artificial tears are helpful for dry eye symptoms and can be self-administered as needed. Preservative-free tear preparations are better tolerated by some patients. For more severe cases, an ophthalmologist can accomplish temporary or permanent occlusion of the lacrimal puncta. Treatment of dry mouth symptoms is more challenging but important to reduce discomfort and the incidence of dental caries. Conservative measures, such as increased oral water intake and chewing sugarless gum, can provide symptomatic relief. Oral pilocarpine (Salagen), 5 mg qid, or cevimelene (Evoxac), 30 mg tid, has been shown to increase saliva production and improve symptoms of oral dryness. Various saliva substitutes are available over the counter. Hydroxychloroquine (see Rheumatoid Arthritis, sec. **II.B.2**) is sometimes prescribed for various manifestations of Sjögren's syndrome. Immunosuppressive agents, such as cyclophosphamide, may be required for systemic vasculitis that affects major organs such as nerves.

Vasculitis

I. The **clinical manifestations of vasculitis** are protean. Fever, weight loss, mononeuropathy, rash, arthritis, abdominal pain, sinusitis, pulmonary hemorrhage, and glomerulonephritis are among the many presenting symptoms. Findings on examination tend to be nonspecific, but skin lesions such as palpable purpura, livido reticularis, and digital gangrene are suspicious for vasculitis. Wrist drop or foot drop is suggestive of mononeuropathy, another important clue to the presence of systemic vasculitis.

A. **Polyarteritis nodosa** exhibits many of the above symptoms but typically presents with hypertension, glomerulonephritis, abdominal pain, and mononeuropathy (commonly wrist drop or foot drop). Onset may be gradual or sudden, and patients are systemically ill.

B. **Giant cell arteritis (GCA)** presents with headache, visual disturbance, tongue and jaw claudication, and scalp tenderness. This is often associated with polymyalgia rheumatica (PMR) [see Polymyalgia Rheumatica and Giant Cell Arteritis (Temporal Arteritis)].

C. **Takayasu's arteritis** affects the aorta and its branches. It occurs most commonly in young Asian women and is often detected by asymmetric pulses or blood pressure measurements. Other symptoms include headache, arm claudication, visual changes, and arthralgias.

D. **Wegener's granulomatosis** presents with the classic triad of upper-airway disease (sinusitis), lower-airway disease (pulmonary hemorrhage), and glomerulonephritis. Limited Wegener's granulomatosis occurs without renal involvement.

E. **Churg-Strauss vasculitis** is classically associated with asthma and systemic eosinophilia. Peripheral neuropathy and pulmonary and cutaneous involvement are common.

F. **Cutaneous vasculitis** may be common to all subtypes of vasculitis and commonly presents with palpable purpura, usually in dependent areas of the lower extremities. Although often associated with systemic diseases, vasculitis may be limited to the skin.

G. **Cryoglobulinemia**, frequently associated with hepatitis C, can present with purpura, arthritis, and glomerulonephritis.

H. **Secondary vasculitis.** Vasculitis may also occur secondary to other rheumatic diseases, such as RA and SLE, and should be suspected when symptoms include cutaneous vasculitis, peripheral neuropathies, or mesenteric ischemia.

II. **Laboratory findings** are nonspecific, but anemia, elevated ESR, and urinalysis abnormalities (proteinuria, hematuria, and cellular casts) are often seen. c-ANCA that truly represents antibody to proteinase-3 is specific for Wegener's granulomatosis. Biopsy of affected tissues, such as skin, muscle, artery, and nerve, can be valuable in establishing the diagnosis. The gastrocnemius muscle and sural nerve are common sources of diagnostic material. Renal biopsy findings tend to be nonspecific (crescentic glomerulonephritis with negative immunofluorescence) and rarely include vasculitis.

III. **Treatment** depends on the specific diagnosis. High-dose corticosteroids (prednisone at 1 mg/kg/day) are usually effective. Cyclophosphamide can also be used, either in a daily oral dose of 1–2 mg/kg/day or a monthly IV dose of 0.5–1.0 g/m². Vasculitis that is limited to the skin does not require potent immunosuppressive treatment.

Polymyalgia Rheumatica and Giant Cell Arteritis (Temporal Arteritis)

PMR and GCA represent a continuum of disease. A patient may have one or both diagnoses, and they can develop in either order. PMR and GCA occur after the age of 50 years, and the incidence increases with age.

I. The classic **history** for PMR is morning stiffness, worse in the neck, shoulder, and pelvic girdle region. The patient may complain of the inability to roll over in bed at night. GCA presents with headache, tongue or jaw claudication, scalp tenderness, and vision loss (typically amaurosis fugax). Systemic symptoms such as fever and weight loss may also occur in GCA.

II. **Physical examination** of patients with PMR is most notable for a profound inability to abduct and elevate the shoulders in most cases. Synovitis, if present, should be minimal. Although an uncommon finding, in GCA, a tender, nodular superficial temporal artery with reduced or absent pulse strongly suggests the diagnosis.

III. **Laboratory tests.** Virtually all patients with PMR or GCA have an **elevated ESR**. The high sensitivity of this test makes PMR/GCA unlikely with a normal ESR. CRP may also be elevated. A temporal artery biopsy should be performed in all patients in whom GCA is suspected. The pathologic findings of granulomatous inflammation with giant cells and fragmentation of the internal elastic lamina confirm the diagnosis, although the diagnosis may occasionally be made with a negative biopsy.

IV. **Treatment** for PMR is oriented toward relieving discomfort and improving quality of life. GCA must be treated aggressively as a systemic vasculitis. Although NSAIDs occasionally are effective for PMR, most patients require prednisone in doses of 10–15 mg/day for relief. Failure of the patient to improve dramatically and rapidly with low-dose corticosteroids should lead to reconsideration of the diagnosis of PMR. Treatment can be tapered over approximately 1 year, although some patients require longer treatment. For suspicion of GCA, high-dose prednisone must be initiated immediately at 1–2 mg/kg/day to prevent the complication of irreversible vision loss. Treatment should not be delayed until a temporal artery biopsy can be performed, because the diagnostic findings on biopsy can still be demonstrated several days after corticosteroid therapy has been started. The dose of prednisone can be tapered slowly over several months, provided that the patient remains asymptomatic. Methotrexate may be an effective steroid-sparing agent in some patients, although the evidence is conflicting.

Polymyositis and Dermatomyositis

I. The cardinal feature of **myositis** is proximal muscle weakness. Typically, patients notice difficulty in getting out of a car, chair, or bathtub; climbing stairs; or using their arms above the head. Distal muscle strength should be normal except in inclusion body myositis, which tends to occur in older individuals. Dysphagia with nasal regurgitation may occur if there is weakness of the striated muscle of the upper esophagus. Dyspnea due to interstitial lung disease and joint pain from inflammatory arthritis may occur, especially in the antisynthetase syndrome (polymyositis with a positive anti–Jo-1 antibody).

II. **Physical examination** should focus on evidence of proximal muscle weakness, a sensitive test of which is the ability to raise the head from the supine position. Standing up from a chair with the arms folded across the chest and rising from a deep squat are other good tests for proximal weakness. Patients with dermatomyositis have typical skin findings such as a heliotrope rash on the eyelids, Gottron's papules on the knuckles, and nail fold capillary abnormalities (see Scleroderma, sec. **I.A**).

III. **Laboratory studies** should include serum muscle enzymes, especially creatine phosphokinase, which is elevated in virtually all cases of inflammatory myopathy. Elevations of AST and aldolase may occur but are less specific for muscle injury. Myositis-associated antibodies (such as anti–Jo-1, anti–MI-2, and anti-SRP) are of academic interest in classifying diseases but have little clinical use. Most patients should undergo electromyography (EMG) to look for the classic myopathic findings of fibrillations, positive sharp waves, and low-amplitude polyphasic motor unit potentials. If the EMG is performed on one side of the body, a muscle biopsy can be done on the contralateral side, corresponding to the most abnormal area on the EMG. The biceps, deltoid, and vastus medialis are the muscles that are easily biopsied.

IV. **Treatment** involves high doses of corticosteroids, approximately 1 mg/kg/day prednisone. Sustained high doses for several months are usually required to control disease activity. Normalization of creatine phosphokinase levels precedes improvement in muscle strength by several weeks. After several months of treatment, it is usually possible to taper the dose of prednisone, often to an every-other-day regimen. Patients whose disease cannot be controlled with corticosteroids can be treated with methotrexate or azathioprine as steroid-sparing agents.

Fibromyalgia

Fibromyalgia is a common cause of musculoskeletal pain. It can be described as a soft-tissue amplification syndrome, in which patients experience diffuse musculoskeletal pain.

Table 22-5. Tender point examination in fibromyalgia

Bilateral occiput
Bilateral lower-cervical spine (C5–C7)
Bilateral trapezius at the midpoint
Bilateral supraspinatus
Bilateral second rib at the costochondral junction
Bilateral lateral epicondyle
Bilateral gluteus
Bilateral greater trochanter
Bilateral knee at the medial fat pad proximal to the joint line

I. A **history** suggestive of fibromyalgia includes diffuse nonarticular pain, sleep disturbance resulting in nonrestorative sleep and fatigue, and accompanying symptoms such as headache, irritable bowel syndrome, paresthesias, and vasomotor symptoms in the hands and feet.
II. **Physical examination** is notable for tenderness to palpation in at least 11 of 18 predetermined tender points (Table 22-5).
III. **Laboratory studies** are normal.
IV. **Treatment** has three primary goals: improve sleep, relieve pain, and enhance physical conditioning. Non–habit-forming medications that aid in sleep include tricyclic antidepressants (e.g., amitriptyline, 10–50 mg qhs), trazodone (25–100 mg qhs), and cyclobenzaprine (10–20 mg qhs). Some of the newer antidepressant medications (such as venlafaxine) may also be beneficial. NSAIDs and other analgesics may bring some relief of pain. An aerobic exercise program is essential and can be supplemented by stretching exercises.

23

Neurologic Disorders

Richard S. Sohn

Approach to the Patient with Neurologic Disorders

I. **Goals.** The physician who cares for patients with disorders of the nervous system has two major targets. First is the **prevention of disability**. This requires expeditious diagnosis and treatment of the nervous system problem because the nervous system has limited potential for recovery and repair. Second is the relief from symptoms.

II. A **diagnosis** needs to be established if treatment is to be effective. The steps in establishing a diagnosis are (1) taking an accurate history, (2) performing a complete neurologic examination, (3) formulating a working hypothesis, and (4) pursuing confirmatory studies.

III. **Studies** may be needed, depending on the working hypothesis.
   A. **Imaging** gives information about the structure of the nervous system. MRI, CT, plain films, angiography, and myelography (injection of radiodense contrast into the subarachnoid space before taking x-rays of the spine) are used.
   B. **Neurophysiologic tests** measure the electrical function of parts of the nervous system.
      1. **EEG** evaluates the electrical activity of the brain. It can detect patterns that are typical for epilepsy and patterns associated with good or poor prognosis in patients with medical coma, for example, after cardiopulmonary arrest. Focal brain disease has characteristics on EEG.
      2. **Electromyography** (EMG) and **nerve conduction times** (NCTs) are usually done together. The EMG can differentiate between nerve and muscle disease and detect irritability of anterior horn cells, nerves, and muscles. NCTs detect focal nerve problems, such as carpal tunnel syndrome (CTS). Slowed nerve conduction is typically seen in demyelinating neuropathy.
   C. **Hematologic** studies can detect underlying conditions such as vitamin B_{12} deficiency or sickle cell disease or trait.
   D. **Biochemical** tests can identify illnesses with neurologic impact such as diabetes. Proton emission tomography gives information about local brain biochemistry.
   E. **Cerebrospinal fluid (CSF) studies** can detect evidence of neoplastic, inflammatory, and infectious disease of the nervous system. CSF protein is elevated in infection, inflammation, and tumors of the nervous system. CSF glucose is decreased in bacterial infections and with meningeal metastases, but not with viral infections. Syphilis staging is influenced by the presence of typical antibodies in the CSF. Cell count can help differentiate between active and chronic inflammatory conditions and between viral and bacterial infections. Immunoglobulin abnormalities are seen in inflammatory diseases such as multiple sclerosis (MS). CSF cultures identify various microbes, and cytology can be examined for malignant cells.

F. **Time** is an overlooked test that allows the physician to determine how the patient's problem changes over weeks to years. Different pathologic entities have very different time courses.

IV. **Treatment** may be (1) lifestyle change; (2) medication; (3) physical, occupational, or speech therapy; (4) referral; (5) hospitalization; and/or (6) symptom relief.

V. **Preexisting neurologic problems** are often exacerbated by a systemic illness such as CHF or infection. A patient with a history of a stroke who is weaker in the same distribution is much more likely to have a urinary tract infection than another stroke.

Headache

Headaches can be divided into two groups, primary and secondary. In primary headache, the headache is the disease. In secondary headache, the headache is a symptom of another illness, for example, brain tumor, meningitis, or hemorrhage.

I. **Secondary headaches** may be caused by many disease processes and vary depending on the underlying pathologic cause. **Warning signs and symptoms** of the presence of a secondary headache include sudden onset, worsening of headache, onset of headache after age 50 years, altered level of consciousness, papilledema, meningeal signs, fever, focal neurologic signs (weakness, dysconjugate eyes, unequal pupils, sensory loss, visual field loss, language disturbance, asymmetric reflexes, or extensor plantar reflexes), and thickened, poorly pulsatile scalp arteries. Signs that precede a headache and resolve before or during the headache suggest classic migraine rather than a secondary headache syndrome.

A. **Intracranial causes** include subdural hematoma, intracerebral hematoma, subarachnoid hemorrhage, arteriovenous malformation, brain abscess, meningitis, encephalitis, vasculitis, obstructive hydrocephalus, postlumbar puncture, and cerebral ischemia and infarction. Headaches from intracranial disease do not follow any one stereotype.

B. **Extracranial causes** include sinusitis, disorders of the cervical spine, temporomandibular joint syndrome, giant cell arteritis (see Chap. 22), glaucoma, optic neuritis, and dental disease.

C. **Systemic causes** include fever, viremia, hypoxia, hypercapnia, severe systemic hypertension, allergy, anemia, caffeine withdrawal, and vasoactive chemicals, including nitrates and carbon monoxide.

D. **Studies** should be considered if there is clinical suspicion of an underlying illness causing the headaches (Table 23-1).

II. **Migraine headaches**

A. **History.** Migraines are typically recurrent, severe, unilateral, pulsating, or throbbing and are associated with nausea, vomiting, sensitivity to light, noise, movement, and odors. They can be preceded by an **aura**, commonly visual, marked by zigzag colored lines. Family history is frequently present. Migraines are seen in women approximately three times more frequently than in men, and the first episode typically occurs before the age of 30 years.

B. **Acute treatment of migraines**

1. **Nonnarcotic analgesics.** Aspirin, acetaminophen, and nonsteroidal anti-inflammatory drugs (NSAIDs) may abort a migraine if taken early.

2. **Combination analgesics,** such as butalbital-acetaminophen-caffeine with or without codeine, are often used as **abortive agents** when simple agents fail. Other nonspecific analgesics that are used for migraine include oxycodone or hydrocodone combined with acetaminophen, and butorphanol, often used as a nasal spray. With the use of these drugs, there is significant danger of inducing medication rebound headache and of true addiction. **The use of abortive agents more often than**

Table 23-1. Headache investigation studies

Study	Looking for	Possible diagnoses
CT	Masses, blood clots, subarachnoid blood, infarction, altered ventricular size	Primary or secondary tumors, subdural or epidural hematomas, SAH, stroke, hydrocephalus, Arnold-Chiari malformation
MRI	Same as CT	More sensitive and specific
Lumbar puncture	RBCs, WBCs, protein elevation, glucose elevation or depression, cerebrospinal fluid pressure	SAH, meningitis, encephalitis, benign intracranial hypertension
Angiography	Aneurysm, abnormal arteriovenous connections, variation of arterial diameter	Aneurysm, arteriovenous malformation, vasculitis
Cervical spine films	Misalignment, loss of disk height, spurs, fracture, lytic or blastic lesions	Degenerative joint disease, metastatic tumor
Erythrocyte sedimentation rate	Elevation	Vasculitis, giant cell, and others

SAH, subarachnoid hemorrhage.

three times/week for more than 2 weeks in a row should raise the suspicion of possible medication overuse and rebound headaches.

3. **Isometheptene mucate, 65 mg; dichloralphenazone, 100 mg; and acetaminophen, 325 mg** (Midrin) are effective in helping some migraine patients. The mechanisms of action of the components are the following: Isometheptene causes mild vasoconstriction, dichloralphenazone causes sedation, and acetaminophen produces analgesia.

4. **Ergotamine** is a vasoconstrictive agent that is effective in aborting migraines, particularly if administered during the prodromal phase. Ergotamine should be taken at symptom onset in the maximum dose tolerated by the patient; nausea often limits the dose. The initial oral dose is 2–3 mg PO, and an additional 1–2 mg can be given 30 minutes after the initial dose. Rectal preparations are better absorbed than oral agents. Rectal (2 mg) administration should be tried in patients who are unresponsive to oral delivery or when emesis prevents its use. Dosages should be limited to less than 16 mg/wk. Toxicity includes angina pectoris, limb claudication, and ergotamine headache and dependency.

5. **Triptans** work selectively on the 5-hydroxytryptamine 1b–d receptors. They are the **agents of choice** in treating migraine headaches. Best results are obtained the earlier in the migraine that they are taken. Five triptans are available in the United States.

   a. **Sumatriptan** is available orally, subcutaneously, and intranasally. At the onset of symptoms, 25–50 mg PO is taken and can be repeated in 2 hours to a maximum dose of 200 mg PO/day. Subcutaneously, 6 mg is injected and can be repeated in 1 hour to a maximum dose of 12 mg SC/day. The spray is 20 mg intranasally and can be repeated in 2 hours to a maximum of 40 mg intranasally/day.

   b. **Rizatriptan**, 5–10 mg PO, is taken at the onset of symptoms and can be repeated in 2 hours. An orally disintegrating tablet is available that is convenient if nausea and vomiting are prominent. The maximum dose is 30 mg/day.

    c. Zolmitriptan, 2.5 mg PO, is taken at the onset of symptoms and can be repeated in 2 hours to a maximum dose of 10 mg/day.

    d. Naratriptan, 1.0–2.5 mg PO, is taken at the onset of symptoms. Naratriptan has a longer half-life than the other triptans, and the dose should not be repeated for 4–6 hours. The maximum dose is 5 mg/day.

    e. Almotriptan, 12.5 mg PO, is taken at the onset of symptoms and can be repeated in 2 hours to a maximum dose of 25 mg/day.

    f. Adverse reactions include chest pressure, facial burning, dizziness, and BP elevation. These are uncomfortable but are rarely dangerous. These symptoms may be less bothersome to a patient if another triptan is taken. Chest and neck tightness, diaphoresis, and sedation are slightly more common with injected sumatriptan than with the orally and nasally administered preparations. These symptoms are secondary to esophageal spasm. Myocardial and brain infarction have rarely been seen in patients after taking a triptan.

    g. Contraindications to the use of the triptans are
        (1) Known or suspected coronary artery disease
        (2) Known or suspected peripheral vascular disease
        (3) Pregnancy and lactation
        (4) Basilar migraine (with brainstem signs or symptoms, or both, other than nausea and vomiting) and hemiplegic migraine (with objective paralysis)
        (5) Use of another triptan, ergotamine, or dihydroergotamine (DHE) within 24 hours
        (6) Uncontrolled hypertension
        (7) Use of a monoamine oxidase inhibitor (MAOI)
        (8) Prior sensitivity to the agent under consideration. Some patients are able to tolerate one triptan, whereas another causes significant adverse reactions.

    h. Triptans are for the acute and not the prophylactic treatment of migraine headaches only.

    i. Triptan failures. A particular triptan should not be considered a failure until a patient has not obtained relief after three tries. Frequently, patients experience relief with one triptan after having had no response to another drug in this class. Patients in whom all the triptans fail need to have diagnoses other than migraine considered. Some of the "triptan failures" may respond to DHE.

  6. DHE is a potent intracerebral arteriovenous shunt constrictor with minimal peripheral arterial constriction.

    a. Dosage and administration. DHE, 1 mg IV/SC, can be very effective for the treatment of an acute migraine attack. Metoclopramide, 10 mg IV, or prochlorperazine, 10 mg IV, is given 15–20 minutes before DHE to reduce the nausea and vomiting that are often induced by the drug. Metoclopramide and prochlorperazine each have intrinsic migraine abortive activity. The maximum dose of DHE is 2 mg/day IV or 3 mg/day SC. **DHE 45 nasal spray** allows patients to use this drug at home. Because of the instability of DHE in oxygen, the sprayer that is used for administration must be assembled immediately before use. A dose of intranasal DHE is one spray in each nostril, repeated in 15 minutes. Patients need to be cautioned not to sniff or to put their heads back after the drug has been administered.

    b. Intractable migraine (status migrainosus) can be treated with DHE, 1 mg IV q8h (*Neurology* 1986;36:995, *Neurol Clin* 1990;8:587). Premedication with either metoclopramide, 10 mg, or prochlorperazine, 10 mg, is given 15–20 minutes before DHE to reduce the risk of nausea and vomiting.

    c. Contraindications to DHE are
        (1) Known or suspected coronary artery disease

  (2) Known or suspected peripheral vascular disease

  (3) Pregnancy and lactation

  (4) Basilar migraine (with brainstem signs and/or symptoms other than nausea and vomiting) and hemiplegic migraine (with objective paralysis)

  (5) Use of a triptan or ergotamine within 24 hours

  (6) Uncontrolled hypertension

  (7) Use of an MAOI

  (8) Prior sensitivity to DHE

C. Nonpharmacologic migraine prevention is an important component in treatment strategies. **Avoidance of migraine triggers** can reduce the risk of headache. Foods such as chocolate, cheese, nuts, citrus, alcohol (especially red wine and beer), nitrates, nitrites, and fresh baked goods are often associated with migraine. Caffeine withdrawal can precipitate migraine, as can too much or too little sleep. Menses and oral contraceptives can worsen migraine, and pregnancy and menopause often help. Patients should be encouraged to keep a **food and activity diary** to correlate triggers to their pattern of migraine. **Regular exercise**, via increase in endorphins, can be helpful in migraine reduction, as well as the use of sunglasses, avoidance of flashing lights, and relaxation/meditation.

D. Migraine prophylactic medications are indicated when migraines occur more than twice a month, when abortive medications are not effective, or when associated symptoms are distressing or disabling.

  1. Beta-blockers, such as propranolol, 20–40 mg PO bid, or timolol, 10 mg PO bid, are effective in preventing recurrent migraines.

  2. Valproic acid, 250 mg PO bid/tid, is useful in migraine and cluster headache prophylaxis. Valproic acid is contraindicated during pregnancy. Other antiepileptic drugs have shown effect in preventing migraine, including **topiramate**, 75 mg/day, and **zonisamide**, 100 mg/day.

  3. Tricyclic antidepressants, such as nortriptyline, 25–75 mg PO qd, may prevent tension and migraine headaches.

  4. Methysergide, 2–4 mg PO qd, is effective in the prevention of migraine and cluster headache. Retroperitoneal, pleural, and endocardial fibrosis are severe but reversible complications of chronic methysergide treatment. The incidence is 1 in 5000 cases. A drug holiday should be given every 6 months.

  5. The **calcium channel blocker** verapamil SR, 240 mg PO qd, may be effective in the prevention of migraine and cluster headaches.

  6. Selective serotonin reuptake inhibitors such as fluoxetine, 20–40 mg PO qd, may be useful.

E. Menstrual migraine may be reduced by the use of transcutaneous estradiol 0.05-mg patches. Three patches are usually needed for each menstrual period. The first one should be applied 2 days before the expected onset of vaginal bleeding. The patch should be worn for 3 days and changed to a fresh one on day 4 and again 4 days later. The patches should not be placed near the breast to avoid breast enlargement. Naratriptan, 1.0–2.5 mg PO bid for 1 week, starting a few days before the beginning of the period can also be helpful but is much more expensive.

III. Cluster headaches are more common in men than in women (6:1 male-female); are excruciatingly painful; are unilateral, orbital, periorbital, or temporal in location; and are associated with unilateral autonomic dysfunction (lacrimation, ptosis, miosis, nasal congestion, or conjunctival injection). Patients are often restless because of the severity of this kind of pain. Alcohol and nitrates are known precipitants of cluster headaches. Periodicity is a hallmark of cluster headaches, with pain often recurring daily at about the same hour. **Acute treatment with oxygen** at 5–7 L/min can often terminate an individual attack within 10 minutes. **Sumatriptan**, 6 mg SC, or **DHE**, 1 mg IV/SC/IM, may abort an attack. Preventive treatment is often difficult. It is not easy to be certain that the medical interventions have been effective because cluster headaches often resolve spontaneously. Corticosteroids (prednisone, 30–60 mg/day); lithium carbonate, 300 mg bid or tid; verapamil SR, 240–480 qd; valproate, 250 bid/tid; and methysergide, 4 mg qd, have all been reported to be beneficial. Once a patient is free of attacks for 1–2 months, the medication should be tapered.

IV. **Tension headaches** are the most common type of headache, with >90% of the population having them at some time in their lives. They are usually symmetric and posterior and have the sensation of pressing or squeezing. They are without associated nausea, vomiting, photosensitivity, and phonosensitivity. Tension headaches are usually self-limited and respond well to simple over-the-counter analgesics (e.g., acetaminophen, NSAIDs). Relaxation is often helpful. Preventive medications are not as effective as for migraines. **Depression** is a common cause of long-standing, treatment-resistant daily headaches. Specific inquiry should be made about vegetative signs of depression.

V. **Medication overuse or rebound.** Chronic daily headaches are usually the result of the daily or almost daily use of abortive headache agents. These headaches are poorly localized and often poorly described. They worsen with physical or mental exertion, or both. They are resistant to migraine and other headache-specific agents, abortive as well as preventative. On occasion when the patient is deprived of the offending agent, frank withdrawal symptoms can develop. A large number of the patients who experience this type of headache see many doctors and purchase medications from many pharmacies at the same time. They request more and more medication, sooner and sooner. **Treatment** depends on elimination of the offending agents. This is difficult as an outpatient, in most cases.

   A. **The patient is hospitalized**, and all analgesics, triptans, and so forth need to be discontinued. DHE, 1 mg IV q8h, preceded by 15–20 minutes with 10 mg of either metoclopramide or prochlorperazine, is given until the patient is headache free for 12 hours.

   B. **A short course of corticosteroids** can be helpful in reducing headache when patients discontinue analgesics. Appropriate prophylactic agents need to be started at this time, along with education about nonpharmacologic steps to reduce migraine.

   C. **Patient education** regarding the proper use of abortive medications is critical. If a patient uses an abortive agent more than three times/week, his or her physician needs to be called to consider altering the prophylactic regime and avoid the reappearance of drug overuse-rebound headaches.

Tremor

Tremor is the most common movement disorder that is seen in general medical practice. It is a repetitive, often regular, usually involuntary oscillatory movement that can involve part or almost all of the body. Tremor may be caused by (1) drugs (β agonists for asthma, antidepressants, valproate, and others), (2) hyperthyroidism, (3) heredity, and (4) Parkinson's disease (PD).

I. **Parkinson's disease** is the result of loss of pigmented neurons in the substantia nigra, located in the mesencephalon.

   A. **Symptoms of PD** and complications of treatment are commonly not volunteered by patients. Physicians should be vigilant to screen for and treat these conditions.

      1. **Tremor** is typically 3 Hz (sec^{-1}) and pill rolling or dough kneading in appearance. The tremor is usually asymmetric and is worse at rest than it is with activity.

      2. **Gait and balance difficulty** may be more disabling than tremor. Restriction of mobility and impaired postural reflexes with subsequent falls are common.

3. **Bradykinesia** (slowness of movement) can make a simple act such as dressing extremely difficult and slow.
4. **Dysphagia** can be a life-threatening problem because of the risk of aspiration.
5. **Hypophonia** (soft speech) results in problems in communicating. Drooling is a potential source of embarrassment.
6. **Dementia** is seen more commonly in PD. It is often difficult to differentiate the dementia of PD from Alzheimer's dementia. The differentiation is important because of the varied medical treatments (see Chap. 30).
7. **Depression** is common and should be screened for and treated. Most antidepressants are well tolerated by patients with PD (see Chap. 29).
8. **Constipation** is frequently encountered. It is often made worse by certain drugs, such as the anticholinergic agents. A combination of a bulk laxative and a colonic stimulant is often effective.
9. **Drowsiness** is made worse by nearly all of the medications that are used to treat PD with the exception of selegiline.

B. **Treatment of PD** is appropriate when the manifestations of the disease place the patient at risk of injury. If problems with balance or walking, or both, increase the risk of falls and injury, treatment should be started. Similarly, if symptoms such as tremor make it difficult to perform ordinary tasks such as dressing, bathing, or eating, or are an embarrassment that prevents social activities, treatment is needed. PD is a progressive disease, and medication may need to be increased as it progresses. At this time, there is no evidence that early treatment prevents or decreases ultimate disability. Rehabilitation services, physical therapy, occupational therapy, and speech therapy can help people learn how to walk safely, use eating utensils, and perform activities of daily living.

1. **Anticholinergics** are primarily effective in the treatment of tremor. **Trihexyphenidyl**, 2 mg PO tid, and **benztropine**, 1 mg PO tid, are often helpful in decreasing tremor amplitude. Dry mouth, constipation, urinary retention, and memory impairment are common side effects.
2. **Amantadine**, 100 mg bid, is useful for the treatment of tremor. It has anticholinergic activity and an effect on dopamine reuptake. Amantadine can cause livedo reticularis, confusion, and nausea. It usually provides better tremor control with fewer unpleasant side effects than do the anticholinergic agents.
3. **Dopaminergic agents** have the potential to ameliorate all of the manifestations of PD. Potential adverse effects include nausea and vomiting, orthostatic hypotension, mental status changes (particularly visual hallucinations), dyskinesias, on-off periods, sedation, and constipation. Most of these respond to a change in dosage or adjustment of the times of administration.
   a. **Levodopa** (L-dopa), combined with **carbidopa** in fixed-ratio preparations, is the most widely used and most efficacious of the agents that are currently available. Carbidopa is added to L-dopa to reduce many of the peripheral adverse effects of L-dopa, such as nausea, vomiting, and orthostatic hypotension. The usual starting dose of **carbidopa–L-dopa is 25/100 PO tid**. Other available formulations are 10/100 and 25/250. Sustained-release carbidopa–L-dopa is also available in 25/100 and 50/200. The sustained-release form may reduce the risk of dyskinesias and on-off effects, which are the fairly sudden onset and cessation of the effect of dopa without apparent cause. Sustained-release carbidopa–L-dopa usually provides smoother control, especially as the disease advances.
   b. **Direct-acting dopamine agonists** are used to help reduce the occurrence of end-of-dose failure and on-off episodes. Their early use may protect against dyskinesias. Several dopamine agonists are available,

including bromocriptine, pergolide, pramipexole, and ropinirole. One should start with very low doses and adjust as needed.

4. **Enzyme inhibitors** work by preventing the breakdown of L-dopa. This allows for a reduction in the L-dopa dose and prolongs the therapeutic effect, reducing on-off phenomena and end-of-dose failure.

   a. **Selegiline** is an inhibitor of MAO-b at 5 mg PO bid. At higher doses, the selectivity for MAO-b is lost, and dietary guidelines for nonselective MAOI must be observed. Selegiline may have a neuroprotective effect by reducing neurotoxic oxidative products of dopamine, although the data are controversial. Selegiline does not retard the progression of PD.

   b. **Tolcapone**, 100 mg tid, a catechol methyltransferase inhibitor, is also useful. Liver functions need to be monitored monthly for the first 2 months and quarterly thereafter.

C. **PD-related diseases**

1. **Many drugs can induce PD.** Neuroleptics and antiemetics are the most common. Drug-induced PD rarely responds to dopaminergic agents but does respond to anticholinergic drugs.

2. Several **degenerative diseases** of the nervous system have PD as one of their manifestations. This group includes striatonigral degeneration, Shy-Drager syndrome, and olivopontocerebellar degeneration. Unfortunately, there is no effective treatment for these disorders, as dopaminergic agents and anticholinergic agents do not have beneficial effects.

II. **Essential tremor** usually has a frequency of 8–12 Hz. The amplitude usually increases and the frequency decreases with age. No anatomic or biochemical cause exists for essential tremor. **Inheritance** is autosomal dominant. Approximately 50% of those with essential tremor have affected first-degree relatives with the same illness. Caffeine, β agonists, nicotine, excess thyroid hormone, and stress can exacerbate the tremor. Many patients report that alcohol reduces tremor.

A. **Beta-blockers** (propranolol, 20 mg PO bid) may help in reducing symptoms. The dose is increased until the desired degree of control or mild adverse reactions (bradycardia, orthostatic changes, decreased exercise tolerance, or fatigue) are seen.

B. **Primidone** can also control essential tremor. The usual starting dose is 50 mg PO bid and can be increased by 50–100 mg/day every 2–3 weeks until the desired degree of control is obtained. Sedation often limits the dose titration.

C. **Thyroid function** should be checked in patients with new-onset tremor to rule out hyperthyroidism.

III. **Other movement disorders** are seen much less commonly than tremor. Patients with these conditions may be difficult to treat, and early referral to a movement disorder specialist is recommended.

A. **Dystonia** is a state of abnormal (either hypo- or hyper-) tonicity in the muscles that can cause twisted posture of any part of the body, usually secondary to a more widespread neurologic disorder. Dystonia can be caused by drug (neuroleptic) administration or withdrawal. Botulin toxin injection and surgical procedures on the basal ganglia may be beneficial.

B. **Chorea**, as the name suggests, is the presence of dance-like movements. Chorea can also be induced by neuroleptics. Huntington's is the most common degenerative neurologic disorder associated with chorea. Haloperidol, 1–5 mg/day, may be effective in controlling symptoms.

C. **Athetosis** is best described as twisting and writhing in appearance. No medical therapy is effective in controlling symptoms.

D. **Cerebral palsy** manifests as a combination of dystonia, chorea, and athetosis. It is the result of intrauterine injury or difficulties at delivery.

E. **Hemiballismus** is perhaps the most dramatic abnormal movement, in which unilateral limb flailing occurs. Hemiballismus is almost always the result of an infarct or hemorrhage in the subthalamic nucleus. Haloperidol, 2–5 mg/ day, can control the movements partially. A benzodiazepine hypnotic is frequently needed.

Neuromuscular Disorders

Neuromuscular disorders are diseases of the peripheral nervous system. The symptoms of which a patient complains and the change of these symptoms over time are important clues to the diagnosis. Depending on the patient's complaint and the examination findings, localization to anterior horn cell, nerve, neuromuscular junction, or muscle may be found. The Washington University Neuromuscular page can be found at http://www.neuro.wustl.edu/neuromuscular.

I. **Symptoms**
   A. **Weakness** is frequently a prominent complaint of patients with neuromuscular problems. Strength is usually graded as the following: 5, full power; 4, some weakness against resistance; 3, able to move against gravity; 2, movement with gravity removed; 1, muscle contraction without joint movement; and 0, no muscle contraction.
   B. **Numbness** or sensory loss is also commonly seen in this group of patients. The distribution of sensory loss and the particular sensory modalities that are involved need to be determined.
   C. **Pain** is commonly seen in neuromuscular disorders. The type and location of pain, and ameliorating or exacerbating factors, or both, are important diagnostic clues. Sometimes the pain is caused by nerve disease, distorting sensations. Pain can also occur when the muscle is inflamed.

II. **Physical examination** includes muscle power, muscle appearance (atrophy, hypertrophy, abnormal contractions), muscle tenderness, sensory examination, evaluation of reflexes, the presence or absence of Tinel's sign, and/or nerve hypertrophy.

III. **Diagnostic tests** can further help in localization to one of a combination of structures that are involved in a patient's illness. With this information, the differential diagnosis is narrowed.
   A. **EMG** studies the electrical characteristics of muscle. A needle electrode is placed into the muscle, and observation of the electrical activity is recorded. Characteristic patterns are seen in normal muscle, muscle with faulty nerve supply, muscle with recovering nerve supply, and muscle that is intrinsically sick.
   B. **NCTs** are a measure of how fast a nerve conducts messages. Motor and sensory conduction times are measured. NCTs can determine if a neuropathy is axonal (involving the nerve itself) or demyelinating (damaging the myelin sheath).
   C. **Somatosensory evoked potentials** measure the rate of conduction of sensory input in the spinal cord and brainstem.
   D. **Laboratory studies** such as sedimentation rate and antinuclear antibody titer can help determine if the muscle disorder is part of a systemic disease. CSF examination can reveal an elevated protein that is associated with inflammatory demyelinating neuropathies.

IV. **Illnesses with prominent weakness**
   A. **Myasthenia gravis (MG)** is an autoimmune disorder that involves antibody-mediated disruption of neuromuscular junction receptors and is often associated with thymus tumors. It is more common in women than in men, and it tends to occur in young women (third decade) and older men (fifth to sixth decade). The clinical course is variable; spontaneous remissions and exacerbations occur.
      1. **History** is typical for muscle weakness with exercise that is relieved with rest. Muscles that are innervated by cranial nerves are most commonly affected early. Diplopia, ptosis, dysphagia, and respiratory

difficulties are common presenting complaints. Many patients with MG have either a personal or family history of other autoimmune diseases.

2. **Diagnosis** is usually evident from the history and physical examination. Blood **acetylcholine receptor antibody level** is a highly sensitive and very specific assay and is the diagnostic test of choice. The **Tensilon test** often produces a marked temporary improvement in strength, but its use as a diagnostic test is limited by a high incidence of false positives.

3. **Treatment of MG** follows no specific protocol. Decisions should be made with regard to symptoms, lifestyle, and response to treatment.

   a. **Thymectomy** is an effective treatment for generalized MG and produces complete remission in many patients. However, it is controversial in children, in adults older than 60 years of age, and in pure ocular MG. A **thymoma** is an absolute indication for surgery at any age.

   b. **Cholinesterase inhibitors** can produce symptomatic improvement in all forms of MG. **Pyridostigmine**, 15–60 mg PO tid–qid, should be titrated to the minimum amount that provides relief of symptoms.

   c. **Immunosuppressive drugs** are typically added when additional benefit is needed after cholinesterase inhibitors. **Prednisone**, 50–80 mg PO qd, is frequently used to achieve rapid improvement, but hospitalization is recommended because initial exacerbation of weakness often occurs. **Azathioprine**, 1–2 mg/kg PO qd, is an alternative choice for treatment, but onset of benefit may require months of treatment. **Cyclosporine, cyclophosphamide**, and intravenous **immune gamma globulin** may be beneficial in selected refractory patients.

4. **Myasthenic crisis** is a life-threatening exacerbation of the disease. Airway protection and ventilatory support are the mainstays of therapy.

B. **Tick paralysis** is acute muscular weakness caused by the bite of the female of more than 30 different species of ticks. Paralysis lasts for as long as the tick remains attached. Treatment is removal of the offending parasite. A careful search, including hairy parts of the body, is needed to exclude this as a cause of weakness.

C. **Guillain-Barré syndrome** typically presents with a rapidly progressive, symmetric ascending weakness. Sensory complaints are often present, with few sensory findings on examination. Tendon reflexes are decreased to absent. Paralysis is usually maximal by 3–7 days. The autonomic nervous system is frequently involved. Typically, CSF protein is elevated; cell count is normal. Hospitalization is required for (1) airway and ventilatory protection, (2) dysautonomia detection and correction, and (3) frequently, plasmapheresis or treatment with immune gamma globulin.

D. **Other causes of acute weakness** include acute intermittent porphyria, acute alcoholic myopathy, botulism, arsenic exposure, and postdiphtheritic paralysis.

E. **Chronic weakness** without sensory signs or symptoms is almost always the result of disease of muscle. These are almost always slowly progressive and symmetric, with proximal weakness greater than distal. Unfortunately, they are largely untreatable. Duchenne's, myotonic, motor neuron disease (amyotrophic lateral sclerosis), and fascioscapulohumeral dystrophies, to name a few, are members of this group. Disorders of mitochondria can cause a similar pattern of weakness and are often associated with the involvement of other organ systems. Several inflammatory muscle disorders are known, most commonly polymyositis. These usually respond to corticosteroids. Some of these are associated with systemic diseases such as collagen vascular disease. Others may be related to specific muscle component antibodies.

V. Illnesses with weakness and numbness are usually the result of abnormality of nerve.

    A. Polyneuropathy is usually symmetric. Damage to either the axon itself or the myelin sheath can result in poor conduction of impulses: sensory, motor, or autonomic. Toxins (alcohol, certain chemotherapeutics, phenytoin, and organic phosphates) are common causes. Elimination of the offending agent allows the nerves, in most cases, to heal. Polyneuropathies are associated with **systemic illnesses** such as diabetes, vitamin B_{12} and vitamin E deficiencies, renal failure, hepatic failure, amyloidosis, and systemic cancer. Resolution of the neuropathy depends on control of the underlying condition. Several hereditary polyneuropathies are known. At present, there are no effective treatments. Physical and occupational therapy can help to ameliorate some of the disabilities from which these patients suffer. Chronic inflammatory demyelinating polyneuropathy, an autoimmune polyneuropathy with motor and sensory manifestations and an elevated CSF protein, has spontaneous exacerbations and remissions. When acutely active or reactivated, chronic inflammatory demyelinating polyneuropathy is treated like Guillain-Barré syndrome. Long-term immunosuppression with corticosteroids, azathioprine, or cyclosporine is often needed. AIDS is associated with a polyneuropathy, which may be the result of the HIV infection itself, opportunistic infections, or drugs that are used for treatment.

    B. Mononeuropathies are usually asymmetric. A named nerve (e.g., median nerve) is the structure involved. EMG and NCT can be very helpful in differentiating between a nerve root and a nerve problem. Mononeuropathies can have "mechanical" or "medical" causes. A systemic illness, such as diabetes, can make nerves more susceptible to trauma with resulting mononeuropathy.

        1. Bell's palsy is weakness of one side of the face, upper and lower, without apparent cause. Many patients complain about facial numbness; however, sensory loss is not found on the face. Further questioning regarding numbness frequently reveals that the patient really has a heavy or strange facial sensation. The neurologic examination is otherwise normal. Pain behind the ear on the affected side and alteration of taste and hearing (hyperacusis) are common. Corneal protection with an eye patch is the mainstay of therapy. If the patient has corneal irritation, ophthalmologic referral is mandatory. Corticosteroids have been shown to have no effect on the improvement of Bell's palsy and should not be used [*Laryngoscope* 1976;86(8):1111]. Controversy is ongoing concerning the role of herpesvirus in the pathogenesis of Bell's palsy. Acyclovir and famciclovir have both been used in this illness in the absence of supporting studies. Of patients with Bell's palsy, 90% have a spontaneous and complete recovery.

        2. CTS is caused by median nerve entrapment at the wrist (the carpal tunnel). It is characterized by (1) aching in the hand, especially at night; (2) decreased sensation in the lateral $3\frac{1}{2}$ fingers and adjacent palm; (3) weakness of the thenar muscles; and (4) Tinel's sign elicited by percussion of the median nerve at the wrist. A positive sign is an electric-like sensation going into the hand or, less frequently, up the forearm. CTS is frequently the result of repetitive hand movements, and modification of the behavior is essential. Hypothyroidism and excessive pyridoxine consumption should be ruled out as causes of CTS.

            a. NSAIDs can relieve the pain of CTS and are appropriate when no neurologic symptoms or signs are present.

            b. Splints that minimally extend the wrist and limit wrist movements decrease irritation of the median nerve at the wrist, resulting in decreased signs and symptoms as the median nerve heals.

            c. Corticosteroids injected around the median nerve at the wrist can reduce local swelling and allow the median nerve to heal.

    d. Surgical decompression of the carpal tunnel reduces mechanical pressure on the median nerve, allowing healing by removing the irritant. Surgery should be pursued when progressive weakness, intractable pain, or both are present. Confirmation of diagnosis by NCT is essential before surgery.

  3. Tardy ulnar palsy is compromise of the ulnar nerve at the elbow and is most commonly caused by pressure on the nerve where it comes through the ulnar groove. Sensory loss is usually limited to the $1^1/2$ medial fingers and the adjacent palm. The interossei and abductor digiti quinti are often weak. Tinel's sign may be present over the ulnar nerve at the elbow. Treatment consists of careful attention to the position of the elbow. Avoiding pressure on the medial elbow removes the common irritant and allows healing. The use of an elbow cushion, especially at night, is useful to help eliminate pressure on the ulnar nerve. In rare refractory cases, surgical correction is necessary. The ulnar nerve is transposed from the ulnar groove to the antecubital fossa to eliminate nerve irritation or compression, or both.

  4. Radial nerve palsy is caused by pressure by a hard object such as a chair back on the nerve as it wraps around the humerus. The salient feature of radial palsy is wrist drop. When the wrist is constantly flexed, finger dexterity is markedly impaired. A wrist cock-up splint may be needed to facilitate finger function until recovery has taken place. Loss of sensation over the anatomic snuffbox is seen. Spontaneous recovery usually occurs, and avoidance of the offending behavior prevents recurrence.

  5. Meralgia paresthetica occurs when the lateral cutaneous nerve of the thigh is impaired as it comes over the pelvic brim. Patients with meralgia paresthetica complain of burning and tingling on the lateral aspect of the thigh. Loss of cutaneous sensation is found in the lateral-anterior area of the thigh, corresponding to the distribution of the lateral cutaneous nerve. Power and reflexes are normal. Diabetics are especially susceptible. Topical capsaicin and tricyclic antidepressants can decrease the discomfort but are rarely needed. Weight loss and avoidance of tight belts and waistbands are of benefit.

  6. Leg-crossing palsy is the result of compression of the common peroneal nerve as it comes around the head of the fibula. Foot drop is characteristic, with occasional loss of sensation on the web between the first and second toes. Compression of the nerve between the head of the fibula and the knee when the legs are crossed is the most common cause. Reflexes are normal, and back pain is absent. Spontaneous recovery is the rule, especially if care is taken to avoid crossing the legs. An ankle-foot orthosis ankle brace is sometimes needed to support gait until the nerve recovers.

  7. Trigeminal neuralgia (tic douloureux) causes sharp, lancinating facial pain. The pain lasts for a few seconds at a time and recurs up to hundreds of times a day. It is one of the most painful neurologic syndromes. The pain is most common in the third division of the trigeminal nerve, with movement of pain from the mouth to the ear. The second division is the next most frequently involved, with pain going from the nose to the eye. The first division is least commonly involved, with forehead pain. Stimuli such as face washing or speaking can trigger paroxysms of pain. Incidence increases with age. The neurologic examination, including facial sensation, is normal. Treatment consists of (1) antiepileptic drugs (phenytoin, 300 mg PO qd; carbamazepine, 200 mg PO tid; or valproate, 500 mg PO tid); (2) baclofen, 20 mg PO tid; (3) radiofrequency neurolysis; and (4) microvascular decompression of the nerve near the junction with the pons.

VI. Nerve root irritation can be the cause of pain and/or weakness and/or numbness. Degenerative joint disease with or without disk herniation is most commonly responsible. The pain of nerve root disease is typically burning and is influenced by body position. Conservative treatment with NSAIDs, exercise, improved body mechanics, and local injections is effective. Surgical treatment is indicated when a progressive neurologic deficit is present (see Chap. 21).

Dizziness

Dizziness is a nonspecific term that is used by patients to describe a variety of sensations. A detailed history and physical examination are essential in reaching an accurate diagnosis. A sensation of movement may be present (**vertigo** is a hallucination of movement), implicating a vestibular problem. A feeling of lightheadedness or impending fainting implicates a failure of generalized perfusion. Falling or unsteadiness suggests a problem with proprioception. A combination of these symptoms is frequently seen. No effective pharmacologic treatment is available for dizziness.

I. **Dizziness of labyrinthine origin** is usually vertiginous and episodic. Coexisting auditory symptoms and signs are common and indicate cochlear pathology as well. The dizzy sensation is often inducible by movement when it is of vestibular origin. Oscillopsia is often present.
   A. **Acute vestibular neuronitis or labyrinthitis** is of acute onset without auditory or other neurologic signs or symptoms. Acute labyrinthitis is self-limited. No specific treatment is available. Antihistamines (meclizine, 12.5–25.0 mg PO qid) may prevent nausea and vomiting but rarely help vertigo. IV fluids and antiemetics are sometimes necessary.
   B. **Ménière's disease** can cause severe repetitive episodes of vertigo and progressive hearing loss. It results from increased endolymphatic pressure. Surgical treatment, endolymphatic sac decompression, or partial or complete nerve section may be required. "Vestibular neuronitis" is monophasic, whereas Ménière's disease is recurrent and has associated auditory phenomena.
   C. **Benign positional vertigo** is symptomatic when the patient experiences rapid head movement. Each attack is brief. The diagnosis is made by having the patient seated with the head turned 45 degrees to the left. The patient is then rapidly made supine with the head kept turned. A test is considered positive when nystagmus is present on right gaze. After becoming supine, the patient may have a 5- or 10-second latency of nystagmus. Repeat with the patient's head turned right to test for left gaze nystagmus. The down ear when nystagmus occurs is the one that has a disintegrated otolith, the cause of the illness. The best treatment is the **Epley maneuver**. For this technique, the patient is supine, with the head over the end of the examination table. Turn the head with the pathologic ear up. Then, gradually turn the head until the damaged ear is down. Specialist referral is appropriate when these remedies for vestibular problems are ineffective.
   D. **Tumors** of nerve, such as schwannoma, dermoid, epidermoid, and metastatic tumors, can involve the eighth nerve and can cause dizziness, usually associated with auditory signs or symptoms, or both. Treatment is surgical, radiation, or a combination.
   E. **Toxic damage** to the eighth nerve with agents such as aspirin or aminoglycosides can cause vertigo.
   F. **Chronic and acute ear infections** can induce vestibular dizziness. Treatment is with antibiotics directed at the infection.
   G. **Vascular disease** is often blamed for vestibular symptoms in the elderly, but it is very difficult to make the diagnosis in the absence of other signs and symptoms of posterior circulation disease. Small end-organ vessels may be involved.

II. **Other types of dizziness** are extraordinarily difficult to localize to neural structures. Drugs such as alcohol, tranquilizers, anticonvulsants, antidepressants, hypnotics, antihistamines, and antihypertensives all can induce dizziness. A component of this dizziness is often vestibular. Reduction of the dose or elimination of the intoxicant is curative. Poor systemic perfusion from arrhythmia, hypotension, or heart failure can produce a "dizzy" sensation. Sleep deprivation, poor vision, or poor diabetic control can also result in unpleasant sensations that are sometimes reported by the patient as dizziness. Treatment of dizziness of these causes is difficult and rarely successful unless the underlying problem can be controlled.

Seizures

I. **Seizures** are the behavioral manifestation of abnormal brain electrical discharges. Depending on the area of the brain that is involved, various seizure types occur. A single seizure does not qualify a patient for a diagnosis of epilepsy.
   A. **Structural abnormalities that cause seizures** include (1) primary or secondary CNS tumors, (2) CNS infections (e.g., bacterial meningitis, herpes encephalitis), (3) CNS inflammatory processes (CNS lupus), (4) cerebral infarction, and (5) acute or pre-existing brain injury (e.g., trauma, hemorrhage).
   B. **Nonstructural precipitants of seizure** include (1) drugs in current use (e.g., cyclosporine, normeperidine, beta-lactam antibiotics), (2) withdrawal of drugs (e.g., alcohol, benzodiazepines, barbiturates, antiepileptic drugs), (3) drug intoxication (e.g., cocaine, theophylline), (4) electrolyte abnormalities (e.g., hypocalcemia, hyponatremia), (5) hypoglycemia, (6) uremia, (7) anoxia, and (8) acute febrile illness.
   C. **An etiology** of a seizure can often be found but cannot be corrected. Scars from old strokes or brain trauma or genetic forms of epilepsy, with or without definable metabolic derangement, are but a few. Very often an etiology of a seizure or of epilepsy cannot be found. If the cause of seizures cannot be found or is not correctable, medication is needed.
II. **Antiepileptic drugs** are very helpful in preventing recurrent seizures, but they are not always indicated. The patient who has a clearly defined correctable cause is better served by correcting the problem. A seizure or two occurring with an acute head injury in the absence of other evidence of brain injury usually does not require antiepileptic drugs. The single seizure without apparent cause poses a difficult problem. It is reasonable to wait for another seizure before starting anticonvulsant medication. Of patients who have had a single seizure, 30–40% will not have another.
   A. **Primary generalized epilepsy** is best treated with valproate, 250–1000 mg PO tid, or lamotrigine. Lamotrigine is started at 25 mg PO qd and slowly increased to 150–200 mg PO bid to avoid serious cutaneous reactions. The types of seizures that are primary (no other neurologic disorder is present) are absence attacks or petit mal and some generalized tonic-clonic seizures, for example, those associated with myoclonus, starting in childhood or adolescence.
   B. **Secondary generalized epilepsy**, tonic-clonic seizures that are secondary to another brain problem, such as tumor, glial scar from a stroke, or a degenerative disease, is treated with phenytoin, 300 mg PO qd; carbamazepine, 200 mg PO tid; and less commonly with valproate. These seizures start from a diseased part of the brain, rapidly spreading to involve the entire brain.
   C. **Simple partial epilepsy**, commonly called **focal seizure**, starts from a damaged part of the brain and does not spread much, if at all. It may manifest as focal clonic movement of a body part, speech arrest, staring into space, unresponsiveness without falling, and/or automatisms. Focal seizures

respond to the drugs for secondary generalized epilepsy (first choice) or the drugs for primary generalized epilepsy and, at times, gabapentin, up to 2 g/day (second choice).

D. Pharmacologic notes. Dosages are for average-sized adults and in many cases need to be adjusted. Phenytoin and carbamazepine are available in immediate and slow-release formulations. One should be sure of medications the patient is using before determining dosage intervals. Monotherapy is the goal. Antiepileptic drug blood levels need not be monitored in patients with good control of seizures and no evidence of toxicity. CBC and liver function tests may need to be monitored in some patients who are receiving antiepileptic agents.

III. Driving privileges are a problem for the patient who has had a seizure or has epilepsy. Although the risks to the patient and the community are clear enough, patients often see restriction of their mobility as being unfair.

A. A **seizure-free interval** of 6 months is reasonable before the patient is allowed to operate a motor vehicle.

B. **State reporting requirements vary.** In some jurisdictions, the patient is required to report the condition to the state agency that issues driver's licenses; in some states, it is the physician's obligation. In those states that do not require physician notification of the epileptic problem, a report by the physician could be constituted as a breach of patient confidentiality.

C. **Restriction of other potentially dangerous activities,** such as the use of firearms, working on ladders, swimming alone, tub baths, and so forth, may be advisable until it is clear that the patient's seizures are well controlled.

Multiple Sclerosis

MS is a demyelinating disease. If the illness in a particular patient is characterized by flare-ups with either return to normal function or plateaus, it is referred to as **relapsing and remitting disease**. If the illness is relentlessly progressive, it is referred to as **chronic progressive disease**.

I. **Diagnosis** depends on attacks at different locations in the nervous system at different times. Historical information is invaluable. The neurologic examination gives information about what neural structures are functioning abnormally. **The most commonly affected areas in the nervous system include** (1) optic nerve (decreased visual acuity, decreased color sensitivity, eye pain), (2) periventricular white matter (sensory loss, weakness, and spasticity), (3) corpus callosum (usually without symptoms), (4) cerebellum (ataxia), (5) brainstem (diplopia, ataxia, sensory loss, weakness, and spasticity), and (6) spinal cord (sensory loss, weakness, and spasticity).

A. **Imaging and electrodiagnostic studies.** Without an abnormality on at least one of the following studies (especially MRI), it is highly improbable that the patient has MS.

1. **MRI** shows areas of demyelination and differentiates between old lesions and active lesions.

2. **Visual evoked potential** demonstrates abnormal function of the optic nerve, sometimes not previously suspected.

3. **Brainstem auditory evoked potential** reveals abnormality of auditory pathways.

4. **Somatosensory evoked potential** reveals abnormalities in spinal cord and intracranial sensory pathways.

B. **CSF abnormalities** that are seen in MS include elevated immunoglobulin G, increased immunoglobulin G synthetic rate, and positive oligoclonal bands.

II. **Acute exacerbations** include a problem in an area of the nervous system that was not previously involved or worsening of an old lesion because of increased demyelination at that site. This should be distinguished from a **flare-up of old**

lesions caused by systemic illness such as infection. The latter needs treatment of the systemic problem.

- **A. Mild exacerbations** need no specific therapy because the probability of spontaneous resolution is high.
- **B. Moderate to severe exacerbations** may also spontaneously resolve but usually warrant treatment to limit the duration of morbidity. Corticosteroids are quite effective in limiting the duration of an exacerbation. Methylprednisolone, 250 mg IV, is given q6h for 3–5 days, followed by tapering oral prednisone over approximately 3 weeks. Dexamethasone, 16 mg PO daily for 4 days, 12 mg daily for 4 days, 8 mg daily for 7 days, 4 mg daily for 7 days, and then 4 mg every other day for three doses is also effective. Physical therapy, occupational therapy, and speech therapy are frequently needed.

III. Chronic treatment. All of the agents used to prevent the progression of MS are administered by injection. No controlled studies have been published that directly compare the three agents.

- **A.** Two **interferon-beta preparations** [1a (Avonex) and 1b (Betaseron)] have been shown to reduce the appearance of white matter lesions on T2 MRI images, an indicator of plaque activity, and to reduce the relapse rate in relapsing and remitting disease. They are being investigated for use in chronic progressive disease. Administration of interferon-beta is frequently followed by flu-like symptoms, which respond to NSAIDs.
- **B. Glatiramer** is a polypeptide that has been shown to reduce the appearance of the T2 MRI lesions only. No controlled studies have shown a salutary effect of glatiramer on patient disability ratings over time.

IV. The urinary tract requires special attention in patients with MS. Infection occurs fairly frequently and can be fatal. MS patients may not have the typical symptoms of dysuria, urgency, and frequency because of impairment of sensation. Neurogenic bladder can be the result of MS and can create secondary health care problems for the MS patient. Neurogenic bladders can be divided into two types:

- **A. Nonemptying.** The patient with this type of bladder dysfunction has stasis of urine in the bladder, which raises the risk of urinary infection and of upper urinary tract damage. The bladder that cannot empty is better treated with intermittent, often self-performed catheterization than with an indwelling catheter.
- **B. Nonstoring.** Patients who are wet much of the time run the risk of skin breakdown. Nonstoring bladders are the result of upper neurologic tract lesions. Men with a bladder that cannot store urine can often be satisfactorily managed with a condom catheter. The condom needs to be removed frequently and the penis cleaned and dried to prevent maceration. Many patients with nonstoring bladders can be kept dry with the use of anticholinergic drugs such as **oxybutynin**, 5 mg PO tid, which then produces the ability to store urine. Sometimes the bladder is converted to a nonemptying one, with the need for intermittent catheterization.

Sleep

I. Sleep hygiene is a set of behaviors that is designed to promote good sleep. Regularity is indispensable. People who go to bed and get up at the same time every day usually enjoy more restful nights than do those with erratic sleep patterns. Rotating work shifts are frequently the major obstacle to regular sleep schedules. Avoidance of stimulation by exercise, spicy food, tobacco, and, surprisingly, alcohol (rebound stimulation) within approximately 3 hours of bedtime improves sleep. The bedroom should be at a comfortable temperature. The sound level, silence, or music, according to taste, help sleep onset and maintenance. The level of illumination is also a matter of personal preference. Nighttime garb should be comfortable. Limitation of the use of the bed for sleep and sex will improve sleep. Watching TV, reading, writing letters, and so forth should be done elsewhere. If sleep does not come in a reasonable period of time, one should get out of bed and do something else out of the bedroom.

II. **History.** The most valuable source of information about an individual's sleep is a roommate or bed partner. Inquiry should be made about snoring with or without apnea, leg movements, myoclonus, and so forth. From the history, the presence of difficulty initiating and maintaining sleep, disorders of excessive somnolence, combinations of the two, or other disturbances of sleep can frequently be determined. Sleep physiology measurement, polysomnography, and/or multiple sleep latency tests are useful in confirming the clinical diagnosis and are essential in regulating some forms of therapy such as continuous positive airway pressure.

III. **Difficulty initiating and maintaining sleep**
  A. **Poor sleep hygiene** is often the cause of poor sleep. Attention to the details in sec. I often results in improved sleep.
  B. **Sleep apnea** can interrupt sleep hundreds of times/night. The cause is obstruction of the airway. People with short, wide necks are prone to this disorder. Many of them also have low-hanging soft palates. They invariably snore and can be observed to cut off the flow of air during sleep. They are rarely, if ever, aware of having awakened from sleep. Diagnosis is usually made from the history and examination. Polysomnography is confirmatory and is used to titrate continuous positive airway pressure or bilevel positive airway pressure. Drugs that suppress rapid eye movement (REM) sleep (barbiturates, tricyclic antidepressants, etc.) are occasionally helpful. Surgical treatment with resection of the uvula and part of the soft palate or tracheotomy is rarely needed. Nonobstructive or central sleep apnea is much less common and is more difficult to treat.
  C. **Periodic leg movements** can also interrupt sleep. As with sleep apnea, the patient is usually not aware of having been awakened. The bed partner, also as with sleep apnea, is frequently awakened by the abnormal process and often has bruises to show as a result of trauma sustained during the night. Dopamine agonists (carbidopa–L-dopa 25/100) or opioid agonists (tramadol, 50 mg) can significantly reduce the abnormal leg movements and improve sleep.

IV. **Disorders of excessive somnolence**
  A. The most common cause of **daytime sleepiness** is poor nocturnal sleep, which may be the result of one of the causes of poor sleep discussed above or the result of not scheduling enough sleep time.
  B. In **narcolepsy**, REM sleep intrudes into consciousness at inopportune times. REM sleep often occurs immediately on falling asleep, skipping the usual progress through stages I, II, III, IV, III, II, REM. The clinical consequences of this abnormal occurrence of REM are inappropriate daytime sleepiness, cataplexy, sleep paralysis, hypnagogic hallucinations, and poor nocturnal sleep. Stimulants such as methylphenidate, 10 mg daily or bid, can be given. If possible, stimulants should be omitted on the weekends.
  C. Many drugs that are not thought of as being sedatives have CNS depressant effects and can cause sleepiness. Prominent among these are antihistamines (types 1 and 2), antihypertensive agents, antidepressants, and antiepileptic drugs.

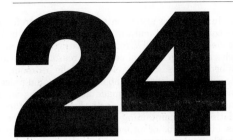

Women's Health

Kathryn M. Diemer and
Karen S. Winters

Osteoporosis

Osteoporosis is defined as a disease of low bone mass and microarchitectural deterioration of bone tissue that leads to enhanced bone fragility and a consequent increase in fracture risk (*Am J Med* 1993;94:646–650). It can have serious consequences on quality of life. Only one-third of patients who experience a hip fracture are able to return to their prefracture level of function, and half of all women who have a hip fracture spend time in a nursing home. The 1-year mortality after a hip fracture has been reported as high as 27% [*J Bone Joint Surg* 1978;60(7):930–934]. Osteoporosis is clinically silent until the first fracture occurs; therefore, it is imperative that those at risk for this disease are recognized early and that steps are taken to prevent bone loss and fracture.

I. **Approach to the patient with suspected osteoporosis**
   A. **History.** Risk factor screening is a useful tool in the evaluation of patients with osteoporosis, as it allows the physician to recognize factors that can influence bone density and fracture risk (Table 24-1). Essential historical information includes the following:
      1. **Height** at age 30 years and any loss of height
      2. **Medications**, including heparin, thyroid medications, diuretics, hormone replacement/birth control pills (BCPs), phenytoin/phenobarbital, prednisone, calcium, calcitonin, vitamins, raloxifene, alendronate, or risedronate
      3. **Dietary history**, specifically dairy products, lactose intolerance, vegetarian or other restrictive diets, or caffeine intake
      4. **Fractures** as an adult
      5. **Family history** of fractures, dowager's hump, or osteoporosis
      6. **Physical activity**
      7. **Menstrual history**
      8. **Pain** and functional limitations of activities of daily living
   B. **Physical examination.** A complete physical examination should be performed on each patient, with emphasis on the accurate measurement of height and weight. A spinal examination should be included, noting evidence of kyphosis, pain, and muscle spasm. A breast examination and education on self-examination should be performed on any woman in whom estrogen replacement is being considered. Gait stability and fall risk should be assessed.

II. **Bone densitometry** has improved the diagnosis and treatment of osteoporosis. It allows the clinician to diagnose low bone mass before fracture occurs. Bone mass measurement is an accurate predictor of fractures (*N Engl J Med* 1995;332:767–773).
   A. **Indications for bone mineral densitometry**
      1. **Bone Mass Measurement Act of 1998**
         a. **Postmenopausal women deciding whether to begin estrogen replacement therapy (ERT)** or other osteoporosis therapy

Table 24-1. Risk factors for an osteoporotic fracture or low bone density

Low bone mineral density	Bilateral oophorectomy
Advanced age	Prolonged amenorrhea
Female sex	Prolonged calcium deficit
History of fracture as an adult	Use of corticosteroids
Family history of an osteoporotic fracture	Excessive caffeine intake (>190 mg/day)
Caucasian or Asian ethnicity	History of gastric surgery
Sedentary lifestyle	Excessive alcohol intake
Smoking	Inability to rise from a chair (reduced muscle strength)
Low body weight (<127 lb)	
Early menopause (before age 45 yrs)	

Source: Osteoporosis: Review of the evidence for prevention, diagnosis, and treatment and cost-effectiveness analysis. *Osteopor Int* 1998;18(4):16–20.

        b. Radiologically suspected osteopenia
        c. Chronic glucocorticoids (≥ 7.5 mg/day for ≥ 3 months)
        d. Primary hyperparathyroidism
        e. Serial monitoring to follow therapy
    2. National Osteoporosis Foundation guidelines
        a. Women age 65 years or older regardless of additional risk factors
        b. Postmenopausal women younger than 65 years old with at least one additional risk factor
        c. Postmenopausal women who seek treatment for fractures
        d. Women considering osteoporosis therapy whose decision might be influenced by bone mineral density (BMD) testing
        e. Women taking hormone replacement for a prolonged period
  B. Bone mineral densitometry techniques. All bone mass measurement techniques are valuable for making the diagnosis of osteoporosis and predicting fracture risk. The most widely available methods are single x-ray absorptiometry, dual x-ray absorptiometry, quantitative computed tomography, and ultrasound densitometry. The techniques vary in terms of precision, cost, radiation exposure, and ability to follow serial changes. The most common method of measuring bone mass and currently the "gold standard" is dual x-ray absorptiometry.
  C. Diagnosis of osteoporosis using bone densitometry (T scores and Z scores). For the diagnosis of osteoporosis, the bone density of a patient is compared to the mean young adult normal reference range (the T score). The World Health Organization has developed diagnostic criteria for osteoporosis using T scores (Table 24-2). The –2.5 or less standard deviation was chosen because more than half of osteoporotic fractures occur below that level. Z scores, which compare a patient's BMD to that of age-matched controls, are also reported on bone mass measurement. If the Z score is more than two standard deviations below age-matched subjects, a cause other than age-related bone loss should be considered, and a secondary cause of osteoporosis should be sought.
  D. Using bone densitometry for following response to treatment. Serial measurements can be used to monitor the effect of treatment or the clinical course of a specific medical condition. The usefulness of serial measurements is dependent on the precision error of the measuring device used. Change in any biologic test should be at least 2.8 times the precision of the technique to be 95% confident that the change is real and not due to a measurement error in the machine. For example, if a densitometer has a 1% pre-

Table 24-2. World Health Organization criteria for the diagnosis of osteoporosis[a]

T score	Category
<–1 SD from peak bone mass	Normal
–1 SD to –2.5 SD from peak bone mass	Low bone mass/osteopenia
≤ –2.5 SD from peak bone mass	Osteoporosis
≤ –2.5 SD with fragility fracture	Severe osteoporosis

SD, standard deviation.
[a]Diagnostic guidelines developed for postmenopausal women.

cision error, there should be at least a 2.8% change to be confident that this change is real.

III. **Laboratory studies** should be limited and directed by the history and physical examination.

A. **Comprehensive biochemical profile** allows simple screening for secondary causes, that is, calcium-phosphorus ratio for hyperparathyroidism, total protein-albumin ratio for myeloma, and screening for liver and kidney disease.

B. **Thyroid-stimulating hormone (TSH)** should be measured in patients with symptoms of hyperthyroidism or those who are receiving thyroid replacement.

C. **25-Hydroxyvitamin D** screens for body stores of vitamin D.

D. **Additional studies** can be considered for those with very low bone mass or those who continue to lose bone despite antiresorptive therapy, including: (1) parathyroid hormone (PTH) battery, (2) 24-hour urine for calcium excretion, (3) serum protein electrophoresis (SPEP), (4) cortisol levels, (5) estradiol levels in women, (6) testosterone levels in men, and (7) bone biopsy.

IV. **Patient education** is essential for the prevention and treatment of osteoporosis.

A. **Fall prevention**

1. **Home hazards.** Inspect and remove throw rugs, loose carpets, slippery floors, cords and wires, or anything that can cause a patient to slip.

2. **Furniture.** Inspect for unstable furniture and clutter that can obstruct mobility.

3. **Lighting.** Assure adequate lighting, especially at night.

4. **Bathroom.** Grab bars for the toilet, placement of nonslip surfaces in the shower.

5. **Properly fitting shoes.**

6. **Outdoor surfaces.** Irregular sidewalks, ice or snow, uneven surfaces.

7. **Postural hypotension.**

8. **Hip protectors** were shown to reduce hip fractures significantly in ambulatory but frail elderly adults [*N Engl J Med* 2000;343(21):1506–1513].

B. **Exercise** should be encouraged in patients with osteoporosis as allowed by their functional status.

1. **Weight-bearing exercise**, such as walking, jogging, basketball, dancing, and cycling, should be initiated at least three times/week.

2. **Avoid unsafe forces**, including flexion and forward bending of the vertebral column, as they can increase the risk of a compression fracture. Rotation of the spinal column also increases compressive forces on the spine.

V. **Diet therapy** is essential in the prevention and treatment of osteoporosis. The calcium intake for postmenopausal women should be 1200–1500 mg/day. Increasing calcium intake is essential for bone health. Examples of the elemental calcium content of various foods include the following: 8-oz glass of milk contains 300 mg, 1 oz of Swiss cheese contains 270 mg, and 1 cup of cooked broccoli contains 100 mg [*JAMA* 1994;272(24):1942–1948].

A. Calcium supplements. Calcium carbonate is acceptable for most patients for supplementation. It is cheap and has relatively few side effects. Guidelines for calcium supplement use include the following:

  1. **Calcium is best absorbed in small amounts.** Consider dividing the daily dose if greater than 500 mg.
  2. **Synthetic calcium supplements are optimal.** Oyster shell calcium, dolomite, and bone meal can contain heavy metal contaminants [*Nutr Rev* 1994;52(3):95–97].
  3. **Eating calcium-fortified foods** should be encouraged.

B. Vitamin D (800 IU PO qd) is beneficial for patients with osteoporosis. Ambulatory men and women older than the age of 65 years who were given calcium carbonate and vitamin D had a significant reduction in nonvertebral fractures [*N Engl J Med* 1997;337(10):670–676].

VI. Medications for the treatment of osteoporosis. It is important to emphasize the importance of calcium and vitamin D supplementation with the administration of antiresorptive and anabolic therapy. All of the studies that cited the efficacy of estrogens, bisphosphonates, calcitonin, and selective estrogen receptor modulators included calcium and vitamin D supplementation.

A. Estrogen replacement therapy (ERT)

  1. **Effect on BMD.** ERT has been shown to slow bone loss following menopause or increase it by as much as 6% [*JAMA* 1996;246(17):1389–1396]. ERT is approved by the U.S. Food and Drug Administration for the prevention of osteoporosis.
  2. **Fracture reduction.** Numerous observational studies support estrogen therapy as effective in the reduction of vertebral fractures by as much as 50–80%. A study of osteoporotic fractures suggested that women who started ERT within 5 years of menopause and used ERT for more than 10 years had a relative risk for wrist fractures of 0.25 and a relative risk for hip fractures of 0.27 (*Ann Intern Med* 1995;122:9–16). No double-blinded placebo-controlled trials have focused on hormone replacement and fractures.
  3. **Dosing recommendations** (see Menopause and Table 24-3).

B. Alendronate is a bisphosphonate that has been approved for the treatment of osteoporosis.

  1. **Effect on BMD.** Alendronate has been shown to improve BMD in the spine by 8.8% and in the hip by 5.9% after 3 years of therapy (*N Engl J Med* 1995;333:1437–1443).
  2. **Fracture reduction.** Women with osteoporosis treated with alendronate therapy for 3 years (2 years of 5 mg and 1 year of 10 mg) had a reduction in vertebral fractures by 47% and hip fractures by 51% [*Lancet* 1996;348(9041):1535–1541].
  3. **Patient instructions.** Alendronate is poorly absorbed from the GI tract and should be taken on an empty stomach with an 8-oz glass of water. The patient should not eat anything for 30 minutes and must remain upright.
  4. **Side effects.** Esophageal irritation and esophageal ulcers have been reported with alendronate [*N Engl J Med* 1996;335(14):1016–1021] and can be minimized by giving the patient proper dosing instructions.
  5. **Recommended dosage** for the treatment of osteoporosis in men and women is **alendronate, 10 mg PO qd or 70 mg PO once weekly**. The dosage for the prevention of osteoporosis in postmenopausal women is 5 mg/day or 35 mg once weekly. The dose for the treatment of corticosteroid-induced osteoporosis is 5 mg/day, except in postmenopausal women not receiving estrogen, for whom the recommended dosage is 10 mg/day.

Table 24-3. Estrogen and progestin formulations

Estrogen	Brand name and strength		
	Name	Strength (mg/day)	Administration frequency
Estradiol transdermal system	Alora	0.05, 0.075, 0.1	Twice weekly
	Climara	0.025, 0.05, 0.075, 0.1	Once weekly
	Esclim	0.025, 0.0375, 0.05, 0.075, 0.1	Twice weekly
	Estraderm	0.05, 0.1	Twice weekly
	Vivelle	0.025, 0.0375, 0.05, 0.075, 0.1	Twice weekly
	Vivelle-Dot	0.0375, 0.05, 0.075, 0.1	Twice weekly
Estradiol tablets	Estrace, 0.5 mg, 1 mg, 2 mg		
Estrogens, conjugated tablets	Premarin, 0.3 mg, 0.625 mg, 0.9 mg, 1.25 mg, 2.5 mg		
Estrogens, esterified tablets	Estratab, 0.3 mg, 0.625 mg, 2.5 mg		
	Menest, 0.3 mg, 0.625 mg, 1.25 mg, 2.5 mg		
Estropipate tablets	Ogen, 0.625 mg, 1.25 mg, 2.5 mg		
	Ortho-Est, 0.625 mg, 1.25 mg		
Ethinyl estradiol tablets	Estinyl, 0.02 mg, 0.05 mg		
Synthetic conjugated estrogens, A tablets	Cenestin, 0.625 mg, 0.9 mg		

Progestin	Brand name and strength		
Progesterone capsules	Prometrium, 100 mg		
Medroxyprogesterone tablets	Cycrin, 2.5 mg, 5 mg, 10 mg		
	Provera, 2.5 mg, 5 mg, 10 mg		
	Amen, 10 mg		
	Curretab, 10 mg		
Norethindrone	Aygestin, 5 mg		

Estrogen/progestin combination products	Generic name and strength		
Prempro	0.625 mg conjugated estrogen + 2.5 mg medroxyprogesterone		
	0.625 mg conjugated estrogen + 5 mg medroxyprogesterone		
Premphase	Pack contains 14 tablets each of 0.625 mg conjugated estrogen and 0.625 mg conjugated estrogen + 5 mg medroxyprogesterone		
Femhrt	5 μg ethinyl estradiol + 1 mg norethindrone		

(continued

Table 24-3. (continued)

Activella	1 mg estradiol + 0.5 mg norethindrone
Ortho-Prefest	Pack contains 15 tablets each of 1 mg estradiol and 1 mg estradiol + 0.09 mg norgestimate
CombiPatch	0.05 mg estradiol + 0.14 mg norethindrone
	0.05 mg estradiol + 0.25 mg norethindrone

Topical estrogens preparation	Commercial name	Administration frequency
Conjugated equine estrogen	Premarin cream	1 g contains 0.625 mg
Dienestrol	Ortho-dienestrol	0.01% cream
Estradiol vaginal ring	Estring	One ring/vagina q90day
Estradiol vaginal tablets	Vagifem	25 mcg estradiol
Micronized estradiol	Estrace cream	1 g contains 0.1 mg

C. **Risedronate** is a bisphosphonate that has been approved for the treatment of osteoporosis.
   1. **Effect on BMD.** Risedronate has been shown to improve BMD in the spine by 4–6% and the hip by 1–3% [*JAMA* 1999;282(14):1344–1352].
   2. **Fracture reduction.** The Vertebral Efficacy with Risedronate Trial (VERT) showed a 41–49% reduction in spinal fractures and a 39% reduction in nonvertebral fractures [*JAMA* 1999;282(14):1344–1352, and *Ost Int* 2000;11:83–91]. Women 70–79 years old with confirmed osteoporosis had a 40% reduction in hip fractures with 5 mg/day [*N Engl J Med* 2001;344(5):333–340].
   3. **Patient instructions.** Risedronate is poorly absorbed from the GI tract and should be taken on an empty stomach with an 8-oz glass of water. The patient should not eat anything for 30 minutes and must remain upright.
   4. **Recommended dosage** for treatment and prevention of postmenopausal osteoporosis is **risedronate, 5 mg PO qd**. The dose for the prevention and treatment of corticosteroid-induced osteoporosis is 5 mg/day. A 35-mg once-weekly dose may be available soon.
D. **Raloxifene** is a selective estrogen receptor modulator. The mixed agonist/antagonist effects of selective estrogen receptor modulators on the estrogen receptor were first noted with women who were being treated for breast cancer with tamoxifen. Tamoxifen was noted to have positive effects on BMD and serum lipids, but endometrial hyperplasia developed (*Am J Med* 1995;99:636–641).
   1. **Effect on BMD.** Treatment with raloxifene has been shown to improve BMD of the femoral neck and spine by 2.1% and 2.6%, respectively, compared to placebo [*JAMA* 1999;282(7):637–645].
   2. **Fracture reduction.** In the Multiple Outcomes of Raloxifene Evaluation (MORE) trial, 7705 women were assigned to receive raloxifene at 60 or 120 mg. Vertebral fractures were reported to be reduced by 38–52% (*JAMA* 1999;282:637–645). No data support reduction in hip fractures at this time.

3. **Additional benefits.** The MORE trial revealed a 70% reduction in the development of invasive breast cancer in patients who were treated with raloxifene. The drug had no effect on the endometrium [*N Engl J Med* 1997;337(23):1641–1647]. Total serum cholesterol and low-density lipoprotein cholesterol levels decreased significantly without change in high-density lipoprotein or triglycerides. Total cholesterol decreased by 6.6% [*JAMA* 1999;282(23):2189–2197].

4. **Side effects** include hot flashes and leg cramps. Raloxifene is similar to estrogen in the risk of thrombosis and thromboembolic disease.

5. **Recommended dosage** for the prevention and treatment of postmenopausal osteoporosis is **raloxifene, 60 mg PO qd**.

E. **Calcitonin.** Salmon or human calcitonin can be given as an SC injection or as a nasal spray.

1. **Effect on BMD.** Calcitonin improves BMD by 1–2% in patients who are treated with calcitonin, 200 IU nasal spray qd.

2. **Fracture reduction.** The Prevent Recurrence of Osteoporotic Fracture (PROOF) trial showed a reduction of vertebral fractures by 36% with the nasal spray in women who were 5 years postmenopausal with vertebral fractures. However, 59% of participants withdrew prematurely; therefore, results of this study should be interpreted cautiously. No significant reduction in hip fractures occurred [*Am J Med* 2000;109(4):267–276].

3. **Additional benefits.** Calcitonin has an analgesic effect when given in the treatment of compression fractures [*Calcif Tissue Int* 1991;49(suppl 2):S9–S13].

4. **Recommended dosage** for the treatment of women greater than 5 years postmenopausal with low bone mass is one spray (200 IU) in one nostril daily. The patient should alternate nostrils each day. The SC dose is 100 IU/day.

F. **Parathyroid hormone (PTH)**, 20–40 µg SC, has been studied in women who were ambulatory, were at least 5 years postmenopausal, and had at least one moderate or two mild atraumatic vertebral fractures. When given intermittently, PTH acts as an anabolic agent primarily stimulating bone formation. Bone density improved in the spine and hip but not in the shaft of the radius. After a median treatment period of 21 months, there was significant reduction in vertebral fractures by 65–69% and nonvertebral fracture by 35–40%. Calcium levels were elevated in 11% of the 20-µg group, in 28% of the 40-µg group, and in 2% of the placebo group; therefore, calcium levels may need to be monitored in patients who are treated with parathyroid injections [*N Engl J Med* 2001;344(19):1434–1444]. PTH is expected to be available in 2002 for the treatment of osteoporosis.

VII. **Corticosteroid-induced osteoporosis**

A. **Skeletal effects of corticosteroids** are related to dose and to duration of therapy.

1. **Daily prednisone** doses of 7.5 mg/day or greater can result in significant bone loss. Lower doses can also have an effect on bone metabolism.

2. **Alternate-day regimens have not been shown to be protective on bone loss.**

3. **Bone densitometry** should be considered on any patient who is presently receiving corticosteroids or if long-term therapy is initiated.

B. **Treatment recommendations**

1. **Patients who are on corticosteroids** should receive adequate calcium intake (1500 mg/day) and vitamin D (800 IU).

2. **Alendronate** has been shown to prevent bone loss in patients receiving corticosteroid therapy and to reduce the risk of fractures in postmenopausal women who are taking steroids [*N Engl J Med* 1998;339(5):292–299].

3. **Calcitonin and calcitriol** (0.6 µg/day) have been shown to prevent corticosteroid-induced bone loss in the lumbar spine [*N Engl J Med* 1993;328(24):1747–1751].

4. **Risedronate** has been shown to maintain or increase bone density of the lumbar spine, femoral neck, and trochanter in patients receiving corticosteroids. It has also been shown to decrease vertebral fractures by 70% (*Calcif Tissue Int* 2000;67:277–285).

VIII. Osteoporosis in men. If a male patient presents with a fracture that is associated with mild to moderate trauma, BMD testing should be performed, and a search for secondary causes of bone loss should be considered.

A. History and physical examination should evaluate for risk factors for osteoporosis including possible drugs that could affect BMD, such as corticosteroids, anticonvulsants, history of alcohol ingestion (more than 100 g/day), or nicotine use.

B. Laboratory studies should include SPEP, CBC, calcium, inorganic phosphate, albumin, creatinine, alkaline phosphatase, PTH battery, TSH, testosterone, 25-hydroxyvitamin D, 24-hour urine collection for calcium and creatinine excretion, and cortisol levels [*Endocr Rev* 1995;16(1):87–116, and *Am J Med* 1993;95(suppl 5A):225–285].

C. Causes of hypogonadism, such as Kleinfelter's syndrome, hyperprolactinemia, anorexia nervosa, and hemochromatosis, should also be considered. Bone biopsy may be needed if no etiology is found.

D. Treatment should be directed toward adequate calcium intake, modification of risk factors, and treatment of a secondary cause, if found. Testosterone has been shown to improve BMD in men with low testosterone levels [*Bone* 1996;18(2):171–177]. Alendronate has been shown to maintain BMD in men with osteoporosis [*N Engl J Med* 2000;343(9):604–610]. Alendronate, 10 mg PO qd, is approved for increasing bone mass in men with osteoporosis. The 70-mg once-weekly dose is also an alternative. Risedronate has been shown to reduce vertebral fractures and increase the bone mass in men treated with corticosteroids (*Calcif Tissue Int* 2001;69:242–247). In a small study of 23 men, PTH has been shown to increase bone mass significantly in men with idiopathic osteoporosis (*Calcif Tissue Int* 2001;69:248–251).

Menopause

Menopause is the permanent cessation of menses due to the decline of ovarian function. The average age at menopause is 51 years. Other causes of amenorrhea should be considered: excessive weight loss, concurrent medical illnesses, and pregnancy.

I. Symptoms associated with menopause

A. Hot flashes affect approximately 75% of menopausal women. They occur most frequently at night and are due to estrogen deficiency. It is believed that estrogen withdrawal lowers the temperature set point in the hypothalamus to reduce the body thermostat. As a result, vasodilatation of the vessels in the hands and upper body occurs so that the heat in the central organs is lost at the periphery (*Ciba Found Symp* 1995;191:171–186). Hot flashes are not synonymous with estrogen deficiency. Other causes of hot flashes should be considered, such as pheochromocytoma, carcinoid, pregnancy, and panic disorder. **Estrogen is the most effective treatment.** It should be continued for at least 2 years and then gradually titrated to prevent the return of hot flashes. Other treatments for women who cannot or will not take estrogen include the following:

1. **Environmental changes**, including keeping the room cool and dressing in layers, may make hot flashes more tolerable.
2. **Clonidine at 0.1 mg/day** decreases hot flashes by 25%; higher doses have increased side effects.
3. **Methyldopa, 250 mg PO tid**, has also been shown to reduce symptoms.
4. **Progestins.** Medroxyprogesterone and megestrol acetate may decrease the flush.
5. **Androgens** decrease hot flush in men but not women.

6. **Phytoestrogens** are weak estrogens of plant origin found in cereals seeds, and nuts that may decrease symptoms [*Ann Intern Med* 1999;131(8):605–616].

7. **Vitamins** B$_6$, E, and C and **beta-blockers** may have some benefit.

8. **Venlafaxine** has been shown to be effective in reducing vasomotor symptoms [*Ann Oncol* 2001;12(3):301–310].

B. **Vaginal atrophy** presents with dyspareunia, vaginal dryness, itching, and irritation. Topical and oral estrogen is useful for symptoms associated with vaginal atrophy.

C. **Urinary symptoms.** The terminal urethra is embryonically related to the vagina. As it becomes thinner, there is more risk of infection and incontinence. Dysuria without evidence of infection is due to the thinning of the epithelium, allowing urine in close contact with the sensory nerves. Also, the normal urethral pressures created by the urethra and surrounding tissues are decreased. Topical estrogen in some studies has been shown to reduce the incidence of urinary tract infections and improve symptoms of urinary incontinence [*Lancet* 1999;353:571–580, and *Ann Intern Med* 1999;131(8):605–616].

II. **Estrogen Replacement Therapy (ERT)**

A. **Indications** for ERT include the treatment and prevention of menopausal symptoms and prevention of osteoporosis. **ERT should not be initiated for secondary prevention of cardiovascular disease until further research is performed that supports its use** (*JAMA* 1998;280(7):605–613). Primary prevention is controversial and should be individualized to each patient.

B. **Contraindications to ERT** include the presence of breast or endometrial cancer or other estrogen-dependent neoplasms, active thrombophlebitis history of thromboembolic event, undiagnosed vaginal bleeding, active liver disease, and pregnancy. In patients with hypertriglyceridemia, transdermal estrogen should be used.

C. **Evaluation** before starting ERT should include a thorough history and physical examination, lipid studies including triglyceride levels, mammography, and Papanicolaou (Pap) smear. Laboratory confirmation of menopause is not usually necessary but would reveal an elevated follicle-stimulating hormone (FSH; >50 mIU/ml) and a low estradiol (<50 pg/ml). It is unusual to identify menopause in regularly menstruating women.

D. **Regimens for ERT** (Table 24-3)

1. **Women without a uterus** should receive continuous estrogen without progestin.

2. **Women with a uterus** have several options. Unopposed estrogen is not recommended due to the increased risk of hyperplasia and endometrial cancer.

a. **Combined continuous regimen.** Estrogen and progestin are both taken daily. The patient can expect irregular bleeding for the first 6 months. After this time, 75% of patients are amenorrheic. The 1-year compliance rate has been estimated to be 60–86%. Endometrial biopsy is indicated for heavier than normal bleeding, bleeding for more than 5 days, any change in the bleeding pattern, and if bleeding persists after 12 months of therapy.

b. **Combined cyclic regimen.** Estrogen is taken daily, and the progestin is taken on days 1–12 of each month. The patient can expect to bleed from day 9–15. The advantage is a predictable bleeding pattern. An endometrial biopsy is indicated if there is bleeding before the ninth day or heavier than usual bleeding.

E. **Side effects of estrogen** include abdominal bloating, cramps, breast tenderness, hypertriglyceridemia (oral estrogen), breakthrough bleeding weight changes, enlargement of benign tumors of the uterus, dry eyes, and skin changes.

F. **Side effects of progestins** include breakthrough bleeding, edema, weight changes, rash, insomnia, and somnolence. In the Postmenopausal Estrogen Progestin Intervention (PEPI) Trial, patients who received conjugated equine estrogen and progestin did not improve high-density lipoprotein cholesterol as much as those treated with estrogen only [*JAMA* 1995;273(3):199–208].

III. **Promotion of a healthy lifestyle** should be encouraged. Postmenopausal women are at increased risk for cardiovascular disease and osteoporosis. All postmenopausal women should be encouraged to exercise regularly, eat sensibly with a low-fat diet that is rich in fruits and vegetables, have adequate calcium intake of 1500 mg/day, avoid smoking, and follow up regularly with their primary care physician. Women on hormone replacement therapy should be advised that there may be a higher risk of breast cancer and they must have regular breast examinations and mammograms [*N Engl J Med* 1997;336(5):1769–1775].

Cervical Cancer Screening

Cervical cancer screening has reduced the incidence of invasive cervical cancer by 95%. Half of the women in the United States with invasive cervical carcinoma have never had a Pap smear, and another 10% have not had a Pap smear in 5 years (*Am J Obstet Gynecol* 1998;179:544–556). **Risk factors** for cervical cancer include smoking, multiple sex partners, sexual activity at an early age, and sex with a "high-risk" partner, characterized by multiple sex partners or a partner who has developed genital neoplasia [*J Clin Pathol* 1998;51(12):96–103].

I. **Screening** for cervical cancer with a Pap smear should begin when a woman becomes sexually active or at the age of 18 years. Screening should continue yearly, and if all Pap smears are negative and the patient is considered low risk, the frequency of Pap smears can be reduced to every 1–3 years. The American College of Physicians and the U.S. Preventive Services Task Force suggest that screening can cease in women older than age 65 years who have had regular testing with no prior abnormal results.

II. **Human papilloma virus** (HPV) appears to be the link between sexual activity and cervical neoplasia. Evidence of HPV infection is consistently found in 90% of cervical cancers. The most common clinical manifestation of HPV infection is condyloma acuminata; the majority of these lesions are caused by nononcogenic form of HPV—types 6b and 11. Other HPV types are associated with cervical neoplasia, such as HPV 16, 18, 45, and 56, which are found in 50–80% of the high-grade squamous intraepithelial lesions. Intermediate-risk HPV types (31, 33, and 35) have been associated with all grades of intraepithelial neoplasms and occasionally with cancer [*J Clin Pathol* 1998;51(2):96–103].

III. **Anatomy.** The normal cervix is covered with squamous epithelium, which is continuous with the squamous epithelia of the vagina. The endocervical canal is lined with columnar epithelium, and the squamous and columnar epithelium normally meet at the external os. The columnar epithelium can extend further onto the ectocervix resulting in "cervical ectopy." It is at the squamocolumnar junction that most cervical intraepithelial neoplasias arise.

IV. **Classification.** Cervical intraepithelial neoplasias are usually divided into categories based on cytologic grades. The Bethesda system is the currently recognized reporting system. Included in this system is the pathologist's interpretation of the smear, including the presence of benign cellular changes or evidence of cellular atypia, or both. Infectious processes such as *Trichomonas*, *Candida*, *Actinomyces*, or cellular changes associated with herpes simplex virus are reported. Reactive (but benign) changes associated with inflammation, atrophy, radiation, or intrauterine contraceptive device are also reported. The four categories of squamous cell abnormalities are atypical squamous cells of undetermined significance (ASCUS), low-grade squamous intraepithelial lesions (LSIL), high-grade squamous intraepithelial lesions (HSIL), and squamous carcinoma.

A. **ASCUS** lesions should be further qualified, if possible, as to whether a reactive or premalignant process is favored. As the majority of ASCUS lesions regress, these patients can be monitored, and only if these lesions persist should ablative therapy be considered. In patients with vaginitis, the infection should be adequately treated and a repeat smear should be done in 3 months. The postmenopausal woman with severe atrophic vaginitis should be instructed to use topical estrogen until the vaginal mucosa is estrogenized; the smear should then be repeated [*Am J Obstet Gynecol* 1996;175(4):1120–1128]. Patients with ASCUS designation should have repeat Pap smears every 4–6 months; when they have three consecutive negative reports, they can be monitored according to routine screening. If a second ASCUS report occurs in the 2-year follow-up period, they should be referred for culposcopy. If the ASCUS is qualified as favoring a neoplastic process, the patients should be managed as if they had an LSIL (*Semin Surg Oncol* 1999;16:217–221).

  B. LSIL lesions include changes associated with HPV infection as well as mild dysplasia (formerly known as **CIN 1**). Most cytology specimens with LSIL revert to normal without therapy; however, a small percentage develop a precancerous process. Patients who are deemed reliable for regular follow-up can be followed with Pap smears every 3–6 months. If the abnormality persists, the patient should be referred for culposcopic examination and biopsy. After three consecutive negative smears, the patient can be returned to a routine screening protocol. If there is concern about compliance and follow-up, the patient should be referred for culposcopy.

  C. HSIL encompasses moderate and severe dysplasia as well as carcinoma in situ. Women with high HSIL should undergo culposcopy and directed biopsy [*JAMA* 1994;271(23):1866–1869].

V. Treatment options for cervical intraepithelial neoplasias include cryotherapy, laser vaporization, and the loop electrosurgical excision procedure. Each has risks and benefits related to ease of use, effectiveness, complication rate, ability to screen for higher-grade lesions, and costs. Treatment decisions should be made with the recommendation of a clinician who is skilled in these procedures.

Breast Masses and Nipple Discharge

I. Breast masses

  A. Risk factors for breast cancer include female gender, increasing age, first-degree relative (mother or sister) with breast cancer (highest risk is if the relative was premenopausal and the cancer was bilateral), previous breast cancer, late age of first pregnancy, and nulliparity [*U.S. Prevention Services Task Force Guide to the Clinical Preventive Services* (2nd ed.) Baltimore: Williams & Wilkins, 1996].

  B. History. The patient should be questioned for any associated symptoms, such as pain and nipple discharge. Menstrual history should be obtained, and she should be questioned to determine the possibility of pregnancy. Medications should be reviewed, and any history of trauma should be obtained. An accurate family history should be elicited. If a history of breast, ovarian, colon, or prostate cancer is found in numerous family members, genetic counseling should be considered.

  C. Physical examination should include inspection and palpation of the breast with the patient seated and then lying flat. The breasts should be observed for skin dimpling or changes in contour. The nipple should be inspected for spontaneous discharge. The axillary and supraclavicular area should be palpated for any evidence of a mass or enlarged lymph nodes. The breast should be palpated gently, including the nipple, areola, and breast tissue. The breast should be palpated circumferentially to the axilla. The nipple should be closely evaluated for discharge, and the character of the discharge should be noted. A ductal carcinoma may present with an isolated spontaneous serosanguineous discharge.

D. **Differential diagnosis** for a discrete nodule includes fibroadenoma, cysts, fibrocystic changes, malignancy, and trauma. A dominant nodule remains unchanged throughout the menstrual cycle. In fibrocystic disease, the palpable nodules frequently feel cystic and are subject to change during the menstrual cycle. Benign nodules have characteristics such as easy mobility, regular borders, and a soft or cystic feel. However, physical examination alone cannot exclude malignancy; therefore, other diagnostic tests are indicated.

E. **Management**

1. **Women younger than age 30 years** with a breast mass and no other symptoms could be observed through one menstrual cycle, and if it resolves, no further treatment is indicated. If the mass is mobile, nontender, and smooth, it is most likely a fibroadenoma and should be removed electively. Any persistent mass requires evaluation by a surgeon experienced in breast disease.

2. **Women aged 30–50 years.** It should be determined if the mass is cystic or solid by ultrasound. If cystic, it could be observed for one cycle, or a needle aspiration can be performed. If the mass completely resolves with fluid aspiration, no further intervention is required. If it does not completely resolve with needle aspiration or it is a solid lesion, a surgical consultation and a mammogram should be obtained. If the mammogram is negative and the mass is persistent, the mass should be surgically excised, as **a negative mammogram does not exclude malignancy.** Any persistent mass requires evaluation by a surgeon experienced in breast disease.

3. **Women older than age 50 years.** A mammogram should be obtained, and the patient should be referred for consultation with an experienced breast surgeon. Mammograms in women older than age 30 years have a false-negative rate of 8–10%. Fine-needle aspiration or needle-core biopsy can be performed on solid lesions by a surgeon or a radiologist, with adequate specimens obtained in 60–85% of instances. Negative cytology on a solid lesion does not rule out malignancy, and further evaluation should be considered. If a mass does not completely disappear or if the fluid that is aspirated is bloody or rapidly reaccumulates, an open biopsy is indicated.

F. **Recommendations for mammography** (Appendix C)

1. **U.S. Preventative Services Task Force** recommends that women aged 50–69 years be screened every 1–2 years with mammography alone or with clinical breast examination (CBE).

2. **American Cancer Society, National Cancer Institute, American College of Obstetrics and Gynecology.**
   a. **Ages 40–49 years:** annual CBE, mammography every 1–2 years
   b. **Ages 50+ years:** annual CBE and mammography

3. **American College of Physicians** recommends mammography every 2 years in women aged 50–74 years.

II. **Nipple discharge** can be classified as galactorrhea, physiologic, or pathologic.

A. **Galactorrhea** is bilateral, milky, involves multiple ducts, and is not associated with pregnancy or lactation. It is very unusual for nulligravid women to secrete breast milk spontaneously, although this may occur in girls as they enter puberty. Breast secretions can be demonstrated in 25% of normal women who have been pregnant; this percentage is even higher when breast massage is performed. Galactorrhea suggests an effect of prolactin either through drugs, pituitary tumors, or an endo-crine effect. Drugs that are associated with galactorrhea include oral contraceptives, tricyclic antidepressants, methyldopa, reserpine, and antiemetics.

B. **Physiologic** nipple discharge is usually bilateral and serous. It is believed to be a consequence of local breast stimulation or irritation in women with hormonally primed breast tissue (either by pregnancy or oral contracep-tives). Gonadal function is preserved. Avoiding breast stimulation should resolve this condition.

C. **Pathologic** nipple discharge is usually unilateral and localized to a single duct. It is spontaneous, intermittent, and persistent. The fluid can be sero-sanguineous, bloody, greenish, or clear. The most common cause of unilat-eral discharge is intraductal papilloma, followed by mammary duct ectasia and fibrocystic disease. Of pathologic nipple discharge, 11% is due to malig-nancy. Increasing age correlates with an increased risk of malignancy [*Am Surg* 1996;62(2):119–122].

D. **History and physical examination.** The history should include questioning in regard to menstrual pattern, recent pregnancy, infertility, medications, symptoms of hypothyroidism, breast stimulation, and presence of head-aches or visual complaints. Any medications associated with galactorrhea should be stopped, and pregnancy should be ruled out. Physical examina-tion should include a complete breast examination and evaluation for signs of hypothyroidism.

E. **Diagnostic evaluation.** If fluid is expressed, it should be evaluated for occult blood. Mammography should be obtained in patients with a patho-logic discharge or if a mass is palpated. A negative mammogram does not exclude malignancy. Galactography (cannulation of the secreting duct fol-lowed by injection of contrast material) can be considered to identify intra-ductal lesions. A prolactin level and TSH should be performed if galactorrhea is present. Very high concentrations of prolactin are associ-ated with prolactinomas. Prolactinomas that are greater than 10 mm in diameter are associated with extremely high prolactin levels (>1000 ng/ml). Excluding pregnancy, a prolactin level of greater than 300 ng/ml is almost always the result of a prolactinoma. Microadenomas may produce lower prolactin levels. Patients with galactorrhea, menstrual irregulari-ties, and otherwise unexplained elevations of prolactin should have imag-ing of the sellar region; MRI with gadolinium enhancement is the procedure of choice, although CT is a reasonable alternative [Evaluating Galactorrhea. In AH Goroll, AG Mulley Jr (eds), *Primary Care Medicine* (3rd ed). Philadelphia: Lippincott, 1995:550–552].

F. **Treatment**

1. **Galactorrhea.** Patients with normal periods and normal prolactin levels do not require treatment. These patients should be followed regularly. If the patient is receiving a medication that is associated with galactor-rhea, the dose can be decreased and the patient followed.

2. **Prolactinoma.** Microadenomas have an excellent prognosis; 80–90% regress or remain unchanged, and only 10% continue to grow. If the patient is symptomatic, medical therapy with a dopamine agonist can be started (see Chap. 17, Hyperprolactinemia). Surgical therapy is considered in those patients who do not tolerate or do not respond to medical therapy. Macroadenomas are also treated with dopamine agonists. In many instances, medical therapy alone controls symp-toms and shrinks the adenoma. Surgery is required for vision loss or refractoriness to bromocriptine therapy [*Ann Med* 1998;30(5):452–459].

3. **Patients with pathologic discharge** should be referred for evaluation by a surgeon who is experienced with diseases of the breast. Mammog-raphy should be performed.

Table 24-4. Causes of dyspareunia

Medical

    Diabetes—fragile mucosa

    GI disease—colitis, inflammatory bowel disease

    Bladder symptoms—cystitis, urinary tract infection

    Prior abdominal surgery

Gynecologic

    Childbirth—cervical, uterine, and ligamentous damage; episiotomy; nerve damage

    Hymenal strands; imperforate hymen

    Uterine fibroids

    Estrogen deficiency

    Sexually transmitted disease—especially herpes simplex virus (HSV), human papilloma virus (HPV)

    Pelvic irradiation

    Prior pelvic surgery

    Vulvodynia—chronic vulvar discomfort

        Infectious—*Candida*, HPV, HSV

        Dermatoses—eczema, contact dermatitis

        Vulvar vestibulitis—exquisite pain in the area between the labia minora without apparent cause

Psychosocial factors

    Current or past abuse

    Relationship factors

    Depressive symptoms

    Life stresses

Dyspareunia, Pelvic Pain, and Dysfunctional Uterine Bleeding

I. **Dyspareunia** is recurrent genital pain associated with intercourse. Clinically, it can be described as superficial, vaginal, and deep. Superficial dyspareunia is pain associated with attempted penetration. It is usually related to vaginal or perineal irritation or anatomic factors. Vaginal dyspareunia is generally associated with lubrication problems or vaginal atrophy. Deep dyspareunia is pain related to thrusting that is often associated with pelvic disease, anatomic distortion, or difficulty with relaxation. Dyspareunia should also be classified as primary or secondary. The key to the diagnosis of dyspareunia frequently is found within the history. Medical conditions, gynecologic causes, and psychological causes should be considered (Table 24-4).

    A. **Physical examination** should include evaluation of the external genitalia for signs of infection, atrophy, Bartholin's gland infection, or a hymenal ring. A "Q-tip" test of the vestibule (touching the vestibule gently with a cotton swab to elicit focal tenderness) should be performed to rule out vulvar vestibulitis. Using only the index finger, vaginal structures are palpated and assessed for tenderness or masses. The bimanual examination is performed to assess uterine size and position, evidence of adnexal masses, cervical motion tenderness, or tenderness over the bladder suggesting cystitis. A rectovaginal examination can detect nodularity suggesting endometriosis. A speculum examination detects vaginal discharge, cervical abnormalities, or evidence of HPV [*Int J Impot Res* 1998;10(2):S117–S120].

B. **Diagnosis and treatment.** Laboratory testing should be guided by history and physical examination. A gonorrhea and *Chlamydia* culture should be performed. Treatment is directed by the findings of the history and physical examination. The patient should discontinue all feminine hygiene products, as these can cause irritation. Treatment of any infectious cause, if present, should be initiated. Hormone replacement therapy should be initiated for vaginal atrophy. Most cases of vulvar vestibulitis resolve on their own, although some patients need therapy. Treatment with 2% lidocaine in an emollient base to the affected area may be beneficial. For patients who do not respond to conservative therapy, surgical excision is recommended for those with severe pain that lasts longer than 2 years. For vaginal strictures, dilatation can be performed. Psychosocial issues also should be addressed.

II. **Pelvic pain** may be a frustrating disease for patients and physicians. It has many possible etiologies, including other organ systems. The patient should be cautioned that the excessive use of narcotics may lead to drug dependency. A thorough history and physical examination should be performed. Appropriate laboratory testing may be helpful. A 3-month trial of oral contraceptives and nonsteroidal anti-inflammatory drugs may offer relief. (Refer to Table 24-5 for possible etiology.)

III. **Dysfunctional uterine bleeding** is defined as any marked change from a patient's usual pattern that should be considered abnormal if there is no obvious cause. Normal menses occur every 28 days (mean), with the range from 21 to 35 days. The normal duration is 2–7 days, with normal blood loss of 20–80 ml. Menarche averages age 13 years, and menopause averages age 51 years.

A. **Etiologies.** Oral contraceptive pills, breakthrough bleeding, chronic anovulation, endometrial hyperplasia, and atrophic endometrium are common causes of dysfunctional uterine bleeding. The most common cause in adolescents is anovulation. When ovulation does not occur, there is continual stimulation of the endometrium, and no progesterone is produced. Less common causes in adolescents are lower genital tract infections or foreign body, or both; malignancy; and systemic disease. In reproductive-aged women, the most common cause is pregnancy and its complications. Less frequent causes are anovulation, leiomyomas, infections, polyps, and cervicitis. Cancers are infrequent but need to be ruled out. Chronic anovulation may also be associated with thyroid or prolactin disorders, premature ovarian failure, adult-onset congenital adrenal hyperplasia, or polycystic ovary syndrome. Some common causes of hypothalamic anovulation are weight loss or gain, eating disorders, stress, chronic illness, and excessive exercise. Anovulatory bleeding can be thought of as estrogen breakthrough bleeding (*Postgrad Med* 2001;109:137). In perimenopausal/postmenopausal women, the likelihood that abnormal bleeding is due to malignancy increases with age. Approximately 5% of premenopausal and 20% of postmenopausal women with abnormal bleeding have endometrial cancer; cervical cancer occurs in about 4–5% of these women. Atrophic endometrium is benign and seen in approximately 25% of cases [*Obstetrics, Gynecology and Infertility* (4th ed). Palo Alto: Scrub Hill Press, 1998:97].

B. **Evaluation.** A history and physical examination, including pelvic examination and pap smear, should be performed. Pregnancy should be ruled out regardless of the patient's stated sexual history. Clotting studies, CBC, TSH, and urinalysis may be helpful pending response to treatment. Consider endometrial biopsy and ultrasound in premenopausal women with abnormal bleeding for 2 months and in all postmenopausal women. Biopsy may require referral to a gynecologist.

Table 24-5. Causes of pelvic pain

Gynecologic	Musculoskeletal
Extrauterine	Coccydynia
Adhesions	Disk problems
Chronic ectopic pregnancy	Degenerative joint disease
Chronic pelvic infection	Fibromyositis
Endometriosis	Hernias
Residual ovary syndrome	Herpes zoster
Uterine	Myofascial pain
Adenomyosis	Nerve entrapment syndromes
Chronic endometritis	Osteoporosis
Intrauterine device	Scoliosis/lordosis/kyphosis
Pelvic congestion	Strains/sprains
Urologic	**Other**
Detrusor hyperactivity	Abuse (physical or sexual)
Interstitial cystitis	Heavy metal poisoning
Stone	Porphyria
Urethral syndrome	Psychiatric disorders
Suburethral diverticulitis	Psychosocial stress
GI	Sickle cell disease
Cholelithiasis	Sleep disturbances
Constipation	Somatiform disorders
Chronic appendicitis	Substance abuse
Diverticular disease	Sympathetic dystrophy
Enterocolitis	
Gastric/duodenal ulcer	
Inflammatory bowel disease	
Irritable bowel disease	
Neoplasm	

Source: American College of Obstetricians and Gynecologists. Chronic pelvic pain. *ACOG Technical Bulletin*, No. 223, May 1996. Copyright 1996, American College of Obstetricians and Gynecologists, with permission.

    C. Treatment. Women who desire contraception are best managed with the oral contraceptive pill. If no bleeding occurs in 2 months, medroxyprogesterone should be started to prevent endometrial buildup. Consider dilatation and curettage or hysteroscopy. For mild to moderate bleeding, moderate-dose estradiol as BCPs with 35–50 µg ethinyl estradiol should be prescribed. Take one bid or tid for 7 days, then one every day for at least 3 months. For severe hemorrhage, 25 mg conjugated estrogen (Premarin) IV can be administered over 30 minutes and can be repeated every 4 hours for 24 hours [*Obstetrics, Gynecology and Infertility* (4th ed). Palo Alto: Scrub Hill Press, 1998:97] or 1.25 mg PO every 4–6 hours for 24 hours, then oral contraceptive as above (*Postgrad Med* 2001;109:137).

Infertility

Infertility is the inability to conceive after 1 year of unprotected intercourse. After both partners have been assessed, female factor infertility accounts for 30%, male infertility accounts for 30%, and combined or unexplained causes account for 40% of couples' infertility [*Mayo Clin Proc* 1998;73(7):681–688].

I. **Female partner evaluation.** The American Society of Reproductive Medicine recommends assessment after 1 year of infertility in women younger than 35 years and after 6 months of infertility for women older than 35 years.

   A. **History.** A medical history should be obtained on every patient to determine medical conditions that could affect fertility. The woman should also be questioned for any conditions that could affect pelvic anatomy, such as pelvic inflammatory disease (PID), surgeries, or use of an intrauterine device (IUD). A history of an abnormal Pap smear with a resultant ablative treatment may result in cervical stenosis. Excessive physical exercise or weight loss of greater than 10% over 1 year may result in anovulation. Neuroleptic, antidepressant, and hypotensive drugs can cause hyperprolactinemia. Previous abdominal surgery, "complicated appendectomy," and gynecologic surgeries all predispose to adhesion formation. Menstrual history helps determine if the woman is ovulating. A menstrual cycle length of 21–35 days is considered normal. Some women can identify ovulatory discomfort or mittelschmerz. A change in the cervical mucus noticed during midcycle also suggests ovulation. Some women have monitored basal body temperature or have charted ovulation with an ovulation predictor kit, which is available commercially. The most likely time for ovulation is 14 days before the next anticipated menstrual period, and sexual intercourse on alternate days during this time frame is optimal. For secondary infertility, details of previous pregnancies, including abortions, miscarriages, and ectopic and molar pregnancies, should be recorded.

   B. **Physical examination.** The presence of hirsutism or acne suggests a hyperandrogenic state of ovarian or adrenal origin. Galactorrhea suggests hyperprolactinemia. Obesity or abdominal striae may suggest Cushing's disease or polycystic ovarian disease. A pelvic examination may reveal a pelvic mass that would require further evaluation or nodularity in the cul de sac, suggesting endometriosis. An enlarged uterus suggests fibroids.

   C. **Laboratory evaluation.** A progesterone level drawn 1 week after expected ovulation that is greater than 3–5 ng/ml confirms ovulation [*Mayo Clin Proc* 1998;73(7):681–688]. If the menstrual cycle is irregular, pregnancy should be ruled out, and a TSH, FSH, and prolactin level should be performed. If the patient has hirsuitism, dehydroepiandrosterone sulfate and testosterone levels should be measured. Circulating FSH levels that exceed 40–50 IU/L on two occasions at least 2 weeks apart suggest premature ovarian failure. Measurement of serum FSH on cycle day 3 indicates ovarian age and predicts pregnancy success rates in women who have in vitro fertilization. By extrapolation, achievement of pregnancy under ordinary circumstances also may be predicted. Patients with an FSH level of less than 15 mIU/ml have good pregnancy rates; women with levels of 15–24 mIU/ml have borderline pregnancy rates, and those with levels of greater than 25 mIU/ml have poor pregnancy rates (*N Engl J Med* 1993;329:1710–1715).

II. **Male partner evaluation**

   A. **History.** The male partner should be questioned about his general health, alcohol or drug use, and whether he has ever fathered a child. A history of testicular injury, mumps orchitis, or cryptorchidism and ongoing medical treatments, such as cancer chemotherapy, anabolic steroids, and hot tub use, should be elicited.

   B. **Physical examination.** The male partner should be examined for testicular size, any testicular masses, or varicocele.

C. **Laboratory evaluation.** Semen analysis: should be collected in a clean specimen container after 2–3 days of abstinence. Normal values: volume >2 ml, sperm concentration >20 million/ml, motility >50% with forward progression or 25% with rapid progression, >50% normal forms, leukocytes <1 million/ml.

III. **Female partner anatomy.** If semen analysis is normal, hysterosalpingography should be performed to assess the female anatomy. This is performed 7–11 days after the onset of menses to avoid exposure to a pregnancy.

IV. **Treatment.** The primary care physician may consider initiating treatment on selected patients. For women whose history suggests irregular ovulation or anovulation (this could be confirmed with an ovulatory predictor kit), clomiphene citrate could be considered. Bromocriptine mesylate (Parlodel) could be used for patients with hyperprolactinemia.

V. **Referral to a specialist.** If a couple has not conceived after 3 years of stopping contraception, the chance of a spontaneous pregnancy in the next year is less than 25% (*BMJ* 1998;316:1438–1441). A woman older than 35 years of age has limited time for the investigations that are necessary for evaluation for assisted conception (i.e., in vitro fertilization); therefore, she should be referred early. Other women who should be referred early include those who are amenorrheic, those with a history of significant pelvic infections, those who do not become pregnant after 3 months on clomiphene, and those who are ovulatory but have not conceived. Men with an abnormal semen analysis should be referred to a urologist who specializes in infertility.

VI. **General considerations.** A woman who is planning to conceive should adopt a healthy lifestyle. She should be counseled to consider a regular exercise program and to avoid nicotine, alcohol, and any illicit drugs. She should discuss with her primary care physician the safety of any prescription medications. She should be encouraged to take prophylactic folic acid while trying to conceive and during the first 12 weeks of the pregnancy. Pregnancy rates are reduced in women who are obese. Weight reduction should be advised for those women with a body mass index of over 30 (*Fertil Steril* 1996;48:905–913).

Birth Control Options

I. **Oral contraceptives.** Prevention of ovulation by suppression of FSH and luteinizing hormone (LH) requires estrogen and progesterone. Estrogen affects FSH, and progesterone affects LH. Combination pills contain estrogen (ethinyl estradiol) and one of the several progestogens. Progestogen has the predominant effect on the endometrium and also causes cervical mucus thickening. Progesterone alone can prevent implantation. Two third-generation progesterones are available in the United States: norgestimate and desogestrel. These claim to be less androgenic, therefore decreasing hirsutism and acne. Progesterone decreases circulating free testosterone by increasing sex hormone–binding globulin. Two types of BCPs are available in the United States: monophasic and multiphasic. The monophasic BCPs have fixed dosage of hormones in the active pills (first 3 weeks of pack). The multiphasic BCPs contain varying dosages of one or both hormones during the first 3 weeks. Multiphasic BCPs were developed to simulate the hormonal changes of normal menses more closely. No convincing evidence has been found that they cause fewer adverse effects or other known advantages. Some BCPs have a small iron supplement during the placebo week (4th week of pack). The menses, withdrawal bleeding, should occur during the early to middle of the fourth week (*N Engl J Med* 1989;320:777–787).

A. **Absolute contraindications** include (1) pregnancy, (2) smokers older than age 35 years, (3) previous or active thromboembolic disease, (4) active liver disease, (5) undiagnosed uterine bleeding, (6) estrogen-dependent neoplasm, and (7) hepatoma.

B. Relative contraindications include hypertension, migraine headaches, active gallbladder disease, sickle cell anemia, and hyperlipidemia.

C. Advantages

1. Excellent form of contraception (unintended pregnancy rate = 0.1–3.0%).
2. Decreased dysmenorrhea.
3. Decreased incidence of PID.
4. Decreased incidence of ovarian and endometrial cancer.
5. Decreased incidence of benign breast disease.
6. Decreased menstrual flow.
7. Treatment for endometriosis.
8. Treatment for hyperandrogenic states/hirsutism.
9. Treatment for acne. Two randomized studies have shown that BCP-containing norgestimate improves acne. Another trial indicates that levonorgestrel or norethindrone may improve acne [*Obstetrics, Gynecology and Infertility* (4th ed). Palo Alto: Scrub Hill Press, 1998:86].

D. Risk of cancer. Endometrial and ovarian cancer occur much less frequently in users of oral contraceptives (up to 40% reduction). The evidence from several large studies supports no increased risk of breast cancer in users. No good evidence has been shown that cervical cancer is more frequent in users.

E. Adverse effects include nausea, breast tenderness/enlargement, and spotting. Nausea may be offset by taking the pill with a meal or before bedtime or switching to a pill with decreased estrogen content. Breast tenderness and menses irregularity (spotting) usually subside within the first 3 months of beginning the pill. If spotting persists and/or becomes troublesome to the user, it is recommended that the pill be changed to one with a higher estrogen content.

F. Management. Start on the first Sunday of the cycle for monophasic and usually the first day of menses for multiphasics. The woman is protected from pregnancy after 5 days. If one pill is missed, take the missed pill as soon as possible. Take the next pill at the usual time. If two pills are missed during the first 2 weeks, take two pills as soon as possible, then two pills the next day. Return to the usual schedule but use a backup method that month. If three pills are missed any time during the month, start a new pack without a pill-free interval and use a backup method for at least 7 days. A backup method should consist of a barrier contraceptive such as a condom or diaphragm.

G. Emergency postcoital oral contraception. The appropriate candidate is a reproductive-aged woman within 72 hours of unprotected coitus or often with failure of barrier contraception. The safety of use has been confirmed in several large multicenter trials. The failure rate is less than 2%, and pregnancy rate is reduced by 75%. By 21 days after treatment, 98% of patients menstruate. The standard regimen is a combination pill that contains 0.05 mg ethinyl estradiol and 0.50 mg norgestrel (Ovral). Two pills are taken 12 hours apart. This may be offered with an antiemetic. Each dosage of the combination pill should contain at least 0.1 mg ethinyl estradiol and 1.0 mg norgestrel or levonorgestrel, and other alternatives include Lo-Ovral (4 white pills; repeat in 12 hours) and Triphasil/Trilevlen (4 yellow pills; repeat in 12 hours) [*Obstetrics, Gynecology and Infertility* (4th ed). Palo Alto: Scrub Hill Press, 1998:89].

H. Minipills contain only the hormone progestin and are taken daily like combined BCPs. These pills may be slightly less effective than combined oral contraceptives. They can decrease menstrual bleeding and cramps and lower the risk of endometrial and ovarian cancer and PID. Progestin-only pills are a good option for mothers who are breast-feeding, as the quantity and quality of breast milk should not be affected. They also are a good option for women with high BP or intolerance to estrogen.

II. Barrier contraception

A. **Diaphragm.** This provides a barrier to cervical entry by spermatozoa. It is a safe method with rare side effects. Urinary tract infections may occur two times as commonly. A decreased rate of sexually transmitted diseases (STDs) has been reported. A spermicide should be used with the diaphragm. Successful fitting, usually by a gynecologist, is crucial and must be assessed annually. The diaphragm can be inserted no longer than 6 hours before intercourse and can be removed 6–24 hours after intercourse.

B. **Cervical cap.** This has comparable effectiveness to the diaphragm. It may be more difficult to place. Four sizes are available. It should be used with spermicide and can remain in position for up to 36 hours without reapplication of spermicide. It can be inserted 20 minutes to 4 hours before intercourse.

C. **Condoms.** Use should be encouraged for individuals with multiple sex partners. Inconsistent use accounts for most failures, but failures may result from breaking or coming off during coitus. Oil-based lubricants should not be used with condoms, as the condom may become weak, causing it to break. Natural skin condoms do not protect against HIV and other STDs.

D. **Spermicides.** These have been proven to decrease the risk of STDs. They should be applied 10–30 minutes before coitus. It is recommended that another method be used, as there is a high failure rate [*Obstetrics, Gynecology and Infertility* (4th ed). Palo Alto: Scrub Hill Press, 1998:89].

E. **Female condom.** This was approved by the U.S. Food and Drug Administration in April 1993. It consists of a lubricated polyurethane sheath shaped similarly to the male condom. The closed end, which has a flexible ring, is inserted into the vagina, while the open end remains outside, partially covering the labia. It is available without a prescription and is intended for single use. It should not be used with a male condom because it may slip out of place.

III. Other hormonal contraception

A. **Norplant** is a subdermal implant system of long-acting, low-dose, reversible progestin (levonorgestrel). The mechanism of action is suppression of LH surge at the pituitary and hypothalamic level, thickening of cervical mucus, and suppression of endometrial maturation. Advantages are that Norplant is highly effective, rapidly reversible, can be used in patients who are unable to take estrogen, and compliance efforts are low. Disadvantages include irregular bleeding in up to 80% of patients, no reduction of STD risk, and the requirement of surgical insertion/removal. Absolute contraindications are active thromboembolic disease or thrombophlebitis, undiagnosed uterine bleeding, acute liver disease, benign or malignant liver tumors, and known or suspected breast cancer.

B. **Depo-Provera** is an injectable contraceptive, medroxyprogesterone acetate (150 mg), given every 3 months. The mechanism of action is similar to that of Norplant. Injection should be given within 5 days of menses for maximal effectiveness. The advantages are that it is highly effective, has less bleeding abnormalities but a higher rate of amenorrhea when compared to Norplant, and a minimization of user compliance. Disadvantages are a delay in return to fertility but no permanent effect, weight gain (5 lb/year), slight reversible bone loss, and the fact that the majority of women experience irregular and possible heavy bleeding for the first 3 months. Treatment of associated bleeding irregularity includes a trial with ibuprofen, 800 mg tid for 5 days, and if bleeding persists, a trial with ethinyl estradiol, 20 mg for 10–21 days; if bleeding persists, consider another method of contraception.

C. **Lunelle** is a newly approved monthly injectable contraceptive, a combination of medroxyprogesterone acetate (25 mg) and estradiol cypionate (5 mg) in suspension. It is reported to be as effective as BCPs, with a failure rate of less than 1%/year. Lunelle must be given within the first 5 days of the start of the normal menstrual period. It must be given monthly, every 28–30 days and no later than 33 days after the last injection. Side effects include irregular bleeding, weight gain of more than 10 lb, fluid retention, and breast pain/tenderness. Return to fertility may be slightly delayed.

IV. Other methods of contraception

  A. IUD. The mechanism of action is a sterile inflammatory reaction to a foreign body, and it primarily prevents fertilization. The copper-releasing Paragard T 380A is effective for 10 years. Candidates are parous women with no history of STD, PID, or ectopic pregnancy who are in a stable monogamous relationship. The U.S. Food and Drug Administration approved an IUD called **Mirena** that releases synthetic progestin-levonorgestrel over a period of 5 years. Amenorrhea and progestin-related adverse effects can occur [*Med Lett* 2001;43(1096):78].

  B. Tubal ligation requires gynecology expertise.

Vaginitis

The presence of vaginal discharge is not always abnormal. Symptoms are usually nonspecific. The vagina has 25 bacterial species, and pH is usually 4.0 due to lactobacilli. Semen, menses, and ectropion may alter the pH. Fifty percent of vaginitis is from bacterial vaginosis, 25% from *Trichomonas* vaginitis, and 25% from *Candida* vaginitis.

I. Bacterial vaginosis is characterized by malodorous vaginal discharge, with or without vaginal pruritus. Usually, there is no external genital irritation or dysuria. The discharge is a homogeneous, nonviscous, milky-white fluid that coats the vagina and cervix. It is thought to result from a polymicrobial alteration in the normal vaginal flora, a dramatic reduction in lactobacilli with marked increase in anaerobes, an overgrowth of *Gardnerella* species, or genital mycoplasmas. It may be cultured from 30–70% of healthy asymptomatic women.

  A. Diagnosis. The presence of "clue cells" (epithelial cells that have lost their sharp margins and have a granular appearance because of the adherence of bacteria over the surface) is an accepted criterion for diagnosis. The pH should be greater than 4.5. Another common test ("Whiff test") involves the amine (fishy) odor released when the vaginal discharge is alkalinized by mixing with 10% KOH (potassium hydroxide). No cultures are needed in clinical diagnosis.

  B. Treatment. Metronidazole is the most effective antimicrobial, with cure rates greater than 90%. Standard treatment is metronidazole, 500 mg PO bid for 7 days. Alternative treatments are metronidazole ER, 750 mg PO qd for 7 days; metronidazole, 2 g PO and repeat in 48 hours; and Metrogel, one application intravaginally every night for 5 nights. Patients should be advised to avoid alcohol consumption during treatment with metronidazole due to a possible disulfiram-type reaction. Alternatives are clindamycin cream 2% intravaginally for 7 nights or clindamycin, 300 mg PO bid for 7 days. The treatment of sexual partners remains controversial. *Gardnerella* vaginalis has been found in the urethra of more than 9% of male partners of affected women. No data about the effect of treatment of the partner are available. Some physicians prefer to treat partners only if bacterial vaginosis fails to respond or recurs. It is unknown if abstinence or condom use affects recurrences.

II. Trichomonas vaginitis. *Trichomonas vaginalis* is a contagious parasite that causes profuse, purulent, malodorous, sometimes foamy vaginal discharge. Pruritus may be present. The "strawberry cervix" caused by cervical petechiae is a characteristic manifestation. It is often found in the presence of other STDs. Many women (25–45%) are asymptomatic. pH greater than 4.5 and Whiff test may be positive. *T. vaginalis* may also cause urethritis in men.

  A. Diagnosis can be made by microscopic detection of motile trichomonads on examination of a saline wet prep or vaginal or urethral secretions. The slide should be examined soon after preparation to detect motility. Organisms are detected in 60–70% of infected women. The reliability of the Pap smear is quite variable.

B. Treatment. Standard treatment is single-dose metronidazole (2 g PO) or 500 mg PO bid for 7 days. Patients should be warned not to drink alcohol during the course of treatment. The cure rate is approximately 90%. Most physicians advocate treating all patients who have detectable organisms to reduce the sexual transmission of the organism. Treatment of male sexual partners of infected women is usually recommended.

III. Vulvovaginal candidiasis. This "yeast infection" is suggested by the presence of vulvovaginal soreness, dyspareunia, vulvar pruritus, external dysuria, and thick or "cheesy" vaginal secretions. Speculum examination may reveal candidal plaques adherent to the vaginal mucosa with erythema or edema of the introitus. The vaginal pH is usually less than 4.5. Factors that predispose to colonization and infection include diabetes, steroid therapy, pregnancy, antibiotics, obesity, BCPs, and immunosuppressant drugs. Ten to twenty percent of women normally have yeast colonized in the vagina; 75% of women have at least one episode of *Candida* vaginitis, and 45% have two or more episodes during their lifetime.

A. Diagnosis can be made by inspection of the typical vaginal lesions or by observation of fungal elements (budding yeast and pseudohyphae) in a KOH preparation. Cultures are not recommended. It is justifiable to treat an apparent or suspected candidal vulvitis even with a negative KOH prep (only 40–80% sensitive).

B. Treatment is with one of the imidazole antifungal drugs, such as miconazole, clotrimazole, butoconazole nitrate (Femstat), terconazole (Terazol), or ketoconazole (Nizoral), single dose to 3–7 days. Most come in cream or suppository for intravaginal use. If the woman is menstruating, she should not use tampons, which may absorb the drug. Single-dose fluconazole (Diflucan), 150 mg PO, is an expensive but very effective alternative. Treatment of asymptomatic male partners is not indicated except in some cases of recurrent candidiasis. Recurrent candidal infections are common and can be distressing. All predisposing factors should be addressed. Alternative treatment strategies include daily acidophilus versus acidophilus taken for 5 days beginning 1–2 days before menses, allowing the patient to self-diagnose and treat, monthly oral prophylactic treatment for 5 days beginning at menses, or continual oral daily or monthly prophylaxis.

Premenstrual Syndrome or Premenstrual Dysphoric Disorder

More than 200 signs and symptoms can be associated with premenstrual syndrome, and none is diagnostic. The symptoms are not an exacerbation of another underlying psychiatric disorder and interfere seriously with the quality of life.

I. Diagnosis must have at least one of the following: marked affective lability, depressed mood/feelings of hopelessness, marked anxiety, persistent and marked anger or irritability, and limited to 2 weeks before menses. The patient must have four other symptoms of depression, such as decreased interest, lethargy, difficulty in concentrating, marked changes in appetite, and a marked change in sleep. Premenstrual dysphoric disorder (PMDD) is distinguished from the much more common premenstrual syndrome by the pattern and severity of symptoms and the degree of impairment; symptoms must be severe enough to interfere with occupational and social functioning (Table 24-6) (*Primary Care in Obstetrics and Gynecology*. New York: Springer, 1998:462).

Table 24-6. Differential diagnosis of premenstrual syndrome and premenstrual dysphoric disorder

Endocrinologic

Hyperprolactinemia/panhypopituitarism

Adrenocorticotropic hormone–mediated disorders

Anorexia nervosa/bulimia

Thyroid disorders

Adrenal disorders

Pheochromocytoma

Hyperandrogenism

Gynecologic

Dysmenorrhea

Pelvic inflammatory disease

Endometriosis

Breast disorders

Perimenopause

Idiopathic edema

Psychiatric/psychological disorders

Unipolar affective disorders

Bipolar affective disorders

Anxiety neurosis

Personality disorders

Substance abuse

Psychosocial problems

Neurologic disorders

Migraine headaches

Seizure disorders

Other

Allergies

Chronic fatigue syndrome

Source: JS Sanfilippo, RP Smith. *Primary Care in Obstetrics and Gynecology.* New York: Springer, 1998:464, with permission.

II. **Treatment.** Recommendations include calcium, 1 g/day, and multivitamin; increased fiber, which offers some GI relief; mild diuretics, which may help with fluid retention; nonsteroidal anti-inflammatory drugs for dysmenorrhea and mastalgia; and BCPs. Consider serotonin selective reuptake inhibitors or buspirone. Use caution regarding benzodiazepines because of increased addictive potential. Fluoxetine and other serotonergic antidepressants taken continuously are effective in some women for treatment of PMDD. Limited data suggest that they might be effective even if taken only for the 2 weeks before menses.

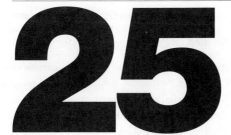

Men's Health

Jason S. Goldfeder,
Geoffrey S. Cislo, and
Michael E. Lazarus

Disorders in men's health range from life-threatening malignancies and organ-threatening emergencies to benign processes that primarily affect quality of life. Traditionally, many of these conditions have received little attention from primary care physicians because of limited understanding, embarrassment, and reluctance to initiate discussion on the part of both patients and physicians. Advances in pharmacologic therapy now allow primary care physicians to provide initial treatment, reserving urology referrals for men who fail therapy or have urgent indications.

Prostate Cancer Screening

Prostate cancer is the most common noncutaneous malignancy in men and is the second most common cause of cancer mortality after lung cancer. The introduction of available screening tests has led to intense debate and varying societal recommendations.

I. **The screening controversy.** Several conflicting arguments exist for and against routine screening for prostate cancer.
   A. **Epidemiology.** Approximately 200,000 new cases and 40,000 deaths are attributed to prostate cancer each year in the United States. However, prostate cancer primarily affects older men who will likely die of other causes, and it ranks last after nonmelanoma skin cancer in years of life lost/patient dying.
   B. **Stage shift.** Early detection and treatment are the only ways to decrease mortality, as prostate cancer is incurable once it has spread outside the capsule. Screening has increased the frequency of locally confined and potentially curable cancer at the time of diagnosis from 30% to 70%. Consequently, the 5-year survival rate for men with newly diagnosed prostate cancer has increased from 61% to 87% over approximately the last 30 years (*Cancer* 1997;80:1857). However, this early detection may be nothing more than a **lead-time bias**, as men who would otherwise never be diagnosed or have any sequelae of prostate cancer are having it detected earlier.
   C. **Screening tests** for prostate cancer (see sec. II) are readily available, inexpensive, easy to perform, and have little associated morbidity. However, the tests have limited sensitivity and specificity, and 25% of men older than 50 years have an abnormality on digital rectal examination (DRE) or prostate-specific antigen (PSA) testing that necessitates further invasive and expensive testing.
   D. **Potential benefits and risks of treatment.** The benefit of treatment in clinically localized prostate cancer has not been definitively proven. In men with well and moderately differentiated cancers, observation alone is associated with high prostate cancer–specific survival rates (*N Engl J Med*

Table 25-1. Processes that affect prostate-specific antigen (PSA) besides prostate cancer

Increase PSA	No effect on PSA	Decrease PSA
Age	Alpha-blocker therapy	Finasteride therapy
Benign prostatic hyperplasia	Cystoscopy	Prostate resection
Prostate biopsy	Routine digital rectal exam	
Prostatitis	Testosterone replacement	
Recent ejaculation	Urethral catheterization	
Urinary tract infection		
Vigorous prostate massage		

1994;330:242). The primary treatment modalities, radical prostatectomy and radiation therapy, are associated with significant rates of complications, including erectile dysfunction (ED), urinary incontinence, and urethral or rectal injury.

E. **Lack of proven efficacy.** No long-term prospective trial has proven that screening for prostate cancer decreases its morbidity or mortality. Multi-center prospective clinical trials are ongoing to assess the overall benefit of screening and the difference in outcome between initial surgery and observation in men with clinically localized prostate cancer. Because of the long-term nature of these trials, results are not expected until near 2010. Therefore, clinical controversy will likely continue for the next decade.

II. **Screening tests**

A. **An abnormal DRE** has a positive predictive value for cancer of 15–30% (*Ann Intern Med* 1997;126:480).

B. **PSA** is considered abnormal if it is greater than 4.0 ng/ml, but it is a continuum, as the risk of prostate cancer increases significantly even within the normal range. The sensitivity of this cutoff is 70–80%, but the specificity is low, as multiple conditions besides cancer can elevate PSA (Table 25-1). **A routine DRE does not clinically change the results of PSA testing** (*JAMA* 1992;267:2227). PSA values of 4–10 ng/ml and greater than 10 ng/ml have positive predictive values for cancer of 20–25% and 40–60%, respectively.

1. **PSA velocity,** the rate of change in PSA over time, is abnormal when greater than 0.75 ng/ml/yr. It is most reliable when determined at the same laboratory over at least 2 years.

2. **Percent free PSA,** the ratio of free circulating to bound PSA in serum, is lower in men with prostate cancer than in those with benign prostatic diseases. It is most useful in deciding which patients with a mildly elevated PSA (4–10 ng/ml) should undergo biopsy. An **upper cutoff of 25%** significantly decreases the number of false-positive biopsies while maintaining a high level of sensitivity (*JAMA* 1995;274:1214).

3. **PSA density,** the PSA divided by prostate volume, and **age/race-specific reference ranges** either require additional cost or have less clear benefit on cancer detection rates and are **not recommended.**

III. **Screening recommendations. The decision as to whether to screen for prostate cancer should be individualized,** as the lack of evidence from clinical trials has led the different major societies to have very different recommendations on screening. See Fig. 25-1 for a rational approach to prostate cancer screening.

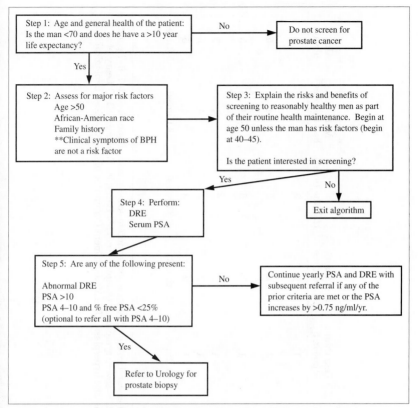

Fig. 25-1. Prostate cancer screening algorithm. BPH, benign prostatic hyperplasia; DRE, digital rectal examination; PSA, prostate-specific antigen.

Benign Prostatic Hyperplasia

Benign prostatic hyperplasia (BPH) occurs as a consequence of α-adrenergic–mediated stromal smooth-muscle contraction and glandular epithelial hyperplasia. Histologic evidence of BPH is found in 80% of patients (*J Urol* 1984;132:474), with clinical symptoms in 25–45% of men older than 70 years.

I. **Diagnosis and evaluation.** Patients with BPH classically have the triad of lower urinary tract obstructive and irritative symptoms, an enlarged prostate on DRE, and abnormal urodynamic testing. There is, however, no universally accepted definition or diagnostic criterion.

   A. **History and physical examination. The American Urological Association Symptom (AUAS) Index** (Fig. 25-2) is a questionnaire that should be administered to all men with BPH. The AUAS Index score is used to classify symptom severity, guide treatment recommendations, and follow response to therapy (AHCPR Publication No. 94-0582, 1994). The prostate should be palpated for nodules and an estimation of its size, with 40 ml the cutoff for a large prostate. Men with enlarged prostates are at increased

During the past month, how often have you…	Not at all	Less than 1 time in 5	Less than half the time	Half the time	More than half the time	Almost always
1. Had the sensation of not emptying your bladder completely after you finished urinating?	0	1	2	3	4	5
2. Had to urinate <2 hrs after you finished urinating?	0	1	2	3	4	5
3. Found you stopped and started several times when you urinated?	0	1	2	3	4	5
4. Found it difficult to postpone urination?	0	1	2	3	4	5
5. Had a weak urinary stream?	0	1	2	3	4	5
6. Had to push or strain to begin urination?	0	1	2	3	4	5
7. Typically needed to get up to urinate from the time you went to bed at night until the time you got up in the morning?	None	1 (time)	2 (times)	3 (times)	4 (times)	5 (times)

Fig. 25-2. American Urological Association Symptom Index. American Urological Association symptom score = sum of questions 1–7. 0–7 points = mild symptoms; 8–19 points = moderate symptoms; 20–35 points = severe symptoms. (Adapted from MJ Barry, FJ Fowler Jr, MP O'Leary, et al. The American Urological Association Symptom Index for benign prostatic hyperplasia. The Measurement Committee of the American Urological Association. *J Urol* 1992;148:1549.)

risk of experiencing complications and undergoing prostate surgery (*Urology* 1999;52:473).

B. Laboratory evaluation
1. **Urinalysis and serum BUN/creatinine** should be obtained to rule out infection and assess for complications (hematuria, renal insufficiency).
2. **PSA testing serves two potential purposes.**
   a. **Screening for prostate cancer is optional,** as its prevalence is not increased despite the fact that PSA is elevated in 25–30% of men with BPH. Percent free PSA testing should be considered in men with a PSA of 4–10 (see Prostate Cancer Screening, sec. **II.B.2**).
   b. **PSA is predictive of prostate size,** as PSA values of greater than 1.6, 2.0, and 2.3 correlate with 70% sensitivity and specificity to prostates greater than 40 ml in size in men in their 50s, 60s, and 70s, respectively (*Urology* 1999;53:581).
3. **Supplemental urodynamic testing and radiographic studies** are unnecessary in routine cases. Renal imaging (ultrasound or intravenous pyelography) should be performed in patients with complications such as hematuria, recurrent urinary tract infections (UTIs), or unexplained chronic renal insufficiency. Urodynamic testing (peak flow rate and pressure volume studies) should be reserved for patients with an unclear diagnosis, suspected neurogenic bladder dysfunction, or moderate to severe disease that fails to respond to initial therapy.

II. Treatment. The major factors to consider in determining the choice of therapy are the man's AUAS Index score and prostate size. Other factors to consider are his age, concomitant hypertension, current medications, sexual history, and the degree to which his symptoms are affecting his quality of life.
   A. Watchful waiting without treatment is recommended for patients with mild symptoms and is an option for those with moderate symptoms who are not too bothered. Patients should minimize evening intake of fluids and avoid medications with anticholinergic or sympathomimetic properties [including antihistamines, tricyclic antidepressants, or decongestants]. Many patients with mild symptoms have no change or improve without treatment.
   B. Pharmacologic therapy is recommended for patients with moderate symptoms who request treatment and for those with severe symptoms.
   1. **Terazosin and doxazosin are α_1-blockers** that relax smooth-muscle cells in the prostate and lead to a rapid dose-related improvement in symptoms. Symptomatic improvement is maintained with long-term therapy (*Urology* 1995;45:406), but α_1-blockers **do not** decrease prostate size, the rate of urinary retention, the need for surgery, or PSA. α_1-Blockers are effective in men with small and large prostates. These agents are good choices for men with concomitant hypertension that requires treatment. Terazosin and doxazosin decrease BP by approximately 10–15/10–15 mm Hg in men with elevated BP but have no clinically significant effect on BP in normotensive patients (*J Urol* 1997;157:525). Treatment is initiated at night with dose titration over 2–3 weeks to minimize side effects. **Terazosin** is titrated from $1 \rightarrow 2 \rightarrow$ 5 mg PO qhs and can subsequently be increased to 10–20 mg PO qhs. **Doxazosin** is titrated from $1 \rightarrow 2 \rightarrow 4$ mg PO qhs and can be subsequently increased to 8–16 mg PO qhs. Common side effects are dizziness, orthostatic hypotension, and fatigue.
   2. **Tamsulosin is a uroselective α_{1A}-blocker** with pharmacologic activity that is limited to the prostate without systemic effects on BP. It is a good choice for men who want rapid symptom relief but are prone to orthostasis. The dose is 0.4–0.8 mg PO qd, and dose titration and nocturnal dosing are unnecessary. Common side effects are ejaculatory problems and dizziness.
   3. **Finasteride is a 5α-reductase inhibitor** that reverses epithelial hyperplasia and shrinks the prostate by approximately 20–25%. Symptomatic

improvement is sustained long term, and it is the only drug that has been shown to decrease the rate of urinary retention and need for prostate surgery (*N Engl J Med* 1998;338:557). However, finasteride is **only effective in men with enlarged prostates greater than 40 ml in size** (*Urology* 1996;48:398). PSA can predict which patients are candidates for treatment with finasteride (see sec. **I.B.2.b**). The **symptomatic response to finasteride is delayed**, and 6–12 months are needed to achieve maximal symptomatic improvement. The dose is 5 mg PO qd. The only common side effects are sexual, including ED, decreased libido, and ejaculatory dysfunction. After 6 months of therapy, finasteride decreases PSA by approximately 50%. **PSA retains its ability to be used as a screening test for prostate cancer provided that the PSA value is doubled** (*Urology* 1998;52:195), whereas percent free PSA is unchanged by treatment.

   4. **Several different forms of herbal therapy**, including saw palmetto (*serenoa repens*), *pygeum africanum*, cernilton, and β-sitosterols, are available and self-prescribed by patients to treat BPH. These agents have been shown to be effective in the short term (*JAMA* 1998;280:1604), but their mechanism of action and long-term efficacy are unknown. **Saw palmetto** (160 mg PO bid) is the most commonly used herb in the United States.

   5. **Combination therapy** with an α_1-blocker and finasteride makes theoretical sense for men with large prostates and is frequently attempted but is of unproven efficacy. Although further studies are ongoing, combination therapy has not yet been shown to be more effective than alpha-blocker treatment alone (*N Engl J Med* 1996;335:533).

C. **Urologic referral**
   1. **Indications for referral to urology** include complications such as recurrent hematuria or UTIs, bladder stones, acute urinary retention and chronic renal insufficiency with hydronephrosis, moderate or severe symptoms that are refractory to medical therapy, a rectal examination or PSA suspicious for prostate cancer, and an unclear diagnosis when urodynamic testing may be helpful.
   2. **Transurethral resection of the prostate (TURP)** has a much greater benefit on reducing symptoms than medical therapy and remains the gold standard. TURP results in retrograde ejaculation and ED in a significant percentage of patients, and approximately 20% have unsatisfactory results and require further therapy. As TURP removes only central prostatic tissue, it does not eliminate the chance of developing prostate cancer.
   3. Several new **minimally invasive surgical procedures** have been introduced as alternatives to TURP.

Prostatitis

The prostatitis syndromes are classified by their acuity of presentation and findings on urinalysis and culture before and after prostatic massage. Only 5–10% of cases are due to bacterial causes (*Urology* 1997;49:809).

I. **Acute bacterial prostatitis**
   A. **Diagnosis.** Patients present with symptoms of a UTI (dysuria, frequency, urgency) and systemic symptoms such as fever, malaise, and lower-abdominal or back pain. The prostate is enlarged, warm, and tender, but **vigorous massage is contraindicated** to avoid causing bacteremia. Urinalysis and culture are positive, most often for *Escherichia coli* or other gram-negative organisms. An abdominal ultrasound or CT scan should be considered in men who do not respond to treatment to rule out a prostatic abscess.

Table 25-2. Diagnostic prostate massage results

Type of prostatitis	Prostate examination	Postmassage urinalysis	Postmassage culture
Acute bacterial (5%)	Warm, boggy, enlarged, tender	Vigorous massage contraindicated	Vigorous massage contraindicated
Chronic bacterial (5–10%)	Can be mildly tender and boggy or can be normal	Positive[a]	Positive[b]
Inflammatory chronic nonbacterial (50–60%)	Usually normal	Positive[a]	Negative
Noninflammatory chronic nonbacterial (prostatodynia) (30–40%)	Usually normal	Negative	Negative

[a]A positive urinalysis is >10–15 WBC/high-power field.
[b]A positive culture has a colony count that is at least 10-fold greater than the premassage culture.

   B. Treatment
   1. Patients typically **respond well to antibiotics, but prolonged courses are needed**. Potential regimens include trimethoprim-sulfamethoxazole, 1 DS tablet PO bid; doxycycline, 100 mg PO bid; ciprofloxacin, 500 mg PO bid; or levofloxacin, 500 mg PO qd for **4 weeks**. Severely ill patients with suspected bacteremia require admission for IV antibiotics.
   2. **Supportive care** with analgesics, stool softeners, and vigorous oral hydration may be beneficial.
   3. Patients with urinary retention who require drainage must have a suprapubic catheter placed, as urethral catheterization increases the risk of bacteremia.
 II. Chronic prostatitis syndromes (Table 25-2)
   A. History. Patients with the three chronic prostatitis syndromes present with similar symptoms, classically a triad of recurrent voiding symptoms, pain (pelvic, perineal, inguinal, back, penile, or scrotal), and ejaculatory symptoms (pain, hematospermia).
   1. Patients with **chronic bacterial prostatitis** are usually older, frequently have a history of recurrent UTIs, and may have a history of acute prostatitis.
   2. Patients with the two **chronic nonbacterial prostatitis syndromes** are often younger and do not have a history of recurrent UTIs. The predominant pain and predilection to occur in younger men distinguish it from BPH. Chronic nonbacterial prostatitis is the most common urologic diagnosis in men younger than 50 years of age.
   B. Diagnosis. The prostate examination is often normal in men with each of the chronic prostatitis syndromes. A diagnostic prostate massage comparing a midstream urine specimen with one after a vigorous prostate massage is the test of choice to correctly diagnose the three syndromes (Table 25-2).
   C. Treatment
   1. **Chronic bacterial prostatitis.** Prolonged courses of 8–12 weeks of antibiotics, preferably with a fluoroquinolone, are recommended. α_1-Blockers (see Benign Prostatic Hyperplasia, sec. **II.B.1–2**) may provide additional symptomatic relief. Patients with frequent recurrences require suppressive therapy with three times/week or daily

treatment with either ciprofloxacin, 100 mg PO qd, or trimethoprim-sulfamethoxazole, one single-strength tablet PO qd.

2. **Treatment of both types of chronic nonbacterial prostatitis is difficult** and often prolonged. Recommendations are based primarily on clinical experience, as controlled trial data is limited (*Ann Intern Med* 2000;137:367).

   a. Patients with **inflammatory chronic nonbacterial prostatitis** should receive a trial of 4–6 weeks of antibiotics (doxycycline, erythromycin, or a fluoroquinolone), with continuation for 12 weeks if improvement occurs because of anecdotal evidence that links the syndrome to atypical pathogens. Repetitive prostate massage two to three times/week, α_1-blockers, nonsteroidal anti-inflammatory drugs, and lifestyle changes (minimizing spicy foods, alcohol, and caffeine) may all be helpful.

   b. Treatment options for **noninflammatory chronic nonbacterial prostatitis (prostatodynia)** include α_1-blockers, nonsteroidal anti-inflammatory drugs, muscle relaxants such as diazepam, and anticholinergic agents (*Urology* 1998;51:362).

Erectile Dysfunction

ED is the **consistent** inability to attain or maintain an erection that is satisfactory for successful intercourse (*JAMA* 1993;270:83). Patients with isolated episodes of erectile failure should be reassured and do not require further evaluation or treatment. Prevalence increases with advanced age (*J Urol* 1993;151:54). ED frequently has a negative impact on quality of life in men who are too embarrassed to raise the issue with a physician.

I. **Diagnosis and evaluation**

A. **History and physical examination**

1. A detailed **sexual history** should assess the severity, onset, duration, progression, and situational nature of the problem to confirm that the patient has erectile failure and not a problem with libido or ejaculation. A gradual progressive onset of ED with absence of nocturnal or morning erections suggests an **underlying medical cause**. ED that develops suddenly is likely either **psychogenic** or due to a **medication**.

2. **Risk factors** for ED should be reviewed (Table 25-3).

3. The **physical examination** should assess for evidence of vascular or neurologic disease and stigmata of hypogonadism (small testicles, gynecomastia).

4. The **potential cardiovascular risk of intercourse** to the patient should be assessed, given the strong association between ED and coronary artery disease. Patients who can safely exercise to a level of 5 metabolic equivalents (see Chap. 2, Table 2-2) are at low risk for coronary ischemia during intercourse. Stress testing should be considered in sedentary men with multiple cardiac risk factors who cannot safely exercise to this level and in those with worrisome symptoms before the initiation of therapy or resumption of intercourse (*Circulation* 1999;99:168).

B. **Routine laboratory evaluation** should include serum glucose, renal function, and lipid analysis. Thyroid-stimulating hormone and liver function tests should be performed if the initial history or physical examination is suggestive of thyroid or liver disease.

C. **Routine testosterone assessment in patients with ED is controversial.** Hypogonadism is the cause of ED in 5–10% of patients, but only approximately one-third of these patients improve with testosterone replacement (*J Urol* 1997;158:1764). Testing with morning total and free serum testosterone is initially recommended only for patients with low libido or evi-

Table 25-3. Common risk factors for erectile dysfunction

Category	Examples
Vascular disease	Coronary artery disease, diabetes, hyperlipidemia, hypertension, peripheral vascular disease
Neurologic disorders	Multiple sclerosis, Parkinson's disease, spinal cord injury, stroke
Endocrine disorders	Hyperprolactinemia, hyperthyroidism, hypothyroidism, primary hypogonadism (testicular), secondary hypogonadism (CNS)
Chronic medical disorders	Chronic renal insufficiency, cirrhosis, COPD
Psychogenic	Anxiety disorder, depression, marital/relationship discord
Urologic disorders	Advanced prostate cancer, colorectal, bladder, or prostate surgery, pelvic trauma/fracture, Peyronie's disease, radiation therapy
Medications	Antihypertensives (especially thiazide diuretics, beta-blockers, clonidine), psychiatric medications (anticholinergics, MAO inhibitors, phenothiazines, SSRIs, TCAs), antiandrogens (cimetidine, digoxin, estrogens, finasteride, ketoconazole, LHRH agonists, spironolactone)
Illicit substances	Alcohol, amphetamines, cocaine, marijuana, opiates, tobacco

COPD, chronic obstructive pulmonary disease; LHRH, luteinizing hormone-releasing hormone; MAO, monoamine oxidase; SSRIs, selective serotonin reuptake inhibitors; TCAs, tricyclic antidepressants.

dence of hypogonadism. Testing should otherwise be deferred until patients have failed oral pharmacologic therapy. Abnormal initial testosterone levels should be repeated for confirmation along with serum luteinizing hormone, follicle-stimulating hormone, and prolactin to determine the source of hypogonadism.
   D. Urologic testing with nocturnal penile tumescence or vascular studies is unnecessary in the primary care setting.
II. Treatment
   A. General approach. In 80–90% of men, erectile function should be able to be restored with some form of therapy. Attempts should be made to improve uncontrolled risk factors, such as diabetes and hypertension, and to decrease the use of tobacco, alcohol, and other illicit substances. If possible, potentially contributing medications should be stopped or have their doses decreased.
   B. Reassurance may be curative in young men with psychogenic ED. Referral to a psychologist for **marital or couples counseling** may be helpful as an adjunctive form of therapy for psychogenic ED that has failed to respond to oral pharmacologic therapy.
   C. Sildenafil is a selective phosphodiesterase-5 inhibitor that potentiates the natural erectile response. **Sexual stimulation is required** for it to assist in an erection. It is effective in all forms of organic and psychogenic ED (*N Engl J Med* 1998;338:1397), but response rates are lower in patients with complete ED, diabetes, and after radical prostatectomy.
      1. Dosage and administration. Sildenafil should be taken **30–60 minutes before anticipated intercourse**. The usual starting dose is 50 mg PO prn. Men who are older than 65 years of age, have advanced renal (creatinine clearance <30) or liver disease, or who are taking cytochrome

P-450 CYP3A4 inhibitors should start at 25 mg PO prn. The dose can be increased to 100 mg PO prn, as efficacy is dose related, with an overall response rate of 65–80%. **Sildenafil should be taken no more than once/day.** It should initially be prescribed in small quantities (four to ten) tablets. Sildenafil should not be used in combination with other treatments for ED. **Sildenafil should not be prescribed to women.**
2. **Dose-related side effects** include headache, flushing, dyspepsia, diarrhea, nasal congestion, and visual disturbances. Sildenafil causes an equivalent small transient decrease in BP in normotensive patients and those who are receiving stable antihypertensive drug regimens (*Am J Cardiol* 1999;83:21C). **Sildenafil is absolutely contraindicated in patients who are taking or have access to any form of nitrates (oral, transdermal, sublingual) due to potentially fatal hypotension.** All forms of nitrates should be avoided for 24 hours after a dose of sildenafil. Sildenafil should be used with caution in men with a history of myocardial infarction, stroke or significant arrhythmia within 6 months, current unstable angina, poorly controlled heart failure or hypertension, and anatomic deformities of the penis.
D. **Yohimbine** is an α_2-blocker with limited efficacy, particularly in organic ED (*J Urol* 1996;156:2007). It must be taken continuously at a dose of 5.4 mg PO tid. Its use should be limited to patients with mild to moderate and primarily psychogenic ED who have contraindications to or intolerable side effects from sildenafil who decline more invasive forms of therapy. Yohimbine is the cheapest, but least effective, form of pharmacologic therapy.
E. **Testosterone replacement is only indicated for patients with documented hypogonadism.** Currently, there are no safe and effective oral forms of testosterone.
1. **Intramuscular injections** of **testosterone enanthate** or **testosterone cypionate** are initiated at dosages of 150–200 mg IM every 2–3 weeks.
2. **Testosterone patches** provide more physiologic doses of hormone replacement and are available as **Testoderm**, 4–6 mg applied qd to the shaved scrotum; **Testoderm TTS**, 5 mg; and **Androderm**, 2.5–7.5 mg applied daily to non–hair-bearing areas.
3. **Androgel**, 5–10 g/day, is a topical gel that is applied to dry areas.
F. **More invasive nonsurgical treatment options include intracorporeal and intraurethral injections of alprostadil and external vacuum constriction devices.** Intracorporeal injections and vacuum devices are very effective but suffer from high dropout rates. These forms of therapy should be deferred to a urologist unless the primary care physician has undergone appropriate training in the administration of these modalities, which require office-based patient education and training.
III. **Indications for referral to urology** include a history of pelvic trauma, abnormal genital examination, contraindications to or intolerable side effects from oral pharmacologic therapy, and failure of oral therapy in patients who wish to try a more invasive modality. Priapism is an indication for an emergent urology consult.

Testicular Masses

Patients with testicular masses may present with a painless lump or scrotal discomfort, ranging from a dull ache that worsens with exercise to severe testicular pain. Benign causes (sec. **II**) include fluid collections, infection (e.g., acute orchitis, focal or subacute orchitis, or postinflammatory scarring), infarction (idiopathic or secondary to torsion), and cysts. Malignant causes (sec. **III**) include primary testicular cancer and extratesticular malignancies such as leukemia or lymphoma. Patients may note masses spontaneously or through a regimen of testicular self-examination.

I. **Testicular examination**
   A. **Patients should be instructed in monthly self-examination of the testes.**
      The scrotum is most relaxed, and the testes most easily palpated, after a
      warm bath or shower. Using both hands, gently roll each testis between the
      thumb and first two fingers. Feel for hard fixed areas, lumps, and nodules. A
      normal testis is freely movable within the scrotum. Be consistent in your
      examination to notice any changes in size, shape, or firmness of the testi-
      cles. No matter how the mass is discovered, the duration of symptoms and
      related complaints should be ascertained. The physical examination can
      preliminarily differentiate the various etiologies of testicular masses.
   B. **The testes** should be palpated for masses, volume, tenderness, and cryp-
      torchidism. A testicle that is less than 4 cm long is considered small. All
      masses and swellings should be transilluminated. Solid tumors do not trans-
      mit light, whereas a hydrocele glows a soft red color. If a testicle cannot be
      palpated within the scrotum, the inguinal canals and lower abdomen should
      be examined.
   C. **The epididymis, spermatic cord, and vas deferens** are examined next. The
      epididymis is located posterior to the testicle. Have the patient perform the
      Valsalva maneuver while standing. Feel for a mass of dilated testicular veins
      in the spermatic cord, forming a varicocele above and behind the testis.
   D. The **inguinal canals** should be explored for hernias or cord tenderness.
      Inflammation of the cord structures can cause inguinal or scrotal pain, with
      a normal testis.
   E. Evaluate men for the presence of **gynecomastia**, as 30% of Leydig cell
      tumors produce testosterone, which is converted to estrogen. Rarely, testic-
      ular tumors present with disseminated disease, such as supraclavicular lym-
      phadenopathy or abdominal masses from retroperitoneal lymph node
      spread or as a result of a tumor that arises within an undescended intra-
      abdominal testis.
II. **Benign causes of testicular masses**
   A. A **hydrocele** is a collection of peritoneal fluid between the parietal and vis-
      ceral layers of the tunica vaginalis, surrounding the testicle. A communicat-
      ing hydrocele allows peritoneal fluid to pass between the peritoneal cavity
      and the layers of the tunica vaginalis. A noncommunicating hydrocele rep-
      resents an imbalance in the secretory and absorptive capacities of the layers
      of the tunica vaginalis. This is most often due to injury or infection with
      resultant inflammatory reaction. A hydrocele may also accompany a testicu-
      lar neoplasm or torsion.
      1. **History.** Men present with a painless scrotal swelling that can be trans-
         illuminated. The swelling may be small and soft on awakening but
         worsens during the day, becoming large and tense.
      2. **Management** may require aspiration of the fluid to be able to palpate
         the testis carefully. A scrotal ultrasound should always be considered if
         the diagnosis is in question, as a reactive hydrocele may occur with a
         testicular neoplasm. Generally, no therapy is needed except in the set-
         ting of either discomfort from a bulky mass or a tense hydrocele, which
         decreases circulation to the testis. Tense or uncomfortable hydroceles
         should always be aspirated.
   B. A **varicocele** is an abnormal tortuosity and dilation of the pampiniform
      venous plexus and internal spermatic vein. Varicoceles are found in 20% of
      men and are usually asymptomatic. It constitutes the most common surgi-
      cally correctable cause of male factor infertility (30% of infertile men).
      1. **Evaluation.** Most varicoceles occur on the left side as the left testicular
         vein drains into the left renal vein, whereas the right testicular vein
         drains directly into the large inferior vena cava. Patients generally
         report a mass that lies posterior to and above the testis. The sudden
         onset of a left-sided varicocele in an elderly man may be indicative of a
         renal cell carcinoma and should be evaluated with a renal ultrasound.

Sudden development of a right-sided varicocele may occur with inferior vena cava obstruction. The venous dilation is commonly decreased when the patient is supine and increases when he is upright. Examine the patient in both positions. Have him perform the Valsalva maneuver when standing, which accentuates the dilation. Classically, one feels a "bag of worms" above the testicle.

2. **Management.** Not all varicoceles are associated with infertility, and not all need to be corrected. If the patient has an abnormal semen analysis and is infertile, or if the patient is symptomatic with a dull ache or feeling of heaviness in the testicle, the varicocele should be treated. Therapy consists of surgical ligation or sclerotherapy of the pampiniform plexus.

C. A **spermatocele** is a painless cystic mass separate from the testis. Spermatoceles are typically located superior and posterior to the testis, freely movable, and transilluminate easily. Aspiration of the contents usually reveals dead sperm. No treatment of the mass is indicated unless it becomes bothersome.

III. **Malignant testicular masses**

A. **Primary testicular cancer.** A painless testicular mass is pathognomonic of a primary testicular tumor but only occurs in a minority of patients. Most present with diffuse testicular pain, swelling, hardness, or some combination of these findings. Because infectious epididymitis or orchitis is more common than a tumor, a trial of antibiotics is often undertaken. If testicular discomfort does not abate or findings do not revert to normal within 2–4 weeks, a testicular ultrasound is indicated. Testicular cancer accounts for only 1% of all cancers in men but is the most common cancer in men 15–34 years of age. A significantly increased number of testicular cancers are found in patients with cryptorchidism, with neoplasms developing in the undescended and the contralateral descended testis [*N Engl J Med* 1997;337(4):242].

B. **Evaluation.** Physical examination and history may help generate a hypothesis as to the etiology of a testicular mass. The following **tumor markers** may be useful in supporting a diagnosis.

1. **α-Fetoprotein** (α-FP) is produced by nonseminomatous germ cell tumors (embryonal carcinomas and yolk sac tumors). An elevated α-FP may be seen at any stage, although 40–60% of patients with metastases have increased serum concentrations.

2. **β-Human chorionic gonadotropin** is increased in seminomatous and nonseminomatous tumors. Elevations occur in 40–60% of patients with metastatic nonseminomatous germ cell tumors and 15–20% of patients with metastatic seminomas.

3. **Lactic dehydrogenase** elevation is nonspecific but has prognostic value in patients with advanced germ cell tumors. It is increased in 60% of patients with nonseminomatous germ cell tumors and 80% of those with seminomatous germ cell tumors.

4. **Imaging.** Testicular **ultrasound** is a highly reliable way of differentiating intratesticular from extratesticular lesions and should be the initial imaging study of choice. Germ cell tumors are typically intratesticular and may produce one or more hypoechoic masses or show diffuse abnormalities with microcalcifications. **CT scans and MRI** demonstrate a mass that is relatively isointense to the surrounding normal testicular parenchyma on T1-weighted images and exhibits brisk and early enhancement after IV gadolinium.

C. **Management** should be with urologic consultation. For lesions that are likely malignant, a radical orchiectomy with ligation of the spermatic cord at the internal ring is required. The primary lymphatic and vascular drainage of the testis is to the retroperitoneal lymph nodes and the renal or great vessels, respectively. Therefore, direct testicular biopsy through the scrotum is contraindicated. The staging workup includes CT scans of the abdomen and pelvis and a chest x-ray. Lesions that are likely benign are followed by serial physical examination and imaging.

D. **Testicular mass with extratesticular malignancy.** Lymphomas and leukemia are the most common extratesticular malignancies to involve the testicles. Lymphoma accounts for 1–7% of all testicular tumors and is a frequent cause of testicular enlargement in men older than 50 years of age. Involvement is bilateral in 50% of cases either simultaneously or successively. Leukemic infiltration (50% have bilateral involvement) is usually seen in children, as the testis is the most common site of relapse of acute leukemia. Gray-scale sonography of lymphomatous and leukemic testicular involvement reveals diffuse or multifocal decreased echogenicity, which can be more subtle and ill defined than the typical well-circumscribed hypoechoic mass of primary testicular cancer.

Priapism

Priapism is a prolonged (>6 hours), usually painful, penile erection that is not initiated by sexual stimuli. It results from a disturbance in the normal regulatory mechanisms that initiate and maintain penile flaccidity.

I. **Low-flow, or ischemic, priapism** is due to decreased penile venous outflow. The etiology includes sickle cell disorders, tumor infiltrates, and oral or injected medications. It can also be idiopathic.

II. **High-flow, or arterial, priapism** produces painless, persistent semirigid to rigid erections that may still increase in tumescence in response to sexual stimuli. It results from increased arterial inflow into the cavernous sinusoids, which overwhelms venous outflow. The etiology is usually groin or straddle trauma that causes injury to the internal pudendal artery or its branches. This establishes a direct arterial-to-cavernous shunt that bypasses the normally regulatory helicine arteries.

III. **Management.** Patients with priapism should be emergently managed in consultation with a urologist. Therapeutic options range from local infiltration of β agonists to surgical intervention.

Androgenetic Alopecia

Androgenetic alopecia is a hereditary thinning of the hair that is induced by androgens in genetically susceptible men. It is also known as **male pattern hair loss** or **common baldness**. Thinning of the hair usually begins between 12 and 40 years of age, and approximately half the population expresses this trait to some degree before the age of 50 years. The pattern of inheritance is polygenic. The onset is gradual, and the condition slowly develops over years. **Topical minoxidil** is a potassium channel opener and vasodilator; in vitro, it is able to increase survival time and delay senescence of cultured keratinocytes. After topical application, minoxidil increases the duration of the anagen phase, leading to production of hairs that are progressively thicker and longer. Minoxidil lotion 2% or 5%, 1 ml, should be applied twice/day to the affected scalp. Twice-daily application has no systemic side effects. The percentage of patients who show cosmetically acceptable hair regrowth after 1 year ranges from 40% to 60%, depending on patient selection. Patients are more likely to respond to minoxidil treatment if they have vertex baldness with a diameter smaller than 10 cm and alopecia of less than 5 years' duration. Minoxidil seems to be poorly effective in the frontotemporal region. Adverse effects include allergic contact dermatitis and reversible hypertrichosis. **Oral minoxidil** provides no added benefit over topical minoxidil, and in view of the potential side effects, it should not be used. Helpful references include *BMJ* 1998;317:865, *N Engl J Med* 1999;341:964, and *J Am Acad Dermatol* 1998;39:578.

   I. **Medical treatment** includes topical and systemic agents (see also Chap. 26, sec. **XIV**).

   II. **Surgical options** including hair transplantation, scalp flaps, and excision of bald scalp with or without tissue expansion are options to treat advanced androgenetic alopecia.

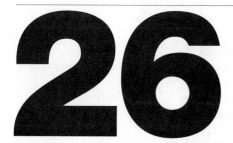

Dermatology

Michael P. Heffernan

Any compromise to the skin and its functions can lead to disfigurement, discomfort, and/or disability. Each year in the United States, a skin problem develops in one in three people. Of outpatient visits to physicians, 10% are for a skin disorder, and two-thirds of these visits are to nondermatologists. Skin disease accounts for 5% of inpatient admissions. Skin signs are also a valuable diagnostic and prognostic marker of internal disease.

Skin disorders often cause temporary or permanent disfigurement and social distress; patients often benefit from education and social support. Support foundations for patients with skin disorders can be accessed through the American Academy of Dermatology (888-462-3376 or **http://www.aad.org**).

Ask your patients to disrobe and put on a gown. Very few patients are embarrassed or bothered by this, and most people expect to put on a gown when they go to the doctor. Approach patients with the assumption that everything you see on the skin is pathology, and try to convince yourself why it should not be biopsied.

The American Cancer Society recommends that everyone be educated in the ABCDs (asymmetry, border irregularity, colors, diameter), practice monthly skin checks, and have total body skin examinations performed by their physician every 3 years from age 20 years to 40 years and yearly after age 40 years.

I. **Approach to the dermatologic diagnosis.** The key to selecting the appropriate dermatologic therapy lies in making the correct diagnosis.
   A. **Classify lesion** (Table 26-1)
   B. **Problem-oriented dermatologic algorithm** (Appendix 26-1)
   C. **Problem-oriented disease groups** (Appendix 26-1 and 26-2)

II. **Office microscopy.** Timely clinical information can be obtained through three simple office microscopic tests. These techniques are best learned through repetition.
   A. **Potassium hydroxide (KOH) prep.** Anything that scales may be tinea. The scales are collected in the center of a microscope slide; one drop of 10–20% KOH ± dimethyl sulfoxide (DMSO) is added, and a coverslip is placed. One should scan at 4–10× for the presence of hyphae, which is diagnostic of a dermatophyte infection. The presence of short "pseudohyphae" and spores is pathognomonic for yeast, especially useful for diagnosing tinea versicolor. Tinea capitis can be confirmed by KOH identification of spores within (endothrix) or around (ectothrix) the hair follicle. Dermatophyte infection can also be confirmed by a fungal culture, which grows in 1–6 weeks.
   B. **Tzanck prep.** Anything that blisters may be herpes; either herpes simplex virus (HSV) or varicella-zoster virus (VZV). Clean the vesicle with an alcohol swab. Unroof the vesicle, push aside the fluid, scrape the base, and apply to a microscope slide. Allow to air dry for 1 minute; apply Giemsa, Wright, or Tzanck stain for 1 minute; gently rinse; and apply a coverslip. Scan at 4–10× for multinucleated giant cells and acidophilic intranuclear inclusions. HSV and varicella infection can be confirmed by direct fluorescent antibody testing, which provides results in 2–24 hours, or by viral culture, which grows in 1–2 days for HSV and 5–7 days for VZV. Specimens for direct fluorescent antibody and viral culture are obtained from the vesicle base.

Table 26-1. Lesion classification

Primary lesions are induced by disease

Macule	<1-cm area of circumscribed color change, not palpable
Patch	>1-cm macule
Papule	<1-cm palpable mass
Plaque	>1-cm papule
Nodule	>1-cm spherical papule
Vesicle	<1-cm fluid-filled papule
Bulla	>1-cm fluid-filled papule
Pustule	Pus-filled papule
Wheal	Edematous papule or plaque

Secondary lesions are induced by the patient

Excoriation	Linear erosions
Lichenification	Skin thickening, hyperpigmentation, and accentuated skin markings

---

C. **Scabies prep.** Anything that itches may be scabies. The majority of mites are found in decreasing order at the hands, wrists, elbows, genitalia, buttocks, and axillae. Identify a burrow(s), apply a drop of mineral oil, and scrape away the epidermis. Apply the scraped material on a microscope slide and examine under low power for mites, ova, or scybala (feces). Examination of multiple burrows increases the diagnostic yield.

III. **Dermatologic therapies.** Skin disorders are characterized by pruritus, inflammation, alterations in hydration, and susceptibility to irritation. Identification and treatment of specific underlying conditions always should be attempted.

A. **Dry skin care.** Almost all itchy skin conditions are improved by the following regimen: short (<5 minutes) cool baths or showers, using mild nondrying soaps (Dove, Oil of Olay, Cetaphil). Pat the water off. Do not scratch or rub. Apply medications only to the area of dermatitis 1–2 times/day. Apply thick moisturizers (Vaseline or Aquaphor ointments; Eucerin or Cetaphil creams; Keri or Lubriderm lotions) as often as needed.

B. **Wet skin care.** Excessive moisture in intertriginous areas requires careful drying followed by application of a powder or dry dressing of absorptive material. In severe cases with maceration, exudation, and erosion, drying dressings such as Domeboro's should be applied. The skin surfaces should be kept separated with absorptive materials.

C. **Antipruritics.** Pruritus and burning can lead to uncontrolled scratching and can perpetuate an underlying condition. Topical agents can be used to control symptoms. Camphor 1–3% and menthol provide a cooling sensation. Phenol 0.25–2.00% causes local hypoesthesia; it is not to be used on raw or ulcerated skin. Topical anesthetics (benzocaine), antihistamines [diphenhydramine (Benadryl)], and neomycin are best avoided due to a high rate of contact dermatitis. Systemic antihistamines (H_1-receptor antagonists) are most useful in the treatment of urticaria but are also helpful in pruritic skin disorders.

D. **Protection.** Cotton and rubber gloves can be used to avoid excessive contact with water or chemical irritants. Cotton absorbs palmar sweat and should be cleaned or changed frequently. Barrier creams and ointments may prevent contact of irritating chemicals with sensitive skin but are not substitutes for mechanical barriers.

Table 26-2. Commonly used topical glucocorticoids

Low strength
    Hydrocortisone 1%, 2.5% (class 7)
    Desonide 0.05% (class 6)
Medium strength
    Fluocinolone acetonide 0.025% (class 5)
    Triamcinolone acetonide 0.1% (class 4)
High strength
    Fluocinonide 0.05% (class 2)
Highest strength
    Betamethasone dipropionate 0.05% (class 1)
    Clobetasol propionate 0.05% (class 1)

Note: Class 6–7 is indicated for facial use. Class 1–5 is indicated for palmar/plantar areas or severe/resistant lesions.

    E. Topical steroids (Table 26-2)
        1. Base. Ointments and creams are more lubricating than gels, lotions, and solutions. Ointments are more occlusive and therefore more potent. A lubricating ointment is best for dry dermatitis, whereas a cream would be more appropriate for a weeping dermatitis. Lotions, gels, and solutions are easy to use in hairy areas, including the scalp.
        2. Strength. Lower-strength (class 6–7) topical steroids are indicated for facial use. Higher-strength (class 1–5) topical steroids are used for palmar/plantar areas or for severe/resistant lesions. Topical steroids can cause skin atrophy, striae, and suppression of the pituitary-adrenal axis. Side effects tend to occur with repeated application or application to the face, neck, axillae, perineum, or inframammary folds. Accurate diagnosis obviates the need for combination agents such as Lotrisone (a weak azole antifungal and a high-strength topical steroid).
        3. Dosage. Applications should be performed bid. When a cream or ointment is used, 1 g covers the face and 30 g covers the body of an adult.
        4. Occlusion. Occlusion with plastic wrap increases the potency of the products but should be reserved for severe resistant lesions. Occlusion increases the risk for side effects and folliculitis.
    F. Skin cancer prevention (see sec. **XXVIII**)
IV. Dermatitis
    A. Contact dermatitis is an inflammatory cutaneous reaction caused by direct cutaneous exposure to an irritant or allergic substance.
        1. Irritant contact dermatitis accounts for 80% of cases. This is a nonallergic reaction of the skin due to chemical or physical agents. Mild irritants require repeated or prolonged contact to cause dermatitis (e.g., soaps, detergents, and solvents). Irritant dermatitis produces erythema and blisters with oozing that later evolve into a dry, thickened fissured pattern. Strong irritants can cause dermatitis following a single exposure (e.g., strong acids or alkali), and blistering, erosion, and ulceration can develop.
        2. Allergic contact dermatitis accounts for 20% of cases. This is a form of delayed hypersensitivity (type IV reaction) that develops in sensitized individuals. Mild dermatitis produces redness, vesiculation with oozing, and crusting. More severe reactions produce edematous and vesiculobullous reactions. The distribution and pattern of the dermatitis provide the chief clue to the diagnosis and may suggest the offending

source. Patch testing may identify the offending allergen. Among the common sources of allergens are

  a. Plants (e.g., *Rhus*: poison ivy, poison oak): vesicular dermatitis with a distinctly linear pattern

  b. Metals (nickel, chrome): produce dermatitis under watchbands, jewelry, clasps, or hooks on clothes, etc.

  c. Rubber: shoes, elastic waistbands, gloves, condoms, etc.

  d. Topical medications: neomycin, benzocaine, ophthalmic preparations

  e. Cosmetics: hair dyes, perfumes and fragrances, formaldehyde-containing preservatives in makeup, mascara, lipstick, etc.

  f. Other: adhesives, printing inks, antibacterials in cutting oils, etc.

  3. Mild dermatitis is treated with topical steroids, topical/systemic antipruritics, and avoidance of the offending chemical or allergen. Severe, disabling blistering reactions are treated with prednisone, 0.5–1.0 mg/kg tapered over 10–21 days, antipruritics, and drying agents.

B. Chronic dermatitis (e.g., atopic or stasis dermatitis, dyshidrotic eczema) is characterized by lichenification, scaling, intense pruritus, and hyperpigmentation. Scratching worsens it. Effective therapy includes emolliation, reduction of pruritus, and control of inflammation. Frequent use of emollients, systemic antihistamines, and topical steroid ointments are beneficial. Successful treatment of stasis dermatitis requires reduction of lower-extremity edema. Systemic steroids reduce symptoms for the chronic dermatitides, but these are best avoided, as the symptoms return and often flare with weaning of the systemic steroids.

C. Seborrheic dermatitis is more severe in patients with HIV or Parkinson's disease. In adults, erythema with fine white or greasy scale is seen on the scalp (dandruff), eyebrows, eyelids, nasolabial folds, ears, sternal area, axillae, inframammary folds, and perineum. Antiseborrheic shampoos, such as selenium sulfide, zinc pyrithione, tar, or 2% ketoconazole, are used at least every other day for 10–15 minutes. For the face or trunk, ketoconazole cream or 1.0–2.5% hydrocortisone cream bid is used.

V. Psoriasis is characterized by erythematous plaques with silvery scale on elbows, knees, scalp, and trunk with nail pitting and arthritis that may progress to generalized erythroderma. Psoriasis tends to worsen with lithium, beta-blockers, and after systemic steroids. Guttate psoriasis is characterized by small erythematous papules on the trunk associated with strep throat; it may respond to penicillin or amoxicillin.

A. Mild to moderate psoriasis is treated topically with emolliation (see sec. **III.A**), topical steroids (see sec. **III.E**), calcipotriene (Dovonex), tazarotene (Tazorac), tar derivatives, or ultraviolet B (UVB). Calcipotriene and tazarotene are more expensive than topical steroids but less likely to cause skin atrophy and tachyphylaxis. Calcipotriene, a vitamin D_3 analogue, can cause hypercalcemia if it is used on more than 10% of the body. Tazarotene, a synthetic retinoid, can cause burning, erythema, and desquamation.

B. Scalp psoriasis is treated topically with tar shampoo and steroid solutions. Prominent scale needs to be removed before other treatments will work.

C. Severe psoriasis may require phototherapy or systemic agents (methotrexate, acitretin, cyclosporine). This therapy is for patients who are incapacitated by their disease and resistant to less toxic forms of treatment. It is best provided under the care of a dermatologist.

VI. Pityriasis rosea is characterized by thin atrophic pink papules, minimal trailing scale, and a Christmas tree distribution. The herald patch is a larger pink plaque with atrophic center. Pityriasis rosea is mildly pruritic and resolves in 6–12 weeks. Treatment includes sunlight, phototherapy, topical steroids, and antipruritics.

VII. Lichen planus is characterized by pruritic, purple, polygonal papules that favor the volar wrists, ankles, and genitals. Wickham's striae or erosions are found on the buccal mucosa. Occasionally, lichen planus is associated with hepatitis and angiotensin-converting inhibitors. Treatment is with topical steroids, occlusion when possible, emolliation, and antipruritics.

VIII. **Thermal burns.** A dermatitis of varying intensity may be caused by the action of excessive heat on the skin. If the heat is extreme, the skin and underlying tissue may be destroyed.

   A. A **first-degree burn** congests superficial blood vessels, causing erythema that may be followed by desquamation (e.g., sunburn). Treatment includes prompt cold application and emolliation.

   B. A **second-degree burn** causes edema and vesicles. Treatment includes prompt cold application and emolliation. Vesicles should not be opened unless they are tense and painful, when drainage under aseptic technique is recommended.

   C. A **third-degree burn** causes full-thickness necrosis of the skin. Severe second- and third-degree burns benefit from specialized teams of physicians. Third-degree burns require skin grafting and heal with scarring.

IX. **Ulcers**

   A. Of **leg ulcers**, 90% are the result of venous insufficiency, 5% result from arterial disease, and 5% are due to miscellaneous causes, including diabetic microangiopathy, pyoderma gangrenosum, malignancies, and infections. Diagnosis of the miscellaneous causes is often aided by skin biopsy.

   B. **Venous ulcers** tend to occur on the lower medial aspect of the legs in areas of preceding stasis dermatitis. Treatment aims to improve venous return with leg elevation and compression hose. Wet-to-dry dressings provide excellent débridement for 2–3 days, but longer use can interfere with wound healing. Most wounds improve with being kept clean, covered, and moist. This is often best achieved with occlusive dressings.

   C. **Arterial ulcers** tend to occur over the lateral malleolus and are often painful. Treatment includes local wound care and improving arterial blood flow.

X. **Blistering disorders**

   A. **Pemphigus vulgaris** is characterized by flaccid bullae that break easily, leaving denuded areas that increase in size by progressive peripheral detachment. Oral lesions are almost always present and may be the first manifestation. Before corticosteroids became available, the mortality of this disease was 80%. **Pemphigus foliaceus** is characterized by flaccid bullae that usually arise on an erythematous base and superficial erosions that may accumulate thick scales. Oral lesions tend not to occur. Pemphigus foliaceus has a better prognosis than pemphigus vulgaris. **Both diagnoses** are made by skin biopsy with direct immunofluorescence, indirect immunofluorescence. **Treatment** is prednisone, 1–2 mg/kg/day, or alternatively, steroid-sparing agents, such as gold, cyclophosphamide, azathioprine, and mycophenolate mofetil.

   B. **Bullous pemphigoid** is characterized by large tense bullae that leave denuded areas. It occasionally presents as urticarial or dermatitic plaques and often occurs in elderly patients. It has a better prognosis than pemphigus. Pemphigoid gestationis characteristically occurs during pregnancy and presents on distended abdominal skin. **Diagnosis** is made by skin biopsy with direct immunofluorescence, indirect immunofluorescence. **Treatment options** are systemic steroids, topical steroids, steroid-sparing agents, tetracycline, and niacinamide.

   C. **Dermatitis herpetiformis** presents with markedly pruritic, eroded, and crusted papules and vesicles that are symmetrically distributed on the extensor elbows, knees, and buttocks. It presents in the second or third decade. Many patients have gluten-sensitive enteropathy (celiac disease). **Diagnosis** is made by skin biopsy with direct immunofluorescence. **Treatment** options include a gluten-free diet, which may be effective, but strict adherence is required. Dapsone, 50–150 mg/day, is another option.

   D. **Erythema multiforme** is an acute, self-limited, often recurrent eruption characterized by "targetoid" lesions of the skin (erythema multiforme minor). It favors the palms and soles. Erythema multiforme is strongly associated with

HSV, *Streptococcus*, *Mycoplasma*, or other infections. **Diagnosis** is made by skin biopsy. **Treatment** consists of symptomatic and supportive care.
  E. **Stevens-Johnson syndrome** presents with a flu-like prodrome, skin sloughing, and mucous membrane erosions of the mouth, eyes, genitalia, and lips with hemorrhagic crusts. It has a strong association with medications: penicillins, sulfonamides, phenytoin, allopurinol, and trimethoprim-sulfamethoxazole. **Diagnosis** is made by skin biopsy. **Treatment** consists of elimination of suspected drugs and supportive care. Systemic steroids are controversial and may contribute to secondary infections.
  F. **Toxic epidermal necrolysis** presents with a flu-like prodrome that is **rapidly** followed by skin pain, exanthem or targetoid lesions, and widespread skin sloughing. It is strongly associated with medications: penicillins, sulfonamides, phenytoin, allopurinol, trimethoprim-sulfamethoxazole. Mortality is 20–25%. **Diagnosis** is made by skin biopsy. **Treatment** includes elimination of suspected drugs; supportive care with maintenance of fluid and electrolyte balance (often in the burn unit); and prevention of secondary infections. Systemic steroids are controversial and may contribute to secondary infections, and there have been case reports of cyclosporine or IV immunoglobulin being helpful.
XI. **Insect bite reactions** (see Chap. 12)
  A. Reactions to insect bites are usually triggered by a toxin or an allergen injected into skin by the offending arthropod.
    1. **Bees, wasps, and yellow jackets.** A normal response consists of a painful red wheal with central punctum; the wheal fades in hours. A persistent local reaction with intense swelling around the bite area may arise. In individuals with immediate systemic allergy, anaphylaxis may develop. Rarely, affected persons may manifest a delayed systemic allergic reaction that shows up as urticaria, polyarthritis, and lymphadenopathy.
    2. **Ants.** Fire ant stings produce wheals with two hemorrhagic puncta; they usually evolve into pustules within hours.
    3. **Mosquitoes.** Pruritic wheals develop within hours of the bite.
    4. **Fleas** produce grouped urticarial papules, some with puncta, frequently on the legs.
  B. **Treatment**
    1. If insects are **attached to the skin**, they should be flicked (not squeezed) off the skin. Alternatively, they can be removed with fine forceps.
    2. **Ticks** are best removed by grasping them as close to the skin as possible with forceps and with a steady upward pull. Protect the hands by wearing gloves to avoid contamination by infectious organisms. Do not "squeeze" the tick or apply hot matches, nail polish, and so forth. Clean the wound with soap, water, or mild disinfectant solution. The patient should report fever or unusual rashes to a physician.
    3. Ice, cold compresses, and phenolated calamine lotion are **soothing agents**.
    4. **Topical steroids and oral antihistamines** may be useful for itching and inflammation.
    5. **Anaphylactic reactions** require emergency treatment (see Chap. 12).
XII. **Drug reactions** (see Chap. 12)
XIII. **Urticaria** (see Chap. 12)
XIV. **Hair disorders.** The number of hairs on the normal scalp is 100,000. The average daily loss of hairs from the scalp is 100.
  A. **Alopecia**
    1. **Scarring alopecia** occurs when hair follicles are scarred and hair loss from it is permanent. Causes include:
      a. Infections: bacterial, fungal (tinea capitis), and viral
      b. Neoplasms (primary and metastatic)
      c. Physical and chemical agents
      d. Autoimmune disorders [discoid lupus erythematosus (DLE), lichen planopilaris]

2. **Nonscarring alopecia.** The follicular unit remains viable and hair regrowth may resume

   a. **Androgenetic alopecia** (see Chap. 25) has a genetic predisposition, with an interaction between circulating androgens and androgen receptors in hair follicles. Vellus hairs gradually replace terminal hairs. Androgenic alopecia affects 25% of patients older than 25 years of age and 50% older than 50 years of age. Male pattern usually begins with bitemporal recession. Female pattern is usually more diffuse, with sparing of the frontal hairline. Men can be treated with 1 ml 5% minoxidil (Rogaine) bid or 1 mg finasteride (Propecia) daily. These agents cause some hair regrowth but are more effective at preventing further hair loss. Hair loss rapidly returns to normal on discontinuation. In women, there is no benefit to finasteride, and 2% minoxidil bid appears to be as effective as the 5% solution. Facial hypertrichosis is a more common side effect in women.

   b. **Alopecia areata** is characterized by rapid, complete hair loss in one or more oval patches. The scalp is most often affected, but any hair-bearing area may be involved. Hairs taper proximally to an attenuated bulb, producing "exclamation point hairs." Alopecia areata is considered to be an autoimmune disorder; spontaneous regrowth often occurs within 6 months. Intralesional Kenalog, 3–10 mg/ml every 4–6 weeks, is used for persistent or rapidly enlarging patches.

   c. **Telogen effluvium** is characterized by abrupt, diffuse hair loss over the entire scalp that results in decreased hair density. Anagen hairs are prematurely pushed into the telogen phase of the hair cycle (usually 2–4 months after the initiating event). Hair loss can continue for a subsequent 120–400 days, but then regrowth occurs. Causes include pregnancy, febrile illness, surgery, crash diets, systemic anticoagulant therapy, and stressful life episodes. Treatment consists of reassurance and should be directed at eliminating the underlying cause.

   d. **Anagen effluvium** is a widespread loss of anagen hairs from actively growing follicles due to arrest of cell division. It often manifests as acute, severe hair loss. Causes include cytotoxic agents for cancer chemotherapy, thallium, boron, and radiation therapy. Treatment consists of reassurance.

3. **Trichotillomania** is excessive and repeated manipulation of hair by the patient that results in hair breakage. It typically produces a well-circumscribed area of broken hairs and alopecia. Treatment should be directed at discussing the nature of the problem with the patient, who may unknowingly persist in manipulating the hair. Extreme cases may require psychiatric evaluation and medication.

4. **Other causes of alopecia**

   a. **Endocrine** (see secs. **XX.A.1** and 2)

   b. **Oral contraceptives** (OCPs) may initiate androgenic alopecia in predisposed women and telogen effluvium may develop 2–4 months after anovulatory agents are discontinued.

   c. **Nutritional causes of alopecia** that should be considered include Kwashiorkor, marasmus, zinc deficiency, essential fatty acid deficiency, and malabsorption.

XV. **Nail disorders** are associated with systemic disease or congenital conditions, or can be the result of infection, injury, repeated trauma, or improper trimming.

   A. **Clubbing.** Lovibond's angle between the proximal nail fold and the distal nail plate is greater than 180 degrees (normal is 160 degrees). It is often, but not always, associated with systemic disease.

      1. **Pulmonary disease** accounts for 80% of acquired clubbing; causes include parenchymal lung neoplasms, pulmonary infections (chronic

bronchitis, pneumonia), mediastinal tumors (lymphoma, mesothelioma, fibrosarcoma), emphysema, and pulmonary fibrosis.

2. Other causes include cardiovascular disease (cyanotic congenital heart disease, subacute bacterial endocarditis, CHF); GI disease (cirrhosis, inflammatory bowel disease, neoplasms, ascaris); and miscellaneous causes [arsenic, phosphorus, or mercury intoxication; systemic LE (SLE); Graves' disease (thyroid acropathy); hereditary; and idiopathic].

B. Koilonychia, or spoon-shaped nails, is associated with hematologic disorders (Plummer-Vinson syndrome, polycythemia vera); metabolic disorders (acromegaly, hyperthyroidism, hypothyroidism, malnutrition, porphyria); and traumatic/occupational disorders (acid/alkali, thermal burns, frostbite, petroleum, thioglycolate).

C. Leukonychia striata are transverse white bands in the nail. Traumatic leukonychia striata are due to occupational trauma and manicuring. Discontinuous parallel, horizontal white bands are present in the nail plate but usually do not span the entire plate. Leukonychia striata are likely to be asymmetric and do not involve all nails. **Mee lines** are homogeneous white bands that span the nail plate. All nails are involved. Common causes include arsenic, carbon monoxide, cardiac failure, chemotherapy, Hodgkin's disease, leprosy, renal failure, and sickle cell anemia. **Muehrcke lines** are paired white transverse lines spanning the nail plate that temporarily disappear with pressure, and associated with chronic hypoalbuminemia.

D. Beau lines are characterized by a universal transverse depression spanning the nail plate that is associated with any systemic disease (chemotherapy, sepsis) that causes a temporary cessation of nail growth. The insult can be dated by measuring the distance between the proximal nail fold and the leading edge of the depression (fingernails grow 0.1–0.15 mm/day).

E. Onycholysis is distal separation of the nail plate from the nail bed. Common causes include trauma, drug reactions, contact dermatitis, and psoriasis.

F. Onychomycosis (sec. **XXI.C.3**).

G. Terry nails are a prominent erythematous band at the distal portion of the nail bed (<20% of the nail bed is involved). The nail plate is normal. They are associated with cirrhosis, renal failure, and healthy patients (especially children). **Half and half nails** are red, pink, or brown transverse distal bands. They are found in 15% of patients with chronic renal failure.

H. Ingrown nails can be congenital, a result of injury, or other pressures between the nail and soft tissues. Erythema, edema, concomitant infection, and pain can accompany an ingrown nail. When severe pain or a paronychia (see below) is present, removal of the offending nail is usually necessary. This can be done chemically, surgically, or with a laser. Patients with diabetes or vascular insufficiency may have poor wound healing and require close follow-up after nail removal.

I. Paronychia are pockets of localized infection at nail margins. They may be acute or chronic (through occupational exposure). Culture are positive for *Staphylococcus* (acute) or *C. albicans* (chronic). Daily saline soaks and a topical antibiotic can be prescribed. Treatment is directed at local wound care and eliminating inciting causes, and systemic therapy may be required (see Chap. 19, Fungal Infections, sec. **I.E**).

XVI. Pigment disorders

A. Vitiligo is characterized by depigmented patches, often symmetric, around the eyes, nose, mouth, ears, genitals, and dorsal hands. It can be segmental or become generalized. It is rarely associated with autoimmune diseases. Recommendations include broad-spectrum sunscreens and observation for cutaneous malignancies. Treatment includes topical steroids, psoralen ultraviolet A (UVA) photochemotherapy (PUVA), and punch grafts and is best performed under the care of a dermatologist.

B. Melasma is characterized by pigmented patches on the forehead, cheeks, lips, and extensor forearms. It is commonly seen with OCPs and pregnancy.

Changing OCP has little effect. Treatment includes broad-spectrum sunscreens, topical hydroquinones, and tretinoin.

XVII. Skin signs of autoimmune disease

A. LE is a multisystem disorder. It can range from a relatively benign but disfiguring cutaneous eruption with no internal involvement to a severe systemic disease that is potentially fatal (see Chap. 22).

1. **LE-specific skin disease**
   a. **Chronic cutaneous LE.** DLE is characterized by erythema, scaling, hypopigmentation, follicular plugging, scarring, and telangiectasias. The two forms are localized and widespread. Widespread discoid lesions occur above and below the neck. SLE will develop in 5% of DLE patients, whereas 20% will have discoid lesions, often widespread.
   b. **Subacute cutaneous LE** is nonscarring and rarely atrophic with prominent photosensitivity. Most patients are antinuclear antibody positive and anti-Ro/SS-A positive. Of patients with subacute cutaneous LE, 50% possess criteria for SLE. **Acute cutaneous LE** is characterized by malar rash, DLE lesions, photosensitivity, and oral ulcers.
2. **Treatment.** Cutaneous LE often responds to the therapy for the systemic disease. The cutaneous disease responds to broad-spectrum sunscreens, antimalarials, and topical steroids. Prednisone has shown little benefit.

B. Dermatomyositis combines an inflammatory myopathy with characteristic cutaneous findings (see Chap. 22). Dermatomyositis sine myositis has characteristic skin findings without evidence of myopathy.

1. **Cutaneous manifestations. Pathognomonic signs** include a **heliotrope rash**, a violaceous hue over the eyelids, and **Gottron's papules** over the bony prominence/knuckles. Other cutaneous findings include periungual telangiectasias, photosensitivity, poikiloderma, calcinosis cutis (more common in children), cuticular hypertrophy, and splinter hemorrhages.
2. **Treatment.** The cutaneous disease often responds to the therapy for the systemic disease. The cutaneous disease responds to broad-spectrum sunscreens, antimalarials, topical steroids, and methotrexate.

C. Scleroderma is characterized by thickening or hardening of the skin associated with increased dermal or subcutaneous sclerosis, or both.

1. Classification
   a. **Localized** cutaneous disease, which includes morphea, linear scleroderma, and facial hemiatrophy.
   b. **Systemic disease**
      (1) Limited scleroderma **(CREST): c**alcinosis, **R**aynaud's phenomenon, **e**sophageal dysmotility, **s**clerodactyly, **t**elangiectasia
      (2) **Diffuse scleroderma** (progressive systemic sclerosis)
   c. **Cutaneous manifestations** include generalized sclerosis, acrosclerosis/sclerodactyly, calcinosis cutis, pruritus, nail fold capillary changes, mat-like telangiectasias, Raynaud's phenomenon, rhagades and taut facies, and salt and pepper dyspigmentation.
   d. **Treatment.** Cutaneous sclerosis and pruritus respond somewhat to PUVA.

D. Vasculitis (see Chap. 22). Most cases of palpable purpura are a skin-limited leukocytoclastic vasculitis but can be associated with the systemic vasculitides. Fifty percent are idiopathic. Potential causes include: infections (hepatitis, *Streptococcus*, respiratory infections); drugs (acetylsalicylic acid, sulfonamides, penicillin, barbiturates, amphetamines, propylthiouracil); and autoimmune diseases (SLE, rheumatoid arthritis, cryoglobulinemia).

1. Appropriate **evaluation** includes history, physical examination, urinalysis, and skin biopsy with direct immunofluorescence. Laboratory work to be considered includes guaiac, CBC, erythrocyte sedimentation rate, chest x-ray, hepatitis panel, and cryoglobulins.

      2. Treatment is aimed at removing the offending agent and most cases are self-limited. Prednisone improves the cutaneous disease but does not change the course. Most patients are treated with rest, nonsteroidal anti-inflammatory drugs, or colchicine.

XVIII. Erythema nodosum is characterized by tender, symmetric subcutaneous nodules, commonly on the shins. It is often a self-limited process, lasting 3–6 weeks. It commonly presents in young women; 50% of cases are idiopathic. **Causes** include drugs (OCPs, sulfonamides, trimethoprim-sulfamethoxazole, salicylates, phenacetin, iodides, and bromides); infections (bacterial, deep fungal, viral); bowel disease (ulcerative colitis, Crohn's, and infectious colitis); and pulmonary disease [*Streptococcus*, tuberculosis, sarcoid (Lofgren's syndrome)]. Appropriate **evaluation** includes history, physical examination, skin biopsy, CBC, purified protein derivative, and chest x-ray. The major pitfall is failure to identify the underlying cause. **Treatment** is aimed at removing the offending agent. Initial therapy is nonsteroidal anti-inflammatory drugs. Alternate therapies include oral potassium iodide, indomethacin, or colchicine. Steroids, intralesional or systemic, should only be considered once infections have been excluded and for recalcitrant cases.

XIX. Skin signs of internal malignancy

    A. Cutaneous metastases. The overall incidence of metastasis to skin is low (2–8%). Metastatic carcinoma appears as firm, flesh-colored, red or blue nodules. The trunk and scalp are the most frequent sites. The source of cutaneous metastases tends to be the same tumors that are most frequent in the general population. The most likely source of occult skin metastasis is the lung, ovary, and kidney.

    B. Lymphoreticular and hematologic malignancies may affect the skin by producing metastasis or paraneoplastic phenomena. Leukemia cutis or lymphoma cutis can resemble carcinomatous skin metastasis and appear as firm papules, nodules, or plaques. It is more likely to be hemorrhagic or plum colored. Gingival hypertrophy and bleeding are common with leukemia.

    C. Mycosis fungoides (cutaneous T-cell lymphoma) may present with erythematous patches, plaques, nodules, tumors, generalized erythroderma, or its leukemic variant, Sézary syndrome. It should be considered in patients with persistent patches or plaques. Diagnosis is confirmed with biopsy. Treatments include PUVA, topical mechlorethamine, and interferon-alpha.

XX. Skin signs of endocrinologic disorders

    A. Thyroid (see Chap. 17)

        1. Hyperthyroidism is associated with fine thin hair that may progress to diffuse alopecia; fine velvety skin with increased warmth and sweating; palmar erythema; and diffuse hyperpigmentation. **Graves' disease** is associated with ophthalmopathy (exophthalmos, lid puffiness, proptosis), pretibial myxedema, thyroid acropachy (characterized by clubbing), soft-tissue swelling of the hands and feet, and periosteal new bone formation.

        2. Hypothyroidism is associated with cretinism or congenital hypothyroidism; generalized myxedema; xerosis, keratoderma; cold pale skin; carotenemia; dull, coarse, brittle hair that may progress to alopecia; loss of lateral third of eyebrows; and thin, brittle, slow-growing nails.

    B. Diabetes mellitus (see Chap. 18)

        1. Diabetic dermopathy is characterized by atrophic hyperpigmented patches on the shins.

        2. Necrobiosis lipoidica diabeticorum is characterized by well-circumscribed, yellow-brown, shiny plaques with pronounced epidermal atrophy and telangiectasia, commonly seen on the shins.

        3. Granuloma annulare is characterized by dermal papules arranged in an annular pattern, usually arising on the distal extremities.

C. **Xanthomas and lipoprotein disorders** (see Chap. 5)
   1. **Eruptive xanthomas** arise in crops and exhibit an inflammatory acnei-form appearance; they may be mistaken for pustules. Patients are at risk for acute pancreatitis. Plasma triglycerides are markedly increased; cholesterol is normal. Etiologic factors include genetic lipoprotein lipase deficiency, ethanol abuse, estrogens, or retinoids.
   2. **Tendon xanthomas** are subcutaneous nodules that affect the tendons with normal-looking overlying skin; they may be mistaken for rheuma-toid nodules. If plasma cholesterol is increased, the most likely cause is familial hypercholesterolemia. Patients are at risk for atherosclerosis and coronary disease.
   3. **Xanthelasma** is the most common but least specific type of xanthoma. It arises in the periocular area, especially on the eyelids. Fifty percent have increased plasma cholesterol.

XXI. **Fungal skin infections** (see Chap. 19)
   A. **Candidiasis** (see Chap. 19)
   B. **Tinea versicolor** is characterized by thin scaly papules and plaques on the trunk, extremities, and face. KOH examination reveals spores and pseudohyphae (macaroni and meatballs). Tinea versicolor is difficult to culture.
      1. **Treatment.** Tinea versicolor is not responsive to griseofulvin or systemic allylamines such as terbinafine (Lamisil).
         a. **Selenium sulfide** 2.5% shampoo is used every day for 15 minutes for 7 days, then weekly, and more often if needed. Medicated Head & Shoulders and Selsun Blue contain less selenium sulfide and need to be used more frequently.
         b. Apply any **topical azole antifungal cream** bid for 2 weeks after the rash resolves.
         c. **Ketoconazole**, 400 mg PO, which is to be repeated in 1 week. The medication is excreted in sweat. Exercise $1^1/2$ hours after ingestion and leave sweat on for as long as possible without bathing.
   C. **Dermatophyte infections.** Primary treatment is topical/systemic azoles or allylamines or griseofulvin. These infections are unresponsive to nystatin.
      1. **Tinea capitis** is characterized by scaling alopecia with broken hairs. Posterior cervical lymphadenopathy often develops. No benefit is found in Wood's lamp examination. Tinea capitis is rarely seen in patients older than 15 years old. Kerions, boggy nodules that often drain pus, can develop and they are best treated with a 2-week course of cepha-lexin (Keflex; 20–40 mg/kg/day), prednisone (1 mg/kg/day), and griseo-fulvin (5–20 mg/kg/day) for 6–8 weeks.
         a. **Differential diagnosis (DDx)**
            (1) **Alopecia areata** is characterized by round patches of nonscal-ing alopecia, often associated with nail pitting. Key finding: no scale.
            (2) In **seborrheic dermatitis**, the scale can be fine white to yellow greasy. It often involves the hairline, ears, eyebrows, perinasal area, and central chest. Key finding: no alopecia.
         b. **Diagnostic test.** KOH examination of scale reveals hyphae; examina-tion of broken hairs reveals endospores. Fungal culture should be done.
         c. **Treatment.** Tinea capitis requires systemic therapy.
            (1) **Griseofulvin**, 5–20 mg/kg/day for 4–8 weeks. Take with a fatty meal. Can cause photosensitivity.
            (2) Often recommend 2.5% **selenium sulfide** or 2% **Nizoral shampoo** qod to decrease the chance of spreading the disease. Children are no longer infectious once on treatment and therefore can return to school.
      2. **Tinea pedis and manuum** is relatively uncommon in children and is pro-gressively more common with age. It usually involves the soles with "moc-

casin" distribution scaling. Interdigital pruritus, scaling, and maceration occur. Occasionally, localized blisters develop on the arch of the foot. It never involves both hands and both feet ("2 foot, 1 hand syndrome"). DDx includes dyshidrotic eczema with localized blisters. Patients often give a history of hyperhidrosis and pruritic vesicles along the sides of the fingers. Caution patients to wear slippers while showering in a public area. **Treatment** includes keeping the area clean and dry, use of drying powders PRN, and use of topical or oral antifungal agents as appropriate.

3. **Onychomycosis.** As a treatment option, terbinafine, 250 mg PO qd, may be more effective for onychomycosis. Fingernail infections should be treated for 6 weeks and toenail infections for 12 weeks. The optimal clinical effect, seen some months after cessation of treatment, is related to the rate of outgrowth of healthy nail. Liver function tests should be monitored during therapy. Alternately, itraconazole may be beneficial, 200 mg PO bid for 7 days, followed by a 3-week hiatus with two treatment cycles for fingernails and three treatment cycles for toenails. Onychomycosis can also be treated with removal of the nail and destruction of the nail matrix.

4. **Tinea cruris** is characterized by advancing scaly, annular erythematous plaques. It can have central clearing, hyperpigmentation, or lichenification and may have pustules at the leading edge. It is often present on the bilateral buttocks and never involves the penis or scrotum. The DDx includes intertrigo/candidiasis that favors the creases, with satellite pustules and bright red plaques. It often involves the scrotum. Erythrasma is characterized by hyperpigmented patch with fine scale. Coral red fluorescence is seen on Wood's lamp examination if the patient has not bathed recently.

5. **Tinea corporis.** Tinea corporis is characterized by advancing scaly, annular, slightly raised erythematous lesions. It may be pustular at the margins or hypopigmented centrally. Trunk and extremities are the most common areas. **Diagnosis** is usually clinical, but can be confirmed with a KOH prep demonstrating hyphae. **Treatment** involves keeping the area clean and dry. Initial topical therapy includes antifungal creams such as Clotrimazole 1% bid for up to 1 month. In severe cases, treatment with an oral antifungal agent (clotrimazole, terbinafine) may be required. For patients with revurrent, severe, or unresolving infection, referral to a dermatologist may be necessary. Consider diabetes mellitus or HIV in an adult with this diagnosis.

6. **Tinea faciei** is often annular. If inflamed, it has often been contracted from animals. **Majocchi's granuloma**, or fungal folliculitis, has multiple pustules within a patch of tinea corporis. Diagnosis is often confirmed by skin biopsy when folliculitis fails to respond to antibiotics. Just as with tinea capitis, it requires griseofulvin for 2–4 weeks.

XXII. Bacterial skin infections (see Chap. 19)

XXIII. Viral skin infections

A. **Warts** are intraepidermal tumors caused by infection with the human papilloma virus.

1. **Common warts (verruca vulgaris)** are flesh to brown colored and hyperkeratotic. Acral areas, especially the hands, are most frequently involved, but all skin and mucous membranes may be involved.

2. **Filiform warts** are finger-like slender projections that arise particularly on the face or neck.

3. **Flat warts (verruca plana)** are small, 1- to 3-mm flesh- to tan-colored papules on the face, neck, and extensor upper extremities. They may be distributed in a linear pattern (koebnerization).

4. **Plantar warts** are common warts that involve the thick skin of the sole.

5. **Condyloma acuminata** are warts that grow on moist areas, especially the genital or perianal skin. These genital warts are the most common type of sexually transmitted disease.
6. **Treatment.** Warts may resolve spontaneously or recur after apparent cure. Multiple treatments are usually necessary.
   a. Keratolytic preparations: salicylic acid (DuoFilm, Occlusal)
   b. Other topical agents: tretinoin (Retin A), fluorouracil, or podophyllum
   c. Surgical destruction: cryosurgery using liquid nitrogen, carbon dioxide laser, or electrodesiccation and curettage
B. **Molluscum contagiosum** are intraepidermal tumors that are also caused by viruses. They are discrete flesh to pearly white waxy papules, 1–5 mm in size, with a central dell or umbilication. Like warts, they are also transmitted through close physical contact. They are commonly found on the face and flexures in children and on the genital area, lower abdomen, and thighs in adults. Mollusca resolve spontaneously in immunocompetent individuals. HIV patients often require more aggressive therapy and referral to a dermatologist is appropriate.
C. **HSV** (see Chap. 19)
D. **VZV** (see Chap. 19)

XXIV. **Skin infestations** (see Chap. 19)
XXV. **Acne vulgaris** tends to develop around puberty and resolves later. Acne is an inflammatory condition with an infectious component. It may be improved by OCPs but worsened by medroxyprogesterone (Depo-Provera).
A. **Papular acne** is characterized by open comedones (blackheads) and closed comedones (whiteheads). It is responsive to comedolytics (see sec. **XXV.D**).
B. **Inflammatory acne** is characterized by inflammatory papules and pustules. It is responsive to comedolytics and topical/systemic antibiotics.
C. **Nodulocystic acne** is characterized by deep-seated nodules and results in scarring. It is responsive to systemic antibiotics or isotretinoin (Accutane).
D. **Comedolytics**
   1. **Benzoyl peroxide 2.5, 5, 10%, wash or gel.** Use higher concentrations and gels in patients with oily skin.
   2. **Retin A (tretinoin) 0.025, 0.05, 0.1% cream; 0.0025, 0.01% gel.** Wash face 1 hour before bedtime, pat dry, wait 1/2 hour, apply small quantity (pea sized). Avoid corners of eyes, nose, and mouth. Wait 1/2 hour so as not to rub off on pillow. Gel preparation or higher concentration can be drying. In addition, can predispose to photosensitivity.
E. **Topical antibiotics**
   1. **Erythromycin solution or pledget** 1–2 times/day
   2. **Clindamycin (Cleocin T) solution, lotion, or pledget** 1–2 times/day
F. **Systemic antibiotics**
   1. **Erythromycin,** 250–1000 mg/day
   2. **Tetracycline,** 250–1000 mg/day on an empty stomach, 1 hour before or 2 hours after meals. Not to be consumed with milk products.
   3. **Doxycycline,** 50–200 mg/day. Photosensitizing
   4. **Minocycline,** 50–200 mg/day. Can develop blue discoloration of the skin when given for longer than 1 year at 100 mg bid.
G. **Isotretinoin,** 1 mg/kg/day for 20 weeks. For severe nodulocystic acne, check monthly liver function tests, lipid panel. This drug is only for women who are willing to undertake appropriate contraception. Due to teratogenicity, monthly pregnancy tests must be checked. There is an increased risk for *Staphylococcus* infections and pyogenic granulomas. Other side effects include severe dryness and photosensitivity. It should only be prescribed by a physician who is familiar with its use.

XXVI. **Acne rosacea** is an association of inflammatory papules, pustules, and telangiectasias that can result in rhinophyma. It usually does not start in those younger than age 25 years. Acne rosacea does not respond to comedolytics. Sunscreen should be used and the "flushers" (sunlight, alcohol, hot spicy foods, hot beverages) avoided. **Treatment** should include topical antibiotics [metronidazole (MetroGel) bid or Cleocin T bid] or systemic antibiotics such as tetracycline, 250–1000 mg/day, or doxycycline, 50–200 mg/day.

XXVII. **Skin cancer.** Half of all primary cancers in the United States are basal cell carcinoma (BCC) and small cell carcinoma (SCC) of the skin. Melanoma has the fastest rising incidence among solid tumors.

A. **Skin cancer prevention.** Patients should be advised to avoid sun exposure between 10 a.m. and 3 p.m. A good rule of thumb is that if their shadow is shorter than they are, they should seek the shade. Sunscreens are useful adjuncts to long sleeves and wide-brimmed hats for fair-skinned people or patients with dermatoses induced by ultraviolet light. Sunscreens for UVB with an SPF 15–30 are sufficient for routine use. For certain light-sensitive disorders (e.g., SLE) and photosensitizing drugs (e.g., tetracycline, sulfonamides, thiazides, quinolones), combination sunscreens [UVA and UVB] are necessary. All sunscreens should be applied **30–60 minutes before exposure** and should be **reapplied** after bathing, swimming, or excessive sweating. Allergic and photosensitivity reactions occur to para-aminobenzoic acid (PABA), especially in patients who are sensitive to benzocaine, procaine, thiazides, and sulfonamides. Titanium dioxide and zinc oxide are opaque sunscreens that shield against UVA and UVB. They are particularly useful on the nose and lips.

B. **BCC** is a pearly, telangiectatic eroded papule that is usually on the face or trunk. It has a low metastatic potential. BCC is caused by chronic sun exposure. Patients have a 50% risk of developing a second primary within 5 years. Examination is needed every 6–12 months.
   1. **Diagnosis** is made by shave or punch biopsy.
   2. **Treatment.** Excision with 2- to 4-mm margins. Electrodesiccation and curettage, x-ray therapy, and monthly skin self-exams. For other preventive measures, refer to sec. **XXVII.A.**

C. **SCC** is characterized by red scaly papules or nodules on the face, hands, and arms. Metastasis occurs in less than 1–5/100 cases. It is due to chronic sun exposure. The risk of a second primary is high. Regular physical examination of the skin and the regional nodal basin is needed. Precursor lesion: actinic keratosis.
   1. **Diagnosis** is made by shave or punch biopsy
   2. **Treatment.** Excision with 4-mm margins and monthly skin self-exams. For other preventative measures, refer to sec. **XXVII.A.**

D. **Actinic keratosis** is a premalignant lesion found on the face, ears, neck, and dorsal hands. It is a discrete raised papule with rough keratotic scaly texture. On palpation it has a "rough sandpaper" feel. **Treatment** is with cryosurgery with liquid nitrogen or 5-fluorouracil (Efudex) bid for 2–4 weeks and monthly skin self-exams. For other preventative measures, refer to sec. **XXVII.A.**

E. **A seborrheic keratosis** is characterized by benign hyperkeratotic epidermal papules; it is commonly found in middle-aged and elderly patients and sometimes confused with skin cancer.
   1. A seborrheic keratosis usually starts as small, flesh, tan, or yellow waxy papules that become dark brown or black with a greasy verrucous surface and a well-defined border. The waxy look and superficial location give them a "stuck-on" appearance. Larger lesions often have white or black "dots" on the surface, which are called keratin pearls or horn cysts. Seborrheic keratoses often arise on the face, chest, and back. **Dermatosis papulosa nigra** is a form with multiple, small, darkly pigmented papules that is seen on the cheeks and periorbital areas of black, Hispanic, and Asian patients.
   2. The crucial **diagnostic** decision to make is to distinguish between seborrheic keratoses and skin cancers (particularly melanoma), because

seborrheic keratosis has **no malignant potential**. If the diagnosis cannot be made clinically, a biopsy is indicated.

    3. Treatment is with cryosurgery (liquid nitrogen), curettage, or scissors excision. Most seborrheic keratoses, however, do not require treatment or are treated for cosmetic reasons.

F. Melanoma can develop anywhere. In Caucasian men, the back is the most common location, whereas in Caucasian women, the legs and back are most common. The palms, soles, and nail beds are most common in Asians, Hispanics, and African-Americans. The depth of invasion (Breslow depth) provides prognostic information. Key points include the following:

    1. ABCDs. **A**symmetry; **b**order irregularity; **c**olors: black, gray, red, white, blue; **d**iameter greater than 6 mm

    2. Diagnosis. Any concerning or changing lesion should receive excisional or incisional biopsy.

    3. Treatment. Definitive surgery. Referral should be made to a dermatologist, oncologist, or surgical oncologist. Patients should perform monthly skin self-examinations. (For other preventive measures, refer to sec. **XXVII.A**).

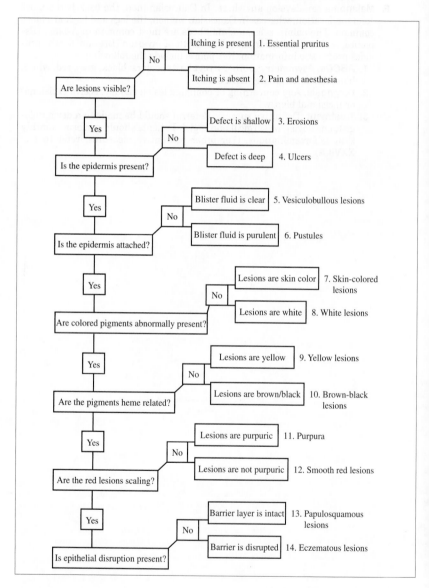

Appendix 26-1. Problem-oriented dermatologic algorithm. [Modified from PJ Lynch, *Dermatology* (3rd ed). Philadelphia: Williams & Wilkins, 1994:89–105. Reprinted with permission.]

Appendix 26-2
Problem-Oriented
Disease Groups

I. Group 1: Essential pruritus
Pruritus secondary to systemic disease, pruritus secondary to (almost) inapparent skin disease, pruritus of psychogenic origin.

II. Group 2: Pain, dysesthesia, and anesthesia
Postherpetic neuralgia (herpes zoster), localized chronic pain syndromes, delusions of parasitosis. Miscellaneous: leprosy, trigeminal neuropathy, reflex sympathetic dystrophy, diabetic neuropathy, erythropoietic protoporphyria, Fabry's disease.

III. Group 3: Erosions (with or without crust)
Roofed vesiculobullous and pustular lesions, erosive candidiasis, impetigo, neurotic excoriation without eczematous disease, burns and other traumatic erosions, toxic epidermal necrolysis, staphylococcal scalded skin syndrome.

IV. Group 4: Ulcers
Stasis ulcers; pressure (decubitus) ulcers; neuropathic ulcers; traumatic ulcers: excoriation and factitial disease; pyoderma gangrenosum; miscellaneous ulcerations: ulcerated malignancy, herpes in the immunosuppressed, deep fungal and mycobacterial disease.

V. Group 5: Vesiculobullous lesions
A. Vesicular disease
Herpes simplex; herpes zoster; dyshidrosis (pompholyx); vesicular tinea pedis; dermatitis herpetiformis; miscellaneous: Sweet's disease, Grover's disease, pityriasis lichenoides, insect bites, id reactions, hand-foot-and-mouth disease, pemphigoid gestationis, molluscum contagiosum.

B. Bullous disease
Bullous impetigo; poison ivy, poison oak; burns and traumatic (frictional) bulla; erythema multiforme (bullous type); pemphigoid; pemphigus; miscellaneous: fixed drug, epidermolysis bullosa acquisita, epidermolysis bullosa simplex, immunoglobulin A bullous disease, necrotizing fasciitis, porphyria cutanea tarda.

VI. Group 6: Pustules
Acne (acne necrotica, chloracne, perioral); rosacea; bacterial folliculitis (hot tub folliculitis); fungal folliculitis; candidiasis; miscellaneous: subcorneal pustular dermatosis, pustular psoriasis, acral pustular dermatosis, hidradenitis suppurativa, stye, chalazion, gonococcemia, Crohn's disease, Behçet's disease, hemorrhagic pustules of neutrophilic vasculitis, pseudopustules.

VII. Group 7: Skin-colored lesions
A. Smooth skin-colored lesions
Dermal nevi; skin tags and soft fibromas; epidermoid (sebaceous) cysts; lipomas; neurofibromas; scars; warts: genital and flat; molluscum contagiosum; BBC; miscellaneous: ganglion cysts, mucinous cysts, closed comedones, sebaceous hyperplasia, striae, edema and lymphedema, syringomas, nevus sebaceous.

B. Scaling skin-colored lesions
Xerosis (xerotic eczema, asteatotic eczema, ichthyosis vulgaris); warts: verruca vulgaris, paronychial warts, and plantar warts; corns and calluses; actinic keratoses; SCC (keratoacanthoma); miscellaneous: keratoderma, tinea pedis, disseminated superficial actinic porokeratosis, stucco keratosis, ichthyosis vulgaris, epidermal nevus, elephantiasis nostra verrucosa.

VIII. Group 8: White lesions
A. White papules
Milium; keratosis pilaris; miscellaneous: molluscum contagiosum, sebaceous gland hyperplasia, lichen nitidus.

B. White patches and plaques
Tinea versicolor; pityriasis alba; vitiligo; miscellaneous: postinflammatory hypopigmentation, lichen sclerosis et atrophicus (LS&A), morphea, white spots of scleroderma, tuberous sclerosis, idiopathic guttate hypomelanosis, halo nevus, atrophie blanche.

IX. Group 9: Yellow lesions
A. Smooth yellow lesions
Xanthelasma; necrobiosis lipoidica diabeticorum; miscellaneous: papular xanthomas, sebaceous gland hyperplasia, nevus sebaceous, juvenile xanthogranuloma, mastocytoma, cysts, solar elastosis, keratoderma, primary amyloidosis, carotenemia, jaundice.

B. Rough-surfaced yellow lesions. These are invariably crusted lesions; as such, they should be reclassified with group 3 (erosions) or group 14 (eczematous lesions).

X. Group 10: Brown/black lesions
A. Brown/black macules and papules
Seborrheic keratosis; dermatofibroma; freckles; lentigines; nevijunctional, compound, and intradermal; nevidysplastic; melanoma; miscellaneous: skin tags, dermatosis papulosa nigra, open comedones, actinic keratoses, angiokeratoma, flat warts, genital warts, bowenoid papulosis, pigmented BCC, urticaria pigmentosa, acanthosis nigricans.

B. Brown/black patches
Birthmarks and café au lait patches; giant congenital pigmented nevus; chloasma (melasma); miscellaneous: tinea versicolor, postinflammatory hyperpigmentation, Becker's nevus, lentigo maligna, lentigo maligna melanoma, acral lentiginous melanoma, morphea, atrophoderma of Pasini and Pierini, generalized hyperpigmentation.

XI. Group 11: Purpuras
A. Nonpalpable purpura
Petechiae (drug reaction, stasis change, benign pigmented purpura); ecchymoses (actinic purpura, steroid purpura, trauma); miscellaneous: primary amyloidosis, disseminated intravascular coagulation, necrosis, scurvy, Langerhans cell histiocytosis, black dot toes and heels, bacteremia, leukemia, coagulation disorders.

B. Palpable purpura
Leukocytoclastic vasculitis; miscellaneous: bacteremia, fungemia, Langerhans cell histiocytosis, pseudopurpura (cherry angiomas, angiokeratomas, Kaposi's sarcoma, pyogenic granuloma).

XII. Group 12: Smooth red lesions
A. Red macules and patches
Flushing; intertrigo; telangiectasia; spider angioma; port-wine vascular malformation; SLE; miscellaneous: erythrasma, candidiasis, cherry angioma (early), stork bite, rosacea, pityriasis rosea, livedo reticularis, viral exanthem, poikiloderma of Civatte, secondary syphilis, seborrheic dermatitis, toxic shock syndrome, Kawasaki's disease, erythromelalgia.

B. Red papules
Insect bites; hemangioma; cherry angiomas and telangiectasias; spider angiomas; pyogenic granuloma; granuloma annulare; miscellaneous: secondary syphilis, Grover's disease, pityriasis rosea, scabies (nodular), sarcoid, urticaria, lichen planus, pityriasis lichenoides.

C. Red nodules
Furuncle; inflamed epidermoid cyst; erythema nodosum; hidradenitis suppurativa; miscellaneous: sarcoid, lymphoma, lymphomatoid papulosis, pseudolymphomas, panniculitis, large-vessel vasculitis, cystic acne, erythema multiforme, Sweet's disease.

D. Solid red plaques
Urticaria; cellulitis (erysipelas, necrotizing fasciitis); erythema multiforme (classic, atypical); Sweet's syndrome; miscellaneous: fixed drug eruption,

Bowen's disease, superficial BCC, erythema nodosum, lipodermatosclerosis, cutaneous T-cell lymphoma (CTCL).

E. Annular red plaques

Granuloma annulare; miscellaneous: gyrate erythemas, LE (subacute cutaneous), CTCL, tinea corporis and cruris, pityriasis rosea (herald patch), lichen planus, secondary syphilis, sarcoid.

XIII. Group 13: Papulosquamous lesions

A. Macules and papules

Pityriasis rosea; lichen planus; secondary syphilis; pityriasis lichenoides; miscellaneous: psoriasis (guttate), rubeola, rubella, eczematous id reaction, follicular eczema.

B. Patches and plaques

Psoriasis (Reiter's syndrome); tinea corporis, pedis manuum, cruris; LE (discoid and subacute cutaneous); CTCL (parapsoriasis and mycosis fungoides); miscellaneous: pityriasis rubra pilaris, Darier's disease, Bowen's disease, superficial BCC, lichen striatus, inflamed linear epidermal nevus, erythrasma, Hailey and Hailey disease.

XIV. Group 14: Eczematous lesions

A. Prominent excoriation

Atopic dermatitis (neurodermatitis, lichen simplex chronicus, infantile eczema); dyshidrotic eczema; stasis dermatitis; miscellaneous: scabies, dermatitis herpetiformis, eczematized papulosquamous disease (psoriasis, tinea corporis and cruris) external otitis, id reactions, exfoliative erythroderma.

B. Minimal excoriation

Seborrheic dermatitis (perioral dermatitis); irritant contact dermatitis; allergic contact dermatitis; xerotic eczema (asteatotic eczema, winter itch); miscellaneous: tennis shoe foot, impetigo, lichen striatus, Hailey and Hailey disease, Darier's disease, Paget's disease, nummular dermatitis.

C. Eczematous reaction patterns

Nummular eczema; autoeczematization; exfoliative erythroderma; eczema of specific regions, hands, feet, anogenital, ear, scalp.

XV. Regional disease groups

A. Scalp and hair

Tinea capitis; alopecia areata; telogen effluvium; androgenetic alopecia; miscellaneous: thyroid disease, drug reactions, syphilis, LE, lichen planopilaris, folliculitis decalvans, pseudopelade, trichotillomania.

B. Fingernails and toenails

Onychomycosis; onycholysis; paronychia; ingrown nails; clubbing; miscellaneous: psoriasis, lichen planus, clubbing, warts, mucinous cyst, periungual fibromas.

C. Lips and mouth

White lesions: lichen planus, LE, candidiasis, syphilis, leukoplakia; geographic tongue; black hairy tongue; oral erosions and ulcers: aphthous ulcerations (cold sores), herpes simplex, erythema multiforme, pemphigus, cicatricial pemphigoid; cheilitis: chapped lips, actinic cheilitis, angular cheilitis; miscellaneous: fissured tongue, mucocele, cheek chewing.

D. Ears and eyelids

External otitis; blepharitis; stye; chalazion; chondrodermatitis nodularis; vitiligo.

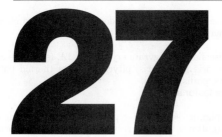

Ophthalmology

Linda M. Tsai and
Stephen A. Kamenetzky

Evaluation of the Patient with Ocular Disease

A careful history and physical examination are essential for correct diagnosis and treatment. The key to the initial evaluation is to also determine the need for referral to an ophthalmologist and to identify the ocular problem as acute, subacute, or chronic. This will dictate the timing for further evaluation and follow-up care (Table 27-1).

I. **Clinical history** should start with subjective ocular complaints and include change in vision, pain, diplopia, flashes or floaters, crusting, discharge, tearing, redness, and photophobia. Care should be taken to differentiate between eyelid and eyeball complaints if possible. Onset of symptoms differentiates between acute (hours), subacute (days), and chronic (weeks to months). Severity of symptoms should also be noted. Symptoms should be evaluated as transient versus constant and monocular versus binocular. Associated constitutional symptoms, such as nausea, vomiting, headache, weakness, numbness, and dizziness, should be elicited.

  A. **Medical history** is very important and should be carefully documented. History of hypertension (HTN), diabetes mellitus (DM), vascular disease, autoimmune disease, thyroid disease, temporal arteritis/polymyalgia rheumatica, and CNS disorders is important. Medications such as anticoagulants, systemic steroids, and thyroid supplementation should be noted.

  B. **Ocular history** should include trauma and previous eye surgery, amblyopia (lazy eye), cataract, glaucoma, age-related macular degeneration (ARMD), high myopia, dry eye, and blepharitis (eyelid disease).

  C. **Family history** of glaucoma, cataracts, ARMD, HTN, DM, and vascular disease should be noted. **Social history**, especially noting alcohol and tobacco use and living conditions, is important. **Occupational history** giving exposure to chemical substances, foreign bodies, and sunlight can be contributory.

II. **Physical examination** is preferably performed with slit lamp but can be done with a penlight.

  A. Measuring **visual acuity** is the most important assessment of visual function. This should be tested in each eye with a distance chart and glasses if the patient needs them. Near visual acuity can also be checked if a distance chart is not available. Reading glasses should be used if required. Patients whose vision is reduced below that measurable with an eye chart should be checked to see if they can count fingers, see hand motion, or see light. No light perception is **absolute blindness**. **Legal blindness** is defined as best-corrected visual acuity of less than 20/200 in the better eye.

    1. **Pinholing** may resolve refractive error and is useful in the patient who is not optimally corrected. This works for near vision and distance vision, but it generally does not resolve vision to better than 20/25.

Table 27-1. Referral guide for primary care physicians

See immediately or send to emergency room (EMERGENCY)

Chemical burns

Acute decrease of visual acuity to 20/100 or less, with suspicion of central retinal artery occlusion or temporal arteritis

Severe pain

Evidence of orbital cellulitis

Evidence or suspicion of penetrating injury to the globe, eyelid laceration, orbital fractures

See ophthalmologist within 24 hours (ACUTE)

Corneal abrasion/contact lens

Acute decrease in vision

Mild to moderate pain

Preseptal cellulitis

Conjunctival or corneal foreign body

Hyphema

Acute visual field loss

Flashes of light or floaters

See ophthalmologist within 1 week (SUBACUTE)

Red eye with no vision loss

Red eye with no pain

2. **Driver's license requirements** vary from state to state but generally require best-corrected binocular visual acuity to be 20/70 or better for daytime driving and 20/40 or better for nighttime driving. Visual field requirements are approximately 140 degrees binocularly. **Reading** is generally difficult below the 20/40 acuity range.

3. **Accommodation** is the ability of the ciliary muscle to contract to make the lens shape more convex to focus at near. In younger patients, **near card vision** is generally equivalent to distance visual acuity due to high accommodative ability. **Decreased accommodation** presbyopia in patients who are older than 40 years of age leads to the need for additional convergence power for near vision (reading glasses).

B. **Pupil evaluation** should include comparison of size and shape of pupils in light and dark conditions. Reactivity to light and accommodation should be noted. The presence of an **afferent pupillary defect (APD)** (**Marcus-Gunn** pupil) is evidence of optic nerve disease or significant retinal damage and should be carefully evaluated in every patient with decreased visual acuity.

C. **External examination of eyelids** can reveal evidence of erythema, edema, or eyelid lesions. **Ptosis** can be congenital or due to trauma, cranial nerve (CN) involvement, or senile involution. **Proptosis** can be seen with thyroid eye disease and orbital tumors. **Enophthalmos** can be seen after orbital trauma and rarely in breast cancer metastasis.

1. **Lymphadenopathy**, especially preauricular, should be checked for, especially in conjunctivitis, orbital tumors, and infections.

2. **Blepharitis and meibomianitis** are difficult to evaluate without a slit lamp examination but may be a significant cause of burning, itching, and eyelid crusting.

Table 27-2. Performing basic tests

I. **Upper eyelid eversion.** Have the patient look down. While using a cotton swab on the upper two-thirds of the upper eyelid as a fulcrum, flip eyelid over using eyelashes. To flip the eyelid back over, continue having the patient look downward and pull eyelashes back down.

II. **Confrontation visual fields.** Have the patient cover one eye. Make eye contact with the patient and explain that you want him/her to stare at your nose while you check the peripheral vision. Hold various fingers in the four main quadrants, making sure not to hold the fingers out too far into the periphery or behind the nose. Note: You are looking for a *large* peripheral defect such as quadrantanopias, hemianopsias, and significant visual field constriction. Minor field defects should be quantified with Goldmann or Humphrey visual field testing in the office.

III. **Amsler grid.** This checks the central 10 degrees of vision only. Have the patient look at the center dot of the grid monocularly. While looking at the dot, have the patient note if the grid lines are straight. Have the patient mark areas where lines are distorted, broken, or missing. Make sure that the patient's fixation is not moving while attempting to delineate defects.

IV. **Fluorescein staining.** Use fluorescein strip to stain corneal epithelium. Have patient look up, put stain on the medial portion of the bottom eyelid, and have the patient blink. Under a cobalt blue or Wood's light, abrasions and ulcers will appear green.

D. **Ocular motility** is important to evaluate for CN palsies, gaze palsies from supranuclear etiologies, restrictive disorders after trauma, thyroid eye disease, and underlying strabismus from childhood disease. Patients' complaints of **diplopia** often differentiate acute, new-onset disease from chronic congenital disease. **Nystagmus** may also be noted and patients should be sent for subspecialty evaluation unless it is long standing.

E. **Visual fields** (Table 27-2) should be evaluated to detect major visual field defects such as a hemianopsia or quadrantanopia. **Confrontation** is standard in the primary care office. A **Humphrey** (computer-generated) or a **Goldmann visual field** can be obtained to quantify visual field loss, especially in diseases such as glaucoma, anterior ischemic optic neuropathy (ION), and optic neuritis.

F. **Anterior segment examination** can be performed with a penlight or a slit lamp.

1. **Conjunctiva** should be evaluated to rule out foreign body and laceration in trauma. Generalized injection in viral and bacterial **conjunctivitis** is also associated with discharge. Uncomplicated conjunctivitis rarely causes pain. Perilimbal injection is common with **iritis**, with associated symptoms of photophobia, pain, and blurred vision. Occasionally, **pterygia** and **pinguecula** can be seen.

2. The **cornea** is usually clear but can be cloudy and opaque in situations such as high eye pressure, decompensated corneal endothelium, scars from previous infection and trauma, and infiltrates from current infections. Foreign bodies and corneal abrasions may be noted under slit lamp examination. Any involvement of the cornea often leads to symptoms of **photophobia, pain,** and **foreign body sensation.** Immediate relief of pain after instillation of topical anesthetic suggests a corneal etiology.

3. **Anterior chamber** pathology is difficult to assess without a slit lamp. Suspicion of blood (**hyphema**) and inflammation (**iritis**) after trauma or spontaneously should be immediately referred for evaluation. **Hypopyon,** a layering of white blood cells, is extremely suggestive of intraocular infection (endophthalmitis) or severe inflammation and needs prompt referral as well.

4. **Iris** shape may be irregular after surgery or trauma. Pigmented lesions may be melanoma and should be referred for specialty evaluation, especially if changing in size or color.
5. The **lens** is usually clear but may have a whitish or yellowish appearance with cataracts. After cataract surgery, the pupil may have a reflective quality from the lens implant.

G. **Intraocular pressure (IOP)** can be quantified with tonometry or qualitatively checked with palpation. It varies diurnally and tends to be highest in the morning. It is not directly related to BP or environmental factors such as stress or pain. Although **glaucoma** is multifactorial in nature, it is believed that most open-angle glaucoma can be treated by either decreasing inflow of aqueous humor (medications) or increasing outflow from the anterior chamber (medications, laser, or surgery).

H. Most **fundus** examinations in the office setting do **not** require dilation. They are performed to assess retinal vascular health and to rule out papilledema and retinal or vitreous hemorrhage. Pharmacologic dilation is usually performed with phenylephrine hydrochloride 2.5% or tropicamide 1%, or both, and causes decreased accommodation for approximately 4–6 hours. Cyclopentolate 1% is often used in children in place of tropicamide and may last for 1–3 days. The patient should not be dilated without the direction of an ophthalmologist if there is the suggestion of a shallow anterior chamber (may induce angle-closure glaucoma), if the patient is undergoing neurologic observation, or if there is any question of an APD.

I. Additional testing, such as **upper eyelid eversion, confrontation visual fields, Amsler grid testing, and fluorescein staining of the cornea**, can be performed when indicated (Table 27-2).

Prescribing Ophthalmic Medications

Some basic classes of medications can safely be prescribed.

I. **Oral antibiotics** are not frequently used but are indicated in certain situations. In preseptal cellulitis or complicated chalazion with no evidence of **orbital cellulitis** (diplopia, pain with eye movement, decreased vision), a 10-day course of cephalexin (Keflex), 250 mg qid, is used. Progression to orbital cellulitis is an emergency and should be referred immediately, because it may require hospitalization and parenteral antibiotics. For eyelid disease such as **blepharitis** and **meibomianitis**, often in association with **rosacea**, a course of minocycline, 100 mg qd, or tetracycline, 250 mg tid, for 2–6 weeks may be helpful.

II. **Topical antibiotics** are often used for conjunctivitis and abrasions. Sulfacetamide 10% (1 drop qid for 5 days), trimethoprim-polymyxin B (Polytrim; 1 drop tid for 5 days), and tobramycin (1 drop qid for 5 days) are used most often. Allergic reactions are possible, and drops should be discontinued if local irritation occurs. Topical sensitivity is very common with neomycin, and it should be avoided.

III. **Artificial tears/artificial tear ointment** are available over the counter and are very useful for symptoms of dry eyes (foreign body sensation, redness, tearing with exposure, variable vision). If the patient has a history of sensitivity or if using drops more than four times/day, preservative-free artificial tears should be considered.

IV. **Topical steroids** can lead to increased IOP, glaucoma, cataracts, and possible worsening and/or masking of clinical symptoms. They should not be used without consultation with an ophthalmologist. Antibiotic/steroid combinations should also be considered in this class.

V. Topical antihistamines/decongestants are available over the counter as well as by prescription. Over-the-counter medicines such as Ocuhist and Visine should only be used for a few days at a time. Prescription antihistamines, such as olopatadine hydrochloride (Patanol; 1 drop bid), levocabastine hydrochloride (Livostin; 1 drop bid), azelastine hydrochloride (Optivar, 1 drop bid) and ketotifen (Zaditor; 1 drop bid), are available for daily use but are quite expensive.

Ophthalmologic Emergencies in the Office

I. A **chemical burn** is one of the rare true emergencies in ophthalmology.
  A. Treatment begins with immediate flushing of the eye with water or normal saline for at least 10 minutes. This can be performed while the history is taken. If possible, the active ingredients of the chemicals should be noted. The pH of the eye should be taken a few minutes after the eye has been flushed, before instilling any ophthalmic drops, and it should be 7.0. This should be checked twice 2–3 minutes apart. If the pH is not 7.0, the eye must be flushed again and pH rechecked. Rarely, a retained foreign body causes continued release of the chemical and needs to be removed. This is particularly common with alkali burns.
  B. Acid burns often leave the eye red and irritated but usually do not result in serious injury. **Alkali burns** are especially dangerous because the eye may appear white and quiet while deeper damage is done due to greater intraocular penetration of alkaline solution.
  C. Referral to an ophthalmologist when the patient's condition is stable is required for evaluation and treatment of chemical damage.
II. Angle-closure glaucoma is a rare disease that occurs when the anterior chamber is anatomically narrow and the dilated iris closes off the outflow of aqueous humor, causing an acute rise in IOP. Symptoms include severe pain, decreased vision, colored halos, corneal edema, and headache. Nausea, vomiting, and abdominal pain may also occur. Extremely high IOP results (possibly up to the 70s), and patients are at risk for vascular occlusions and glaucomatous damage to the optic nerve. An ophthalmologist manages the IOP initially with medications, but the definitive treatment is a laser peripheral iridotomy, which should be performed as soon as possible; it is also done on the unaffected eye for prophylaxis.
III. Retinal detachment typically presents with constant photopsia (flashing lights), floaters, and a shade over part of the vision in one eye. Partial detachments may not affect central visual acuity dramatically, but those that involve the central macular area with significant decreased visual acuity can be associated with an APD. Similar symptoms of acute onset of floaters and occasional flashes but no vision loss may be seen with acute **posterior vitreous** detachment. These patients need an extensive dilated retinal examination by an ophthalmologist to evaluate the status of the retina carefully and to rule out a small retinal hole, tear, or peripheral detachment.

Acute Vision Loss

Acute vision loss (within 24 hours) with or without pain should be evaluated immediately. Occasionally, patients will not have noticed vision loss in an eye until the other eye is covered (see Chronic Vision Loss). Vision loss that is transient and returns to baseline vision may also be confused with acute vision loss (see Transient Vision Loss).

I. **Vascular occlusion** may lead to devastating, painless vision loss. Often seen in people with previously diagnosed vascular disease, it may also occur in younger patients and requires evaluation for embolic (for arterial occlusion) or thrombotic (for venous occlusion) disease.

   A. In a **central retinal artery occlusion**, the patient presents with severe painless vision loss and on fundus examination may have evidence of pallor, vascular **"boxcarring,"** and a **"cherry-red spot"** as the normal macular appearance contrasts with generalized retinal ischemia. Irreversible damage has been shown to occur after 90 minutes of occlusion, and therefore patients should be sent to the emergency room or for referral immediately. As an emergency measure in the primary care office, the physician can attempt to compress the eye with the heel of the hand, pressing firmly for 5 seconds, then releasing for 5 seconds over a period of 5 minutes. This is designed to cause rapid changes in IOP and dislodge the embolus before irreversible retinal damage occurs. An ophthalmologist can use more invasive techniques such as anterior chamber paracentesis.

   B. A **central retinal vein occlusion** presents with a painless ophthalmoscopic picture of optic nerve swelling, venous engorgement, retinal hemorrhage, and cotton-wool spots, often described as **blood and thunder**. Although visual prognosis is poor, follow-up ophthalmologic care is imperative, as there is a high incidence of neovascularization of the retina and iris, which may lead to neovascular glaucoma and intractable pain. This may require treatment with laser photocoagulation.

   C. **Branch artery and vein occlusions** vary in their effect on visual acuity and should also be referred. They are painless and frequently present with loss of a portion of the visual field. Branch vein occlusions may cause secondary macular edema, which can be treated with laser photocoagulation.

   D. **Ischemic Optic Neuropathies (IONs)** are often associated with HTN, DM, vascular disease, and temporal arteritis (rare) and are discussed in Neuro-Ophthalmology.

   E. **Medical evaluation** for vascular disease varies according to etiology, and retinal vessel occlusions occur most commonly in patients with hypertension and diabetes mellitus. **Retinal arterial disease** may require carotid Doppler and cardiac echography. **Retinal venous disease** may be associated with thrombotic disease and hypercoagulable states, such as cryoglobulinemia, multiple myeloma, sickle cell disease, polycythemia vera, and lymphoma-leukemia. CBC, protein C and S, anticardiolipin, and evaluation for polyproteinemia may be required.

II. **Media opacities**

   A. **Cataracts** are the most common cause of media opacity but are usually gradual in onset (see Chronic Vision Loss).

   B. **Corneal edema** is usually associated with pain, a hazy appearance of the cornea, and decreased vision. If gradual, it may be due to underlying corneal disease. Acutely, it may be secondary to increased IOP as in angle-closure glaucoma or rubeosis irides. Inflammation, infection, or opacity of the cornea may be difficult to differentiate from corneal edema with penlight examination.

   C. **Vitreous hemorrhage** may occur after trauma or with any condition that may cause abnormal retinal neovascularization. Often seen in diabetes, vein occlusions, retinal holes or breaks, and occasionally ARMD, it should be evaluated and followed by an ophthalmologist. Laser treatment may be needed after the blood has resorbed. Unresolved hemorrhage may require surgical removal. **Terson's syndrome** (vitreous and retinal hemorrhage in association with subarachnoid hemorrhage due to trauma and coagulopathies) is rare.

III. **Retinal detachment** should be included in the differential diagnosis (see Ophthalmologic Emergencies in the Office, sec. **III**).

IV. **Optic neuritis** is associated with pain on eye movement and APD (see Neuro-Ophthalmology, sec. **I.A.**)

Chronic Vision Loss

I. **Cataract** is the most common cause of media opacity and is usually gradual in onset (over months to years). Changes in the lens thickness occur with cataract development and initially can be corrected by a change in glasses. Cataracts are a normal part of aging; they may not interfere with visual function and may not require surgical removal.

  A. **Symptoms** that occur as the lens opacifies may include decreased night vision, difficulty with glare, difficulty with reading, and decreased distance acuity. Rarely, patients complain of double vision and decreased color vision and brightness in the affected eye.

  B. The **indication for elective surgical cataract removal** is that it affects activities of daily living. Rarely, the cataract may need to be removed if it causes a secondary glaucoma or if it interferes with monitoring other ocular diseases such as macular degeneration, diabetes, or glaucoma. Elective cataract surgery is performed under local or topical anesthetic as an outpatient and can be offered to any patient who is visually or topical impaired and in stable medical health. Anticoagulants required for medical care may not need to be discontinued. A recent history and physical are required. Ancillary tests such as CBC, ECG, chest x-ray, and Chem-7 may be needed for review.

II. **Age-related macular degeneration (ARMD)** is a chronic, often progressive disease that affects central vision. Often bilateral, it may be asymmetric.

  A. **Risk factors** include family history, race (Caucasian), and age.

  B. The Age-Related Eye Disease Study demonstrated that in patients with moderate to severe ARMD, treatment with vitamins and antioxidants reduced the rate of progression to severe vision loss. Progression is usually slow, but sudden profound vision loss can occur if a subretinal neovascular membrane develops with hemorrhage and scarring.

  C. Home monitoring with an **Amsler grid** (Table 27-2) is recommended for early detection of central distortion.

III. **Glaucoma** is the second most important cause of blindness in the United States (after cataracts) and is the single most important cause of blindness in African-Americans. Most patients with glaucoma are asymptomatic, and many can lose significant peripheral vision before having any visual symptoms.

  A. **Risk factors** for open-angle glaucoma include HTN, DM, age, race (African-American), and family history.

  B. **IOP** is determined by the rate of production of aqueous humor by the ciliary body and the outflow of this fluid through the trabecular meshwork. Most normal eyes have an IOP of approximately 20 mm Hg or lower. IOP has diurnal variation, and the pressure is usually highest in the morning. Gradual increases of IOP are tolerated well without visual complaints or pain. Acute rises of IOP, as in acute-angle closure, are associated with corneal edema, pain, injection, tearing, and a mid-dilated pupil.

  C. The optic nerve has a depression in the center that is called the **cup of the optic disc**. The ratio of the size of the cup to total nerve head diameter is the cup disc ratio (CDR). Normal CDR is up to approximately 0.5 but may vary between individuals. Monitoring of optic cup enlargement, especially with concomitant IOP monitoring, is a way to quantify the severity of the progression of glaucoma.

  D. **Frequency of visits** is dictated by the IOP control and the severity of disease. General follow-up is usually every 6 months, with visual field testing every year.

  E. **Medical management.** Glaucoma medications either decrease aqueous humor production, facilitate outflow of fluid, or both. Aqueous humor suppressants include beta-blockers [timolol, levobunolol, carteolol, betaxolol hydrochloride (Betoptic)], α_2 agonist (apraclonidine, iopidine), and carbonic anhydrase inhibitors (dorzolamide, oral acetazolamide). Those that facilitate outflow include prostaglandin analogs [latanoprost ophthalmic solution (Xalatan), travoprost (Travatan), bimatoprost (Lumigan)], miotics (pilocarpine), and epinephrine derivatives (dipivefrin). They all can have significant systemic side effects, and inquiries regarding their usage should be part of a careful medical history.

F. **Laser trabeculoplasty** is usually performed with an argon laser and is done as an office procedure. It works by increasing aqueous humor outflow. It can be done a maximum of two times to each eye, and its result may be transient.

G. **Surgical intervention** for glaucoma is a trabeculectomy (a glaucoma "filter" surgery) and is performed on an outpatient basis. It creates a new outflow passage from the eye, which is covered by conjunctiva, bypassing the trabecular meshwork.

Transient Vision Loss

I. **Amaurosis fugax** is transient monocular vision loss due to transient retinal arterial occlusion. The occlusion is usually caused by a cholesterol or platelet embolus but can result from vasospasm.

A. Often described as a **"shade or curtain coming over the vision"** that lasts a few minutes, it is most common in patients over the age of 50 years or those with a history of vascular disease. A full ophthalmologic examination must be performed by an ophthalmologist to rule out impending vascular occlusion.

B. The **most common site of an atheroma** is from the **carotids** or the **heart**. Evidence of a **Hollenhorst plaque** (cholesterol plaque visible in the retinal vasculature) may be seen on physical examination.

C. **Medical evaluation**, including carotid Doppler, cardiac echography, and basic hematologic workup, should be performed to rule out systemic disease, even in the absence of Hollenhorst plaques.

II. **Ophthalmic migraines** are transient episodes that usually cause at least 5–15 minutes of obscuration of vision. **Fortification** (jagged "lightning bolts") and **scintillating scotomas** (blind spot centrally with hazy edges) are characteristic, but colored lights and other visual symptoms can occur. Visual acuity should return to baseline completely after the episode, but headache or mild nausea may follow. A history of migraine may or may not be present. Often ophthalmic migraines develop in patients who previously had migraine headaches. History should be taken to rule out concomitant neurologic symptoms carefully. Both eyes are usually affected, although it may be sufficiently asymmetric as to appear to be monocular. Ophthalmologic evaluation is important to rule out retinal diseases.

Ocular Manifestations of Systemic Disease

I. **DM** is the leading cause of new cases of blindness in working-age Americans. The likelihood of developing retinopathy is directly related to the length of time a person has the disease. Approximately 5 years after the diagnosis, 23% of patients have diabetic retinopathy; after 15 years, 80% have retinopathy. These statistics are similar for type I and type II, with a slightly lower incidence in type II.

A. **Preventive care** is the cornerstone for decreasing visual morbidity.

1. Stricter glucose control has been shown to decrease the rate of development and severity of diabetic retinopathy.

2. Diabetic retinopathy often develops without producing visual symptoms, and therefore **yearly follow-up** is required once diabetes has been diagnosed. If retinopathy develops, more frequent visits may be indicated.

B. Clinical trials by the National Eye Institute have shown that with early detection and treatment, the incidence of severe vision loss can be decreased by 50%. Panretinal and focal argon laser photocoagulation are **treatments** for diabetic retinopathy that may be recommended to decrease the progression of retinopathy. Surgical vitrectomy is occasionally required for nonclearing vitreous hemorrhages.

C. **Decrease in visual acuity** due to diabetic retinopathy may not be directly related to the severity of the underlying systemic disease. Patients with mild non–insulin-dependent DM may have significant retinopathy. If present, reduced acuity may be due to macular edema, macular ischemia, vitreous hemorrhage from neovascularization, optic neuropathy, optic nerve damage from neovascular glaucoma secondary to rubeosis, or retinal detachment from neovascularization and retinal membrane formation. Visual acuity is not often recoverable, but laser treatment, surgical vitrectomy, or both, are recommended to stabilize the process.

II. Hypertensive changes in the retina can be chronic or acute.

A. **Chronic changes** are more common and are characterized by arteriolar sclerosis and arterial/venous nicking. An **acute rise in BP** (usually diastolic greater than 120 mm Hg) may cause exudates, cotton-wool spots, flame-shaped hemorrhage, and, rarely, retinal edema. **Malignant HTN** is rare but presents with optic disc swelling and is usually bilateral.

B. **Management** includes control of systemic BP. A sudden decrease in BP may cause decreased perfusion of retinal and choroidal circulation, as well optic nerve infarction. This is postulated to occur overnight. Systemic BP medication is best taken in the morning to prevent these transient hypotensive events.

III. Thyroid disease/Graves' disease is an autoimmune disease associated with hyperthyroidism. However, it may appear or progress in patients who are clinically euthyroid or hypothyroid. Tobacco usage has been associated with higher incidence of ocular complications. Most common manifestations include **eyelid retraction, proptosis, and corneal dryness**. Serious involvement of extraocular muscles causes restrictive myopathy with **diplopia**. Rarely, **compression of the optic nerve** within the orbit causes decreased vision with an APD and may require parenteral steroid therapy, radiation treatments, or surgical decompression. These patients should be referred for ophthalmologic consultation.

IV. Sarcoidosis is a chronic disease most common in African-American women aged 20–40 years. Focal noncaseating granulomas are histologically characteristic and can be found in affected conjunctiva and the lacrimal gland. Other symptoms from sarcoidosis include anterior or posterior uveitis, retinal inflammatory disease, and even optic nerve and motility disease. Dry eye is common, especially over the age of 40 years. Conjunctival biopsy performed under topical anesthesia can give a positive tissue diagnosis, but only has a high yield if a discrete granuloma is present.

V. AIDS is a disease in which depression of the immune system can lead to opportunistic infections. Common ocular manifestations include cotton-wool spots, cytomegalovirus (CMV) retinitis, and Kaposi's sarcoma of the eyelids. Also common are herpes zoster (shingles) ophthalmicus, herpes simplex keratitis, conjunctival microangiopathy, toxoplasmic uveitis, and CNS involvement. Yearly examination after diagnosis of AIDS is recommended, and patients should be closely monitored when CD4 counts drop below 500. CMV retinitis is rare in patients with CD4 counts greater than 50.

Ocular Trauma

I. Corneal abrasions are common and often present with significant redness, pain, photophobia, and lid swelling.

A. **Topical anesthetics** can be used to aid examination of the eye but should **never** be used for treatment, as they may cause epithelial toxicity and decreased healing. Evaluation can be aided with fluorescein staining and observation with cobalt blue–filtered light.

B. **Careful documentation** of mechanism of injury, vision, and size of abrasion should be made.

C. **Treatment** should include antibiotic eye drops (usually sulfacetamide 10%, 1 drop qid for 1 week, or tobramycin 0.3%, 1 drop qid for 1 week) or antibiotic ointment [polymyxin B sulfate (Polysporin Ophthalmic), 1/8-in. strip bid, or erythromycin, 1/8-in. strip bid]. Ketorolac (1 drop qid for 1 week) may be used. If it is clear that the injury has recently occurred (within a few hours), there is no evidence of infection, and there is no retained foreign body, the eye may be patched. Any corneal haze or evidence of nonhealing abrasion should be re-evaluated by an ophthalmologist.

II. **Foreign body/rust ring** in the eye can be carefully removed with either a wet cotton tip or needle under direct visualization using a slit lamp. A burr drill is occasionally used to remove rust rings. After the foreign body is removed, the eye should be treated with topical antibiotics (see sec. **I.C**). Eversion of the eyelid should be performed to rule out retained foreign bodies under the eyelid.

III. **Laceration of the cornea, conjunctiva, and eyelid** is common after penetrating and blunt trauma. A thorough eye examination including dilation must be performed by an ophthalmologist to rule out concurrent ruptured globe or other trauma.

IV. **Traumatic iritis** is common 2–3 days after blunt trauma and may present with decreased vision, photophobia, and dull pain. Patients should usually be referred to an ophthalmologist, as they may need to be treated with topical steroids. Traumatic iritis must be differentiated from bleeding (microhyphema) and infection.

V. **Hyphema** (visible blood in the anterior chamber) may lead to decreased vision, photophobia, and a dull achiness around the eye. Usually it is a result of direct trauma to the eye, but it can be caused by abnormal blood vessels (secondary to tumors, diabetes, chronic inflammation, intraocular surgery, and so forth). It should be evaluated and followed by an ophthalmologist to rule out additional ocular involvement and manage possible complications such as rebleeding in the eye and increased IOP. Hyphema is often treated with dilation and topical steroid medication but may require surgical washout if medical management is insufficient. The status of sickle cell disease/trait should be noted, as it affects the clearance of RBCs from the anterior chamber through the trabecular meshwork.

VI. **Orbital fractures** are often seen with blunt trauma. A thorough eye examination must be performed to rule out ruptured globe or other trauma.

A. **Fractures** should be **treated** with cephalexin, 250 mg PO qid for 10 days. Emphasis on no nose blowing and oxymetazoline tid for 3 days aids in decreasing the risk of extension of sinus disease into the orbit.

B. Fractures are usually re-evaluated 1 week after initial trauma. Indications for fracture repair from an ophthalmologic standpoint are (1) diplopia in primary gaze, (2) significant enophthalmos, and (3) unstable orbit. Many fractures are treated conservatively and are never surgically repaired.

VII. **Ruptured globe** is the most serious complication of ocular trauma. If there is any indication of prolapsed uvea, full-thickness laceration of the cornea or sclera, or distortion of the globe, the eye should be covered with a metal shield and the patient sent for ophthalmologic evaluation. This is usually done in the emergency department, and adjunctive radiologic studies such as CT of the orbit may be helpful to evaluate the globe and rule out an intraocular foreign body. If ruptured globe is suspected, no drops should be given.

VIII. **Contact lens** use often leads to minor trauma to the cornea. Contact lens wearers should be evaluated yearly to assess the health of the eye. Abrasions are common but should be evaluated because a higher incidence of infection/ulceration is associated with contact lens use. Contact lens wear should always be discontinued if the eye is red until a full evaluation can be done.

Neuro-Ophthalmology

Optic nerve disease is often detectable on careful pupillary examination by finding an APD.

I. **Papillitis or optic disc edema** is a general term that describes acute inflammation of the optic nerve with disc elevation, edema of the nerve fiber layer, distortion of the retinal vasculature, and an APD.

 A. **Optic neuritis** is a disease of younger patients and, although often idiopathic, may be associated with multiple sclerosis. It is an inflammation of the optic nerve and may involve the optic disc (with hyperemia and optic disc swelling) or be retrobulbar (with no apparent optic disc changes). Vision may be reduced to bare light perception and it is often associated with pain with ocular movement. Treatment consists of either parenteral steroids or supportive care. Oral steroids have not been shown to be effective. Visual prognosis after a single event is good. Additional diagnostic tests include visual field testing and color vision testing. These patients should be followed by an ophthalmologist and referred to a neurologist for imaging.

 B. **ION** is a common etiology for papillitis and vision loss in the older adult. It is due to underlying vascular disease and often leaves a permanent altitudinal visual field loss.

 C. **Giant cell arteritis or temporal arteritis** should always be considered when an ION develops, especially in a patient over the age of 60 years. Concomitant symptoms of malaise, weight loss, anorexia, scalp tenderness, jaw claudication, or shoulder/limb girdle weakness should be documented. Because this is a systemic disease that may lead to bilateral blindness within a few days, early diagnosis and a high level of suspicion are required. In any patient with ION, retinal arteritic occlusion, or even ophthalmoplegia, an erythrocyte sedimentation rate should be obtained immediately. If it is elevated to greater than 40 (or if there is a high suspicion of disease) treatment with systemic steroids (60 mg PO qd) should be initiated, and a temporal artery biopsy should be performed promptly for histologic diagnosis.

 D. **Papilledema** is optic nerve swelling from increased intracranial pressure, often seen in hydrocephalus, tumors, and pseudotumor cerebri. In papilledema, both optic nerves normally are involved. Visual acuity and pupillary reflexes occasionally are normal. Patients may complain of transient obscurations in their vision.

II. **Pupillary disorders** in the absence of trauma are often localizing symptoms of neurologic disease. Asymmetry of pupil size in dark or light, dilated pupils, and tonic pupils (unreactive pupils) should be evaluated. An APD is never normal and needs to be referred for further evaluation.

III. **Motility** abnormalities may suggest an acute or chronic CN palsy (III, IV, or VI) or extraocular muscle disorder. Acute changes are usually accompanied by complaints of diplopia, which may be horizontal or vertical in nature. Chronic changes may be asymptomatic. Medical conditions such as thyroid eye disease, also referred to as **Graves' disease** (even with normal levels or low levels of thyroid-stimulating hormone); idiopathic inflammatory pseudotumor (ocular myositis); myasthenia gravis; demyelinating disease (multiple sclerosis); and cerebellar dysfunction may manifest with abnormal eye movements.

IV. **Visual field defects** may occur from retinal and optic nerve disease but may also reflect intracranial disease. Lesions anterior to the optic chiasm (e.g., retina, glaucoma, optic neuritis) produce lesions in one eye only. Pituitary adenomas at the optic chiasm may produce bitemporal field loss. Behind the optic chiasms (e.g., damage to the optic tracts, radiations, or the occipital cortex), lesions produce homonymous hemianopsias or other homonymous defects. Stroke is the most common cause of homonymous hemianopsia.

V. **Intracranial aneurysm** is rare but may present with CN defects. Involvement of CN 3, 4, 5, and 6 should suggest cavernous sinus pathology. Pupil-involving CN 3 defects can be seen in posterior communicating artery aneurysms, and magnetic resonance angiography may be helpful in diagnosis. Diabetic or microvascular ischemic third nerve palsy usually spares the pupil.

Red Eye

Referring to hyperemia or bleeding of the superficial vessels of the conjunctiva, episclera, or sclera, the red eye may or not be associated with pain. However, it does not usually cause significantly decreased visual acuity.

I. **Infections** are a common etiology, and **viral and bacterial conjunctivitis** are associated with redness, mattering, mucous discharge, and tearing. Although topical antibiotics are useful, topical corticosteroids should **not** be used without consultation by an ophthalmologist. **Blepharitis** is caused by mild eyelid infections, which can lead to a foreign body sensation (especially in the morning) and dry eye. **Herpes simplex keratitis** can lead to corneal ulceration and scarring and should be referred to an ophthalmologist.

II. **Keratoconjunctivitis sicca ("dry eyes" or "tear film dysfunction")** is common, especially in cases of lagophthalmos (incomplete closure) with Bell's palsy, thyroid disease, rheumatologic diseases, contact lens wear, and age. Often a decrease in the protein or oil component of the tears due to eyelid disease (rosacea, blepharitis, meibomianitis) leads to a decrease in the quality, not quantity, of tears. Patients may even complain of tearing with extreme sensitivity to air, light, and prolonged usage of eyes, especially with near vision. A trial of artificial tears with carboxymethocellulose along with eyelid scrubs is often recommended. Symptoms of dryness may be worsened by some systemic medications (antihistamines, antidepressants, or hormone replacement).

III. **Subconjunctival hemorrhage** can be seen after inadvertent trauma or straining. Usually self-limited, it does not affect vision and is generally painless. Patients may have mild eye irritation due to increased corneal dryness. Treatment involves cool compresses and artificial tears prn. The patient should be questioned about other bleeding episodes or bruising, use of anticoagulants and aspirin, and HTN. Anticoagulants do not need to be discontinued for an isolated subconjunctival hemorrhage. If multiple episodes occur, or if other systemic symptoms are present, a hematologic workup may be indicated.

IV. **Traumatic abrasions and laceration** of the cornea or conjunctiva lead to redness of the eye. The history is important in these cases, and referral may be needed for treatment and follow-up. Minor abrasions can be treated with topical antibiotics, but referral is indicated if symptoms do not resolve within 24 hours.

V. **Iritis or iridocyclitis** is the inflammation of the iris or ciliary body, or both. A perilimbal distribution of redness is often present. This pattern is most common after trauma or with anterior uveitis.

VI. **Seasonal allergies** are common. For occasional use, over-the-counter antihistamines are reasonable, but for chronic use, new prescription medications are more effective (see Prescribing Ophthalmic Medications).

VII. **Episcleritis** is usually localized inflammation of the episclera. It may be associated with mild pain and often resolves with topical steroid treatment. It should be noted that episcleral redness blanches with phenylephrine, which helps to distinguish it from scleritis, a much more serious inflammation. **Scleritis** is treated with systemic steroids, and patients need to be monitored carefully for the development of scleral thinning and possibly perforation. Scleritis may indicate a serious systemic disease such as a collagen vascular disorder.

VIII. **Acute angle-closure glaucoma** is an uncommon form of glaucoma due to the sudden and complete occlusion of the trabecular meshwork with iris. Associated with corneal edema, mid-dilated pupil, and pain, this is a serious condition and should be **referred to an ophthalmologist immediately**.

IX. **Injected pterygium/pinguecula** is from conjunctival degeneration/abnormal growth on the conjunctiva that becomes inflamed. It can contribute to corneal dryness.

Tearing

Tearing is a common complaint but may be a nonspecific symptom of various underlying disorders. Subjective complaints are often enough to warrant an ocular evaluation. Quantitative measure of basal and reflex tearing is made by Schirmer's testing.

I. A common etiology is **reflex tearing**. This may be due to environmental and occupational irritants, pain, corneal foreign body or abnormality (infection, abrasion) and irritation caused by underlying tear film disorder. Poor blink due to diseases such as Bell's palsy and Parkinson's disease leads to underlying corneal keratopathy with tearing.

II. **Tear duct disorder** can cause overflow tearing due to inadequate drainage. In younger patients, blockage from nasal mucosal swelling, infections, and anatomic defects is common. In the older population, eyelid malpositions such as ectropion and entropion keep the puncta from its correct position against the globe. In addition, patients with poor and infrequent blink have decreased muscle tone to force drainage of tears toward the puncta.

III. **Conjunctivitis** is a common cause of tearing, often associated with itching, discharge, and redness. Viral conjunctivitis is more common, often self-limiting, and may be associated with other viral systemic symptoms. Treatment with topical antibiotics for bacterial conjunctivitis (usually more purulent) and to cover for suprainfections in viral conjunctivitis is reasonable, but the patient should be instructed to call if there is any loss of vision or symptoms do not resolve in a few days.

IV. **Anterior uveitis** (inflammation of the anterior chamber) may be associated with significant tearing, perilimbal injection, and photophobia. It is occasionally associated with systemic disease, and recurrent episodes require a medical evaluation, which includes CBC, antinuclear antibody, rheumatoid factor, human leukocyte antigen-B27, tuberculosis test, angiotensin-converting enzyme level, or chest x-ray.

External Eye and Eyelid Problems

I. **Blepharitis** refers to the chronic inflammation and infection around the eyelashes. The usual organisms involved are common skin pathogens (gram-positive *Staphylococcus* and *Streptococcus*). Patients complain of symptoms in the morning of burning, foreign body sensation, and blurring of vision. Treatment includes warm washcloth soaks and massage before bed and in the morning. **Meibomianitis** is inflammation and infection around the oil glands in the eyelids by the eyelid margin that leads to burning, irritation, and chalazion (see sec. **III**). Blepharitis associated with rosacea may require additional treatment with oral antibiotics such as minocin or tetracycline.

II. **Eyelid lesions** that may be **malignant** include basal cell, squamous cell, and sebaceous cell carcinomas. The length of time that a lesion has been present, plus any history of recent change in size or shape, should be determined. Any lesions of concern should be referred for further evaluation and possible biopsy for histopathologic diagnosis.

III. **Chalazion** is acute inflammation from a plugged Meibomian gland in the eyelid. It is the most common eyelid lesion. The mainstays of **treatment** are warm compresses with gentle massage along with topical or oral antibiotics, or both. Conservative treatment should be carried out for 2–3 weeks. If the lesion has not completely resolved and is no longer actively inflamed, surgical incision and drainage or injection of chalazion with intralesional steroids may be recommended.

IV. **Ptosis (drooping of eyelids)** is a common condition that may occur from congenital disease, neurologic disease, or involutional changes with aging. If the upper eyelid appears to interfere with the superior field of vision, or if the patient is symptomatic, surgical intervention is possible. **Dermatochalasis** refers to excess eyelid skin that may cause symptoms similar to those of ptosis. Blepharoplasty is the treatment for symptomatic dermatochalasis.

V. **Ectropion (eyelid turned outward) and entropion (eyelid turned inward)** are malpositions of the eyelid on the globe that can lead to tearing and exposure keratitis. In entropion, the eyelashes may cause keratopathy and corneal abrasions/ulcerations due to direct trauma.

VI. **Dacryocystitis** is infection of the tear sac from inadequate drainage of tears. It presents with redness, pain, and swelling in the inferomedial part of the lower eyelid. Acutely, oral antibiotics are necessary (cephalexin, 250 mg PO qid for 10 days). Surgical **dacryocystorhinostomy** is usually required after the inflammation has resolved because recurrences are likely. In a dacryocystorhinostomy, a new drainage passage is created from the tear sac to the nose.

28

Otolaryngology

James Hartman

Cerumen Impaction

I. **Introduction.** Cerumen is composed of desquamated skin and adnexal gland lipid secretions in the external auditory canal (EAC).

II. **Risk factors**
   A. Age: 60 years and older
   B. Obstruction of EAC by hair proliferation or narrowing secondary to scarring from chronic infection
   C. Foreign bodies, such as hearing aids or earplugs, or the use of cotton-tipped applicators in the EAC
   D. Anatomic anomalies such as narrow EACs, as is common in Down syndrome

III. **Physical findings.** The appearance of cerumen is typically a thick amber to brown waxy clump that obstructs a percentage or all of the EAC.

IV. **Management.** Accumulations of cerumen can be resolved by manual removal, irrigation, or chemical dissolution.
   A. **Manual disimpaction** can be completed by using a cerumen curet during inspection with an otoscope. Care must be taken to avoid contact with the sensitive bony EAC.
   B. **Irrigation** can be used to flush cerumen from the ear canal with a large syringe with the patient sitting up. The water should be approximately body temperature and directed toward the superior wall of the EAC until the impaction is extruded. An emesis basin placed beneath the ear catches the irrigant. Irrigation is **contraindicated** when a history of perforation exists, infection is present or recurrent, or the patient has had a mastoidectomy. Excessive force induces pain and may result in EAC lacerations or tympanic membrane (TM) perforation.
   C. **Dissolution** involves instilling chemical solvents, resulting in thinning of the cerumen and its egress from the EAC. Over-the-counter preparations are available, but plain hydrogen peroxide instilled 4–5 drops at a time is also effective. When cerumen is particularly dry, irrigation can be facilitated by placing 4 drops of triethanolamine polypeptide oleate (Cerumenex) into each EAC several days before irrigation.
   D. **Alternative remedies**, such as burning an ear candle to draw the wax out of the EAC, are on the market. This has not proved to be effective and may result in burns of the external ear.
   E. **Referral to an otolaryngologist is appropriate** for use of binocular microscope and otologic instruments when the cerumen is severely impacted. Other factors that make referral appropriate include TM perforation, a history of TM or mastoid surgery, EAC stenosis, or pain with other attempts at removal.

Hearing Loss

I. **Introduction.** Ten percent of Americans have some degree of hearing loss (*N Engl J Med* 1993;329:1092).
   A. **Causes** of hearing loss are numerous and may be congenital, infectious, traumatic, toxic, neoplastic, vascular, immunologic, neurologic, metabolic, or hereditary. Hearing loss is subtyped into sensorineural, conductive, or mixed based on audiometric measures.
   B. **Risk factors** for hearing loss vary with age. In children, low-birth-weight intrauterine infections, meningitis, and a family history are risk factors. In adults, unprotected noise exposure, head trauma, exposure to ototoxins (such as aminoglycosides), or radiation to the head is associated with a greater risk of hearing loss.
   C. **Differentiation** of hearing loss into several types aids in diagnosis.
      1. **Conductive loss** is caused by a disturbance of the mechanism that transmits sound waves from the environment to the cochlea.
      2. **Sensorineural loss** represents a dysfunction of the cochlea, auditory nerve, or auditory pathway of the CNS.
      3. **Mixed hearing loss** involves dysfunction in both pathways. It results from a single source such as chronic otitis media (OM), cholesteatoma, temporal bone trauma, or otosclerosis, or may be the result of several conditions over the course of a patient's life [*Clinical Otology* (2nd ed). New York: Thieme Medical Publishers, 1997:159].
   D. **Diagnosis**
      1. **History** that is important to elicit is whether hearing loss is unilateral or bilateral, age at onset, and course of hearing loss (i.e., sudden, progressive, or fluctuating). Associated symptoms may include tinnitus, dizziness, aural fullness, otalgia, or otorrhea. History should include past ear infections or surgery, head trauma, the presence of other illnesses, and ototoxic exposures such as noise or medications. Commonly implicated medicines include aminoglycosides, vancomycin, cisplatinum, nitrogen mustard, furosemide, ethacrynic acid, salicylates, and quinine [Ototoxic Drugs. In B Bailey (ed). *Head and Neck Surgery—Otolaryngology Release* (2nd ed). Philadelphia: Lippincott, 1993:2165–2168].
      2. **Physical examination** includes the assessment of normality of anatomy as well as abnormal findings. Inspection of the EAC and TM can be performed with otoscope or microscope.
         a. The normal TM is pearly gray and transparent. In the EAC, identification of cerumen, blood, pus, fungus, granulation tissue, heratinaceous debris, or foreign body may be noted and removed. Polyps, osteomas, exostoses, or tumors may be found and prevent visualization of the TM. TM mobility can be assessed by pneumatic otoscopy (gentle insufflation of the EAC with a rubber bulb attached to the otoscope). Inspection of the TM may reveal TM scarring, perforation, atrophic segments, or retraction pockets. Middle-ear serous fluid appears amber, pus looks white, and hemotympanum is reddish blue. Masses may be seen and appear white (cholesteatoma) or red (glomus tumor).
         b. **Tuning fork testing** suggests conductive or sensorineural hearing loss (SNHL). The Weber and Rinne tests are used together.
            (1) The **Weber** test places the vibrating fork in the midline of the head. The sound is perceived louder in the ear with conductive loss or in the better-hearing ear with SNHL.
            (2) The **Rinne** test places a vibrating fork on the mastoid and then over the EAC. The sound is louder with the fork on the mastoid

with conductive hearing loss (CHL) and louder over the EAC when conductive loss is **not** present.

3. **Audiologic testing** is the measure of choice with suspected hearing loss. This examination includes testing of pure tone thresholds for air and bone conduction in a soundproof booth.

    a. **SNHL** is identified when the two thresholds match.

    b. **Conductive** hearing is present if air thresholds are below bone thresholds.

    c. **Speech discrimination** measures a patient's ability to perceive and repeat words.

    d. **Tympanometry** measures TM mobility and is reduced with middle-ear fluid, infection, or mass.

    e. **Acoustic reflex testing** determines the intactness of a reflex arc passing through the cochlear nerve brainstem, facial nerve, and stapedial muscle. Abnormal reflex tests suggest cochlear nerve or brainstem pathology such as an acoustic neuroma or meningioma.

4. **Laboratory testing** is directed at uncovering systemic disease that results in hearing loss.

    a. **Sedimentation rate.** When the sedimentation rate is elevated, inner-ear antigen-specific tests can reveal autoimmune SNHL, a condition that is reversible with high-dose steroid therapy.

    b. **Other tests** include thyroid function tests, fasting glucose, cholesterol and triglycerides, and the fluorescent treponemal antibody absorption test (FTA-Abs).

    c. Congenital or acquired syphilis can result in hearing loss, and therefore a **positive FTA-Abs** should be followed by a **VDRL test** to determine active infection. When hearing loss is associated with positive syphilis serology, neurosyphilis should be suspected and a lumbar puncture performed for cerebrospinal fluid testing.

5. **Radiologic evaluation** uses high-resolution CT when temporal bone pathology or trauma is suspected. MRI with gadolinium as contrast is used for suspected pathology of the cochlear nerve, brainstem, or brain.

II. **Management.** The diagnosis of hearing loss is best accomplished using the above assessments in collaboration with an otolaryngologist.

  A. **CHL** etiologies are treated by the removal of obstructive wax, debris, or lesions; evacuation of the fluid in OM; or microsurgical repair of anatomic defects, such as TM perforation, ossicular chain disruption, or cholesteatoma.

1. **Otosclerosis** is another common cause of CHL that may also cause progressive sensorineural hearing loss. It occurs as uncontrolled new bone formation in the otic capsule, resulting in fixation of the stapes.

    a. **History.** The disease is passed on by autosomal dominant transmission with incomplete penetrance and is most prevalent in Caucasians and women as young adults. The disease process is accelerated by pregnancy.

    b. **Examination.** Otologic examination is usually normal.

    c. **Diagnosis.** Diagnosis is established when progressive conductive loss occurs in a young or middle-aged adult with a positive family history.

    d. **Treatment.** Treatment is surgical, with replacement of the stapes by prosthesis or aural amplification by hearing aid to compensate for the loss.

2. **Cholesteatoma** is defined as a squamous epithelium pocket or sac filled with keratin debris within the middle ear or mastoid. It manifests with bone destruction secondary to enzymatic activity at a bone interface and often becomes chronically infected, causing fetid drainage.

    a. **Types** of cholesteatomas include congenital (an epithelial cyst in the mastoid air cells or middle ear without communication with the external ear); primary acquired (develops from perforation of the flaccid portion of the TM); and secondary acquired (develops from a progressive retraction pocket of an atrophic TM).

    b. Diagnosis is typically made after referral to an otolaryngologist by otoscopic examination or with binocular microscopy. The extent of disease is best delineated by audiometric testing and temporal bone CT.

    c. Treatment involves surgical removal of the cholesteatoma and repair of the damaged TM or ossicles.

B. SNHL etiologies are treated based on a specific diagnosis. Most SNHL is not reversible, but several exceptions are known. Accurate diagnosis is essential.

    1. Slowly progressive SNHL (presbycusis) is a nontreatable hearing loss that is secondary to aging and persistent noise exposure.

      a. Treatment

        (1) Rehabilitation with hearing aid evaluation and fitting by an otolaryngologist or audiologist. Patients who are most likely to benefit from a hearing aid have moderate to severe loss that impairs their understanding of conversational speech. In general, bilateral amplification is recommended, as patients are more likely to understand speech, justifying the extra cost.

        (2) Use noise protection strategies (earplugs) when exposure to loud noises is anticipated (i.e., weapons firing, power tools, lawnmowers, or vacuuming).

        (3) Profound loss is best treated by implantable hearing aids or cochlear implantation, but assistive listening devices are also helpful for enhancing face-to-face communication, telecommunications, and alerting devices.

    2. Fluctuating or rapidly progressive SNHL may occur with a handful of conditions and is sometimes reversible.

      a. Ménière's disease. The pathogenesis of Ménière's disease is believed to be an increase in fluid pressure of the endolymph in the inner ear.

        (1) Symptoms include unilateral fluctuating SNHL, tinnitus, recurrent attacks of vertigo, and a sense of aural fullness.

        (2) Diagnosis is achieved by exclusion of other etiologies in the differential and by evidence of SNHL fluctuation on serial audiograms. Alternating remissions and exacerbations of symptoms are common, but after several years the vertigo has a tendency to subside and hearing loss stabilizes at the moderate to severe level.

        (3) Treatment. Unpredictability of remissions renders the analysis of treatment difficult.

          (a) Diet. The mainstay of treatment is a regimented diet, avoiding salt, coffee, nicotine, alcohol, and theophylline.

          (b) Medical. The implementation of hydrochlorothiazide diuretics is appropriate if diet control fails. Dyazide, 25 mg/day, is recommended. Referral to an otologist for local instillation of aminoglycosides (gentamicin) into the middle ear has shown promise for ending the vertiginous spells and sparing hearing (*Arch Otorhinolaryngol* 1978;221:149).

          (c) Surgical. When the severity of vertigo impairs quality of life, referral to an otolaryngologist for surgical therapy should be considered.

      b. Acoustic neuroma is a schwannoma of the eighth cranial nerve.

        (1) Symptoms. Progressive growth results in **unilateral** progressive SNHL and in some cases ataxia.

        (2) Diagnosis is confirmed by a slowed neural conduction in the cochlear nerve on auditory brainstem response audiometry or an enhancing mass in the internal auditory canal on MRI with gadolinium contrast.

        (3) Treatment consists of surgical extirpation by skull base otolaryngologists and neurosurgeons or, more recently, by gamma knife obliteration in controlled studies.

   c. **Autoimmune inner-ear disease** is the most responsive etiology of
   rapidly progressive SNHL.
      (1) **Symptoms.** It presents with bilateral SNHL and progressive loss
      in at least one ear over days to months. Half of the patients com-
      plain of dizziness, and 15% have other autoimmune disorders.
      (2) **Diagnosis.** It can be differentiated from multiple sclerosis (MS) by
      an MRI with gadolinium, which is normal in autoimmune inner-ear
      disease. The diagnosis is confirmed when inner-ear antibodies are
      found on serologic tests (*Laryngoscope* 1990;100:516, and *Laryngo-
      scope* 1988;98:251).
      (3) **Treatment** consists of prednisone (1 mg/kg/day to a maximum of
      60 mg/day) for 4 weeks, at the end of which time an audiogram is
      repeated. Responders are continued until recovery plateaus and
      then are decreased to 10 mg/day for 6 months. Nonresponders
      are tapered off prednisone over 14 days. The degree of response
      is variable, and for patients who are not able to tolerate cortico-
      steroids, methotrexate or cyclophosphamide can be used.
   d. **Perilymphatic fistula (PLF)** occurs when perilymph of the inner ear
   is exposed to the middle ear and thus results in dysfunction of the
   inner ear.
      (1) **Symptoms.** Patients note sudden or fluctuating hearing loss, with
      tinnitus and vertigo, and may reveal antecedent trauma to the head.
      (2) **Diagnosis** is achieved with referral to an otolaryngologist for an
      otologic examination that reveals a positive fistula test, in which
      a pneumatic otoscope is used to apply positive pressure to the
      TM, resulting in vertigo and nystagmus. High-resolution tempo-
      ral bone CT is recommended in patients with a history of head
      trauma or in children to rule out a congenital malformation as
      the source of PLF.
      (3) **Treatment** is initially conservative, with bed rest, head elevation,
      and avoidance of straining. If symptoms persist or progress, sur-
      gical exploration of the middle ear is performed to search for a
      perilymph leak. If a leak is found, it is patched with fascia.
   e. **Idiopathic causes** should be treated with a 10-day course of prednisone, 1 mg/kg/day up to 60 mg/day, and then tapered over 14 days,
   with repeat audiometry 2 weeks into treatment.
3. **Sudden SNHL** is defined as 30 dB or more of SNHL over at least three
   contiguous audiometric frequencies occurring in 3 days or less. It is usually unilateral and thought to be most often secondary to a viral etiology, although a vascular interruption etiology is known to exist.
   a. **Symptoms.** Patients present complaining of sudden deafness with
   associated tinnitus. Vertigo is mild or absent in most. Sudden SNHL
   is a medical emergency and requires prompt treatment to effect a
   recovery of hearing.
   b. **Diagnosis** is confirmed with a sensorineural loss on an audiogram.
   c. **Treatment.** The only proven effective treatment is the administration
   of corticosteroids as quickly as possible (*Laryngoscope* 1984;94:664).
   Prednisone, 60 mg/day, should be initiated for 1 week and then
   tapered anytime within 4 weeks of the sudden loss. Vasodilators and
   anticoagulants have not proved to be effective. The use of antiviral
   agents is currently being investigated.

Tinnitus

I. **Introduction.** Fifty million Americans have tinnitus, for which 20% seek clinical
assistance. Tinnitus is a perception of sound that is not related to any external

sound. It is classified into two types. **Objective tinnitus** is the perception of sound arising from sounds within the body that an examiner can also perceive. It is secondary to acoustic energy that is created by turbulent blood flow through vessels near the ear. **Subjective tinnitus** cannot be heard by an examiner. It is the elevated spontaneous discharge rates that occur in auditory cortex neurons in response to acoustic trauma or after aspirin consumption. The description of subjective tinnitus varies, including ringing, buzzing, hissing, whooshing, or cricket sounds.

    A. Symptoms. Most often, patients complain of sleep disturbance or impaired concentration, but anxiety or depression is also commonplace.

    B. Risk factors include acoustic trauma. Exposure to intense sound or a blast injury frequently causes transient tinnitus, but chronic exposure (often job related) results in noise-induced hearing loss and permanent tinnitus (*Audiology* 1981;20:72). Medical side effects from aspirin (acetylsalicylic acid), nonsteroidal anti-inflammatory drugs (NSAIDs) in high doses, or aminoglycoside antibiotics are known to induce transient tinnitus.

II. Diagnosis

    A. History. The characteristics of tinnitus may distinguish between objective and subjective tinnitus. **Objective tinnitus** is pulsatile in nature, is often unilateral, and may be enhanced by exertion. **Subjective tinnitus** is not pulsatile and is prevalent in quiet times. Associated otologic symptoms include hearing loss, dizziness, and aural fullness.

    B. Physical examination

        1. Otoscopy may reveal a hair, dollop of cerumen, or foreign body (including insects) in contact with the TM. Removal solves the problem.

        2. Auscultation can reveal the sound of pulsatile tinnitus when listening over the mastoid, the infra-auricular region, or the carotid artery. Possible causes include glomus tumors, aberrant carotid arteries, arteriovenous malformations, or carotid bruits.

        3. The **Queckenstedt test** may suggest a glomus tumor or benign venous hum by altering acoustic noise from blood flow in the lesion or internal jugular vein. This is done by first impressing the ipsilateral vein while the patient listens for a decrease in tinnitus. Then, the contralateral internal jugular vein is compressed to see if tinnitus is increased. Finally, both internal jugular veins are compressed to see if the tinnitus is eliminated.

    C. Testing centers on the assessment of hearing loss by standard audiometry.

    D. Radiography

        1. For unilateral pulsatile tinnitus, a CT of the neck and temporal bone is indicated to rule out jugulare or a glomus tympanicum tumor.

        2. For subjective tinnitus that is severe, assessment by MRI with gadolinium is indicated to search for an aberrantly located posteroinferior cerebellar artery in the internal auditory canal.

        3. When pulsatile tinnitus is associated with carotid bruits, Doppler ultrasound is recommended to evaluate carotid flow.

III. Management

    A. Objective tinnitus. For vascular anomalies such as **venous hum** or an **aberrant carotid artery**, reassurance alone or masking with competitive sounds from a radio or sound machine is usually adequate. Vascular lesions (specifically **glomus tumors** or **arteriovenous malformations**) usually require resection.

    B. Subjective tinnitus

        1. Avoidance therapy includes the minimization of aspirin or NSAID use, avoiding extreme noise, and the tight control of blood pressure when tinnitus is linked to hypertensive episodes.

        2. Adaptation

            a. It is helpful to provide reassurance to the patient that no medical problem is the source and that deafness is not a likely sequela of the tinnitus. A brief explanation of how competing environmental sounds can mask the tinnitus is useful. Common choices for masking include soft music on the radio, television, or a room fan.

   b. **Masking** devices are sometimes necessary to provide relief from intractable tinnitus. These are essentially sound generators worn like a hearing aid that produce low-level broadband noise and are available from audiologists.

   c. **Tinnitus retraining therapy** administered by an audiologist results in significant improvement in 80% of patients. This regimented therapeutic approach uses a combination of counseling to enhance the patient's understanding of the problem, as well as sound therapy, several hours a day, which suppresses the tinnitus for a prolonged period.

3. Medical treatment

   a. Neurontin, 300–600 mg three times/day, may suppress unrelenting tinnitus.

   b. Currently, the use of prostaglandin agonists or calcium channel blockers is under investigation.

   c. Controlled studies using gingko biloba demonstrated no benefit (*Audiology* 1994;33:85).

4. Future correction is likely to become available as auditory neuron regeneration is accomplished by using nerve growth factors.

Vertigo

I. **Dizziness** is a sensation that is perceived as an impairment of spatial orientation. It may be typed based on the specific perception that the patient experiences. Examples include dysequilibrium (unsteadiness), presyncope (lightheadedness), intoxication (detachment), and vertigo (the illusion of movement, either of self or the environment). Five percent of Americans older than 65 years of age are impaired by dizziness, and it is the most common complaint from patients older than 75 years of age who present to primary care physicians. The daunting task of evaluating dizziness requires knowledge of the physiology of balance and the hundred-plus diseases that can present with this symptom.

II. **Pathophysiology**

   A. Components of the vestibular system include (1) structures that provide sensory input (labyrinth, eyes, deep receptors in the cervical spine, and proprioceptors in the lower limbs), (2) central processing (brainstem, cerebellum, and cortex), and (3) motor output (ocular and peripheral). Dysfunction in the vestibular system or interruption in their blood supply results in dizziness.

   B. The **otologic components** of the vestibular system are found in the semicircular canals, utricle, and saccule.

      1. **Physiology.** Each component is oriented to detect head movement in a specific plane. Its receptors are tonically active, even at rest. This spontaneous activity increases or decreases when the head turns. For example, before turning, the activity is equal, and there is a sense of balance. Turning to the right results in increased neural firing in the right horizontal semicircular canal and decreases firing in the left horizontal canal. When the difference is perceived, the brain interprets this as head rotation, and this results in compensatory eye movements and postural adjustments. The CNS constantly compares all the sensory input of the vestibular system.

      2. **Pathology.** If one component's input is inaccurate relative to the others, the discrepancy is perceived as dizziness. In the above example, if a per-

son has a right vestibular irritant, at rest he or she has an increased activity from the right and a normal activity on the left. The discrepancy between the two sides is interpreted as head rotation, but visual and kinesthetic information are interpreted as no motion. These discordant data result in a perception of dizziness [Ménière's Disease and Other Peripheral Vestibular Disorders. In *Otolaryngology Head and Neck Surgery* (3rd ed). St. Louis: Mosby, 1998:2672–2673].

   3. Adaptation. Importantly, the CNS has the ability to adapt to a discordance, thereby compensating for the dizziness and reattaining a sense of balance.

III. Diagnosis

A. Introduction. The pattern of presentation is critical to identify the etiology; thus, a well-taken history is essential. The first step is to differentiate the type of dizziness experienced. This allows the physician to narrow dramatically a list of more than 100 major diseases down to a few possible causes. Common examples from each category follow: vertigo—vestibular neuritis, benign paroxysmal positional vertigo (BPPV), Ménière's disease, MS, or postconcussion vertigo; dysequilibrium—peripheral neuropathy, extrapyramidal disorders, or cerebellar atrophy; presyncope—cardiac arrhythmias, hypotension, hypoglycemia, or anxiety reactions; intoxication—CNS depressants [alcohol, benzodiazepines, antihistamines, or tricyclic antidepressants (TCAs)]. After dizziness is subtyped, the history is focused on its characteristics. The rest of this section reviews this approach for vertigo.

B. History

   1. Duration

   a. Spells that last for seconds suggest BPPV.

   b. Spells that last for minutes to hours are seen with Ménière's disease, otic syphilis, or Cogan's syndrome.

   c. Longer spells that last for days to weeks are seen in vestibular neuronitis.

   d. Vertigo of variable duration occurs with PLF, temporal bone trauma, barotrauma, or familial vestibulopathy.

   2. Recurrence and frequency. Single episodes occur with vestibular neuritis, otic syphilis, and OM. Recurrent attacks occur with BPPV, Ménière's disease, MS, autoimmune inner-ear disease, migraine, or otic syphilis.

   3. Impact of motion

   a. Influence by motion occurs with Ménière's disease, syphilis, migraine, and vertebrobasilar ischemias.

   b. Initiated by motion, BPPV classically is related to rolling over or turning and looking up.

   c. MS can produce vertigo in either category.

   4. Exacerbating factors include certain foods or sound exposure.

   5. Associated symptoms

   a. Hearing loss

   (1) When associated with tinnitus, Ménière's disease is suspected.

   (2) When progressive sensorineural loss occurs, a PLF is suspected.

   b. Brainstem dysfunction. Complaints of dysarthria, diplopia, and paresthesias suggest vertebrobasilar insufficiency or Wallenberg's syndrome (lateral medullary syndrome or brainstem infarction).

   c. Anxiety attacks present with dyspnea, hyperventilation, and palpitations.

   6. Concomitant ear conditions may be a factor. Otorrhea or prior ear surgery may indicate cholesteatoma. Head trauma or barotrauma suggests a PLF.

   7. Medications such as **ototoxic drugs** (i.e., aminoglycosides), **anticoagulants** (resulting in hemorrhage in the labyrinth), and **intoxicants** (alcohol) may be causative.

C. Clinical evaluation

1. **Physical examination.** The neurotologic examination evaluates the components of the vestibular system as well as hearing and cranial nerve function.

   a. **Cardiac**

      (1) Auscultation of the heart and neck to find arrhythmias or bruits should be performed.

      (2) Postural vital signs to rule out orthostatic hypotension should be obtained.

   b. **Neurologic.** Assessment of gait, deep tendon reflexes, and cerebellar function should be performed.

   c. **Ocular.** Examination of the eyes looking for spontaneous or gaze nystagmus or diplopia is essential.

   d. **Otologic**

      (1) Otoscopy should include a fistula test to see if vertigo and nystagmus are induced with insufflation of air into the EAC.

      (2) A Dix-Hallpike positioning test may reveal nystagmus after a change in head position. Maintaining open eyes and the head turned 45 degrees to one side with the patient sitting, quickly lay the patient on their back with the head hanging slightly off the bed. Observe for the onset of nystagmus for 1 minute. Then have the patient sit up, and repeat the maneuver with the head turned 45 degrees to the other side. Onset of nystagmus suggests BPPV that originates from the down-turned ear.

   e. **Psychological.** A hyperventilation test to elicit dizziness for comparison to the patient's symptoms can be done when anxiety is suspected.

2. **Laboratory evaluation.** Several tests quantitate vestibular function and are particularly useful in identifying the etiology behind a dizziness complaint.

   a. **Electronystagmography (ENG)** records eye motion during vestibular and oculomotor manipulation. It can measure unilateral or bilateral labyrinthine hyper- or hypofunction or disorders of oculomotor control.

   b. **Caloric testing** induces nystagmus with warm- and cold-water irrigation of the EAC. This measures labyrinth function independent of the other side.

   c. **Rotary chair** measures vestibular response to angular acceleration and is useful to assess patients who are suspected of having bilateral hypofunction or cerebellar abnormalities.

   d. **Posturography** uses a "balance booth" to alter proprioceptive and ocular sensory input to search for dysfunction with these systems or with central processing.

IV. Management

A. Supportive measures

1. **Vestibular sedation** can be accomplished with oral meclizine, 12.5–25.0 mg PO tid–qid, resulting in a decrease in intensity of symptoms.

2. **Physical therapy** can be applied to help adapt to many vestibular disorders either at home (Cawthorne exercises) or in the hands of a trained balance therapist.

3. **Safety warnings** should be issued. Patients should avoid driving and heights (ladders or standing on chairs) until symptoms resolve. The most common etiologies and their treatment are now reviewed.

B. Disease-specific treatment

1. **BPPV.**

   a. **Pathogenesis** results from dislodged otoconia in the semicircular canals.

b. **Symptoms.** BPPV is the most common cause of vertigo. Short-lived recurrent vertigo is induced by positional change. BPPV may follow head trauma or vestibular neuritis.

c. **Physical examination.** Nystagmus with the Dix-Hallpike maneuver is latent, fatigues, and reverses with a return to the seated position.

d. **Testing.** ENG helps confirm the diagnosis.

e. **Therapy.** Referral to an otolaryngologist for an otolith repositioning procedure is appropriate. The procedure involves head rotation while vibrating the temporal bone, using gravity to facilitate this repositioning (*Otolaryngol Head Neck Surg* 1980;88:599).

2. **Ménière's disease** (idiopathic endolymphatic hydrops).

a. **Pathogenesis.** Ménière's disease is secondary to overaccumulation of endolymph in the labyrinth.

b. The **differential diagnosis** includes otic syphilis, which is known for fluctuating SNHL and single or recurrent vertigo attacks, and delayed endolymphatic hydrops, in which vertigo attacks follow a previous profound hearing loss. Cogan's syndrome is an autoimmune disorder characterized by interstitial keratitis, SNHL, vertigo, and negative syphilis serology.

c. **Symptoms.** Episodic attacks of vertigo, fluctuating SNHL, tinnitus, and aural fullness. The condition is usually unilateral, and the course is highly variable. The vertigo is unrelated to head movement or postural change.

d. **Physical examination.** Horizontal, direction-varying nystagmus is present only during attacks.

e. **Testing.** ENG or calorics can demonstrate vestibular hypofunction.

f. **Treatment**

(1) **Medical therapy.**

(a) Avoidance by preventing the endolymph accumulation. This includes restriction of sodium, caffeine, and alcohol.

(b) Diuretics can be used to reduce the volume of endolymph. A daily Dyazide tablet is usually effective.

(c) Symptomatic treatment includes antivertiginous medications (meclizine, 12.5–25.0 mg PO tid or qid prn).

(2) Surgical treatment is indicated when medical therapy fails.

(a) Chemical labyrinthectomy has become effective. Gentamicin is instilled into the middle ear and is effective for controlling vertigo 83% of the time with a 10% risk of advancing SNHL (*Am J Otol* 1993;14:278).

(b) Hearing-conserving endolymphatic sac operations are well tolerated and resolve vertigo 50–75% of the time.

(c) Vestibular neurectomy is 95% effective but requires a craniotomy.

3. **Vestibular neuritis.** Severe persistent vertigo and nausea that last days to 12 weeks.

a. **Pathogenesis.** Vestibular neuritis follows a viral infection, leading to the belief that symptoms arise from a viral neuritis. If the inflammatory process results in SNHL as well, the diagnosis is instead labeled **viral labyrinthitis**.

b. **Symptoms.** One ear is affected, and motion exacerbates symptoms. Gradually, definite improvement occurs until the patient is fully recovered.

c. **Physical examination.** Horizontal nystagmus may be present at rest.

d. **Testing.** Caloric testing usually reveals a significant decrease in responsiveness of the involved ear, but does recover.

e. **Treatment.** Management is supportive, with antivertiginous medication (meclizine, 12.5–25.0 mg PO tid–qid) tapered over 4–8

weeks. Early ambulation and vestibular exercises are also recommended.
4. **Traumatic vertigo** includes PLF and postconcussion vertigo. PLF is addressed in Hearing Loss, sec. **II.B.2.d**. Postconcussion vertigo follows closed head trauma.
   a. **Pathogenesis** is secondary to intralabyrinthine hemorrhage.
   b. **Symptoms.** Variable intensity and chronic dysequilibrium. Recovery usually occurs over several weeks.
   c. **Physical examination** and testing are normal.
   d. **Treatment** is supportive with antivertiginous medication and vestibular rehabilitation therapy.
5. **Familial vestibulopathy** is an autosomal dominant disease.
   a. **Symptoms** include sudden attacks of vertigo that last minutes and chronic dysequilibrium. Attacks are induced by stress, and no change in hearing occurs.
   b. **Testing.** Caloric testing reveals bilateral hypofunction, and rotary chair testing is abnormal.
   c. **Treatment.** Vertigo can be eliminated with administration of acetazolamide (*Neurology* 1994;44:20).

Otitis

Otitis is subdivided into otitis externa (OE) or OM based on its anatomic location.
I. Otitis externa
A. **Introduction. Otitis externa** is defined as inflammation of the EAC, with acute OE being the most common infection. It is particularly common after swimming ("swimmer's ear") or after local trauma with a foreign body. **Differential diagnosis** includes otomycosis, cerumen impaction, seborrheic dermatitis of the EAC, furuncles, and perichondritis (painful inflammation of the auricle). Pain usually precedes the development of vesicles in herpes zoster oticus, and facial nerve paresis confirms the Ramsay Hunt syndrome. OE is classified into three stages: preinflammatory, acute inflammatory, and chronic inflammatory (>6 weeks) (*Diseases of the External Ear: An Otologic-Dermatologic Manual.* New York: Grune & Stratton, 1980). Cultures of purulent secretions in acute OE typically reveal *Pseudomonas aeruginosa, Staphylococcus aureus*, or fungi.
B. **Diagnosis**
   1. **Symptoms.** Itching or pain, hearing loss, and/or fetid drainage. The complaints are almost always unilateral and usually follow a precursor event or recent travel in a tropical environment. Pain is the most common complaint and ranges from dull achiness to an intense incapacitating level. Fever may occur when the inflammation is severe.
   2. **Physical examination** of an ear with acute OE reveals a normal auricle but tenderness with tragal manipulation. The EAC skin is erythematous, and induration ranges from mild to severe, in which the canal lumen obstructs secondary to edema. The lumen contains moist desquamated debris, serum, or seropurulent secretions. The TM appears lusterless or erythematous or may not be visible secondary to narrowing of the lumen. In severe cases, temporomandibular joint (TMJ) tenderness and cervical lymphadenopathy may be found.
C. **Management** attempts to reverse the precipitating factors and eliminate infection and inflammation.
   1. **Débridement.** The EAC should be cleansed with suction under binocular microscopy and kept free from water exposure and digital manipulation.
   2. **Topical antibiotics** with or without steroids should be applied for 1 week. Commonly used preparations include Cortisporin Otic suspension (3

drops tid); gentamicin ophthalmic solution (3–4 drops tid); or ofloxacin otic solution (5 drops bid). When otomycosis is present, 5 drops tid of a 2% buffered acetic acid solution [Vosol (Wallace); Domeboro (Burroughs-Wellcome)] should be applied after EAC cleaning.

3. **Oto-wick** (Merocel sponge, Xomed) **placement** is indicated when OE is severe, because the EAC lumen may become occluded secondary to induration, and this impedes the access of drops. In such cases, the Oto-wick should be gently inserted with fingers into the EAC to provide a conduit for the antibiotic drops. As the edema recedes, the wick should be removed, usually in 48–72 hours.

4. **Pain control** often necessitates the use of oral analgesics, including narcotics for 2–3 days.

5. **Referral** (within 48 hours) to an otolaryngologist allows for complete débridement, which expedites the recovery.

D. **Complications** may occur secondary to the choice of drops or the OE.

1. **Contact dermatitis.** Neomycin preparations cause contact dermatitis and apparent worsening of the OE in 5% of patients. The application of a steroid otic suspension resolves the dermatitis. Dexamethasone otic solution, 3–4 drops tid, should be used for 7 days.

2. **Malignant OE** is the most feared complication of OE. It is an aggressive invasive infection of *Pseudomonas aeruginosa* in the EAC that affects cartilage or bone. It is most likely to affect the elderly, diabetics, or the immunosuppressed. Oral antipseudomonal antibiotics should be added to the treatment regimen for these patients to try and prevent this invasive infection. Findings consist of severe worsening ear pain with purulent drainage, spiking fevers, and possible cranial nerve palsies. Culture of the drainage should be performed. Nuclear imaging or temporal bone high-resolution CT can be performed. Hospital admission for daily EAC débridement and intravenous antipseudomonal antibiotics is indicated.

II. **OM**

A. **Introduction. OM** is defined as an inflammatory process in the middle-ear space and can be present in various stages along a continuum. It is characterized by middle-ear effusion, pain, and redness of the TM. It occurs in adults in 1 of every 200 upper-respiratory infections (URIs).

1. **Risk factors** include recent URI, smokers in the home, and nasopharyngeal colonization by *Streptococcus pneumoniae, Haemophilus influenzae,* or *Moraxella catarrhalis.*

2. **Types.** Recurrent acute OM denotes episodes of acute OM that frequently recur after complete clearance of effusion between episodes. OM with effusion is the presence of serous fluid in the absence of clinical symptoms other than hearing loss. Chronic OM with effusion occurs when OM with effusion persists for longer than 30 days.

B. **Diagnosis**

1. **Symptoms.** Fever follows a preceding URI and includes ear pain, hearing loss, fever, and irritability.

2. **Physical examination**

a. **Acute OM.** Otoscopy reveals erythema and bulging of the TM, with serous or purulent fluid in the middle ear. TM mobility is reduced with pneumatic otoscopy. Myringitis is a variant of acute OM in which inflammation of the TM occurs but effusion is absent and the TM mobility is normal. In severe cases of acute OM, necrosis of a portion of the TM occurs, resulting in a pinpoint perforation and otorrhea.

b. **Chronic OM with effusion.** Otoscopy finds a retracted hypomobile TM with serous fluid in the middle ear.

3. **Testing**

a. **Audiometry** reveals a mild to moderate CHL and a flattened tympanogram.

    b. Tympanocentesis for culture is rarely necessary but may be help-ful in immunocompromised patients, patients whose symptoms fail to respond, or patients in whom complications of acute OM, such as intracranial infection, develop [Acute Otitis Media and Otitis Media with Effusion. In *Pediatric Otolaryngology Head and Neck Surgery* (3rd ed). St. Louis: Mosby, 1998:468]. This should be done by an otolaryngologist.

C. Treatment

  1. Acute OM

    a. Oral antibiotic therapy for 10 days is the standard treatment in the United States. Amoxicillin is the first-line agent, 500 mg tid. Alter-natives include trimethoprim-sulfamethoxazole DS bid or erythro-mycin, 500 mg tid. If penicillin resistance is common or no response to therapy occurs, a second-line drug is chosen, such as amoxicillin-clavulanate, 875 mg bid; cefuroxime, 250 mg bid; loracarbef, 200 mg bid; or clarithromycin, 500 mg bid.

    b. Adjunctive therapy includes the use of oral or topical decongestants, or both; pseudoephedrine, 60–120 mg orally bid; and oxymetazoline, 2 puffs in each nostril bid for 5 days only. However, pseudoephedrine should be avoided in patients with hypertension or heart disease. Antihistamines should be avoided because of their sludging effect on secretions.

    c. Myringotomy (an incision to open the TM) offers little value unless pain is severe or complications occur.

    d. Follow-up is necessary to ensure resolution of the effusion. If symp-toms and signs have resolved and only the effusion remains, repeat-ing or extending courses of antibiotics has no additional effect. The postinflammatory change is gradual, and only half of ears with effu-sion clear by 2 weeks; 90% clear by 6 weeks. Repeat examination should occur at approximately 6 weeks after the diagnosis is made. If, on the other hand, symptoms persist, early follow-up to assess adequacy of response is necessary.

  2. Recurrent acute OM

    a. Prophylaxis

      (1) Antibiotic prophylaxis is effective at preventing acute OM, but its routine use has fallen out of favor because of promotion of resis-tance in common pathogens.

      (2) Surgical prophylaxis by the insertion of tympanostomy tubes is effective and is recommended for recurrent acute OM (*Pediatrics* 1995;96:712).

  3. OM with effusion (essentially asymptomatic effusion) is treated in a manner identical to acute OM (see sec. **II.C.1**).

  4. Chronic OM with effusion

    a. Medical therapy has not been shown to be effective.

    b. Surgical therapy is effective and should be used when effusion has persisted for 6–12 weeks.

      (1) Myringotomy alone has proved disappointing because of rapid closure. Current studies are under way for laser tympanostomy.

      (2) Insertion of tympanostomy tubes is the gold standard treatment for chronic OM with effusion.

      (3) Adenoidectomy has been confirmed effective in the treatment of OM by reducing eustachian tube (ET) reflux of colonized nasopharyngeal secretions; tonsillectomy is not effective (*N Engl J Med* 1987;317:1444). Adenoidectomy is reserved for those with recurrent chronic OM with effusion.

      (4) Complications of surgical therapy exist but do not outweigh the benefits.

Eustachian Tube Dysfunction

I. Introduction

A. Pathophysiology. The ET performs three physiologic functions: ventilation of the middle ear, protection from reflux of nasopharyngeal secretions, and drainage of the middle-ear space. Interference with any one of these functions by obstruction or abnormal patency can result in a disturbance of the middle ear [Diseases and Disorders of the Eustachian Tube—Middle Ear. In *Otolaryngology* (3rd ed). Philadelphia: Saunders, 1991:1289–1315]. Obstruction interferes with the ventilation and drainage functions of the ET. Abnormal patency diminishes the protective function of the ET by more easily allowing reflux of nasopharyngeal secretions to the middle ear.

B. Risk factors for eustachian tube dysfunction (ETD).

1. Patients with **cleft palates** or **craniofacial syndromes** such as Down or Turner's syndrome are at great risk.
2. **Intrinsic mechanical obstruction** occurs from allergy or ciliary dyskinesia or after radiation therapy to the head or neck.
3. **Extrinsic mechanical obstruction** results from recurrent adenotonsillitis or congenital cholesteatoma.
4. American Indians and Eskimos have a **genetic predisposition** to have abnormally patent ETs.
5. **Perforation of the TM** also increases patency of the ET.

II. Clinical presentation and management.

Most ETD results in some form of OM for which the patient seeks medical attention (see Otitis, sec. **II.C**). ETD can result in other clinical scenarios, with varying degrees of symptoms.

A. Atelectasis

1. **Pathogenesis.** Chronic obstruction may weaken the TM and cause it to retract into the middle-ear space.
2. **Symptoms.** TM retraction results in a CHL and occasionally mild vertigo. Recurrent serous OM develops with URIs.
3. **Physical examination** reveals a thinned sunken-in TM and readily visible incudostapedial joint of the ossicles.
4. **Complications.** This may result in an acquired cholesteatoma.
5. **Treatment** simply requires interruption of the persistent negative pressure; therefore, a myringotomy is performed and a tympanostomy tube inserted. The TM often reverts to normal while the tube remains in place.

B. Fluctuating obstruction

1. **Pathogenesis.** Inflammatory conditions of ET mucosa may wax and wane. Typical examples include upper-airway allergy, sinusitis, or pharyngitis.
2. **Symptoms.** Patients typically complain of pressure or discomfort in the ear; popping, clicking, or squeaking in the ear; an increased perception of their heartbeat (consistent with a CHL); and an increase in tinnitus. A history or evidence of palatal trauma or trigeminal nerve injury should be excluded. Less frequent complaints include ear pain or vertigo.
3. **Physical examination.** Otoscopy may discover a retracted TM but usually is normal. When chronic ET obstruction develops, it should prompt a search for an underlying cause. Nasal or nasopharyngeal obstruction secondary to inflammation, polyps, or neoplasm should be eliminated as a source by flexible endoscopic examination. Tuning fork testing occasionally reveals a mild CHL, but an audiogram is more sensitive at detecting this. Tympanograms detect even subtle negative middle-ear pressure. Finally, clinical investigation to rule out myasthenia gravis should be considered when appropriate, as this disorder has presented with ETD.

4. Treatment
   a. **Medical therapy** should be directed toward resolving the underlying inflammatory disorder, as well as ET inflammation. Typical remedies use topical oxymetazoline, 2 puffs in both nostrils bid for 5 days only, oral decongestants (pseudoephedrine, 60–120 mg/day bid prn), topical nasal and oral steroid preparations, and antibiotics. When allergy is suspected as the source, treatment with topical nasal steroids or oral antihistamine/decongestant combinations is recommended.
   b. **Autoinflation.** When symptoms persist despite medical therapy, frequent autoinflation of the middle ear may be useful (accomplished by Valsalva with the nose pinched and mouth closed).
   c. **Surgical therapy.** Myringotomy and placement of a tympanostomy tube in the otolaryngologist's office may be necessary.
C. A **patulous ET** may be noted in adolescents or adults but rarely in children.
   1. **Pathogenesis.** It may occur after significant weight loss.
   2. **Symptoms.** Patients present complaining of hearing their own breathing in the ear (autophony). This often disappears when the patient lies down.
   3. **Physical examination.** Otoscopy reveals motion of the TM, medially with inspiration and laterally with expiration, and is exacerbated by forced respiration. Because venous engorgement may relieve the patency when patients are supine, the ear should be examined with the patient in the sitting position. Oral inspection may reveal palatal contractions for palatal myoclonus, which can give rise to a patulous ET.
   4. **Testing.** Tympanometry is confirmatory.
   5. **Treatment.** Management depends on the severity of the disturbance. Most often reassurance alone satisfies a patient's concern. When symptoms are chronic and annoying, TCAs may be useful, and attempts to narrow the ET are indicated when the patient continues to suffer, but they carry the risk of complications.

Otalgia and Facial Pain

I. **Introduction. Otalgia** literally translates as ear pain and is classified into primary (otogenic) and secondary (referred). In more than 50% of patients who complain of ear pain, it is referred from a non-ear source [*Otolaryngology* (3rd ed). Philadelphia: Saunders, 1991:1237]. The source of otogenic otalgia can be infections, trauma, allergy, neoplasms, foreign bodies, or cerumen. Infection can involve the auricle (perichondritis), the meatus (furuncles or herpes zoster oticus), the EAC (OE), the TM (myringitis), or the middle ear (OM or mastoiditis). Referred otalgia can be either acute or chronic. Acute etiologies are usually infectious or traumatic, whereas chronic sources are more often inflammatory, neurologic (including headache), neoplastic, or cervicogenic. Due to the complexity of otalgia etiologies, **early referral** to otolaryngologists and neurologists is mandatory. If no etiology can be found, a head CT should be obtained to rule out intracranial pathology. If normal, empiric therapy should be initiated with NSAIDs or TCAs. If the patient still does not respond, he or she should be referred to a pain management clinic where medical blockade and behavioral therapy are used.
II. **Clinical presentation and management**
   A. **Otogenic otalgia** (see Otitis)
   B. **Referred otalgia**
      1. **Acute**
         a. Common **oral sources** of acute referred otalgia include dental or periodontal infection or impacted teeth. Nondental oral sources are

numerous, including herpetic gingivostomatitis, herpes zoster, aphthous stomatitis, erosive lichen planus, and glossitis. Dental sources require antibiotics (clindamycin, 300 mg tid for 7 days) and dental evaluation.

b. **Facial sources** include maxillary sinusitis, infectious rhinitis, parotitis, and the acute phase of TMJ arthralgia. Sinusitis should be treated with antibiotics (amoxicillin, 500 mg tid for 10 days) and decongestants (pseudoephedrine, 60 mg bid for 10 days) and an oxymetazoline (2 puffs in each nostril bid for 5 days only). TMJ arthralgia is best controlled with NSAIDs (ibuprofen, 600 mg tid for 14 days), bruxism splints, and jaw rest.

c. **Disorders of the pharynx** that also cause otalgia include tonsillitis or peritonsillar abscess, posttonsillectomy pain, and acute pharyngitis. Tonsillitis also requires antibiotic therapy, either penicillin VK, 500 mg qid for 7 days, or clindamycin, 300 mg tid for 7 days.

d. **Laryngeal inflammation** from reflux or laryngitis is also a possible source. Reflux laryngitis is best managed with antireflux medication [ranitidine hydrochloride (Zantac), 150 mg bid] or a proton pump inhibitor such as pantoprazole, 40 mg qa.m., and reflux control strategies.

e. **Visceral sources** include acute viral thyroiditis, angina, or aortic aneurysms. Although viral thyroiditis can be managed with NSAIDs such as ibuprofen, 600 mg tid, suspected angina or aortic aneurysms require appropriate evaluation [Otalgia. In *Clinical Otology* (2nd ed). New York: Thieme Medical Publishers, 1997:438].

2. **Chronic etiologies**

a. **Inflammatory orofacial disorders** may result in referred otalgia. These are classified as nonarticular or articular causes:

   (1) Nonarticular etiologies include **myofascial pain dysfunction (MPD)** secondary to hyperactivity of the muscles of mastication. It is characterized by sudden onset with local trigger points in tender muscles [*Rheum Dis Clin North Am* 1989;15(1):31]. The area of involvement is diffuse. It is most likely to affect women between the ages of 30 years and 60 years. Besides otalgia, pain can be located in the jaw, temple, frontal or occipital region, or teeth. This syndrome may be palliated by NSAIDs or nonaddictive muscle relaxants (methocarbamol, 500 mg qid; carisoprodol, 350 mg PO qid; or chlorzoxazone, 500 mg PO tid or qid). Finally, TCAs such as nortriptyline, 25 mg tid, are frequently effective. Bite appliances, physical therapy, and nerve block injections may also be helpful. Occasionally, psychiatric evaluation may be necessary to control anxiety or depression linked to the chronic pain.

   (2) **Articular disorders** include internal disk derangement, TMJ arthritis, ankylosis, and condylar dislocation. They are characterized by pain exacerbated by function (mastication), TMJ clicking, and decreased range of motion. These disorders can best be evaluated and managed by oromaxillofacial (OMF) surgeons or otolaryngologists. Treatment includes NSAIDs, splints, and judicious use of surgery in the TMJ.

b. **Neurologic causes** are well-known sources of chronic otalgia and facial pain.

   (1) Most common of these is **trigeminal neuralgia** (tic douloureux). It is characterized by episodic attacks of severe sharp pain in the distribution of a branch of the trigeminal nerve. The attacks last seconds to minutes and are triggered by light touch of the face or oral cavity. Pinching a trigger area is unlikely to start an attack, in contrast to MPD. The physical examination is normal (*Neurol Clin* 1989;2:385). This neuralgia can be managed medically for most patients. Choices include baclofen, 10–20 mg PO tid; car-

bamazepine, 100–600 mg PO bid; clonazepam, 0.25–0.50 mg PO bid or tid; or valproic acid, 10–15 mg/kg PO qid. TCAs and NSAIDs are also useful. Neural blockade is often helpful if response to medical therapy is inadequate. This can be obtained by referral to a neurosurgeon or pain clinic.

  (2) **Postherpetic neuralgia** is persistent severe pain and can persist beyond the vesicular eruptions in the distribution of involved cranial nerves. It may primarily involve the ear or be referred from other facial locations. It often requires the use of narcotics to control the pain. TCAs may also be helpful, as can antineuralgic medications, which are used for trigeminal neuralgia as well. Sympathetic nerve blockade may also bring relief.

  (3) **Headaches** represent a complex diagnostic challenge, but several broad categories of headache are known to be associated with referred otalgia and facial pain. Tension headaches have a known propensity for referred otalgia, whereas vascular headaches (migraine and cluster) do not (see Chap. 23 for headaches). These headaches can usually be managed with NSAIDs, muscle relaxants, and applications of heat and massage. Occasionally, refractory pain requires nerve blockade or lidocaine and steroid injection into trigger points. These can be obtained by referral to a neurosurgeon or pain clinic.

  c. **Other causes.** Neoplastic causes of otalgia can occur in any location previously discussed and patients must receive a thorough examination of the head and neck, including the upper-aerodigestive system. Cervicogenic causes of otalgia arise from inflammation of cervical nerve roots, vertebral joints, disks, ligaments, or muscles.

Temporomandibular Joint Disorders

I. **Introduction.** TMJ disorders afflict 10 million Americans. These disorders encompass two major groups of patients: those with true TMJ dysfunction and those with inflammation of masticatory muscles, termed **MPD syndrome**.

II. **Clinical presentation and management.** TMJ disorders are divided into several categories. It is generally geared toward the relief of pain and the restoration of normal function. Therapy for each condition is specific.

A. **Arthritis** is the most common condition to affect the TMJ.

  1. **Degenerative arthritis** typically affects older adults gradually. They have mild pain and minimal limitation of opening. A secondary form follows trauma or chronic clenching from MPD syndrome. It affects younger adults and causes severe pain and restricted jaw movement. Both are typically unilateral. TMJ radiography frequently reveals erosion of the articular surface or osteophyte formation. Treatment includes the administration of NSAIDs; ibuprofen, 600 mg tid, or celecoxib (Celebrex), 200 mg PO bid; a soft diet; and limitation of jaw opening. If bruxism (chronic teeth clenching or grinding) is present, a bite appliance can be used. This is available through orthodontists or OMF surgeons. Surgical recontouring of the articular surface is reserved for refractory chronic cases.

  2. **Traumatic arthritis** follows acute mandibular trauma without fracture. Joint pain and limitation of opening increase during the early inflammatory period. Radiographs may show widening of the joint space due to edema or hemorrhage. Therapy consists of NSAIDs as in degenerative arthritis, soft diet, limitation of jaw opening and application of heat.

3. **Rheumatoid arthritis** generally starts in other joints first. When the TMJ is involved, pain is bilateral. Swelling, limitation of motion, and anterior open bite are common. Radiographs demonstrate destruction of the articular surface of the condyle, and the joint space is obliterated. Treatment is the same as for rheumatoid arthritis in other joints (see Chap. 22). NSAIDs, oral steroids, and jaw exercises are appropriate for mild cases; severe cases may require hydroxychloroquine, gold, or penicillamine. Surgery is reserved for when ankylosis develops (*Oral Surg* 1986;61:119).

B. **Traumatic injuries**

   1. **Fractures** frequently involve the condylar process. Patients complain of preauricular pain and trismus following a blow to the head or fall to the ground. Radiographs usually reveal a fracture at the base of the condylar process. They are managed by referral to an OMF surgeon or otolaryngologist for maxillomandibular fixation (jaw wiring) or open reduction and internal fixation.

   2. **Dislocations** typically follow trauma or forced opening. During dislocation the mandible is fixed in the open position with only posterior molars making contact. Three clinical scenarios exist: a single acute episode, chronic recurrent episodes, or chronic persistent dislocation. Typically, only the patient with an acute episode experiences pain. Treatment requires referral to an OMF surgeon. Acute dislocation is managed by manual reduction under anesthesia. Chronic recurrent dislocation can be treated with sclerotherapy injected into the TMJ or by surgical repair of the joint capsule. Chronic persistent dislocation can be reduced manually or by temporal myotomy.

C. **Internal derangement** of the intra-articular disk may be secondary to trauma or bruxism or spasm accompanying MPD syndrome; it is usually unilateral. Anterior disk displacement that reduces with mouth opening is characterized by clicking but not pain. Displacement that reduces and has no pain requires no treatment. If pain is present, the use of NSAIDs, muscle relaxants, or a bite appliance is indicated. Anterior disk displacement without reduction on attempted mouth opening is characterized by locking the mandible closed. Patients complain of significant pain, and examination reveals clicking and extreme resistance to passive opening. Disk adhesion to the articular surface of the glenoid fossa is characterized by rigid limitation of opening to approximately 20 mm. Increasing pain occurs as opening excursion increases. All are managed by referral to an OMF surgeon.

D. **Neoplasia** is a rare cause of TMJ symptoms but is occasionally responsible. Pain is variable, but progressive limitation of motion is seen. Radiographs reveal an enlarged condyle or bony destruction. An MRI demonstrates a mass, and biopsy elicits a diagnosis. Referral to an otolaryngologist or OMF surgeon for surgical resection as the primary treatment of benign and of malignant tumors is necessary. Reconstruction of the defect is attempted at the time of resection.

Epistaxis

I. **Introduction.** Epistaxis (nasal bleeding) can be a single prolonged episode or multiple minor episodes. The incidence of epistaxis is greatest in older patients. Nasal bleeding is more common during winter months due to decreased humidity and frequent URI. The vascular anatomy of the nose and clinical experience have led to the division of epistaxis into anterior and posterior locations. Greater than 80% of the time, the location of epistaxis is easily visible in the front of the nose and is designated as anterior. This usually involves an area of anterior septum known as **Kiesselbach's plexus**, where multiple vessels anastomose (*Laryngoscope* 1969;79:969).

II. **Causes** are divided into local and systemic etiologies.
A. **Local causes**
1. **Mechanical or traumatic causes** may result in mucosal lacerations and epistaxis. This is usually short lived and responds to nasal pinching for 10 minutes in an upright position. Chronic trauma from recurrent nasal picking may result in anterior ulceration and bleeding. Other sources of chronic mucosal trauma include administration of steroid nasal sprays and recurrent use of intranasal cocaine. Occasionally, epistaxis may occur weeks after head trauma with the formation of a traumatic aneurysm. Bleeding is recurrent and heavy and may be fatal.
2. **Septal deformities** may cause turbulent airflow, resulting in excessive drying and subsequent epistaxis. These deformities include deviations, spurs, and perforations.
3. **Inflammation** may result from URIs, sinusitis, nasal allergy, or exposure to toxic inhalants.
4. **Neoplasms**, benign or malignant, of the nose, sinuses, or nasopharynx may result in recurrent bouts of epistaxis. Recurrent bleeds require endoscopic evaluation by an otolaryngologist of the entire internal nose to search for tumor as a possible etiology. An office biopsy may be contraindicated due to risk of severe hemorrhage. Head CT and MRI establish the diagnosis [Refractory Posterior Epistaxis. In *Current Therapy in Otolaryngology—Head and Neck Surgery* (6th ed). St. Louis, Mosby, 1998:331–335].
B. **Systemic causes. Coagulation abnormalities** should be suspected when easy bruisability, prolonged bleeding after surgery or laceration, and a positive family history are present. Acquired coagulopathies may be drug induced, or systemic disease may result in a coagulopathy. Hereditary hemorrhagic telangiectasia (Osler-Weber-Rendu disease) is an autosomal dominant disease characterized by diffuse mucocutaneous telangiectasias. A positive family history is found in 80% of patients. The telangiectasias may also occur in the lung, bowel, CNS, or liver. Frequent bleeds require transfusion (*Laryngoscope* 1991;101:977). Treatment of hereditary hemorrhagic telangiectasia focuses on reasonable limitation of hemorrhage and elimination of the need for recurrent transfusion. General measures use humidity, topical moisturizers (Ocean Saline Spray or Ponaris Nasal Emollient), and iron replacement. Repetitive laser photocoagulation with the neodymium:yttrium-aluminum-garnet laser can provide hemostasis (*Oper Tech Otol Head Neck Surg* 1994;5:274).
III. **Evaluation and management**
A. **Evaluation** begins with a history to discern severity, location, duration, and frequency of bleeding as well as the presence of other nasal symptoms including obstruction or rhinorrhea. The general history should investigate traumatic injuries, underlying medical conditions, medications, use of tobacco or alcohol, and family history. Anterior rhinoscopy is facilitated by applying topical nasal decongestant spray [phenylephrine (Neo-Synephrine) 0.25%, 2 puffs each nostril]. Endoscopes are used to visualize the remaining mucosal surfaces to identify posterior epistaxis and to search for tumors. Laboratory testing is appropriate to assess severity of blood loss or coagulopathy. CT or MRI is indicated to evaluate neoplasms.
B. **Treatment of anterior epistaxis** should occur with the patient seated, adequate light, suction, cautery, and packing materials available. On removal of clots, topical 4% lidocaine and phenylephrine are sprayed into the nose. If bleeding is not active, a suction or cotton-tipped applicator can gently

abrade likely source vessels on the anterior septum to identify the bleeding site.

1. **Cautery** comes in two forms, chemical and electrical. Silver nitrate on applicator sticks provides an effective chemical cauterization with only a mild burning sensation when applied to bleeding vessels. Electrocautery is available from a hand-held concept cautery and is also very effective; however, because it is associated with greater pain, it may require the injection of a local anesthetic. After cautery, a piece of absorbable oxidized cellulose (Surgicel) is placed over the newly created eschar to provide additional protection, and the patient is advised to apply saline spray every 2 hours while awake and to practice epistaxis precautions for 5 days. Epistaxis precautions include avoidance of nose blowing, nasal picking, heavy lifting or straining, and aspirin or NSAIDs. If bleeding recurs, pinching the nasal tip firmly closed for 10 continuous minutes usually stops the bleeding, allowing the patient to seek attention again in a nonemergent fashion.

2. **Packing** is indicated when cauterization fails but is generally achieved by referral to an otolaryngologist. First, expandable compressed sponges (Merocel) are easily inserted with minimal discomfort to tamponade anterior bleeding rapidly, but they sometimes fail to apply adequate pressure. If they fail, an inflatable balloon or Vaseline gauze should be inserted instead. This gauze is 1/2 in. by 72 in. and is layered on the floor of the nose, progressing upward until the nose is entirely filled. This is moderately painful to undergo but can be tolerated after topical anesthesia. Once epistaxis is controlled by packing, the packing should be removed 2 or 3 days later and the nose inspected. Mild pain medications should be given for comfort, and oral cephalexin, 500 mg tid, should be administered until the packs are removed to prevent toxic shock syndrome secondary to *Staphylococcus aureus* colonization.

3. Treatment of epistaxis due to **underlying coagulopathy** is aimed at correcting the coagulopathy and obtaining hemostasis without further traumatizing the nasal mucosa. Consultation of an otolaryngologist for placement of a hemostatic-like substance, microfibrillar collagen (Avitene) or oxidized cellulose, over the bleeding site can accomplish the latter goal during the correction of the coagulopathy [Epistaxis. In *Otolaryngology Head and Neck Surgery* (3rd ed). St. Louis: Mosby, 1998:856].

C. **Treatment of posterior epistaxis** follows a stepwise approach in the hands of an otolaryngologist.

1. **Packing** traditionally uses a gauze sponge pulled into the nasopharynx via strings through the nostrils. This is combined with an anterior pack and left in place for 3 days. However, this is cumbersome and painful. Now, inflatable balloons (Storz epistaxis catheter or Applied Therapeutics Inc. Rapid RHINO catheter) are available that insert easily and can be gradually filled with water by a syringe until bleeding stops. Patients who require posterior packing should be admitted for observation and pulse oximetry, as nocturnal hypoxic episodes may occur. Pain control usually requires oral or intramuscular narcotics and occasional benzodiazepines to sleep. Cephalexin, 500 mg tid, should be given until the packs are removed to prevent toxic shock syndrome secondary to *S. aureus* colonization.

2. **Endoscopic cautery** has become an effective means of controlling posterior epistaxis because the fiberoptic nasal endoscopes provide excellent visualization of the mucosal surface of the nose, allowing for accurate localization of the bleeding source. The procedure is best tolerated in the operating room with anesthesia. This method is 90% effective (*Arch Otol Head Neck Surg* 1992;118:966).

3. **Arterial embolization** is particularly useful when bleeding is too heavy for visualization with endoscopes, the patient is too ill for anesthesia, or surgical intervention fails. The major risks from embolization are rare but include cerebrovascular accident.
4. **Arterial ligation** is a 75–100% effective technique of obtaining epistaxis control (*Laryngoscope* 1988;98:760). The specific vessels to ligate depend on the location of the likely bleeding site. Occasionally, bilateral ligation is necessary.

Nasal Fractures

I. **Introduction.** Nasal fractures are the most common injury to the facial skeleton, comprising up to 50% of all facial fractures. The resulting deformity may alter appearance and the airway function of the nose. Males are twice as likely to sustain a nasal fracture. Two age groups are most likely to present with a fractured nose: young adults secondary to altercations or sports injuries and the elderly secondary to falls. Nasal fractures can be classified as lateral or frontal impact injuries.
II. **Diagnosis** is best made in the otolaryngologist's office but can be established in the emergency room as well.
   A. **History** should discern the type of impact to the nose, as the mechanism of injury helps predict the extent of injury. The appearance of the nose before the injury should be ascertained. Information regarding nasal obstruction, loss of smell, epistaxis, and clear rhinorrhea should be obtained.
   B. **Physical examination** after nasal trauma includes inspection of external and internal surfaces. Changes in dorsal contour should be noted. Periorbital ecchymosis (black eyes) strongly suggests nasal fracture. Early posttraumatic edema may obscure subtle deformities up to 4 days after the injury [Nasal Fractures. In *Otolaryngology Head and Neck Surgery* (3rd ed). St. Louis: Mosby, 1998:869]. Palpation of the nasal pyramid may reveal tenderness, mobility, or step deformities. Internal examination requires adequate light for visualization with a nasal speculum and removal of clots and crusts by suction or bayonet forceps. The septum should be evaluated for dislocation, swelling, or possible septal hematoma contributing to nasal obstruction. When clear rhinorrhea has been reported, endoscopic inspection of the apex of the nose should be performed, and the fluid should be collected and tested for beta-2 transferrin in an attempt to identify a cerebrospinal fluid leak.
   C. **Radiographic evaluation**, a standard emergency room practice, is largely unnecessary, as it fails to have an impact either on management or outcome in adults or children (*Arch Emerg Med* 1993;10:293). If other facial fractures are suspected, a noncontrast facial CT should be obtained.
III. **Management**
   A. **Acute care.** Control of bleeding is preeminent after nasal trauma. Fortunately, pinching the nostrils firmly for 10 minutes usually gains hemostasis. If not, packing may be required. Internal swelling that results in obstruction may respond to topical decongestants such as oxymetazoline (Afrin), 2 puffs in each nostril bid used for 3–5 days.
   B. If a **septal hematoma** is suspected, referral to an otolaryngologist for direct aspiration should occur. This is performed with a large-bore needle after intranasal administration of topical anesthesia. Then, anterior nasal packs should be placed bilaterally to prevent reaccumulation of blood. Unrecognized hematomas may devascularize the septal cartilage, resulting in necrosis, then cosmetic deformity (saddle nose) or septal perforation.
   C. **Referral** should be made to an otolaryngologist for reduction of the fracture, but due to posttraumatic swelling closed reduction of fractures is recommended at between 3–7 days. Open reduction may be necessary when attempts at closed reduction fail or when severe septal deviation occurs.

Aphthous Stomatitis

I. **Introduction.** Recurrent aphthous ulcerations, also known as **canker sores**, are usually small ulcers that typically involve nonkeratinized mucosa. Young adults are the age group that is most often affected. Ulcers may be single or multiple and vary in the frequency of recurrence. Three categories are described. Minor aphthae are the most common and are limited in size up to 10-mm ulcerations. Major aphthous ulcers are larger, even 2–3 cm in size. Finally, herpetiform ulcerations are aphthous ulcers that mimic herpes simplex infection. Multiple 1- to 2-mm ulcers are clustered in one nonkeratinized mucosal area. The etiology is unknown, but several factors are suggested as causative or contributory; these include the L form of alpha streptococcus, cell-mediated hypersensitivity to oral mucosa, and an inherited predisposition. Associated factors include hormonal changes, vitamin B_{12} or folic acid deficiency, gluten-sensitive enteropathy, and stress (*Oral Surg Oral Med Oral Pathol* 1992;74:79).

II. **Diagnosis**

   A. The **differential diagnosis** of aphthous stomatitis includes primary herpetic gingivostomatitis, traumatic ulcerations, Behçet's syndrome, and primary syphilis.

   1. **Primary herpetic gingivostomatitis,** a herpes simplex virus, usually type 1, results in a few mildly painful ulcers with or without systemic symptoms of viremia (fever, malaise, headache, and cervical adenopathy). Vesicles form several days after symptoms, then ulcerate, and the gingiva is inflamed. Typically, multiple 1- to 3-mm lesions are seen, last 1–2 weeks, and do not recur. The diagnosis can be confirmed by exfoliative cytology or viral culture.

   2. **Traumatic ulcerations** are usually single and attributable to an initial injury that the patient recalls. These lesions are irregularly shaped and resolve in 1–2 weeks unless recurrent bite injury occurs.

   3. **Behçet's syndrome** occurs when two or more signs are present, including aphthous-like ulcerations of oral mucosa, genital ulcers, and uveitis (which presents with photophobia).

   4. **Primary syphilis lesions** (chancres) can occur orally after exposure to *Treponema pallidum*. An ulcerated papule develops that is painless. Significant cervical adenopathy is usually present. Diagnosis can be confirmed by a silver stain or a biopsy specimen [Oral Mucosal Lesions. In *Otolaryngology Head and Neck Surgery* (3rd ed). St. Louis: Mosby, 1998:1542].

   B. **Clinical presentation.** Classic locations for ulcers include buccal, labial, ventral tongue, or soft-palate mucosa. The ulcers are oval and have a central depression with a white fibrinous pseudomembrane and an erythematous border. The ulcer is painful and does not involve keratinized mucosa (gingiva and hard palate). Systemic symptoms are lacking, and adenopathy rarely develops. Healing usually occurs within 10 days for minor aphthae but 2–4 weeks for major aphthae. Because the major ulcerations tend to cycle very frequently, patients are rarely free of them. In the herpetiform variety, lesions recur and viral cultures are consistently negative.

III. **Management.** Treatment depends on the severity of the disease. Small isolated lesions require no treatment or application of topical over-the-counter anesthetic preparations (Ambucil or Oragel) for discomfort. Abrading the ulcer with a toothbrush may increase local blood flow and accelerate healing. This usually requires that a topical anesthetic be applied first. Topical steroid gels (fluocinonide gel, 0.05%, applied 2–4 times/day) or rinses (betamethasone syrup, 0.6 mg/5 cc for swish and spit) may also speed up healing. Moderate to severe cases may require prescription anesthetic agents such as benzocaine 20% (Hurricane Gel) or oral steroids [methylprednisolone (Medrol) dose pack]. Recurrent ulcerations may respond to oral tetracycline elixir, 250 mg in 5 cc for swish and swallow tid for 10 days, to eradicate L forms of alpha streptococcus. Ulcerations that persist for longer than 2 weeks should be considered for biopsy.

Hoarseness

I. **Introduction. Hoarseness** (dysphonia) is a nondescript term that is intended to mean an impairment in the sound of one's voice. Risk factors for voice disruption include smoking, voice abuse, gastroesophageal reflux disease (GERD), and cervical or mediastinal surgery. Disruption of muscular or epithelial layers, or both, of the vocal cords results in dysphonia. Both layers may be destroyed with invasion by malignancy or fibrosis from radiation therapy.

II. **Diagnosis.** Voice evaluation begins with a detailed history, physical examination, and perceptual evaluation, and it continues with audio-video documentation and sometimes objective measures.

   A. The **history** should solicit information about the character of the hoarseness, the onset and duration, and the course, as well as associated symptoms, the patient's voice-use patterns, and social habits (smoking). Any history of neck trauma or radiation therapy should be divulged.

   B. **Physical examination** must include the entire ear, nose, and throat in addition to the larynx. Assessment of hearing, sinus function, and oral cavity disease may reveal clues to the etiology of hoarseness. Visualization of the larynx can be readily achieved by indirect mirror inspection or flexible fiberoptic laryngoscopy. The mirror examination gives a true-color reflection of the larynx by positioning the mirror against the soft palate, avoiding contact with the base of the tongue to prevent gagging and retracting the tongue forward while a light is reflected against the downward-angled mirror. The fiberscope, passed through the nose to the pharynx, is well tolerated and allows thorough examination of the larynx structure and function (phonation). Consideration of general health is appropriate to realize the impact of respiratory conditions or neuromuscular disorders on phonation.

   C. **Perceptual evaluation** of the voice includes a description of vocal quality, pitch of the spoken voice, range of the voice, ability to sustain phonation, and estimation of the severity of impairment.

   D. **Videolaryngoscopy** attaches a camera to the fiberscope so that videotaping of the examination can occur. Audio recordings are also obtained. These allow detailed analysis and create a permanent record. Pulsed light can be flashed onto the vocal cords during phonation to create the illusion of slow motion. This technique, called stroboscopy, is particularly useful in assessing the mucosal vibration.

   E. **Objective measures** of phonation include aerodynamic and acoustic measures. These are useful in assessing glottic competency and patency as well as analyzing the severity of impairment (Hoarseness. In *Otolaryngology—Head and Neck Surgery*. Philadelphia: Saunders, 1992:701–702).

III. **Management.** The application of the above methods to derive a diagnosis generally falls into the hands of a voice team, typically comprised of an otolaryngologist and speech therapist. Then team members can implement disease-specific therapy.

   A. **Acute laryngitis,** the most common malady that results in hoarseness, is most often secondary to mucosal edema from a URI or may follow an episode of vocal abuse. The vocal cords are erythematous and edematous, and the mucosal wave is severely impaired. The impairment is short lived (less than 2 weeks) but may be severe for several days. If a URI initiates the dysphonia, treatment with humidity, hydration, and voice rest is indicated. If the hoarseness persists for 5 days, antibiotics, such as amoxicillin, 500 mg tid for 7 days, are appropriate, and a methylprednisolone dose pack can be used to expedite recovery of the voice. Voice rest usually corrects edema secondary to vocal abuse. If hoarseness persists after no more than 2 weeks of antibiotic therapy, referral to an otolaryngologist is indicated.

B. Chronic laryngitis is created by long-term inflammatory conditions such as smoking, GERD, and chronic sinusitis. The voice is usually deeper than normal, and frequent throat clearing is evident with GERD. Inspection reveals mild to moderate edema and thick mucus on the vocal folds' surface, but minimal erythema. Posterior laryngeal erythema or hyperkeratosis is common when GERD is present. The mainstay of treatment is eliminating the inciting problem and maintaining proper hydration.

C. Vocal fold nodules are bilateral calluses that form in response to repeated forceful closure, as occurs with screaming, speaking too loudly, throat clearing, and chronic coughing, and prevent full closure of the vocal cords. The voice is deep, coarse, and sometimes breathy with limited pitch range. The treatment is to eliminate the abusive patterns of voice use and is directed under the care of a speech therapist. Rarely, nodules persist after therapy and require microscopic removal.

D. Vocal fold polyps are usually unilateral fleshy growths on the surface of the vocal fold. They generally result from vocal abuse or smoking. When smoking is the etiologic agent, the polyps are more often bilateral. Occasionally, they can be large enough to cause gradual airway obstruction, but typically voice changes similar to those found with nodules are the sole presenting complaint. Microscopic excision of the polyp is the treatment of choice.

E. Vocal cord malignancy presents with a variety of complaints, including mild to severe hoarseness, dysphagia, otalgia, and varying degrees of airway obstruction, usually in smokers. Symptoms are progressive over several months. The appearance ranges from a white plaque on the surface of the vocal cord to an irregular exophytic mass. Biopsy confirms the diagnosis. Treatment involves surgical resection or radiotherapy; either is highly effective for early disease.

F. Laryngeal papillomatosis can occur in adults when human papilloma virus, types 6 or 11, infests epithelium in the border between ciliated and squamous cells. The virus is likely transmitted to the fetus during vaginal births of mothers with active condylomas. The risk of transmission is 1 in 400 (*Laryngoscope* 1986;68:795). The lesions can be removed by laser ablation to palliate symptoms, but they usually recur over several months to a year.

G. Vocal fold paralysis results from temporary or permanent interruption of the vagus nerve or its branch, the recurrent laryngeal nerve. This can occur after cervical or thoracic surgery (the most common etiology), trauma, forceps delivery, aortic aneurysm, congestive heart failure, or cerebrovascular accident or secondary to neoplasm along the course of the vagus or recurrent laryngeal nerve. Loss of neural innervation prevents adduction (closure) of the vocal fold and arytenoid cartilage; thus, contact between the cords for phonation is lost. The voice is, therefore, breathy and weak, with fewer words/breath. The patient is unable to project (speak loudly) or cough vigorously and occasionally has mild aspiration. Over time, atrophy of the vocalis muscle occurs, resulting in worsening of symptoms if the injury is permanent. Otherwise, recovery of some function may develop between 6 and 12 months. The laryngoscopy reveals a lateralized immobile vocal fold that is flaccid. When the cause is unknown, evaluation should include CT of the neck and superior mediastinum to rule out neoplasm, as well as referral to an otolaryngologist. Treatment consists of repositioning the immobile vocal fold to the midline by placing an implant or injecting the vocal cord with fat or collagen. Speech therapy is helpful to control potentially damaging compensatory mechanisms (Speech Pathology: Evaluation and Treatment of Disorders. In *Otolaryngology—Head and Neck Surgery*. Philadelphia: Saunders, 1992:132–133).

H. Vocal fold bowing, presbylaryngia, results when vocalis muscle atrophy occurs as a result of decreased usage and aging. The patient is chronically soft spoken. The voice is breathy and weak and often trails off to inaudible levels. Projection is lost, but cough is mildly weakened or intact. Laryngoscopy reveals normal mobility but bilateral concavity of both vocal folds that results in a persistent gap during phonation. Speech therapy can often restore some muscle bulk and improve vocal performance. Rarely, bilateral vocal cord medialization is required for restoration of adequate voice.

I. **Spasmodic dysphonia,** a focal dystonia of adductor or abductor muscles in the larynx, results in spasms that interrupt phonation. Patients complain of a choked-off sound to the voice. Spoken numbers and words beginning with "h" are common triggers. Because stress frequently exacerbates the severity, and patients sound as if they are on the verge of crying, they are often misdiagnosed with psychiatric disorders. Yet psychiatric medications have no impact on the dysfunction. Examination reveals vocal fold spasm that results in interruption of phonation. Injection of the affected muscles with botulinum toxin (Botox) can prevent the spasms and restore adequate phonation temporarily. Repeat injections are required every 4–5 months.

Globus Pharyngeus

I. **Introduction.** Globus pharyngeus is a foreign body sensation in the throat, commonly caused by GERD. Other common causes include mechanical injury or true foreign bodies, infectious causes, or neoplasms. Thirty percent of Americans have GERD, and it manifests in many different ways, from occult disease to severe erosive esophagitis. Risk factors for globus include risk factors for GERD, including hiatal hernia, obesity, pregnancy, and smoking, as well as a diet with bony meats, chips, or extremely hot liquids and risk factors for neoplasia, including smoking and ethanol ingestion.

II. **Pathophysiology.** GERD allows inflammation of the laryngeal and pharyngeal mucosa as a result of direct exposure to the acid in the refluxed fluid. This mucosal swelling is perceived as a sensation of a foreign body. Infectious causes can also result in mucosal inflammation and globus, as can mucosal burns from scalding coffee or soup. Traumatic ingestions of bone or chips can abrade mucosa, resulting in local irritation and a feeling of a retained foreign body, or can become lodged and remain as a foreign body. Neoplasms cause globus through growth in the throat or local mucosal ulceration.

III. **Diagnosis**

   A. **GERD** that causes globus is typically associated with a rare or absent history of indigestion. Symptoms of reflux are not volunteered but may be elicited on questioning (see Chap. 14). Often patients know of a pre-existing hiatal hernia or reveal occasional use of antacids. Physical examination must include pharyngolaryngoscopy, which is best accomplished by referral to an otolaryngologist for fiberoptic endoscopic examination. Diagnostic evaluation may use two tests, barium esophagraphy and 24-hour esophageal pH probe monitoring [Gastroesophageal Reflux Disease. In *Otolaryngology Head and Neck Surgery* (3rd ed). St. Louis: Mosby, 1998:2414–2417]. Please see Chap. 14 for further discussion of diagnostic evaluation of GERD.

   B. **Infectious causes** of globus are usually acute and associated with symptoms that are attributable to the primary infection (e.g., sore throat-pharyngitis, hoarseness-laryngitis, and productive cough–bronchitis). Indirect pharyngolaryngoscopy most often reveals diffuse erythema or moderate vocal cord edema.

   C. **Traumatic ingestion** is always time linked to the offending swallow. An immediate sense of irritation is noted, and the patient typically is convinced that a foreign body is still present. Attempts to clear the foreign body with swallowing liquid or bread fail to help. Pharyngolaryngscopy is usually normal, although a focal area of inflammation is occasionally seen. Palpation of the base of the tongue with a gloved finger reveals no foreign body. However, a true foreign body can occur and always results in globus. Fish bones are the most common objects to become lodged and are usually located in the lingual tissue at the base of the tongue. Because pharyngolaryngoscopy may miss the foreign body, palpation of the base of the tongue is necessary. When no foreign body is found and the examination is unrevealing, soft-tissue cervical x-rays may reveal a bony foreign body or air in the soft tissues.

   D. **Neoplasms** are the most feared cause of globus. This fear is what usually motivates patients to seek evaluation for chronic globus. A careful physical examination can confirm the existence or absence of a tumor. When a tumor is not found, a barium swallow or esophagoscopy should be obtained to evaluate the esophagus. When this, too, is normal, reassurance should be provided to the patient and follow-up examination performed in several weeks if symptoms persist.

IV. **Management**
   A. **GERD** therapy, whether empiric or proven necessary, typically involves antireflux medication and strategies (see Chap. 14).
   B. **Infectious causes** of globus respond to antimicrobial therapy. Topical anesthetics (Chloraseptic spray) and saline gargles help with discomfort.
   C. **Traumatic ingestion** without a retained foreign body is best treated with reassurance and topical anesthetics (Chloraseptic spray) or occasionally oral narcotics or sucralfate, 1 g PO qid. Antibiotics are not necessary unless air is seen on a soft-tissue radiograph of the neck. Resolution of symptoms usually occurs within 7–10 days; however, if globus persists, a follow-up examination is indicated. If a foreign body is discovered, removal should be attempted either in the office after administering topical anesthesia (4% lidocaine) or in the operating room under general anesthesia.
   D. **Therapy** for neoplasms is tumor and location specific and beyond the scope of this section.

Evaluation of a Neck Mass

I. **Introduction.** Patients of all ages can present with neck masses secondary to numerous possible conditions. Neck masses can be classified based on their etiology. Broad categories include congenital, inflammatory, neoplastic, and traumatic causes [Differential Diagnosis of Neck Masses. In *Otolaryngology Head and Neck Surgery* (3rd ed). St. Louis: Mosby, 1998:1686–1687].
   A. **General considerations** can narrow the differential diagnosis to an exact diagnosis or a select few possibilities. These factors include the patient's age and the location of the mass in the neck. Patients can be grouped into three age categories: pediatric (up to 15 years), young adult (16–40 years), and older adult (older than 40 years). Within each age group, the incidence of congenital, inflammatory, and neoplastic disease is known. In young adults, inflammatory masses are more common than congenital or neoplastic masses. In older adults, neoplasms are more common, followed by inflammatory masses and then congenital masses.
   B. The **location** of a neck mass is particularly helpful in differentiating congenital masses. Thyroglossal duct cysts and dermoids occur in the midline, and branchial cleft cysts are found in the anterior triangle of the neck. When inflammatory or neoplastic causes are suspected, the location of the mass may point to the source of infection or primary tumor. For example, upper-jugular nodes suggest oral cavity or oropharyngeal disease; submandibular nodes occur with sinus, oral cavity, and lip disease; midjugular nodes are found with hypopharyngeal or laryngeal disease; and supraclavicular nodes present with disease below the clavicles.

II. **Clinical presentation and management**
   A. **Congenital masses** may become evident through natural growth or remain indolent until inflammation secondary to a URI results in enlargement and

the onset of symptoms. Initially, control of local infection, if present, is achieved with antibiotic therapy. Incision and drainage are best avoided to facilitate later resection. Hemangiomas should be observed in infants and toddlers, as most resolve spontaneously. Those that persist as well as all other congenital masses that persist require surgical excision to be cured.

B. Inflammatory masses are mostly comprised of two categories: lymphadenitis and sialoadenitis, depending on the involved structures. Infectious lymphadenopathy comprises the majority of neck masses.

   1. Lymphadenitis is most often infectious in nature, either reactive to a local or systemic infection (tonsillitis and dental infections or mumps and AIDS, respectively) or directly involved by infection itself (bacterial lymphadenitis, tuberculous lymphadenitis, or cat-scratch disease). However, inflammatory lymphadenopathy can occur in the absence of infections, as seen in sarcoidosis. When bacterial infection, either at a primary site or within the node, is suspected, oral antibiotics (amoxicillin-clavulanate, 875 mg bid for 7–14 days) are indicated and usually resolve the mass. If a granulomatous infection is suspected, excisional biopsy for diagnosis is recommended. Culture of biopsy tissue may identify pathogens and guide antibiotic selection. Cervical lymph node hyperplasia is extremely common in HIV-positive patients and does not require biopsy **unless** a single node is greater than 3 cm, is enlarging, or has become painful. These patients have increased incidence of lymphoma, Kaposi's sarcoma, and squamous cell carcinoma.

   2. Sialoadenitis most often is secondary to infection that directly involves the parotid or submandibular gland, although reactive lymphadenopathy within the parotid may also occur. Infection usually begins with obstruction to salivary outflow secondary to dehydration and sludging or an intraductal stone. Sialoadenitis is best treated with antistaphylococcal antibiotics such as dicloxacillin, 500 mg qid for 7–10 days, as well as hydration, sialogogues (lemon drop candy), local massage, and heat. If a stone is present, it should be extracted by an otolaryngologist to re-establish salivary flow. Occasionally, chronic infection persists and the gland requires resection by an otolaryngologist for control of symptoms.

C. Neoplastic masses are further classified as benign or malignant. Benign tumors (pleomorphic adenomas and thyroid adenomas) and malignancies (lymphoma and thyroid cancer) that arise from anatomic structures in the neck usually have no clear etiology. Metastatic tumors (squamous cell carcinoma and adenocarcinoma) arise in cervical lymph nodes secondary to migration via lymphatic channels from primary tumor sites. These masses are generally treated by resection in the hands of an otolaryngologist. Several notable exceptions include lymphoma, metastatic adenocarcinoma from nonthyroid sources, and some sarcomas. These are usually treated with a combination of chemotherapy and radiation therapy.

D. Traumatic masses arise after injury to existing structures.

   1. Classically, traumatic pseudoaneurysms develop after injury to an arterial wall. Gradually, the arterial pressure dilates the adventitia until an aneurysm becomes apparent as a mass. Pseudoaneurysms of major vessels require surgical repair or grafting by a vascular surgeon.

   2. When nerves are sectioned, the resulting regrowth of neurons up to the injury site may allow an accumulation of axons into a mass of neural tissue called a neuroma. Neuromas can be eradicated by surgical excision.

III. Evaluation

  A. Historical considerations focus mainly on the developmental time course of the neck mass, a history of growth or fluctuation in size, and associated symptoms, including hoarseness, dysphagia, pain, history of trauma radiation or surgery, and the use of tobacco and alcohol.

  B. Physical examination should first discern the location of the neck mass, its size, its relationship to contiguous structures, its consistency, and the presence of pulses. The rest of the head and neck examination, including all mucosal surfaces of the upper-aerodigestive tract, may reveal additional clues toward etiology and must be examined.

C. Trial therapy with antibiotics is an appropriate diagnostic approach when the history and physical examination suggest an inflammatory source of a neck mass. The course of antibiotics should not exceed 2 weeks, and post-treatment re-examination should be performed to evaluate the response to therapy. If the mass persists, further evaluation is necessary.

D. Diagnostic testing involves two major categories: biopsy and imaging.

1. **Biopsy** remains the definitive test for obtaining a diagnosis and should be performed if the history and physical examination do not reveal the etiology of a mass. This is safely achieved with a fine-needle aspiration of the mass, which is 85% sensitive in establishing a diagnosis. The aspirated cells are processed and analyzed by a cytopathologist. If the evaluation fails to yield a diagnosis or it raises the suspicion for lymphoma, an open biopsy is indicated.

2. **Imaging** with CT and MRI has replaced most other imaging techniques, and therefore, ultrasound, radionuclide studies, and sialography have very limited usefulness. Either CT or MRI locates the mass and its relationship to the surrounding anatomy, differentiates solid masses from cystic, and identifies vascular masses. CT of the neck with contrast is adequate to obtain this information and is usually preferred over MRI. However, clinical judgment and biopsy reduce the need for even these tests. Their greatest use is in assessing the extent of disease with malignancies. When vascular lesions are suspected, angiography is often helpful to differentiate aneurysms from vascular neoplasms. Positron emission tomographic scans have been used to differentiate malignancies from benign masses by assessing the metabolic activity of the mass.

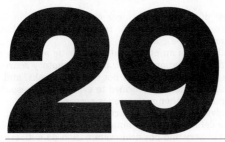

Psychiatric Disorders

John Rogakos and
Susan Boyer

The lifetime risk of developing any mental disorder, including substance abuse, anxiety disorders, mood disorders, and schizophrenia, is 25–30%. Some presentations are obvious, such as mania and psychosis, whereas others, including alcohol dependence and anxiety disorders, can be more subtle. Many patients suffer silently for years unless they are asked about specific symptoms. Some patients present with psychiatric symptoms that are actually part of an underlying general medical condition. Often, because of fear of social stigma and denial, many patients with psychiatric symptoms are more likely to seek help from a primary care physician than from a mental health professional.

Anxiety Disorders

Anxiety disorders are the most common of the psychiatric illnesses. The estimated lifetime prevalence approaches 20% in the general population and between 14% and 66% of patients seen in the primary care setting. Anxiety disorders include (in decreasing frequency) social phobia, generalized anxiety disorder (GAD), panic disorder, and obsessive-compulsive disorder (OCD).

I. **Social phobia** is significant apprehension of social or performance situations resulting in fear of scrutiny or embarrassment. The affected person recognizes that the apprehension is excessive, and it interferes significantly with functioning (i.e., a patient refuses a job promotion because it includes public speaking). The lifetime prevalence is 7%, with females affected more often than males. The onset is typically during the mid-teens, with a lifelong and continuous course that is often related to life demands and stressors.

A. **Differential diagnosis**
   1. **Panic disorder with agoraphobia** is similar to social phobia in that both can involve significant anxiety in public settings. However, social phobia is a primary fear of social settings, whereas panic disorder involves a primary fear of having a panic attack while in a social situation.
   2. **GAD** and social phobia both involve fear of humiliation or embarrassment. GAD does not necessarily involve social anxiety but, instead, nonspecific worry about multiple issues.
   3. **Normal shyness** also involves anxiety about social situations. Only social phobia results in significant impairment or distress (i.e., normal shyness does not cause inability to perform one's job or inability to use public restrooms).

B. **Treatment**
   1. **Propranolol**, 10 mg PO 1 hour before a stressful event to prevent certain physiologic symptoms (i.e., rapid heart beat, tremor, perspiration).
   2. **Lorazepam**, 0.5 mg PO 1 hour before a stressful event.
   3. **Selective serotonin reuptake inhibitors (SSRIs).** If stressful events occur frequently, the patient can be treated with an SSRI (Table 29-1). **Par-**

Table 29-1. Antidepressants

Drugs by class	Initial dose	Incremental change	Dosage range	Side effects	Drug interactions	Comments
SSRIs						
Celexa (citalopram)	10–20 mg	Increase by 10 mg q3wks	20–80 mg	Weight gain[a]	None known	—
Paxil (paroxetine)	10–20 mg	Increase by 10 mg q3wks	10–80 mg	Weight gain[a]	Cimetidine + Paxil increases Paxil; tricyclics + Paxil increases tricyclics	—
Prozac (fluoxetine)	10–20 mg	Increase by 10 mg q3wks	10–80 mg	Insomnia, nausea, initial weight loss[a]	Metoprolol + Prozac increases metoprolol; tricyclics + Prozac increases tricyclics	Long half-life (reduces risk of relapse in less adherent patients)
Luvox (fluvoxamine)	50 mg	Increase by 50 mg weekly	100–200 mg	Weight gain[a]	Tricyclics + Luvox increases tricyclics; propranolol + Luvox increases propranolol; warfarin + Luvox increases warfarin; theophylline + Luvox increases theophylline	Marketed for treatment of OCD
Zoloft (sertraline)	25–50 mg	Increase to 50 mg in 1 wk, then increase by 50 mg q3wks	50–150 mg	Weight gain[a]	Warfarin + Zoloft increases the effect of warfarin; tricyclics + Zoloft increases tricyclics	—

(continued)

Table 29-1. (continued)

Drugs by class	Initial dose	Incremental change	Dosage range	Side effects	Drug interactions	Comments
Others						
Effexor (venlafaxine)	37.5 mg	37.5 mg for 3 days, then 75 mg; increase by 37.5 mg q3wks	75–225 mg	Hypertension (uncommon)	No significant drug interactions have been reported	Indicated for SSRI failures
Remeron (mirtazapine)	15–30 mg	Increase by 15 mg after 3–4 wks	30–45 mg	Sedation, weight gain	None known	15 mg or less for treatment of insomnia; indicated for thin, elderly patients with insomnia
Wellbutrin SR (bupropion)	100 mg	Increase to bid after 1 wk	200–400 mg	Agitation, headache	Carbamazepine + Wellbutrin decreases Wellbutrin	Helpful in smoking cessation; can treat adult ADHD; contraindicated in active eating disorders and seizures; low incidence of sexual side effects; need to bid dose
Serzone (nefazodone)	50 mg bid	Increase by 50 mg q4–7 days	300–600 mg	Sedation, orthostasis, nausea	Hismanal + Serzone increases Hismanal; Halcion + Serzone increases Halcion; Xanax + Serzone increases Xanax; Digoxin + Serzone increases Digoxin	Low incidence of sexual side effects

TCAs

Amitriptyline, imipramine, doxepin, desipramine	25 mg	Increase by 25 mg weekly	150–300 mg	Dry mouth, constipation, urinary retention, sedation, and cardiac conduction delays	—	—
Nortriptyline			75–150 mg	—	—	—
MAOIs		Initiation not recommended in primary care setting			Decongestants, vasoconstrictors, meperidine, dextromethorphan, SSRIs contraindicated	Tyramine-free diet
Nardil (phenelzine)	—	—	—	—	—	—
Parnate (tranylcypromine)	—	—	—	—	—	—

ADHD, attention deficit hyperactivity disorder; MAOIs, monoamine oxidase inhibitors; OCD, obsessive-compulsive disorder; SSRIs, selective serotonin reuptake inhibitors; TCAs, tricyclic antidepressants.

[a]Sedation versus insomnia, headache, anorgasmia, rare syndrome of inappropriate antidiuretic hormone secretion.

oxetine, for example, can be initiated at 10 mg PO qd for 4–6 weeks and increased by 10-mg increments as necessary every 4–6 weeks, up to 40 mg/day. The dose equivalent for sertraline is 25 mg PO qd, up to 150 mg/day.

    4. Consider referral to a psychiatrist if treatments are unsatisfactory. Referral to a psychologist for cognitive/behavioral therapy may also be helpful.

II. GAD is worry about multiple events or activities that occurs on most days for a period of at least 6 months. The lifetime prevalence is 5%, with females affected twice as often as males. Onset is typically within the first 30 years of life, with half experiencing onset during childhood and adolescence. The course is chronic and fluctuating, often worsening during times of increasing life demands and stressors.

  A. Differential diagnosis

    1. Panic disorder and GAD both involve impairment as a result of excessive worry. Panic disorder is limited to fears specific to experiencing a panic attack.

    2. Depression is similar in that anxiety, sleep disturbance, and fatigue are prominent features of both. However, in depression, patients tend to experience more severe mood disturbance (as opposed to occasional demoralization about stress), greater occupational disturbance, guilt, hopelessness, and possible suicidal ideation. GAD tends to involve more prominent vigilance and hyperventilation.

    3. Hypochondriasis also involves excessive worry but is limited to excessive fear of serious disease despite medical evidence to the contrary.

    4. Somatization disorder also involves anxiety but is limited to multiple physical complaints.

    5. Endocrine dysregulation, including hyper- and hypothyroidism, hypoglycemia, pheochromocytoma, and hyperparathyroidism.

    6. Cardiopulmonary diseases, including CHF, pulmonary embolism, cardiac arrhythmias, and chronic obstructive pulmonary disease.

    7. Neurologic disorders, including complex partial seizures, delirium, and stroke, each with associated signs and symptoms.

    8. Substance abuse, including amphetamines, caffeine, pseudoephedrine (diet pill), benzodiazepine withdrawal, and alcohol withdrawal.

  B. Treatment

    1. SSRIs. Initiate a starting dose of an SSRI (Table 29-1) once/day with food. The dose should be doubled after 1 week and increased every 3–4 weeks until symptom relief or side effects occur. Effective doses often are higher than for treatment of major depression.

    2. Buspirone, 5 mg PO bid for 1 week, then doubled weekly to a maximum of 20 mg tid. Improvement occurs over 4–6 weeks. This is a nonbenzodiazepine, nonsedating, non–habit-forming medication.

    3. Bupropion, sustained-release 100 mg PO once in the morning for 1 week, then bid. Improvement usually occurs within 4–6 weeks. The dose may be increased to 150 mg bid if results are unsatisfactory. Contraindications include seizure disorder and active eating disorders.

    4. Benzodiazepines, such as lorazepam, 0.5 mg PO bid; clonazepam, 0.25–0.5 mg PO bid; or diazepam, 5 mg PO bid/tid (diazepam should be avoided in the elderly), can be used to treat severe acute anxiety symptoms in the short term (2–4 weeks), especially in conjunction with any of the above medications, which have a delayed therapeutic effect. Patients should be cautioned about driving until they are well familiar with the effects and should be especially careful to avoid the use of alcohol.

III. Panic disorder is defined as the presence of recurrent unexpected panic attacks followed by at least 1 month of persistent concern about having another panic attack. A panic attack is a discrete period of intense fear or discomfort that develops abruptly and reaches a peak within 10 minutes. Symptoms include palpitations, sweating, fear of choking, chest discomfort, fear of dying or losing control, and derealization. The lifetime prevalence is 3.5%, with a female-male ratio of 3:1. Age of onset varies but is typically between late adolescence and mid-30s. The course is chronic, with waxing and waning symptoms. Follow-up studies suggest that 6–10 years after treatment, 30% remitted, 45% improved but remained symptomatic, and 25% were unchanged or worse.

A. Differential diagnosis

1. **Social phobia** involves fear that stems from social exposure itself and does not involve having panic attacks. In panic disorder, the fear is limited to experiencing a panic attack in a social context.

2. **Somatization** is similar to panic disorder in that somatic complaints of palpitations, dyspnea, chest pain, nausea, and other vague physical symptoms commonly occur. In somatization disorder these complaints are but a few of a multitude of symptoms, both psychiatric and somatic, involving several organ systems and are not necessarily brought on by social situations.

3. **Major depression** and panic disorder both can involve ruminative worries and feelings of demoralization about one's condition. Panic disorder and major depression can coexist. They are dissimilar in that in major depression, patients tend to experience more severe mood disturbance, anhedonia, hopelessness, unrealistic guilt, and possible suicidal ideation.

4. **Endocrine dysregulation,** including hyperthyroidism and hypoglycemia.

5. **Cardiopulmonary diseases,** including CHF, pulmonary embolism, cardiac arrhythmias, and chronic obstructive pulmonary disease.

6. **Substance abuse,** including amphetamines, caffeine, pseudoephedrine (diet pill), benzodiazepine withdrawal, and alcohol withdrawal.

B. Treatment

1. **Patient education** that panic disorder is a well-known and described occurrence, that people do not die from panic attacks, and that treatments are effective can provide much relief in and of itself. One should ask about pregnancy before starting medications. Reducing alcohol and caffeine, avoiding diet pills, and increasing exercise are very helpful. The definitive treatment for panic disorder is with SSRIs, which tend to be nonsedating, are non–habit forming, and are safe for long-term use. However, they typically require to 2–4 weeks of consistent daily use for effectiveness.

2. **Benzodiazepines.** A short course (i.e., 2–4 weeks) of lorazepam, 0.5–1.0 mg PO bid, or clonazepam, 0.25–0.5 mg PO bid, should quickly blunt the intensity of attacks, especially to bridge the gap in the onset of efficacy of SSRIs. Sedation is a common side effect, and patients should be cautioned against driving during the first few days of treatment.

3. **SSRIs.** One should initiate a starting dose of an SSRI (Table 29-1) once/day with food. The dose should be doubled after 1 week. After 2–4 additional weeks, if response is limited, the dose should be doubled again.

4. If **agoraphobia** is prominent, referral to psychology for cognitive-behavioral therapy is recommended.

IV. OCD involves recurrent intrusive thoughts and/or performance of obligatory repetitive acts that are severe enough to be time consuming or cause marked distress or significant impairment. At some point, the person has recognized that these obsessions or compulsions are excessive or unreasonable, and usually is embarrassed by this. The lifetime prevalence is 2.5%, with males and females equally affected. Onset is usually adolescence or early adulthood. The course is typically chronic, with periods of waxing and waning severity. Exacerbation of symptoms may be related to stress, with variable response to treatment ranging from excellent to fair. Fifteen percent of patients show progressive deterioration, and 5% have an episodic course with minimal or no symptoms between episodes.

A. Differential diagnosis

1. **Hypochondriasis** is similar to OCD in that patients can experience recurring anxiety regarding health matters. However, the anxiety of

hypochondriasis is limited to a fear of disease and is not recognized by the patient as excessive.
2. **Delusional disorder** is similar in that patients can become overfocused regarding particular issues. However, in delusional disorder, beliefs are fixed, not considered unreasonable at any time, and typically are not considered intrusive by the patient.
3. **Behavior disorders** (i.e., "compulsive" gambling, drinking, or stealing) and OCD both involve repeated maladaptive behavior. In behavior disorders the activity is initially pleasurable with negative consequences, whereas in OCD the activity is usually considered burdensome but needed to reduce anxiety.
4. **Eating disorder** is similar in that it also results in repetitive behavior. However, the fear of gaining weight is not considered excessive/intrusive by the patient with an eating disorder.

B. Treatment
1. **Referral to psychiatry and psychology** is warranted due to the complicated course, the usual only partial response to medications, and the benefit of behavioral interventions.
2. **SSRIs** (Table 29-1). Treatment typically requires higher doses (up to three- to fourfold higher than in treatment of depression or other anxiety disorders) and a longer trial before response, often 3 months or longer.
3. **Clomipramine**, 25 mg PO qhs, is a second-line or augmenting agent when treatment with SSRIs is inadequate.

Mood Disorders

I. **Major depression** is an episode of at least 2 weeks of consistently depressed mood or loss of interest in personally interesting activities with several of the following: decreased energy, feelings of worthlessness/guilt, poor concentration, recurrent thoughts of death or suicidal ideation, and change of appetite, weight, sleep, or psychomotor activity. The lifetime prevalence is 20%, and females are affected twice as often as males. Average age of onset is in the mid-20s. The course is variable, with 50–60% of patients with one major depressive episode experiencing a recurrence. With each episode, the chance of a recurrence continues to increase. Five percent to 10% of patients eventually experience a manic episode, and 10% die by suicide.

A. Differential diagnosis
1. **Normal sadness and crying**, often described as "depression," is a universal human experience. However, some experiences such as illness or loss can precipitate a major depressive episode in some patients. **The defining difference in major depression is the duration of low mood, preoccupation with guilt/worthlessness, impairment in function, presence of physical symptoms (changes in appetite, sleep, energy), and recurring thoughts of wanting to die.** Rather than attempting to assess the appropriateness of the response to the experience (i.e., is it "normal" for a patient with cancer to be sad?), the clinician should look for the presence of these core symptoms that define major depression and treat accordingly.
2. **Adjustment disorder with depressed mood** is similar in that it, too, may present with a depressed mood. However, an adjustment disorder always is related to a preceding stressor, does not carry the same suicide risk, does not reach the same degree of severity of impairment, and symptoms typically resolve with resolution of the stressor. Experiencing a life stressor does not rule out the presence of major depression. Clinicians are guided by assessment for defining symptoms regardless of the stressor.

3. **Dysthymic disorder** is similar in that it also involves low mood. It is dissimilar in that patients do not reach the degree of severity of major depression, and the mood disturbance tends to be more chronic in dysthymic patients (i.e., years).

4. **Bipolar depression** is similar in that depressive episodes look identical. It is dissimilar in that bipolar patients have experienced at least one manic episode, and antidepressant treatment of depression in bipolar disorder can precipitate a manic episode. Bipolar disorder eventually declares itself in up to 10% of patients who were previously thought to have experienced major ("unipolar") depression.

5. **Dementia** and major depression both can present with prominent cognitive symptoms in elderly patients. The premorbid functioning in a non-demented depressed patient is typically normal, with an abrupt decline that is temporally associated with the depression and not the gradual decline related to dementia.

6. **Bereavement** is a normal reaction to the death of a loved one, frequently with significant overlap of symptoms with depression. In bereavement, the usual course of resolution is within 2 months. Major depression is only diagnosed if symptoms persist beyond 2 months, if the patient becomes preoccupied with guilt and low self-esteem, or if the patient becomes actively suicidal.

7. **Endocrine dysregulation**, including hypothyroidism and hyperthyroidism (especially in the elderly).

8. **Neurologic disorders** include multiple sclerosis, Parkinson's disease, dementia, and cerebral vascular disease.

9. **Substances**, including beta-blockers, corticosteroids, contraceptives, cimetidine, cocaine withdrawal, and alcohol.

B. **Treatment**
1. **Suicide assessment** (see Suicide, sec. II).
2. **Assess the patient for substance abuse or dependence** (see Substance-Related Disorders).
3. **Patient and family education.** The patient and family should be made aware that major depression is a medical illness and not a sign of weak character. The negative thoughts and sadness are part of the illness and should abate with treatment. Patients should be instructed that antidepressants are not "happy pills" or "addicting" but over time help them to fight depression so that they feel like their normal selves again. Antidepressants do not exert their effects on a "pill-for-pill" basis (i.e., like benzodiazepines). Therefore, (1) the effect does not wear off after each dose, (2) taking extra medication on a bad day does not help one to feel better, and (3) skipping medication on a good day, although unlikely to be noticeable that day, may jeopardize the long-term recovery. A full course of antidepressant therapy for a first episode is 7–12 months duration. Second episodes of depression and relapses require chronic antidepressant therapy.
4. **Pharmacotherapy** (Table 29-1).
   a. **SSRIs** are currently the initial drugs of choice for treating major depression.
   b. **Bupropion** is not associated with sexual side effects and tends not to cause weight gain. It is also an initial drug of choice. Contraindications are seizure disorders and active eating disorders.
   c. **Mirtazapine** tends not to produce sexual side effects. Weight gain with mirtazapine may occur, and sedation, which may be bothersome to some patients, may be helpful in others who experience distress from insomnia.
   d. **Tricyclic** antidepressants are very effective but, because of increased risks of side effects relative to newer agents, are no longer first-line treatments.

  5. Treatment of an underlying general medical disorder tends to optimize the outcome in depression.

II. **Mania (bipolar disorder)** is a distinct period of uncharacteristically elevated or irritable mood. Symptoms include uncharacteristic grandiosity, decreased need for sleep, flight of ideas, pressured speech, and excessive indulgence in high-risk activities. Symptoms must be present for 1 week, or less if severe enough to warrant hospitalization. The lifetime prevalence is 1%, with males and females equally affected. Onset typically is in the early 20s but can occur at any age. Onset before adolescence is very rare. Males often present initially with mania, and females typically present with mania after several depressive episodes. Social stress or sleep deprivation may precipitate an episode. Escalation of symptoms usually occurs over a few days and can be characterized by mood lability (severe mood swings; not to be confused with rapid cycling, explained below) and possible development of psychosis. Duration, if the patient is not treated, is a few weeks to several months, often followed by a depressive episode. The course is usually one of return to normal functioning between episodes, with an average of four episodes every 10 years. Five percent to 15% of patients develop rapid cycling, which is the presence of four or more episodes/year, associated with a more severe course of illness.

A. **Differential diagnosis**
  1. **Substances** including corticosteroids, levodopa, cocaine, amphetamines, and, occasionally, alcohol intoxication.
  2. **Schizophrenia** and mania are similar early in the course of illness, with prominent mood disturbances and the presence of psychosis. They are dissimilar in that typical onset in schizophrenia is over months, whereas mania is over days. In schizophrenia psychosis is more prominent, and a return-to-baseline mental state is not as common. Family history may be helpful in determining the diagnosis.
  3. In **personality disorders** (antisocial and borderline personality), patients may also appear impulsive and irritable, complain of mood swings or auditory hallucinations, or tell their physician that they are bipolar or "manic-depressive." Furthermore, lithium, valproate, and carbamazepine are sometimes used to dampen impulsivity in these patients, and their use may cause patients with personality disorders to be mistakenly diagnosed with bipolar disorder. Personality symptoms are chronic characteristic traits that date back to childhood or early adolescence, and mood instability in these individuals tends to be short lived (i.e., minutes to hours). In bipolar disorder, the derangement is uncharacteristic of the patient's baseline behavior.
  4. **Endocrine dysregulation,** such as hyperthyroidism, may be present with agitation that resembles mania.
  5. **Neurologic disorders** such as multiple sclerosis and frontal lobe injury.

B. **Treatment** of patients who are suspected of having bipolar disorder should be referred to a psychiatrist for management.
  1. **In the acute phase,** an antipsychotic (haloperidol, 5–20 mg PO qd; olanzapine, 10–20 mg PO qd) and a benzodiazepine (clonazepam, 1–2 mg PO bid; lorazepam, 2 mg IM for severe agitation) are typically used. A mood stabilizer, the usual definitive, long-term treatment, is started but usually requires several days to weeks to produce an effect.
  2. **Lithium** is an effective mood stabilizer. Treatment is started at 300 mg PO tid; a serum drug level is checked every 5 days, and the dose is titrated to a level of 0.8–1.2 µg/ml. A baseline ECG, electrolytes, BUN, creatinine, thyroid-stimulating hormone, and beta–human chorionic gonadotropin (in a woman of childbearing years) should be checked before therapy is started. Once the patient's condition is stabilized, the dose should be consolidated to qhs if possible. Common side effects include nausea, diarrhea, sedation, polyuria, polydipsia, weight gain, and

fine tremor. Arrhythmias are uncommon, with a higher incidence in patients with sick sinus syndrome. Hypothyroidism has also been associated with lithium use and is usually reversible. Renal complications are rare, but BUN and serum creatinine should be monitored every month for the first 3 months and then every 6 months subsequently. Symptoms of toxicity include vomiting, severe diarrhea, coarse tremor, ataxia, convulsions, and coma and are usually related to rises in plasma concentration. Nonsteroidal anti-inflammatory drugs and thiazide diuretics may increase lithium levels.

3. **Valproate** is a commonly used mood stabilizer. Treatment is started at 250 mg PO tid; a serum drug level is checked every 5 days, and the dose is titrated to a level of 60–100 µg/ml. A baseline CBC and liver function tests should be checked before therapy is started, then monthly for 3 months, then every 6 months. Side effects include transient nausea, sedation, and tremor. Elevation of liver enzymes occurs in 40% of patients and is usually asymptomatic. Rare, fulminant hepatitis occurs at a rate of 1 in 50,000 patients, most of these being people aged <10 years or on multiple antiepileptic agents [*Goodman and Gilman's the Pharmacological Basis of Therapeutics* (9th ed.) New York: McGraw-Hill, 1996:477]. Valproate raises the level of phenobarbital and sometimes phenytoin.

4. **Carbamazepine** is another mood stabilizer. Treatment is started at 200 mg PO bid; a serum drug level is checked every 5–7 days, and the dose is titrated to a level of 8–12 µg/ml. A baseline CBC and liver function tests should be checked initially and periodically thereafter. Common side effects include sedation, visual effects (diplopia, blurring), ataxia, and nausea. Most of these tend to abate and can be minimized by slow titration. Aplastic anemia is rare, approximately 1/200,000, and evidence of efficacy of monitoring CBCs to reduce risk is unclear [*Goodman and Gilman's the Pharmacological Basis of Therapeutics* (9th ed.) New York: McGraw-Hill, 1996:473]. Although transient leukopenia develops in 10% of patients, persistent WBC suppression that requires discontinuation of treatment develops in only 2%. The syndrome of inappropriate antidiuretic hormone secretion is an uncommon reaction. Carbamazepine tends to induce liver enzymes and reduces the levels of various medications (some oral contraceptives, valproate, phenytoin, primidone).

5. **Refractory mania** may respond to electroconvulsive therapy, clozapine, or other adjunctive antipsychotics.

6. **Education** includes discussion that medication adherence is critical and that inconsistent adherence may lead to a more refractory course of illness. Good sleep hygiene and building a family support system are critical components to therapy. Families are often able to detect subtle signs of early deterioration and can be instrumental in warning the physician to take necessary steps to prevent or mitigate an impending manic episode.

Suicide

Suicide is the ninth leading cause of death in the United States. Ninety-five percent of patients are thought to have had a psychiatric illness at the time of suicide, with major depression accounting for half and alcohol dependence and other substance dependence accounting for another third. Most of these patients had never been seen by a mental health professional, but had seen their primary care physician within 1 month of their deaths.

I. **Risk factors for suicide**

A. **Sex.** Male-female ratio is 3:1 for completed suicide.

   B. Age. The peak age for men is 75 years and older. Women's peak age is the late 40s to early 50s.
   C. Psychiatric illness. Bipolar depression, major depression, substance disorder, schizophrenia, borderline and antisocial personality disorder, and panic disorder all increase risk.
   D. Recent release from psychiatric hospitalization.
   E. Family history of completed suicide, especially violent suicide (i.e., gunshot as opposed to overdose).
   F. Marital status. The divorced or widowed are at increased risk.
   G. Race. Caucasians have the highest risk.
   H. Social stressor or major loss.
   I. Personal history of suicide attempts.
   J. Medical illness (AIDS, Huntington's chorea, end-stage renal disease) in which an increased incidence of major depression is likely the mediating factor.
   K. Access to firearms.
II. **Assessment.** Ask something like, "Often people who feel depressed and fatigued think about wishing they could die. Furthermore, some people actually think about ways they can make that happen. Have you had thoughts like these?" **Asking if patients are suicidal does not cause them to be suicidal.** All patients with depressed mood should be asked whether they have considered suicide, have attempted suicide in the past, or have a family history of suicide. A family history of suicide is a red flag, especially violent suicide, such as hanging, jumping, and gunshot in which the act was clearly not ambivalent. Assess the degree of intent, including the plan and urgency of enacting the plan.
III. **Suicide prevention**
   A. Not all suicides are preventable.
   B. Screening for and aggressively treating an underlying psychiatric disorder carries the highest chance of suicide prevention.
   C. Any patient with suicidal ideation beyond a passive death wish should be referred to a psychiatrist.
   D. Any patient with a suicide plan and means should be hospitalized. This may involve involuntary commitment to the hospital if the patient is not cooperative or is too impaired to participate in informed decision making. Commitment laws vary from state to state but generally provide for and require physicians to protect their patients in these circumstances. If in doubt, the clinician should consult with a psychiatrist for guidance regarding the commitment process.

Insomnia

Up to one-third of Americans experience distress from a sleep disorder. Insomnia may be a normal human experience (i.e., one to several nights), a persistent but isolated symptom (primary insomnia), or one of several symptoms of an illness.
I. **Causes of insomnia**
   A. General medical conditions, such as chronic pain, pulmonary insufficiency, hypo- or hyperthyroidism, or renal failure, may cause insomnia.
   B. Poor sleep hygiene. Varying sleep/wake times, daytime napping, watching TV in bed, and even small amounts of alcohol or caffeine in the evening can disrupt sleep in sensitive individuals. Good sleep hygiene becomes more important as people age because their sleep becomes lighter.
   C. Major depression may manifest as early-morning awakening with inability to fall back asleep but can also be present with initial or middle insomnia.
   D. Alcohol. Use and withdrawal both produce sleep disturbance.

   E. **Substances.** Caffeine, amphetamines, cocaine, ephedrine, tobacco (>1 pack/day), or benzodiazepine withdrawal may cause insomnia.
   F. **Sleep apnea** is typically 30+ episodes of cessation of breathing/night, approximately 10 seconds each episode. Common complaints include depression, unrefreshing sleep, fatigue and sleepiness during the day, and concentration problems. The bed partner may report snoring or temporary cessation of breathing, during the night.
   G. **Nocturnal myoclonus** is lower limb movement that disrupts rapid eye movement sleep. Common symptoms include depression, anxiety, sleepiness/fatigue, depression, and poor concentration.
II. **Treatment**
   A. **Treat any underlying disorder** that is contributing to insomnia.
   B. Help the patient **establish good sleep hygiene** and relaxation techniques.
   C. **Pharmacologic** treatment for primary insomnia
      1. **Antidepressants.** Mirtazapine, 7.5–15.0 mg PO qhs; trazodone, 50–150 mg PO qhs (rare risk of priapism requiring immediate treatment); or amitriptyline, 10–25 mg PO qhs are non–habit-forming antidepressants that often aid in sleep.
      2. **Zolpidem,** 2.5–10.0 mg PO qhs for a short course (2–4 weeks), is beneficial.
      3. **Benzodiazepines.** Lorazepam, 0.5–1.0 mg PO qhs and temazepam, 15–30 mg PO qhs, are useful for short courses of therapy (i.e., 2–4 weeks). Patients with chronic insomnia can be referred to psychiatry or a sleep disorders clinic. Longer-acting benzodiazepines with active metabolites (diazepam, flurazepam) should be avoided in the elderly because the metabolites accumulate over long periods of time and can produce insidious cognitive deficits, increase fall risk, and promote daytime sleepiness.
      4. **Antihistamines.** Diphenhydramine and hydroxyzine can be helpful in selected cases but tend to produce daytime sedation and are especially risky in the elderly due to their tendency to produce disorientation, orthostasis, and urinary retention.

Eating Disorders

I. **Anorexia nervosa** is characterized by the inability to maintain a minimum of 85% of ideal body weight and amenorrhea in premenopausal women. The two types are (1) **restricting** (during the current episode the person has dieted, exercised, and/or used laxatives/stimulants without regularly engaging in binge-eating or purging behavior) and (2) **binge eating/purging**. Prevalence in females in late adolescence and early adulthood is 0.5–1.0%. Data concerning the prevalence in males is limited but thought to be less than in females. Mean age of onset is 17 years, with possible bimodal peaks at 14 and 18 years. Onset is rare over age 40 years. The natural history is variable: Some recover fully after one event, some have a fluctuating pattern, and others chronically deteriorate. Hospitalization may be required to restore weight and correct fluid and electrolyte imbalances. The long-term mortality is >10% of individuals who are admitted to university hospitals. Death most commonly results from starvation, suicide, or electrolyte imbalance. Associated findings include amenorrhea, hypotension, hypothermia, and bradycardia. Laboratory evaluation may reveal leukopenia, electrolyte abnormalities, mild anemia, elevated cholesterol, elevated liver function tests, low T_3, and low to normal T_4.
II. **Bulimia nervosa** is defined by recurrent episodes of binge eating characterized by eating an amount of food that is larger than most people would consume given the same circumstances and a sense of lack of control over eating during the episode. Unlike anorexia, patients with bulimia are able to maintain at or above

85% of ideal body weight. In purging type, patients regularly engage in self-induced vomiting or the misuse of laxatives, diuretics, or enemas during the current episode. In nonpurging type, patients use other compensatory behaviors, such as fasting or exercise. Prevalence among adolescent and young adult females is 1–3%; prevalence among males is one-tenth that in females. Bulimia nervosa usually begins in late adolescence or early adult life, frequently during or after an episode of dieting. The course may be chronic, with waxing and waning episodes. Associated findings include substance abuse or dependence (33%), electrolyte abnormalities, enlarged parotid gland, and eroded dental enamel. In a 3-year follow-up, fewer than one-third of patients were in remission, more than one-third had some improvement in their symptoms, and one-third had a poor outcome. Prognosis appears to be associated with degree of electrolyte imbalance, amylasemia, salivary gland enlargement, and dental caries.

III. **Differential diagnosis**
  A. **General medical conditions**, including GI disease, occult malignancies, and HIV.
  B. **Major depression** may also cause significant weight loss. However, weight control is not a focus in major depression.
  C. **Schizophrenia** may also cause weight loss. Patients with schizophrenia do not fear gaining weight but may not be eating due to a delusion that their food is poisoned or because they are so impaired by their psychosis that their general care is neglected.
  D. **Social phobia** is similar in that patients may avoid eating in public places. It is dissimilar in that with social phobia the focus is general public scrutiny and not an inherent concern regarding calories and weight.
  E. **OCD** is similar in that patients may exhibit obsessions and compulsions related to food. It should be diagnosed only if the patient exhibits additional obsessions and compulsions in addition to food and body image.

IV. **Treatment** includes a comprehensive plan with individual and family therapy with a mental health professional and a dietitian who specializes in eating disorders. Education regarding the effects of starvation, vomiting, and laxatives on the body, dietary misconceptions, and how profoundly people are influenced by cultural phenomena is important. Encourage (1) throwing out scales, (2) a 0.5-lb/week weight gain, (3) three meals/day of moderate caloric intake (even if binge eating), (4) recording intake, and (5) limiting exercise. If weight falls below goal or medical instability occurs, hospitalization may be necessary. Medications may have some benefit, but their role is modest and should be initiated by a psychiatrist. Antidepressants typically produce no benefit unless the patient has another underlying mental disorder (i.e., depression). Appetite stimulants can actually exacerbate the eating disorder and should be used judiciously.

Substance-Related Disorders

"Substance" refers to a drug of abuse, a medication, or a toxin. **Substance dependence** is a maladaptive pattern of substance use that leads to clinically significant distress as manifested by tolerance, withdrawal, unsuccessful efforts to cut down, and use of the substance despite knowing its adverse effects. Substance dependence can be applied to every class of substance except caffeine. **Substance abuse** is a maladaptive pattern of substance use manifested by recurrent and significant adverse consequences related to the repeated use of the substance. Unlike substance dependence, the criteria do not include tolerance, withdrawal, or a pattern of compulsive use but are instead limited to the harmful consequences of repeated use.

I. Alcohol dependence carries a 15% lifetime prevalence, with a male-female ratio of 3:1. Peak age of onset ranges between the 20s and the mid-30s. The course is variable and frequently is characterized by episodes of remission and relapse.

   A. Screening should be performed on all patients regardless of age, sex, race, or background (see Chap. 1, Screening for Disease, sec. **VIII**). Suggestive history includes variable and mild hypertension, a history of pancreatitis without gallstones, and complaints of insomnia or anxiety. Suggestive laboratory findings include elevated AST relative to ALT and macrocytic anemia.

   B. Treatment

    1. Confrontation may be useful to take advantage of the patient's chief complaint (i.e., insomnia, decreased sexual performance, depression) to educate patients as to how alcohol may contribute to the problem. The level of persistence of the physician, rather than exceptional confrontational skills is more closely correlated with positive results. Incorporating family support can be of great help.

    2. Detoxification. In the absence of a severe medical disorder or combined drug abuse, detoxification consists of rest, adequate nutrition, and multivitamins, especially thiamine. Mild withdrawal includes insomnia and anxiety and can usually be treated and monitored in a "social detoxification" residential/brief stay setting. Agitation or vital sign changes warrant inpatient hospitalization and treatment with a benzodiazepine.

    3. Rehabilitation may consist of individual or group therapy. The patient, alternatively, may be referred to Alcoholics Anonymous.

    4. Pharmacotherapy. Naltrexone, an opioid antagonist, 50 mg PO qd, in the context of a rehabilitation program can reduce rates of relapse. Drinking while on naltrexone is not associated with increased health risks. Disulfiram, 250 mg PO qd, may be helpful in very well-informed, motivated patients who understand that the risk of drinking while taking this medication can be life threatening.

II. Amphetamine, cocaine, and hallucinogen-related disorders do not typically involve medically dangerous withdrawal syndromes. Therefore, treatment involves referral to Narcotics Anonymous, regular follow-up, and persistence in asking about use and Narcotics Anonymous attendance. Hospitalization is warranted only if repeated attempts at abstinence are unsuccessful or the patient's environment directly and repeatedly leads to relapse.

III. Opioid-related disorders do not typically involve medically dangerous withdrawal; however, withdrawal symptoms are usually so uncomfortable that hospitalization is often needed for detoxification.

   A. Methadone/opiate detoxification requires a specific license and inpatient hospitalization.

   B. Nonopiate detoxification regimen

    1. Clonidine, 0.1–0.3 mg PO tid, can help attenuate withdrawal (doses >1.0 mg/day are not recommended for outpatients).

    2. Ibuprofen, 800 mg PO q8h for musculoskeletal pain.

    3. Lomotil, 10 ml or 2 tablets PO qid for diarrhea.

    4. Lorazepam, 1–2 mg PO q8h for insomnia/anxiety.

Schizophrenia

Schizophrenia is a chronic mental disorder, marked by decline in social function over weeks to months, increasing social withdrawal, and development of psychotic signs: delusions (fixed false beliefs), hallucinations, disorganized thinking/speech, and disorganized behavior. Lifetime prevalence is 1% with equal female-male ratio. Onset is typically the early 20s in men and the late 20s in women and rarely before adolescence. Onset after 45 years of age occurs in 10% of cases and usually accompanies a chronic premorbid history of social isolation and mistrust of others. Symptom escalation is gradual, usually with a prodromal phase of declining function and increasing isolation, declining hygiene, perhaps transient affiliation with fringe groups (i.e., cults, extremist groups), and occasionally (more often in men) mild antisocial activity (theft of small items). Eventually, active psychotic symptoms occur. Often, residual symptoms persist, with amotivation, blunted affect, and cognitive deficits ("negative symptoms") with periodic active psychotic episodes with hallucinations and delusions ("positive symptoms"). However, the course can vary from virtual remission between episodes to continuous refractory active symptoms.

I. **Differential diagnosis**

   A. **Delirium** also can present with agitated disorganized behavior and hallucinations. The onset of delirium is rapid (minutes to hours), with disorientation to time and place a defining feature. Hallucinations are often visual in delirium. Onset of active psychosis in schizophrenia is typically over weeks without disorientation. Hallucinations in schizophrenia are usually auditory.

   B. **Dementia** may also include psychosis; however, this typically occurs late in the course, with concomitant impairment of orientation. In schizophrenia, orientation is typically intact. The clinician should obtain information about longitudinal course of function from the family.

   C. **Substance-related disorders**, including cocaine, amphetamine, and phencyclidine, may cause acute psychosis with intoxication.

   D. **General medical conditions** are numerous and include Wilson's disease, CNS tumors, and complex partial seizures.

   E. **Bipolar disorder** involves prominent mood disturbance and the presence of psychosis, frequently early in the course. It is dissimilar in that, typically, the onset of schizophrenia is over weeks, whereas in mania onset is over days. A family history of schizophrenia versus bipolar disorder can be helpful.

   F. **Psychotic depression** presents with prominent mood and psychotic features. However, in schizophrenia mood symptoms tend to play a minor overall role, with a history of prominent psychosis in the absence of mood disturbance. Psychosis in psychotic depression is accompanied by depressive symptoms throughout its history.

   G. **Personality disorders** are similar to schizophrenia in that individuals with antisocial personality can present with a chief complaint such as "I'm hearing voices telling me to kill myself and hurt others," especially in the emergency room for secondary gain. People with borderline personality, especially under stress, can describe hearing voices or seeing things (i.e., "dead bodies floating in front of me") as a way of expressing vivid thoughts. Brief (i.e., minutes to hours) stress-associated paranoid thinking can also develop. This is dissimilar in that visual hallucinations are uncommon in schizophrenia. Patients with schizophrenia rarely complain of hallucinations or delusions even though they are clearly hallucinating or delusional—that is, because they lack insight that this is abnormal, they do not complain or may be unable to verbalize this.

   H. **Somatization disorder** involves multiple physical (somatoform) complaints and may also present with multiple psychiatric (psychoform) complaints. Descriptions of hallucinations tend to be vivid and of multiple senses (i.e., "I see my dead grandmother in front of me and telling me to run away" or "I see horses and hear hoof beats"). Associated signs of schizophrenia (delusions, cognitive and/or affective blunting, disorganized thoughts) are missing. Patients with schizophrenia typically do not complain of hallucinations and sometimes have difficulty in articulating hallucinatory experiences as such.

   I. **Normal human experience**, such as hearing one's name called or single word utterances or visual or auditory hallucinations while falling asleep (hypnagogic) or awakening (hypnopompic), are not considered psychotic.

II. **Treatment**

   A. **Referral to a psychiatrist** is recommended in all cases of suspected schizophrenia.

B. **Family education** should include discussion of schizophrenia as a chronic illness and the importance of medication adherence to an overall better outcome. Family support is important because patients often chronically lack insight into their illness and are unmotivated to take medications because of multiple side effects. **Amotivation** often is part of the illness, and the patient should not be blamed for an apparent lack of effort. Patients often require gentle encouragement to maintain hygiene and attend community organizations and vocational rehabilitation. Highly charged emotional and conflict-ridden environments tend to lead to poor outcomes and increase the risk of relapse.

C. **Referral to community support** organizations that promote socialization and vocational training for people with serious mental illness is essential.

D. **Pharmacotherapy**

1. **New-generation (atypical) antipsychotics** are usually the standard of care. These include risperidone, olanzapine, quetiapine, ziprasidone, and clozapine. Advantages include fewer motor and cognitive side effects than traditional antipsychotics. Disadvantages include higher risk of weight gain and possible hyperglycemia. Dietetic education, monitoring of weight, and diabetes screening should be a routine part of care. Clozapine use carries a 1% risk of **agranulocytosis** and requires weekly monitoring of WBC counts for the first 6 months of treatment and every 2 weeks thereafter. Generally, atypical antipsychotics are safe and effective, with few drug interactions.

2. **Typical antipsychotics** include haloperidol, fluphenazine, trifluoperazine, and thiothixene. Haloperidol and fluphenazine are available in depo injectable forms, which are particularly useful for patients who are nonadherent to oral medication regimens. This permits treatment by injection every 2–4 weeks. Also, these drugs generally do not interact adversely with other medications.

Somatoform Disorders

The hallmark of somatoform disorders is the presence of physical symptoms that are not fully explained by a general medical condition, substance disorder, or another mental illness. These disorders are not feigned and include somatization, conversion, hypochondriasis, and pain disorders.

I. **Somatization disorder** is a pattern of recurring, multiple, clinically significant somatic complaints, including multiple pain symptoms, GI, sexual, and neurologic. These begin before age 30 years, are not intentionally feigned, and cannot be fully explained by any known general medical condition or the direct effects of a substance. Somatization disorder occurs in 1–2% of females and approximately 0.1% of males. The course is chronic but fluctuating, with diagnostic criteria typically met before age 25 years.

A. **Differential diagnosis**

1. **General medical conditions** that can present with multiple vague complaints should be ruled out (hyperparathyroidism, acute intermittent porphyria, multiple sclerosis, systemic lupus erythematosus, etc.). Somatization should be considered when symptoms involve multiple organs, early onset with chronic course without physical signs or structural abnormalities, and absence of characteristic laboratory abnormalities.

2. **Schizophrenia** may also cause patients to be preoccupied with somatic delusions. However, individuals with somatization can respond to reassurance because their somatic complaints are not fixed false beliefs (i.e., delusions).

3. **Anxiety disorders** may also involve multiple physical symptoms. However, patients with panic disorder typically experience physical symp-

toms only during a panic attack. Patients with GAD do not limit their worry to physical complaints.

4. **Depressive disorder** may produce symptoms of headaches, GI disturbance, or unexplained pain. These tend to remit with treatment of depression.

5. **Hypochondriasis** also involves excessive preoccupation with physical problems. However, a patient with hypochondriasis is focused on having a deadly disease and not on particular symptoms.

6. **Conversion disorder** is similar in that physical complaints have no objective medical findings. It is dissimilar because it typically involves only one or two physical complaints, usually neurologic, and is often preceded by a stressor.

7. **Factitious disorder and malingering** patients also may express multiple somatic complaints. However, these individuals intentionally feign symptoms. The difference between factitious disorder and malingering is that in factitious disorder the patient purposefully feigns symptoms for the sole purpose of assuming the patient role, whereas malingering is for some external benefit.

B. Treatment. Because there is no cure, management is the key. This includes establishing the primary care physician as the patient's main and, if possible, only physician; setting up brief, regularly scheduled visits every 4–6 weeks; and performing at least a partial physical examination during each visit directed at the organ system of complaint. The physician should understand symptoms as emotional communications rather than a warning for a new disease and avoid diagnostic tests, laboratory evaluations, and operative procedures unless they are clearly indicated.

II. Conversion disorder is the presence of symptoms affecting voluntary motor or sensory function, not intentionally produced, that cannot be fully explained by a general medical condition or the direct effects of a substance. Prevalence estimates vary from 11–500/100,000, with a female-male ratio of 2:1. Risk factors include lower socioeconomic status, rural background, and lower medical and psychological sophistication. Symptoms occur more commonly on the left than on the right side of the body, especially in women. Onset is from late childhood to early adulthood and is typically acute. Recurrence is common. Individuals often undergo numerous medical examinations, diagnostic procedures, surgeries, and hospitalizations that expose them to increased risk of morbidity. Factors associated with a good prognosis are acute onset, the presence of clearly identifiable stress at the time of onset, a short interval between onset and beginning of treatment, good premorbid health, no ongoing compensation litigation, and above-average intelligence. Symptoms of paralysis, aphonia, and blindness are associated with a better prognosis than tremor and seizures.

A. Differential diagnosis. The eventual emergence of medical, neurologic, or other psychiatric disorders is highly likely to account for the "conversion symptoms" (i.e., degenerative diseases, psychosis in up to one-half of patients initially thought to have conversion disorder). Conversion disorder is a diagnosis of exclusion; a psychiatrist cannot rule out conversion disorder.

1. **General medical conditions.** Because of the neurologic nature of symptoms, conditions in the differential diagnosis include myasthenia gravis, periodic paralysis, brain tumor, multiple sclerosis, optic neuritis, partial vocal cord paralysis, Guillain-Barré, Parkinson's disease, degenerative diseases of the basal ganglia, and subdural hematoma.

2. **Psychiatric disorders** (see sec. I.A). Studies performed on patients who were admitted to psychiatry units for conversion disorder reveal that 25–50% have clinically significant mood disorders or schizophrenia. Treating a coexistent psychiatric disorder, if present, may be associated with remission of the conversion symptom.

B. Treatment. Most conversion symptoms remit spontaneously or after behavioral treatment and a supportive environment. The physician should reassure the patient that all tests to rule out dangerous or fatal causes are being conducted. It is not helpful to argue with the patient about the cause of the symptom (i.e., that the physical disability is the representation of a psychological problem). Referral to a psychiatrist does not replace the need for continued regular primary care follow-up for the symptoms. Patients are highly sensitive to suggestions that "this is all in my head." Therefore, it should be communicated that the referral is for the purpose of helping the patient to cope with the stress of having such a difficult medical problem and that the primary physician will continue to follow closely. This is especially comforting to both the patient and doctor if a medical cause is eventually found.

III. **Hypochondriasis** is preoccupation with the fear of developing or having a serious disease, despite medical reassurance to the contrary. In a 6-month period, 4–6% of the general population has a hypochondriacal disorder; risk is not influenced by social position, education, marital status, or other demographic descriptors. Age range of onset is wide and most common between 20 and 30 years of age. The course is chronic, with waxing and waning of symptoms. Fifty percent of patients show improvement, with good indicators being high socioeconomic status, the presence of other treatable conditions (i.e., depression), acute onset, and the absence of a personality disorder or comorbid general medical disease.

A. **Differential diagnosis**

1. **General medical conditions** include early stages of neurologic conditions (multiple sclerosis, myasthenia gravis), endocrine conditions (thyroid or parathyroid disease), and multiple system diseases (systemic lupus erythematosus).

2. Patients with **somatization** disorder are concerned about their multiple symptoms and are relatively indifferent to the possibility of serious underlying disease. Individuals with hypochondriasis typically do not have multiple symptoms.

3. **Psychotic disorder** is dissimilar because in patients with hypochondriasis, somatic preoccupations do not reach delusional proportions. They can entertain the idea that the feared disease is not present.

4. **OCD** involves obsessions and compulsions that are not restricted to concerns about illness (i.e., checking that the doors are locked).

B. **Treatment** includes attention to any comorbid psychiatric conditions that, if treated, may help to decrease the severity of hypochondriasis. Regularly scheduled follow-up visits may be beneficial. Patients may initially be resistant to psychiatric referral; however, after medical workup is completed, they may accept referral for psychiatric care if it is framed in the context of help with stress associated with their medical problems.

IV. **Pain disorder** involves pain in one or more anatomic sites, not intentionally produced, that causes significant distress, with psychological factors judged to play an important role in the onset, severity, exacerbation, or maintenance of the pain. The patient's preoccupation with pain is consuming and to some extent disabling. It is relatively common; in any given year, 10–15% of adults have some form of work disability due to back pain alone. The female-male ratio is 2:1. Age of onset is variable, with a peak incidence in the fourth and fifth decades, especially in those with blue-collar occupations. A good prognostic indicator is participation in regularly scheduled activities (i.e., work) despite the pain and resistance in allowing pain to determine lifestyle. An additional diagnosis of pain disorder should be considered only if the pain is an independent focus of clinical attention, leads to clinically significant distress, and is in excess of what is usually associated with the other medical disorder. The clinician should acknowledge the patient's pain and predicament at each visit, but the major focus should be on regaining function. Guidelines for discontinuing a particular treatment should be set at the onset (i.e., no improvement in 6 months may be grounds for a change in treatment). Treatment should be multidisciplinary, including individual therapy, pain management, treatment of other underlying psychiatric disorders, and general health maintenance. Regimens, including nonsteroidal anti-inflammatory drugs, tricyclics, nerve blocks, visual imaging, relaxation, or hypnosis, may be benefical, and reduce opioid need or use.

Violence

Nearly 12 million women will be abused by a current or former partner sometime during their lives (*American Medical Association Treatment Guidelines on Domestic Violence*. Washington, DC: American Medical Association, 1992). In 1997, more than 32,000 Americans died by gunfire, a death rate by a consumer product second only to motor vehicle accidents (*National Vital Statistics Report* 47 1999;19:68). In 1998, only 30% of victims of firearm homicides were killed by strangers, and 50% of female victims were killed by their husbands or boyfriends (*Supplementary Homicide Report*. Washington, DC: Federal Bureau of Investigation, 1998). In 1997, homicide was the leading cause of death among African-Americans aged 15–24, and nearly nine of ten victims were killed by firearms (*National Vital Statistics Report* 47 1999;19:69).

I. **Handguns and violence**
   A. **Screening (acronym "GUNS")**
      1. Do you or anyone at home own a hand**G**un?
      2. Are you around the **U**se of alcohol or other drugs?
      3. Do you feel a **N**eed to protect yourself? Have you recently moved your gun closer to you (i.e., into a bedroom or from closet to bed)?
      4. Do any of these **S**ituations apply to you:
         a. Have you seen or been involved in acts of violence?
         b. Have you experienced sadness, depression, or mental illness?
         c. Do you have school-aged children or adolescents in your home?
   B. **Recommend safe storage of guns** to patients. Guns should never be kept loaded, guns and ammunition should be locked in separate places, a gun should always be treated as if it were loaded, and children should never be allowed the possibility of access to guns.
II. **Domestic abuse** typically follows a cyclical pattern involving a tension-building phase, acute battering incident, and period of kindness or contrition followed by repetitive and increasingly destructive episodes.
   A. **Screening.** All women who seek care in emergency departments should be asked directly about partner violence, regardless of marital status or current relationships. The Massachusetts College of Emergency Physicians proposed the following acronym "RADAR" to screen.
      1. **R**emember to ask routinely about violence.
      2. **A**sk questions ("At any time has your partner hit, kicked, or otherwise hurt or frightened you?"). Interview patients in private at all times.
      3. **D**ocument findings. Information about suspected domestic violence in a patient's chart may be used by the judicial system.
      4. **A**ssess the patient's safety. Ask if it is safe to return home. Find out if there are any weapons accessible, children in danger, or escalating violence.
      5. **R**eview options. Let patients know where help is available. Tell them about shelters, support groups, and legal advocates.
   B. **Abuse and children.** Any recent history of suspected child abuse, even if the child is not your patient, must be reported to the Division of Family Services. Because physicians are mandated reporters, they are legally obligated to report any safety concerns and are immune from repercussions for doing so. A reasonable statement to make would be, "It sounds like there's a great deal of stress at home. It also sounds like the kids are being involved, and I know you would rather get help than continue to see them hurt. I'm going to call Family Services and have a social worker come out to be helpful." Assuring concerned parent(s) that Family Services' primary goal is to keep families together whenever possible can also be helpful.

30

Geriatrics

David B. Carr

Primary care providers are frequently faced with an aging patient population. Many of them work in the nursing home setting or at residential care centers, or both. Identifying and evaluating geriatric syndromes such as dementia and incontinence, addressing polypharmacy, preventing injury and disability, maintaining function, and discussing advance directives are just a few of the important priorities in providing care to the older adult.

Health Screening and Geriatric Syndromes

I. **Preventing disability and maintaining function.** General guidelines for health screening are covered elsewhere in this manual (see Appendix C). The decision to screen for various diseases in the older adult is often complicated by limited life expectancy with advanced age, the presence of comorbid illness, the reluctance of the patient to undergo testing, and the paucity of literature that would demonstrate efficacy of screening in late life. However, it should be noted that the average 85-year-old woman has a life expectancy well past 5 years, which is often within the range of survival rates quoted for many cancer treatments. In addition, the common causes of morbidity and mortality in advanced age remain atherosclerosis, cancer, injury, dementia, infections, and adverse drug events. Thus, the decision to perform screening and health maintenance in the older adult should focus on a variety of health issues while remaining individualized for each patient. Smoking cessation has been found to be beneficial and bestow health benefits despite advanced age. Primary prevention of hypercholesterolemia in patients older than age 70 years is still controversial, but secondary prevention has been demonstrated to decrease rates of myocardial infarction and death in the older adult. The role of weight training and aerobic activity in maintaining cognitive or physical health, or both, is imperative, and these interventions should be discussed and encouraged with older adult patients.

II. **Geriatric syndromes.** Common geriatric syndromes or disorders in the outpatient setting that should be identified may include dementia (see Dementia), delirium, depression (see Chap. 29), falls (see Injury Prevention), incontinence (see Chap. 20), malnutrition (see Chap. 3), impotence (see Chap. 25), sensory deprivation, and polypharmacy (see Pharmacotherapeutics in the Older Adult). These conditions may be identified by the clinician, patient, or family. However, many of these syndromes are not identified or evaluated unless the primary care physician systematically screens for them. Clinicians should inquire about the presence of these syndromes with their older adult patients and caregivers during office visits. Selected screening measures should also be incorporated in yearly health examinations for patients older than age 65 years. These may include medication reviews, screening for hearing impairment (by questionnaire or screening audiometry) and visual impairment

Table 30-1. Short Blessed screening test for cognitive impairment

Cognitive screen	Maximum error	Error score × weight[a]	=	Subscore
1. What year is it now?	1	_____	4	_____
2. What month is it now?	1	_____	3	_____
Repeat this phrase after me and remember it:				
John Brown, 42 Market Street, Chicago				
No. of trials to learning: _____				
3. About what time is it without looking at your watch? (within 1 hr)	1	_____	3	_____
Response _____				
Actual time _____				
4. Count backward from 20 down to 1	2	_____	2	_____
Mark correctly sequenced nos.				
20 19 18 17 16 15 14 13 12 11 10 9 8 7 6 5 4 3 2 1				
5. Say the months of the year in reverse	2	_____	2	_____
Mark the correct months				
D N O S A JL JU MY AP M F J				
6. Repeat the name and address I asked you to remember.	1	_____	2	_____
John Brown, 42 Market Street, Chicago[b]				
		Total weighted error score[c]		_____

[a]Scoring: 0 = no errors, 1 = 1 error, 2 = 2 or more errors.
[b]An answer of either Market or Market Street is acceptable.
[c]A total weighted error score of 9 or greater indicates a need for further assessment.
Source: R Katzman, T Brown, P Fuld, et al. *Am J Psychiatry* 1983;140:734–739, with permission.

(Snellen eye chart or Rosenbaum pocket chart), identifying the presence or risk for falls or motor vehicle crashes (see Injury Prevention), screening for dementia (Table 30-1) and depression, discussing and documenting advance directives, and identifying a surrogate decision maker. In addition, many of these screens can serve as a baseline and can be repeated during future examinations to determine response to treatment.

III. Assessment of function. Many disorders come to the attention of the physician if they are impairing job performance or function at home. Diagnoses such as dementia require the new onset of functional impairment. Improvements in functional status are often used as a marker of treatment success. In addition, a review of the activities of daily living can assist in targeting additional assistance that may be needed at home. Thus, clinicians should be prepared to quickly assess and document the presence of functional impairment. Two mnemonics for basic and instrumental activities of daily

Table 30-2. Activities of daily living

Instrumental activities of daily living	Basic activities of daily living
Shopping	**D**ressing
Housework	**E**ating
Accounting	**A**mbulation
Food preparation	**T**oileting/incontinence
Transportation/driving	**H**ygiene/grooming

Source: KC Fleming, JM Evans, DC Weber, DS Chutka. Practical functional assessment of elderly patients: a primary care approach. *Mayo Clin Proc* 1995;70;890–910.

living are listed in Table 30-2. The presence of functional impairment due to any illness should be documented and monitored for further changes in function over time.

IV. **Geriatric assessment** is a holistic approach to patient care and focuses on the physical, functional, social, and psychological health of the individual along with providing assistance to caregivers. These assessments are typically performed in the outpatient or hospital setting by a geriatrician, gerontological nurse specialist, and/or social worker. The role of the social worker may include locating a chore worker to assist the caregiver, finding a durable power of attorney, providing financial information, assisting with Medicare or Medicaid eligibility, counseling, referral to state and local area agencies on aging, addressing advance directives, or recommending relocation to assisted living or long-term care centers. Geriatric assessment can be performed in the outpatient setting by the primary care clinician in conjunction with a social worker or a geriatric case manager who can be consulted in difficult cases. Geriatric evaluations should include the physical, functional, social, and psychological assessment of patients in the context of their current environment. These assessments can assist patients and their families regarding the myriad of issues that can affect the independence of frail older adults in the community.

Dementia

I. **Changes in cognition with aging.** Healthy older adults demonstrate an age-related reduction in working memory, where information must be stored or held while performing other cognitive activities. This in turn may correspond to frequent complaints by elderly persons concerning poor retrieval of names and limited capacity to keep several items in mind simultaneously. Age-associated deficits also have been reported for language, psychomotor speed, and visuospatial abilities. In healthy older persons, these changes typically do not interfere substantially with usual activities or social or occupational performance. The maintenance of functional ability in everyday activities is a major clinical feature that distinguishes cognitively healthy aging from dementia. The use of a brief cognitive screen may assist the primary care physician in identifying older adults with significant cognitive impairment (Table 30-1).

II. **Dementia** can be simply defined as a memory and cognitive disorder that impairs an individual's function and/or social relationships. *Diagnosis and Statistical Manual IV* criteria for diagnosing a dementing illness include memory impairment (impaired ability to learn new information or to recall learned information) and at least one of the following: apraxia (impaired ability to carry out motor activities despite intact motor function), agnosia (failure to

Table 30-3. Indications for brain imaging in the diagnostic workup of dementia

Sudden onset of symptoms

Age <60 yrs

CNS complaints (headaches, blurred vision)

Early onset of gait disorder/incontinence

History or current diagnosis of cancer

Subacute course

Focal neurologic signs/symptoms

Use of anticoagulation

Head trauma/falls

Weight loss/depression

Reprinted from Supplement: Management of Dementing Disorders Conclusions from the Canadian Consensus Conference on Dementia, 15 June 1999;160(12 Suppl):S1–S15, by permission of the publisher. © Canadian Medical Association.

recognize or identify objects despite intact sensory function), disturbances in executive functioning (planning, organizing, sequencing), aphasia (disturbance in language), judgment and problem solving, and orientation. In addition, the cognitive deficits must cause significant impairment in social or occupational functioning and represent a decline. The mnemonic **DEMENTIA**—**D** (drugs), **E** (emotional disorders), **M** (metabolic disorders), **E** (eye and ear disorders), **N** (nutritional deficiencies), **T** (tumor/trauma), **I** (infection), **A** (arteriosclerosis)—is often used to identify the presence of potentially treatable causes of cognitive decline. Diagnostic tests such as vitamin B_{12} and a thyroid-stimulating hormone level may be justifiable in all patient evaluations. The decision to pursue a rapid plasma reagin (RPR), EEG, and/or a lumbar puncture in the evaluation of dementia should be individualized and based on the clinical index of suspicion as raised by history and physical examination. The indications for obtaining a brain-imaging study are listed in Table 30-3. In general, an MRI study is preferred when focal deficits are found on the neurologic examination. A CT scan without contrast may be appropriate for more chronic cases that have a nonfocal presentation, such as ruling out a subdural hematoma or assessing ventricular size when considering normal-pressure hydrocephalus. The pretest probability of the disease should guide the test selection, rather than using a "blanket" approach.

A. Dementia of the Alzheimer's type (DAT)
  1. **Demographics.** DAT may affect as many as four million people in the United States. It is largely a disease of the elderly, increasing exponentially after age 70 years to achieve prevalence rates up to 47% of those older than age 85 years. Because the percentage of the population older than 80 years of age will double by 2010, the burden of DAT to society will increase to enormous proportions.
  2. **Diagnosis.** The clinical hallmark of DAT is the gradual onset and progression of memory loss and other cognitive functions. The diagnosis is greatly facilitated with information from a collateral source or caregiver that the cognitive changes represent a decline from a prior level of performance and are sufficient to interfere with everyday function. Short-term memory impairment often is manifested by repetition, misplacement of items, and missed appointments. Incomplete or absent recall of recent events increasingly occurs, and eventually remote memory also is impaired. Behavioral changes of passivity, lack of interest, and withdrawal are frequent. The initial changes often are subtle, and

the diagnosis is frequently missed. Functional performance, however, declines, as evidenced by impaired driving, financial imprudence, and inability to produce a complete meal. Impairment of language, constructional ability, praxis, recognition, judgment, and abstraction can occur throughout the course of the illness. Currently, no validated test is available for the diagnosis of DAT. Rather than simply a diagnosis of exclusion, however, the characteristic onset and course of memory and other cognitive deficits increasingly make DAT a diagnosis of inclusion. Laboratory and neuroimaging procedures are usually obtained for screening for the presence of other diseases that can contribute to cognitive impairment. Apolipoprotein E genotype testing is currently only recommended for research purposes.

3. **Treatment.** Care of the Alzheimer's patient usually focuses on assisting the caregiver(s), treatment of behavior, or drug treatment for the symptoms of cognitive impairment.

   a. **Caregiver stress.** For any dementing illness, the patient and family should be informed of the disease, the extent to which it is treatable, the degree of disability, the prognosis, and the areas of cognition that are intact. The social and psychological needs of the caregiver should be assessed. Future changes regarding levels of care should be discussed. Referral to a geriatric assessment center, a geriatric case manager, local support services, and especially the Alzheimer's Association should be considered to assist the family. Legal issues, such as identifying a durable power of attorney, should be pursued along with a discussion of advance directives. Assisted living and nursing home placement may be appropriate during the course of the illness. Community aging services may be available to assist in the home.

   b. **Pharmacotherapy for cognitive impairment.** The pharmacologic therapies for DAT remain limited.

      (1) Cholinesterase inhibitors. Donepezil (5 mg PO qd for 1 month; increase to 10 mg PO qd if tolerated), **galantamine** (4 mg PO bid for 1 month and increase to 8 mg bid if tolerated), **rivastigmine** (6–12 mg/day with bid dosing after titrating up slowly from 3 mg bid), or **tacrine** (40–160 mg/day qid dosing) can be initiated for the treatment of DAT in the early stages of the disease. The patient should be committed to at least a 3-month trial, because it may take some time for these drugs to take effect. The beneficial cognitive effects of these agents, if present, are usually modest. Some patients and family members desire to stay on the medication as long as there is no observed progression of symptoms. Side effects are infrequent and are related to excess cholinergic activity, such as diarrhea, urinary frequency, muscle cramps, nausea, and hypersalivation. However, tacrine can cause liver inflammation, and liver function monitoring should be performed every 2 weeks when initiating therapy.

      (2) Vitamin E. In one study (*N Engl J Med* 1997;336:1216–1222), vitamin E appeared to delay the onset of disability and/or nursing home placement. Although the dose used for this study was 1000 IU bid, vitamin E at 400 IU bid is recommended by many dementia experts as an adjunct to delay progression of cognitive impairment.

      (3) Other agents. Gingko biloba cannot be recommended at this time because of limited data regarding efficacy. Estrogen and nonsteroidal anti-inflammatory drugs have not yet been shown to be effective for secondary prevention, and further study is still needed to determine whether they will play a role in primary prevention. Many urban centers have Alzheimer's Disease Research Centers that may include participation in research trials, which

Table 30-4. Environmental or behavioral interventions for managing difficult behaviors in dementia

Educate about dementia and agitation

Talk to patients/distract attention

Identify specific precipitants to behavior

Experiment with targeted changes to schedule

Separate disruptive and noisy persons from quieter persons

Control door access; use safety latches to prevent egress

Provide reassurance and verbal efforts to calm

Reduce isolation

Encourage the joining of support groups

Provide a predictable routine for the patient

Structure the environment

Provide orienting stimuli

Provide bright enough daytime lighting

Use a night light in bedroom during sleep

should be encouraged. These centers can also serve as resources for diagnosis and education.

c. **Treatment of behavior.** Many behaviors in patients with dementia are difficult to manage. These may include wandering, anxiety, psychosis, delusions, disruptive vocalization, combativeness, or insomnia.

(1) **Diagnosis.** The mnemonic **DRNO** [**D** (describe the behavior), **R** (reason for the behavior), **N** (nonpharmacologic approach), **O** (order medication as a last step)] may provide a useful systematic approach to address difficult behaviors in the DAT patient. The goal is to describe specifically the unwanted behavior and then to determine the reasons for the behavior (e.g., pain, hunger, need for elimination, etc.). Nonpharmacologic approaches based on structuring the environment and behavioral interventions should be attempted first and are listed in Table 30-4.

(2) **Treatment.** Medications are the last line of therapy and should be prescribed for short-term use (weeks to months). Pharmacologic agents that are recommended for use in demented patients depend on the primary behavioral problem. Psychotropic drugs for behavior should be used on an as needed basis. Any routine use of these drugs should be short term with periodic trials to taper or discontinue their use. Insomnia (trazodone, 50 mg PO qhs; temazepam, 7.5 mg PO qhs; zolipidem, 5 mg PO qhs), anxiety (buspirone, 5–15 mg PO tid; lorazepam for short-term acute anxiety), and psychosis (haloperidol, 0.5–2.0 mg in divided doses; risperidone, 0.25–2.0 mg in divided doses) may be used safely if given for a brief period of time. Newer atypical or novel antipsychotic agents (olanzapine, quetiapine) are expensive, may be sedating, and should be used in those individuals with concomitant extrapyramidal disease or intolerance to other agents. However, if long-term neuroleptic therapy is desired, these agents should be considered because of a lower incidence of tardive dyskinesia (*BMJ* 1999;174:23–30). Anticonvulsants appear to work on gamma aminobutyric acid receptors (valproic acid, carbamazepine) and may be useful in these

settings. Clinicians should be aware of the side effects for these drugs and educate their patients and family members accordingly.

B. Vascular dementia and atypical dementias

   1. The diagnosis of vascular dementia may be difficult, because there are no universally accepted criteria or consensus on the amount of infarcted brain volume at specific anatomic sites that are necessary to establish a dementing illness. In addition, most clinicopathologic studies indicate that it is more likely to have a diagnosis of DAT with vascular disease than to have an isolated vascular dementia alone. Nevertheless, focal areas of injury appear to be highly associated with the onset and development of DAT (*JAMA* 1997;227:813–817). A clinical determination can usually be made as to whether focal or global cerebral insult was present based on the patient's history and clinical examination. Symptoms or signs of an ischemic vascular dementia include abrupt onset, a step-wise deterioration, an early onset of gait or incontinence problems, emotional lability, somatic complaints, focal findings on clinical examination, and infarcts identified on brain-imaging studies. Risk factors include hypertension, atrial fibrillation, and advanced age. Currently, there is no treatment for the improvement of symptoms. Management focuses on prevention of additional brain injury by modifying vascular risk factors such as cessation of smoking, control of diabetes and hypertension, daily aspirin use, and anticoagulation with warfarin if not contraindicated for atrial fibrillation. The utility of additional agents on preventing cognitive impairment, such as 3-hydroxy-3-methylglutaryl coenzyme A reductase inhibitors, or drugs that may enhance blood flow, such as pentoxifylline, requires further study.

   2. Other non-Alzheimer's type dementia. A growing number of primary degenerative dementias are increasingly recognized but are beyond the scope of this chapter. In summary, dementias that are associated with extrapyramidal signs (diffuse Lewy body disease, progressive supranuclear palsy, cortical basal ganglionic degeneration); early onset of gait disorder or incontinence, or both (normal-pressure hydrocephalus, vascular dementia); or a subacute course (Jakob-Creutzfeldt disease, viral encephalopathy) should be referred to a neurologist for further evaluation.

Pharmacotherapeutics in the Older Adult

Many older adults have multiple medical problems and are taking numerous medications. It is important for the clinician to have a basic knowledge of pharmacokinetic and pharmacodynamic changes with aging and a systematic approach to medication prescribing.

I. Factors that affect drug metabolism. The duration that a particular drug exerts its effect in any patient is based on the volume of distribution (Vd) of the drug, the metabolism of the drug (hepatic function), the clearance (renal function), or a combination of factors, all of which can change with aging. The time for a drug to decline to one-half of its concentration is known as the **drug's biologic half-life**. The half-life is directly proportional to the Vd and inversely proportional to the clearance. Vd is determined by the degree of plasma protein binding and by the patient's body composition.

II. Age-related changes in drug metabolism

   A. Changes in body composition. The proportion of adipose tissue increases with aging. This increase results in a larger Vd and longer half-life, and therefore lipophilic medications such as benzodiazepines have a longer duration of action. Total body water decreases by 15% in those older than 80 years of age. The Vd for hydrophilic drugs, such as lithium, cimetidine, and ethanol, is decreased, resulting in higher drug concentrations. Elderly persons have on average a decreased lean body mass. Digoxin, which binds to muscle adenosine triphosphatase, may have a decreased Vd, meaning that toxicity can occur at lower doses. The concentrations of plasma proteins such as albumin also tend to decline in older adults. This results in a reduced protein-bound form of many drugs and greater amount of free drug levels. Examples include digoxin, theophylline, phenytoin, and warfarin. Most drug level determinations measure total (protein-bound and free levels) drug concentrations. Thus, total drug levels may not accurately reflect drug activity.

B. Changes in hepatic and renal metabolism. In general, there is a decrease in the number of hepatocytes and liver mass with age. Drugs that have a large first-pass effect in the liver, such as beta-blockers, nitrates, calcium channel blockers, and tricyclic antidepressants, may be effective at lower doses. Phase I (cytochrome P-450) oxidation declines on average with aging, and doses of medications such as benzodiazepines should be reduced. Knowledge about cytochrome P-450 drug interactions has grown and should be reviewed by all prescribing clinicians (*Sci Med* 1998;1:16–25). Medications that are primarily excreted by the kidney often need to be adjusted by estimating creatinine clearance by age and body weight (see Chap. 20). Examples such as aminoglycosides, digoxin, atenolol, vancomycin, lithium, acyclovir, and amantadine require dose reductions in older adults.

C. Changes in pharmacodynamics. End-organ responsiveness to a drug at the receptor level may be changed with age. Changes in receptor binding, a decrease in receptor number, or altered translation of a receptor-initiated cellular response into a biochemical reaction may be responsible. Consistent findings in the literature include (1) a decreased response to beta-blockers and (2) increased sensitivities to benzodiazepines, opiates, warfarin, and anticholinergics. Thus, clinicians need to be aware that dose adjustments in these drugs may be necessary.

III. Steps in preventing polypharmacy and drug toxicity

A. Reducing medications. Older adults may be treated by several physicians and obtain their medications at several pharmacies. The initial step in assessing polypharmacy is to identify all prescription and over-the-counter drugs. The patient and, if necessary, a family member should bring in all medications each visit for review. All drugs should be recorded by generic name, and unnecessary medications should be discontinued. The clinical indication should be identified for all drugs. The side effect profile should be reviewed, and safer medications should be substituted.

B. Starting new medications. Before a new drug is started, risk factors for adverse drug reactions, such as advanced age, liver or kidney disease, or use of multiple medications, should be identified. A review of the specific allergic reaction to any medications should be done, and drugs that have cross reactivity, such as sulfa and celecoxib, should be identified. It is imperative to make a firm diagnosis (e.g., DAT) before drug therapy is initiated. Attempts should be made to manage medical conditions (e.g., hypertension) without drugs when possible. The individual clinical status of each patient (e.g., chronic renal insufficiency) needs to be reviewed. The clinician should establish a therapeutic goal and an appropriate time frame for treatment duration. Generic medications are preferred for their lower cost. Choosing a once-a-day drug, starting at a low dose, and titrating slowly are sound principles when adjusting medications.

C. Compliance (see Chap. 1). The risk of medication errors increases dramatically with the number of medications taken by the patient. Several steps to improve compliance when ordering medications are suggested: (1) Drug regimens should be simple; (2) use the same dosage schedule with other drugs and time their administration with a daily routine such as a meal;

(3) instruct relatives and caregivers on drug regimens and enlist others, such as home health nurses and pharmacists, to assist with appropriate delivery; (4) be sure that the patient can afford the medication, has transportation to the pharmacy, and can open the container; and (5) encourage the use of aids, such as pillboxes, calendars, and an updated medication record. Reviewing the patients' knowledge of the reason they take each medication and inquiries about adverse drug reactions on each visit are essential aspects of successful prescribing.

Injury Prevention

Injury is the fourth leading cause of death in the older adult population. Common causes of injuries include falls and motor vehicle crashes. Burns, accidental poisoning, smoke inhalation, and hypothermia in demented patients are not uncommon. These safety issues should be addressed for all older adults, with special attention paid to patients with DAT and their caregivers.

I. Falls are important to identify and prevent in the elderly population. Osteoporosis should be considered and treated if identified (see Chap. 24). A family history of fracture, or a patient history of fracture, falls, gait difficulties, or balance impairment, should be discussed. In addition, a lower-extremity mobility screen such as the "up and go" test should be considered for older adults (*J Am Geriatr Soc* 1991;39:142–148). Focusing on lower-extremity muscle strength, gait, and balance tests appear to be a powerful predictor of disability in the older adult (*N Engl J Med* 1995;332:556–561).

   A. Risk factors for falls. To prevent falls and subsequent injury, a thorough review of the patient and environment is needed to target recommendations (*Am Fam Physician* 2000;61:2159–2168). Common intrinsic factors for falls in older adults include gait and balance disorders, proximal muscle weakness, dizziness, sedating drugs, postural hypotension, and visual impairment. Common causes of these disorders include dementia, Parkinson's disease, cerebrovascular accidents, peripheral neuropathy, alcohol use, deconditioning, arthritis, cataracts, glaucoma, orthostatic hypotension from dehydration or drugs, foot abnormalities, and psychotropic medications. Many of these conditions are amenable to treatment or intervention. Syncope, seizures, vestibular dysfunction, acute illnesses, arrhythmia, subclavian steal, and carotid sinus hypersensitivity should be considered but are less common. Extrinsic factors are very common. A review of the household environment for improper lighting, throw rugs, uneven steps, low-lying tables, and grab bars for the bathroom is imperative.

   B. Treatment and prevention. A thorough search for intrinsic and extrinsic risk factors as described above is the first step in prevention. A home occupational therapy assessment can assist with management of extrinsic risk factors. Physical therapy is often helpful in gait and balance training, evaluation for an assistive device, and muscle strengthening when indicated. Identifying and treating the cause of postural hypotension and visual impairment are often necessary. There is growing interest in hip protectors to prevent hip fractures from falls. These devices may become readily available as more randomized controlled trials are completed. A thorough examination of the older adult for occult fractures on presentation after a fall is mandatory. Plain films may be negative for a fracture in the initial evaluation of a geriatric patient who has a painful joint after falling. A high clinical index of suspicion for a nondisplaced fracture should be maintained. A low threshold should exist for repeating films or obtaining a bone scan or MRI.

II. Motor vehicle crashes. Driving concerns in the older adult may come to the attention of the primary care physician for several reasons. Patients may have insight into their driving skills and may question their own ability to drive safely. A concerned family member or friend may have observed unsafe driving behaviors. Finally, the department of motor vehicles may have raised some concerns and referred the individual to the physician for an evaluation of driving competency.

A. Risk factors. The initial assessment begins with the driving history. Inquiries about crashes, tickets, near misses, or becoming lost in previously familiar environments should be addressed to the patient and, if possible, a friend or family member. Information from a collateral source who has driven with the patient may be beneficial. A review of medications that have the potential to sedate the older driver should be sought, with efforts at drug reduction or substituting safer alternatives. A search for diseases that have the potential to increase crash risk should be pursued and may include dementia, psychiatric disorders, stroke, sleep apnea, arthritis, alcohol use, sensory deprivation, seizures, diabetes, or heart disease. Vision, hearing, attention, visuospatial skills, judgment, muscle strength, and flexibility should be assessed. Efforts should be made at stabilizing or improving these illnesses or physiologic variables when possible. Counseling older drivers to use safety restraints, refrain from drinking alcohol when driving, obeying the speed limit, avoiding cellular phones, and considering a refresher course for driving such as the 55 Alive program (sponsored by the American Association of Retired Persons) are all important issues in motor vehicle crash prevention.

B. Evaluation and prevention. Referral may be necessary if the primary care physician is unsure as to whether the patient is safe behind the wheel. Occupational therapists who have experience in assessing older drivers can be invaluable in the evaluation process with on-the-road tests or by recommending and implementing adaptive equipment. In the event that the clinician makes a recommendation to stop driving, this information should be communicated in a professional and sensitive manner and documented in the medical record. It is helpful if alternate modes of transportation are discussed. Patients may refuse to stop driving despite the advice of their physician or family, or both. DAT drivers may lack insight into their own safety risk. Therefore, removing the car from the premises, hiding the car keys, changing the locks, filing down the ignition key, or disabling the battery cables may be necessary. Letters can be written to the department of motor vehicles and may be ethically appropriate. Some states have laws that grant physicians civil immunity from reporting unsafe drivers or have mandatory reporting requirements. Physicians should be aware of state and local requirements for reporting and obtain legal advice before breaching confidentiality.

Nursing Home Care

I. Pressure sores

A. Risk factors. The most common causes for wounds in older adults are pressure and friction. Risk factors include malnutrition, immobility, vascular insufficiency, and other systemic illnesses. Moisture from urinary or fecal incontinence, friction (pulling the patient across bed sheets), and shearing forces (patients sliding down a bed with the head elevated) can combine to damage tissue further. Once the pressure on tissue exceeds intracapillary pressure (10–30 mm Hg), tissue ischemia can occur.

B. Prevention. Pressure should be removed by frequent position changes, mobility and exercise, massage, and/or physical therapy. Keeping the skin dry, preventing friction, and avoiding sheering forces can assist in prevention and healing. Topical creams and lubricants can be helpful to treat dry skin, provide a skin barrier, and increase blood flow to the area with application.

C. **Treatment.** Nutrition is critical, and calorie or protein supplements, or both, may be helpful adjuncts to promote healing of wounds. Some data suggest that vitamin C and zinc supplementation may be of benefit in refractory cases. Foley catheters should be avoided but may be necessary to prevent contamination of nonhealing wounds. Dressings and gels, such as hydrocolloids (DuoDerm, Tegasorb) and hydrogels (IntraSite, Solosite), that cover the wound bed and provide a surface on which epithelial cells can migrate are often helpful for stage II (partial-thickness) or stage III (full-thickness skin loss with damage to the subcutaneous tissue) wounds. Topical enzymatic débridement agents with collagenase and/or sharp mechanical débridement can be used to remove black eschar, with the goal of promoting granulating tissue, which promotes healing. Wet-to-dry dressings can be used for noninfected wounds. However, if not changed routinely, they simply remove migrating epithelial tissue and inhibit further healing. Alginates (Kaltostat) are very absorbent and can be helpful in exudative wounds.

D. **Complications.** Topical antibiotic creams are generally not used for routine wound care unless the area is infected. Polysporin, silver sulfadiazine, or mupirocin (the latter for methicillin-resistant *Staphylococcus aureus*) can be helpful in reducing bacterial counts. Systemic antibiotics should be used in cellulitis or deep-seated infections with sepsis. Osteomyelitis should be considered in nonhealing wounds that continue to drain or are exudative. Finally, support mattresses that use foam, air, or water can also assist in prevention or healing. Deep wounds into the muscle or bone (stage IV) or multiple nonhealing wounds may benefit from an air-fluidized bed or low–air-loss bed. However, their cost and size may be prohibitive. Consultation with general or plastic surgeons to assist in wound healing, which could include débridement or flap procedures, or both, to close the wound may be necessary.

II. **Malnutrition and artificial nutrition and hydration**

A. **Definitions.** A simple method of identifying protein-calorie undernutrition in the older adult is to follow serial weights. In general, weight loss is significant if there is a 5% loss of body weight in 1 month, 7.5% loss in 3 months, or 10% loss in a 6-month period of time. The clinician should not count weight loss that is due to diuresis or volume status. Frequent weights and early assessment by a dietitian in the long-term care setting are appropriate. Physical examination findings and laboratory assessment are discussed in Chapter 3.

B. **Differential diagnosis.** Weight loss and anorexia have a multitude of causes in the older adult and are often multifactorial. They include the use of "therapeutic diets," such as a salt-restricted or diabetic diet, cachexia from advanced end-organ disease (CHF/chronic obstructive pulmonary disease), malabsorption, cancer, or thyroid disease. Zinc deficiency, acute or chronic illnesses, alcoholism, medications, nonconducive environment, poor food preparation and presentation, and ethnic preferences may also contribute. Difficulty in feeding due to hand and upper-extremity disability, cognitive impairment, psychosis, oral or dental disease, or ill-fitting dentures is not uncommon. The mnemonic **MEALS ON WHEELS** may be helpful to the clinician in identifying reversible causes for protein-energy malnutrition in the long-term care setting (Table 30-5).

C. **Treatment.** If patients are unable to sustain themselves from a nutritional standpoint after evaluation of reversible causes of weight loss have been identified and treated, input from a dietitian and the judicious use of nutritional supplements may be in order. Despite these efforts, the use of artificial nutrition and hydration may need to be addressed. It is important that the risks and benefits of tube feedings (typically administered after pursuing percutaneous gastrostomy or percutaneous endoscopic gastrostomy) are discussed with the patient or surrogate decision maker, or both. Tube feedings can assist with providing adequate calories, are helpful in preventing dehydration, and may assist in the prevention and treatment of pressure sores. Gastrostomy feeding tubes are typically helpful in cases in which there is anticipated functional improvement (e.g., cerebrovascular acci-

Table 30-5. Reversible causes for protein-energy malnutrition

Medications (e.g., digoxin, theo-phylline)	**W**andering and other dementia-related behaviors
Emotional problems (depression)	**H**yperthyroidism/hypercalcemia/hypoadrenalism
Anorexia tardive/alcoholism	**E**nteric problems (malabsorption)
Late-life paranoia	**E**ating problems
Stones (cholelithiasis)	**L**ow-salt, low-cholesterol diets
Oral problems	**S**wallowing disorders
Nosocomial infections (tuberculo-sis, *Helicobacter pylori*, *Clostridium difficile*)	

Source: JE Morely. Anorexia of aging: physiologic and pathologic. *Am J Clin Nutr* 1997;66: 760–773. Reprinted with permission © American Society for Clinical Nutrition.

dent). However, there is a paucity of data to indicate that gastrostomy feeding tubes prevent respiratory infection, improve morbidity, or delay mortality in the patient with advanced DAT (*JAMA* 1999;282:1365–1370).

III. Ethics
   A. Advance directives. Many physicians are well versed with the use of advance directives in the hospital setting. It is imperative in the outpatient and long-term care setting that advance directives are discussed openly with the frail older adults and their family members. In addition, many patients or surrogate family members, or both, desire to avoid CPR, intubation and/or ventilation, ICU treatment, dialysis, or tube feedings based on quality-of-life issues or futility of treatment. Even if questions such as code status cannot be decided before an acute event, it is of the utmost importance to identify a surrogate decision maker for the patient. A legal document such as a durable power of attorney is preferred, because guardianship is often a lengthy process that is difficult to expedite. Usually, a family member or friend can be identified who can assist in making difficult decisions.
   B. Informed consent and decision-making capacity. When discussing options or interventions with a patient, it is important to follow the steps of informed consent. This likely includes the nature and purpose of the test or procedure, the risk and benefits, the probable outcome of the intervention or refusal of the plan, and any additional alternatives to the diagnostic test or procedure (*Emerg Med Clin North Am* 2000;18:233–242). Decision-making capacity of the patient should be assessed, because many individuals have cognitive impairment or behavioral problems. Steps for assessing capacity include the ability to communicate choices, understand and retain relevant information, appreciate the situation and its consequences, and manipulate information rationally (*Psychol Med* 1999;29:437–446).

Resources

American Geriatric Society, http://www.americangeriatrics.org
Administration on Aging, http://www.aoa.dhhs.gov
Alzheimer's Disease Education and Referral Center, http://www.alzheimers.org
Family Caregiver Alliance, http://www.caregiver.org

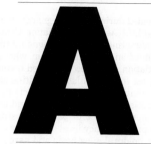

Medical Therapeutics of Pregnancy

Angela L. Brown

Pregnancy may exacerbate or reactivate a pre-existing medical condition, or it may predispose the body to the initial activation of disease processes that may have been dormant for years. In addition, there are dynamic physiologic changes in multiple organ systems. Medical illnesses and their therapies during pregnancy not only have significant effects on the mother, but on the fetus as well, leading to spontaneous abortions, fetal demise, congenital abnormalities, or premature labor. As more women delay the age of childbearing, the risk of encountering women with chronic medical illnesses will increase, as will the number of medical complications.

The U.S. Food and Drug Administration's Pregnancy Categories (modified)

A	Studies show no risk to the fetus in any trimester.
B	Studies are limited, but there is no evidence of risk in humans.
C	Animal studies have shown increased risk to the fetus. Human studies are not available or inadequate. Potential benefits must justify the potential risks to the fetus.
D	Positive evidence of risk to the human fetus. In certain cases, the benefit of use may outweigh the risk.
X	Contraindicated in pregnancy.

I. **Asthma** is the most common pulmonary complication of pregnancy. Oxygen consumption increases 25% during pregnancy. The clinical course of asthma during pregnancy is variable, but the history in prior pregnancies and severity of the disease before pregnancy are good predictors. The more severe the disease before pregnancy, the more likely it will worsen, although one-third of patients may actually experience improvement of symptoms during their pregnancy. The overall management goals of asthma in pregnancy are effective management of symptoms to avoid fetal hypoxia, while minimizing any drug-related risks to the fetus.

A. **Treatment** of asthma during pregnancy is no different from that of prepregnancy. The most severe symptoms are experienced between 29 and 36 weeks of gestation. Exposure to known asthma treatment modalities have no known adverse outcomes on the fetus. Aerosolized therapy is the preferred method of drug delivery due to the decreased chance of a systemic effect.

1. β_2 **agonists** should be used as first-line therapy. Terbutaline is preferred.

2. **Inhaled anti-inflammatory agents, corticosteroids, and cromolyn sulfate** can also be added to the therapeutic regimen. Oral steroids and theophylline should be added as deemed appropriate. Inhaled triamcinolone is teratogenic and should not be used.

3. **Smoking cessation** is recommended for all patients (see Chap. 1 for recommendations).

4. **Parenteral epinephrine** should be avoided during early pregnancy due to the risk of congenital malformations (*JAMA* Asthma Information Center: http://www.ama-assn.org/special/asthma/treatment/updates/pregnant.htm).
5. **Immunotherapy** can be safely continued in pregnant women who are already receiving immunotherapy. Initiation is not recommended because the risk of a systemic reaction is highest during initiation. Routine skin testing should be deferred due to the potential risk of systemic reactions.
B. During **labor** and **delivery**, only 10% of patients report symptoms and usually only one-half of those require treatment. In 73% of patients postpartum, the severity of asthma reverts to its prepregnancy level (*J Allergy Clin Immunol* 1988;81:509–517). During labor, epidural anesthesia and narcotics should be used with caution. Given its bronchoconstrictor properties, prostaglandin F_2 should be avoided. Patients who have been receiving steroids during the past year should be given stress doses, hydrocortisone, 100 mg every 6–8 hours.

II. **Hypertension.** High BP places the mother and baby at risk for complications. Hypertension may be related to lifestyle choices: poor dietary habits, obesity, smoking, or alcohol or other drug use. Hypertension during pregnancy is a concern, as damage to smaller blood vessels can occur and affect the blood flow to the uterus. The complications may be directly related to the severity of the hypertension before pregnancy. If the BP has been generally well controlled, the chances for a good outcome are favorable. If the hypertension before pregnancy is severe (>160/100), development of preeclampsia is great. Complications may include seizures, strokes, or abruptio placentae in the mother and growth retardation and premature birth for the baby.
A. **Classification**
1. **Chronic hypertension.** Hypertension that is present before pregnancy or that is diagnosed before the twentieth week of gestation. This also includes hypertension that is diagnosed for the first time during pregnancy and does not resolve in the postpartum period.
2. **Preeclampsia-eclampsia.** Increased BP associated with proteinuria after 20 weeks' gestation. Women with a rise of 30 mm Hg systolic or 15 mm Hg diastolic warrant close follow-up. **Eclampsia** refers to the sudden onset of seizures with or without the other manifestations of preeclampsia.
3. **Preeclampsia superimposed on chronic hypertension.** The prognosis for the mother and fetus is worse than with either condition separately.
4. **Gestational hypertension.** BP elevation detected for the first time after midpregnancy without proteinuria. If preeclampsia has not developed and the BP has returned to normal by 12 weeks postpartum, this state would be considered transient hypertension.
B. **Treatment of chronic hypertension.**
1. Women with **mild BP elevation**, systolic BP of 140–179 mm Hg, or diastolic BP of 90–109 mm Hg are at low risk for cardiovascular complications and for adverse maternal and neonatal outcomes. Withholding pharmacologic therapy should be considered given that the BP usually decreases during the first half of pregnancy.
2. For women with **more elevated BPs**, antihypertensive therapy is initiated. Methyldopa is the preferred drug. Labetalol and nifedipine are also considered safe to use. Side effects include drowsiness or postural hypotension. In general, women who were controlled on antihypertensive therapy before pregnancy can be kept on the same agents, with the exception of angiotensin-converting enzyme inhibitors and angiotensin II receptor blockers, which are **contraindicated** in pregnancy. Beta-blockers are indicated for the treatment of hypertension in women with Marfan's syndrome or coarctation of the aorta. Diuretics can decrease maternal intravascular volume and are not indicated as first-line therapy.
C. **Treatment of preeclampsia.** In mild cases, outpatient monitoring is possible if the patient is reliable and has rapid access to health care personnel; how-

ever, hospitalization is usually indicated. Delivery is the only definitive treatment modality. It is generally accepted that treatment should be initiated when diastolic levels are persistently 105–110 mm Hg. Intravenous hydralazine or labetalol are used as first-line therapy. The short-acting form of oral nifedipine is no longer recommended. Caution should be exercised when using any calcium antagonist with magnesium sulfate. Intravenous magnesium sulfate should be given during labor, delivery, and postpartum to prevent seizures in women with preeclampsia or to prevent recurrence of seizure in women with eclampsia. Sodium nitroprusside may be indicated in rare cases if other drugs fail.

 D. Treatment of gestational hypertension. A woman with gestational hypertension need not be treated unless she has evidence of preeclampsia. Gestational hypertension may be a predictor for later development of primary hypertension.

III. Diabetes. During pregnancy, the placenta produces several hormones that counteract the effects of insulin. The body must produce more (as much as 30% more) to do the job. Gestational diabetes occurs in 2–5% of all pregnancies and is one of the most common complications of pregnancy. These patients are at increased risk for development of type 2 diabetes and should be screened at least every 3 years postpartum. Birth defects are more common in diabetic patients. In mild diabetes, the increased blood glucose level crosses the placenta and raises the blood glucose and insulin levels in the fetus, resulting in large babies.

 A. Risk factors. Women at increased risk of gestational diabetes include those older than 30 years of age, those who have a family history of diabetes, or those who have had a very large (over 9 1/2-lb) baby or a stillborn.

 B. Preconception. For diabetic women planning to conceive, regimens should be switched to insulin with the goal of achieving a normal hemoglobin A_{1c} for 1–2 months before conception. Women with pre-existing diabetes who take oral medications to control their blood glucose levels need to switch to insulin before conceiving and during pregnancy, as the oral medications may pose a risk of birth defects.

 C. Treatment. Insulin is the treatment of choice when needed. Metformin and acarbose are category B. Hemoglobin A_{1c} should be checked before conception and during the first trimester. The rate of malformation is approximately 22% for hemoglobin A_{1c} of greater than 8.5. Ophthalmology evaluation should be encouraged during the first and third trimesters.

IV. Thromboembolic disease. Prophylactic therapy should be initiated in women with a history of thromboembolism during a previous pregnancy or while using hormonal contraception. Prophylaxis and treatment center around heparin and low-molecular-weight heparins, neither of which cross the placenta. Acute events should be treated with intravenous heparin followed by subcutaneous dosing. Enoxaparin has been used at doses of 1 mg/kg bid for acute events and 40 mg qd for prophylaxis. Warfarin therapy is contraindicated during the antepartum period but is appropriate for postpartum women who require continued anticoagulation.

V. Analgesics should be used with some caution as some medications may not be acceptable for use during different trimesters. Full-strength aspirin is considered category D, but baby aspirin is category A. Indomethacin use is acceptable during the first trimester (category A) but should be avoided during the second and third trimesters. Ibuprofen and other NSAIDs are category C and should be avoided if possible. Acetaminophen is relatively safe for use as it is category B. Codeine and oxycodone are Category A and safe to use; however, they should be used cautiously before delivery because of neonatal depression. Meperidine use is similar to that of codeine except for its relative safety during the first trimester.

VI. Gastroenterology. Antacids, milk of magnesia, and psyllium are category A and safe to use. Docusate is category B. Loperamide and lactulose may also be used. Ranitidine is the only H_2-blocker that is category A and safe to use.

Cimetidine, famotidine, and nizatidine are category C. The proton-pump inhibitors omeprazole (Prilosec) and lansoprazole (Prevacid) are category C. Misoprostol (Cytotec) should be avoided. Metoclopramide (Reglan) is category C. The antiemetic drug prochlorperazine is used with relative safety.

VII. Allergic rhinitis. Immunotherapy, intranasal cromolyn, and intranasal steroids should be considered first-line agents for therapy. First-generation antihistamines are preferred over second-generation agents, although neither has been identified as a human teratogen. Loratadine and cetirizine are considered pregnancy category B, and fexofenadine is category C. Antihistamines should be used cautiously as they can precipitate a withdrawal syndrome in the neonate if use is constant during pregnancy. Oral decongestants are pregnancy category C and should be used for short-term, acute relief only. Intranasal/ophthalmic decongestants, ophthalmic antihistamines, and inhaled/intranasal corticosteroids are all pregnancy category C. Mast cell stabilizers are category B.

VIII. Epilepsy. Although most anticonvulsants are teratogenic, careful preconception and prenatal management allow women with epilepsy to have at least a 90% chance of having a healthy baby (*Ann Pharmacother* 1998;32:794–801). Because the risk of major malformations increases with the number of anticonvulsants used together, the regimen should be streamlined as much as possible; monotherapy with an agent that best controls epileptic episodes in the mother is encouraged. Ideally, the changes should be made before conception to taper to the lowest effective dose. Consideration should be given to gradual withdrawal of medications (with the goal of eliminating all anticonvulsants during pregnancy) for those patients with no seizure activity for several years. Increased doses of medications may be needed during pregnancy to compensate for the increased estrogen levels (may decrease seizure threshold) or increased drug clearance and plasma volume. Folic acid supplementation (4 mg/day) should begin several months prior to conception as neural tube defects are associated with carbamazepine and valproic acid.

IX. Antibiotics (Table A-1)

A. Pneumonia. Penicillins, cephalosporins, erythromycin, and azithromycin are the drugs of choice for covering community-acquired pneumonias in pregnancy, of which *Streptococcus pneumoniae* is the most common organism. Amantadine and ribavirin are both used for treatment of influenza in pregnancy. Varicella should be treated with acyclovir. Trimethoprim-sulfamethoxazole is the treatment of choice for *Pneumocystis carinii* pneumonia (PCP) in pregnancy. Its use increases the risk of neonatal kernicterus; however, the overall consequences of PCP outweigh the risk to the neonate.

The **influenza vaccine** should be given to pregnant women who are at high risk during the second or third trimesters of pregnancy. **Pneumococcal vaccines** can be given as well. **Varicella, measles, mumps, and rubella vaccines** should **not** be given to pregnant women. However, varicella immunoglobulin can be given within 72–96 hours of exposure to varicella. **PCP prophylaxis** with trimethoprim-sulfamethoxazole should be given, and continued into the third trimester, to pregnant women who are HIV positive.

B. Urinary tract infections. All pregnant women should be screened during the first trimester with routine urinalysis and culture if indicated. Acceptable antimicrobial agents include ampicillin, cephalosporins, gentamicin, and sulfonamides. Of note sulfonamides should be used in the first and second trimester. Trimethoprim should be avoided in the first trimester due to its mechanism of folate antagonism. Women with pyelonephritis should be hospitalized and treated with IV antibiotics until they have been afebrile for 48 hours.

C. Tuberculosis. Women should undergo screening with a PPD following the same guidelines as used with nonpregnant individuals. A positive reaction should be followed by a chest x-ray, shielding the uterus. Active tuberculosis during pregnancy should be treated with a three-drug regimen of isoniazid, rifampin, ethambutol, and supplemental pyridoxine. Few data are

Table A-1. Antibiotics: U.S. Food and Drug Administration Pregnancy Categories (modified)

A	B	C	D	X
No antibiotics listed	Penicillins (all)[a,m]	Clarithromycin[c,m]	Fluoroquinolones[g]	Erythromycin estolate[b]
	Penicillin plus beta-lactamase inhibitors[m]	Gentamicin[d]	Tetracyclines[j]	Streptomycin
		Imipenem		Pyrazinamide
	Cephalosporins (all)[m]	Vancomycin[e]		Ethionamide
		Trimethoprim[i]		Cycloserine
	Erythromycin[b,m]	Nitrofurantoin[m]		
	Azithromycin[m]	Isoniazid[k]		
	Clindamycin	Rifampin		
	Spectinomycin	Zidovudine		
	Aztreonam	Chloramphenicol[l]		
	Metronidazole[f]	Acyclovir[m]		
	Sulfonamides[h]			
	Ethambutol			

[a]Considered "safest" antibiotics to use during pregnancy.

[b]Drug of choice for infections with *Legionella*, *Mycoplasma*, and *Chlamydia* in pregnancy. The estolate formulation is contraindicated due to the risk of hepatotoxicity in the fetus.

[c]For treatment and prophylaxis of *Mycobacterium avium* complex in women who are HIV positive.

[d]Given with ampicillin for spontaneous bacterial endocarditis prophylaxis, chorioamnionitis, or pyelonephritis. Given in combination with clindamycin to treat mixed aerobic and anaerobic pelvic infections.

[e]Drug of choice for *Clostridium difficile* and methicillin-resistant *Staphylococcus aureus* and *Enterococcus* in penicillin-allergic patients.

[f]Second and third trimesters only. Use with caution in lactation (mutagenic and carcinogenic effects in some species).

[g]Cause irreversible arthropathy in immature animals.

[h]May cause neonatal hyperbilirubinemia with kernicterus or hemolytic anemia in fetus born to glucose-6-phosphate dehydrogenase–deficient mother.

[i]May be indicated for *Pneumocystis carinii* pneumonia prophylaxis in HIV-positive pregnant women.

[j]Cause decidual teeth discoloration. Not recommended during lactation (bone and teeth deposition).

[k]Not recommended during lactation (hepatotoxicity).

[l]May cause vascular collapse in second and third trimester. Not recommended during lactation (gray baby syndrome).

[m]Compatible with lactation.

available on the teratogenicity of pyrazinamide; therefore, its use is generally not recommended.

D. Sexually transmitted diseases. All pregnant women should be screened at the initial prenatal visit, with repeat screening of women at high risk in the third trimester. Refer to Table A-2 for specific therapeutic regimens.

E. Treatment of HIV. Limited data suggest that pregnancy does not accelerate the course of HIV disease. All pregnant women with HIV infection should be offered zidovudine after the fourteenth week of gestation to decrease the perinatal transmission rate. Initiation of antiretroviral therapy should follow the guidelines outlined for nonpregnant patients except that medication should be started after the first trimester. The same applies to prophylactic regimens.

Table A-2. Treatment of sexually transmitted diseases

Disease	Treatment
Chlamydia	Azithromycin, 1 g PO × one dose
	Erythromycin base, 500 mg PO qid × 7 days
	Erythromycin ethylsuccinate, 800 mg PO qid × 7 days
	Amoxicillin, 500 mg PO tid × 7 days[a]
Gonorrhea	Ceftriaxone, 125 mg or 250 mg IM × one dose
	Cefixime, 400 mg PO × one dose
	Spectinomycin, 2 g IM × one dose
Syphilis	
Primary, secondary, or early latent disease of less than 1 yr's duration	Benzathine penicillin G, 2.4 million units IM × one dose
Late latent or disease of unknown duration	Benzathine penicillin G, 2.4 million units IM weekly for 3 wks
Neurosyphilis	Aqueous penicillin G, 2–4 million units IV every 4 hrs for 10–14 days
Concomitant HIV infection	Aqueous penicillin G, 2.4 million units IM weekly for 3 wks
Herpes simplex virus	
Uncomplicated	Not recommended due to safety concerns about acyclovir
Severe or life-threatening disease	Acyclovir, 200 mg PO five times a day × 7–10 days or 400 mg PO tid × 5–7 days
Suppressive therapy	Acyclovir, 400 mg PO bid[b]
Trichomonas vaginitis	Metronidazole, 2 g PO × one dose or 500 mg bid × 7 days
Bacterial vaginosis	Metronidazole 0.75% gel, one applicatorful intravaginally once/day × 5 days
	Clindamycin 2% cream, one applicatorful intravaginally once/day × 5 days
	Metronidazole, 500 mg PO bid × 7 days
	Clindamycin, 300 mg PO bid × 7 days
Hepatitis B	
Sexual exposure	Hepatitis B immune globulin within 14 days of exposure, 0.06 ml/kg IM
Other routes of exposure	Two doses of immune globulin at monthly intervals followed by vaccination with either Recombivax HB, 10 μg at 0, 1, and 6 mos; or Energix-B, 20 μg IM at 0, 1, 2, and 12 mos

[a]Repeat test in 3 wks to verify eradication.
[b]Valacyclovir and famciclovir are pregnancy category B but are not approved for recurrent outbreaks in pregnant women.

F. HIV-positive women should be **screened** for tuberculosis, hepatitis, and sexually transmitted diseases. Papanicolaou smears should be done and repeated as necessary because of the high incidence of abnormality in this population.

X. Medications and lactation. In general, most medications are compatible with breast-feeding. It is important to choose drugs that appear in small amounts in the breast milk and avoid drugs that are long acting to decrease risk of accumulation in the child. If possible, schedule maternal administration so that the least amount of medication possible is in the milk at the time of nursing. Observe the child for changes in feeding, sleep, and wake patterns.

References

Brown HL, Bobrowski R. Anticoagulation. *Clin Obstet Gynecol* 1998;41(3):545–554.

Dashe JS, Gilstrap LC. Antibiotic use in pregnancy. *Obstet Gynecol Clin North Am* 1997;24(3):617–629.

Eplin MS, Clark SL. Outpatient management of asthma during pregnancy. *Clin Obstet Gynecol* 1998;41(3):555–563.

Jackson SL, Soper DE. Sexually transmitted diseases in pregnancy. *Obstet Gynecol Clin North Am* 1997;24(3):631–643.

Magee LA, Ornstein MP, von Dadelszen P. Fortnightly review: management of hypertension in pregnancy. *BMJ* 1999;318(7194):1332–1336.

Mason E, Rosene-Montella K, Powrie R. Medical problems during pregnancy. *Med Clin North Am* 1998;82(2):249–269.

Mazzotta P, Loebstein R, Koren G. Treating allergic rhinitis in pregnancy. Safety considerations. *Drug Safety* 1999;20(4):361–375.

Perloff D. Hypertension and pregnancy–related hypertension. *Cardiol Clin* 1998;16(1):79–101.

Riley LE. Pneumonia, tuberculosis, and urinary tract infections in pregnancy. *Curr Clin Top Infect Dis* 1999;19:181–197.

Witlin AG, Sibai BM. Hypertension. *Clin Obstet Gynecol* 1998;41(3):533–544.

Working group report on high blood pressure in pregnancy. NIH Publication No. 00-3029. Bethesda, MD: NIH, 1990, 2000 (revised).

Yankowitz J, Niebyl JR. *Drug Therapy in Pregnancy* (3rd ed). Baltimore: Lippincott Williams & Wilkins, 2001.

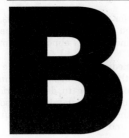

B Drugs and Renal Failure

Way Y. Huey
and Daniel W. Coyne

Medication	Route	Adjusted dosing interval (hrs) or % dose >50 GFR (ml/min)	10–50 GFR (ml/min)	<10 GFR (ml/min)	Supplement dose after specific dialysis
Analgesics—nonnarcotic					
Acetaminophen	H	4	6	8	HD
Aspirin	H, R	4	4–6	A	HD
Celecoxib	H	N	N	N	N
Diclofenac	H	N	N	N	N
Ibuprofen	H	N	N	N	N
Indomethacin	H, R	N	N	N	N
Ketoprofen	H	N	N	N	N
Ketorolac (IM)	H, R	N	N	50%	N
Nabumetone	H	N	N	N	N
Naproxen	H	N	N	N	N
Oxaprozin	H	N	N	N	N
Piroxicam	H	N	N	N	N
Rofecoxib	H	N	N	N	N
Sulindac	H, R	N	N	50%	N
Tramadol	H, R	N	12	12	N
Analgesics—opioid					
Codeine	H	N	75%	50%	N
Meperidine	H	N	75%	50%	N
Morphine	H	N	75%	50%	N
Antiarrhythmics					
Amiodarone	H	N	N	N	N
Bretylium	R, H	N	25–50%	A	?
Digoxin*	R	24	36	48	N
Disopyramide*	R, H	75%	15–50%	10–25%	HD
Flecainide*	R, H	N	50%	50%	N
Lidocaine*	H, R	N	N	N	N
Mexiletine	H, R	N	N	50–75%	HD
Moricizine	H	N	N	50–75%	N

Medication	Route	Adjusted dosing interval (hrs) or % dose			Supplement dose after specific dialysis
		>50 GFR (ml/min)	10–50 GFR (ml/min)	<10 GFR (ml/min)	
Procainamide*	R, H	4	6–12	12–24	HD
Propafenone	H	N	N	50–75%	N
Quinidine*	H, R	N	N	N	HD, PD
Sotalol	R	N	30%	15%	N
Tocainide*	R, H	N	N	50%	HD
Antibiotic drugs					
Aminoglycosides					
Amikacin*	R	8–12	12	>24	HD, PD
Gentamicin*	R	8–12	12	>24	HD, PD
Tobramycin*	R	8–12	12	>24	HD, PD
Antimycobacterial drugs					
Clofazimine	H	N	N	N	N
Cycloserine	R	12	12–24	24	N
Ethambutol	R	24	24–36	48	HD, PD
Ethionamide	H	N	N	50%	N
Isoniazid	H, R	N	N	N	HD, PD
Pyrazinamide	H, R	N	N	50%	HD, PD
Rifabutin	H	N	N	N	N
Rifampin	H	N	N	N	?
Cephalosporins					
Cefadroxil	R	12	12–24	24–48	HD
Cefazolin	R	8	12	24–48	HD
Cefdinir	R	12	24	48	HD
Cefepime	R	12	16–24	24–48	HD
Cefixime	R	12–24	75%	50%	N
Cefonicid	R	N	50%	25%	N
Cefoperazone	H	N	N	N	N
Cefotaxime	R, H	6–8	8–12	24	HD
Cefotetan	R	12	24	24	HD, PD
Cefoxitin	R	8	8–12	24–48	HD
Cefpodoxime	R	12	16	24–48	HD
Cefprozil	R	12	16	24	HD
Ceftazidime	R	8–12	24–48	48	HD
Ceftibuten	R	24	50%	25%	HD
Ceftizoxime	R	8–12	12–24	24	HD
Ceftriaxone	R, H	N	N	24	N
Cefuroxime	R	8	8–12	24	HD
Cephalexin	R	8	12	12	HD, PD
Cephalothin	R	6	6–8	12	HD, PD

| Medication | Route | Adjusted dosing interval (hrs) or % dose | | | Supplement dose after specific dialysis |
		>50 GFR (ml/min)	10–50 GFR (ml/min)	<10 GFR (ml/min)	
Cephradine	R	6	50% q6h	25% q6h	HD, PD
Loracarbef	R	12	50%	3–5 days	HD
Penicillins					
Amoxicillin/ clavulanate	R, H	8	8–12	12–24	HD
Ampicillin	R, H	6	6–12	12–24	HD
Ampicillin/ sulbactam	R, H	6–8	12	24	HD
Carbenicillin	R, H	8–12	12–24	24–48	HD, PD
Dicloxacillin	R, H	N	N	N	N
Mezlocillin	R, H	4–6	6–8	8–12	HD
Oxacillin	R, H	N	N	N	N
Penicillin G	R, H	N	75%	25–50%	HD
Piperacillin	R	4–6	6–8	12	HD
Piperacillin/ tazobactam	R, H	6	8	12	HD
Ticarcillin	R	8	8–12	24	HD
Ticarcillin/ clavulanate	R, H	3.1 g q4– 6h	2g q6–8h	2g q12h	HD
Quinolones					
Ciprofloxacin	R	N	12–24	24	N
Enoxacin	R	N	50%	50% q24h	N
Gatifloxacin	R	N	50%	50%	HD, PD
Levofloxacin	R	8–12	24	48	N
Lomefloxacin	R	N	75%	50%	N
Moxifloxacin	H	N	N	N	N
Norfloxacin	R	N	12–24	A	N
Ofloxacin	R	N	12–24	24	N
Other antibacterial drugs					
Azithromycin	H	N	N	N	N
Aztreonam	R	N	50–75%	25%	HD, PD
Chloramphenicol	R, H	N	N	N	N
Clarithromycin	R, H	N	75%	50%	N
Clindamycin	H	N	N	N	N
Dirithromycin	H	N	N	N	N
Doxycycline	R, H	12	12–18	18–24	N
Erythromycin	H	N	N	N	N
Imipenem	R	N	50%	25%	HD
Meropenem	R	N	50% q12h	50% q24h	HD
Metronidazole	R, H	N	N	50%	HD

Medication	Route	>50 GFR (ml/min)	10–50 GFR (ml/min)	<10 GFR (ml/min)	Supplement dose after specific dialysis
Pentamidine	?	N	N	24–48	N
Quinupristin/ dalfopristin	H	N	N	N	N
Sulfamethoxazole	R, H	12	18	24	HD
Tetracycline	R, H	12	12–18	18–24	N
Trimethoprim	R, H	12	18	24	HD
Vancomycin* (IV)	R	6–12	24–48	48–96	N
Antifungal drugs					
Amphotericin B	N	24	24	24–36	N
Fluconazole	R, H	N	50%	25%	HD
Flucytosine	R	6	24	24–48	HD, PD
Itraconazole	H, R	N	N	50%	N
Ketoconazole	H	N	N	N	N
Miconazole	H	N	N	N	N
Terbinafine	R, H	N	?	?	?
Antiviral drugs					
Abacavir	H	N	N	N	?
Acyclovir (IV)	R	6	24	48	HD
Acyclovir (PO)	R	N	12–24	24	HD
Amantadine	R	12–24	24–72	72–168	N
Amprenavir	H	N	N	N	?
Cidofovir	R	N	A	A	?
Delavirdine	H	N	?	?	?
Didanosine	R	12	24	48	N
Efavirenz	H	N	N	N	?
Famciclovir	R	8	12–24	48	HD
Foscarnet	R	25 mg/kg q8h	15 mg/kg q8h	6 mg/kg q8h	HD
Ganciclovir	R	12	24	24	HD
Indinavir	H, R	8	?	?	?
Lamivudine	R	12	24	33% q24h	?
Nelfinavir	H	N	N	N	?
Nevirapine	H	N	?	?	?
Rimantadine	H	N	N	50%	?
Ritonavir	H	N	N	N	?
Saquinavir	H	N	N	N	?
Stavudine	H, R	N	50% q12–24h	?	?
Valacyclovir	R	8	12–24	50% q24h	HD
Zalcitabine	R	8	12	24	?
Zidovudine	H	N	N	N	HD

Medication	Route	>50 GFR (ml/min)	10–50 GFR (ml/min)	<10 GFR (ml/min)	Supplement dose after specific dialysis
Anticoagulants					
Antithrombin agents					
Argatroban	H	N	N	N	?
Dalteparin	R	N	?	?	N
Enoxaparin	R	N	?	?	N
Heparin	H	N	N	N	N
Lepirudin	R	N	15–50%	A	?
Warfarin	H	N	N	N	N
Platelet glycoprotein IIb/IIIa–receptor antagonists					
Abciximab	—	N	N	N	N
Eptifibatide	R	N	50%	A	A
Tirofiban	R	N	50% if CrCl <30	50%	N
Cardiovascular agents					
Angiotensin-converting enzyme inhibitors					
Benazepril	H, R	N	75%	50%	N
Captopril	R, H	N	N	50%	HD
Enalapril	R	N	75%	50%	HD
Fosinopril	H	N	N	N	N
Lisinopril	R	N	50%	25%	HD
Moexipril	R, H	N	50%	50%	?
Quinapril	H, R	N	75%	50%	N
Ramipril	R, H	N	50%	50%	HD
Trandolapril	R, H	N	25–50%	A	N
Angiotensin II–receptor antagonists					
Candesartan	GI	M	50%	50%	N
Irbesartan	H	N	N	N	N
Losartan	H	N	N	N	N
Telmisartan	H	N	N	?	N
Valsartan	R	H	N	N	?
β-Adrenergic antagonists					
Acebutolol	R, H	N	50%	25%	N
Atenolol	R	N	50%	25%	HD
Betaxolol	H, R	N	N	50%	N
Bisoprolol	H, R	N	50%	25%	N
Carteolol	R	24	48	72	?
Carvedilol	H	N	N	N	N
Labetalol	H	N	N	N	N
Metoprolol	H	N	N	N	HD
Nadolol	R	N	50%	25%	HD

Medication	Route	>50 GFR (ml/min)	10–50 GFR (ml/min)	<10 GFR (ml/min)	Supplement dose after specific dialysis
Penbutolol	H	N	N	N	N
Pindolol	H, R	N	N	N	?
Propranolol	H	N	N	N	N
Sotalol	R	N	24–48	?	?
Timolol	H	N	N	N	N
Calcium channel antagonists					
Amlodipine	H	N	N	N	N
Diltiazem	H	N	N	N	N
Felodipine	H	N	N	N	N
Isradipine	H	N	N	N	N
Nicardipine	H	N	N	N	N
Nifedipine	H	N	N	N	N
Verapamil	H	N	N	50–75%	N
Diuretics					
Acetazolamide	R	6	12	A	—
Bumetanide	R, H	N	N	N	—
Furosemide	R	N	N	N	—
Indapamide	H	N	N	N	—
Metolazone	R	N	N	N	—
Spironolactone	R	6–12	12–24	A	—
Thiazide	R	N	N	A	—
Torsemide	H, R	N	N	N	—
Other antihypertensives					
Clonidine	R	N	N	N	N
Doxazosin	H	N	N	N	N
Hydralazine (PO)	H	8	8	8–16	N
Methyldopa	R, H	8	8–12	12–24	HD, PD
Minoxidil	H	N	N	N	HD
Nitroprusside	N	N	N	N	N
Prazosin	H, R	N	N	N	N
Terazosin	R	N	N	N	N
CNS agents					
Antidepressants					
Amitriptyline	H	N	N	N	N
Doxepin	H	N	N	N	N
Fluoxetine	H	N	N	N	N
Imipramine	H	N	N	N	N
Nortriptyline	H	N	N	N	N
Paroxetine	H	N	N	N	N
Sertraline	H	N	N	N	N

Adjusted dosing interval (hrs) or % dose

| Medication | Route | Adjusted dosing interval (hrs) or % dose | | | Supplement dose after specific dialysis |
		>50 GFR (ml/min)	10–50 GFR (ml/min)	<10 GFR (ml/min)	
Trazodone	H	N	N	N	N
Venlafaxine	H	N	75%	50%	N
Anticonvulsants					
Carbamazepine*	H, R	N	N	75%	N
Ethosuximide*	H, R	N	N	75%	HD
Phenobarbital*	H, R	N	N	12–16	HD, PD
Phenytoin*	H	N	N	N	N
Primidone*	H, R	8	8–12	12–24	HD
Valproic acid*	H	N	N	75%	N
Sedatives					
Alprazolam	H	N	N	N	N
Chlordiazepoxide	H	N	N	50%	N
Diazepam	H	N	N	N	N
Flurazepam	H	N	N	N	N
Lorazepam	H	N	N	N	N
Midazolam	H	N	N	50%	N
Temazepam	H	N	N	N	N
Zolpidem	H	N	?	?	N
Other psychoactive drugs					
Buspirone	H, R	N	N	25–50%	HD
Chlorpromazine	H	N	N	N	N
Haloperidol	H	N	N	N	N
Lithium*	R	N	50–75%	25–50%	HD, PD
Others					
Antidiabetic drugs					
Acarbose	GI	N	A	A	N
Acetohexamide	H	12–24	A	A	N
Chlorpropamide	?	24–36	A	A	N
Glimepiride	H, R	N	N	N	N
Glipizide	H, R	N	N	N	N
Glyburide	H, R	N	A	A	N
Metformin	R	A	A	A	N
Pioglitazone	H	N	N	N	N
Repaglinide	H	N	N	?	?
Rosiglitazone	H	N	N	N	N
Tolazamide	H	N	N	N	N
Tolbutamide	H	N	N	N	N
Antihistamines					
Azatadine	H	N	N	N	N

Medication	Route	>50 GFR (ml/min)	10–50 GFR (ml/min)	<10 GFR (ml/min)	Supplement dose after specific dialysis
Cetirizine	H, R	N	50%	50%	?
Fexofenadine	H, R	N	24	24	?
Loratadine	H	N	48	48	N
Antilipemic drugs					
Cholestyramine	N	N	N	N	N
Clofibrate	H	6–12	12–24	24–48	N
Fluvastatin	H	N	N	?	N
Gemfibrozil	R, H	N	50%	25%	N
Lovastatin	H	N	N	N	N
Pravastatin	R, H	N	N	50%	N
Simvastatin	H	N	N	50%	N
GI drugs					
Cimetidine	R	6	8	12	N
Famotidine	R, H	N	N	50%	?
Mesalamine	H	N	N	?	N
Metoclopramide	R, H	N	75%	50%	N
Misoprostol	R	N	N	N	N
Nizatidine	H	N	24	48	N
Omeprazole	H	N	N	N	?
Ranitidine	R	N	18–24	24	HD
Other drugs					
Alendronate	R	N	A	A	?
Allopurinol	R	N	50%	10–25%	?
Colchicine (PO)	R, H	N	N	50%	N
Dipyridamole	H	N	N	N	?
Etidronate	R	N	A	A	?
Finasteride	H, R	N	N	N	N
Glucocorticoids	H	N	N	N	N
Nitrates	H	N	N	N	N
Pentoxifylline	H	N	N	N	N
Risedronate	R	N	A	A	?
Terbutaline	H, R	N	50%	A	?
Theophylline	H	N	N	N	HD, PD
Ticlopidine	H	N	N	N	?
Tiludronate	R	N	A	A	?

Heading: Adjusted dosing interval (hrs) or % dose

A, avoid use; CrCl, creatinine clearance; GFR, glomerular filtration rate; H, hepatic; HD, hemodialysis; N, none; PD, peritoneal dialysis; R, renal; %, percentage of normal dose; ?, no data.
*Serum levels should be used to determine exact dosing.
Source: G Aronoff, W Bennett, J Berns, et al. *Drug Prescribing in Renal Failure: Dosing Guidelines for Adults* (4th ed). Philadelphia: American College of Physicians, 1999; CR Gelman, BH Rumack, AJ Hess (eds), *Drugdex System.* Englewood, CO: Micromedex, Inc, 1999; and GK McEvoy (ed), *American Hospital Formulary Service Drug Information.* Bethesda, MD: American Society of Health-System Pharmacists, 2000.

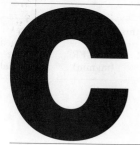

Simplified
Screening
Schedule

Megan E. Wren and
Mary V. Mason

This table is based on widely accepted recommendations from major organizations; other expert groups recommend alternative schedules with less frequent screening (see text references for details). These are general guidelines that apply only to **asymptomatic** individuals at **average risk** for the disease; individuals with risk factors may need more aggressive screening. Screening in the elderly should be an individualized decision based on patient preference, estimated life expectancy, and comorbid conditions.

Target condition	See text	Source	Screening recommendations			
			Ages 20–39 yrs	Ages 40–49 yrs	Ages 50+ yrs	
Breast cancer	Chap. 24	ACS	Self-breast exam q1 mo; clinical breast exam q3 yrs	Self-breast exam q1 mo; clinical breast exam q1 yr; mammography q1 yr	Self-breast exam q1 mo; clinical breast exam q1 yr; mammography q1 yr	
		USPSTF	—	—	Age 50–69: mammography q1–2 yrs ± clinical breast exam	
Colorectal cancer	Chap. 13, 14	ACS	—	—	FOBT q1 yr and/or flex sig q5 yrs or DCBE q5 yrs or colonoscopy q10 yrs	
		USPSTF	—	—	Offer FOBT q1 yr or flex sig (frequency unspecified)	
Skin cancer	Chap. 26	ACS	Skin exam q3 yrs	Skin exam q1 yr	Skin exam q1 yr	
		USPSTF	Insufficient evidence to recommend for or against screening			
Prostate cancer	Chap. 25	ACS	—	Age 45+ yrs in African-Americans or +FHx: "offer" PSA and DRE q1 yr	"Offer" PSA and DRE q1 yr	
		USPSTF	Routine screening not recommended			
Cervical cancer[a]	Chap. 24	ACS	Pap q1 yr; if 3 normal, frequency can be decreased "at physician's discretion"			
		ACP	Pap q1–3 yrs; annually if sexually active or on oral contraceptives			
		USPSTF	Pap at least q3 yrs			
Testicular cancer	Chap. 25	ACS	Testicular exam q3 yrs	Testicular exam q1 yr	Testicular exam q1 yr	
		USPSTF	Insufficient evidence to recommend for or against screening			

(continued)

Screening recommendations

Target condition	See text	Source	Ages 20–39 yrs	Ages 40–49 yrs	Ages 50+ yrs
Ovarian cancer	Chap. 24	ACS	Pelvic exam q3 yrs	Pelvic exam q1 yr	Pelvic exam q1 yr
		USPSTF	Insufficient evidence to recommend for or against screening		
Lung cancer	Chap. 10		General screening not currently recommended		
Hypertension	Chap. 4	JNC VI	Measure BP q1–2 yrs		
Hyperlipidemia	Chap. 5	NCEP		Fasting lipid profile q5 yrs	

ACP, American College of Physicians (http://www.acponline.org/sci-policy/guidelines/); ACS, American Cancer Society (www.cancer.org); ADA, American Diabetes Association (www.diabetes.org); DCBE, double-contrast barium enema; DM, diabetes mellitus; DRE, digital rectal examination; FBS, fasting blood sugar; FHx, family history; flex sig, flexible sigmoidoscopy; FOBT, fecal occult blood testing; JNC VI, Joint National Committee on Prevention, Detection, Evaluation, and Treatment of High Blood Pressure, 6th Report (http://www.nhlbi.nih.gov/guidelines/hypertension/jncintro.htm); NCEP National Cholesterol Education Program (http://www.lipidhealth.org/ or http://www.nhlbi.nih.gov/guidelines/cholesterol/index.htm); Pap, Papanicolaou's test; PSA, prostate-specific antigen; USPSTF, U.S. Preventive Services Task Force (http://odphp.osophs.dhhs.gov/pubs/guidecps/).

Individualized screening can be considered for patients with risk factors for the following conditions or symptoms:

DM (see Chap. 18): FBS q3 yrs in high-risk patients (overweight: body mass index >27 kg/m^2), age older than 45 yrs, impaired glucose tolerance, history of gestational DM or delivery of babies weighing more than 9 lb, family history of DM, and patients of certain ethnic groups (e.g., African-Americans, Hispanic-Americans, Native Americans, Asian-Americans, Pacific Islanders)

Thyroid disease (see Chap. 17): Consider thyroid-stimulating hormone in older women, especially if subtle symptoms of thyroid disease exhibited

Osteoporosis (see Chap. 24): Risk groups include women who are Caucasian or Asian-American, or have low body weight, or who have had a bilateral oophorectomy before menopause

Visual acuity (see Chap. 27): In the elderly

Glaucoma screening (see Chap. 18): In African-Americans age older than 40+ yrs, Caucasians age 65+ yrs, those with diabetes, severe myopia, or +FHx glaucoma
[a]No testing required for patients who have had a hysterectomy in which the cervix was removed, unless the hysterectomy was performed for cancer.

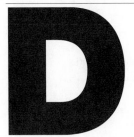

Reportable Diseases

American College of
Preventive Medicine

I. Surveillance

A. Reporting. Clinicians are required to report cases (and suspected cases) of selected diseases and conditions to their local, county, or state public health department to aid in disease surveillance efforts at the local, state, and national levels. State health officials, the Centers for Disease Control and Prevention (CDC), and the Council of State and Territorial Epidemiologists (CSTE) develop a list of recommended diseases and conditions for national surveillance. States and territories have varied reporting requirements [*JAMA* 1999;282(2):164–170].

B. Benefits. The information gathered from disease surveillance helps to protect the health of patients and communities in many ways. Major benefits include (1) prompting interventions to prevent further disease transmission (or to reduce the morbidity or mortality associated with the condition) when cases or clusters of cases are identified; (2) assessing the health impacts of events, habits, or patient characteristics; (3) monitoring the effectiveness of disease prevention and control interventions; (4) identifying population groups or geographic areas at high risk for disease; and (5) contributing to the development of hypotheses and studies about risk factors for disease causation, propagation, or progression [*J Public Health Manag Pract* 1996;2(4):16–23].

II. Diseases

A. According to a CSTE survey, the 35 diseases and conditions listed in Table D-1 were reportable (mostly by clinicians, some by clinical laboratories) in at least 90% of U.S. states and territories in January 2001.

B. In 2000, the 28 additional diseases and conditions listed in Table D-2 were recommended by the CSTE and the CDC for national surveillance.

C. A full listing of state and territorial disease **reporting requirements** is available on the Internet at http://www.cste.org/Surveys/NNDSSQ9.htm and http://www.cste.org/Surveys/NNDSSQ10.htm; however, public health reporting requirements change often. For the most up-to-date reporting requirements in their area, clinicians should contact their public health department.

Table D-1. Reportable diseases and conditions, 2001

AIDS	Cholera
Anthrax	Cryptosporidiosis
Botulism	Diphtheria
Brucellosis	*Escherichia coli* O157:H7
Campylobacteriosis	Gonorrhea
Chlamydia trachomatis	*Haemophilus influenzae*, invasive

(continued)

Table D-1. (continued)

Hepatitis A	Plague
Hepatitis B	Poliomyelitis, paralytic
Hepatitis C	Rabies, human
HIV infection, adult (≥13 yrs)	Rubella
HIV infection, pediatric (≤13 yrs)	Salmonellosis
Legionellosis	Shigellosis
Lyme disease	Syphilis
Malaria	Tetanus
Measles/rubeola	Trichinosis
Meningococcal disease	Tuberculosis
Mumps	Typhoid fever
Pertussis	

Table D-2. Diseases and conditions recommended for national surveillance, 2000

Chancroid	Hepatitis; non-A, non-B
Coccidioidomycosis	Listeriosis
Cyclosporiasis	Psittacosis
Ehrlichiosis, human granulocytic	Q fever
Ehrlichiosis, human monocytic	Rabies, animal
Encephalitis, California serogroup	Rocky Mountain spotted fever
Encephalitis, Eastern equine	Rubella, congenital syndrome
Encephalitis, St. Louis	Streptococcal pneumonia, drug resistant
Encephalitis, Western equine	Streptococcal toxic shock syndrome
Enterohemmorhagic *Escherichia coli* (EHEC)	Streptococcus, invasive, Group A
	Toxic shock syndrome
Hansen disease (leprosy)	Tularemia
Hantavirus pulmonary syndrome	Varicella (deaths only)
Hemolytic-uremic syndrome, post-diarrheal	Yellow fever

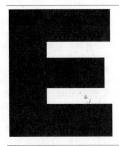

Impairment and Disability Evaluation

Bradley A. Evanoff and
H. Bryan Rogers

I. **Impairment and disability.** During their careers, most physicians are asked to evaluate a patient's ability to work following the onset of an injury or disease or for the purposes of job placement. Physicians may also serve as advocates for their patients who experience employment difficulties due to a physical impairment.

A. **Americans with Disabilities Act (ADA).** Physicians should be familiar with Title 1 of the ADA, which Congress passed in 1990. It is designed to protect individuals with disabilities against discrimination in the workplace. The ADA explicitly defines who is protected and what the employer or physician must do to ensure that an individual's rights are not violated. It defines a **disability** as "a physical, mental, or emotional impairment that substantially limits one or more major life activities." The act states that a qualified individual with a disability must be offered the same opportunities for employment or advancement as an individual without a disability if the person has "the skills, education, and overall qualifications needed to perform the essential job functions" as described by the employer.

B. **Accommodations.** Changes to company policies, procedures, and workplace design may be necessary to offer "reasonable accommodation" to an otherwise qualified individual who cannot perform some fundamental activities of the job due to a disability, unless these changes constitute an "undue hardship" to the employer. Physicians who advocate for their patients should be aware that the ADA considers scheduled time off for medical appointments, alterations to work schedules to accommodate side effects of medications, and purchasing or modifying equipment as forms of reasonable accommodation.

C. **ADA evaluations.** Pre-employment physicals are not permitted under the ADA, but employers may request "preplacement" examinations. A **preplacement examination** can be performed only after an applicant has been offered a position and only if the examination is required of all individuals in similar positions. The purpose of this evaluation is to determine if the employee is able to perform the essential functions of the position and if the applicant has a disability that creates substantial and immediate risk of harm to the applicant or to others in the context of a specific job. Before performing such an examination, the physician should have a job description that details the essential job functions and the work environment. If a disability is identified that prevents the individual from performing the essential job functions, the worker's functional limitations and capabilities should be clearly documented. The physician may also use this as an opportunity to make suggestions as to how the obstacles can be overcome. It is important to note that decisions regarding reasonable accommodation are ultimately the responsibility of the employer and not the physician. Under the ADA, only information about the disability that needs accommodation can be given to the employer; other medical information should not be released.

II. **Disability evaluations.** Physicians may be asked to evaluate disability for patients who are covered under a variety of social insurance programs, including Social Security, worker's compensation, other state and federal programs, or private disability insurance. Physicians may be asked to make determinations of **permanent** disability (when substantial recovery is not expected) or **temporary** disability (e.g., after a hospitalization or work injury when recovery is expected). When asked to do a disability evaluation, the physician must be careful to separate the concepts of impairment and disability.

A. **Impairment** is a loss or decrease in function of a body part or system due to injury or illness, whereas **disability** is the decreased ability to work or function in society that results from the impairment. Different people may have different degrees of disability that result from the same impairment (e.g., amputation of a thumb may be completely disabling for a surgeon but probably not so for a professional soccer player). Age, education, previous job experience, and other factors come into play in determining whether a given impairment is disabling.

B. **Disability definitions.** It is also important to note that different definitions of disability apply in different insurance systems. For purposes of temporary disability, the physician may need to determine when someone can return to his or her usual job. For permanent disability, the question may be whether the patient can return to his or her usual work (relevant with some private disability insurances) or to any gainful work. The Social Security Administration defines disability as "the inability to engage in any substantial gainful activity by reason of any medically determinable physical or mental impairment which can be expected to result in death or has lasted, or can be expected to last, for a continuous period of not less than 12 months." Physicians can readily determine impairment but cannot determine disability without detailed information about what definition of disability is used in a particular insurance or compensation scheme.

C. **Medical examination.** When composing a report for determination of permanent disability, the general outline is the same as for any complete medical evaluation.

1. The patient's **history** is obtained in the first person and is supplemented by medical records, which are generally provided in great quantity. This evaluation should also include social history, family history, and medical history—both pertinent to the current diagnosis for which disability is being sought and for other possible contributing medical diagnoses.

2. The **physical examination** is performed. According to the standards set forth by the requesting agency, the physician's opinion is rendered as to whether the individual is or is not disabled for his or her current employment or sometimes disabled in any way.

3. **Additional studies** are obtained as needed, but they often are not authorized in an unlimited fashion. The examiner must be dependent on evaluations performed in the past by treating physicians. Occasionally, these tests are remote enough in the past that the examiner needs to request further evaluation before he or she can formulate a detailed assessment and opinion regarding the disability status.

III. **Disability determination.** Determinations of permanent partial impairment or a disability rating for worker's compensation injuries must take into account subjective complaints and objective abnormalities. In the present era, settlements under worker's compensation law are usually made between the insurance carrier and the injured employee. If there is any disagreement, legal counsel is usually obtained and may involve additional medical opinions. Therefore, it is extremely important for the examining physician to document all of the subjective complaints, all of the objective abnormalities that are found, and correlate them with available studies and other available opinions. After this evaluation, the examining physician determines a disability rating expressed as a percentage of the body as a whole or a part thereof.

A. **Homunculus.** Determinations of permanent partial impairment are often done on the basis of a homunculus that usually differs from source to source and from state to state. The body is divided extremity by extremity and joint by joint, with a certain number of weeks of worker's compensation benefits being assigned to impairment at each level. In turn, a week of worker's compensation benefits are converted into dollar figures by the settling parties based on a level that is usually predetermined by the state legislature.

B. **Partial impairment.** The American Medical Association's *Guide for the Performance of Permanency Evaluations* is used by the majority of examiners and the majority of states as the basis for determining the percent of permanent partial impairment. Worker's compensation judges and commissions tend to look at three parameters; the physician should consider all of these in formulating a report: objective abnormalities, subjective complaints, and cosmetic results.

C. **Maximum medical improvement.** When an evaluation under worker's compensation law is requested, the physician is asked to determine if the patient has reached maximum medical improvement. The physician is then asked to render an opinion as to whether the patient has achieved as much recovery as can reasonably be expected and whether he or she is in stable condition with regard to the injury and the results of the treatment thereof.

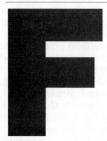

Internet Medicine and Useful Web Sites

Gregory J. Golladay and
Tammy L. Lin

I. Prevalence. The Internet is a growing source of medical information for patients and physicians. Thousands of medically oriented Web sites currently exist, and the number continues to grow. Approximately 50% of patients presenting to clinical encounters have Internet access and approximately 50% of patients with access to the Internet will have searched for medical information related to their presenting complaint. As information technology continues to advance, it promises to influence virtually every aspect of medical care.

II. Resources. A variety of Web resources are at the fingertip touch of a mouse:

   A. E-mail. Many physicians communicate with patients via electronic mail. E-mail can be useful to help clarify unanswered questions, alleviate minor concerns, convey test results, and follow up on previous discussions. It can help make the time between clinic visits and face-to-face time more productive.

   B. Mailing lists. Mailing lists are made up of subscribers who receive e-mail related to a common topic of interest.

   C. Medline, PubMed, Grateful Med, etc. A number of sites (sec. **V**) offer free access to these search tools for researching the most current literature on a given topic. This access is vital, given the increasing emphasis on practicing evidence-based medicine. **Medline Plus** offers information specifically designed for easy patient access (sec. **V**).

   D. Web sites. Web sites range from national and institutional sites, organizational and commercial sites, and personal Web pages. Many physicians and practices have Web sites to advertise their practices, share contact and referral information, and provide information on a wide array of clinical conditions.

   E. On-line journals. A growing number of printed journals are currently available on-line; many allow full-text articles to be downloaded and printed. A few exclusively electronic journals also exist.

   F. Telemedicine. A few resources exist for on-line consultation and case presentations. Some sites contain self-diagnosis and treatment algorithms for patients. As technology develops and computer access increases, this area promises to benefit underserved areas, foreign countries, and those with physical disabilities.

   G. Continuing medical education (CME). Some Web sites allow physicians and other health care professionals to obtain CME credit on-line, usually for a small fee.

   H. Patient resources. In addition to the sources listed above, patients may access support groups on-line or ask questions of expert physicians through chat rooms and dedicated patient Web sites. Many patients with common or rare illnesses find them helpful. Other resources and information about clinical trials are also available on-line.

   I. On-line pharmacies. Some Web sites offer on-line prescriptions for patients.

III. Problems. The rapid, relatively unregulated expansion of the Internet as a medical information resource has resulted in a number of real and theoretical concerns.

   A. Volume and variability. There are thousands of Web sites dedicated to medically related topics. Web page search matches to a single medical search term (on commonly used search engines) can range from just a few to tens of thousands. Medically oriented sites are growing in number, and the information contained within them is variable in quality and accuracy.

B. **Lack of peer review.** Approximately one-third of medical Web sites have no reference to peer review. Because search engines do not filter for peer review, patients have no way of knowing what information is credible, and it can be difficult even for a wary clinician to discern at times. Factually incorrect information may be present on non–peer reviewed sites at a rate of 6% or more [*Cancer* 1999;86(3):381–390].

C. **Identification of authorship.** Although many medically oriented Web sites attribute authorship, this is by no means uniform.

D. **Accessibility.** Accessing health information using search engines and simple search terms may not be efficient, and finding relevant content is often difficult. Other issues including literacy skills required to comprehend information and coverage of key information on foreign language sites are problematic as well [*JAMA* 2001;285(20):2612–2621].

E. **Financial interest.** Many Web sites have an entrepreneurial bent that is overt or may be subtle. Such financial interest is not subject to disclosure rules as is the case in printed journals.

F. **Dating.** The date of a Web site's posting and updating is typically found on the main Web page, but is not requisite. This makes currency a concern.

G. **Time, billing, documentation.** The growth of the Web as a medical information source takes time in the face-to-face clinical encounter and outside of it. The time taken to answer e-mail or to review Web-based information that a patient brings to the clinical setting has no fee code. Documentation in the medical record of the time taken to respond to electronic patient information requests and the content of such discussions is essential.

H. **Medicolegal.** Medical information dispersal, on-line prescription of medications, and on-line consulting raises issues of liability licensure that have not yet been well-defined. This is particularly concerning for those purchasing medications that may have devastating side effects in certain patient populations or when combined with other medications. Reported fatalities involving the on-line purchase of sildenafil and hydroxyzine underscore this point.

I. **Confidentiality.** Although there is increasing security on the Internet, many resources, such as e-mail, are not uniformly secure. Employers and internet service providers typically can access user e-mail easily. This makes patient confidentiality a concern, particularly when sensitive information (e.g., HIV status) is transmitted electronically. Most sites log user visits and many deposit "cookies" on the user's hard drive so that patterns of usage can be monitored. The shift toward electronic medical records and integration of available services raises concerns. Patient data on electronic medical records is more secure and usually encrypted, but security breaches can occur. Most sites contain a privacy statement on the home page.

J. **Physician insecurity and frustration.** When faced with increasingly informed patients, many physicians feel threatened or burdened by their patients' knowledge, sophistication, and questions. In addition, there is evidence suggesting that teleadvice may be excessively used by chronically ill or frustrated patients to seek information or express disappointment with prior care (*Arch Dermatol* 1999;135:151–156).

K. **Alternative medicine.** Many Web sites contain references to alternative medicine or are solely devoted to it. Patients who search the Internet for medical information may find a great deal of information regarding treatment options that may not coincide with traditional medicine or be harmful.

IV. **Solutions**

A. **Awareness.** Physicians and other health care providers need to be aware of the Internet as an information source for themselves and their patients. If deficient, physicians may seek computer literacy skills, and more emphasis should be placed on the early acquisition of these skills in training. The American Medical Association and other organizations have designed programs specifically geared toward physicians to meet this goal (http://www.ama-assn.org). Physicians should be proactive in the development of accurate, reliable health information on the Web, be prepared to engage patients in discussions regarding information they have gleaned from the Internet, and help guide patients to appropriate, credible, and accessible sites.

B. Quality control

   1. **Designation of authorship, attribution of references, disclosure of ownership and sponsorship, and date of posting or updating** should become more uniform in Web medical information (*JAMA* 1997;277:1244–1245).

   2. **Quality ratings and seals of approval.** Although Web sites have been developed to rate Internet medical information, the expanding, fluid nature of the Internet makes such ratings difficult at best (*JAMA* 1998;279:611–614).

C. Peer review. Peer review should be requisite when medical information is posted on the Web.

D. Partnership. In the age of electronic enlightenment, physicians need to adopt a less paternalistic approach to health care decision making. Patients should feel comfortable discussing information found on the Internet with their physician, especially when decision making is involved.

E. Guidelines for patients. Advice for patients seeking health-related information on the Internet should at least include a check on: accuracy of the material (citations and identifiable primary sources of information, author credentials); currency (date of most recent update); security (posted privacy notice or https://); and sponsorship (identity and reputation of sponsor and any potential conflicts of interest or bias). Receptiveness to informed and inquisitive patients' questions and demands is likely to promote better medical care and patient satisfaction.

V. Selected Web sites (Table F-1)

Table F-1. Selected medical information Web sites

General sites: Contain information on a variety of problems

http://www.health.yahoo.com[a]	http://www.healthcentral.com[a]
http://www.excite.com/health	http://www.nih.gov
http://www.drkoop.com	http://www.medem.com
http://www.mywebmd.com or http://www.webmd.com	http://www.lwwmedicine.com http://www.mdconsult.com
http://www.intellihealth.com	http://www.uptodate.com
http://www.healthatoz.com	http://www.healthfinder.gov
http://www.reutershealth.com	http://www.mayohealth.org[a]
http://www.guideline.gov	http://www.vh.org
http://www.clinicaltrials.gov	http://www.medicinenet.com[a]
http://www.pubmed.gov	

Cardiovascular disease

http://www.americanheart.org	http://www.heartinfo.org[a]
http://www.nhlbi.nih.gov	http://www.bloodpressure.com

Cerebrovascular disease and stroke

http://www.strokeassociation.org[a]	http://www.mayo.edu/cerebro/education/stroke.html[a]
http://www.ninds.nih.gov	http://www.strokecenter.org
http://www.stroke.org	

Pulmonary diseases and allergy

http://www.lungusa.org	http://www.emphysemafoundation.org[a]
http://www.aafa.org	http://www.sleepapnea.org[a]
http://www.aarc.org	http://www.sleepnet.com

(continued)

Table F-1. (continued)

Endocrine disease and diabetes
http://www.niddk.nih.gov
http://www.endocrineweb.com[a]
http://www.diabetes.org

http://www.endo-society.org
http://www.thyroid.org

Rheumatology
http://www.arthritis.org[a]
http://www.lupus.org[a]
http://www.arthritislink.com

http://www.nih.gov/niams/index.htm
http://www.pslgroup.com/ARTHRITIS

Nephrology
http://www.niddk.nih.gov
http://www.aakp.org[a]
http://www.kidneydirections.com[a]

http://www.renalnet.org
http://www.kidney.org

Oncology
http://www.cancer.org[a]
http://www.cancerfacts.com[a]
http://www.oncolink.upenn.edu
http://www.atcancer.com

http://cancer.gov
http://www.dfci.harvard.edu
http://www.mskcc.org

Gastroenterology
http://www.gastro.org
http://www.acg.gi.org

http://www.ccfa.org[a]

Infectious disease/HIV
http://www.thebody.com[a]
http://www.hivinsite.ucsf.edu
http://www.hivatis.org[a]
http://www.hopkins-aids.edu
http://www.aids-ed.org

http://www.cdc.gov/travel
http://www.niaid.nih.gov
http://www.hepnet.com
http://www.who.int
http://www.idsociety.org

Geriatrics, aging, osteoporosis
http://www.alzheimers.org/adear[a]
http://www.aarp.org/healthguide[a]

http://www.aoa.dhhs.gov/elderpage.html[a]
http://www.osteo.org

Women's health
http://www.4women.gov
http://www.womens-health.com[a]
http://www.estronaut.com[a]

http://www.womenshealth.org
http://www.wellweb.com/WOMEN/WOMEN.HTM
http://partnership.hs.columbia.edu[a]

Alternative medicine
http://nccam.nih.gov

http://drweil.com[a]

Nutrition
http://www.eatright.org[a]

http://www.navigator.tufts.edu

On-line pharmacies and related drug information
http://www.drugstore.com[a]
http://www.fd.gov/OC/buyonline

http://talkaboutrx.org[a]
http://pdr.net

On-line journals
http://www.nejm.org
http://www.annals.org

http://www.ama-assn.org
http://www.bmj.org

Note: Some sites may require a fee or registration for access.
[a]Predominately patient-oriented.

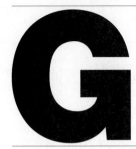

New Immigrant and Refugee Health

Johnetta M. Craig and
Barbara Bogomolov

I. **Patterns of immigration.** Between 1980 and 1995, the number of foreign-born persons residing in the United States grew dramatically, and continued growth of this population is predicted at a similar rate. Census data also demonstrated the uneven effect of immigration. Approximately three-fourths of this population settled in only seven states: California, New York, Texas, Florida, New Jersey, Illinois, and Massachusetts (U.S. Bureau of the Census, Population Division. *The triennial comprehensive report on immigration*, 1999). Every wave of immigration in the United States has introduced unique concepts of health and illness. The culturally competent provider recognizes the value of understanding and incorporating the immigrant patient's world view when delivering care. In addition, the process of immigrating and adjusting to a new culture has both medical and psychosocial implications for risk factors.

II. **Types of residents**
   A. **Legal immigrants** may be sponsored by an American citizen or an agency (governmental or nongovernmental organization), or they may be invited to the country as part of the nation's commitment to the United Nations refugee resettlement activities. Many legal immigrants emigrate for economic reasons.
   B. **Official refugees** may emigrate for reasons of religious or political persecution, economic hardship, war, or natural disasters. Many refugees will have spent time in United Nations–sponsored refugee camps for many months or years before emigration. Refugees are eligible, on arrival in the United States, for Medicaid and continue under coverage for as long as they meet eligibility requirements. Individuals granted asylum are managed as refugees.
   C. **Other immigrants,** including parolees and individuals seeking but not yet granted asylum, are expected to be sponsored and supported by family or agencies and are ineligible in most states for Medicaid by law or common practice for up to 5 years. These immigrants must seek insurance privately or pay out of pocket. Refugees older than 65 years of age are eligible for Medicare.
   D. **Nondocumented residents** may be here for economic reasons or for reunification with family. They have limited access to health care in many regions and are likely to seek services in acute situations only. Many nondocumented individuals fear exposure of their status even though health care providers are not required to report them to the U.S. Immigrant and Naturalization Service (INS) and, in many states, such reporting would be a violation of statutes protecting patient confidentiality.

III. **Immigration examinations.** Immigration status may have a significant impact on the necessary evaluation and management of a foreign-born patient.
   A. **All legal immigrants and refugees** should have undergone the **mandatory** Department of State/INS medical examination. Illegal immigrants may not have undergone any medical evaluation at all. The Centers for Disease Control and Prevention, Division of Quarantine, provides the technical instructions and guidance for physicians who are charged with conducting the medical examination for immigration (http://www.cdc.gov/ncidod/dq/health.htm). The

purpose of the examination is to identify applicants with inadmissible health-related conditions. These conditions include: a communicable disease of public health significance; failure to present documentation of vaccine-preventable diseases; a physical or mental disorder with associated harmful behavior; and drug abuse or addiction. Individuals residing in the United States on temporary visas (tourist, student, and employment) are not required to have the INS medical examination.

B. Permanent residency examination. When legal immigrants file with INS for permanent residency (at 1 year for many immigrants and 5 years for those seeking early naturalization), they must undergo a physical and mental examination by an INS-designated civil surgeon. At this time, additional areas are assessed, including disabilities, substance abuse, mental health, and completion of all basic vaccinations as well as varicella (evidence of previous disease is acceptable if documented by the physician), hepatitis B, and, when indicated by age or pre-existing condition, influenza and pneumococcal pneumonia.

C. Medical examination.

1. Recommended evaluation/laboratory tests

a. Recommended tests include a chemistry panel and nutritional assessment (body mass index); stool for ova and parasites; hepatitis panel; CBC; VDRL and/or rapid plasma reagin; HIV; thyroid-stimulating hormone/T_4 (thyroxine); and purified protein derivative (PPD).*

b. Preventive health assessments are also recommended. Age-appropriate screening should be done for all patients. It is important to note that common screening examinations such as a Papanicolaou smear or visual/hearing assessments may not be routinely done in other countries. In addition, many patients may not be familiar with the concept of preventive screening and interventions if they are not performed in their country of origin.

2. Communicable diseases of public health significance that must be reported to the local, county, or state public health department include tuberculosis, HIV infection, syphilis, chancroid, gonorrhea, granuloma inguinale, lymphogranuloma venereum, and Hansen's disease (leprosy) (see Appendix D).

3. Vaccine-preventable diseases include mumps, measles, rubella, polio, tetanus and diphtheria toxoids, pertussis, influenza type B, and hepatitis B. Other vaccinations against vaccine-preventable diseases recommended by the Advisory Committee for Immunization Practices currently include varicella, pneumococcal pneumonia, and influenza.

IV. General approach to the patient

A. Assess language and cultural barriers and seek the services of a professional medical interpreter whenever possible. The interpreter can be a valuable resource both on-site and via telephone with regard to information on cultural differences. Avoid using family members or children as interpreters.

B. Make effective use of the interpreter by prebriefing when necessary, positioning the patient and the interpreter to allow direct communication (including eye contact where culturally appropriate) between the physician and the patient, and speaking in lay language using first person syntax. The interpreter should be able to provide clues to the meaning of the patient's nonverbal communication.

---

*Current recommendations from the Centers for Disease Control and Prevention are that **prior bacillus Calmette-Guérin (BCG) exposure does not obviate the need for testing and does not have an impact on interpretation of the test result and implementation of isoniazid chemoprophylaxis**. Previous BCG vaccination reduces the predictive value of serial PPD, especially in those recently vaccinated (without known tuberculosis exposure) or those vaccinated multiple times with intradermal BCG (*Ann Intern Med* 1999;131:32–36).

   C. Use lay (rather than medical) terminology. This is particularly important in populations in which learning the language and culture already provide formidable challenges.

   D. Evaluate for impact of gaps in an immigrant's primary country's health care system or the sequelae from time spent in flight and refugee camps (e.g., immunization practices, access to care, preventive services, and standards of treatment for chronic illness in primary country and exposure to risk factors during flight and primary asylum, such as starvation, poor sanitation, and physical/psychological trauma).

   E. Be alert for any symptoms or signs of abuse, torture, depression, acculturation issues, posttraumatic stress disorder, or adjustment difficulties.

V. Special challenges

   A. Noncompliance with a therapeutic regimen may result from many factors such as cultural mismatch between patient and provider regarding the causes of health and illness or distrust of Western medicine or medical providers and fear of deportation (especially when presenting with mental health disorders). The use of nurse or social work case managers with transcultural experience may be very helpful, as is the use of directly observed therapy. Explicit, interpreted oral instructions or translated written instructions for literate patients are very useful. Close follow-up, either by telephone, nursing visits, or scheduled clinic visits, can also be helpful.

   B. Resettlement issues, including transportation, insurance, and other medical and social issues, may be barriers to patients seeking medical care. The sponsoring agency, the local refugee community, and other institution-based resources can often assist with these issues.

   C. Careful documentation of all findings is essential. Documentation of the examination may be used later for legal or asylum proceedings.

   D. Acculturation is a dynamic process that occurs as patients grapple with exposure to different world views and seek an individual balance between original and host cultures. The provider who discovers, rather than assumes, the patient's understanding of such crucial elements as the patient/provider relationship, concept of health/illness, and the art/science of healing will find it easier to establish a therapeutic relationship.

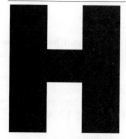

Endocarditis Prophylaxis*

Michael W. Rich

I. Cardiac conditions for which prophylaxis is recommended
A. High-risk category
1. Prosthetic cardiac valves (all types)
2. Prior bacterial endocarditis
3. Complex congenital heart disease
4. Surgically constructed systemic-pulmonary shunts or conduits

B. Moderate-risk category
1. Acquired valvular heart disease (e.g., rheumatic)
2. Hypertrophic cardiomyopathy
3. Mitral valve prolapse with regurgitation or thickened leaflets
4. Bicuspid aortic valve
5. Other congenital cardiac malformations except isolated secundum atrial septal defect, repaired atrial septal defect, repaired ventricular septal defect, and repaired patent ductus arteriosus

II. Procedures for which prophylaxis is recommended in high- and moderate-risk conditions
A. Dental procedures
1. Dental extractions
2. Periodontal procedures
3. Dental implants
4. Root canal surgery beyond the apex
5. Subgingival placement of antibiotic fibers or strips
6. Initial placement of orthodontic bands but not brackets
7. Intraligamentary local anesthetic injections
8. Prophylactic cleaning if significant bleeding is anticipated

B. Respiratory tract
1. Tonsillectomy or adenoidectomy
2. Surgical procedures involving respiratory mucosa
3. Rigid bronchoscopy

C. GI tract (recommended for high-risk patients, optional for moderate-risk patients)
1. Sclerotherapy for esophageal varices
2. Esophageal stricture dilation
3. Endoscopic retrograde cholangiography with biliary obstruction
4. Biliary tract surgery
5. Surgical procedures involving intestinal mucosa

D. Genitourinary tract
1. Prostatic surgery
2. Cystoscopy
3. Urethral dilation

*Adapted from Prevention of bacterial endocarditis. Recommendations by the American Heart Association. *Circulation* 1997;96:358–366.

III. Prophylactic regimens for adults

A. Dental, oral, respiratory tract, or esophageal procedures
   1. Standard prophylaxis: amoxicillin, 2.0 g orally 1 hour before procedure
   2. Unable to take oral medication: ampicillin, 2.0 g IM or IV within 30 minutes before procedure
   3. Allergic to penicillin
      a. Clindamycin, 600 mg orally 1 hour before procedure, **or**
      b. Cephalexin or cefadroxil, 2.0 g orally 1 hour before procedure, **or**
      c. Azithromycin or clarithromycin, 500 mg orally 1 hour before procedure
   4. Allergic to penicillin and unable to take oral medication
      a. Clindamycin, 600 mg IV within 30 minutes before procedure, **or**
      b. Cefazolin, 1.0 g IM or IV within 30 minutes before procedure

B. Other GI and genitourinary procedures
   1. High-risk patients
      a. Ampicillin, 2.0 g IM or IV, and gentamicin, 1.5 mg/kg (not to exceed 120 mg) within 30 minutes of starting procedure, **and**
      b. Amoxicillin, 1 g orally, or ampicillin, 1 g IM or IV 6 hours later
   2. High-risk patients allergic to penicillin
      a. Vancomycin, 1.0 g IV over 1–2 hours, **and**
      b. Gentamicin, 1.5 mg/kg (not to exceed 120 mg) completed within 30 minutes of starting procedure
   3. Moderate-risk patients
      a. Amoxicillin, 2.0 g orally 1 hour before procedure, **or**
      b. Ampicillin, 2.0 g IM or IV within 30 minutes before procedure
   4. Moderate-risk patients allergic to penicillin: vancomycin, 1.0 g IV over 1–2 hours to complete infusion within 30 minutes of starting procedure

Index

Page numbers followed by *f* indicate figures; numbers followed by *t* indicate tables.

Dopamine agonists
  in Parkinson's disease, 517–518
  in periodic leg movements, 527
Dornase alpha in cystic fibrosis, 213
Doxazosin
  in hypertension, 77t
  in prostate hyperplasia, benign, 555
  in urinary incontinence, 455
Doxepin in urticaria, 240
Doxycycline
  in acne
    rosacea, 578
    vulgaris, 577
  in bronchitis, 409
  in chlamydial infections, 426–427, 430
  in diarrhea, 417
  in gastroenteritis, 418
  in malaria, 414
  in pelvic inflammatory disease, 431
  in pneumonia, 410–411
  in prostatitis, 557, 558
  in syphilis, 428
Drawer tests in knee pain, 481, 484
Driving. *See* Motor vehicle use
Dronabinol in cancer
  in anorexia and cachexia, 353
  in nausea and vomiting, 352
Drug-induced disorders
  adrenal failure in, 368
  allergic reactions in, 241–245. *See also*
    Allergic reactions, to drugs
  aplastic anemia in, 242, 329t, 334
  arrhythmias in, 146, 147t
    in digoxin toxicity, 127–128, 150
  chest pain in, 112–113
  constipation in, 268
  cough in, 179, 183
  Cushing's syndrome in, 369
  diarrhea in, 271, 420
  dizziness in, 524
  dyspnea in, 188, 189–190
  dystonia in, 518
  erectile dysfunction in, 558, 559t
  erythema nodosum in, 574
  headache in, 512–513, 516
  hearing loss in, 599
  hematuria in, 442
  hemolytic anemia in, 329t, 334
  hypogonadism of male in, 376
  hypokalemia in, 456, 457
  of kidneys, 451
  of liver, 281–282
  lung disease in, interstitial, 215, 216t,
    217t
  nausea and vomiting in, 261–262, 351
  osteoporosis in, 528
    in corticosteroid therapy, 232, 496,
      529, 531, 534–535
    in men, 535
  Parkinson's disease in, 518
  peptic ulcer disease in, 290, 293–294
  photosensitivity in, 577

  of platelet function, 339
  rhinitis in, 247, 248
  seizures in, 524
  sleepiness in, 527
  Stevens-Johnson syndrome in, 570
  thrombocytopenia in, 335–336, 337t,
    337–338
    in chemotherapy, 336, 352
    in heparin therapy, 170–171, 338
  of thyroid
    function tests in, 360, 360t
    hyperthyroidism in, 360, 363
    hypothyroidism in, 360, 362
  tinnitus in, 603
  torsades de pointes in, 146, 147t
  toxic epidermal necrolysis in, 570
  urinary incontinence in, 453, 455t
  vertigo in, 605
Drug therapy
  compliance with, 2–3. *See also* Compli-
    ance with therapy
  in elderly, 651–653. *See also* Elderly,
    drug therapy in
  interaction with food and nutrients, 57,
    57t–58t
  metabolism of drugs in, 651–652
  perioperative, 33–37
  in renal failure
    avoidance of nephrotoxins in, 451
    dose adjustment in, 664–671
  safety precautions in, 4
Dry eye, 507, 595
  artificial tear preparations in, 507, 587
Dumping syndrome, diarrhea in, 271
Duodenum, peptic ulcer disease of,
    290–294
  chest pain in, 194, 195
  dyspepsia in, 265–267
Dupuytren's contracture, 476
Dust mite allergy, 232
  rhinitis in, 247
Dysbetalipoproteinemia, 91, 96
Dyscrasia, plasma cell, 343
Dysequilibrium, 604, 605
Dyslipidemia in diabetes mellitus, 394t, 400
Dyspareunia, 541t, 541–542
Dyspepsia, 265–267
Dysphagia, 263–265
  in gastroesophageal reflux, 264, 265
    and esophageal strictures, 289
  in Parkinson's disease, 517
Dysphonia, 620–622
Dysphoric disorder, premenstrual,
    549–550, 550t
Dyspnea, 186–194
  in cancer, supportive care in, 354
  in chronic obstructive pulmonary dis-
    ease, 187, 189, 193, 202–203
  in interstitial lung disease, 188, 193, 214
  in pulmonary hypertension, 188, 221
Dysthymic disorder, 633
Dystonia, 518

and energy requirements for various
    activities, 24t
  in heart failure, 122
  hematuria after, 442
  in hyperlipidemia, 92, 94, 95
  in hypertension, 74–75
  in knee pain, 482
  in migraine prevention, 515
  in myocardial infarction, 116, 117
  in neck pain, 461
  in osteoporosis, 530
  in peripheral vascular disease, 161, 162
    and diabetes mellitus, 400
  in plantar fasciitis, 487
  postoperative, 37
    breathing exercises in, 30
  in shoulder pain, 470–471
  in stress testing
    in angina pectoris, 106–107, 117
    in cardiac rehabilitation, 117
    contraindications to, 115t
    in dyspnea, 193
    in myocardial infarction, 115, 115t
  in urinary incontinence, 455
Expectorants, 184
Eye disorders, 584–597
  in corticosteroid therapy, 232
  corticosteroid therapy in, 587
  in diabetes mellitus, 394t, 398–399,
    591–592
  drug therapy in, 587–588
  in dry eye, 507, 595
    artificial tear preparations in, 507, 587
  emergency care in, 588
  evaluation of, 584–587
  external, 596–597
  in glaucoma, 587, 588, 590–591, 595
  in Graves' disease, 363, 592, 594
  in HIV infection and AIDS, 437, 592
  in inflammatory bowel disease, 295
  in motility, 586, 594
  neurologic, 594–595
  red eye in, 595–596
  referrals in, 584, 585t
  retinal. See Retinal disorders
  in sickle cell disease, 331
  in Sjögren's syndrome, 507
  in spondyloarthropathy, 504
  in systemic disease, 591–592
  tearing in, 596
  traumatic, 592–593
    in chemical burn, 588
    red eye in, 595
  vertigo in, 606
  vision loss in, 588–591. See also Vision loss
Eyelid disorders, 583, 596–597
  drug therapy in, 587–588
  examination in, 585
  in thyroid disease, 363, 592
  traumatic, 593

FABERE test in hip examination, 478, 490

Facet joint injections in back pain, 467
Facial nerve palsy, 521
Factitious disorder, 642
Factor V Leiden mutation, 169
Factor VII
  concentrate products, 340t
  deficiency of, 340
Factor VIII
  antibodies to, 341
  concentrate products, 340t, 342
  deficiency of, 340, 341–342
Factor IX
  concentrate products, 340t
  deficiency of, 340, 342
Factors, clotting
  concentrate products, 340t, 342
  deficiency of, 340, 341–342
Fainting, 523
Fallopian tube ligation, 548
Falls
  ankle sprain in, 486
  in dizziness, 523
  in elderly, 653
  hip fracture in, 480
  in osteoporosis, prevention of, 530,
    653
  in Parkinson's disease, 516, 517
  shoulder injury in, 472
Famciclovir
  in herpes simplex virus infections, genital, 429
  in varicella-zoster virus infections,
    412
    in HIV infection and AIDS, 437
Family
  abusive and violent behavior in, 644
  and caregiver stress in Alzheimer's disease, 649
  education of
    in depression, 633
    in mania, 635
    in schizophrenia, 641
  history of
    in colon cancer, 279, 307
    suicidal behavior in, 636
Famotidine
  in gastroesophageal reflux, 287t
  in peptic ulcer disease, 292
Fasciitis
  necrotizing, 432
  plantar, 487–488
Fat, dietary, 49, 51, 92–93
  deficiency of, 39–41
  in diabetes mellitus, 382
  in hyperlipidemia, 92–93
  malabsorption of, 270, 271
  monounsaturated, 51, 93
  polyunsaturated, 51, 93
  replacement products, 52–53
  saturated, 51, 92–93
  in weight-loss diets, 51
Fat pad atrophy, plantar, 488

Nizatidine
    in gastroesophageal reflux, 287t
    in peptic ulcer disease, 292
Nodules
    adrenal, 370
    pulmonary, 199–201
    of thyroid, 367
        in multinodular goiter, 362–363, 364,
            367
    of vocal folds, 621
Noise exposure
    hearing loss in, 601
    tinnitus in, 603
Norethindrone, 532t
Norgestrel in oral contraceptive prepara-
        tions, 546
Nortriptyline, 629t
    in migraine, 515
    in myofascial pain dysfunction, 613
Norwalk virus infections, 271, 300, 419
    foods associated with, 301t, 419
Nose
    bleeding from, 615–618
        in von Willebrand's disease, 342
        in warfarin therapy, 176
    fractures of, 618
5-Nucleotidase serum levels in liver disor-
        ders, 308, 309t
Nursing home care, 654–656
Nutcracker esophagus, 289
Nutrition, 38–69
    and abdominal pain, 257
    allergic reaction to foods in, 228,
        245–246
        and food additives, 240
        urticaria and angioedema in, 239,
            240, 245
    in alopecia, 571
    in anorexia, 637, 638
        in cancer, 353
        in elderly, 655
    assessment of, 38–39
        in elderly, 655
        in periodic health examination, 1, 2
    carbohydrates in, 48–51
        deficiency of, 39–41
        in diabetes mellitus, 382, 396
    in chronic obstructive pulmonary dis-
        ease, 203, 206
    compliance with diet in, 3
    in constipation, 268
    in coronary artery disease, 104
    in diabetes mellitus, 381–382, 391
        in hypoglycemia, 396
        perioperative, 33, 394
        in pregnancy, 398
    dietary supplements in, 57–59
    in diverticular disease of colon, 304
    and drug-nutrient interactions, 57,
        57t–58t
    and dyspepsia, 265–267
    in eating disorders, 638

    in elderly, 655–656, 656t
    energy requirements in, 47–48
    fat in. *See* Fat, dietary
    fiber in. *See* Fiber, dietary
    folic acid in, 41, 42t–43t
        in pregnancy and lactation,
            326, 660
    and foodborne diseases, 301t–302t,
        413–414, 416–421
    functional foods in, 59, 68t, 69
    in gastroesophageal reflux, 287
    in gluten-sensitive enteropathy, 300
    in heart failure, 122
    herbal and botanical products in, 59,
        60t–67t
    history-taking on, 39
    in hyperkalemia, 457, 458
    in hypertension, 75
    in hypokalemia, 456, 457, 458t
    Internet resources on, 46, 59, 69
        in coronary artery disease, 104
    in irritable bowel syndrome, 304–305
    in lactose intolerance, 274
    and lipoprotein levels, 4, 90, 92–95, 101,
        104
    macronutrient deficiency in, 39–41
    in Ménière's disease, 601
    micronutrient deficiency in, 41
    in migraine, 515
    minerals in, 55–57
        deficiency of, 41
    in nephrolithiasis, 448, 449
    and obesity, 38, 41
    in osteoporosis, 530–531
    parenteral, cholestasis in, 320
    poisoning from food in, 420–421
    in pressure sores, 655
    protein in. *See* Protein, dietary
    recommended daily intake in, 41–47,
        42t–46t
        in alternate food plans, 46–47
        food pyramid on, 46, 47f
    in renal failure, chronic, 451
    in smoking cessation, 9
    and swallowing disorders, 263–265
    in travel, precautions in, 413–414
    vitamins in, 53–55
        deficiency of, 41
        recommended daily intake, 2, 41,
            42t–45t, 53
    and vomiting after meals, 261
    in weight-loss diets, 51–53
Nystagmus, 586
    in benign positional vertigo, 523
Nystatin in *Candida* infections, 421

Obesity, 38, 41
    diabetes mellitus in, 400
    in hyperlipidemia and metabolic syn-
        drome, 95
    hypertension in, 83
    screening for, 5

Potassium—*continued*
serum levels of, 456–458
in adrenal failure, 368
in hyperkalemia, 368, 457–458
in hypokalemia, 456–457
urine levels of, 456
Potassium chloride in diabetes mellitus, perioperative, 395
Potassium citrate in nephrolithiasis, 449
Potassium hydroxide preparation in office microscopy, 565
Potassium iodide
in sporotrichosis, 426
supersaturated, in hyperthyroidism, 365, 366
Pott's puffy tumor, 405
Pravastatin, 96–97
Prazosin
in hypertension, 78t, 79
in urinary incontinence, 455
Prednisone
in adrenal failure, 369
in asthma and cough, 182
in cancer
in anorexia and cachexia, 353
in fatigue and malaise, 353
in chronic obstructive pulmonary disease, 204–205
in dermatitis, 568
in gout, 499
in headaches, cluster, 515
in hearing loss, sensorineural, 602
in hemolytic anemia, autoimmune, 333
in hepatitis, autoimmune, 319
in hypercalcemia, 373
in inflammatory bowel disease, 297t, 298–299
in lupus erythematosus, 503
in mononucleosis, 412
in myasthenia gravis, 520
osteoporosis from, 534
perioperative, 36, 369
in *Pneumocystis carinii* pneumonia and HIV infection, 439
in polymyalgia rheumatica, 508–509
in polymyositis and dermatomyositis, 509
in radiocontrast media reactions, 245t
in rheumatoid arthritis, 495–496
in thrombocytopenic purpura, immune, 336
in tinea capitis, 575
in urticaria, 240
in vasculitis, 508
in giant cell arteritis, 161, 509
in venom hypersensitivity, 238
Preeclampsia, 658–659
Pregnancy, 657–663
analgesics in, 659
antibiotic therapy in, 660–663, 661t, 662t
classification of drug risk in, 661t
asthma in, 657–658
bacteriuria in, asymptomatic, 446

classification of drug risk in, 657, 661t
diabetes mellitus in, 380, 397–398, 659
epilepsy in, 660
folic acid intake in, 326, 660
gastroesophageal reflux in, 659–660
heparin therapy in, 171, 659
HIV infection and AIDS in, 661–663
hypertension in, 87, 658–659
hyperthyroidism in, 363, 364, 365, 366
hypothyroidism in, 362
nausea and vomiting in, 262, 660
pneumonia in, 660
in prolactinoma, 375
pyelonephritis in, 447
rhinitis in, allergic, 660
sexually transmitted diseases in, 661–663, 662t
in sickle cell diseases, 333
smoking cessation in, 8, 657
thrombocytopenic purpura in, immune, 336
thromboembolic disease in, 659
tuberculosis in, 434, 660–661
urinary tract infections in, 446, 447, 660
vaccinations in, 11–12, 13, 660
warfarin therapy in, 171, 175, 659
Premature complexes, 139–140
Premenstrual syndrome or dysphoric disorder, 549–550, 550t
Prepatellar bursitis, 485, 498
Presbycusis, 601
Presbylaryngia, 621–622
Preventive health care, 1
periodic examination in, 1–2
Priapism, 563
in sickle cell disease, 332
Primaquine in malaria, 414, 415
Primidone in tremor, 518
Prinzmetal's angina, 112
Probenecid in gout, 500
Procainamide, 148t
Prochlorperazine
in diabetic gastroenteropathy, 399
in hiccups, 265
in migraine, 514
in nausea and vomiting, 263, 351
in cancer, 351, 357
Proctalgia fugax, 275
Progesterone, 532t
in oral contraceptives, 545
Progestins, 532t–533t
in contraceptive preparations
implant system, 547
oral, 545–546
in menopause, 535, 536–537
Proguanil and atovaquone in malaria, 414
Prolactin levels, 373–375
in male hypogonadism, 376
in nipple discharge, 540
in pituitary adenoma, 373–375
Prolactinoma, 373–375
nipple discharge in, 540

nodules of, 621
paralysis of, 621
polyps of, 621
spasm of, 622
Voice, hoarseness of, 620–622
Vomiting, 261–263. *See also* Nausea and vomiting
von Willebrand's disease, 342
Vulvovaginal candidiasis, 427, 549

Waldenström's macroglobulinemia, 343
Warfarin therapy, 166t, 167t, 168, 171–177
in atrial fibrillation, 143, 144, 156, 172
coagulation disorders in, 341
dose adjustments in, 173–174, 174t
drug interactions in, 174, 175, 175t
education of patients in, 172, 173t
generic preparations in, 177
in heart failure, 128
hemorrhage in, 174, 175, 176, 341
initiation of, 172
international normalized ratio in, 171–174, 172t, 174t
and vitamin K therapy, 175–176
monitoring of, 174
patient self-monitoring in, 174
in myocardial infarction, 116, 166t
in pregnancy, 171, 175, 659
in prosthetic heart valves, 137, 167t, 173
in pulmonary hypertension, 225
skin necrosis in, 174–175
in surgical patient, 32
perioperative adjustment in, 34, 35, 176–177
vitamin K in, 175–176, 341
Warm-antibody autoimmune hemolytic anemia, 333
Warts, 430, 576–577
anogenital, 430
Wasting syndromes, 38, 39t
Weakness
in cancer, 353
in neuromuscular disorders, 519–522
Web sites, 680–682, 682t–683t
on alcohol abuse and alcoholism, 5
on allergies, 255, 682t
on asthma, 255
in pregnancy, 658
on cancer, 6, 346, 347t, 683t
and hospice care, 358
on carotid artery disease, 159
on chronic obstructive pulmonary disease, 204
on complementary and alternative medicine, 69, 681
on diabetes mellitus, 403, 683t
on fungal infections
Candida, 421
systemic, 423, 425, 426
on gastrointestinal infections, 416
on heart failure, 122
on hospice care, 358

on immigration examinations, 684
on immunizations, 9
in travel, 13, 415
on lipid disorders, 88
on neuromuscular disorders, 519
on nutrition, 46, 69
in coronary artery disease, 104
and dietary supplements, 59, 69
on otolaryngology, 598
peer review of, 681, 682
on peripheral vascular disease, 162
of pharmacies on-line, 680, 683t
on pharyngitis, streptococcal, 407
on pneumonia, community-acquired, 410
on pulmonary hypertension, 219
on reportable diseases, 675
on travel, 13, 414, 415
Weber test in hearing loss, 599
Wegener's granulomatosis, 507–508
dyspnea in, 187, 191
Weight
in anorexia nervosa, 637
and body mass index, 41
in bulimia nervosa, 638
gain in
in diabetes mellitus, 384–85
in smoking cessation, 9
in heart failure, daily measurement of, 122
loss of, 51–53
in chronic obstructive pulmonary disease, 203
diet programs for, 51–52, 52f
drug therapy for, 52
in dysphagia and odynophagia, 264
in elderly, 655
history of, 39
in hyperlipidemia therapy, 92, 94, 95
in hypertension therapy, 74, 83
in sleep apnea therapy, 209
surgery for, 52
in obesity, 5, 38, 41
in overnutrition, 38
periodic measurement of, 5
in undernutrition, 38
Wenckebach block, 141
Whiplash injury of neck, 459, 463
Wilson's disease, 321
Withdrawal symptoms, 639
from alcohol, 639
in surgical patient, 22
hypertension in, 86
from opioids, 639
Wolff-Parkinson-White syndrome, 145, 146
Women's health issues, 528–550
birth control, 545–548
breast cancer, 538–540
cervical cancer, 537–538
cystitis, 444, 445
dysfunctional uterine bleeding, 542–543
dyspareunia, 541t, 541–542
hypertension, 85
infertility, 544–545